# Inflammatory Disorders of the Skin

ATLAS OF NONTUMOR PATHOLOGY

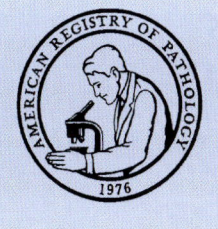

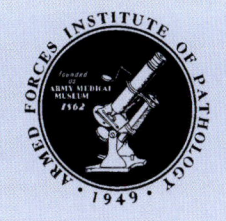

**ARP PRESS**™

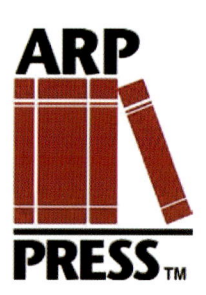

Editorial Director: Mirlinda Q. Caton
Production Editor: Dian S. Thomas
Editorial Assistant: Magdalena C. Silva
Editorial Assistant: Alana N. Black
Copyeditor: Audrey Kahn

ATLAS OF NONTUMOR PATHOLOGY

First Series
Fascicle 10

# Inflammatory Disorders of the Skin

George F. Murphy, MD

Arturo P. Saavedra, MD, PhD

Martin C. Mihm, Jr., MD

*Published by the*
American Registry of Pathology
Silver Spring, MD

2012

# ATLAS OF NONTUMOR PATHOLOGY

**EDITOR**
Donald West King, MD

**ASSOCIATE EDITORS**
William A. Gardner, MD
Leslie H. Sobin, MD
J. Thomas Stocker, MD
Bernard Wagner, MD

**EDITORIAL ADVISORY BOARD**
Ivan Damjanov, MD
Cecilia M. Fenoglio-Preiser, MD
Fred Gorstein, MD
Daniel Knowles, MD
Virginia A. LiVolsi, MD
Florabel G. Mullick, MD
Juan Rosai, MD
Fred Silva, MD
Steven G. Silverberg, MD

**Manuscript Reviewed by:**
Ronald DeLellis, MD
Jack Longley, MD
Bruce Smoller, MD

Available from the American Registry of Pathology
Silver Spring, MD 20910
www.arppress.org
ISBN: 1-933477-24-5
978-1-933477-24-4

Copyright © 2012 The American Registry of Pathology

All rights reserved. No part of this publication may be reproduced or transmitted in any form or by any means: electronic, mechanical, photocopy, recording, or any other information storage and retrieval system without the written permission of the publisher.

## INTRODUCTION TO SERIES

This is the tenth Fascicle of the Atlas of Nontumor Pathology, a complementary series to the Armed Forces Institute of Pathology (AFIP) Atlas of Tumor Pathology, first published in 1949.

For several years, various individuals in the pathology community have suggested the formation of a new series of monographs concentrating on this particular area. In 1998, an Editorial Board was appointed and outstanding authors were chosen shortly thereafter.

The purpose of the atlas is to provide surgical pathologists with ready expert reference material most helpful in their daily practice. The lesions described relate principally to medical non-neoplastic conditions. Many of these lesions represent complex entities and, when appropriate, we have included contributions from internists, radiologists, and surgeons. This has led to some increase in the size of the monographs, but the emphasis remains on diagnosis by the surgical pathologist.

Our goal is to continue to provide expert information at the lowest possible cost. Therefore, marked reductions in pricing are available to residents and fellows as well as to pathology faculty and other staff members purchasing the Fascicles on a subscription basis.

We believe that the Atlas of Nontumor Pathology will serve as an outstanding reference for surgical pathologists as well as an important contribution to the literature of other medical specialties.

Donald West King, MD
William A. Gardner, MD
Leslie H. Sobin, MD
J. Thomas Stocker, MD
Bernard Wagner, MD

## ACKNOWLEDGMENTS

The authors acknowledge the assistance of the following individuals who provided invaluable help and support in the preparation of this work: David Elder, MD, Terry Hadley, MD, Michael Ioffreda, MD, Richard Johnson, MD, and Rosalynn M. Nazarian, MD. Assistance in the preparation of the text and figures was provided by Robert Anolik, MD, and Ms. Diana Whitaker-Menezes. We finally acknowledge the influence of Ramzi Cotran, MD, whose spirit pervades all such endeavors in pathology that seek to marry excellence in scholarship with relevance to practical application.

The authors appreciate the special assistance provided in photomicrography by Andrew Carlson, MD, in clinical photography by Samule Moschella, MD, and the editorial review by Ms. Robin Schanche.

Lastly, Cecilia Lezcano, MD provided outstanding editorial oversight and assistance that served as a major impetus in bringing this endeavor to completion.

This work is dedicated to the memory of Dr. Arlene Herzberg, whose outstanding accomplishments as a surgical pathologist, cytologist, and dermatopathologist were only eclipsed by a personality that radiated warmth and understanding to all who were privileged to have known her.

We also dedicate this volume to Dr. William A. Gardner, whose assistance, advice, and stewardship in no small way made this Fascicle a reality.

**George F. Murphy, MD**
Professor of Pathology, Harvard Medical School
Director of Dermatopathology, Brigham and Women's Hospital
Boston, Massachusetts

**Arturo P. Saavedra, MD, PhD**
Assistant Professor of Dermatopathology, Harvard Medical School
Brigham and Women's Hospital
Boston, Massachusetts

**Martin C. Mihm, Jr., MD**
Clinical Professor of Dermatopathology, Harvard Medical School
Director, Melanoma Program, Department of Dermatology,
Brigham and Women's Hospital
Boston, Massachusetts

## INTRODUCTION

The Fascicle series of the Armed Forces Institute of Pathology (AFIP) has long been a mainstay for the practice of surgical pathology as it relates to the differential diagnosis of neoplastic diseases. Originally conceived as atlases, the Fascicles have flourished to become a marriage between visual and textural materials, with the goal of providing an accessible and practical guide to the surgical pathology of tumors and tumor-like conditions. As such, practicality implies a thematic focus that delineates the "forest from the trees": an organizational infrastructure that is user-friendly; physical attributes conducive to portability; and affordability that promotes accessibility. Experience has indicated that when dealing with tumors of the skin, it is a daunting task to incorporate, into one or two volumes, comprehensive information relevant to the plethora of neoplastic diseases to which the flesh is heir. Faced with the category of non-neoplastic disorders, which encompasses an extraordinary myriad of conditions and their variants, the task is even more challenging, potentially within the realm of impossibility.

To accomplish this goal, it was clear that utilization of all existing resources and extraordinary organization and focus would be mandatory. We were most fortunate when all materials from the first edition of the text, Dermatopathology (1), and its companion Atlas of Dermatopathology (2) were officially transferred from publisher to author for use in other endeavors. There existed significant interest in revised and expanded editions, and this material provided an infrastructure of visual and descriptive information upon which the non-neoplastic Fascicle could be sculpted. Organization, however, remained a challenge through numerous writings and rewritings that spanned almost a decade. We were aware that the basic infrastructure of this new Fascicle would be critical to its conceptual understanding and usability. In time, the philosophy outlined below was formulated, representing the fundamental framework of this new volume.

Disorders of the skin are divided into two general categories, namely, neoplastic and non-neoplastic. The latter is concerned primarily but not exclusively with diseases mediated by inflammatory cells. Because inflammatory skin disorders represent the most common and significant non-neoplastic skin diseases, as well as the most frequently encountered diagnostic hurdle for the practicing pathologist, they are the focus of this Fascicle. The fundamental intent of this Fascicle is to concisely portray many of the more commonly encountered dermatoses in words and images that facilitate practical recognition of these important conditions. Although ideally such a work would be comprehensive in its treatment of individual diseases and in the inclusive scope of disorders discussed, such an approach would generate a more expansive product than has been intended for the Fascicle series. Indeed, other excellent and current sources are readily available for this purpose (3,4). Therefore, this book seeks to summarize and illuminate relevant clinical and pathologic findings for non-neoplastic disorders of skin in the context of recent knowledge and in a manner that promotes practicality.

Certain categories that are already addressed in other texts (e.g., many skin infections, in which the *Pathology of Tropical and Extraordinary Diseases* remains a standard reference (5), and a more restrictive discussion of rare variants and subsets of mainstream conditions) have been de-emphasized or not addressed in this volume. In situations where specific infections are exemplary of diagnostically important or useful patterns (as in nodular/interstitial dermatitis), individual conditions (e.g., types of deep fungal infections) are briefly illustrated and discussed.

The information presented in the pages to follow represents a synthesis of material available in conventional and standard texts dealing with dermatology and dermatopathology as well as the clinical and diagnostic experiences of the authors. This is particularly true regarding the clinical and pathologic input of Dr. Mihm, whose decades of pioneering study of skin disease has generated numerous "pearls" unavailable in most existing resources. Where appropriate, specific references are included to facilitate further reading and for purposes of documentation. We have made efforts to provide current sources, with an emphasis on papers published since 2000. Useful reviews that supplement understanding of specific disorders have been cited. We acknowledge, however, that it was not practical to provide exhaustive comprehensive reference lists. Accordingly, to those who have made the many contributions upon which this work is based, but who could not be cited, we extend both our apologies as well as our gratitude.

Differential diagnosis is important to the pathologist at two levels. First, one must be aware of histologically similar conditions that must be considered in the context of the diagnostic algorithm. Second, knowledge of the clinical differential is of key importance in establishing accurate clinicopathological correlation. For example, neutrophil-rich nodular and interstitial dermatitis of the leg with clinical impression of erythema nodosum may be appropriately diagnosed as Sweet syndrome when one realizes that the former and the latter may at times show similar clinical presentations at this anatomic site. Thus, the differential diagnosis sections consider both clinical and histologic details.

In this work, we have relied heavily on the concept of pattern analysis, as originally taught by Wallace Clark, for the classification of non-neoplastic conditions of skin. This permits the conceptual grouping of dermatitides in the context of architectural patterns. Such an approach is conducive to the development of algorithms to aid in the differential diagnosis. Accordingly, after introductory material that reviews the general aspects of nomenclature, structure, function, and special diagnostic techniques, the main categories of non-neoplastic disorders are broadly defined. These are the inflammatory dermatoses, including those subcategories with and without primary epidermal alterations, and those with primarily adnexal pathology. This approach lends itself to systematic organization and discussion of the various relevant types of non-neoplastic skin disease. For example, spongiotic dermatitis is inflammatory with epidermal changes, in contrast to urticaria, which is inflammatory without epidermal alterations. The diseases in this Fascicle are approached using the following algorithmic schema:

Is it primarily inflammatory or noninflammatory?
    If inflammatory, is there primary epidermal alteration?
1. If there is epidermal change, what type? (spongiosis, retiform, hyperplasia, etc.)
2. If epidermal change is lacking, is the inflammation primarily dermal or subcutaneous?
   a. If primarily dermal, what is the pattern (angiocentric, interstitial, etc.)
   b. If primarily subcutaneous, what is the pattern (septal, lobular, etc.)
3. If epidermal change is lacking, is the inflammation primarily adnexal?
   a. If so, is it follicular, eccrine, or apocrine?

Each category (e.g., spongiotic dermatitis) is discussed in terms of general considerations, molecular pathogenesis, special diagnostic studies, and animal models if relevant. Each specific disorder under each category is next addressed with respect to definition, clinical and histologic features, differential diagnosis, and treatment considerations that may be relevant to pathologic diagnosis (e.g. partially steroid-treated lupus erythematosus).

Recognizing that a Fascicle is used primarily as a rapid and efficient reference to facilitate diagnostic decision making, we remain committed to the importance of visual information in this process. In addition to photomicrographs and graphic illustrations, tables represent a middle ground where text is provided within an architectural matrix that lends itself to visual grouping for purposes of comparisons and contrasts. In this spirit, we have employed tables selectively with the intent of further enhancing the efficiency by which this resource may be applied.

Non-neoplastic diseases of the skin are ubiquitous and numerous. They are responsible for significant morbidity for patients worldwide and account for enormous time consumption and cost within the medical community. If we achieve our goal even in part, this Fascicle will in some way facilitate the diagnosis and treatment of these important conditions in a manner that will benefit patients and clinicians alike. There remains unfinished business, however, in the form of non-neoplastic, noninflammatory disorders, which involve often inherited conditions showing abnormal keratinization, altered dermal-epidermal stability, abnormal dermal matrix elements, or nonphysiologic deposits. While many of these conditions are only rarely encountered, they represent potentially devastating maladies to those afflicted, and also serve as important models for the genetic and molecular bases of skin disease in general. Such diseases could represent the subject of a future skin Fascicle that would bring the trilogy of neoplastic, dermatitic, and non-neoplastic diseases to comprehensive fruition.

## DEFINITIONS AND NOMENCLATURE

Dermatopathology is a unique subspecialty with regard to the colorful, often complex and distinctive lexicon inherent in naming and discussing lesions both at a clinical and histologic level. Understanding the language of dermatopathology is critical to those embarking on the study of dermatopathology, and for this reason, standard texts designed for medical students provide a list of the most relevant terms (4). The dermatopathology lexicon is extensive, and many of the terms used are either ambiguous or defy universal acceptance. For example, dermatology texts vary with regard to the definition of a vesicle versus a bulla, with some citing 0.5 cm and others 1.0 cm as breakpoints in this distinction. The term "parapsoriasis" is another example. While it literally suggests a disorder like psoriasis, which it is not, there is confusion as to whether some forms of this condition actually represent malignancies of T cells rather than dermatoses. The list that follows, however incomplete and potentially flawed, is an attempt to provide some of the essential vocabulary that will be required in order to maximize the utility of the pages that follow.

### Clinical Terms

*Bulla:* An elevated, fluid-filled lesion more than 1 cm in diameter, as in bullous pemphigoid.

*Collarette:* A fine line of scale that closely follows an advancing erythematous border, as in dermatophytosis.

*Crust:* An admixture of serum, inflammatory exudate, and sometimes blood on the cutaneous surface, producing granular, yellow-brown, dried material, as in impetigo.

*Dermal atrophy:* Diffuse or discrete regions of dermal thinning, often associated with a consistency whereby the skin is easily wrinkled upon mechanical manipulation, as in aging or steroid-induced atrophy.

*Epidermal atrophy:* An area of skin where the surface tends to be shiny and where underlying vessels often are abnormally visible.

*Erythroderma:* Cutaneous erythema covering most or all of the body surface, as in generalized seborrheic dermatitis.

*Follicular plugging:* Dilated follicular ostia containing keratotic debris and sometimes melanin, as in a comedone or discoid lupus.

*Furuncle:* A larger (greater than 1 cm) localized collection of acute inflammatory cells within the dermis, often with associated abscess formation.

*Gyrate and circinate:* Lesions that form rounded, polycyclic, arcuate borders, as in erythema annulare centrifugum.

*Hide-bound:* Inability to freely move the dermis over underlying fascial planes, as in progressive systemic sclerosis.

*Macule:* A small (usually less than 1 cm) generally flat zone of hyperpigmentation or erythema, as in a region of petechial hemorrhage.

*Nodule:* A deeply seated indurated lesion with a palpable inferior contour, as in certain lesions of panniculitis.

*Papule:* An elevated, often dome-shaped solid lesion less than 1 cm in diameter, as in acne.

*Patch:* A smaller (less than 1 cm) slightly elevated zone of erythema, often with abnormal scale, as in pityriasis rosea.

*Plaque:* A larger (greater than 1 cm) variably raised, circumscribed lesion, often associated with erythema and scaling, as in psoriasis.

*Poikiloderma:* Flat zones of epidermal thinning (atrophy) imparting a finely wrinkled texture, hyperpigmentation, hypopigmentation, and prominent, dilated vessels visible beneath the epidermal surface, as in some early forms of cutaneous lupus erythematosus.

*Pustule:* A small (less than 1 cm) circumscribed elevation of the skin formed by aggregated acute inflammatory cells, as in folliculitis.

*Telangiectasia:* Prominent, dilated, tortuous blood vessels visible through the superficial dermis and epidermis, as in discoid lupus erythematosus.

*Umbilication:* A central crater or indentation, usually within a papule or nodule.

*Vesicle:* An elevated, fluid-filled lesion less than 1 cm in diameter, as in herpes simplex.

*Wheal:* A rounded or flat-topped, pale pink elevation which usually disappears within 24 hours, as in hives.

## Histologic Terms

*Acantholysis:* Dissolution or dysfunction of intercellular junctions, resulting in rounded, detached keratinocytes, as in pemphigus.

*Acanthosis:* Thickening of the viable epidermal layer, predominantly involving the stratum spinosum, as in psoriasis.

*Apoptosis:* Programmed or pathologically accelerated cell degeneration and death due to endonuclease-mediated nuclear degeneration, as in forms of cytotoxic dermatitis.

*Atrophy:* Thinning of the epidermal layer with loss of rete ridges, as in lupus erythematosus.

*Colloid body:* An anucleate residua of a keratinocyte that has been incorporated into the papillary dermis, as in lichen planus.

*Desmoplasia:* Proliferation of fibroblasts and associated collagen deposition; often in the context of tumor stroma or connective tissue alterations with persistent inflammation or injury (e.g., about vessels in erythema elevatum diutinum).

*Dyskeratosis:* Abnormal or premature keratinization, as in transient acantholytic dermatosis.

*Elastosis:* Abnormal superficial dermal deposition of gray, homogeneous elastin, as in chronic actinic injury.

*Epidermotropism:* The process whereby cells, usually T lymphocytes, migrate into the epidermal layer; such cells are referred to as being epidermotropic.

*Fibrinoid necrosis:* Deposition of pink-purple, granular, refractile fibrin in vessel walls, as in leukocytoclastic vasculitis.

*Hypergranulosis:* Thickening of the stratum granulosum, as in lichen simplex chronicus.

*Hyperkeratosis:* Increased thickness of the stratum corneum, as in a clavus.

*Hypogranulosis:* Thinning or absence of the stratum granulosum, as in psoriasis.

*Impetiginization:* Diffuse infiltration of stratum corneum by neutrophils, serum, and bacteria, as in impetigo.

*Mucinosis:* Infiltration of epithelial intercellular spaces, as in follicular mucinosis, or dermal collagen, as in lupus erythematosus, by stringy, particulate, blue-gray mucopolysaccharides.

*Munro microabscess:* Focal aggregates of neutrophils within parakeratotic stratum corneum, as in psoriasis.

*Necrobiosis:* Mucinous, fibrinoid, or sclerotic degenerative alteration of connective tissue, as in forms of palisaded granulomatous dermatitis.

*Nuclear dust formation:* Fragmentation of neutrophil nuclei (karyorrhexis and karyolysis), often referred to as "leukocytoclasia."

*Parakeratosis:* Retention of keratinocyte nuclei in the stratum corneum, as in psoriasis.

*Pautrier microabscess:* Discrete collection of atypical lymphocytes within a relatively nonspongiotic epidermal layer (seen in cutaneous T-cell lymphoma and mimicked by localized collections of Langerhans cells in some hypersensitivity reactions).

*Pigment incontinence:* Loss of epidermal melanin pigment into superficial dermal macrophages, as in postinflammatory hyperpigmentation or in chronic cytotoxic injury to the basal cell layer.

*Satellitosis:* The process whereby cells, usually T lymphocytes, migrate into the epidermis and aggregate at the periphery of a central cell that is generally undergoing resultant cytotoxic injury, as in acute graft-versus-host disease.

*Sclerosis:* Abnormal collagen deposition, as in scleroderma and lichen sclerosus et atrophicus.

*Spongiform pustule:* Focal collection of neutrophils in the upper stratum spinosum, as in psoriasis.

*Spongiosis:* Epidermal intercellular edema, resulting in widened intercellular spaces and eventually in vesiculation, as in acute eczematous dermatitis.

*Squamatization:* Transformation of normally rounded basal cells to polyhedral cells resembling those of stratum spinosum, as in lichen planus.

*Vacuolar degeneration:* Lucent cytoplasmic vacuoles, often within basal cells, as in erythema multiforme.

## REFERENCES

1. Murphy GF. Dermatopathology: a practical guide to common disorders. Philadelphia: WB Saunders; 1995.
2. Murphy GF, Herzberg AJ. Atlas of dermatopathology. Philadelphia: WB Saunders; 1996.
3. Lever WF, Elder DE, Elenitasas R, Johnson BL Jr, Murphy GF, Xu X, eds. Lever's histopathology of the skin, 10th ed. Philadelphia: Lippincott Williams & Wilkins; 2009.
4. Calonje E, Brenn T, Lazar A, McKee PH. McKee's pathology of the skin, 4th ed. Philadelphia: Elsevier-Saunders; 2012.
5. Binford CH, Ash JE, Connor DH. Pathology of tropical and extraordinary diseases. Washington DC: Armed Forces Institute of Pathology; 1976.

# CONTENTS

1. Structure, Function, and Reaction Patterns .................................... 1
   - Architecture and Cellular Components .................................... 1
   - Regional Anatomy .................................... 1
   - Responses to Injury .................................... 1
      - Keratinocytes .................................... 1
      - Melanocytes .................................... 12
      - Langerhans Cells .................................... 14
      - Merkel Cells .................................... 16
      - Hair Follicles .................................... 17
      - Eccrine Glands .................................... 20
      - Apocrine Glands .................................... 20
      - Basement Membrane Zone .................................... 21
      - Dermal Microvascular Unit .................................... 22
      - Extracellular Dermal Matrix .................................... 24
      - Subcutaneous Fat .................................... 27
   - Special Diagnostic Techniques .................................... 28
      - Histochemistry .................................... 28
      - Immunohistochemistry .................................... 28
      - One-Micron Sections and Electron Microscopy .................................... 29
      - In Situ Hybridization .................................... 29
      - Immunofluorescence .................................... 29
2. Inflammatory Disorders with Primary Epidermal Alterations: Spongiotic Dermatitis ... 35
   - Pathogenesis .................................... 36
   - Diagnostic Studies .................................... 37
   - Allergic Contact and Primary Irritant Dermatitis .................................... 37
   - Actopic Dermatitis .................................... 43
   - Dyshidrotic Eczema .................................... 45
   - Early Psoriasis .................................... 46
   - ID Reaction .................................... 47
   - Spongiotic Arthropod Bite Reaction .................................... 48
   - Spongiotic Drug Eruption .................................... 51
   - Photoeczematous Eruption .................................... 52
   - Seborrheic Dermatitis .................................... 54
   - Erythema Annulare Centrifugum .................................... 55
   - Eczematous Stasis Dermatitis .................................... 58
   - Parapsoriasis, Including Small Plaque and Superficial Digitate Dermatosis Types ... 60

xv

*Inflammatory Disorders of the Skin*

|  | Pityriasis Rosea | 62 |
|---|---|---|
|  | Dermatophytosis | 64 |
|  | Scabies | 65 |
|  | Papular Acrodermatitis of Childhood (Gianotti-Crosti Syndrome) | 67 |
|  | Toxic Shock Syndrome | 68 |
| 3. | Acanthotic Dermatitis (Retiform Epidermal Hyperplasia) | 73 |
|  | Lichen Simplex Chronicus and Prurigo Nodularis | 74 |
|  | Psoriasis | 78 |
|  | Reiter Disease | 87 |
|  | Pustular Psoriasis | 87 |
|  | Follicular Psoriasis | 88 |
|  | Erythrodermic Psoriasis | 88 |
|  | Psoriasis and Acquired Immunodeficiency Syndrome (AIDS) | 89 |
|  | Pityriasis Rubra Pilaris | 89 |
|  | Chronic Seborrheic Dermatitis | 92 |
|  | Pityriasis Rosea | 94 |
|  | Psoriasiform Stasis Dermatitis | 97 |
|  | Hyperkeratosis Lenticularis Perstans (Flegel Disease) | 98 |
|  | Retiform Epidermal Hyperplasia Induced by Mycotic Infection | 100 |
|  | Psoriasiform Reactions to Halogens | 100 |
|  | Interface Dermatitis with Retiform Epidermal Hyperplasia | 103 |
|  | Psoriasiform Nutritional Disorders | 107 |
| 4. | Primary Acantholytic Dermatitis | 113 |
|  | Pathogenesis | 113 |
|  | Special Diagnostic Studies | 113 |
|  | Pemphigus Group | 114 |
|  | Grover Disease (Transient Acantholytic Dermatosis) | 123 |
|  | Darier Disease (Keratosis Follicularis) | 125 |
|  | Benign Familial "Pemphigus" (Hailey-Hailey Disease) | 126 |
|  | Herpetic Blisters | 129 |
| 5. | Nonacantholytic Vesiculobullous and Vesiculopustular Dermatitis | 137 |
|  | General Considerations | 137 |
|  | Pathogenesis | 139 |
|  | Special Diagnostic Studies | 140 |
|  | Animal Models | 142 |
|  | Bullous Pemphigoid | 142 |
|  | Herpes Gestationis | 148 |
|  | Epidermolysis Bullosa Acquisita, Inflammatory Variant | 149 |
|  | Dermatitis Herpetiformis | 153 |

Bullous Disease of Childhood . . . . . . . . . . . . . . . . . . . . . . . . . . . . . . . . . . . . . . . . . 156
Linear IgA Disease . . . . . . . . . . . . . . . . . . . . . . . . . . . . . . . . . . . . . . . . . . . . . . . . 158
Bullous Lesions of Interface Dermatitis . . . . . . . . . . . . . . . . . . . . . . . . . . . . . . . . 158
Staphylococcal Scalded-Skin Syndrome (Ritter Disease) . . . . . . . . . . . . . . . . . . . 159
Inflammatory Vesiculobullous Lesions Due to Ischemia . . . . . . . . . . . . . . . . . . . 162
    Bullous Manifestations of Primary Vasculopathic Injury . . . . . . . . . . . . . . . . 162
    Bulla Due to Physical Agents . . . . . . . . . . . . . . . . . . . . . . . . . . . . . . . . . . . . 162
Subcorneal Pustular Dermatosis (Sneddon-Wilkinson Disease) . . . . . . . . . . . . . 166
IgA Pemphigus . . . . . . . . . . . . . . . . . . . . . . . . . . . . . . . . . . . . . . . . . . . . . . . . . . 167
Pustular Eruptions of Infancy . . . . . . . . . . . . . . . . . . . . . . . . . . . . . . . . . . . . . . . 169
    Erythema Toxicum Neonatorum . . . . . . . . . . . . . . . . . . . . . . . . . . . . . . . . . . 169
    Transient Neonatal Pustular Melanosis . . . . . . . . . . . . . . . . . . . . . . . . . . . . . 169
    Acropustulosis of Infancy . . . . . . . . . . . . . . . . . . . . . . . . . . . . . . . . . . . . . . . 171
Intestinal Bypass Syndrome . . . . . . . . . . . . . . . . . . . . . . . . . . . . . . . . . . . . . . . . 171
Impetigo . . . . . . . . . . . . . . . . . . . . . . . . . . . . . . . . . . . . . . . . . . . . . . . . . . . . . . . 171
Pustular Candidiasis . . . . . . . . . . . . . . . . . . . . . . . . . . . . . . . . . . . . . . . . . . . . . . 172
Pustular Vasculitis . . . . . . . . . . . . . . . . . . . . . . . . . . . . . . . . . . . . . . . . . . . . . . . . 173
Vesiculopustular Eruption of Hepatobiliary Disease . . . . . . . . . . . . . . . . . . . . . . 174

6. Interface Dermatitis (Acute Cytotoxic Dermatitis) . . . . . . . . . . . . . . . . . . . . . . . . . . 181
General Considerations . . . . . . . . . . . . . . . . . . . . . . . . . . . . . . . . . . . . . . . . . . . . 181
Pathogenesis . . . . . . . . . . . . . . . . . . . . . . . . . . . . . . . . . . . . . . . . . . . . . . . . . . . . 181
Pathology . . . . . . . . . . . . . . . . . . . . . . . . . . . . . . . . . . . . . . . . . . . . . . . . . . . . . . 181
Special Diagnostic Studies . . . . . . . . . . . . . . . . . . . . . . . . . . . . . . . . . . . . . . . . . 183
Animal Models . . . . . . . . . . . . . . . . . . . . . . . . . . . . . . . . . . . . . . . . . . . . . . . . . . 183
Erythema Multiforme Group . . . . . . . . . . . . . . . . . . . . . . . . . . . . . . . . . . . . . . . . 183
Toxic Epidermal Necrolysis . . . . . . . . . . . . . . . . . . . . . . . . . . . . . . . . . . . . . . . . 188
Acute Graft-Versus-Host Disease . . . . . . . . . . . . . . . . . . . . . . . . . . . . . . . . . . . . 190
Pityriasis Lichenoides et Varioliforms Acuta . . . . . . . . . . . . . . . . . . . . . . . . . . . 195
Acute Cytotoxic Generalized Drug Eruption . . . . . . . . . . . . . . . . . . . . . . . . . . . . 200
Fixed Drug Eruption (Active Phase) . . . . . . . . . . . . . . . . . . . . . . . . . . . . . . . . . . 200
Interface Dermatitis of Human Immunodeficiency Virus . . . . . . . . . . . . . . . . . . 204
Paraneoplastic Pemphigus . . . . . . . . . . . . . . . . . . . . . . . . . . . . . . . . . . . . . . . . . . 206

7. Lichenoid Dermatitis (Subacute to Chronic Cytotoxic Dermatitis) . . . . . . . . . . . . . . 211
General Considerations . . . . . . . . . . . . . . . . . . . . . . . . . . . . . . . . . . . . . . . . . . . . 211
Pathogenesis . . . . . . . . . . . . . . . . . . . . . . . . . . . . . . . . . . . . . . . . . . . . . . . . . . . . 211
Special Diagnostic Studies . . . . . . . . . . . . . . . . . . . . . . . . . . . . . . . . . . . . . . . . . 211
Animal Models . . . . . . . . . . . . . . . . . . . . . . . . . . . . . . . . . . . . . . . . . . . . . . . . . . 211
Lichen Planus . . . . . . . . . . . . . . . . . . . . . . . . . . . . . . . . . . . . . . . . . . . . . . . . . . . 211
Lichen Nitidus . . . . . . . . . . . . . . . . . . . . . . . . . . . . . . . . . . . . . . . . . . . . . . . . . . . 219

|   |   |   |
|---|---|---|
| | Lichen Striatus | 220 |
| | Chronic Graft-Versus-Host Disease (Epidermal Type) | 225 |
| | Lupus Erythematosus | 226 |
| | Dermatomyositis | 234 |
| | Pityriasis Lichenoides Chronica | 237 |
| | Lichenoid Immune Responses | 237 |
| | Secondary Syphilis | 239 |
| | Lichen Sclerosus (Early/Inflammatory Stage) | 243 |
| | Lichenoid Pigmentary Purpura | 245 |
| 8. | Perforating Dermatitis | 253 |
| | General Considerations | 253 |
| | Kyrle Disease | 253 |
| | Elastosis Perforans Serpiginosa | 254 |
| | Reactive Perforating Collagenosis | 257 |
| | Acquired Perforating Disorder of Diabetes or Renal Failure | 259 |
| 9. | Ulcerative Dermatitis | 261 |
| | General Considerations | 261 |
| | Aphthous Stomatitis/Mucositis | 261 |
| | Pyoderma Gangrenosum | 263 |
| | Ulcerating Infectious Disorders | 266 |
| |     Ecthyma Gangrenosum | 266 |
| |     Streptococcal Ecthyma | 267 |
| |     Anthrax | 268 |
| |     Tularemia | 268 |
| |     Lymphogranuloma Venereum | 270 |
| |     Cat Scratch Disease | 270 |
| |     Chancroid | 271 |
| |     Granuloma Inguinale | 271 |
| |     Primary Syphilis | 271 |
| 10. | Nonvasculitic Angiocentric Dermatitis | 275 |
| | General Considerations | 275 |
| | Pathogenesis | 276 |
| | Special Diagnostic Studies | 276 |
| | Animal Models | 277 |
| | Superficial Variants | 278 |
| |     Urticaria | 278 |
| |     Pruritic Urticarial Papules and Plaques of Pregnancy | 282 |
| |     Dermal Contact Dermatitis | 285 |
| |     Progressive Pigmentary Purpura | 287 |

|     |                                                                              |     |
| --- | ---------------------------------------------------------------------------- | --- |
|     | Reticular Erythematous Mucinosis                                             | 288 |
|     | Morbilliform Viral Exanthem                                                  | 289 |
|     | Superficial and Deep Variants                                                | 294 |
|     | Polymorphous Light Eruption                                                  | 294 |
|     | Erythema Annulare Centrifugum (Deep Variant)                                 | 296 |
|     | Erythema Gyratum Repens                                                      | 296 |
|     | Erythema Chronicum Migrans                                                   | 297 |
|     | Jessner Lymphocytic Infiltrate                                               | 299 |
|     | Still Disease                                                                | 301 |
| 11. | Vasculitic Angiocentric Dermatitis                                           | 307 |
|     | General Considerations                                                       | 307 |
|     | Superficial Vasculitic Variants                                              | 307 |
|     | Cutaneous Necrotizing Vasculitis (Leukocytoclastic Vasculitis)               | 307 |
|     | Septic (Bacterial) Vasculitis and Pustular Vasculitis                        | 313 |
|     | Urticarial Vasculitis                                                        | 313 |
|     | Rocky Mountain Spotted Fever                                                 | 314 |
|     | Superficial and Deep Vasculitic Variants                                     | 314 |
|     | Thrombogenic Vasculopathy                                                    | 314 |
|     | Cutaneous Polyarteritis Nodosa                                               | 315 |
|     | Superficial Migratory Thrombophlebitis                                       | 318 |
|     | Livedo Reticularis, Livedo Vasculitis, and Atrophie Blanche                  | 319 |
|     | Nodular Vasculitis (Early Erythema Induratum)                                | 320 |
|     | Granulomatous Vasculitis                                                     | 320 |
|     | Wegener Granulomatosis                                                       | 322 |
|     | Granuloma Faciale                                                            | 324 |
|     | Erythema Nodosum Leprosum                                                    | 325 |
|     | Erythema Elevatum Diutinum                                                   | 325 |
|     | Lymphocytic Vasculitis Group                                                 | 327 |
|     | Lymphomatoid Papulosis                                                       | 329 |
|     | Angioimmunoblastic Lymphadenopathy Involving the Skin                        | 332 |
| 12. | Nodular/Interstitial Dermatitis                                              | 337 |
|     | General Considerations                                                       | 337 |
|     | Pathogenesis                                                                 | 338 |
|     | Special Diagnostic Studies                                                   | 339 |
|     | Primarily Granulocytic Nodular/Interstitial Infiltrates                      | 339 |
|     | Acute Febrile Neutrophilic Dermatitis (Sweet Syndrome)                       | 339 |
|     | Eosinophilic Cellulitis (Wells Syndrome)                                     | 341 |
|     | Pyoderma Gangrenosum                                                         | 342 |
|     | Infectious Causes of Nodular/Interstitial Granulocytic Infiltrates: Pyoderma | 344 |

## Inflammatory Disorders of the Skin

    Primarily Lymphocytic Nodular/Interstitial Infiltrates . . . . . . . . . . . . . . . . . . . . . . . 347
        Morphea (Early/Inflammatory Stage) . . . . . . . . . . . . . . . . . . . . . . . . . . . . . . . . 347
    Primarily Histiocytic Nodular/Interstitial Infiltrates . . . . . . . . . . . . . . . . . . . . . . . . 350
        Granulomatous Reactions to Drugs and Foreign Substances . . . . . . . . . . . . . . . . 350
        Sarcoidosis . . . . . . . . . . . . . . . . . . . . . . . . . . . . . . . . . . . . . . . . . . . . . . . . . . . 350
        Cheilitis Granulomatosa . . . . . . . . . . . . . . . . . . . . . . . . . . . . . . . . . . . . . . . . . 356
        Cutaneous Crohn Disease . . . . . . . . . . . . . . . . . . . . . . . . . . . . . . . . . . . . . . . . 356
        Granuloma Annulare . . . . . . . . . . . . . . . . . . . . . . . . . . . . . . . . . . . . . . . . . . . 358
        Necrobiosis Lipoidica . . . . . . . . . . . . . . . . . . . . . . . . . . . . . . . . . . . . . . . . . . . 360
        Rheumatoid Nodule . . . . . . . . . . . . . . . . . . . . . . . . . . . . . . . . . . . . . . . . . . . . 362
        Annular Elastolytic Giant Cell Granuloma . . . . . . . . . . . . . . . . . . . . . . . . . . . . 363
        Necrobiotic Xanthogranuloma . . . . . . . . . . . . . . . . . . . . . . . . . . . . . . . . . . . . 365
        Nephrogenic Systemic Fibrosis . . . . . . . . . . . . . . . . . . . . . . . . . . . . . . . . . . . . 367
        Granulomatous and Interstitial Inflammatory Reactions to Infectious Agents . . . 371

13. Panniculitis . . . . . . . . . . . . . . . . . . . . . . . . . . . . . . . . . . . . . . . . . . . . . . . . . . . . . . . 397
    General Considerations . . . . . . . . . . . . . . . . . . . . . . . . . . . . . . . . . . . . . . . . . . . 397
    Pathogenesis . . . . . . . . . . . . . . . . . . . . . . . . . . . . . . . . . . . . . . . . . . . . . . . . . . . 398
    Special Diagnostic Studies . . . . . . . . . . . . . . . . . . . . . . . . . . . . . . . . . . . . . . . . . 399
    Erythema Nodosum, a Septal Panniculitis . . . . . . . . . . . . . . . . . . . . . . . . . . . . . . 399
    Erythema Induratum (Nodular Vasculitis), a Mixed Panniculitis . . . . . . . . . . . . . . . 404
    Panniculitis Due to Connective Tissue Disease . . . . . . . . . . . . . . . . . . . . . . . . . . . 409
        Lupus Profundus, a Mixed Panniculitis . . . . . . . . . . . . . . . . . . . . . . . . . . . . . . . 409
        Connective Tissue Panniculitis . . . . . . . . . . . . . . . . . . . . . . . . . . . . . . . . . . . . . 411
        Panniculitis of Dermatomyositis and Polymyositis, Morphea, and Scleroderma . . 412
    Eosinophilic Fasciitis, with Septal or Mixed Panniculitis . . . . . . . . . . . . . . . . . . . . 414
    Relapsing Febrile Nodular Nonsuppurative Panniculitis (Weber-Christian Disease) 414
    Pancreatic (Enzymatic) Panniculitis . . . . . . . . . . . . . . . . . . . . . . . . . . . . . . . . . . 416
    Sclerema Neonatorum . . . . . . . . . . . . . . . . . . . . . . . . . . . . . . . . . . . . . . . . . . . 416
    Subcutaneous Fat Necrosis of the Newborn . . . . . . . . . . . . . . . . . . . . . . . . . . . . 417
    Lipodermatosclerosis, a Mixed Panniculitis . . . . . . . . . . . . . . . . . . . . . . . . . . . . . 419
    Histiocytic Cytophagic Panniculitis, a Lobular Panniculitis . . . . . . . . . . . . . . . . . . 420
    Eosinophilic Panniculitis . . . . . . . . . . . . . . . . . . . . . . . . . . . . . . . . . . . . . . . . . . 421
    Miscellaneous Panniculitides . . . . . . . . . . . . . . . . . . . . . . . . . . . . . . . . . . . . . . . 422
        Hypogammaglobulinemia . . . . . . . . . . . . . . . . . . . . . . . . . . . . . . . . . . . . . . . . 422
        Migratory Panniculitis . . . . . . . . . . . . . . . . . . . . . . . . . . . . . . . . . . . . . . . . . . 422
        Panniculitis of Rothman-Makai . . . . . . . . . . . . . . . . . . . . . . . . . . . . . . . . . . . . 422
        Alpha-1-Antitrypsin Deficiency . . . . . . . . . . . . . . . . . . . . . . . . . . . . . . . . . . . . 422
        Panniculitis Secondary to Covert Fungal or Mycobacterial Infection . . . . . . . . . . 422

14. **Inflammatory Disorders with Primary Adnexal Alterations: Follicular Conditions** .... 431
    - General Considerations ................................................. 431
    - Pathogenesis ......................................................... 432
    - Special Diagnostic Studies ............................................ 432
    - Animal Models ........................................................ 432
    - Acne Vulgaris ........................................................ 432
    - Infectious Folliculitis .............................................. 436
    - Acne Rosacea ......................................................... 443
    - Keratosis Pilaris, Inflammatory Variant .............................. 444
    - Eosinophilic Pustular Folliculitis ................................... 445
    - Perforating Folliculitis ............................................. 448
    - Alopecia Areata ...................................................... 449
    - Androgenetic (Pattern) Alopecia ...................................... 450
    - Alopecia Mucinosa .................................................... 453
    - Lupus Alopecia ....................................................... 454
    - Lichen Planopilaris .................................................. 457
    - Traumatic and Scarring Alopecia Group ................................ 460
        - Trichotillomania ................................................. 460
        - Traction Alopecia ................................................ 460
        - Follicular Degeneration Syndrome ................................. 460
        - End-Stage Scarring Alopecia ...................................... 460

15. **Apocrine and Eccrine Conditions** ..................................... 467
    - Miliaria Group ....................................................... 467
    - Neutrophilic Eccrine Hidradenitis .................................... 468
    - Hidradenitis Suppurativa ............................................. 469
    - Apocrine Miliaria .................................................... 471

    Index ................................................................. 473

# 1 STRUCTURE, FUNCTION, AND REACTION PATTERNS

## ARCHITECTURE AND CELLULAR COMPONENTS

The normal cutaneous microanatomy is complex, and a thorough understanding of structural-functional relationships is integral to accurate histopathologic diagnosis of both inflammatory and neoplastic skin conditions (1–7). The skin is composed of three layers: the epidermis, the dermis, and the subcutaneous fat. The epidermis is composed of keratinocytes, Langerhans cells, melanocytes, and Merkel cells. The dermis, which is separated from the epidermis by a basement membrane, contains fibroblasts, mast cells, phagocytic and antigen-presenting macrophages, nerve fibers, endothelial cells forming blood vessels, and highly dendritic cells, some of which express coagulation factor XIIIa (dermal dendrocytes), all embedded within an extracellular matrix composed of collagen, elastin, and mucopolysaccharides. Adipocytes predominate in subcutaneous fat. The adnexal epithelium consists of pilar and related sebaceous and smooth muscle structures as well as apocrine and eccrine glands. Table 1-1 summarizes many of the structural/functional relationships inherent to the epidermal and dermal strata.

## REGIONAL ANATOMY

The recognition of regional anatomic characteristics in skin biopsy specimens prevents potential misinterpretation of normal variations as pathology. This is particularly true when evaluating non-neoplastic disorders of the skin, where subtle deviations from the normal thickness or composition of one or more skin layers may contribute to a diagnosis. Table 1-2 summarizes some of the pathologic lesions that regional variation in microanatomy mimic. Detailed information concerning biopsy site must be assessed with correlative clinical information to avoid these common pitfalls when evaluating non-neoplastic conditions.

## RESPONSES TO INJURY

A comprehensive understanding of the structure and function of normal skin and recognition of its extensive, yet finite, repertoire of responses to exogenous and endogenous injury are fundamental to the practice of dermatopathology. Most non-neoplastic disorders of the skin are typified by a constellation of reaction patterns, which collectively permit diagnostic recognition and sometimes even predict etiology. In this section, normal anatomic and functional relationships are briefly reviewed, with specific reference to their diagnostic utility in evaluating commonly encountered pathologic conditions affecting the skin.

### Keratinocytes

**Histology.** *Keratinocytes* are the cells that form the most superficial layers of the skin, the surface epidermis and associated adnexal downgrowths. The keratinocyte is the only cell that is reliably identified by routine light microscopy (melanocytes and Merkel cells within the basal cell layer and Langerhans cells within the mid-epidermis may show slightly different nuclear characteristics, but antibody markers are generally required to confirm their identity). Keratinocytes are responsible for the synthesis of the tough structural protein, keratin, and are important in the synthesis of immunologically active cytokines. Keratinocytes are primary intermediates between the internal fibrovascular milieu of the underlying dermis and the external environment. Keratin is a resilient, protective protein that forms the outermost scaly layer that shields the body from harmful environmental stimuli. Keratinocytes are also recipients of brown melanin pigment produced by nearby melanocytes, a transfer process that allows uniform distribution of this endogenous sunscreen throughout the epidermal layer. Cytokines produced by epidermal keratinocytes are fundamental to the regulation of

Table 1-1

**CUTANEOUS STRUCTURAL/FUNCTIONAL RELATIONSHIPS RELEVANT TO NON-NEOPLASTIC DISORDERS OF THE SKIN**

| Cell/Structure | Primary Function(s) | Pathology | Specific Disorder[a] |
|---|---|---|---|
| Keratinocyte | Keratin protein production<br>Cytokine production<br>Melanin storage/dispersion | Hyperplasia (acanthosis) | Lichen simplex chronicus |
| -Stratum corneum | Surface protection | Parakeratosis | Psoriasis |
| -Stratum granulosum | Permeability barrier | Acantholysis | Pemphigus foliaceous |
| -Stratum spinosum | Intermediate filament assembly | Spongiosis | Contact allergy |
| -Stratum basalis | Replication/renewal (stem cells at rete tips) | Apoptosis | Graft-vs-host disease |
| Melanocyte | Melanin production | Depletion | Vitiligo |
| Langerhans cell | Antigen uptake and presentation | Hyperplasia | Langerhans cell microgranuloma |
| Merkel cell | Unknown in humans | Unknown | Unknown |
| Follicular germ | Trichogenesis | Depletion | Alopecia areata |
| Follicular bulge | Stem cell domain | Depletion | Lichen planopilaris |
| Sweat glands | Temperature regulation | Inflammation | Miliaria |
| Basement membrane | Epidermal-dermal adhesion | Reduplication | Lupus erythematosus |
| Anchoring fibrils | Basement membrane-dermal anchorage | Gene deletion | Epidermolysis bullosa (dystrophic) |
| Fibroblasts | Collagen/elastin production | Abnormal synthesis | Scleroderma |
| Dermal dendrocyte | FXIIIa production, antigen presentation | Proliferation | ? Altered wound healing<br>? Dermal immune reactions |
| Mast cell | Vasoactive mediator production (histamine, cytokines) | Degranulation | Urticaria |
| Histiocyte/macrophage | Particulate uptake, antigen presentation | Melanophage accumulation | Fixed drug eruption |
| Nerve fibers | Sensation, neuropeptide secretion | Idiopathic pruritus, cell maturation and growth | Prurigo nodularis<br>Hair cycle |
| Endothelial cells | Leukocyte adhesion, anti-coagulation | Necrosis | Leukocytoclastic vasculitis |

[a]An example of a non-neoplastic condition in which this pathologic change occurs, usually along with multiple other alterations that, in aggregate, permit diagnosis.

Table 1-2

**REGIONAL MICROANATOMY MIMICKING PATHOLOGIC CHANGES**

| Normal Skin Site | Relevant Normal Feature(s) or Response(s) | Potential Diagnostic Pitfall[a] |
|---|---|---|
| Acral | Compact and thickened stratum corneum | Lamellar ichthyosis |
| Mucosal | Absence of stratum granulosum | Psoriasis |
| Mucosal/paramucosal | Many subepithelial vessels | Reactive angiogenesis |
| Mucosal/paramucosal | Plasma cells | Secondary syphilis |
| Elbow/knee | Slightly verrucous epidermis | Verrucoid lichen simplex chronicus |
| Photoaged skin | Epidermal atrophy | Atrophic interface dermatitis |
| Darkly pigmented skin (any site) | Increased melanophages | Late stage of fixed drug eruption |

[a]Pathologic pitfall based on this single feature; detailed analysis of most biopsies should permit correct diagnosis based on ancillary findings, although it is always advisable to interpret all findings in the context of knowledge of the biopsy site.

**Figure 1-1**

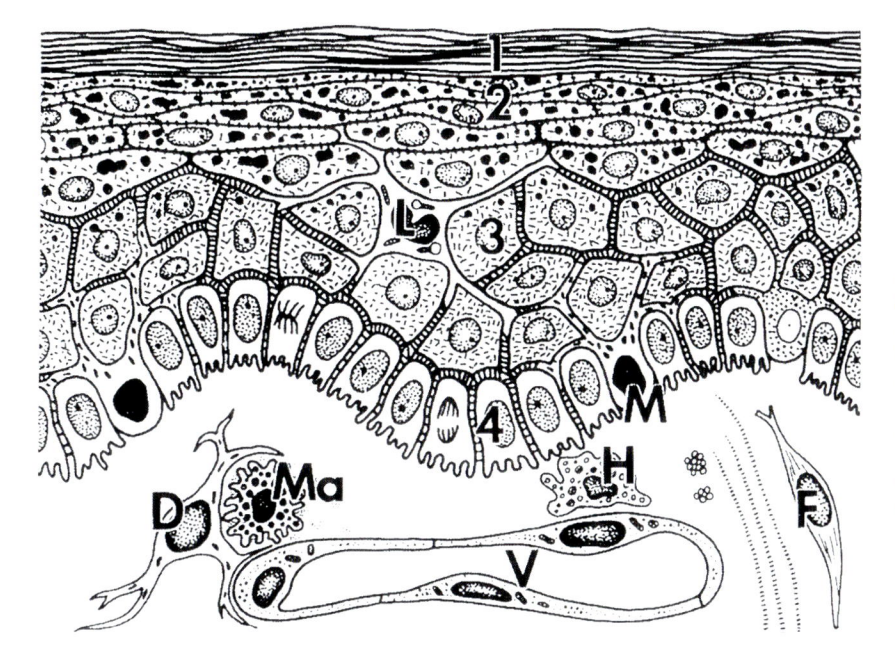

**SCHEMATIC OF SUPERFICIAL SKIN LAYERS**

Schematic diagram of normal epidermal and superficial dermal layers. (1-4 = epidermal strata: stratum corneum, stratum granulosum, stratum spinosum, and stratum basalis, respectively. M = melanocyte; L = Langerhans cell; V = postcapillary venule; H = histiocyte/macrophage; Ma = mast cell; D = dermal dendrocyte; F = fibroblast.)

**Figure 1-2**

**NORMAL EPIDERMIS: HISTOLOGY**

The more melanized stratum basalis shows gradual upward maturation to become stratum spinosum, stratum granulosum, and stratum corneum. The latter forms an acellular "basket-weave" pattern on the epidermal surface of nonacral skin.

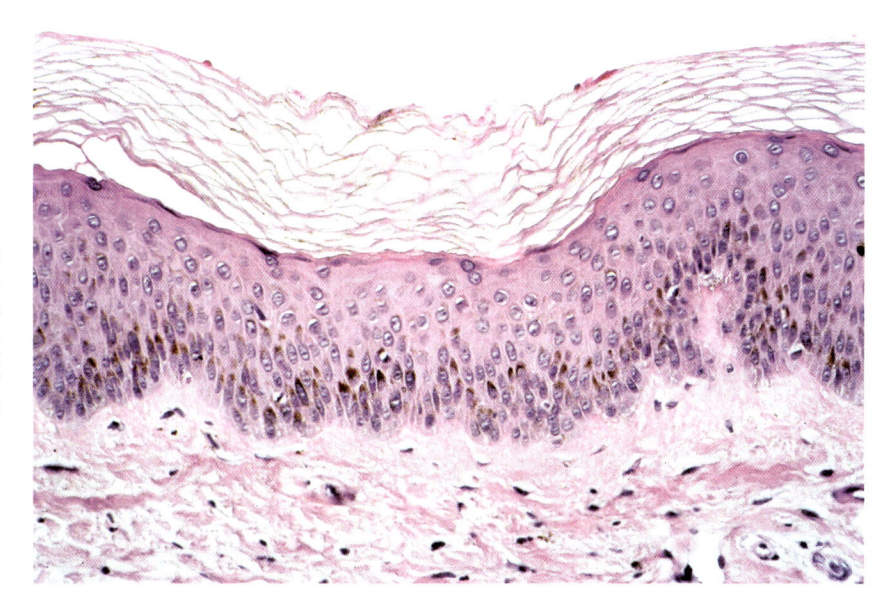

cutaneous inflammatory responses, protecting the body from harmful exogenous antigens and potentially assisting in recognizing endogenous neoantigens on mutated cells.

Schematically, the epidermis may be divided into discrete layers that are integrally associated with the superficial dermis to form a superficial reactive unit (fig. 1-1). At scanning magnification, the epidermis appears as a well-demarcated layer of eosinophilic cells on the surface of the superficial dermis. On closer inspection, the cells that form the uppermost layers of the epidermis are radically different from those that form the lower layers (fig. 1-2). This distinction is the result of epidermal maturation, a phenomenon that results in the genesis of terminally differentiated keratinizing cells that form the most superficial anucleate layer, the *stratum corneum*. The normal stratum corneum from truncal skin has a characteristic basket-weave architectural pattern, which changes dramatically according to normal regional anatomic variation and in

*Inflammatory Disorders of the Skin*

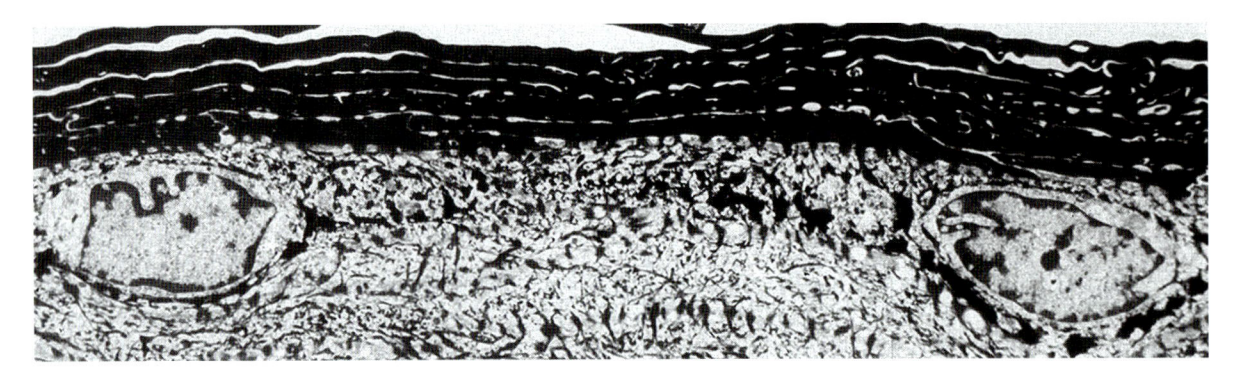

**Figure 1-3**

**NORMAL SUPERFICIAL EPIDERMIS: ULTRASTRUCTURE**

Upon glutaraldehyde fixation the basket-weave configuration is less apparent. The keratohyaline granules directly beneath the stratum corneum define the site of terminal differentiation and cornified envelope formation.

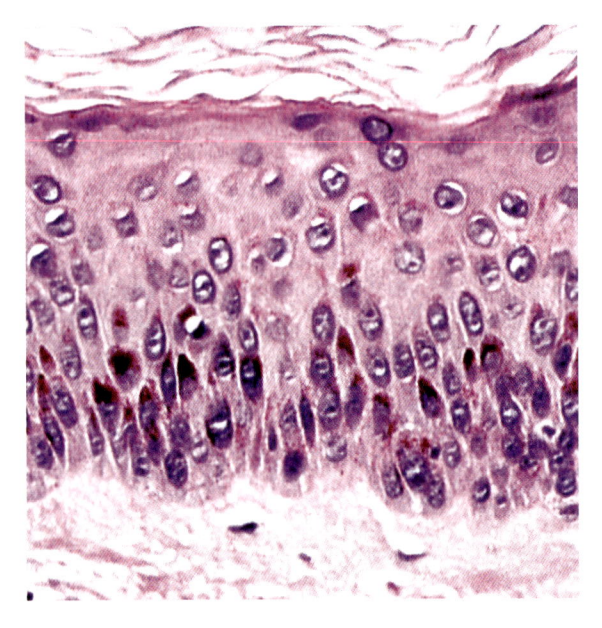

**Figure 1-4**

**STRATUM SPINOSUM**

Note the visible intercellular spaces and the preferential distribution of melanin within the lowermost epidermal layers.

response to injury (fig. 1-2). The cells that form the stratum corneum are flattened, anucleate, keratin-filled plates that fuse to form a protective surface (fig. 1-3).

Directly beneath the stratum corneum is a layer that is normally several cells thick and is composed of nucleated, flattened keratinocytes that are slightly smaller in radial diameter than the cells of the overlying stratum corneum. These small, flattened keratinocytes contain minute, variably shaped, dark blue keratohyaline granules; accordingly, this layer is named the *stratum granulosum* (figs. 1-2–1-3). The cytoplasmic granules contribute to the cell envelope, composed of the protein involucrin, that typifies terminal epidermal differentiation.

The thickest epidermal layer lies immediately below the stratum granulosum and is termed the *stratum spinosum* because of its spiny appearance, due to the prominence of intercellular attachment plaques (desmosomes) that are present throughout all the epidermal layers (figs. 1-4–1-10). The cells composing the stratum spinosum are smaller than those that lie above and have a polyhedral contour. They synthesize keratin proteins that are demonstrated immunohistochemically (fig. 1-11) and that correlate with intracytoplasmic intermediate filaments ultrastructurally (fig. 1-12)

The lowermost epidermal layer is the *stratum basalis*, a single layer of round to vertically ovoid cells (figs. 1-4 and 1-13). These cells rest upon a subjacent basement membrane, which joins the epidermis to the dermis below. Unlike the cells of other layers, the cells of the stratum basalis are capable of continuous replication (8,9), resulting in self-renewal of the entire epidermis on approximately a monthly basis (fig. 1-14). The undersurface of the epidermis forms a honeycomb of rete ridges, which interdigitate with the dermal papillae of the adjacent papillary dermis. Basal cells at the tips of rete ridges at some anatomic sites (e.g., palm) are slow cycling and possess characteristics of stem cells (10), as do

*Structure, Function, and Reaction Patterns*

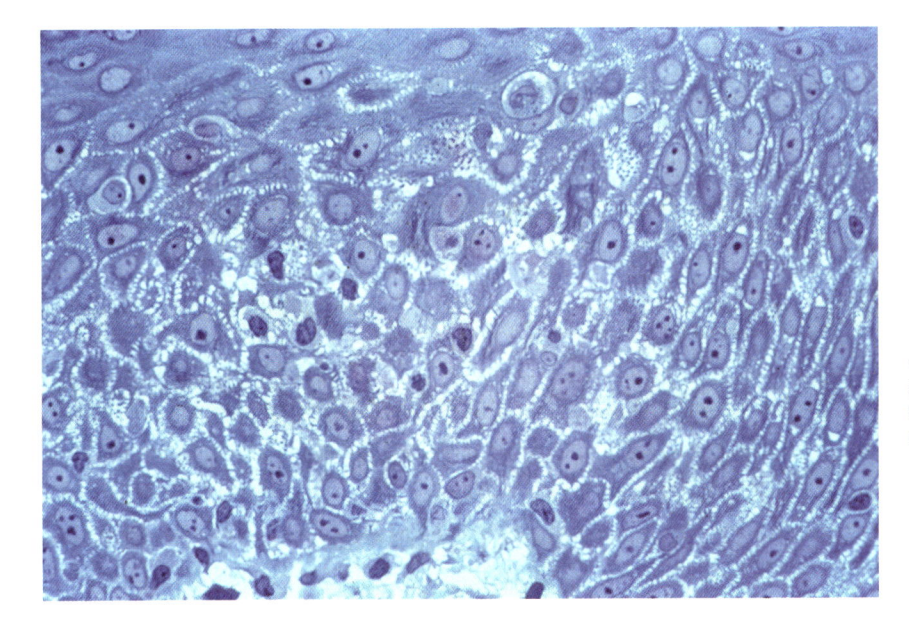

**Figure 1-5**

**ONE-MICRON, PLASTIC-EMBEDDED SECTION OF STRATUM SPINOSUM**

The scattered smaller cells with dark nuclei are T lymphocytes that normally percolate throughout the skin in numbers that exceed those in the peripheral blood.

**Figure 1-6**

**ONE-MICRON, PLASTIC-EMBEDDED SECTION OF STRATUM SPINOSUM**

High magnification of the epidermal layer using this technique shows polyhedral keratinocytes, cytokeratin intermediate filaments, and prominent spiney intercellular connections.

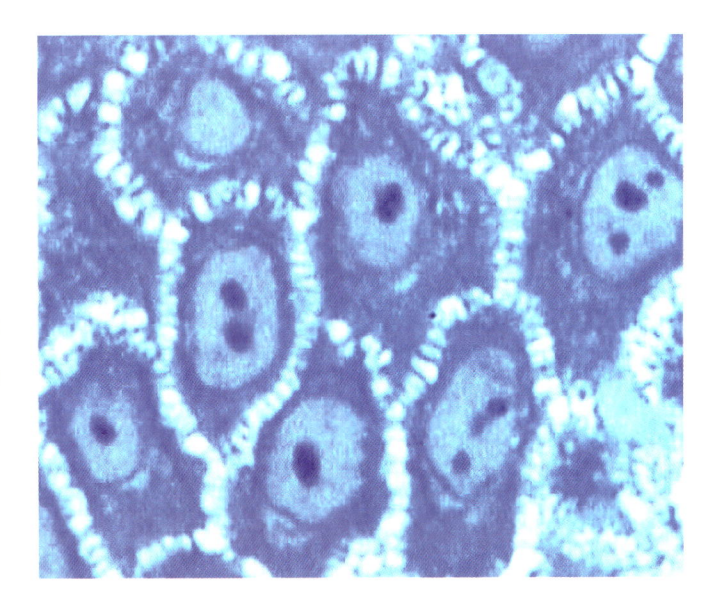

similar cells that form the bulge region of the hair follicle (11) (see below).

The thickness and architecture of the epidermis vary considerably according to body site. The density, morphology, and composition of adnexal downgrowths of the epidermal layer also change according to anatomic location. Diagnostic recognition of these differences is fundamental to determining whether tissue is expressing normal regional variation or true pathologic alteration. All skin specimens must be evaluated within the context of the known anatomy of normal skin at the site of the biopsy. Moreover, normal physiologic alterations also cause confusion. Common examples of this include the universal thinning of the epidermal layer associated with advanced age, a finding that could be interpreted as pathologically relevant atrophy when associated with underlying inflammation, and racially determined

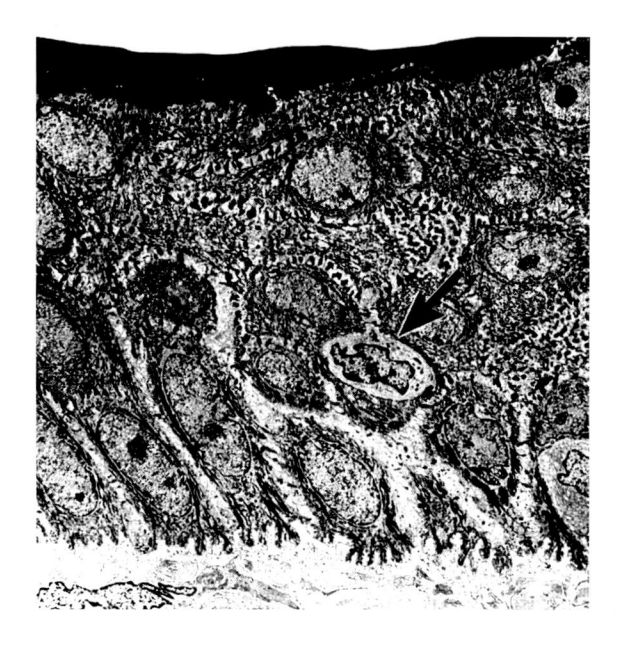

## Figure 1-7
**NORMAL EPIDERMIS: ULTRASTRUCTURE**

The intermediate (cytokeratin) intracytoplasmic filaments as well as spiney intercellular attachments are readily discerned. Nonkeratinocytes (arrow) are also apparent.

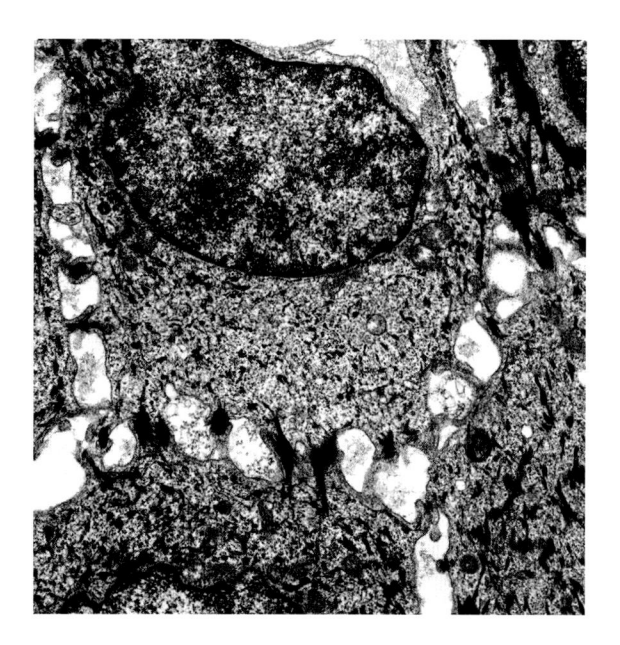

## Figure 1-8
**NORMAL STRATUM SPINOSUM: ULTRASTRUCTURE**

At high magnification, intermediate filaments, also called tonofilaments, are aggregated near dense intercellular bridges, indicating structural integrity between cytoskeletal components and intercellular junctional complexes.

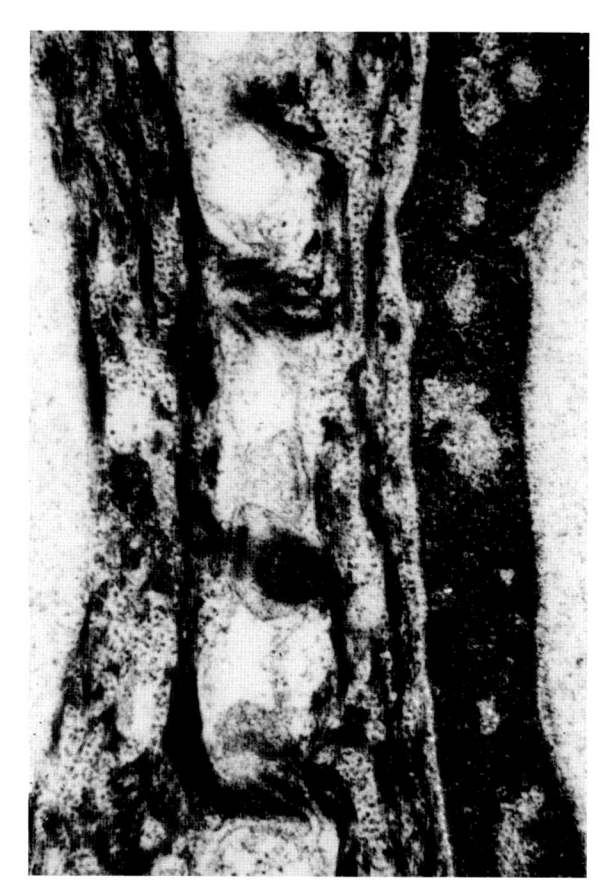

## Figure 1-9
**UNIFICATION OF DESMOSOMES AND INTERMEDIATE CYTOSKELETAL FILAMENTS**

Emanating from each desmosome is a fibrillary tuft of cytokeratin filament that connects to the cytoskeleton.

darkly pigmented skin, which may superficially mimic melanin pigment incontinence after basal cell layer injury.

**Ultrastructure.** The ultrastructural features of the epidermal keratinocyte that are relevant to diagnostic dermatopathology include desmosomes and hemidesmosomes, intermediate filaments, and phagocytized melanosomes. *Desmosomes* are specialized laminated attachment plaques that bind together the plasma membranes of adjacent keratinocytes. Desmosomes consist of two outer, electron-dense, thick bands and three inner thin bands arranged in a parallel array (figs. 1-9, 1-10) (12,13). Between the inner bands is the *glycocalyx*, or intercellular cement substance, which is the presumed site of injury in pemphigus and is chemically associated with the desmogleins.

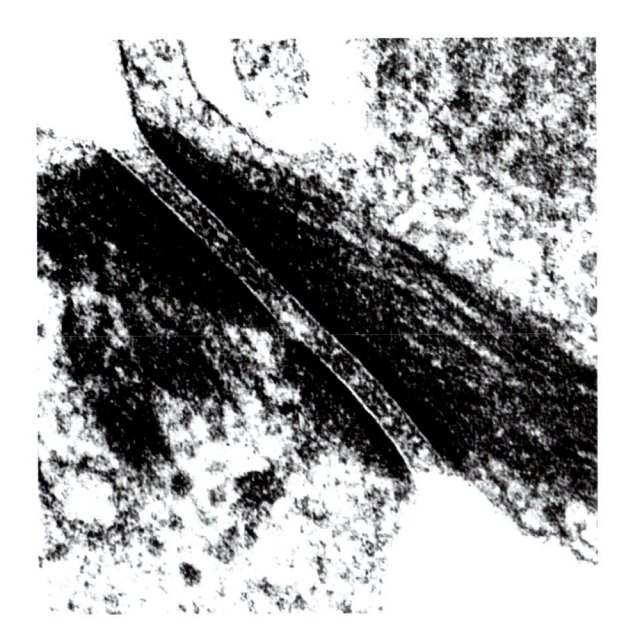

## Figure 1-10

**INTERCELLULAR JUNCTIONAL COMPLEX: ULTRASTRUCTURE**

The desmosomal disk has a laminated internal structure which is sandwiched between aggregated intermediate filaments that belong to two adjacent keratinocytes within the stratum corneum.

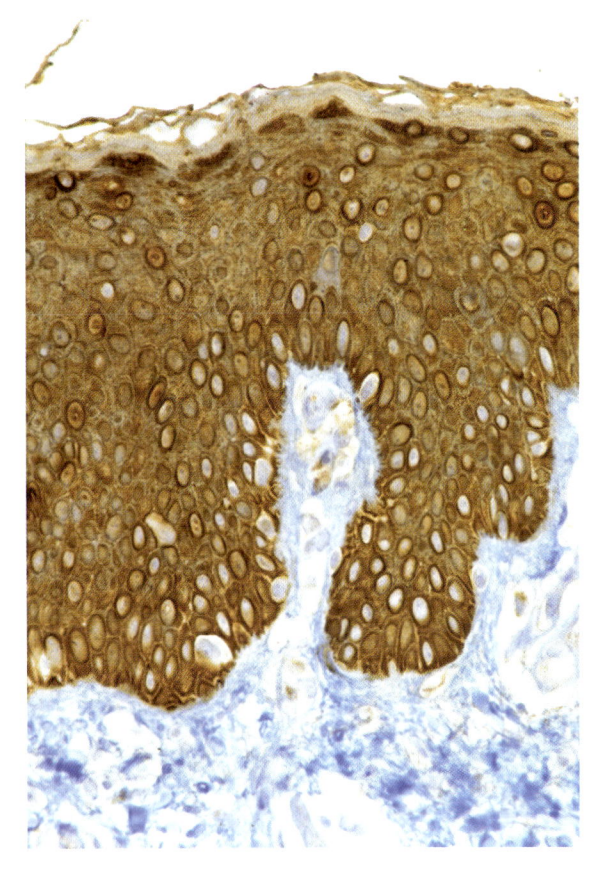

## Figure 1-11

**IMMUNOPEROXIDASE STAINING OF CYTOKERATINS OF VARIOUS MOLECULAR WEIGHTS WITHIN THE EPIDERMAL LAYER**

Because the antibody "cocktail" labels both simple and complex cytokeratins, the staining is diffuse throughout the epidermal layer.

Smaller, structurally less complex *hemidesmosomes* assist in anchoring the inferior surface of the basal cell plasma membrane to the adjacent basement membrane. Although desmosomes cannot be detected by routine light microscopy, their presence may be inferred by the detection of spiny intercellular junctions that routinely become stretched and thus more prominent in the setting of spongiotic dermatitis.

*Intermediate filaments* are also called *tonofilaments* when found in keratinocytes (fig. 1-12). They are synthesized in molecular pairs within the basal cell layer and become progressively larger and heavier within the maturing overlying epidermal layers. These clustered aggregates of cytoplasmic fibrils are 7 to 8 nm in diameter. While many of these filaments are continuous with the attachment plaques of desmosomes, others lie free within the cytoplasm. Most of these filaments represent intracytoplasmic keratin protein, and their distribution throughout the cell results in a cytoskeleton integral to the formation and preservation of cell shape and structure (fig. 1-11). Intermediate filaments are characteristic, although not entirely specific, of keratinocytes, and cells such as Merkel cells may display prominent perinuclear clusters of keratin type intermediate filaments within their cytoplasm.

*Melanosome complexes* are membrane-bound aggregates of melanized, electron-dense melanosomes within the cytoplasm of keratinocytes and macrophages (melanophages). In the normal epidermis, these complexes result from physiologic pigment donation from nearby melanocytes, and they tend to be diffusely distributed within the epidermal layer. The tendency for keratinocytes to package melanosomes in small aggregates, as opposed to solitary organelles, is characteristic of the skin of Caucasians and those of Asian descent, whereas transmitted

# Inflammatory Disorders of the Skin

Figure 1-12

**ULTRASTRUCTURAL CORRELATE OF CYTOKERATIN STAINING**

Loosely aggregated bundles of keratin intermediate filaments are present amid a background of free ribosomes.

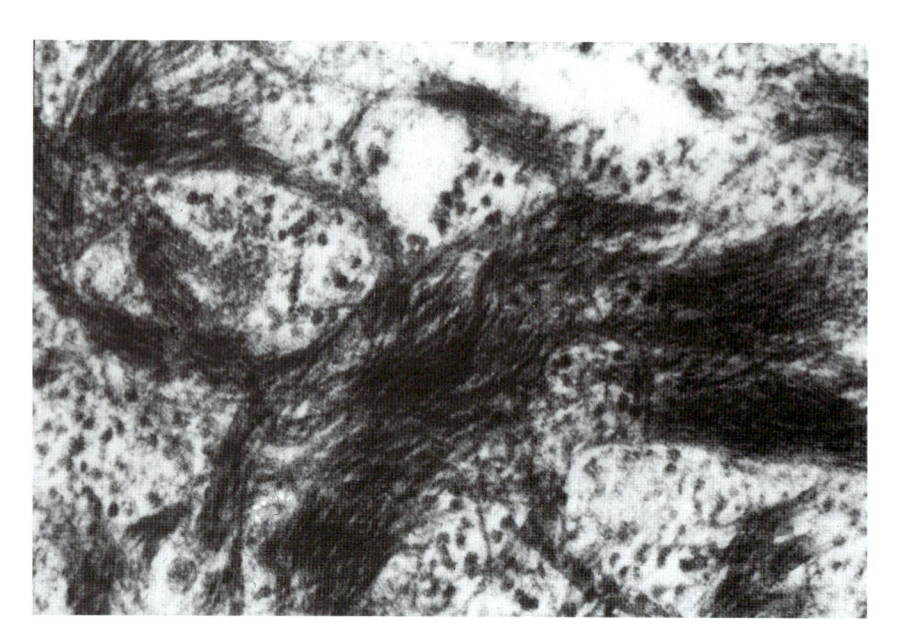

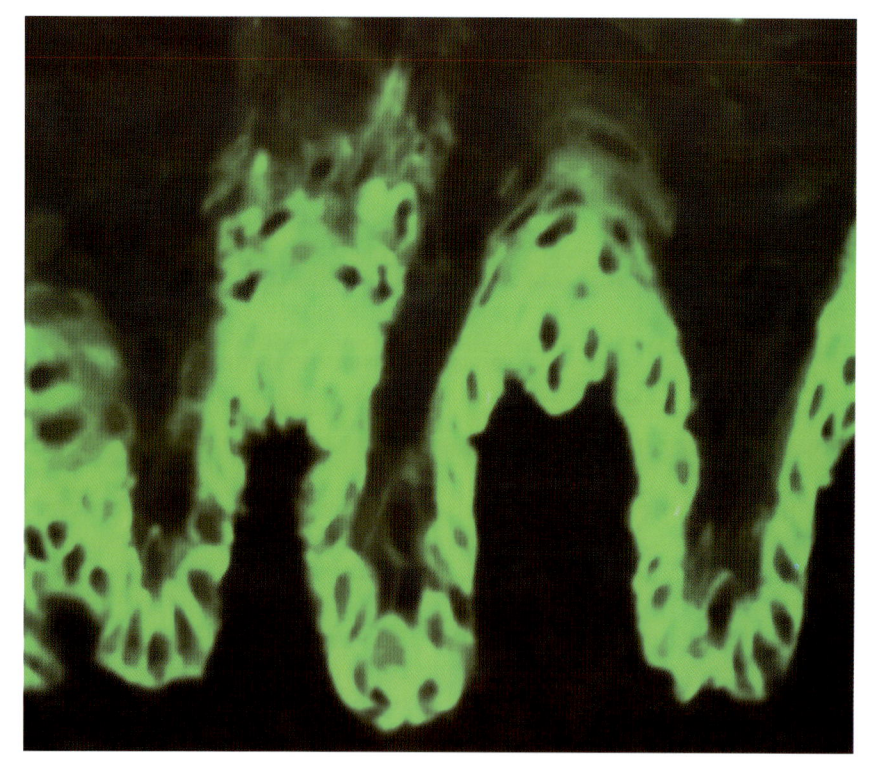

Figure 1-13

**IMMUNOFLUORESCENCE MICROSCOPY OF LOW MOLECULAR WEIGHT CYTOKERATIN (CYTOKERATIN 14)**

There is restriction to the more primitive cells of the basal layer.

melanosomes remain solitary within keratinocytes of individuals of African descent and in Australian aborigines. Ultrastructural detection of melanocytes and melanosomes, and their extent of melanization, may be diagnostically important when evaluating skin disorders that result in clinical hypopigmentation.

**Hyperplasia (Acanthosis).** *Epidermal hyperplasia* may be diffuse or preferentially favor the stratum granulosum, stratum spinosum, or stratum basalis. It is manifested by increased epidermal thickness for body site, by abnormal keratinization, and often but not invariably, by increased numbers of mitotic figures within and above

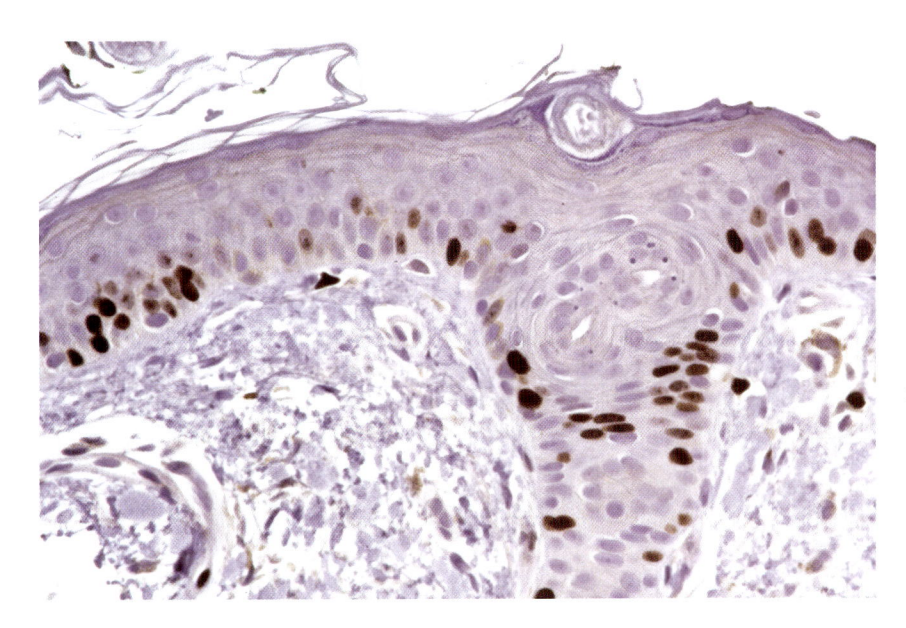

**Figure 1-14**

**LABELING OF REPLICATING EPIDERMAL CELLS BY Ki-67 (MIB-1)**

Cycling cells are normally restricted to the stratum basalis.

the stratum basalis. Epidermal hyperplasia preferentially involving the stratum spinosum and stratum basalis may take the form of endophytic expansion of rete ridges to similar (*regular acanthosis*) or differing (*irregular acanthosis*) horizontal levels within the superficial dermis. Because acanthosis appears to originate in the mitotically active cells associated with the rete ridges, which become accentuated during this process, we refer to disorders showing such alteration as those with *retiform epidermal hyperplasia*.

Accurate characterization of acanthosis is imperative, because it greatly facilitates diagnostic recognition of a number of commonly encountered dermatoses. The regular acanthosis with hypogranulosis of psoriasis, for example, is distinct from the irregular acanthosis with hypergranulosis of lichen simplex chronicus. The features of the latter are separable from chronic active eczematous dermatitis, which also displays spongiosis. Wedge-shaped hypergranulosis with acanthosis is more commonly seen in lichen planus than in rare hypertrophic variants of lupus erythematosus. Acanthosis may be accompanied by reactive atypia (variability in nuclear size and nucleolar prominence in the presence of uniformly finely dispersed chromatin and a delicate nuclear membrane), particularly in the setting of repeated attempts at reepithelialization (e.g., at the edge of an ulcer). The reactive atypia seen in inflammatory and reparative processes must be differentiated from keratinocyte proliferation accompanied by dysplasia (variability in nuclear size and nucleolar prominence in the presence of irregularly coarsely dispersed chromatin and a thickened nuclear membrane as a result of chromatin condensation), as is commonly encountered in actinic keratoses and squamous cell carcinomas (Table 1-3).

**Abnormal Keratinization (Hyperkeratosis and Parakeratosis).** Abnormalities in keratinization are sometimes the most subtle of diagnostic manifestations detectable at the light microscopic level (e.g., in the setting of ichthyosis), or are so grossly visible that a clinically apparent, animal-like cutaneous horn is produced. Normal basket-weave stratum corneum is referred to

**Table 1-3**

**CYTOLOGIC DIFFERENCES BETWEEN REACTIVE KERATINOCYTIC ATYPIA AND DYSPLASIA**

| | Reactive Atypia | Dysplasia |
|---|---|---|
| Nuclear size | Relatively uniform | Variable |
| Nuclear shape | Round to ovoid | Angulated contour |
| Nuclear membrane | Thin, uniform | Thick, irregular |
| Heterochromatin | Delicate, evenly dispersed | Clumped, uneven |
| Nucleolus | Prominent | Prominent |
| Mitotic rate | Often high | Often high |
| Atypical mitosis | Infrequent | Often seen |

as *orthokeratotic scale*. Retention of nuclei into the scale is termed *parakeratosis*, a process that may be exquisitely focal and mound-like, as in pityriasis rosea, or diffuse and confluent, as in untreated active psoriasis. When the stratum corneum is increased in thickness without parakeratosis, the term *hyperorthokeratosis* is used. When the cells that form the layer lie closer together, the modifier *compact* is used. Thus, whereas ichthyosis may show only compact orthokeratotic stratum corneum, lichen simplex chronicus is characterized by a compact hyperorthokeratotic stratum corneum. Although exceptions exist, hyperorthokeratosis is generally associated with underlying hypergranulosis and parakeratosis often is associated with underlying diminution in thickness of the stratum granulosum.

Abnormalities in the stratum corneum do not always correlate with an underlying proliferative defect (e.g., retiform epidermal hyperplasia), because impaired desquamation may also result in retention of altered scale. Recognition of normal stratum corneum overlying an inflammatory infiltrate associated with epidermal injury usually signifies that the lesion is days or hours old (e.g., erythema multiforme) and testifies to the sensitivity of scale as an eventual indicator of even subtle chronic perturbations of underlying epidermal cells (e.g., guttate parapsoriasis). The normal stratum corneum of palm and sole skin would represent strikingly compacted hyperorthokeratosis if found on the trunk, and any form of stratum corneum or stratum granulosum is abnormal in mucosal epithelium.

**Dyskeratosis.** Although epidermal keratinization normally occurs on the skin surface, keratin may be produced prematurely by underlying cells in certain pathologic circumstances. In transient acantholytic dermatosis, individual cells of the uppermost stratum spinosum and stratum granulosum become condensed and develop abnormal keratin-rich cytoplasm in association with acantholysis. Individual keratinocytes prematurely undergoing keratinization acquire cytoplasmic eosinophilia inappropriate for their level within the epidermis. This phenomenon, termed *dyskeratosis*, is different from the cellular degeneration and necrosis that result in cytoplasmic hypereosinophilia due to pH and water shifts or that are usually accompanied by an inflammatory insult and evidence of nuclear degeneration. Dyskeratosis is also different mechanistically from eosinophilic apoptotic cells that arise normally or pathologically as a consequence of endonuclease-mediated DNA fragmentation within the cell nucleus.

**Atrophy.** *Atrophy* is the thinning of the epidermis. It is invariably associated with diminution to absence of the epidermal rete ridges, producing a relatively straight, as opposed to an undulant, dermal-epidermal interface. Some degree of atrophy accompanies normal senescence of the skin, although physiologic thinning may be accelerated by substances such as prolonged or intensified application of potent topical steroids (e.g., as with occlusion). Chronic destruction of the stratum basalis commonly eventuates in epidermal atrophy (e.g., discoid lupus erythematosus). Advanced atrophy may result in a clinically semitransparent, easily wrinkled epidermal layer reduced to only several cell layers in thickness.

**Spongiosis.** The accumulation of plasma fluid in the intercellular spaces of the epidermis results in widened intercellular spaces and a prominent display of stretched intercellular junctions. This spongy appearance is the basis for the term *spongiosis* and permits broad classification of a diverse array of inflammatory dermatoses that share this feature. The prototype of spongiotic dermatitis is allergic contact dermatitis. Pathophysiologically, spongiosis usually occurs in disorders characterized by the increased permeability of superficial dermal venules and the migration of lymphocytes into the epidermis. Retiform epidermal hyperplasia or acanthosis is often seen in combination with spongiosis of subacute to chronic duration (weeks to months). Progression of spongiosis results in traumatic disruption of desmosomes and the formation of fluid-filled intraepidermal vesicles. The absence of spongiosis may be as diagnostically critical as its detection, as is the case in psoriasis, where spongiosis is generally absent, in contrast to acute to chronic allergic contact dermatitis, where spongiotic alterations at least focally persist.

**Acantholysis.** *Acantholysis* is a process whereby desmosomal attachments are lost or compromised, resulting in defective intercellular adhesion within the epidermis. The result generally is blister formation that occurs spontaneously or in association with minor trauma. Acantholytic cells within the stratum spinosum lose their angulated, polyhedral contour and characteristically become rounded. Unlike spongiosis, which mechanically disrupts membrane attachment sites, potentially killing cells that constitute the perimeter of the forming blister, the precisely localized lysis of desmosomal attachment plaques produces an acantholytic cell which may persist for some time as a rounded epithelial cell floating in nutrient-rich plasma filtrate. Pemphigus vulgaris is an example of immunologically mediated acantholysis. Keratinocytes that are genetically or neoplastically altered to produce faulty intercellular attachments also may exhibit acantholysis (e.g., as in Darier disease and in certain invasive squamous cell carcinomas). These acantholytic cells also frequently show associated dyskeratosis (so-called *acantholytic dyskeratosis*). Acantholytic and dyskeratotic cells appear as small, seed-like ovoid cells with densely eosinophilic cytoplasm and pyknotic nuclei ("corps grains") when they occur in the uppermost epidermal layers, or as larger, rounded acantholytic cells with characteristic perinuclear halos ("corps ronds") when they occur in the midepidermis. The extensive acantholysis of squamous cell carcinoma may produce gland-like spaces, resulting in confusion with adenocarcinoma, unless the acantholytic process is accurately recognized.

**Apoptosis.** Although cell replication is balanced, in part, by surface desquamation, keratinocytes are also individually eliminated physiologically by the process of *apoptosis*, or programmed cell death. Apoptosis refers to the death of individual cells within the epidermis, often within the stratum spinosum and basalis. Affected cells show cytoplasmic eosinophilia and nuclear pyknosis. The earliest degenerative alterations involve the nucleus, however. These consist of DNA fragmentation that produces a ladder-like pattern by electrophoresis and that is mediated by endonucleases. Frequently, these cells are in apposition to, or are partially engulfed by, adjacent mononuclear cells, which ultrastructurally are phagocytic macrophages capable of digesting necrotic keratinocytes. Rare apoptotic cells are physiologically normal, especially in involuting follicular epithelium, although their presence is increased after certain forms of radiation and chemotherapy, and during cytotoxic or cytokine-mediated epidermal injury. In the latter scenario, ligation of death receptors at the keratinocyte surface may be responsible for setting into motion an intracellular cascade that eventuates in the activation of caspases. Apoptotic cells may also be incorporated into the superficial dermis, where they appear as anucleated, rounded eosinophilic bodies (colloid bodies) that ultimately are transformed so that they stain for epidermal type amyloid and contain immunoglobulin. Colloid body formation is typical of lichen planus, and may assist in the diagnosis of this condition.

**Cytotoxic Alteration.** *Cytotoxic alteration* refers to degeneration and necrosis of keratinocytes in association with inflammatory infiltrates composed of lymphocytes with cytotoxic capabilities. Some forms of cytotoxic injury involve apoptosis, whereas others (e.g., those due to cell membrane lysis) involve primary extranuclear insult. Acute cytotoxic injury frequently results in vacuolar degeneration of the germinative cells that form the stratum basalis. This finding is of diagnostic significance in disorders such as lupus erythematosus, erythema multiforme, and fixed drug eruptions. Another manifestation of cytotoxic injury is an increased number of apoptotic cells, either singly or in small clusters.

**Satellitosis.** *Satellitosis* occurs when mononuclear cells are radially arranged about apoptotic cells. This finding is of diagnostic significance in acute graft-versus-host disease and certain other forms of cytotoxic dermatitis. Chronic manifestations of cytotoxic injury include epidermal atrophy, abnormalities in stratum corneum formation, and reorganization of the stratum basalis into more angulated, keratinized, polyhedral cells (often referred to as squamatization). The latter feature is a characteristic finding in lichen planus.

**Ischemic Change.** Subtle ischemic injury may produce mild basal cell layer vacuolization or an increase in the number of apoptotic cells within the midepidermis. Marked *ischemia*, on the other hand, may result in full-thickness necrosis of the epidermis as well as blister formation as a result of dermal-epidermal separation. Ischemia must be differentiated from other forms of epidermal injury that result in similar

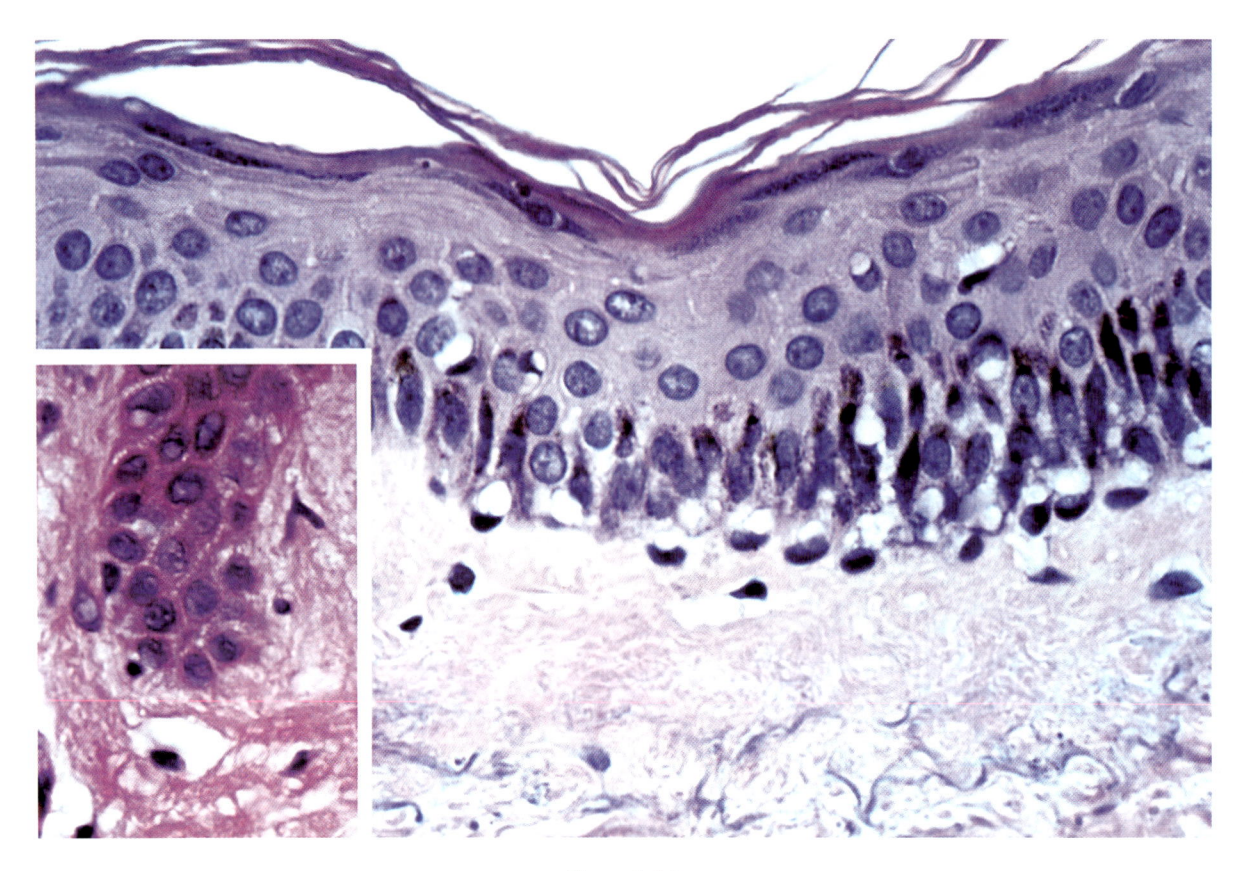

*Inflammatory Disorders of the Skin*

**Figure 1-15**
**EPIDERMAL MELANOCYTE: HISTOLOGY**
Unlike normal melanocytes that are relatively few within the basal layer (1:5-10 ratio to keratinocytes; inset), hyperplastic melanocytes are seen in the basal layer as increased numbers of darkly stained ovoid nuclei surrounded by discrete clear spaces.

zones of full-thickness epidermal necrosis (e.g., second- and third-degree burns). Electrical injury may produce extensive necrosis, although the tendency for keratinocyte nuclei to become elongated and arranged in parallel is a characteristic feature that usually permits diagnostic recognition of this type of insult.

**Hydropic Change.** Swelling of keratinocytes (*hydropic degeneration*) may result from fluid shifts, cytopathic effects of viral infection, or nutritional and metabolic imbalances. The net result is cellular enlargement and cytoplasmic pallor. In human papillomavirus infection of epidermal keratinocytes, cell swelling and associated nuclear changes produce diagnostically important koilocytes within the superficial epidermal layers. Maturational disturbances may result in frank lysis of keratinocytes, resulting in cellular clearing and dyshesion. An example of this phenomenon is epidermolytic hyperkeratosis, in which the lytic defects involving superficial keratinocytes are associated with excessive scale formation and expression of enlarged keratohyaline and trichohyaline granules by the affected cells.

## Melanocytes

**Histology.** In tissue sections stained with hematoxylin and eosin (H&E), *melanocytes* are inconspicuous (14). At high magnification, melanocytes may be detected along the stratum basalis by the clear pericellular spaces that are an artifact of tissue fixation (fig. 1-15). Their detection is facilitated when they are increased in number within the basal cell layer, or when tissue is sectioned thinly (at 1-μm intervals) after embedding in plastic resin. Melanocyte cell bodies contract freely since they are not anchored to adjacent basal keratinocytes by desmosomal attachments. Compared to the larger

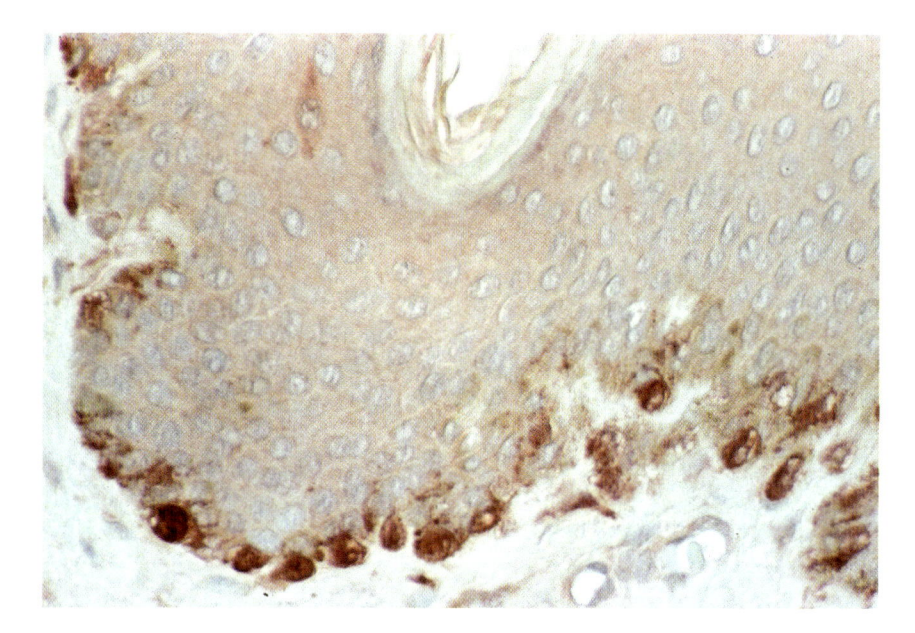

**Figure 1-16**

**S-100 IMMUNOHISTOCHEMISTRY OF HYPERPLASTIC MELANOCYTES CONFINED TO THE EPIDERMAL BASAL CELL LAYER**

Occasional dendrites tortuously coursing among suprabasal keratinocytes are apparent.

and more open nuclei of keratinocytes, melanocytes have small, dense, ovoid nuclei, another distinguishing feature at the light microscopic level. The cytoplasm of melanocytes is pale pink and difficult to visualize in routine preparations. Melanin pigment is infrequently detected by light microscopy. When melanin is observed, particularly in heavily pigmented individuals, it tends to be distributed diffusely throughout the basal keratinocytes of the epidermis.

There is a normal tendency for melanocytes to grow exclusively within the basal cell layer, and suprabasal melanocytes are seldom encountered. There is approximately 1 melanocyte for every 10 basal cells of normal epidermis, although regional variation is common: sun-exposed facial skin, for example, commonly has significantly greater than a 1 to 10 ratio (15). When attempting to determine subtle decreases in melanocyte number (as may occur in evolving vitiligo), it may be helpful to obtain a mirror image sample of control skin for variations related to site, age, and exposure to sunlight. Hyperplastic melanocytes may initially appear to represent vacuolated basal keratinocytes on cursory inspection. Immunohistochemical detection of melanocytes is also a helpful adjunct in determining their density relative to normal skin (fig. 1-16).

**Ultrastructure and Immunohistochemistry.** Melanocytes show an electron-lucent cytoplasm that is free of tonofilaments ultrastructurally. Numerous thin dendrites extend from the cell bodies, insinuating themselves upward between keratinocytes of the stratum spinosum and stratum granulosum. The characteristic feature of melanocytes is a cytoplasmic organelle termed the *melanosome*. This is a 0.3- to 0.8-μm-wide, membrane-bound, ellipsoid structure with a characteristic internal periodicity formed by membranes upon which tyrosinase-dependent melanization occurs (fig. 1-17). As this enzymatic process takes place, melanosomes become progressively electron dense. Eventually, melanosomes are transported to melanocytic dendrites and expelled into the cytoplasm of adjacent keratinocytes, a process known as pigment donation. This mechanism results in the diffuse dispersion of pigment within keratinocytes, which produces an endogenous sunscreen that partially protects against the deleterious effects of ultraviolet radiation. Within keratinocytes, melanosomes of Caucasians and those of Asian descent become packaged, with several melanosomes enclosed within a limiting membrane; within keratinocytes of those of African descent, melanosomes tend to reside as solitary organelles (unpackaged) within the keratinocyte cytoplasm.

There are a number of special diagnostic techniques that facilitate the study of melanocytes. The Fontana-Masson stain renders melanosomes intensely dark gray to black, facilitating their detection by light microscopy in situations in which defective synthesis or

## Inflammatory Disorders of the Skin

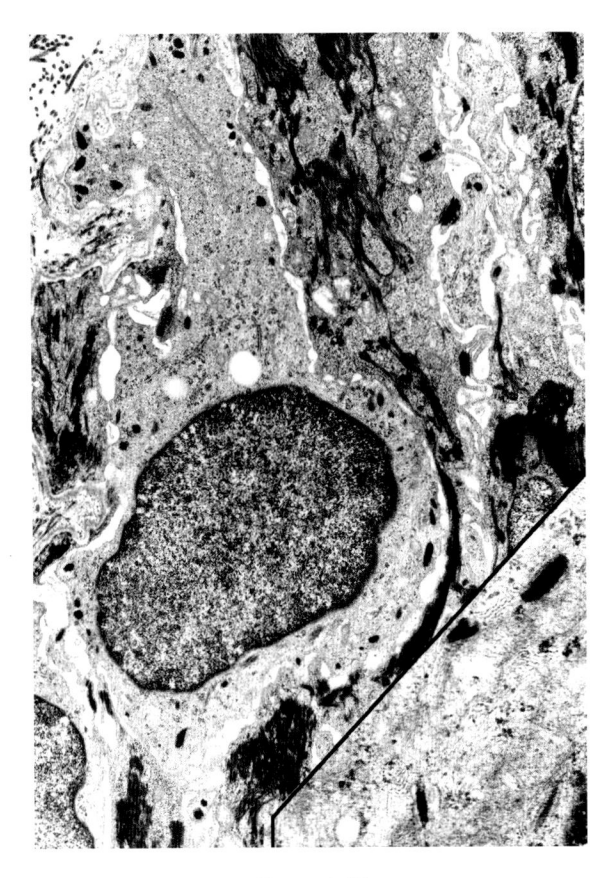

**Figure 1-17**

**MELANOSOMES WITHIN A NORMAL EPIDERMAL MELANOCYTE: ULTRASTRUCTURE**

The cell membrane is separated inferiorly from the underlying papillary dermis by a thin basement membrane zone. The inset (lower right) depicts individual melanosomes at higher magnification.

pigment donation is suspected. The dopa enzyme histochemical stain requires frozen tissue, and is capable of detecting cells and organelles that contain tyrosinase. This approach helps evaluate certain forms of albinism. Although not entirely specific for melanocytes, antibodies to S-100 protein are routinely used for melanocyte enumeration (e.g., in the evaluation of vitiligo) (fig. 1-16). A melanosome-associated antibody, termed HMB45, has become available. This antibody does not react with normal melanocytes or most melanocytic nevi, but with melanoma cells principally of the nonspindle cell type, some melanocytes that have been perturbed by trauma or inflammation, and some melanophages that have ingested melanocyte fragments. Both S-100 protein and HMB45 are applicable to formalin-fixed, paraffin-embedded tissue sections. S-100 protein is sensitive, but not specific (e.g., Langerhans cells also stain within the epidermis). HMB45, while more (albeit not entirely) specific, is only variably expressed by non-neoplastic melanocytes, often upon their activation.

Recently, more specific and reliable immunohistochemical stains for tyrosinase, microphthalmia-associated transcription factor (MITF), and the Mart-1 protein have facilitated melanocyte detection. Tyrosinase is the enzyme intrinsic to the production of melanin; its presence in a cell speaks strongly for melanocytic lineage. MITF is a transcription factor characteristic for melanocytes but also found in certain sarcomas. It also functions as an oncogene when expressed with BRAF protein in tumor progression to melanoma (15a). Its value relates to the intranuclear location of the antigen, thus aiding in the diagnosis of melanomas in which extranuclear biomarkers are equivocal or inconclusive, or to exclude from melanocytic lineage macrophages that express cytoplasm-associated melanocytic markers as a result of phagocytosis. Certain spindle cell sarcomas may be positive for MITF, however, whereas spindle cell melanomas may be negative, emphasizing the need for application of a panel of melanocytic markers when evaluating such lesions (15b). Mart-1 is a transmembrane component of melanocytes and thus is quite specific for melanocytes, nevus cells, and melanoma cells. Mart-1 and the related epitope, Melan-A, are both encoded for by the same gene.

**Pigment Incontinence.** Melanosomes that are liberated as a consequence of melanocyte, or more commonly, keratinocyte, injury are generally phagocytized by dermal macrophages in a process referred to as *melanin pigment incontinence*. This results in the accumulation of melanophages within the superficial dermis, as is prototypically seen in postinflammatory hyperpigmentation (e.g., in the inactive phase of a fixed drug eruption).

### Langerhans Cells

**Histology.** *Langerhans cells* are predominantly located in the mid-portion of the stratum spinosum (fig. 1-18) and, like underlying melanocytes, extend elaborate dendritic processes toward the epidermal surface (fig. 1-19). Langerhans cells are

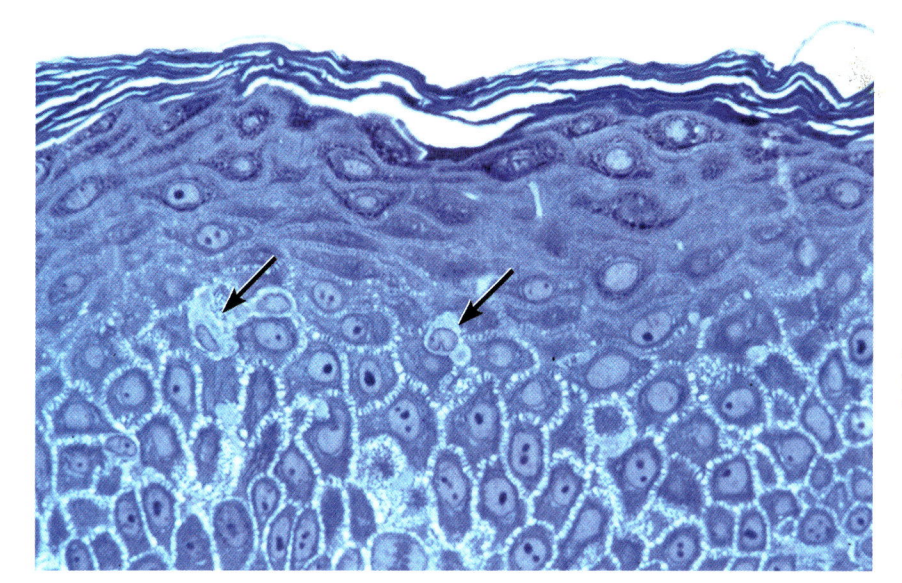

## Figure 1-18
### ONE MICRON-THICK SECTION SHOWING SEVERAL MIDEPIDERMAL "CLEAR" CELLS (ARROWS)
These Langerhans cells are difficult to discern in routinely prepared formalin-fixed, paraffin-embedded sections.

important primarily as antigen presenters to T cells during the evolution of cell-mediated immune responses in skin. These cells are remarkably uniformly distributed in a highly efficient manner that leaves no region of the epidermal surface free of the presence of a nearby patrolling dendrite. Routine H&E-stained sections do not permit detection of Langerhans cells; ultrastructural enzyme histochemical and immunohistochemical methods (figs. 1-19–1-21) are required for their definitive identification. In 1-µm-thick, plastic-embedded sections. Langerhans cells are apparent as midepidermal clear cells, although migrant histiocytes may mimic them (fig. 1-18).

**Ultrastructure and Immunohistochemistry.** On ultrastructural examination, Langerhans cells are characterized by eccentric, frequently infolded nuclei; clear cytoplasm; absence of cell junctions; and the presence of specific cytoplasmic granules termed Birbeck granules (fig. 1-21) (16). Birbeck granules are plate-like disks with variably sized, round vacuoles at one end. In cross section, Birbeck granules frequently appear as tennis racquet-shaped structures with internal zipper-like periodic striations within the handles. Although Birbeck granules are useful in the ultrastructural detection of Langerhans cells and their proliferative counterparts (histiocytosis X cells). They appear to form in association with endocytotic, clathrin-coated pits at the plasma membrane surface. Cells, usually intradermal, with the ultrastructural features of Langerhans cells,

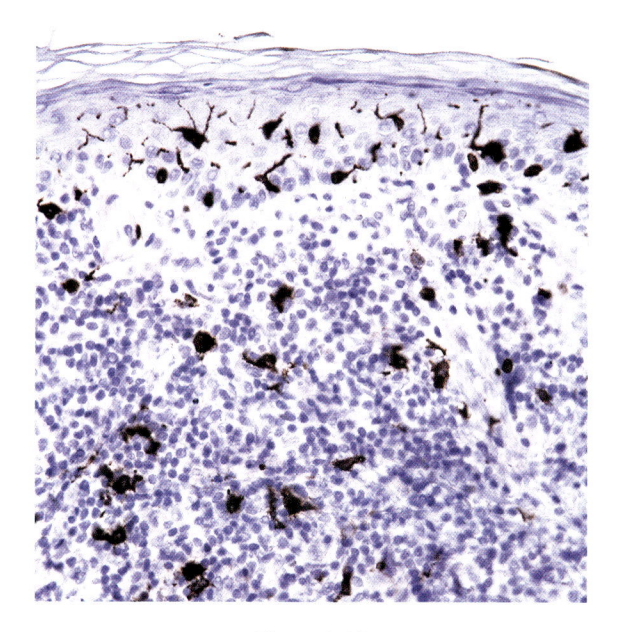

## Figure 1-19
### LANGERHANS CELLS (CD1a IMMUNOSTAINING)
Numerous stained dendritic cells are present within the epidermal layer as well as within the dermis of this inflamed skin site. The involved dermal component signifies active immunologic trafficking.

but without Birbeck granules upon serial sectioning, have been referred to as *indeterminate cells*.

Like melanocytes, Langerhans cells show cytoplasmic reactivity for S-100 protein. They are also characterized by expression of the CD1a cell surface epitope and by ATPase reactivity (figs. 1-19, 1-20) (17,18). CD1a, and more recently,

*Inflammatory Disorders of the Skin*

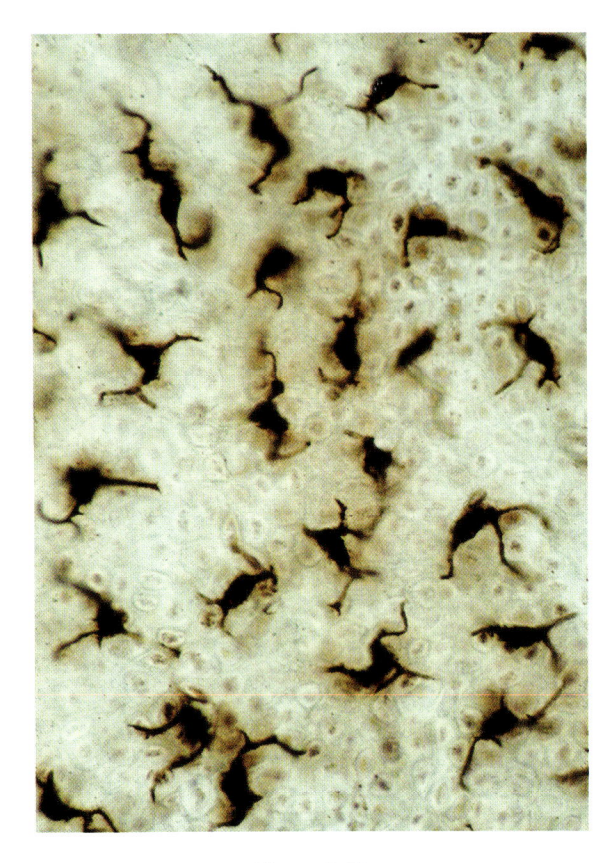

**Figure 1-20**

**IDENTIFICATION OF LANGERHANS CELLS BY ENZYME HISTOCHEMISTRY (ATPase STAIN)**

These highly dendritic cells, here seen in a detached epidermal sheet displayed enface, are evenly interspersed within the epidermal layer for surveillance of environmental haptens and antigens.

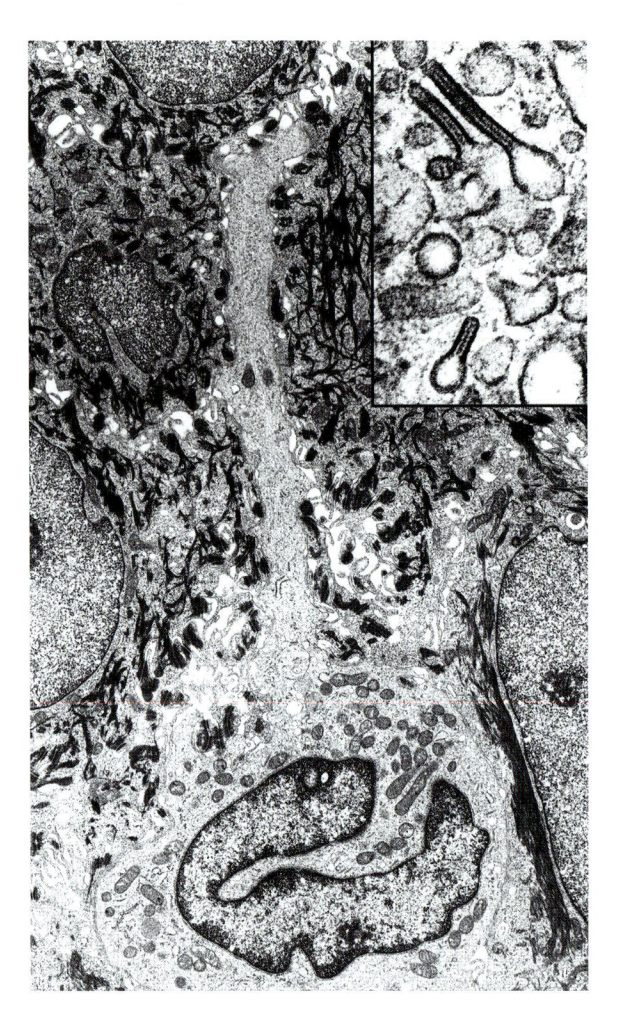

**Figure 1-21**

**LANGERHANS CELL: ULTRASTRUCTURE**

The cell has fairly clear cytoplasm devoid of intermediate filaments, lacks desmosomes, has dendritic extensions, and contains characteristic tennis racquet-shaped organelles termed Birbeck granules (inset).

Langerin, represent highly specific markers for the detection of Langerhans cells in paraffin-embedded sections.

**Langerhans Cell Microgranulomas.** Focal occurrences of Langerhans cell hyperplasia, referred to as *Langerhans cell microgranulomas,* may produce small clusters of Langerhans cells in the superficial epidermis in the setting of florid immune responses and particularly in the setting of allergic contact dermatitis (19). Such clusters must not be confused with Pautrier microabscesses of cutaneous T-cell lymphoma. Tumoral proliferations of Langerhans cells occur in Langerhans cell histiocytosis (histiocytosis X).

## Merkel Cells

*Merkel cells* are poorly understood cells that, in lower vertebrates, probably subserve neurosensory function in association with the pilar apparatus. In humans, these neuroendocrine cells are located individually along the basal cell layer and follicle bulge region, where they are detected only with the use of immunohistochemical or ultrastructural techniques (20,21). Their importance lies in the rare occurrence of primary neuroendocrine, or Merkel cell, carcinoma of the skin, a lesion associated with the incorporation of polyomavirus transcripts (22a). There is no currently known relevance of this cell type to non-neoplastic disorders of the skin, however, and it is mentioned here only for completeness.

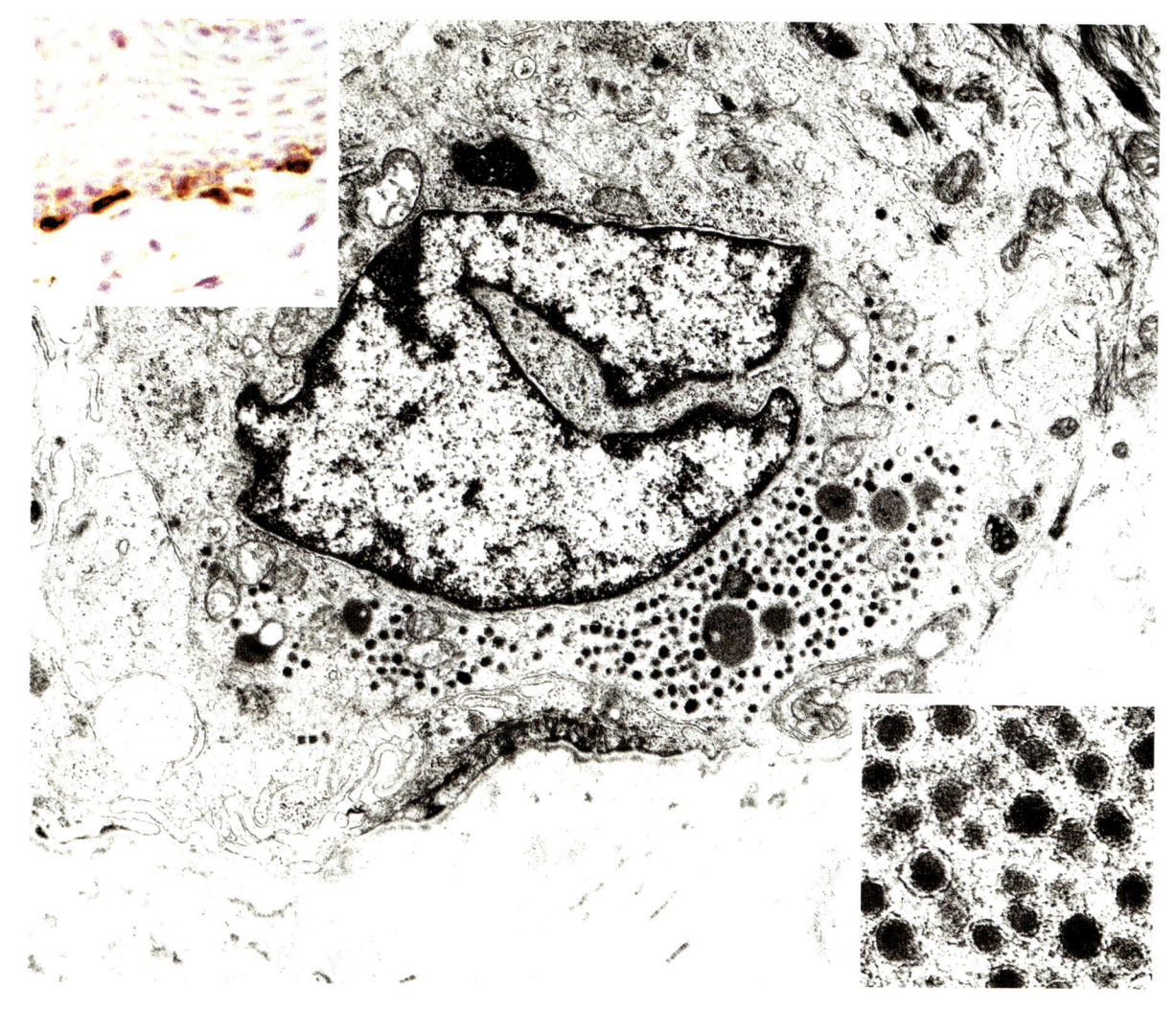

## Figure 1-22

**MERKEL CELL WITHIN NORMAL EPIDERMIS: ULTRASTRUCTURE**

Merkel cells reside within the basal layer and contain characteristic membrane-bound dense-core neurosecretory granules within the cytoplasm (inset, lower right). Their distribution within the basal layer is best appreciated at light microscopic magnification using immunohistochemistry for cytokeratin 20 (inset, upper left).

Merkel cells ultrastructurally contain small, dense core type neurosecretory granules (fig. 1-22). These granules are uniform in size, membrane bound, and considerably smaller than melanosomes and lysosomes. Merkel cells also contain characteristic perinuclear aggregates of keratin type intermediate filaments, and their plasma membranes display desmosomes attached to keratinocytes. Moreover, they are immunoreactive for certain cytokeratins, such as cytokeratin (CK) 20 (fig. 1-22, inset upper left). Unlike epithelial cells, however, Merkel cells contain neuron-specific enolase and occasionally are documented ultrastructurally in apposition to unmyelinated nerve fibers.

### Hair Follicles

*Hair follicles* are specialized downgrowths of the epidermis. Their importance in the diagnostic dermatopathology of non-neoplastic disorders of the skin lies in their involvement in inflammatory and neoplastic diseases (e.g., lupus erythematosus, cutaneous T-cell lymphoma); their participation in certain inflammatory and noninflammatory alopecias; and the emerging recognition that the follicle is an important

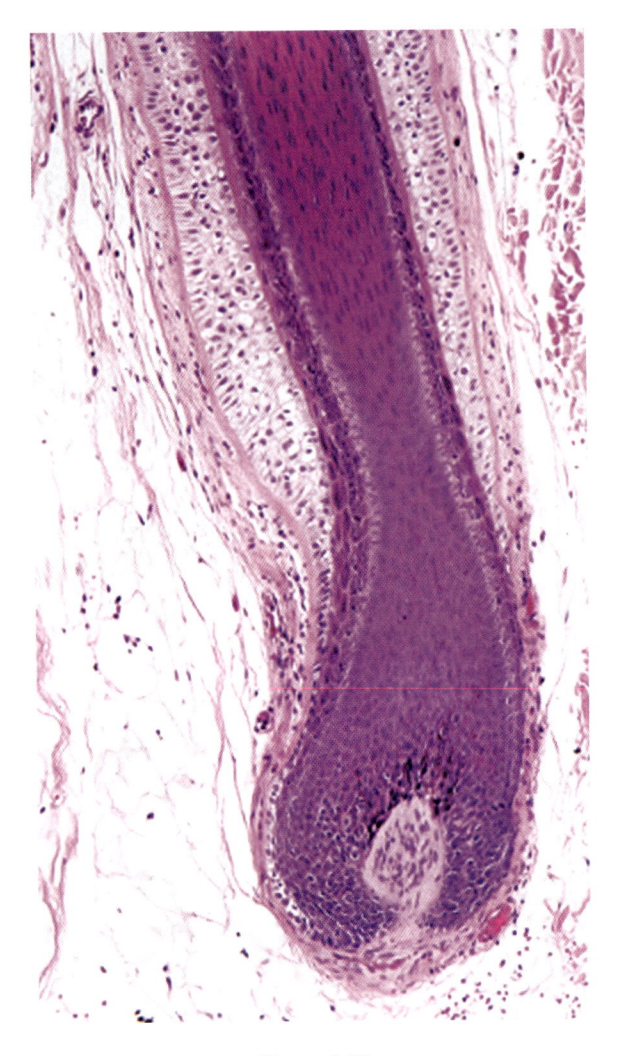

## Inflammatory Disorders of the Skin

**Figure 1-23**
**LOWER PORTION OF AN ANAGEN HAIR FOLLICLE**
Multiple layers originate from the matrix cells of the bulb that surrounds the follicular papilla and that gives rise to the centrally located forming hair shaft within the follicular canal. This bulb extends into the subcutaneous fat, typical of scalp skin.

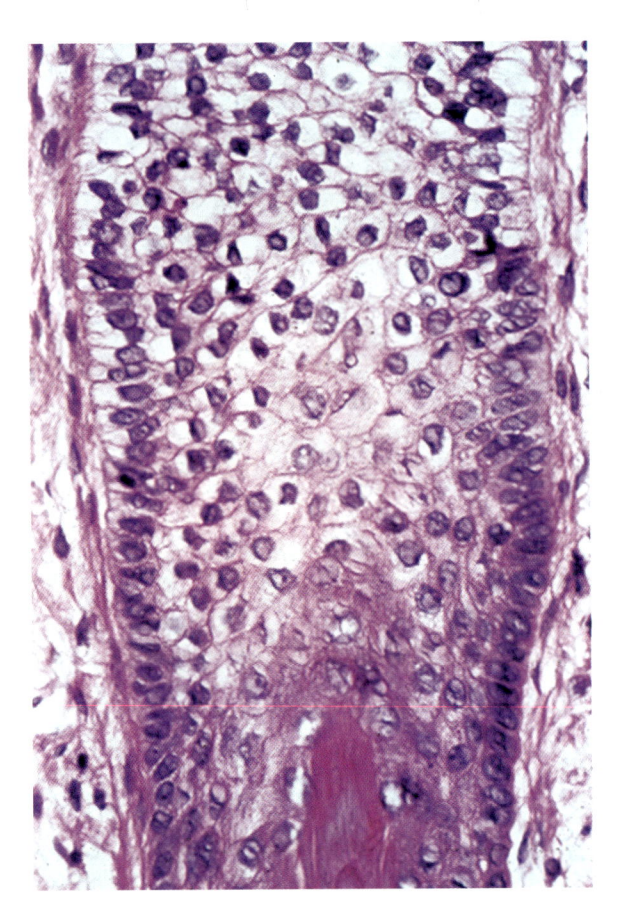

**Figure 1-24**
**HAIR FOLLICLE**
The clear cells represent the highly glycogenated component that forms the outer root sheath.

reservoir of skin-associated lymphoid tissue and epithelial stem cells. Moreover, the relationship of hair follicles to their surrounding dermal structures may provide important regional anatomic clues to the site from which a biopsy specimen has been obtained (e.g., deep follicular extension into subcutaneous fat in scalp skin).

The hair follicle is divided into three parts: the lowermost portion from the follicular bulb to the insertion site of the arrector pili muscle; the midportion represented by the short isthmus that runs between the insertion site of the arrector pili muscle and the sebaceous duct; and the uppermost infundibulum that spans the sebaceous duct and the follicular orifice on the skin surface. The lowermost portion of the follicle is the most complex and is composed of the mast cell–rich follicular papilla; the basaloid hair matrix; the hair medulla, cortex, and cuticle; the inner root sheath; and the outer root sheath (figs. 1-23–1-25). The matrix cells within the anagen bulb are normally replicating, and this may be shown by labeling with tritiated thymidine (fig. 1-26). Other cells in the follicle that are normally dividing include the basaloid component of the sebaceous lobule that is connected by a short and inconspicuous duct to the follicular canal at the level of the lower infundibulum (fig. 1-27).

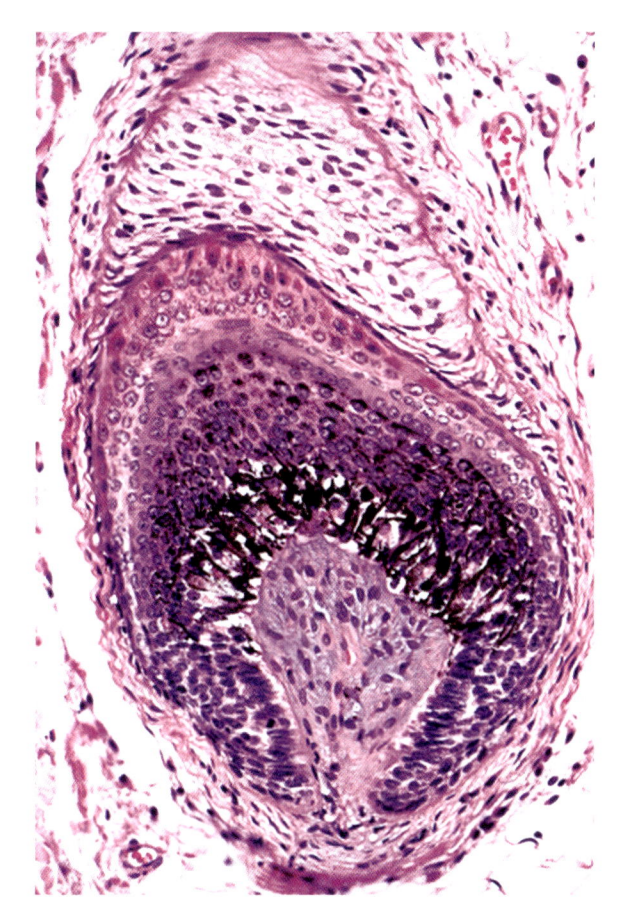

Figure 1-25
HAIR FOLLICLE
The bulb region consists of basaloid matriceal epithelium that contains pigmented melanocytes. It surrounds a central stromal component termed the follicular papilla.

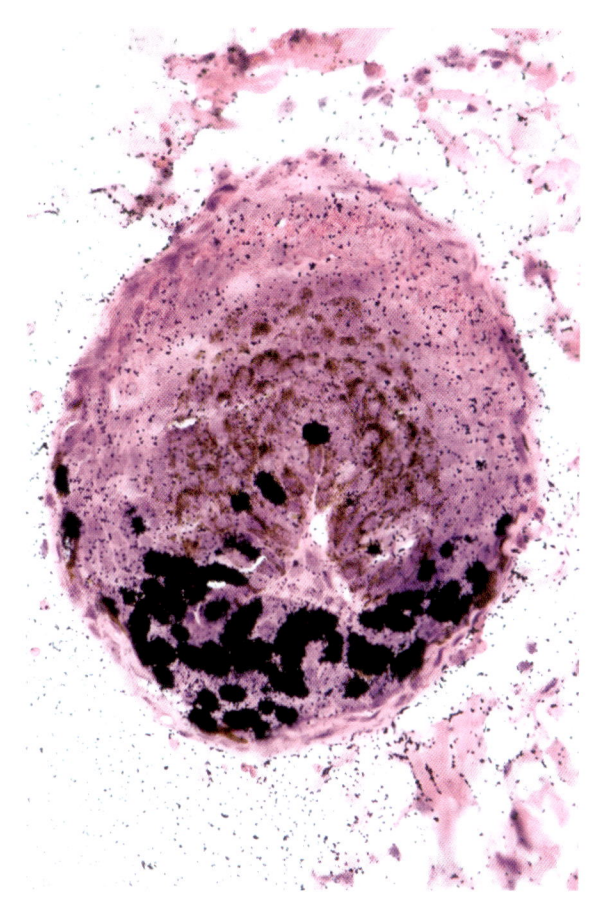

Figure 1-26
TRITIATED THYMIDINE LABELING OF CYCLING CELLS IN ANAGEN HAIR BULB
The marked activity correlates with active hair shaft production during the anagen phase.

The different stages of follicular cycling (anagen, catagen, and telogen) are important because alterations in the ratio of hairs represented in each stage typify certain types of alopecia. *Anagen* is the rapid growth phase of the hair cycle (see fig. 14-1). At this point, the hair follicle is most developed, and often extends deeply into the dermis or subcutaneous fat (fig. 1-23). The follicular papilla, matrix cells, inner and outer root sheaths, sebaceous gland (figs. 1-23–1-25), and follicular infundibular epithelium are maximally developed at this stage. When the follicle begins to involute, the bulb and epithelial column ascend, leaving behind a thin fibrous tract. This intermediate stage of involution is referred to as *catagen*. With the advent of *telogen*, the follicle has retracted maximally along with the mesenchymal papilla, which eventually catches up to the rapidly ascending follicular epithelial column. In normal scalp, the majority of follicles are in the anagen stage. The ratio between anagen, catagen, and telogen hairs in a skin biopsy may assist in determining the cause of alopecia; therefore, these morphologic signposts are noteworthy.

Many follicular inflammatory disorders that result in temporary hair loss tend to involve leukocytic infiltration and injury of the lowermost portion of the anagen follicle (bulb). Conditions that result in permanent hair loss, on the other hand, frequently are characterized by inflammatory infiltrates and cellular injury involving the isthmic/infundibular region of the follicle. The basis of the latter phenomenon may reside in

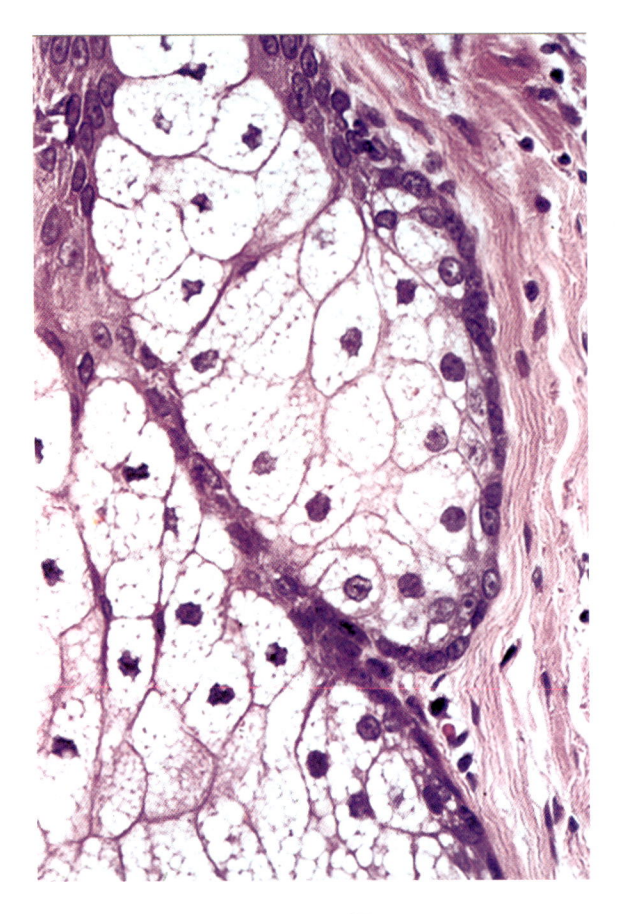

*Inflammatory Disorders of the Skin*

**Figure 1-27**
**SEBACEOUS LOBULE**
At high magnification, the prominently lipidized sebocytes are seen.

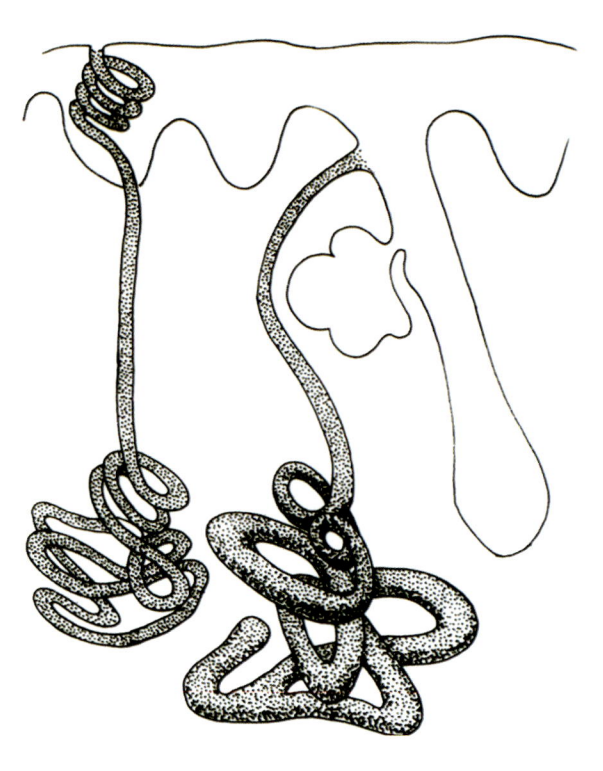

**Figure 1-28**
**SCHEMATIC REPRESENTATION OF ECCRINE (LEFT) AND APOCRINE (RIGHT) SWEAT GLANDS**
The apocrine sweat glands generally originate from follicular infundibula.

the presence of a putative cluster of epithelial stem cells (the bulge) near or at the insertion site of the arrector pili muscle (11). Injury to these cells could eliminate the stem cells necessary for follicular cycling, and thus affect permanent alopecia. Prototypical disorders that correlate with temporary and permanent inflammatory alopecia and preferentially affect the bulb and bulge regions, respectively, are alopecia areata and lichen planopilaris.

## Eccrine Glands

*Eccrine glands* originate as pores on the epidermal surface. For unknown reasons, they form corkscrew-like spiraling ducts (acrosyringia) that course through the epidermal layer (figs. 1-28, 1-29). These ducts are lined by a thin mantle of hyalinized eosinophilic material (cuticle) that stains with periodic acid-Schiff (PAS). The eccrine duct becomes straight as it courses down into the dermis. The terminal eccrine gland is coiled and consists of a single layer of cuboidal epithelial cells. These cells have lighter-staining cytoplasm than the more darkly staining cytoplasm of the cells that compose the eccrine duct (fig. 1-30). The outer mantle of the secretory coil is rimmed by myoepithelial cells embedded in a vascular adventitia replete with unmyelinated nerves and mast cells.

## Apocrine Glands

*Apocrine ducts* generally originate in the upper portion of the hair follicle (fig. 1-28). The apocrine duct, similar to the eccrine duct, communicates with the apocrine gland and secretory coil, the latter of which is composed of cuboidal epithelium showing characteristic "decapitation" secretion (fig. 1-31). *Apocrine glands* are concentrated at specific body sites, such as axillae, the anogenital region, and the periumbilical area.

*Structure, Function, and Reaction Patterns*

**Basement Membrane Zone**

The epidermal-dermal *basement membrane zone* (BMZ) is the structural cement that anchors the epidermal layer to the leathery underlying dermis. The normal BMZ is composed of a thin layer of compacted protein that defines the lower limits of the basal cell layer; this zone can be identified by the PAS stain (fig. 1-32) (22,23).

The BMZ is enriched with specialized structural proteins, such as bullous pemphigoid antigen and laminin. These proteins facilitate normal epidermal-dermal attachment. Ultrastructurally, the BMZ is composed of a dense layer *(lamina densa)*, which is separated from the inferior border of the basal cell plasma membrane by a uniform, thin, clear zone *(lamina lucida)* (fig. 1-33). The lamina lucida is deceptively vacuous; it contains a portion of the bullous pemphigoid antigen and other visually elusive proteins critical to epidermal-dermal bonding. The basement membrane (lamina densa and lamina lucida) is linked to the overlying epidermis by hemidesmosomes and to the underlying dermis by anchoring fibrils that are composed of type VII collagen. Compromised integrity of the structural components of basement membrane may result in specific pathology, as is the case in bullous pemphigoid (bullous pemphigoid antigen [fig. 1-34]) and epidermolysis bullosa dystrophica (anchoring fibrils) (24,25).

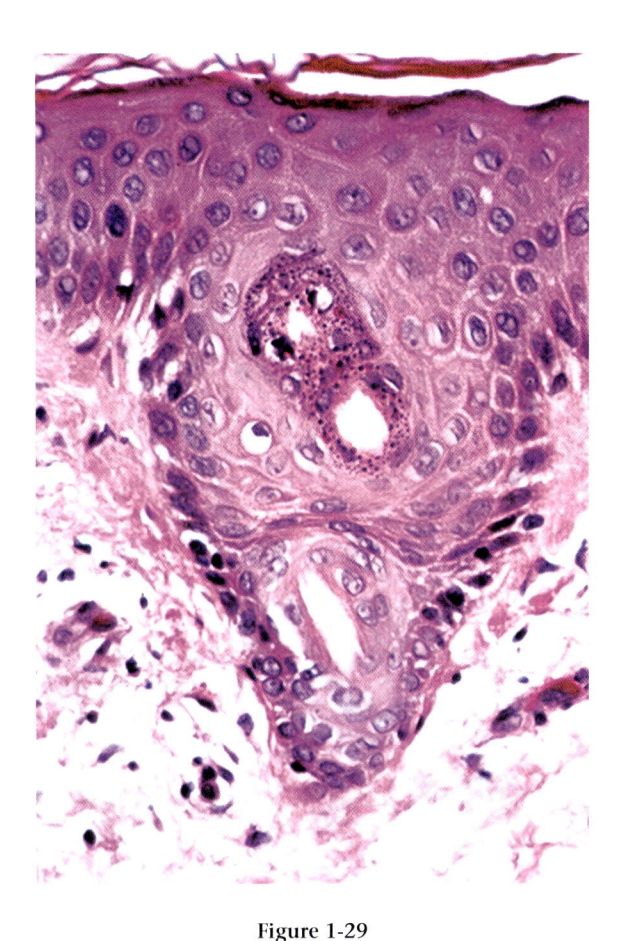

Figure 1-29

**ACROSYRINGIUM**

The duct lumen has a characteristic spiral architecture as it traverses the epidermal layer.

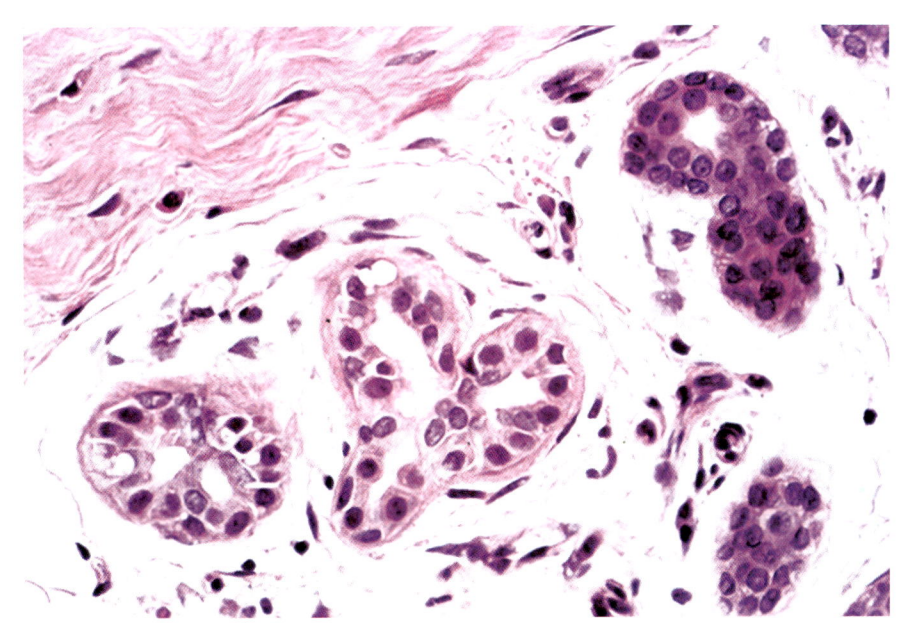

Figure 1-30

**ECCRINE SECRETORY COIL**

The secretory cells have pale cytoplasm in contrast to the cells lining the distal duct (right).

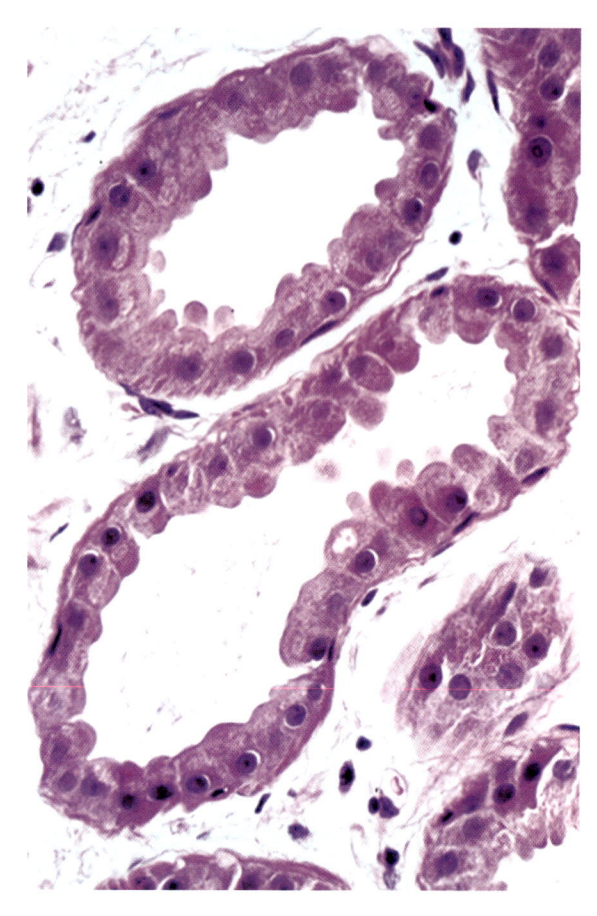

# Inflammatory Disorders of the Skin

## Dermal Microvascular Unit

The *superficial microvascular plexus* separates the papillary dermis from the reticular dermis. This plexus contains postcapillary venules, which are critical targets of inflammatory cells that become adherent to endothelial cells during cutaneous immune responses. From this plexus emanate capillary loops that extend upward into each dermal papilla, supplying nutrients to the nearby avascular epidermal layer (fig. 1-35). These vascular loops may undergo hyperplasia in the setting of chronic stasis dermatitis, and the delicate, felt-like papillary dermal matrix in which they are embedded may transform to vertically oriented strands of collagen as a result of chronic excoriation. The reticular dermis and subcutis are separated by a horizontal plexus of venules and arterioles termed the *deep vascular plexus*. This plexus is linked to its superficial counterpart by vertical vessels that course, often at angles, through the reticular dermis at irregular intervals. Vessels that supply septa that separate lobules of underlying subcutaneous fat communicate with those of the deep vascular plexus.

The dermal microvasculature is surrounded by a sparse complement of immunologically important cells, including factor XIIIa–containing dermal dendrocytes, phagocytic and

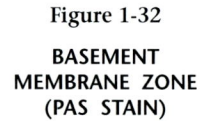

**Figure 1-31**

**APOCRINE SECRETORY COIL**

The glands are larger than those of the eccrine coil and are lined by cells showing "decapitation" secretion.

**Figure 1-32**

**BASEMENT MEMBRANE ZONE (PAS STAIN)**

The periodic acid–Schiff (PAS) stain is used to confirm the pathologic thickening of the basement membrane, as in lupus erythematosus.

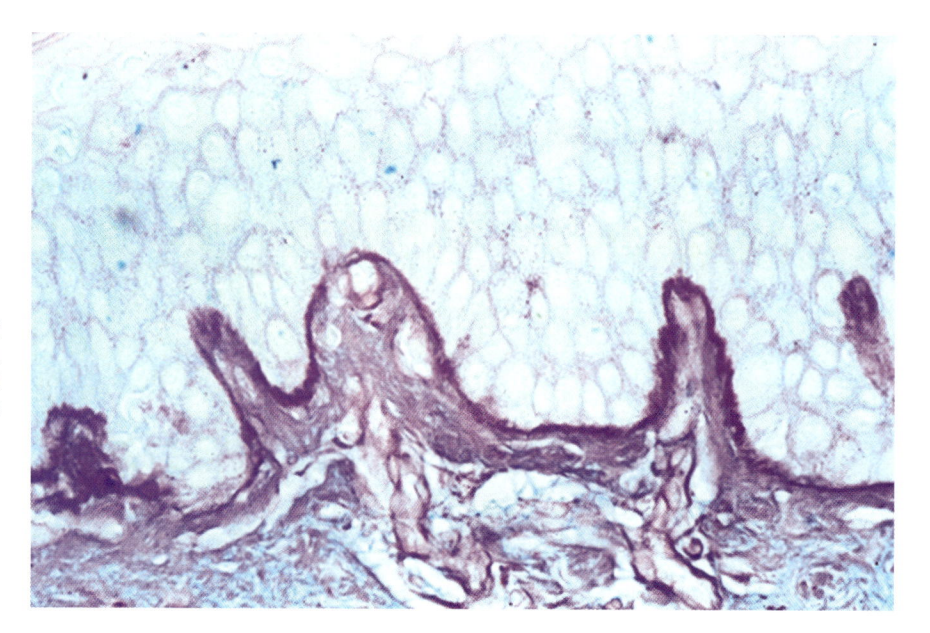

antigen-presenting macrophages, and mast cells (fig. 1-36). Collectively these cells and functionally interrelated structures comprise the *dermal microvascular unit* (DMU). The cellular components of the DMU appear to collaborate to coordinate antigen presentation, cellular inflammation, wound healing, and hemostasis in the immediate perivascular microenvironment (26–37). Mast cells may trigger adhesive events between circulating leukocytes and endothelial cells that result in certain forms of angiocentric cutaneous inflammation. Mast cell activation and degranulation result in the local release of granule mediators, such as histamine, heparin, serine proteinases, and cytokines. Neuropeptide molecules within the unmyelinated axons that surround perivascular mast cells, such as substance P, are capable of rapidly liberating the contents of nearby mast cells, thus setting into motion a cascade of molecular events that eventuate in leukocyte-endothelial adhesion. In addition, small fibers from these neural plexuses innervate the sensory receptors responsible for the critically important sensations of cutaneous pain, pressure, and temperature perception.

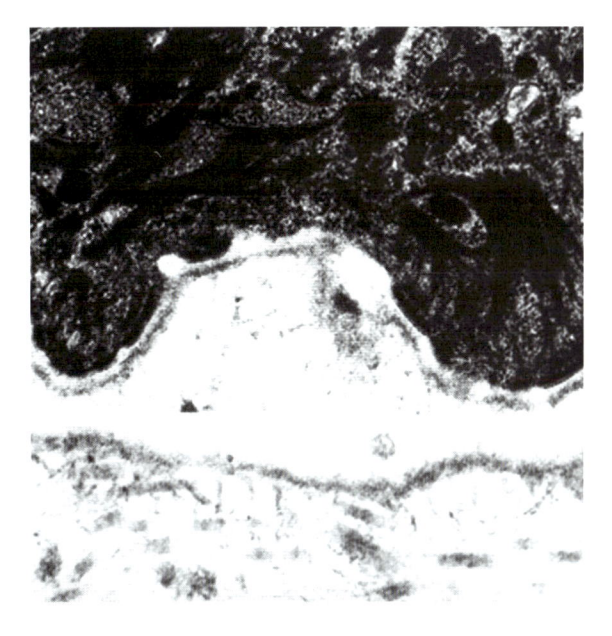

Figure 1-33

DERMAL-EPIDERMAL JUNCTION: ULTRASTRUCTURE

Hemidesmosomes, lamina lucida, lamina densa, and anchoring fibrils are identifiable. The lower panel is higher magnification of the basement membrane and underlying papillary dermis.

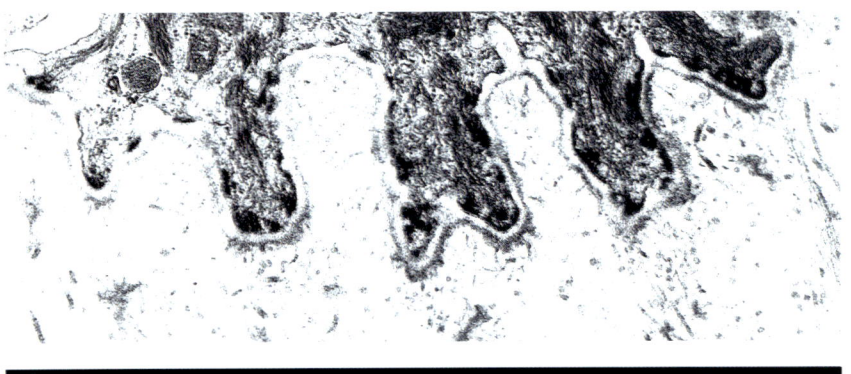

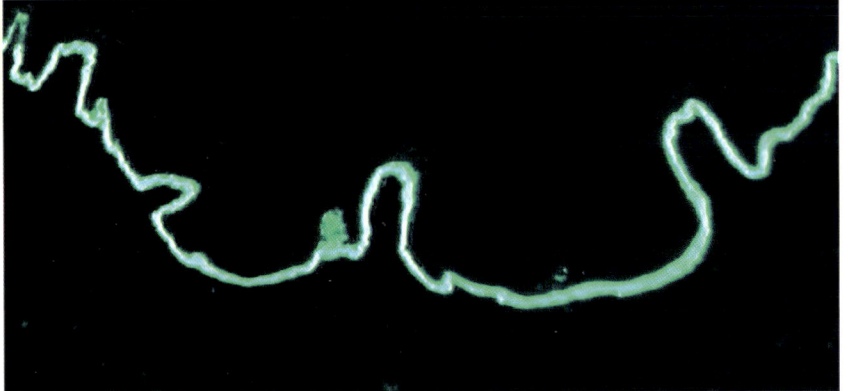

Figure 1-34

COMPARATIVE ULTRASTRUCTURE (UPPER PANEL) AND IMMUNOFLUORESCENCE (LOWER PANEL) OF BASEMENT MEMBRANE

The antibody detected in the lower panel is directed against bullous pemphigoid antigen, and thus decorates proteins concentrated in part in the lamina lucida.

*Inflammatory Disorders of the Skin*

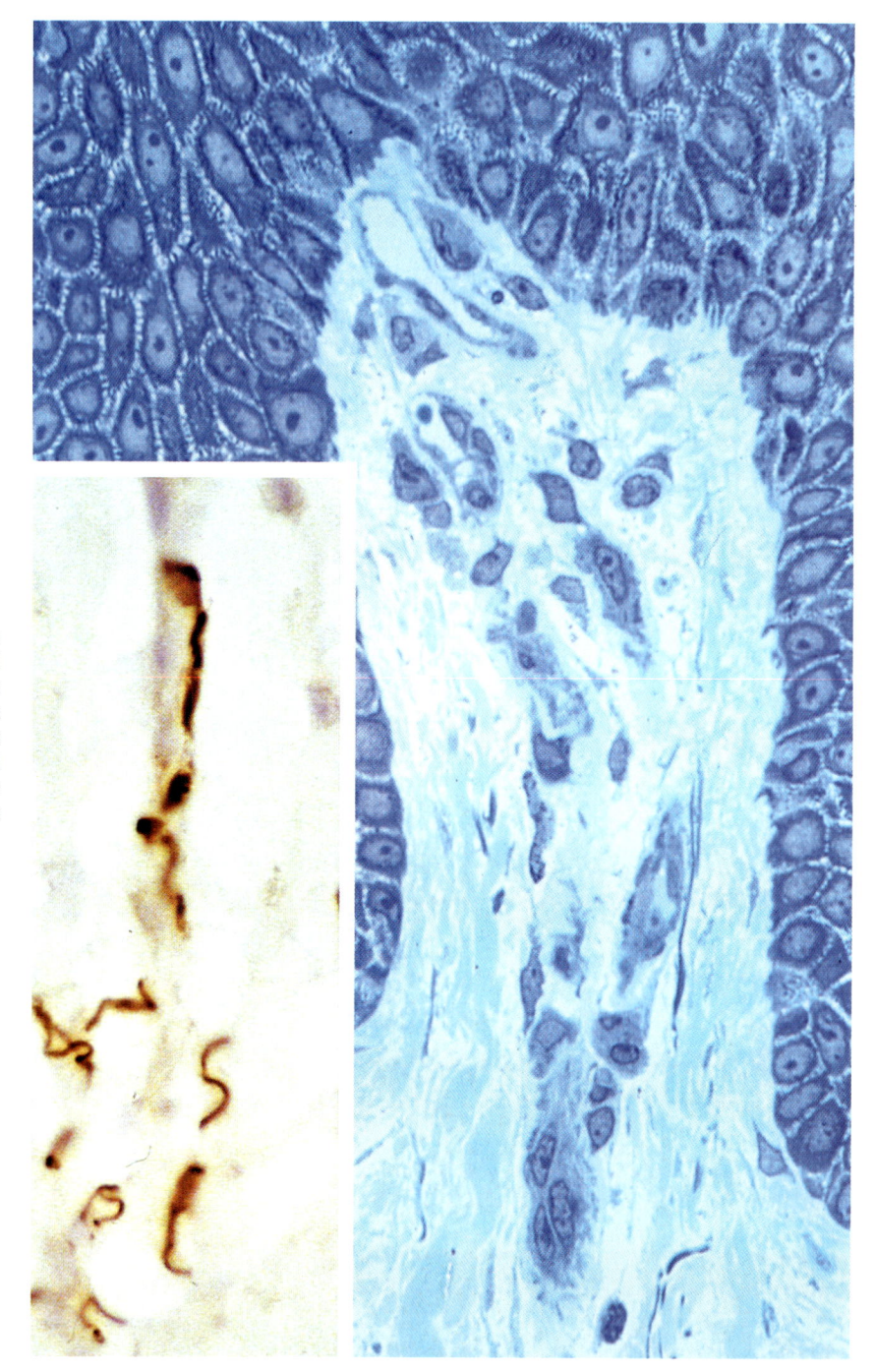

**Figure 1-35**

**DERMAL MICROVASCULAR UNIT, ONE-MICRON SECTION**

A postcapillary venule gives rise to a capillary loop within a dermal papilla. The cells and structures that surround this vessel include an elaborate plexus of nerve twigs that is only appreciated by immunohistochemistry for neural cell adhesion molecule (inset).

### Extracellular Dermal Matrix

The dermis is predominantly composed of the tough structural protein *collagen*, the primary component in animal hide or leather. Fibroblasts, the source of collagen production, are present in low numbers throughout the dermal matrix (38,39). Collagen within the dermis is quite heterogeneous and specialized with regard to its molecular structure (40,41). The papillary dermis is composed primarily of type III collagen, whereas the reticular dermis is composed predominantly of type I collagen (fig. 1-37). Basement membranes about dermal vessels and forming the dermal-epidermal interface contain type IV collagen, whereas anchoring fibrils that tether the epidermal basal lamina to the papillary dermis are composed of type VII collagen (42).

The papillary dermis also contains thin elastic fibers that traverse this layer in vertical array and appear to anchor the epidermis to the underlying superficial reticular dermis (fig. 1-38, top) (43). When these exquisitely delicate and intricate fibers are replaced by coarse, amorphous deposits of abnormal elastin due to chronic sun exposure, diminished recoil and actinic aging (surface wrinkles) ensue. The elastic fibers that normally course through the reticular dermis are thick, branching strands that tend to be horizontally oriented (fig. 1-38, bottom). Pathologic conditions such as pseudoxanthoma elasticum may provoke profound alterations even in these most resilient components of the dermal extracellular matrix, resulting in marked fraying and fragmentation.

An often overlooked but major component of the dermal extracellular matrix is the *mucopolysaccharide ground substance* present between collagen and elastin fibers (figs. 1-39, 1-40) (44). Ground substance is apparent only as minute, particulate, gray-blue particles and strands on routine light microscopy. Ground substance often is appreciated only after it has become markedly increased, as in lupus erythematosus, granuloma annulare, and pretibial myxedema. Special stains helpful for the detection

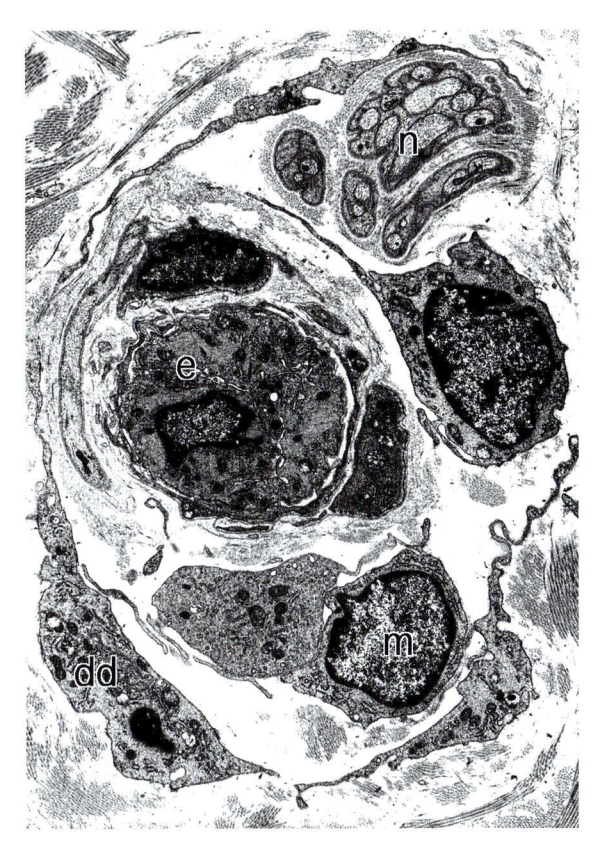

Figure 1-36

**DERMAL MICROVASCULAR UNIT: ULTRASTRUCTURE**

There are activated endothelial cells (e), monocyte/macrophage (m), dermal dendrocyte (dd), and nerve fiber (n).

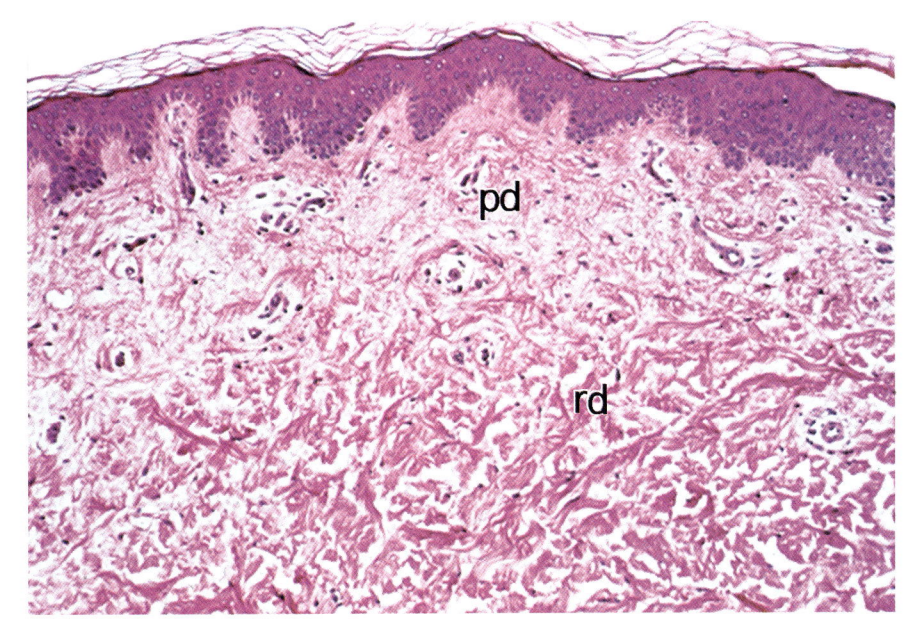

Figure 1-37

**DERMIS: HISTOLOGY**

There is a thin subepithelial layer of delicate collagen (papillary dermis, pd) and a deeper, thicker layer formed by coarse collagen (reticular dermis, rd).

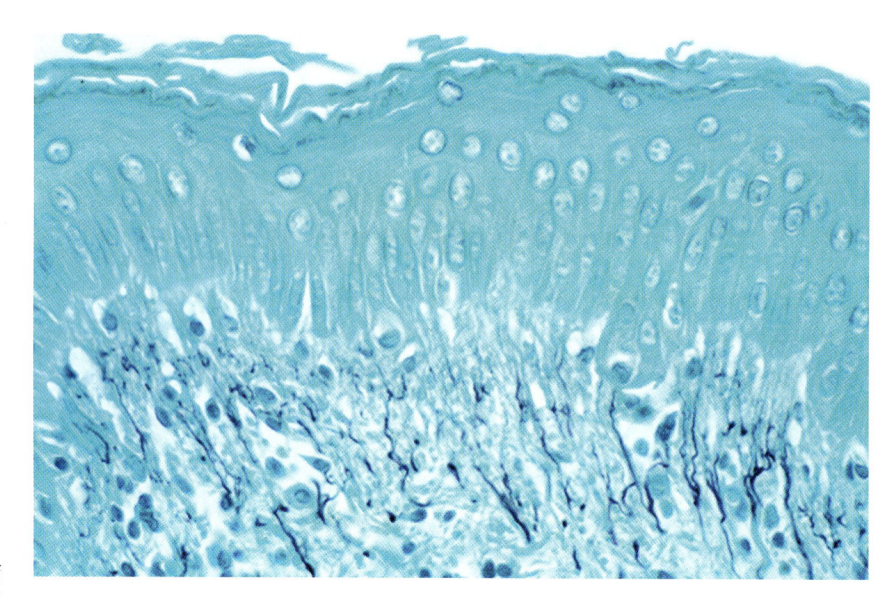

**Figure 1-38**

**ELASTIC FIBER NETWORK OF PAPILLARY (UPPER PANEL) AND RETICULAR (LOWER PANEL) DERMIS**

The thin and delicate fibers of the papillary dermis are oriented primarily perpendicular to the epidermal layer, whereas the thicker strands of the reticular dermis are more horizontal in orientation (histochemical stain for elastin).

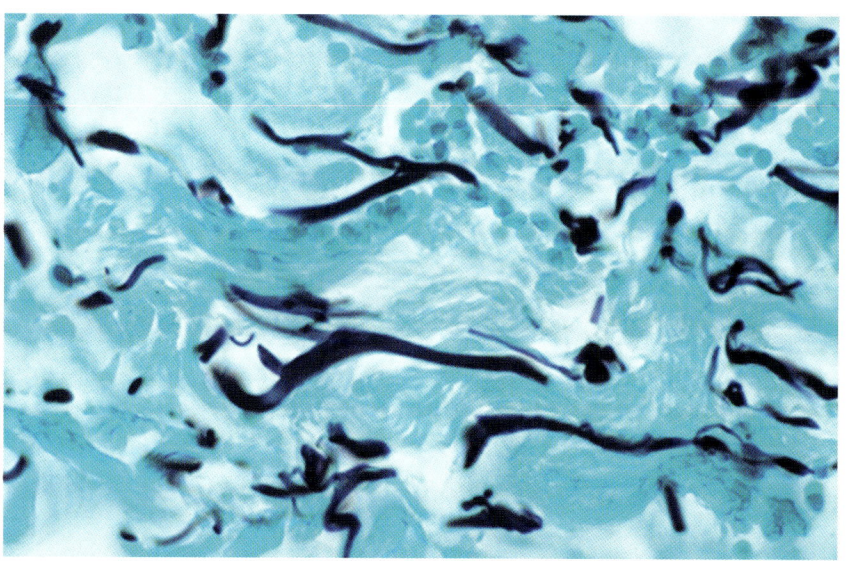

of mucopolysaccharides include Alcian blue (pH 2.5) and colloidal iron, especially for acid mucopolysaccharides, and mucicarmine for those of the neutral type.

Pathologic alterations in the extracellular matrix occur frequently, and their recognition is critical to the formulation of an accurate diagnosis. Collagen fibers are increased in number in the setting of hypertrophic scars, and individual bundles become thickened and hyalinized in the poorly understood, yet common and related condition of keloid formation. Diffuse hyalinization and thickening of collagen, with encroachment on adnexa and subcutaneous fat, are characteristic of scleroderma. In all of these pathologic abnormalities of extracellular matrix and related cells, characteristic clinical lesions evolve, and their histologic identification depends on the recognition of these basic reaction patterns of extracellular matrix proliferation and deposition.

**"Necrobiosis."** Degeneration of extracellular matrix elements occurs commonly, and there are several basic reaction patterns. Mucinous degeneration with necrobiosis is a poor term, because extracellular matrix is not living (bio), and therefore it cannot die (necro). A typical disorder in which this pattern is observed is granuloma annulare. In mucinous degeneration of the extracellular matrix, there is pallor of

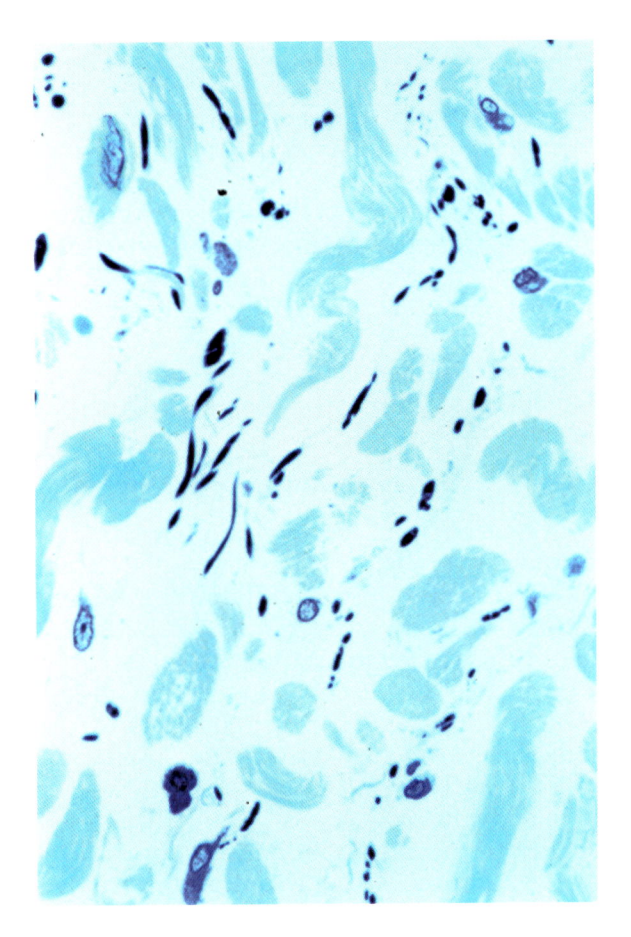

**Figure 1-39**

**DERMAL COMPONENTS IN PLASTIC-EMBEDDED SECTION**

The small darker fibers are elastin, and the larger lighter fibers are collagen. The clear background corresponds to mucopolysaccharides.

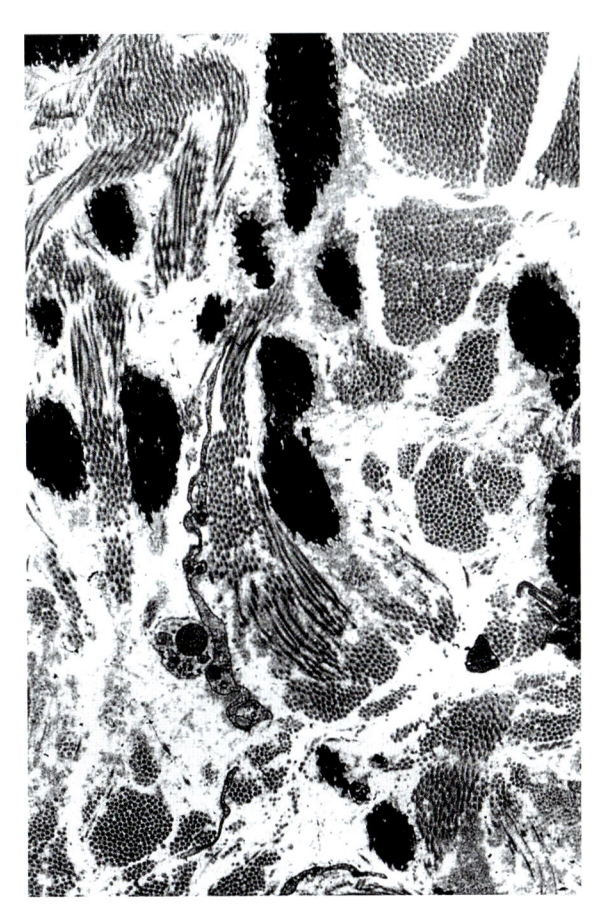

**Figure 1-40**

**DERMAL COMPONENTS: ULTRASTRUCTURE**

Collagen bundles, largely in cross-section, and dark elastic fibers are surrounded by a delicate extracellular matrix composed primarily of mucopolysaccharide ground substance.

collagen fibers associated with mucin deposits manifested as particulate, string-like, pale blue-gray fibers between collagen bundles. Fibrinoid degeneration (necrobiosis) of collagen is characteristically seen in rheumatoid nodules, where zones of collagen acquire a deep red, refractile quality reminiscent of extravasated fibrin. Collagen bundles also may become eosinophilic as a result of exposure to potent proteolytic enzymes, such as those produced by eosinophils. Degeneration of collagen bundles associated with degranulating eosinophils is observed in eosinophilic cellulitis (Well syndrome). In this disorder, irregular arrays of deeply eosinophilic collagen bundles resemble flames, and thus have been termed "flame figures." This feature assists in the recognition of eosinophilic cellulitis, although similar findings may be seen in insect bites, hypereosinophilic syndrome, Churg-Strauss syndrome, and occasionally, severe hypersensitivity reactions containing numerous eosinophils.

## Subcutaneous Fat

The *subcutaneous fat* is both a cushion to prevent mechanical injury and a storage depot for high-potency energy sources. Fat is stored in *adipocytes*, which are enormously distended clear cells that comprise the majority of cells in mature (adult) adipose tissue. Adipocytes are best observed with glutaraldehyde fixation and plastic embedding, in which the intracytoplasmic stores of fat do not dissolve but appear as homogeneous, dense storage globules. Adipocytes are arranged in sheet-like lobules separated by thin, fibrous septa through which nutrient vessels course. These septa anchor the deepest limits of the reticular dermis to the underlying fascia, with an intervening cushion of subcutaneous lobules formed by masses of adipocytes. Degeneration of adipocytes is a consequence of inflammation, as in lupus panniculitis, where these cells undergo coagulative and liquefactive necrosis. Lipids may also crystallize into needle-like arrays in certain disorders, such as subcutaneous fat necrosis of the newborn. Inflammation of the subcutaneous fat may result in septal or lobular panniculitis, and preferential involvement of either of these architectural domains may be of profound diagnostic significance.

## SPECIAL DIAGNOSTIC TECHNIQUES

### Histochemistry

Routine histochemical stains are used for the chemical detection of inorganic substances such as iron, calcium, and silver; polysaccharides (periodic acid-Schiff [PAS] stain, with and without diastase digestion); mucopolysaccharides (Alcian blue stain); mast cell metachromasia (Giemsa reagent); lipids (oil red-O stain); extracellular matrix elements (Weigert elastic stain); organisms (Ziehl-Neelsen stain for acid-fast bacilli); and certain enzymes (dopa reagent). Although these stains provide important information for the evaluation of many skin disorders, they should be used with discretion based on knowledge of specificity and sensitivity. For example, superficial fungi within the stratum corneum are often detected without the aid of a PAS stain, and when required for detection of viable fungi, either a PAS or silver stain, but not both, is usually sufficient. Alternatively, the epidermal basement membrane thickening that accompanies established lesions of lupus erythematosus often requires the PAS stain for visualization, and subtle deposits of dermal mucin in lupus and metabolically induced mucinoses are identified with greater certainty with Alcian blue.

Most of histochemical stains are performed on formalin-fixed, paraffin-embedded tissue sections. Enzyme histochemistry, however, usually requires cryostat sections of fresh frozen tissue. The 3,4-dihydroxyphenylalanine (dopa) stain permits detection of cells with tyrosinase activity, and in the past, has proven useful for the identification and quantification of epidermal melanocytes, as in the diagnostic evaluation of vitiligo. More recently, antibodies that permit antigenic detection in conventionally fixed and embedded tissues have supplanted the need for most applications of enzyme histochemistry. A summary of histochemical reagents commonly employed in the evaluation of non-neoplastic inflammatory disorders of the skin is provided in Table 1-4.

### Immunohistochemistry

Tissue antigens preserved after formalin fixation and paraffin embedding are detected by immunoperoxidase methods using paraffin immunohistochemistry. Immunoperoxidase detection involves incubation of tissue sections with the relevant antibody (usually polyclonal for paraffin immunohistochemistry) to the target antigen (generally cytoplasmic proteins), followed by the application of a biotinylated or peroxidase-linked secondary antibody directed against the target-specific antibody probe. The antigen-bound antibody-antibody complex is identified and localized by using either an avidin-biotin or peroxidase-antiperoxidase enzyme detection system, whereby horseradish peroxidase is linked to the growing "sandwich" of layered antibodies. The complex is then incubated with an enzyme substrate (aminoethyl carbazole or an insoluble chromogen such as diaminobenzidine), which on reaction with peroxidase becomes red or brown at sites of antibody-antigen reactivity. This approach, unlike fluorescence-based methods of antibody localization, produces a permanent record in which the signal does not fade or dissipate over time. Examples of paraffin immunohistochemistry include antibody stains for S-100 protein (melanocytes and Langerhans cells), keratin proteins (epithelial cells), carcinoembryonic antigen (some gland-forming epithelial tumors), chromogranin (neuroendocrine tumors), desmin (smooth muscle), factor VIII–associated antigen (endothelium), alpha-1-antichymotrypsin (histiocytic tumors), and vimentin (mesenchymal and fibroblastic proliferations). In the setting of non-neoplastic disorders of the

Table 1-4

HISTOCHEMICAL STAINS COMMONLY USED FOR NON-NEOPLASTIC SKIN DISORDERS

| Stain | Rationale | Specific Condition |
|---|---|---|
| Periodic acid-Schiff (PAS) | Thickened basement membrane | Discoid lupus erythematosus, fungi/dermatophytes |
| Alcian blue (pH 2.5) and colloidal iron | Acid mucopolysaccharides | Discoid lupus erythematosus, granuloma annulare |
| Giemsa reagent | Mast cell granules | Mast cell degranulation/hyperplasia |
| Methenamine and Grocott silver | Fungi | Deep mycoses |
| Verhoeff-van Gieson/Weigert | Elastic fibers | Pseudoxanthoma elasticum |
| Fite, Ziehl-Neelsen | Acid fast bacilli | Leprosy, mycobacterial infections |
| Brown-Brenn | Bacteria | Cellulitis/folliculitis |
| Warthin-Starry, Dieterle, Steiner | Spirochetes | Primary/secondary syphilis, erythema centrifugum migrans |
| Von Kossa | Calcium | Calciphylaxis |

skin, this approach is often used to determine whether lymphoid infiltrates express T and B cells, as well as macrophage markers consistent with reactive processes (as opposed to clonal infiltrates which may correlate with malignancy [45]). None of these antibodies is entirely specific, and results must be interpreted within the context of a comprehensive panel of reagents. Examples of antibodies that are presently available for the detection of cluster differentiation (CD) antigens and that correlate with specific cell phenotypes and functions include: CD3 (T cells), CD4 (helper T cells), CD8 (cytotoxic/suppressor T cells), CD56 (natural killer [NK]-like cells), CD5 and CD7 (mature T cells), CD68 and CD163 (macrophages), and CD20 (B cells).

### One-Micron Sections and Electron Microscopy

One-micron sections are generated from glutaraldehyde-fixed tissue embedded in plastic resin and sectioned at about one sixth the thickness of conventional paraffin sections. The result is a high-resolution image under high-power lenses that makes possible the detection of subtle nuclear membrane characteristics (e.g., Sézary cells), endothelial activation and microvascular injury (e.g., urticarial vasculitis), and anomalies in organelles (e.g., macromelanosomes) often not possible in routine sections. Diagnostic electron microscopy is well suited to the classification of different forms of epidermolysis bullosa. More recently, however, immunohistochemical and immunofluorescence approaches to the antigenic mapping of BMZ proteins have provided an alternative technique for the classification of various forms of epidermolysis bullosa.

### In Situ Hybridization

In situ hybridization involves the detection of mRNA or DNA when quantities of protein antigen are not present for conventional immunohistochemical evaluation. Typing of human papillomavirus (HPV) is possible using in situ hybridization. The detection of other infectious agents (e.g., human immunodeficiency virus, cytomegalovirus) is also possible, and oncogene expression may also be defined by this technology.

### Immunofluorescence

Direct immunofluorescence is a method of visualizing tissue deposits of immune reactants that have become bound to target cells and matrix molecules in vivo. Antigen is detected in a frozen section of skin from a patient biopsy by the application of fluorescein isothiocyanate (FITC)-labeled antibody of desired specificity. Fresh tissue is generally provided immediately after biopsy on saline-soaked gauze placed on an ice slurry and delivered within 2 hours of biopsy, or alternatively, after placement into Michel transport medium, which preserves immunoreactants for at least several weeks, in our experience. Tissue is gently washed prior to embedding and freezing in a viscous, soluble, embedding medium

## Table 1-5
### USEFUL DIRECT IMMUNOFLUORESCENCE PATTERNS IN SKIN

| Site of Deposit | Character | Disorder | Significance |
| --- | --- | --- | --- |
| Stratum corneum | Loculated, homogeneous mixed immunoglobulins | Acute to subacute spongiotic dermatitis | Loculated serum, scale-crust; nonspecific |
| Stratum corneum | Focal, granular, with parakeratosis | Psoriasis | At Munro microabscesses, ? primary or secondary; nonspecific |
| Intercellular | Fine, uniform, fish-net, restricted immunoglobulins (IgG) | Pemphigus family | Antidesmoglein autoantibodies |
| Intercellular | Coarse, irregular, mixed immunoglobulins | Spongiotic dermatitis | Nonspecific serum leakage |
| Nuclear | Homogeneous, granular, nucleolar | Connective tissue disorders | Autoimmunity (e.g., Ro and La in subacute lupus and B23 in scleroderma); may not have clinical relevance |
| Basement membrane | Linear, C3 predominates[a] | Pemphigoid family | Autoantibody to bullous pemphigoid antigen |
| Basement membrane | Linear, IgG predominates[a] | Epidermolysis bullosa acquisita | Autoantibody to collagen VII in lamina densa and anchoring fibrils |
| Basement membrane | Linear, IgA predominates | Linear IgA disease | Autoantibody to multiple basement membrane components |
| Basement membrane | Granular immunoglobulin and complement | Lupus erythematosus | Membrane attack complex; association with systemic disease when in nonlesional, sun-protected skin |
| Papillary dermis | Granular IgA | Dermatitis herpetiformis | Associated intestinal pathology |
| Microvessels (venules) | Granular C3, IgG | Hypersensitivity, vasculitis | Immune complex-mediated injury |
| Microvessels (venules) | Granular IgA | Henoch-Schönlein purpura | Immune complex-mediated injury |
| Microvessels (venules) | Homogeneous IgG, albumin | Porphyria cutanea tarda | Nonspecific deposition at sites of vascular injury |
| Vessels (arteries) | Granular, segmental | Polyarteritis nodosa | Immune complex-mediated injury |

[a] C = complement; Ig = immunoglobulin.

(e.g., Tissue-Tek O.C.T. Compound, Miles Inc., Elkhart, IN). In a moist chamber, cryostat sections are reacted for 30 minutes with various antisera such as antibodies to immunoglobulin (Ig)G, IgA, IgM, complement, and fibrinogen linked to FITC. After incubation, sections are rinsed in buffer and examined by epifluorescence microscopy. This technique is widely used as an adjunct in the diagnosis of connective tissue diseases and vesiculobullous disorders. With minor modification, the same basic technique is effective for the detection of various infectious agents (Table 1-5).

One of the uses of indirect immunofluorescence is to determine titers of circulating immunoglobulins in the serum of a patient with a bullous disorder such as pemphigus vulgaris and bullous pemphigoid. For this analysis, serum is separated from a sample of venous blood, serially diluted with buffered saline admixed with bovine serum albumen, and incubated with cryostat sections of a target tissue containing the relevant target molecules (e.g., monkey esophagus, normal human skin). Sections are gently rinsed, and FITC-linked antiserum to human immunoglobulin is applied to define sites of in vitro serum antibody binding. By fluorescence microscopy, zones of reactivity are designated as present or absent, and the endpoint is represented by the dilution at which reactivity ceases. A typical report would read "epidermal intercellular immunoglobulin deposition detected to and including a dilution of 1:160." Such a report could be used as an adjunct to diagnosis or for the assessment of disease activity or response to treatment. The linkage between disease activity is generally

Table 1-6

**GUIDELINES FOR DIRECT IMMUNOFLUORESCENCE**

| |
|---|
| Early lesions should be sampled |
| The edges of lesions, particularly when blistering is present, are most useful |
| At least one third of the biopsy specimen should include perilesional skin |
| Never biopsy the base of an ulcer or the center of a blister |
| If the epidermis separates from the dermis, submit both in separate, labeled containers |
| Place specimens immediately into Michel transport medium, never in fixative |
| If transport medium is not available, cover specimen with gauze soaked in physiologic saline, place in ice slurry, and transport immediately to immunofluorescence laboratory for processing |

tighter in pemphigus than in pemphigoid, and occasionally, circulating autoantibodies are detected in individuals without evidence of primary vesiculobullous disease.

An important application of indirect immunofluorescence is the evaluation of epidermolysis bullosa acquisita (EBA). This nonheritable disorder differs clinically from classic forms of epidermolysis bullosa (EB) and resembles an autoimmune disorder more than a primary mechanobullous disorder. Direct immunofluorescence shows deposits of IgG and other immunoreactants in a linear array along the epidermal basal lamina in 25 to 50 percent of patients, a pattern that is indistinguishable from bullous pemphigoid. Differentiation of the two disorders relies on a strategy whereby the substrate for indirect immunofluorescence is normal human skin split along the dermal-epidermal junction via preincubation in 1 mol/L sodium chloride. This results in segregation of the lamina lucida and associated bullous pemphigoid antigen on the epidermal roof, and type IV collagen and lamina densa along the dermal base. When this split substrate is reacted with the patient's serum, bullous pemphigoid antibodies decorate the epidermal side, whereas autoantibodies in EBA localize to the dermal side. Split skin preparations, as well as immunologic mapping of native antigens at sites of blister formation to define the molecular site of the lesion, continue to provide important diagnostic insights into the classification and pathogenesis of commonly encountered vesiculobullous disorders involving the skin.

For direct immunofluorescence, precision and site selection are of critical importance. Table 1-6 contains the guidelines which should be applied.

## REFERENCES

1. Murphy GF. Dermatopathology: a practical guide to common disorders. Philadelphia: Saunders; 1995.
2. Murphy GF, Herzberg A. Atlas of dermatopathology. Philadelphia: Saunders; 1996.
3. Elder D, Murphy GF. Melanocytic tumors of the skin. AFIP Atlas of Tumor Pathology, 4th Series, Fascicle 12. Washington DC: American Registry of Pathology; 2010.
4. Patterson JW, Wick MR. Nonmelanocytic tumors of the skin. AFIP Atlas of Tumor Pathology, 4th Series, Fascicle 4. Washington DC: American Registry of Pathology; 2006.
5. Binford CH, Connor DH. Pathology of tropical and extraordinary diseases, vols. I & II. Washington DC: Armed Forces Institute of Pathology; 1976.
6. Murphy GF, Sellheyer K, Mihm MC Jr. The skin. In: Kumar V, Abbas AK, Fausto N, eds. Robbins and Cotran pathologic basis of disease, 7th ed. Philadelphia: Elsevier-Saunders; 2004:1227-72.
7. Elder DE, Eleneitsas R, Johnson BL, Murphy GF, eds. Lever's histopathology of the skin, 9th ed. Philadelphia: Lippincott Williams & Wilkins; 2005.
8. Van Scott EJ, Ekel TM. Kinetics of hyperplasia in psoriasis. Arch Dermatol 1963;88:373-81.
9. Penneys NS, Fulton JE Jr, Weinstein GD, Frost P. Location of proliferating cells in human epidermis. Arch Dermatol 1970;101:323-7.
10. Lavker RM, Sun TT. Heterogeneity in epidermal basal keratinocytes: morphological and functional correlations. Science 1982;215:1239-41.
11. Cotsarelis G, Sun TT, Lavker RM. Label-retaining cells reside in the bulge area of the pilosebaceous unit: implications for follicular stem cells, hair cycle and skin carcinogenesis. Cell 1990;61:1329-37.
12. Hashimoto K, Lever WF. The cell surface coat of normal keratinocytes and of acantholytic keratinocytes in pemphigus. Br J Dermatol 1970;83:282-90.
13. Odland GF. The fine structure of the interrelationship of cells in the human epidermis. J Biophys Biochem Cytol 1958;4:529-38.
14. Clark WH Jr, Watson MC, Watson BE. Two kinds of "clear" cells in the human epidermis; with a report of a modified DOPA reaction for electron microscopy. Am J Pathol 1961;39:333-44.
15. Cochran AJ. The incidence of melanocytes in normal skin. J Invest Dermatol 1970;55:65-70.
15a. Garraway LA, Widlund HR, Rubin MA, et al. Integrative genomic analyses identify MITF as a lineage survival oncogene amplified in malignant melanoma. Nature 2005;436:117-22.
15b. Granter SR, Wellbaecher KN, Quigley C, Fletcher CD, Fisher DE. Clear cell sarcoma shows immunoreactivity for microphthalmia transcription factor: further evidence for melanocytic differentiation. Mod Pathol 2001;14:6-9.
16. Niebauer G, Krawczyk WS, Wilgram GF. [The Langerhans cell organelle in Letterer-Siwe's disese.] Arch Klin Exp Dermatol 1970;239:125-37. [German]
17. Murphy GF, Bhan AK, Harrist TJ, Mihm MC Jr. In situ identification of T6-positive cells in normal human dermis by immunoelectron microscopy. Br J Dermatol 1983;108:423-31.
18. Chu A, Eisinger M, Lee JS, Takezaki S, Kung PC, Edelson RL. Immunoelectron microscopic identification of Langerhans cells using a new antigenic marker. J Invest Dermatol 1982;78:177-80.
19. Burkert KL, Huhn K, Menezes DW, Murphy GF. Langerhans cell microgranulomas (pseudo-Pautrier abscesses): morphologic diversity, diagnostic implications, and pathogenetic mechanisms. J Cutan Pathol 2002;29:511-6.
20. Moll I. Merkel cell distribution in human hair follicles of the fetal and adult scalp. Cell Tiss Res 1994;277:131-8.
21. Hashimoto K. Fine structure of Merkel cell in human oral mucosa. J Invest Dermatol 1972;58:381-7.
22. Cooper JH. Microanatomical and histochemical observations on the dermal-epidermal junction. Arch Dermatol 1958;77:18-22.
22a. Feng H, Shuda M, Chang Y, Moore PS. Clonal integration of a polyomavirus in human Merkel cell carcinoma. Science 2008;319:1096-1100.
23. Eady RA. The basement membrane. Interface between the epithelium and the dermis: structural features. Arch Dermatol 1988;124:709-12.
24. Eady RA. Babes, blisters, and basement membranes: from sticky molecules to epidermolysis bullosa. Clin Exp Dermatol 1987;12:161-70.
25. Bruckner-Tuderman L, Rüegger S, Odermatt B, Mitsuhashi Y, Schnyder UW. Lack of type VII collagen in unaffected skin of patients with severe recessive dystrophic epidermolysis bullosa. Dermatologica 1988;176:57-64.
26. Yen A, Braverman IM. Ultrastructure of the human dermal microcirculation: the horizontal plexus of the papillary dermis. J Invest Dermatol 1976;66:131-42.
27. Braverman IM, Yen A. Ultrastructure of human dermal microcirculation. II. The capillary loop of the dermal papillae. J Invest Dermatol 1977;68:44-52.

28. Thorgeirsson G, Robertson AL Jr. The vascular endothelium-pathobiologic significance. Am J Pathol 1978;93:803-48.
29. Albelda SM, Oliver P, Romer L, Buck CA. EndoCAM: a novel endothelial cell-cell adhesion molecule. J Cell Biol 1990;110:1227-37.
30. Berger R, Albelda S, Berd D, Ioffreda M, Whitaker D, Murphy GF. Expression of platelet-endothelial cell adhesion molecule-1 (PECAM-1) during melanoma-induced angiogenesis in vivo. J Cutan Pathol 1993;20:399-406.
31. Jones DA, Abbasi O, McIntire LV, et al. P-selection mediates neutrophil rolling on histamine-stimulated endothelial cells. Biophys J 1993;65:1560-9.
32. Thorlacius H, Raud J, Rosengren-Beezley S, Forrest MJ, Hedqvist P, Lindbom L. Mast cell activation induces P-selectin-dependent leukocyte rolling and adhesion in postcapillary venules in vivo. Biochem Biophys Res Commun 1994;203:1043-9.
33. Albelda SM, Smith CW, Ward PA. Adhesion molecules and inflammatory injury. FASEB J 1994;8:504-12.
34. Butcher EC. Leukocyte-endothelial cell recognition, three (or more) steps to specificity and diversity. Cell 1991;67:1033-6.
35. Walsh LJ, Murphy GF. Role of adhesion molecules in cutaneous inflammation and neoplasia. J Cutan Pathol 1992;19:161-71.
36. McEver RP. Selectins: novel receptors that mediate leukocyte adhesion during inflammation. Thromb Haemost 1991;65:223-8.
37. Ioffreda M, Albelda SM, Elder DE, et al. TNFα induces E-selectin expression and PECAM-1 (CD31) redistribution in extracutaneous tissues. Endothelium 1993;1:47-54.
38. Grant ME, Prockop DJ. The biosynthesis of collagen. N Engl J Med 1972;286:194-9.
39. Nigra TP, Friedland M, Martin GR. Controls of connective tissue synthesis: collagen metabolism. J Invest Dermatol 1972;59:44-9.
40. Meigel WN, Gay S, Weber L. Dermal architecture and collagen type distribution. Arch Dermatol Res 1977;259:1-10.
41. Stenn K. Collagen heterogeneity of skin. Am J Dermatopathol 1979;1:87-8.
42. Leigh IM, Eady RA, Heagerty AH, Purkis PE, Whitehead PA, Burgeson RE. Type VII collagen is a normal component of epidermal basement membrane, which shows altered expression in recessive dystrophic epidermolysis bullosa. J Invest Dermatol 1988;90:639-42.
43. Hashimoto K, Dibella RJ. Electron microscopic studies of normal and abnormal elastic fibers of the skin. J Invest Dermatol 1967;48:405-23.
44. Winand R. Biosynthesis, organization and degradation of mucopolysaccharides. Arch Belg Dermatol Syphiligr 1972;28:35-40.
45. Zaravinos A, Mammas IN, Sourvinos G, Spandidos DA. Molecular detection methods of human papillomavirus (HPV). Int J Biol Markers 2009;24:215-22.

# 2 INFLAMMATORY DISORDERS WITH PRIMARY EPIDERMAL ALTERATIONS: SPONGIOTIC DERMATITIS

*Spongiotic dermatitis* represents a diverse group of dermatoses that are often classified clinically as papulosquamous eruptions (Table 2-1) (1–4). Shared by all clinical-pathologic variants is the presence of spongiosis, or widening of the spaces between keratinocytes as a result of intercellular edema, resulting in prominence of the spiney, desmosome-associated cell junctions. The clinical term, *eczema,* often refers to spongiotic dermatitis and covers a variety of disorders.

Spongiotic dermatitis is characterized in the fully evolved lesion by a triad of basic symptoms and signs: an acute vesicular eruption associated with erythema; itching, often striking, with associated excoriation, leading to the second or subacute phase in which there is scaling with weeping, crust formation, and usually a plaque; and finally, a dry lesion that is hyperkeratotic, persistently pruritic, and often reveals an increase in skin markings.

The prototype of spongiotic dermatitis is *allergic contact dermatitis*, a disorder induced by delayed hypersensitivity to a variety of environmental antigens and characterized by discrete acute, subacute, and chronic clinical phases. The acute form is characterized by erythema and induration, and often by the formation of fluid-filled vesicles. Subacute to chronic forms tend to be dominated by excessive scale production. In both acute and subacute phases, spongiosis may give rise to intraepidermal vesicle formation as a result of eventual disruption of intercellular junctions consequent to mechanical stretching. With chronicity (one or more

Table 2-1

**CLINICAL VARIANTS OF SPONGIOTIC DERMATITIS**

| Variant | Clinical Features | Histologic Features |
| --- | --- | --- |
| Allergic contact dermatitis | Sites of antigen contact | Langerhans cell microgranulomas; eosinophils may be numerous |
| Atopic dermatitis | Flexural involvement in childhood | Epidermal hyperplasia; eosinophils may be sparse |
| Nummular dermatitis | Coin-like patches and plaques on arms and legs | Pinpoint microvesicles with mild spongiosis |
| Seborrheic dermatitis | Oily, scaling dermatitis of scalp, facial folds, midback, and chest | Subacute spongiotic dermatitis with scale and rare neutrophils in dermis or in scale at follicular ostia |
| Dyshidrotic eczema | Vesicles on palms and/or soles | Prominent intraepidermal microvesicles in acral skin |
| Id reaction | Association with primary dermatitis, often with fungal or bacterial component or stasis-related | Perivascular lymphoid infiltrate often with numerous eosinophils in dermal infiltrate |
| Pityriasis rosea | Ovoid patches and plaques following skin lines | Mound-like parakeratosis; papillary dermal hemorrhage |
| Small plaque parapsoriasis | Ovoid patches and plaques, resistant to therapy | Mound-like parakeratosis; no hemorrhage |
| Photoallergic dermatitis | Photo distribution | Fading of lymphoid infiltrate from superficial to mid-dermal vessels; endothelial vacuolization |
| Spongiotic drug eruption | Often diffuse involvement | Superficial and deep infiltrate; perivascular eosinophils |
| Spongiotic insect bite reaction | Grouped papulonodules | Wedge-shaped infiltrate; eosinophilic spongiosis; interstitial eosinophils |

weeks), progressive epidermal hyperplasia and increased scale production supervene. The end result of chronically excoriated pruritic forms of spongiotic dermatitis may be lichen simplex chronicus (see Acanthotic Dermatitis).

## PATHOGENESIS

Spongiotic dermatitis is associated with type IV immune responses to contact, injected or systemically administered haptens and protein antigens, infectious agents, and chemical and mechanical irritants (5). Many clinical-pathologic entities associated with spongiosis remain idiopathic. Epidermal Langerhans cells are critical to T-cell sensitization and challenge to antigens, and in both allergic and irritant forms of this disorder, cytokines derived from keratinocytes, mast cells, and mononuclear cells are important driving forces. The earliest alterations in spongiotic dermatitis are now known to involve the degranulation of mast cells located about postcapillary venules, resulting in the liberation of tumor necrosis factor alpha and triggering the expression of endothelial molecules that promote the adhesion of circulating memory T cells (6,7).

The prototypic spongiotic dermatitis, allergic contact dermatitis in its various stages of clinical evolution (8), may be experimentally reproduced and studied as the sequential evolution of a delayed hypersensitivity reaction induced by topical application of potent sensitizers like dinitrochlorobenzene. The initial uptake and presentation of intact antigen or hapten, which combines with endogenous protein to form antigen, are mediated by epidermal Langerhans cells. Langerhans cells take up antigen by endocytosis, then migrate through lymphatics from skin to draining lymph nodes. There, they present processed antigen to helper T cells, which then become sensitized to proliferate and become immunologically activated (e.g., capable of lymphokine production) on re-exposure to the specific antigen (9,10). It may take many repeated exposures to some antigens before sensitization occurs. About 2 weeks after successful sensitization in most cases, the primed T cells are ready to respond when challenged.

Topical challenge by antigen in a previously sensitized individual initiates a complex cascade of events (11–15). Within several hours and possibly within minutes after challenge, dermal mast cells about superficial blood vessels are induced to degranulate, resulting in discharge of their preformed mediators in the vicinity of postcapillary venules (16,17). Endothelial cells contract as a result of the release of mast cell histamine, and mast cell cytokines aid in the induction of endothelial glycoproteins that promote adhesive interactions between circulating sensitized T cells and the vessel surface. Mast cell proteases potentially play a role in facilitating subsequent T-cell diapedesis across the vessel wall, and it is even possible that heparin impedes formation of microthrombi during this process. Once liberated into the skin, the primed antigen-specific T cells respond to the antigen by releasing cytokines, which amplify the inflammatory infiltrate by recruiting even more mononuclear cells.

By 24 hours after challenge, significant numbers of T cells are observed about superficial dermal venules. Until this point, the ongoing tissue changes are unapparent clinically. During the subsequent 2 to 3 days, the progressive movement of T cells into the epidermis, facilitated by lymphokine-mediated induction of adhesive glycoproteins such as intercellular adhesion molecule-1 on keratinocytes, is associated with progressive erythema, spongiosis, and vesiculation. The association of T-cell epidermotropism with spongiosis raises the possibility that factors associated with the induction phases of inflammation (e.g., protease release) and passage of inflammatory cells across the normally intact dermal-epidermal junction, may, in concert, be responsible for the intercellular edema within the epidermal layer. The epidermotropism of early cutaneous T-cell lymphoma may actually represent an intraepidermal T-cell proliferation rather than dermal-epidermal trafficking, hence the relative absence of spongiosis.

The response to injected antigens is probably similar to that of topical antigens, but it is likely that most of the antigenic signals are communicated to T cells by native populations of dermal dendritic immune cells rather than epidermal Langerhans cells. This may be why contact allergy evokes prominent epidermal changes as opposed to predominately dermal alterations that typify delayed hypersensitivity reactions to circulating or injected proteins (e.g., drug eruptions, insect bite reactions). For most disorders of the spongiotic dermatitis group, the exogenous or endogenous antigens that stimulate their respective immune reaction patterns are yet to be discovered. This discussion centers on normal immune responses to proteins perceived as antigenic. In immunocompromised patients, provocative stimuli may differ from those that are antigenic to normal skin, and the patterns, cytologic composition, and time course of hypersensitivity reactions may also vary.

## DIAGNOSTIC STUDIES

In most instances, special studies are not essential for the diagnosis and classification of the various types of spongiotic dermatitis. In situations representing delayed hypersensitivity reactions to infectious agents (e.g., dermatophytes), periodic acid–Schiff (PAS) staining is often confirmatory. Occasionally, spongiotic dermatitis is confused with early cutaneous T-cell lymphoma (so-called spongiotic simulants of mycosis fungoides). In such instances, immunohistochemistry to establish mixed epidermotropism (CD4- and CD8-positive T cells) and mature CD4-positive T-cell phenotype (e.g., positive for CD4, CD5, CD7), as well as polymerase chain reaction analysis to exclude clonal T-cell receptor gene rearrangements, help establish a diagnosis of reactive spongiotic immune response.

There exist numerous animal models for the study of both allergic contact dermatitis and primary irritant dermatitis. These involve primarily rodents, although allergic contact dermatitis has been reproduced in human skin xenografted onto immunosuppressed (SCID) mice (17a).

## ALLERGIC CONTACT AND PRIMARY IRRITANT DERMATITIS

**Definition.** *Allergic contact dermatitis* is a common, pruritic, vesicular to scaling dermatitis elicited as the result of a type IV immune response provoked by topical contact with specific antigenic proteins and haptens (18–41). *Primary irritant dermatitis* (42) shares many clinical and histologic features, although it is elicited by topical exposure to nonimmunologic contactants (e.g., chemical and physical factors). This type of reaction, which shows clinical and pathologic changes similar to allergic contact dermatitis, is due to a variety of external agents, usually an organic or metalloorganic substance.

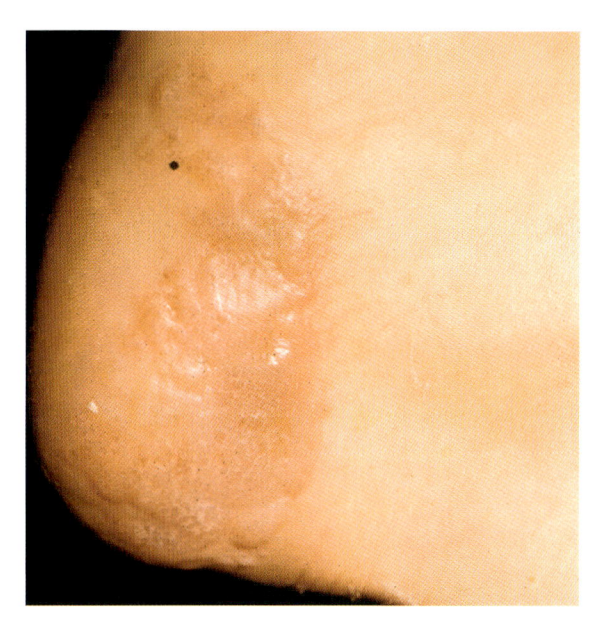

**Figure 2-1**

**ALLERGIC CONTACT DERMATITIS**

An area of erythema with confluent vesicles has developed on the lateral heel as a consequence of antigens present in the tanning of shoe leather.

**Clinical Features.** Allergic contact dermatitis occurs at any age in life but is uncommon in the young. The clinical manifestations vary based on the underlying cause and lesion age (figs. 2-1–2-3). The acute phase consists of well-demarcated patches or, less frequently, edematous plaques, and prominent vesiculation. These vesicles break down and lead to weeping. When the foot is involved (fig. 2-1), the dermatitis is noted in the thinner aspects of the lateral foot and is well-demarcated without involving the thick part of the sole. The subacute phase shows erythema in a well-defined plaque-like lesion, with mild desquamation and scale-crust formation. The chronic plaque at sites of persistent contact reaction is often equivalent to lichen simplex chronicus where irregular acanthosis dominates the clinical picture (see Acanthotic Dermatitis, chapter 3, for additional details).

The arrangement of the clinical lesions in contact dermatitis often follows the area of contact with a specific substance. With poison ivy, for example, the lesion gives rise to linear

## Inflammatory Disorders of the Skin

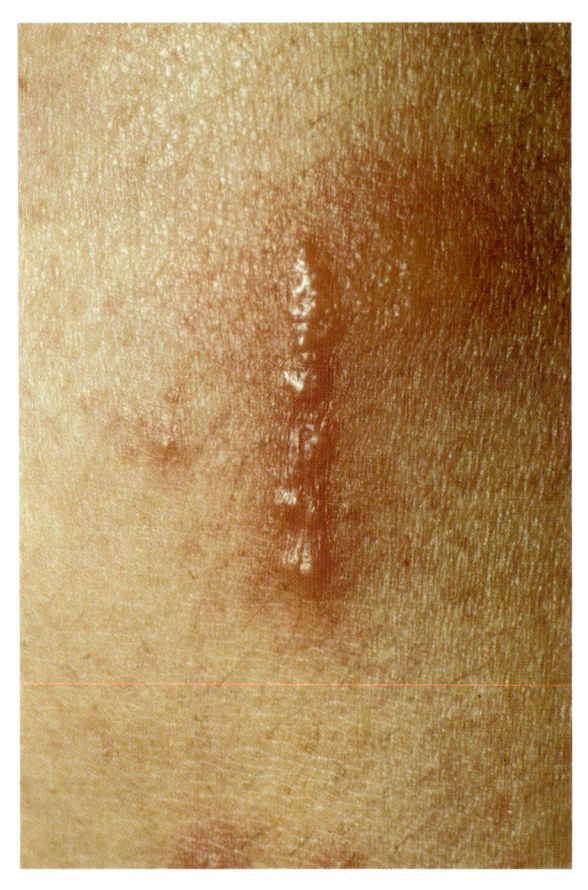

#### Figure 2-2
**ALLERGIC CONTACT DERMATITIS: POISON IVY**
Erythema and vesiculation are linear, a characteristic pattern indicating the site of epicutaneous exposure to the rhus antigen.

vesicles in the acute phase. In the case of nickel, the vesicular reaction and the subsequent evolution occur underneath the site of nickel contact (e.g., as with gold jewelry fortified with nickel alloy). Because of the thickness of the stratum corneum, it is rare for primary contact dermatitis to involve the palms and soles. A reaction to chromates on the dorsum of the foot, for example, will stop at the junction line of the palm or the sole. Once the barrier has been breached, as in irritant dermatitis, then contact allergy may develop and exacerbate the irritant effect. Occasionally, ultraviolet light is an essential cofactor to the development of allergic contact dermatitis, a condition referred to as a *photoeczematous reaction* (18,19).

*Photoeczematous spongiotic dermatitis* results when topically applied substances (e.g., perfumes) or ingested agents (e.g., certain drugs) are rendered antigenic in skin exposed to ultraviolet light, evoking an initially vesicular and eventually scaling dermatitis. Deposition of plant material (e.g., pollen) carried by wind may also elicit this condition upon exposure to sunlight (i.e., *phytophotodermatitis*). Clinically, photoeczematous dermatitis is confined to sites of solar irradiation, and this pattern assists in making the correct diagnosis. Regardless of whether ultraviolet light serves as a cofactor in the development of allergic contact dermatitis, an extraordinary number of environmental agents worldwide may produce contact skin

#### Figure 2-3
**NUMMULAR ECZEMA**
This form of spongiotic dermatitis is characterized by multiple, coin-like, erythematous scaling plaques.

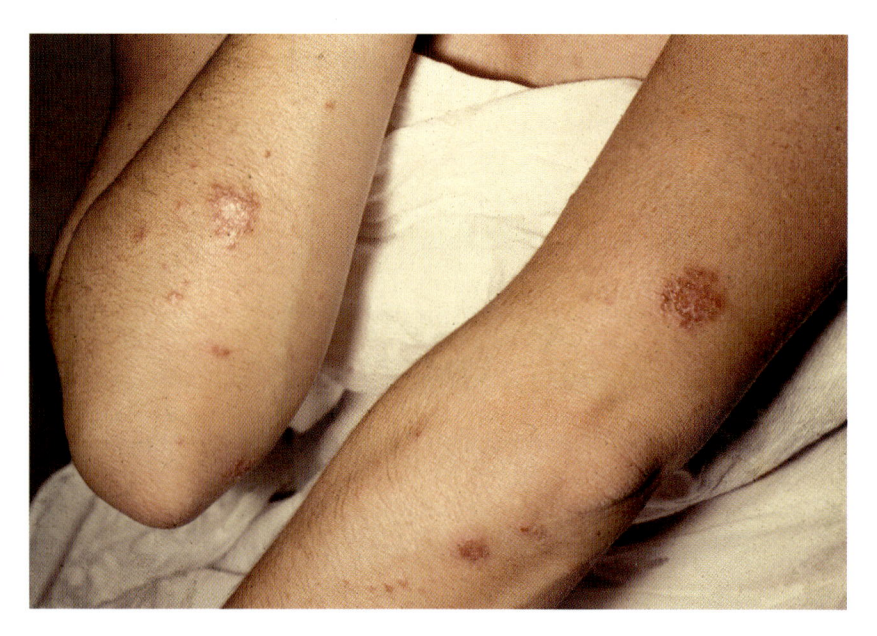

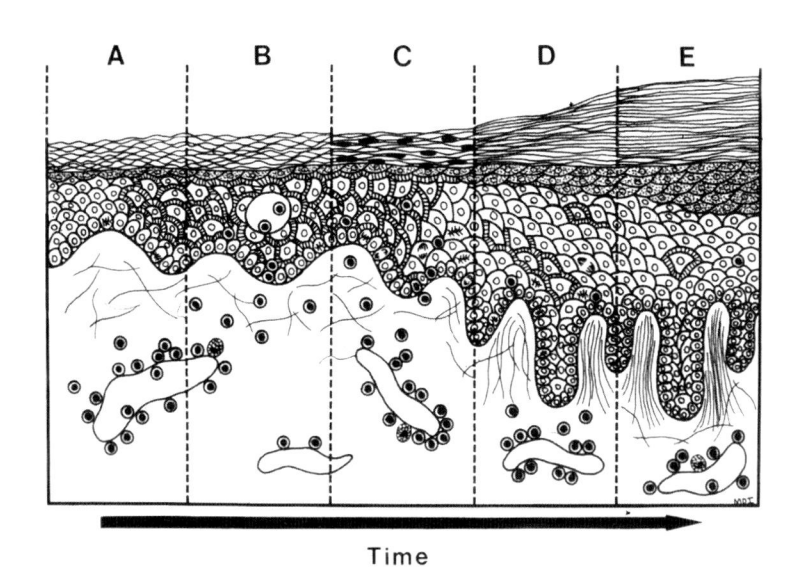

**Figure 2-4**

**SEQUENTIAL EVOLUTION OF SPONGIOTIC DERMATITIS**

In the early stages (A,B), there is progressive widening of the intercellular spaces within the epidermis, resulting in microvesicle formation (B). The perivascular lymphocytic infiltrate persists from the earliest stages of the disorder, even before appreciable spongiosis is noted. In the subacute to chronic stages (C–E), there is progressive acanthosis (retiform epidermal hyperplasia), abnormal scale formation (parakeratosis and compact hyperorthokeratosis), and gradual diminution in the amount of spongiosis. By the chronic stages of the condition (D,E), the histopathology represents acanthotic dermatitis, and could be designated as lichen simplex chronicus.

allergy (20–39), including substances such as preservatives in corticosteroid creams (40,41), the agent of choice used to treat this condition in most patients.

Unlike allergic contact dermatitis, primary irritant dermatitis does not require initial sensitization, although there is considerable overlap in the clinical and histologic appearance of both lesions (42,43). Lesions either sting or are pruritic, and the characteristic evolutionary sequence seen in allergic contact dermatitis is closely mimicked. Clinical patch testing with a broad panel of potentially offending antigens and chemical irritants may be required to define the lesion etiology. The response to an irritant, which may be limited to itching or stinging in affected areas, occurs in most patients within a few seconds after an irritant, such as when methanol-containing chemicals or chloroform is applied. A spectrum of changes occur in the area of contact, from acute vesicular reactions to chapping to chronic eczematous type lesions. The lesions usually heal within a few weeks; complete remission is unusual, however, and usually there is a subacute smoldering state, especially if the irritants persist.

*Atopic dermatitis*, the cutaneous manifestation of atopy, is a form of spongiotic dermatitis that typically begins in childhood, although lesions occur at any time from the first few months of life to old age. Slightly more females are affected than males. The lesion onset is usually during the first 10 years of life and consists of dry skin with variable erythema. In the earliest phase, there may be vesiculation in a poorly defined patch of redness; the subacute phase is chapped scaly skin; and the chronic lesion shows a well-defined plaque with striking lichenification or exaggeration of skin markings with hyperkeratosis. The characteristic chronic manifestations are present in the flexural regions, front and sides of the neck, eyelids, and dorsum of the hands and feet. The lesions are incited by a variety of foods, substances that are inhaled, and bacteria, especially *Staphylococcus aureus*. *S. aureus* contains superantigens that exacerbate symptoms by amplifying the immune response via the T-cell receptor. The lesions usually improve in the summer and become worse in the winter. The patients usually have a familial history of hay fever, allergic rhinitis, or asthma. Typically, immunoglobulin (Ig) E levels are elevated in the serum.

**Pathologic Findings.** The histopathology of allergic contact dermatitis changes with the duration of the lesion (fig. 2-4). At scanning magnification, acute lesions are characterized by a superficial, perivascular lymphocytic infiltrate in the papillary dermis, with variable associated edema, discerned as pallor of the subepidermal collagen bundles (44). The epidermis may be of normal thickness for the anatomic site or show mild irregular acanthosis. Compared to adjacent, uninvolved epidermis, the epithelial

*Inflammatory Disorders of the Skin*

**Figure 2-5**

**EARLY EVOLUTIONARY STAGE OF SPONGIOTIC DERMATITIS**

The epidermal pallor is a result of widening of the intercellular spaces that separate keratinocytes.

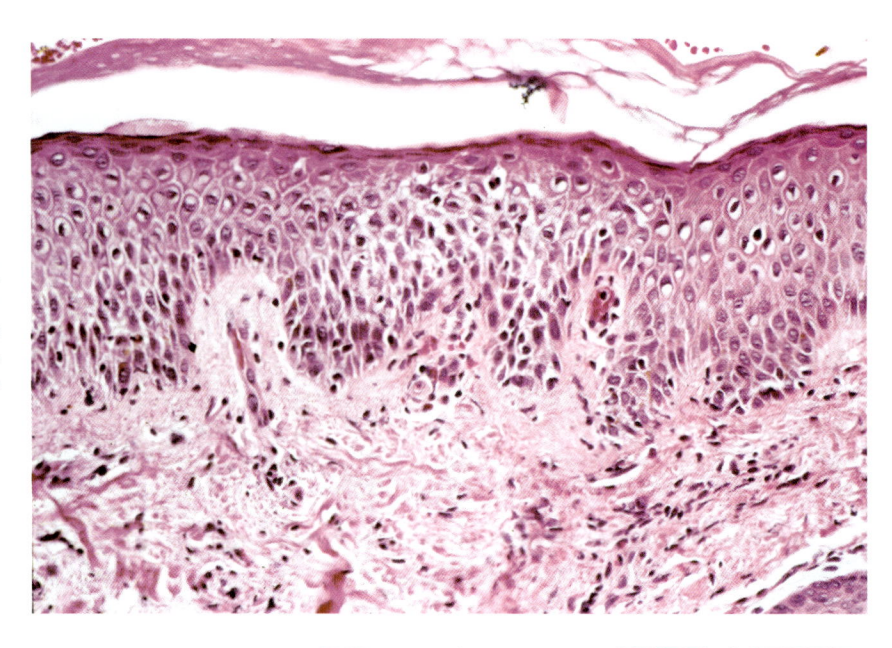

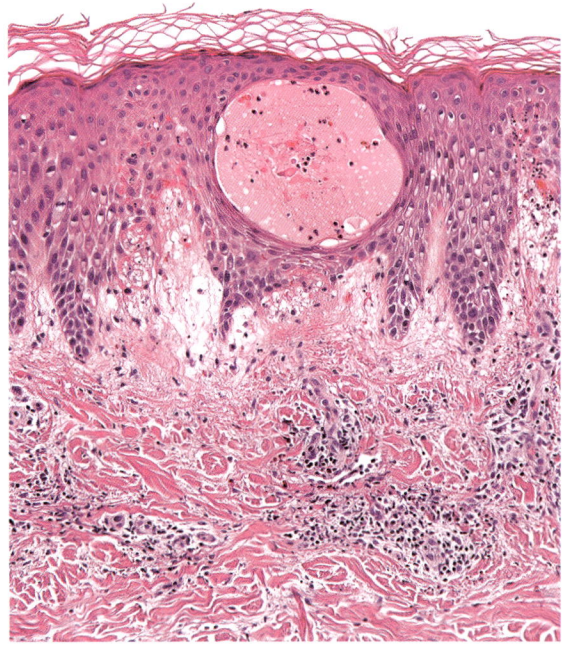

**Figure 2-6**

**ACUTE SPONGIOTIC DERMATITIS**

Intraepidermal vesicle of allergic contact dermatitis. Note the associated superficial dermal edema and normal basket weave stratum corneum indicative of acute onset.

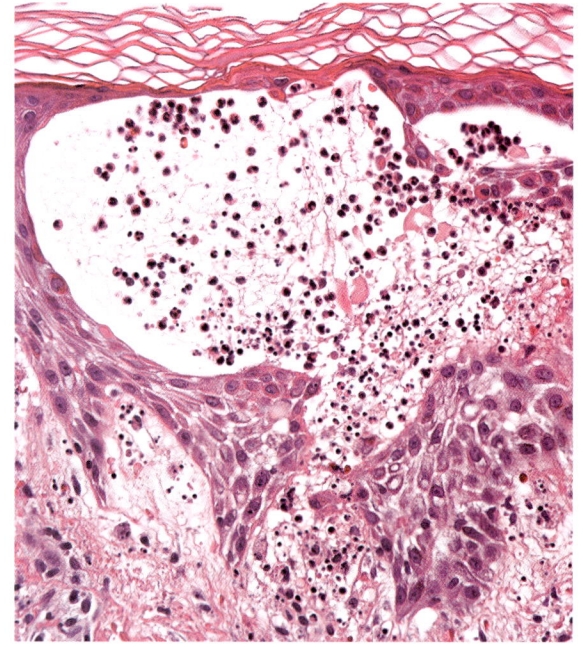

**Figure 2-7**

**SPONGIOTIC DERMATITIS**

An intraepidermal vesicle contains numerous eosinophils, indicative of a hypersensitivity reaction.

layer may demonstrate pallor due to intercellular edema or frank intraepidermal microvesiculation (figs. 2-5–2-9).

Although these changes establish the diagnosis of spongiotic dermatitis, closer inspection at higher magnification is required to determine whether features compatible with allergic contact dermatitis are present (figs. 2-10, 2-11). These include: 1) eosinophils about superficial venules and, occasionally, within the spongiotic

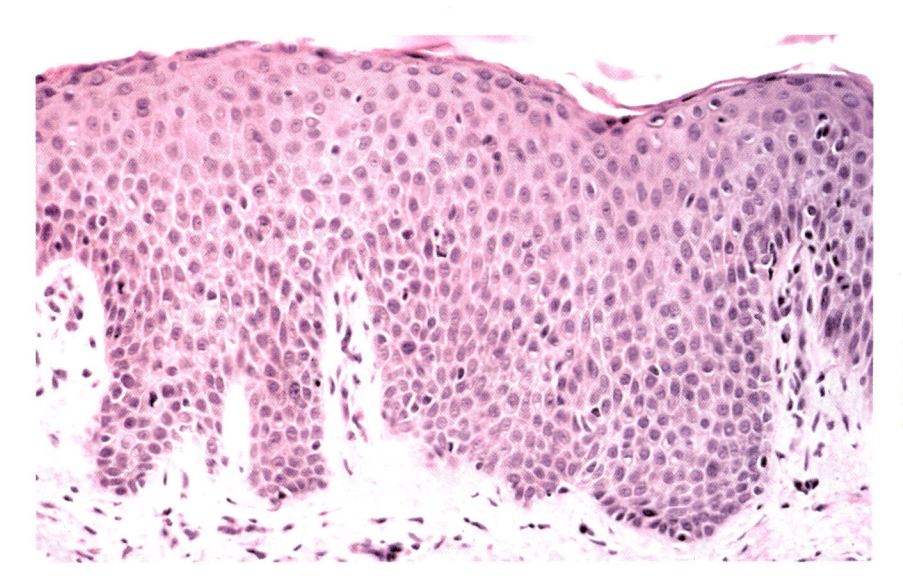

## Figure 2-8
### SUBACUTE SPONGIOTIC DERMATITIS (PRIMARY IRRITANT DERMATITIS)

Although there is diffuse spongiosis, irregular epidermal thickening (acanthosis) has already developed, a typical finding of primary irritant dermatitis.

## Figure 2-9
### ACUTE SPONGIOTIC DERMATITIS, NUMMULAR TYPE

There is diffuse epidermal spongiosis. A discrete intraepidermal microvesicle is forming.

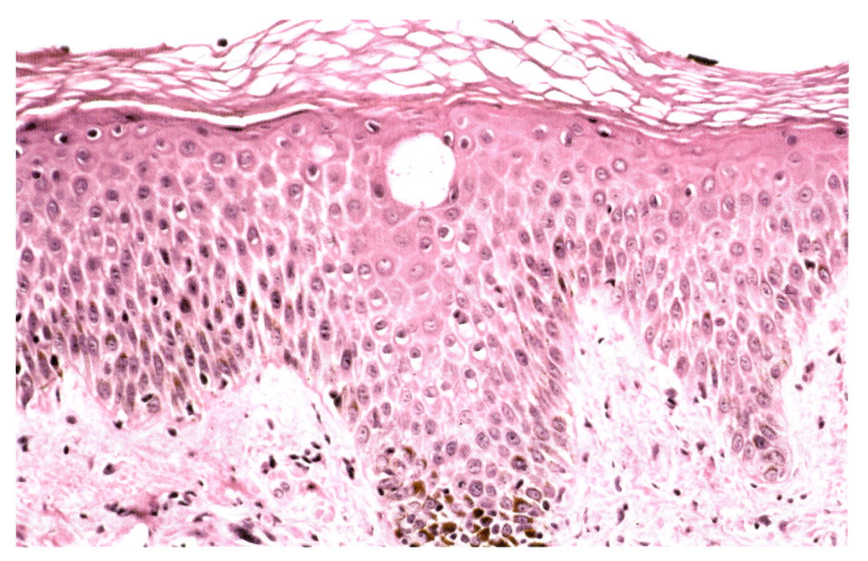

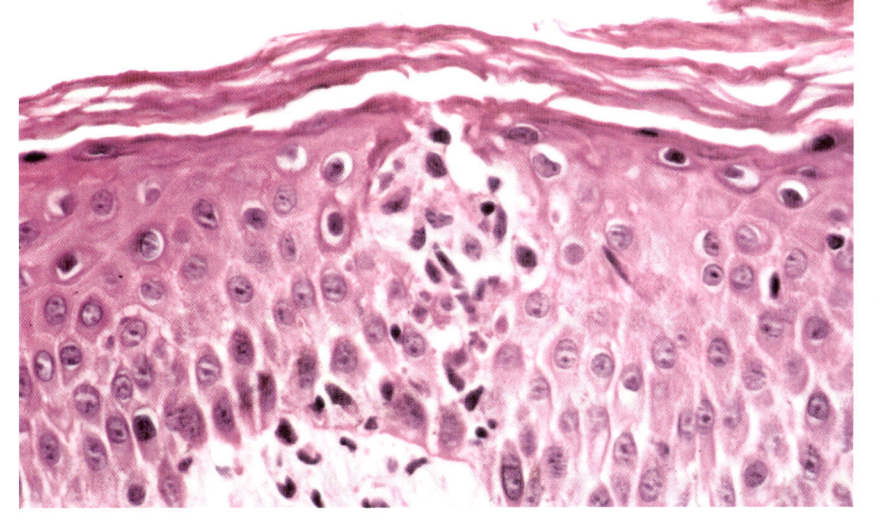

## Figure 2-10
### LANGERHANS CELL MICROGRANULOMA FORMATION IN ACUTE ALLERGIC CONTACT DERMATITIS

In addition to mild spongiosis, there is a subcorneal accumulation of pale histiocytic cells. These cells have abundant cytoplasm and characteristically infolded nuclear contours. Special staining shows them to be Langerhans cells.

**Figure 2-11**

**DERMAL COMPONENT OF ACUTE ALLERGIC CONTACT DERMATITIS**

In addition to superficial dermal edema, evidenced by widening of the spaces between collagen bundles, there is a characteristic perivascular infiltrate of activated lymphocytes with admixed eosinophils.

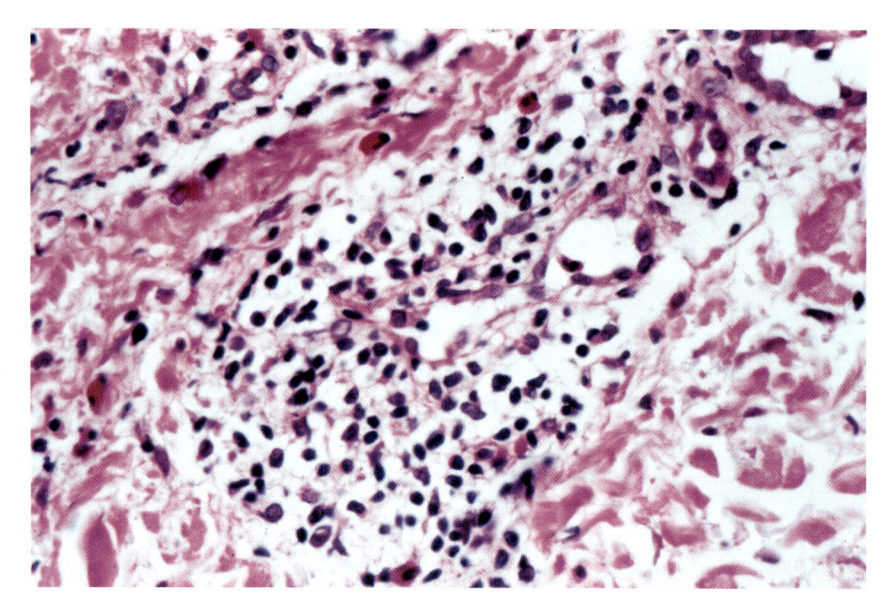

epidermal layer (i.e., eosinophilic spongiosis), in association with epidermotropic lymphocytes (45,46); 2) microvesicles that are usually larger and localized to the upper epidermis or almost replace the epidermis, as opposed to the smaller more scattered vesicles of atopic dermatitis; and 3) intraepidermal microgranulomas consisting exclusively of Langerhans cells or an admixture of Langerhans cells and lymphocytes. Hyperplastic Langerhans cells are larger than lymphocytes, exhibit pale but visible cytoplasm, and have a characteristic infolded nucleus containing scant heterochromatin. The nucleolus usually lies along the nuclear membrane. Stains for CD1a often help confirm the presence of Langerhans cell microgranulomas and differentiate them from Pautrier microabscesses of CD4-positive T cells, as occurs in epidermotropic cutaneous T-cell lymphoma (47,48). Their prominence in certain biopsy specimens relates to immune mechanisms involved in antigen presentation and cytokine regulation of the superficial delayed hypersensitivity response that underlies the histologic reaction pattern of allergic contact dermatitis.

The spongiosis of allergic contact dermatitis may also involve the follicular infundibula, and in the clinical variant, *follicular eczema*, intercellular edema may exclusively affect the pilar apparatus. Certain antigens and haptens, such as nickel, neomycin, and even gentian violet, among others, appear to have a peculiar procliv-ity to stimulate follicular immune responses. In African-American patients, atopic dermatitis may be limited to follicular involvement. This variant may be confused grossly with other follicular diseases (e.g., inflammatory keratosis pilaris). Accordingly, the clinical history is critical and multiple serial biopsy sections may be required, for documentation of follicular spongiosis.

**Differential Diagnosis.** In some patients allergic contact dermatitis cannot be reliably distinguished from primary irritant dermatitis by histology alone, although the presence of eosinophils and Langerhans cell microgranulomas is suggestive evidence in support of the former. Other forms of spongiotic dermatitis may provide clues as to the underlying cause, particularly with respect to the architecture and composition of the dermal component (49). Spongiotic drug and insect bite reactions may also pose problems, although these conditions usually demonstrate a deep as well as superficial dermal inflammatory infiltrate. Eczematous variants of bullous pemphigoid sometimes resemble contact dermatitis, although pemphigoid usually shows degranulating eosinophils intimately associated with the basal cell layer. Severe irritant dermatitis usually shows evidence of apoptosis and necrosis of individual intraepidermal keratinocytes. Due to the necrosis, neutrophils focally migrate into the epidermis and are also scattered along the dermal-epidermal junction. In acute irritant reactions, there is little organized infiltrate around superficial vessels, whereas in repeated irritant reactions, superimposed hypersensitivity may ensue and a dermal infiltrate appear. The differential diagnosis of irritant contact dermatitis includes mainly atopic dermatitis, photodermatitis, allergic contact dermatitis, and injury by thermal burn or ionizing radiation.

In photoeczematous spongiotic dermatitis, a biopsy of involved skin demonstrates, at scanning magnification, a superficial and at least mid-dermal perivascular inflammatory infiltrate composed predominantly of lymphocytes and occasional eosinophils. The infiltrate gradually diminishes in intensity with depth (i.e., grades off), a helpful diagnostic feature. Prominent endothelial cells with vacuolated cytoplasm line involved dermal venules. The overlying epidermal layer shows variable spongiosis and lymphoid epidermotropism. The histologic findings in photoeczematous spongiotic dermatitis are not entirely specific, and validation by an appropriate clinical history is required in the majority of cases to establish an accurate diagnosis. Photo patch testing is used when the gross and microscopic findings fail to reveal definitive alterations.

While the histologic findings in acute allergic contact dermatitis are not entirely specific beyond categorization as spongiotic dermatitis, with chronicity, they become even less diagnostic. This is because epidermal hyperplasia and secondary alterations resulting from excoriation supervene. In general, subacute lesions show focal spongiosis, irregular acanthosis, and an admixture of hyperorthokeratosis and parakeratosis. In chronic lesions, the spongiosis is often minimal, and the histologic changes of lichen simplex chronicus may dominate. Residual eosinophils and foci of epidermal or follicular spongiosis, in concert with the appropriate clinical parameters, suggest a diagnosis of subacute to chronic allergic contact dermatitis. Lesions should be biopsied early in their clinical evolution, avoiding sites of refractory dermatitis that have within 3 to 4 weeks been partially treated with topical corticosteroids, which confounds further the histology of allergic contact dermatitis.

Primary irritant dermatitis and atopic dermatitis (which may represent either true contact allergy or a lowered threshold for irritant change) often mimic the histopathology of allergic contact dermatitis. Indeed, many observers have suggested that it is not possible to differentiate these two conditions based on microscopic alterations. Irritant dermatitis is one of the most profound diagnostic challenges in the spongiotic category of cutaneous reaction patterns. This is because some degree of irritant effect is common to all subacute and chronic forms of pruritic spongiotic dermatitis of identifiable etiology or genetic predisposition (e.g., allergic contact dermatitis and atopic dermatitis). Mechanical irritation or scratching alone may induce dermatitis that, because of the initiation of the scratch-itch cycle, is self-perpetuating. Primary irritant dermatitis should be suspected whenever there is an accompanying clinical history of accessible, previously normal-appearing skin subject to endogenously produced pruritus (e.g., dry, aged skin; presence of hepatobiliary or renal disease) that has become erythematous or develops induration and abnormal scale.

**Treatment and Prognosis.** The treatment of acute allergic contact dermatitis is wet dressings applied with Burrow's solution, if possible every few hours. Topical corticosteroid application is also very helpful (50). In extensive cases, a brief course of systemic corticosteroids is required. For subacute to chronic cases, topical corticosteroids of increased strength are used. Lubricants and emollients are necessary because of the dryness. Any offending or inciting agent must be eliminated.

For primary irritant dermatitis, the principal treatment is avoidance of potentially offending physical or chemical agents by the use of gloves and protective clothing. Immediate washing of the surface after contact is important. Acute lesions are usually soaked with Burrow's solution and chronic lesions treated with topical, or when severe, systemic corticosteroid therapy.

## ATOPIC DERMATITIS

**Definition.** *Atopic dermatitis* is a disorder that goes through a triad of acute, subacute, and chronic changes (51–54). It is associated with much itching and a history of dermatitis, allergic rhinitis, or asthma, either personally or in the family.

**Clinical Features.** The lesions occur from the first few months of life to late age. Females are

*Inflammatory Disorders of the Skin*

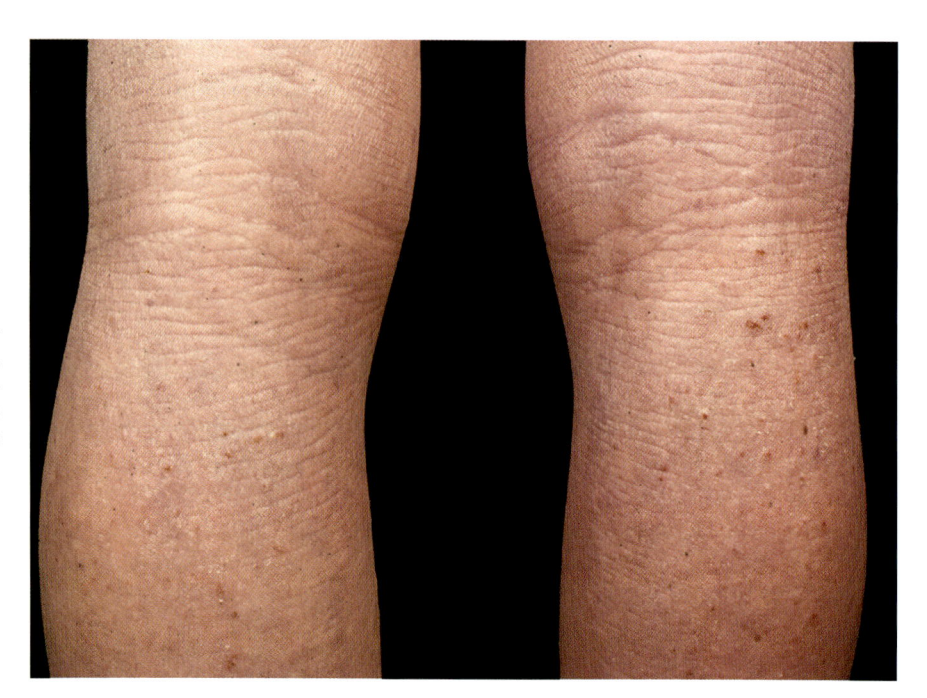

**Figure 2-12**

**ATOPIC DERMATITIS**

The pale erythematous plaques are characteristically present in the flexural areas of extremity skin. The accentuated skin folds and scale patterns are indicative of the chronicity of this condition.

affected slightly more often than males. Onset is usually during the first 10 years of life and consists of dry skin with variable erythema. In the earliest phase, there may be vesiculation in a poorly defined patch of redness. The subacute phase is a chapped scaly patch. The chronic lesion is usually well-defined, with striking lichenification or exaggeration of skin markings and hyperkeratosis. The lesions are characteristic and are present in flexural surfaces, front and sides of the neck, eyelids, and dorsum of the hands and feet (fig. 2-12). The lesions are incited by a variety of foods, substances that are inhaled, and bacteria, especially *Staphylococcus aureus*. Bacteria that contain superantigens exacerbate the symptoms. Lesions usually improve in the summer and become worse in the winter. Patients often have a history of hay fever or asthma. Typically, serum IgE levels are elevated.

**Pathologic Features.** Atopic dermatitis shares many histologic features with allergic contact dermatitis and primary irritant dermatitis. A superficial dermal perivascular and epidermotropic infiltrate of lymphocytes and eosinophils is characteristic. Spongiosis is present, associated acanthosis is often prominent, and microvesiculation may not be apparent (fig. 2-13). The reason for the dominance of the acanthotic alteration over spongiosis in atopic dermatitis may relate to the low-grade chronicity of active lesions.

**Differential Diagnosis.** A variety of dermatoses, including nummular eczema, contact dermatitis, early or excoriated psoriasis, and even early phases of mycosis fungoides, must be differentiated.

**Treatment and Prognosis.** Lesions spontaneously remit but then exacerbate during times of anxiety, such as stress in school in children, the onset of adolescence, or times of grieving (death of a partner or loss of a job) in adults. Acute eczema usually responds to wet soak dressings, topical application of corticosteroids, and sometimes topical antibiotics. In addition, topical immunomodulators may be employed, particularly in children, in an effort to avoid the effects of chronic steroid use. Antipruritic medicines are helpful and include some antihistamines. Trials with various histamine (H)1- and H2-blocker medications usually result in relief. For patients with evidence of superinfection, oral antibiotics are given. For chronic lesions, topical antiinflammatory medications are used with topical emollients and hydration. Topical doxepin has been useful. Systemic corticosteroids are used in some patients. Adults with severe manifestations of the disorder respond to cyclosporine or azathioprine, given for a limited period of time. Oral tacrolimus has been used in recalcitrant cases. Phototherapy with psoralen and ultraviolet A (PUVA) also has been used with some success (55).

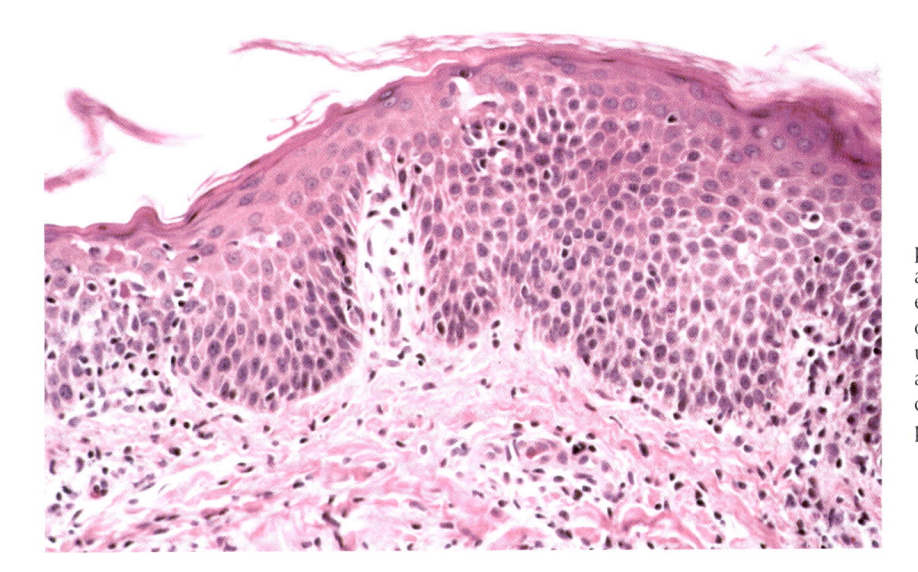

**Figure 2-13**

**ATOPIC DERMATITIS**

Irregular epidermal hyperplasia, multiple foci of spongiosis, and abnormal scale formation evidenced by compact hyperorthokeratosis are present. The underlying dermis is edematous and shows a perivascular lymphocytic infiltrate containing eosinophils.

## DYSHIDROTIC ECZEMA

**Definition.** One of the many examples of misnomers in dermatologic disease, *dyshidrotic eczema* is not a disturbance of eccrine sweat production or a specific eczematous disorder (56,57). Rather, it is a form of pruritic, vesicular, hand and foot dermatitis without apparent external cause. Occasionally, it is associated with atopic disease, dermatophyte infection, or sometimes, severe contact allergy. Superinfected vesicles may form pustules that mimic psoriasis and pustulosis palmaris et plantaris. Dyshidrotic eczema has an acute, chronic, and severe form, which is often dubbed *chronic hand dermatitis*.

**Clinical Features.** The lesions usually occur in the first three to four decades of life, but may occur later in life as well. Men and women are equally affected. The initial outbreak is as strikingly pruritic, usually deep-seated vesicles that have been referred to as "tapioca"-like. These vesicles cluster and extend along the sides of the fingers and the toes in some patients. Eventually, fissures and erosions occur, with crusting; secondary infection is common and can result in lymphangitis. Recurrence is common and may last for weeks, with periods of exacerbation and partial resolution.

**Pathologic Findings.** At scanning magnification, dyshidrotic dermatitis (i.e., hand or foot eczema) consists of well-formed, intraepidermal, spongiotic vesicles beneath the normally thickened stratum corneum of acral skin (fig. 2-14). It is thought that the microvesicles are well-developed as a result of their prolonged retention within the relatively thick epidermal and horny layers that typify the skin of the palm and sole. The inflammatory infiltrate is typically superficial and composed of mononuclear cells, although neutrophils and eosinophils are occasionally present. Lymphoid exocytosis is generally restricted to spongiotic areas. Even with chronicity, intraepidermal serum extravasation may be detected in the stratum corneum overlying a nonspongiotic hyperplastic epidermis.

After a diagnosis of dyshidrotic dermatitis is established, easily identified causes should be excluded. A detailed clinical history should assist in excluding atopic dermatitis. History and patch testing are appropriate screening maneuvers for contact hand and foot allergy, although, as noted above, contact dermatitis is unusual on palms and soles.

**Differential Diagnosis.** Allergic contact dermatitis, pustular psoriasis, atopic dermatitis, and tinea of the hands and feet should be considered and must be excluded. Allergic contact dermatitis may be difficult to rule out without extensive patch testing. Atopic dermatitis is excluded by a careful clinical history and a PAS stain to exclude hyphae within the stratum corneum. Psoriasis may be excluded by the absence of the histologic alterations typical of the acral manifestations of this condition.

**Figure 2-14**

**DYSHIDROTIC ECZEMA**

This spongiotic dermatitis affecting the skin of the palm (note the characteristically thickened and compacted stratum corneum) shows multiple, discrete, fluid-filled intraepidermal microvesicles.

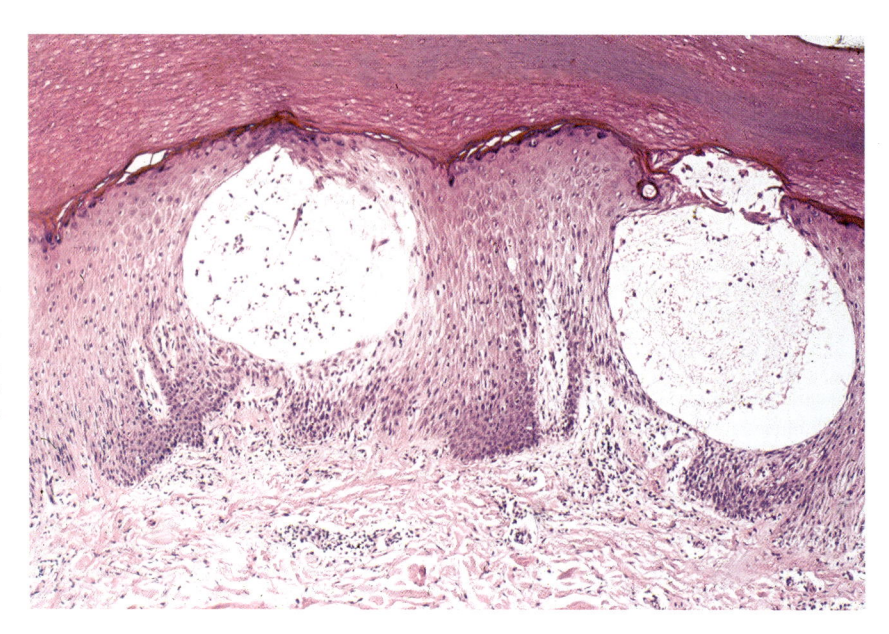

**Treatment and Prognosis.** For acute vesicular lesions, wet dressings with Burrow's solution are helpful. Corticosteroids of high potency may be applied topically, and in some of the more resistant cases, steroids are injected intralesionally. For patients with bacterial superinfection, oral antibiotics must be administered. PUVA therapy is useful in some cases.

## EARLY PSORIASIS

**Definition.** The early form of *psoriasis* is sometimes obscure in its clinical presentation, but it is an early lesion of the psoriatic spectrum that usually does not have the characteristic scale.

**Clinical Features.** The lesions of early psoriasis occur in two forms. The first is *guttate psoriasis*, which is an eruption of small papules over the trunk and upper portion of the extremities. The papules are oval to round and have a drop-like appearance, hence, called guttate. These lesions are often salmon colored and may or may not have superficial scale. The other type of early psoriasis is a *papulosquamous eruption*. This presents on the characteristic surfaces affected by psoriasis as salmon-colored patches which become scaly.

**Pathologic Findings.** Early lesions of psoriasis show inconspicuous retiform epidermal acanthosis, focal parakeratosis, and little or no neutrophils, or alternatively, as in eruptive pustular lesions, prominent accumulation of neutrophils within the uppermost epidermal layers (fig. 2-15). Focal spongiosis within the epidermal layer is often observed, prompting consideration of subacute spongiotic dermatitis, either with or without associated impetiginization (Table 2-2). A valuable finding in establishing a diagnosis of early psoriasis is the presence of dilated and tortuous capillary loops within widened dermal papillae with overlying epidermal thinning. There is focal loss of the granular cell layer beneath the focal parakeratosis. Eosinophils are notably absent within the superficial dermis.

**Differential Diagnosis.** Guttate psoriasis should be differentiated from guttate parapsoriasis, which forms a lenticular or lens-like scale composed of tightly applied parakeratotic nuclei with little or no evidence of significant underlying inflammation. Early psoriasis should be differentiated from eczema, or contact dermatitis, or occasionally, erythema elevatum diutinum in its early form, particularly if salmon-colored plaques are present on the extensor surfaces.

**Treatment and Prognosis.** Topical corticosteroids are useful in early lesions. Emollients may help reduce the itching that may occur in these early lesions. When there are multiple widespread lesions, topical light therapy may be beneficial. Although biologic therapy is reserved for advanced psoriatic disease, it may have a role in disseminated early disease, particularly when

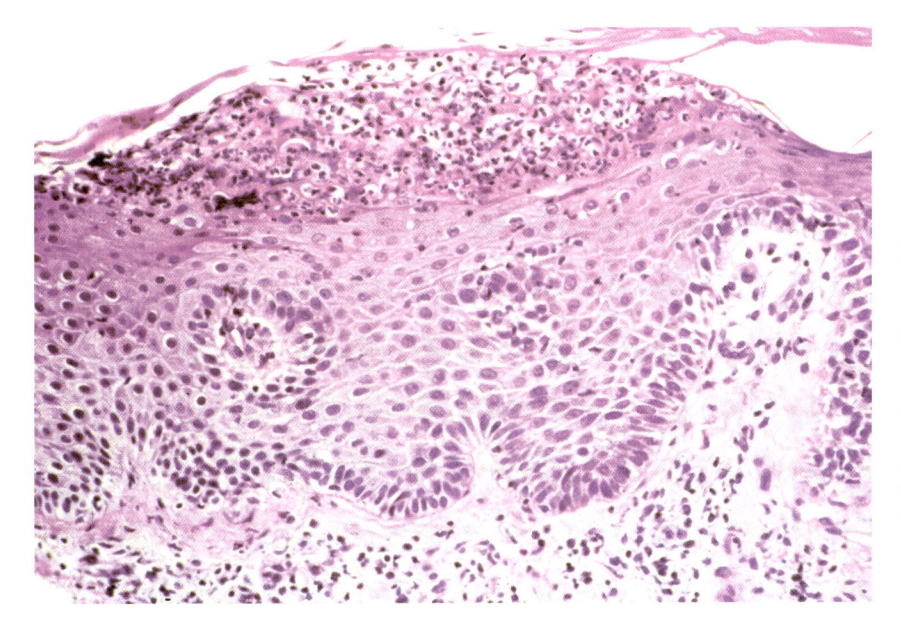

**Figure 2-15**

**EARLY PSORIASIS WITH SPONGIOSIS**

Although the characteristic psoriasiform acanthosis has yet to develop, there is an accumulation of neutrophils within the scale and dilated and ectatic capillary loops within dermal papillae. There is prominent spongiosis within the epidermal rete ridges, a finding that may occur in early and active psoriatic lesions and lead to confusion with impetiginized primary spongiotic dermatitis.

Table 2-2

**DIFFERENTIAL DIAGNOSIS OF SEBORRHEIC DERMATITIS, ALLERGIC CONTACT DERMATITIS, AND EARLY PSORIASIS**

|  | Seborrheic Dermatitis | ACD[a] | Psoriasis |
| --- | --- | --- | --- |
| Spongiosis | Mild | Mild to marked | Focal, mild |
| Hypogranulosis | Absent | Absent | Present |
| Eosinophils | Absent | Present | Absent |
| Lymphoid epidermotropism | Minimal | Mild to marked | Minimal |
| Capillary alterations[b] | Absent | Absent | Present |

[a]ACD = allergic contact dermatitis.
[b]Defined as dilated and tortuous capillary loops within edematous dermal papillae.

associated with arthritic lesions. Other immunosuppressant medications, such as cyclosporine and methotrexate, are helpful in cases where topical steroid application is not feasible.

## ID REACTION

**Definition.** The concept of an *id reaction* is riddled with confusion. Broadly defined, it implies a cutaneous inflammatory or immune response provoked by a distant and seemingly unrelated dermatitis, systemic condition, or infection (58–62). A spongiotic id reaction describes an abrupt hypersensitivity response that occurs in association with primary inflammatory dermatoses such as dermatophytes or stasis dermatitis, and presents as a generalized spongiotic eruption. Perhaps better termed *autosensitization spongiotic dermatitis*, the id reaction may be a manifestation of heightened systemic immunologic responsiveness due to liberation of proinflammatory mediators or products of infectious agents at sites of localized dermatitis.

**Clinical Features.** The id reaction often develops as a widespread response to a localized, inflammatory, often weeping dermatitis, such as severe stasis dermatitis, or in association with an inflammatory dermatophyte reaction. Most commonly, the patient initially develops a papulovesicular eruption on the trunk and extremities. This highly pruritic eruption is considered a hypersensitivity, or id, reaction to the underlying dermatosis. There are certain infections that likewise result in a hypersensitivity reaction to the organism. These id-like reactions to organisms, such as to mycobacteria, are designated *tuberculids* and are often nodular lesions that may have granulomas as part of their response. These may be solid granulomas or palisading granulomas. The latter type of eruption is characteristically not as pruritic or as acutely inflammatory as is the acute papulovesicular id reaction, and it generally is not associated with spongiosis.

**Pathologic Findings.** The histopathology of an id reaction is similar to the acute phase of allergic contact dermatitis. Eosinophils are generally present in the superficial perivascular lymphoid inflammatory component. Because the histopathology resembles that of other forms of acute spongiotic dermatitis, a careful clinical history is required for evaluation and confirmation of an id reaction. One clue to the diagnosis is the very focal nature of the reaction: a well-defined spongiotic dermatitis affecting a few rete ridges is often seen in the id reaction, as compared to the gradual tapering of a contact reaction from central marked involvement to gradual diminution at the edges.

The granulomatous id-like reactions involve a different response to provocative systemic factors, and include epithelioid well-formed granulomas, palisading granuloma annulare-like reactions of the dermis, and mixed neutrophilic and granulomatous interstitial dermal infiltrates.

**Differential Diagnosis.** Drug reactions and disseminated contact dermatitis are entities in the differential diagnosis of the acute id reaction. The palisading granulomatous reaction may generate a differential diagnosis that includes granuloma annulare and necrobiosis lipoidica.

**Treatment and Prognosis.** The basic therapeutic approach is removal of the causative agent, as by treatment of the stasis dermatitis or dermatophyte infection by appropriate measures. If a drug or organism is causative, then the drug should be removed and the organism treated with appropriate antibiotics. For raging acute reactions, oral steroid therapy is sometimes used; this approach is reserved for the most severe inflammatory and pruritic eruptions. Otherwise, topical measures, including emollients and steroid creams, are usually sufficient for therapy.

## SPONGIOTIC ARTHROPOD BITE REACTION

**Definition.** A localized form of spongiotic delayed hypersensitivity reaction may be elicited by the bite or sting of an arthropod. Often referred to as *arthropod bite reaction*, the term *insect bite reaction* is preferred for spongiotic reactions because bites and stings of many members of the phylum Arthropoda do not produce the histology described (e.g., many spiders and crustaceans). Insect bites do not invariably result in localized spongiotic dermatitis, and although the plethora of localized and systemic manifestations that may result is well-described in the literature (63–74), little is yet known regarding the correlation of insect type with the dermatopathology of the resultant immune response.

**Clinical Features.** Spongiotic insect bite reactions are common causes of spongiotic dermatitis in routine dermatopathology practice. The spongiotic component of the reaction is often appreciated only histologically, and accordingly, the initial gross impression ranges from urticaria to pityriasis lichenoides to erythema nodosum and nodose forms of vasculitis. Occasional reactions produce overt vesicles and even bullae.

The clinical lesion is the result of the direct injection of a foreign protein that produces a predominantly dermal delayed hypersensitivity reaction (fig. 2-16). Pruritic papules and nodules are the rule, and secondary changes due to pruritus and excoriation are frequent. The lesions are often linear or clustered, providing important presumptive information concerning the possibility of insect bite. Overtly vesicular lesions may be confused with primary pruritic vesicular dermatitides, including dermatitis herpetiformis.

**Pathologic Findings.** A characteristic feature of spongiotic insect bite reactions at low-power magnification is the tendency to form a wedge-shaped infiltrate within the superficial and deep dermis (fig. 2-17). This infiltrate is angiocentric at the periphery and coalesces toward the center. The overlying epidermis has a small, centrally located, indented zone lined by necrotic cells and inflammatory debris. This is the punctum through which the proboscis or stinger of the insect has injected the offending protein. The adjacent epidermis shows variable hyperplasia and spongiosis, with occasional frank microvesiculation and eosinophilic spongiosis (such as that seen in allergic contact dermatitis). The vesicle may appear intraepidermal or subepidermal, depending on the level of the most severe spongiosis that produced the fluid-filled cavity (fig. 2-17).

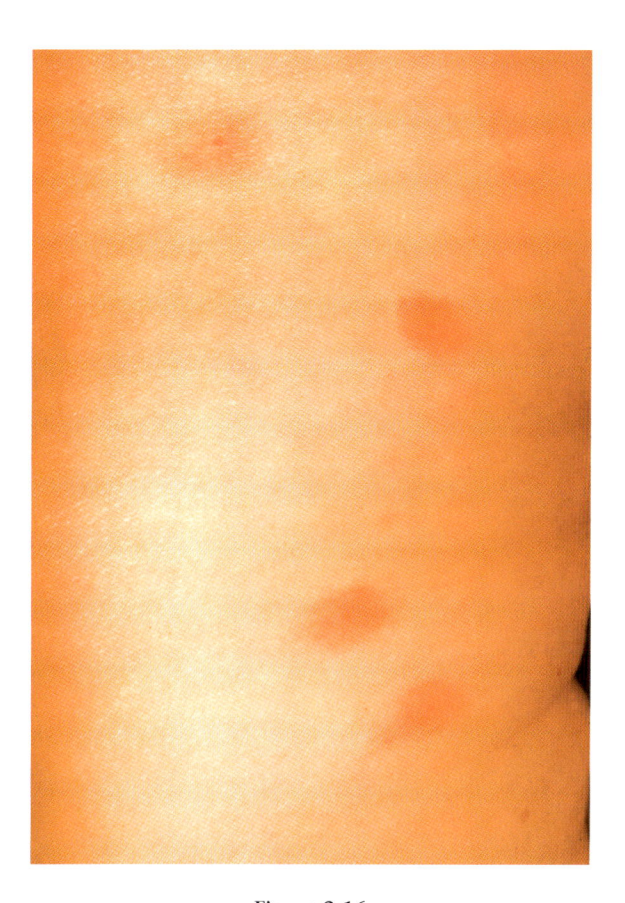

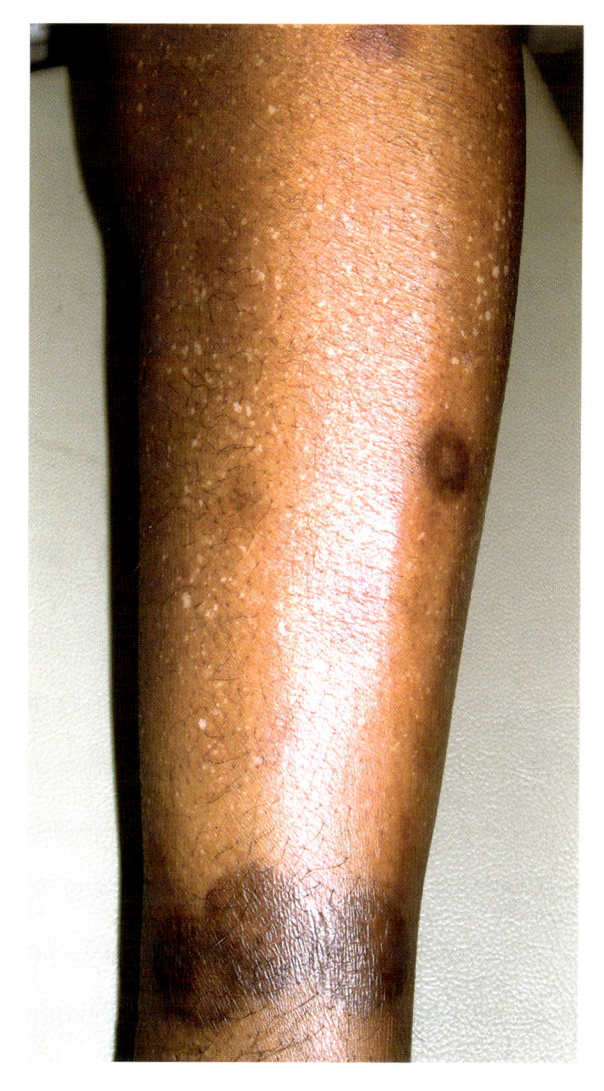

*Inflammatory Disorders with Primary Epidermal Alterations: Spongiotic Dermatitis*

**Figure 2-16**

**SPONGIOTIC INSECT BITE REACTION**

Above: Multiple erythematous plaques are in a vaguely linear distribution, characteristic of insect bites.

Right: In darkly pigmented skin, the epidermal alterations may produce pigment incontinence.

At medium to high magnification, the inflammatory infiltrate is composed of activated lymphocytes, histiocytes, and frequently, large numbers of eosinophils (fig. 2-17D). A helpful diagnostic feature is the tendency for these inflammatory cells to diffusely infiltrate collagen bundles of the intervenular interstitium, often in a fashion similar to the early histiocytic response in granuloma annulare. When degranulating eosinophils are numerous at these sites, they may surround zones of hypereosinophilic, degenerating collagen (i.e., flame figures), similar to that seen in eosinophilic cellulitis (i.e., Well syndrome). In occasional exuberant inflammatory responses to insect bites, focal vasculitis with fibrin thrombus formation or striking dermal mucinosis is detected. Rarely, small granulomatous foci corresponding to birefringent particles of chitinous insect mouth parts are observed. With chronic immunologic stimulation by foreign proteins refractory to proteolytic degradation (i.e., persistent insect bite reaction), benign lymphoid hyperplasia and fibrosis supervene. Such lesions may clinically and histologically mimic lymphoma. Occasionally, in the severe reactions, follicular mucinosis is observed. This change, associated with the reactive atypical lymphocytes of the hypersensitivity reaction, may lead to the mistaken interpretation of the folliculotropic variant of mycosis fungoides.

**Differential Diagnosis.** Spongiotic insect bite reactions must be differentiated from other forms of acute spongiotic dermatitis, including

49

*Inflammatory Disorders of the Skin*

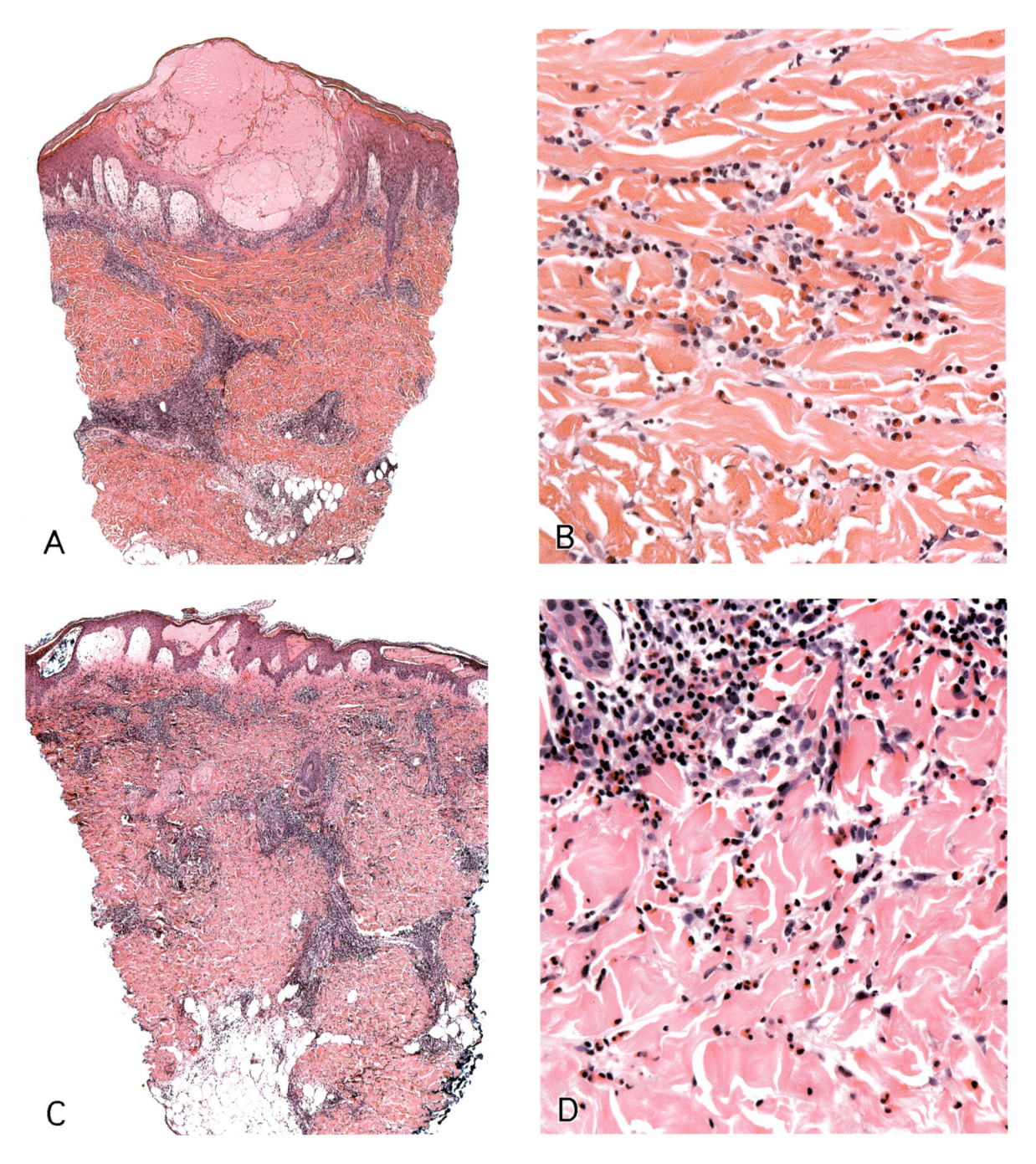

Figure 2-17

**INSECT BITE REACTION**

A: At scanning magnification of vesicular insect bite reaction, the intraepidermal spongiotic vesicle and associated superficial and deep inflammatory infiltrates are readily apparent.

B: At high magnification, the dermal component shows the characteristic interstitial location of responding lymphocytes and eosinophils.

C: Scanning magnification of bullous insect bite reaction shows a forming subepidermal blister as a result of papillary dermal edema and an inflammatory infiltrate that focally extends into subcutaneous fat. The epidermis also shows variable spongiosis.

D: The interstitial component of bullous insect bite reaction shows numerous degranulating eosinophils in a granuloma annulare-like interstitital pattern.

spongiotic drug eruptions, that have a deep perivascular inflammatory component. The finding of interstitial histiocytes and eosinophils, along with the clinical appearance, is often helpful in establishing a diagnosis of insect bite. Although granuloma annulare-like regions, flame figures, and vasculitis may be focally observed in insect bite reactions, the presence of spongiosis separates these situations from true granuloma annulare, eosinophilic cellulitis, and primary vasculitis. Differentiation from pityriasis lichenoides varioliformis acuta is facilitated by the presence of spongiosis as well as the absence of interface changes and scattered keratinocyte necrosis.

**Treatment and Prognosis.** Most spongiotic insect bite reactions are treated symptomatically, using topical measures to decrease pruritus, prevent bacterial superinfection, and diminish inflammation. In cases of severe pruritus, oral antihistamines usually offer relief.

## SPONGIOTIC DRUG ERUPTION

**Definition.** A *spongiotic drug eruption* is one of a variety of cutaneous reaction patterns that may be elicited by ingested or intravenously administered pharmacologic agents (drugs may also provoke urticarial, interface, lichenoid, vasculitic, psoriasiform, and panniculitic eruptions) (75,76).

**Clinical Features.** Any ingested agent capable of being perceived as a foreign antigen in the form of a hapten-protein complex may elicit a spongiotic drug eruption. This form of dermatitis often presents as a diffusely erythematous or morbilliform rash several days after administration of the offending agent (fig. 2-18). In some cases, photoactivation is required to elicit clinical lesions, and this variant is appropriately considered under the category of photoallergic dermatitis. Although spongiotic dermatitis is caused by certain drugs, the gross pathology may be highly variable, ranging from predominantly urticarial to frankly vesicular manifestations. Drug ingestion is associated with a wide range of dermatitides with highly variable histologic patterns, including cytotoxic dermatitis and panniculitis.

**Pathologic Findings.** At scanning magnification, spongiotic drug eruptions appear as superficial and deep perivascular infiltrates associated with variable superficial dermal edema.

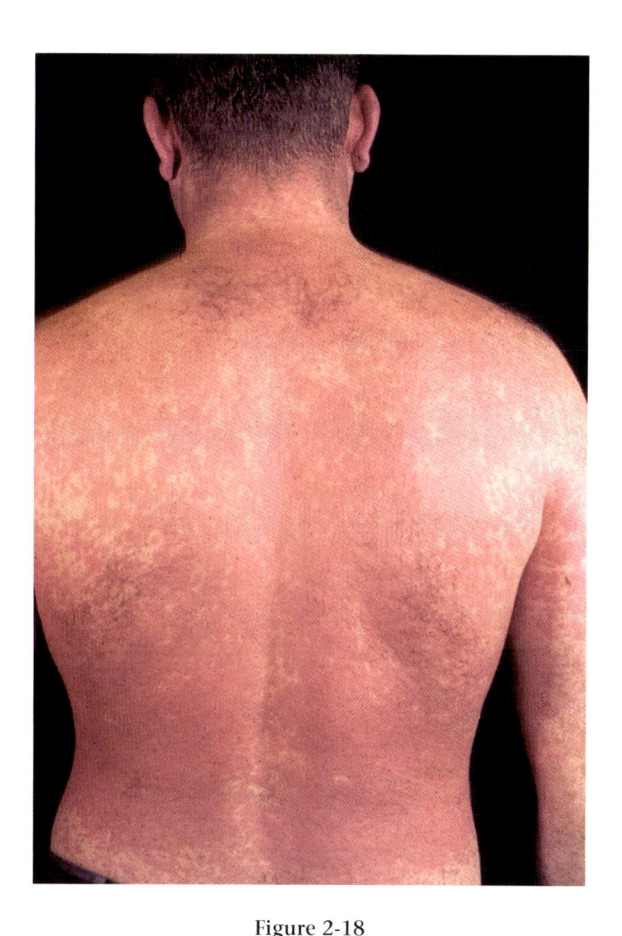

Figure 2-18

**MACULOPAPULAR/SPONGIOTIC DRUG ERUPTION**

Blotchy erythema and coalescing papules affect the skin of the back. This eruption developed as a consequence of antihypertensive therapy.

The spongiosis may be minimal. In contrast to photoallergic dermatitis, the inflammatory components of drug eruptions that develop independent of irradiation generally do not diminish in intensity with extension into the deep dermis (fig. 2-19, top). In fact, vessels of the subcutaneous fat are frequently involved. At higher magnification, eosinophils, in addition to lymphocytes and monocyte-macrophages, are present within the perivascular space (fig. 2-19, bottom). Unlike insect bite reactions, however, eosinophils meandering among bundles of intervascular collagen are not conspicuous. The epidermis may show only minimal areas of spongiosis and lymphoid epidermotropism. The morbilliform drug reaction, on the other hand, is associated with scattered neutrophils and eosinophils in the edematous papillary dermis.

*Inflammatory Disorders of the Skin*

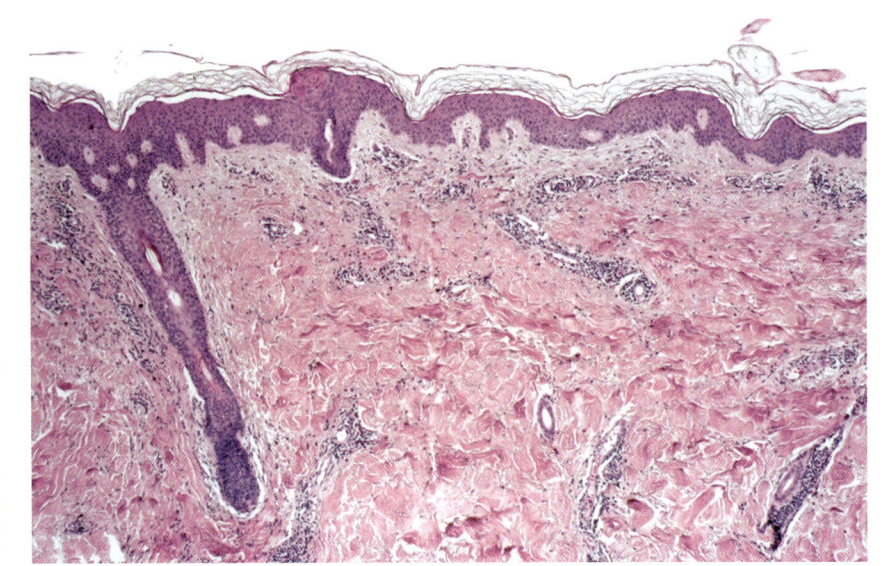

**Figure 2-19**

**SPONGIOTIC DRUG ERUPTION**

Top: At scanning magnification, the epidermal layer shows variable thickening and mild spongiosis. The characteristic inflammatory component is perivascular and involves both the superficial and deep dermis, in contrast to allergic contact dermatitis, where superficial vessels are preferentially involved.

Bottom: Higher magnification of the perivascular inflammatory component shows the activated lymphocytes and numerous eosinophils surrounding the postcapillary venule within the mid-dermis.

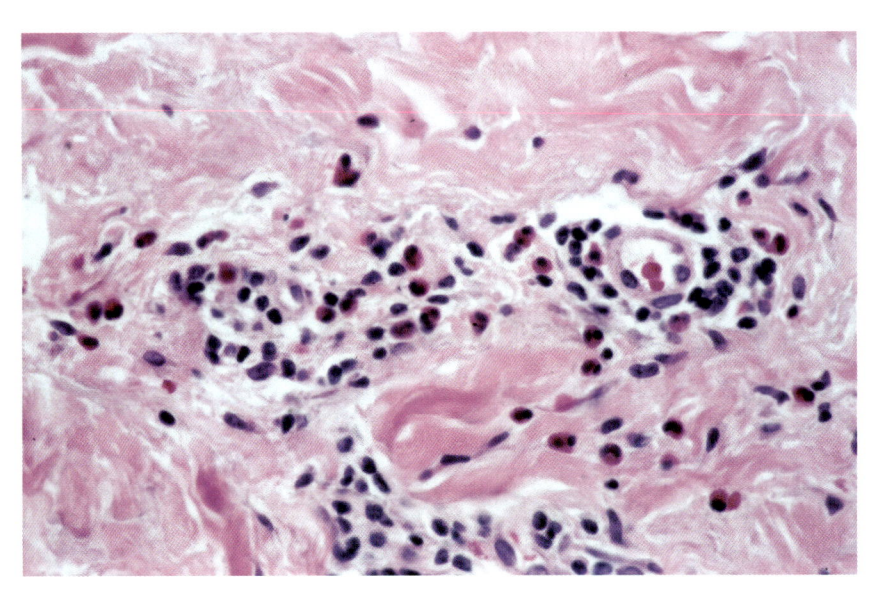

**Differential Diagnosis.** The possibility of spongiotic drug eruption should be considered whenever a biopsy specimen shows a superficial and deep angiocentric inflammatory infiltrate with eosinophils, particularly when spongiosis is minimal. A careful history is required to elicit evidence of a potentially offending agent, particularly because routine and over-the-counter preparations may not be considered and reported by patients (e.g., aspirin, oral contraceptives). The timing of the rash to drug administration is usually several days, about the same time as is required for the development of a delayed-type hypersensitivity reaction after challenge. Although sensitization is required, reactions may develop in some individuals months or even years after repeated use.

**Treatment and Prognosis.** Although systemic and topical immunosuppressive agents may blunt the dermatitis of a spongiotic drug eruption, the treatment of choice is identification and elimination of the offending agent from the therapeutic regimen.

## PHOTOECZEMATOUS ERUPTION

**Definition.** *Photoallergic dermatitis* is one of a number of clinically distinctive photo-induced eruptions, including *polymorphous light eruption and solar urticaria, phototoxic dermatitis*, and *photoallergic spongiotic (photoeczematous) dermatitis*

## Table 2-3
### DIFFERENTIAL DIAGNOSTIC FEATURES OF PHOTO-INDUCED DERMATITIDES

| Type | Clinical | Epidermis | Infiltrate |
|---|---|---|---|
| Photoallergic, spongiotic type | Vesicular, scaling | Spongiosis and rare dyskeratosis | Superficial and mid-dermal; grades off with depth in dermis |
| Phototoxic | Erythema | Extensive dyskeratosis/apoptosis | Minimal; mostly neutrophils |
| Polymorphous light eruption | Papules, plaques | Minimal change; rare dyskeratosis and basal layer vacuolization | Superficial and deep; papillary dermal edema |
| Urticarial | Plaques | Minimal change; rare dyskeratotic cells | Minimal; edema predominates; rare neutrophils, especially within venular lumens |

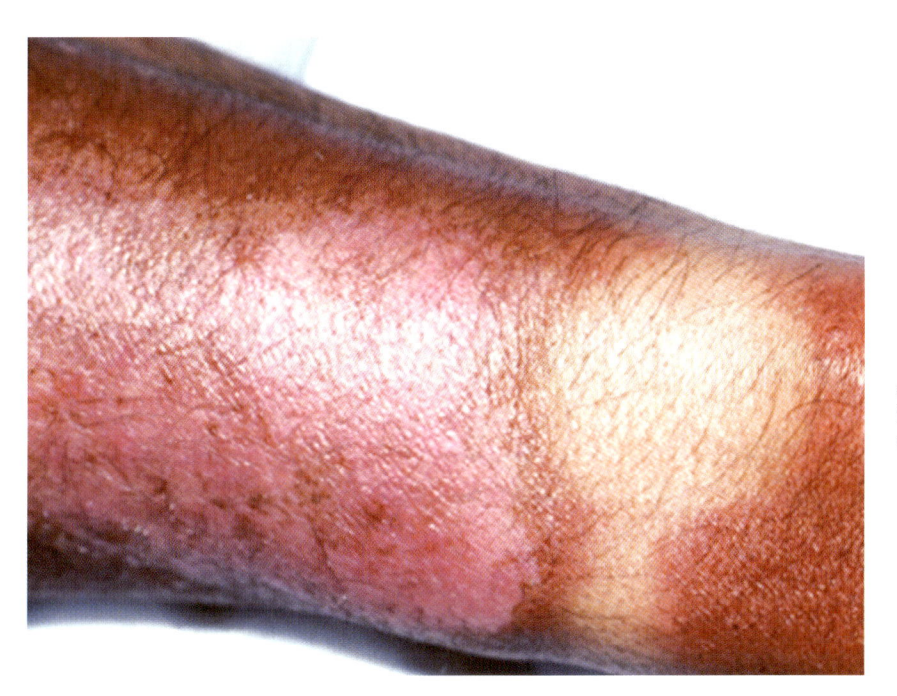

Figure 2-20

**PHOTOECZEMATOUS ERUPTION**

Erythema, fine vesiculation, and early scale formation preferentially involve skin sites exposed to ultraviolet light.

(Table 2-3) (77–82). Whereas polymorphous light eruption and solar urticaria result primarily from angiocentric infiltration with variable papillary dermal edema, and phototoxic dermatitis is a form of exaggerated sunburn, photoallergic spongiotic dermatitis, or *photoeczematous dermatitis*, is akin to a delayed hypersensitivity response with epidermal involvement similar to that seen in allergic contact dermatitis Photoallergic spongiotic dermatitis results when topically applied substances (e.g., perfumes) or ingested agents (e.g., certain drugs) are rendered antigenic in exposed skin by ultraviolet light, evoking an initially vesicular and eventually scaling dermatitis (83–87). Deposition of plant material (e.g., pollen) carried by wind may also elicit this condition upon exposure to sunlight (*phytophotodermatitis*) (88,89).

**Clinical Features.** Photoeczematous eruptions are often suspected by their striking photodistribution (fig. 2-20). Accordingly, exposed skin is preferentially affected, and areas prone to partial photoprotection due to shading (e.g., submental skin) are less severely affected. The clinical differential often involves contact dermatitis, and if vesicles are not prominent, photoexacerbation of lupus erythematosus. The lesions are generally indistinguishable from allergic contact dermatitis, progressing through the evolutionary stages of erythema, vesiculation, and eventual scaling.

**Pathologic Findings.** The epidermal changes of photoeczematous dermatitis are indistinguishable from the various evolutionary phases of other causes of spongiotic dermatitis, except

*Inflammatory Disorders of the Skin*

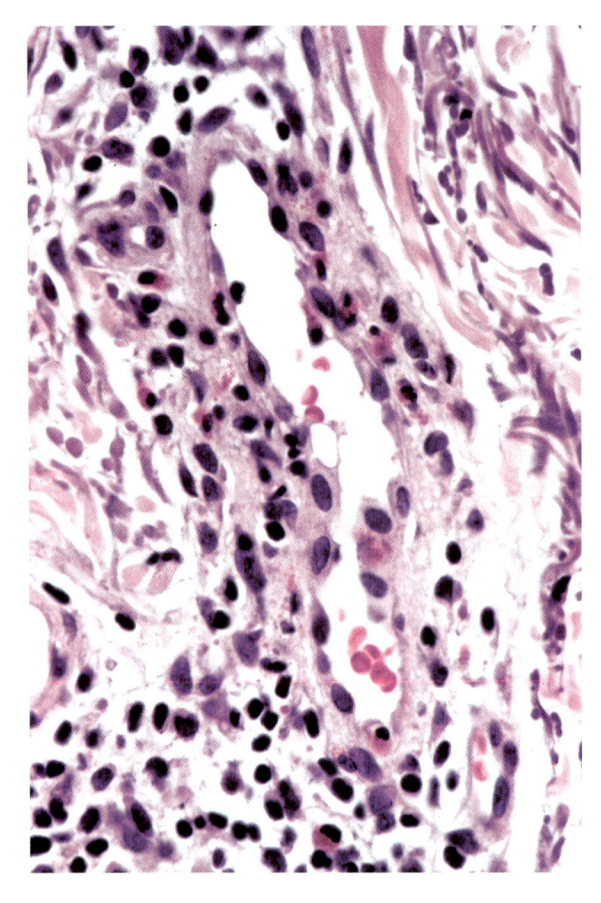

**Figure 2-21**

**DERMAL INFLAMMATORY COMPONENT OF PHOTOECZEMATOUS ERUPTION**

Like the spongiotic drug eruption, there is a perivenular lymphocytic infiltrate containing eosinophils. Foci of hemorrhage are present and marked endothelial activation (bulging) with occasional cytoplasmic vacuolization is typical. The infiltrate tends to dissipate ("grade off") with depth into the dermis.

in most cases, a rare dyskeratotic or apoptotic cell is present in the midspinous layer. At scanning magnification, biopsy of involved skin demonstrates a superficial and at least mid-dermal perivascular inflammatory infiltrate composed predominantly of lymphocytes and occasional eosinophils (fig. 2-21). The infiltrate gradually diminishes in intensity with depth (i.e., "grades off"), a helpful diagnostic feature. Another clue to the diagnosis is the presence of prominent endothelial cells with vacuolated cytoplasm lining involved dermal venules. The overlying epidermal layer shows spongiosis and variable lymphoid epidermotropism.

The histologic findings in photoallergic spongiotic dermatitis are not entirely specific, and validation by appropriate clinical history is required in the majority of cases to establish an accurate diagnosis. Photo patch testing helps when the gross and microscopic pathology fail to reveal definitive alterations.

**Differential Diagnosis.** The differential diagnosis includes other types of spongiotic dermatitis that show a deep as well as superficial perivascular dermal inflammatory component. This includes spongiotic drug eruption and spongiotic insect bite reaction. The latter is distinguishable by a focal interstitial component involving histiocytes and eosinophils. The former usually exhibits diffuse involvement of venules, without the tapering effect of the deeper infiltrate characteristic of light eruptions.

**Treatment and Prognosis.** The treatment is generally directed at identifying the offending antigen that requires photoactivation in order to exert its proinflammatory effect. Avoidance of sun exposure and potent topical blocking agents are also employed.

## SEBORRHEIC DERMATITIS

**Definition.** *Seborrheic dermatitis* is a common cutaneous inflammatory reaction that occurs predominantly in the areas of sebaceous glands. Response to therapy is difficult to achieve in some cases and lesions can be longstanding. In children, a variant is known as "cradle cap."

**Clinical Features.** Seborrheic dermatitis can begin in the first few weeks of life, but most cases occur after age 20 and into mid-late life. The lesions appear gradually, with areas of slight erythema and fine scaling, especially on the scalp, eyebrows, face, anterior chest, and body folds (90,91). As the lesions progress, they tend to coalesce, but can be well demarcated, occurring as a patch or plaque (fig. 2-22). The changes on the scalp are mainly those of scaling, so called "dandruff." On the trunk, the lesions are irregularly shaped, erythematous, and annular to oval.

**Pathologic Findings.** Seborrheic dermatitis is extraordinarily subtle histologically, and unless accompanied by a potentially supportive description of the gross pathology and associated clinical parameters, lesions are commonly assigned the vague and unhelpful diagnosis of "chronic dermatitis." The initial lesion shows a sparse, perivascular, lymphoid infiltrate with a few scattered neutrophils in the dermis but also in the epidermis, with associated slight spongiosis. As the lesions develop, seborrheic dermatitis appears similar to subacute allergic contact dermatitis at low-power magnification, with variable, irregular epidermal hyperplasia overlying a superficial perivascular inflammatory infiltrate (fig. 2-23, top). At high magnification, this infiltrate is typically composed of both mononuclear cells and small numbers of neutrophils. Neutrophils may also be detected within a focally parakeratotic stratum corneum as well as within the dermis (fig. 2-23, bottom). Small aggregates of neutrophils, as well as mounds of parakeratosis, appear at the shoulder of the hair follicle (fig. 2-24). The spongiosis is generally mild, and intraepidermal microvesicles seldom occur. In the lupus-like seborrheic dermatitis that may accompany acquired immunodeficiency syndrome (AIDS), plasma cells and mild basal cell layer vacuolization may be present. Occasionally, the chronic plaques of seborrheic dermatitis show significant retiform epidermal hyperplasia, with significant histologic similarity to lesions of psoriasis (fig. 2-23, top). Such pathology often correlates with an ambiguous clinical picture, accounting for the descriptive term "sebopsoriasis."

**Differential Diagnosis.** Contact dermatitis, atopic dermatitis, psoriasis, and other eczematous processes are entities in the differential diagnosis. Careful assessment for the presence of scattered neutrophils in the dermis and especially adjacent to follicles, with small aggregates on the follicle shoulder, assist in the diagnosis of seborrheic dermatitis. Gram stains are negative for bacteria. There exist chronic, plaque-like lesions on the scalp that are difficult clinically and histologically to distinguish from psoriasis. However, prominent retiform hyperplasia, prominent and dilated capillaries within the papillary dermis, and a marked loss of the granular cell layer favor the diagnosis of psoriasis.

**Treatment and Prognosis.** Shampoo often diminishes the scalp symptoms; nontreated areas of the trunk and face sometimes also respond. Low-potency topical corticosteroid application is often adequate for milder cases; for more severe cases, tar-containing substances, higher strength steroid cream, ketoconazole cream or shampoo, and tar shampoo have proven effective in controlling the lesions (91).

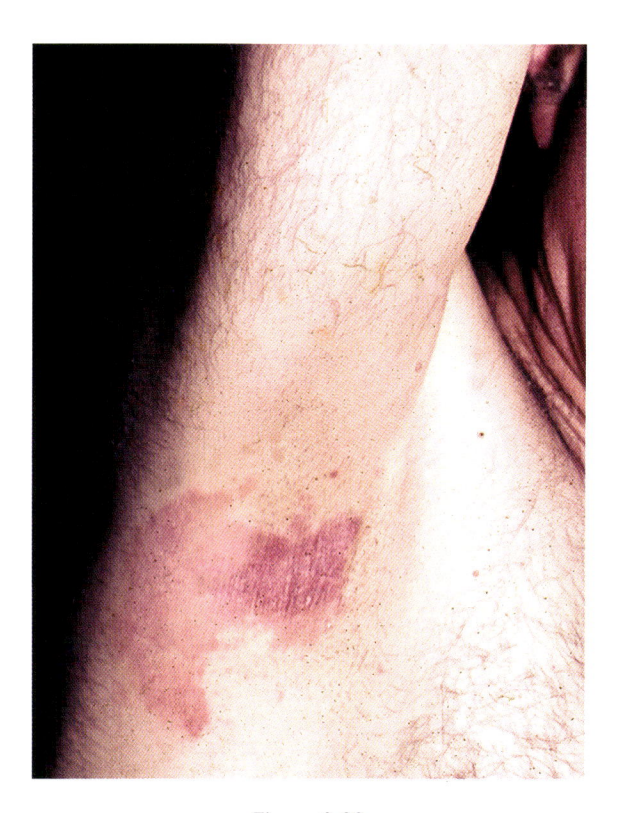

Figure 2-22

**ACTIVE SEBORRHEIC DERMATITIS**

Erythema and scaling involve the facial skin as well as the skin of the chest and axilla (depicted here).

## ERYTHEMA ANNULARE CENTRIFUGUM

**Definition.** *Erythema annulare centrifugum* (EAC) is an eruption of papules, in an annular or arciform array, that slowly spreads in centrifugal fashion. A characteristic light scale is associated with the advancing edge. EAC occurs at any age. Along with erythema chronicum migrans and erythema gyratum repens, it is often referred to as a form of deep figurate or gyrate erythema, although more superficial variants with spongiotic changes may occur, as discussed here. Most cases of EAC are idiopathic, although some are associated with dermatophyte infection (usually on the soles), food allergens, or drugs. Viral infections have been described as causative. Occasionally, the eruption is associated with a malignant neoplasm, with disappearance of the lesion after extirpation of the neoplasm and

*Inflammatory Disorders of the Skin*

**Figure 2-23**

**ACTIVE SEBORRHEIC DERMATITIS WITH SPONGIOTIC COMPONENT**

Top: In addition to irregular acanthosis and a superficial perivascular inflammatory infiltrate, there is parakeratotic scale containing inflammatory cells and multiple foci of intraepidermal spongiosis.

Bottom: At higher magnification, marked edema within the superficial dermis and a mixed inflammatory infiltrate containing occasional neutrophils are seen. The epidermis shows characteristic widening of the intercellular spaces.

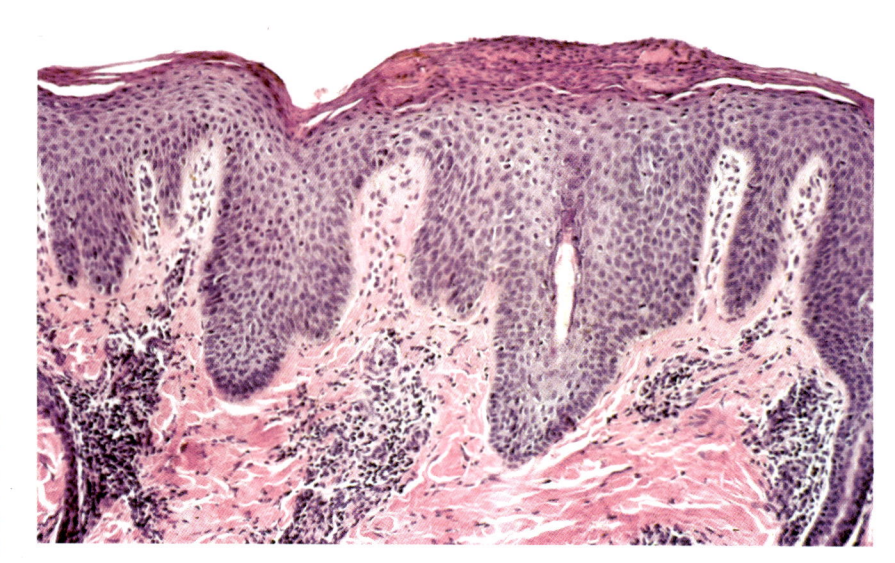

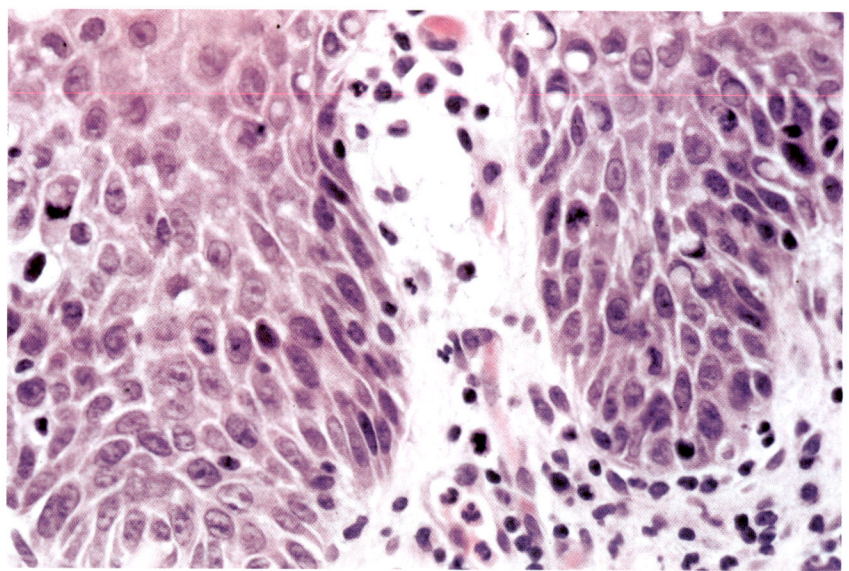

recurrence of the lesion with tumor recidivism. The histologic findings suggest that the process is a predominantly dermal delayed hypersensitivity reaction.

**Clinical Features.** EAC first appears as a reddish urticarial patch or plaque composed of papules (fig. 2-25). The papules slowly extend to form annular or arcuate lesions, which continue migrating a few millimeters each day. An overall width of several centimeters is reached before the lesion ceases to spread. Behind the advancing edge is a scale, termed a "trailing scale." The lesions are often pruritic. The deep variant shows similar evolution, but with a more striking raised border, a thickened scale, and without the symptoms of itching.

**Pathologic Findings.** Scanning magnification reveals a well-defined, perivascular inflammatory infiltrate composed of lymphocytes and occasional rare eosinophils tightly clustered about superficial and mid-dermal vessels (fig. 2-26). Often, the apposition of inflammatory cells to affected vessels is so discrete that the vascular channels so outlined resemble Chinese figure writing, a finding of assistance in recalling the pattern of "figurate erythema." At higher magnification, the tight perivascular cuff of lymphocytes, often referred to as a "coat-sleeve

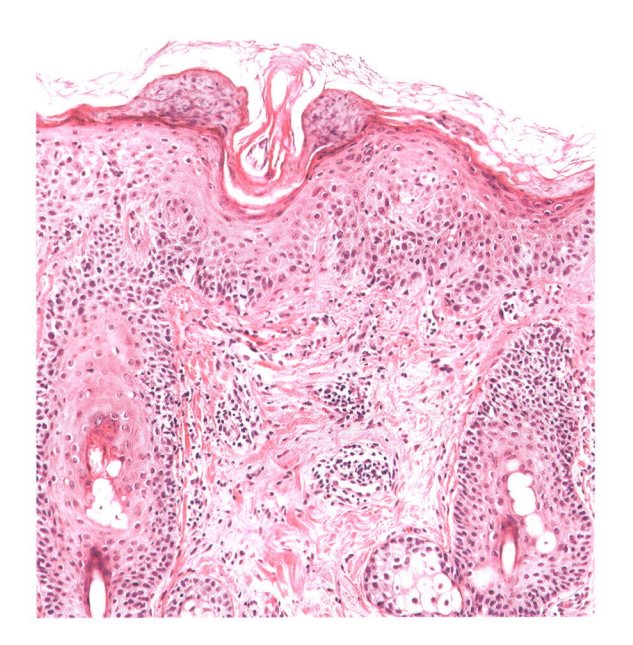

*Inflammatory Disorders with Primary Epidermal Alterations: Spongiotic Dermatitis*

Figure 2-24
**SEBORRHEIC DERMATITIS**
Shoulders of parakeratotic scale associated with a follicular infundibulum are associated with subacute spongiotic changes.

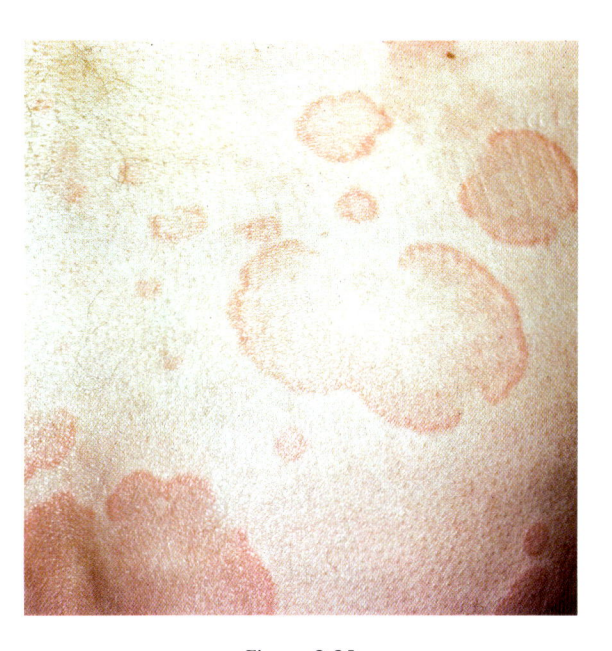

Figure 2-25
**ERYTHEMA ANNULARE CENTRIFUGUM**
There are multiple erythematous polycyclic plaques. Adherent trailing scale is characteristically present at the borders of these annular erythematous lesions.

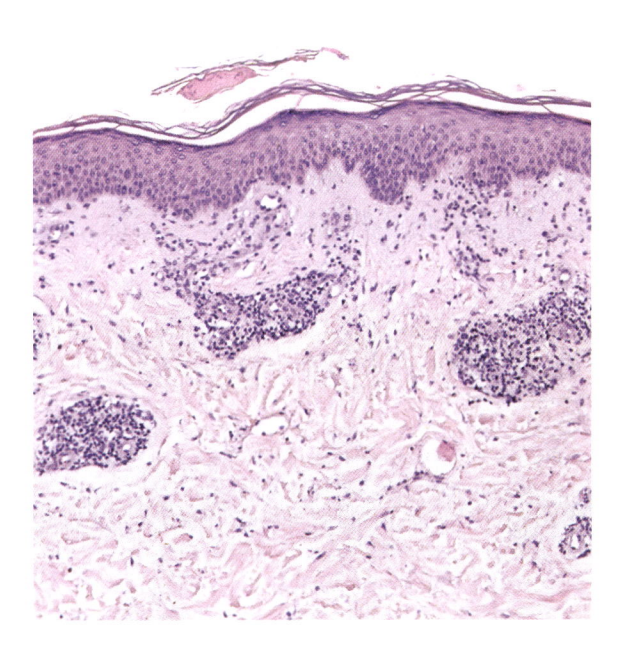

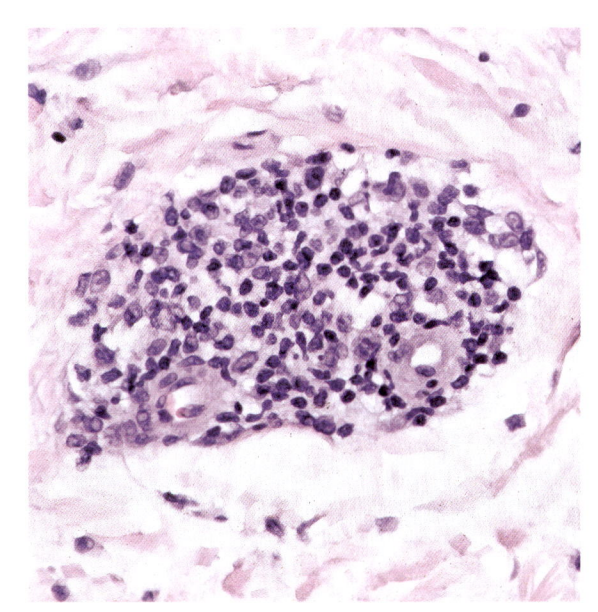

Figure 2-26
**ERYTHEMA ANNULARE CENTRIFUGUM**
Left: The epidermis shows foci of compact hyperorthokeratotic as well parakeratotic scale formation. The epidermis is irregularly thickened and mildly spongiotic. The characteristic finding, however, is the intensely angiocentric perivascular lymphoid inflammatory infiltrate within the underlying dermis, producing a typical "coat-sleeve" pattern.
Right At higher magnification, the tightly compacted cuff-like pattern of lymphoid aggregation involves a postcapillary venule within the superficial dermis.

*Inflammatory Disorders of the Skin*

**Figure 2-27**

**EPIDERMAL CHANGES IN ERYTHEMA ANNULARE CENTRIFUGUM**

The abnormal scale formation, irregular acanthosis, and foci of spongiosis are changes virtually indistinguishable from other forms of subacute spongiotic dermatitis.

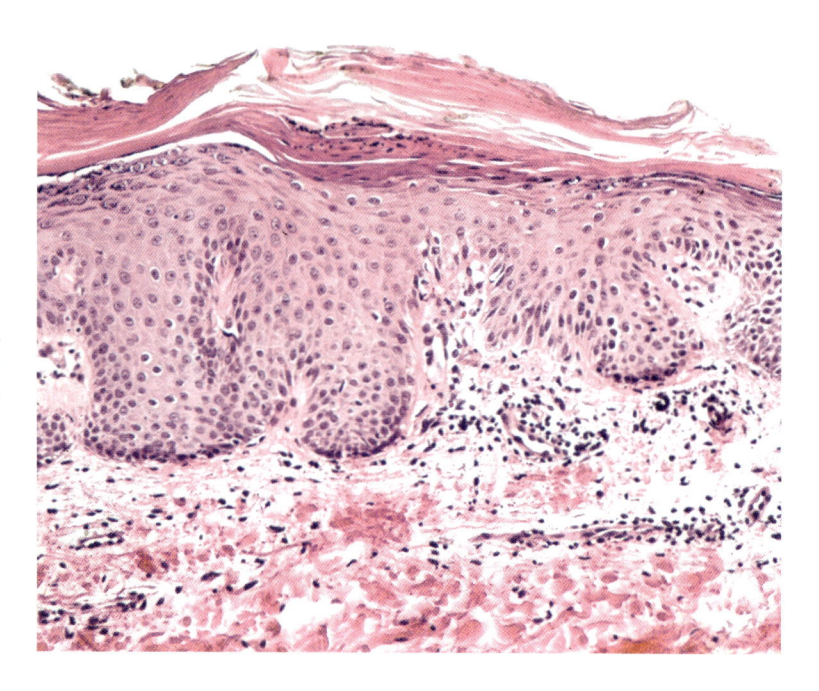

infiltrate," is better appreciated. The overlying epidermis may be unaffected, although if the region of the clinical lesion showing the trailing scale is biopsied, focal parakeratosis and mild epidermal hyperplasia and spongiosis are usually observed (fig. 2-27). As described above, a deeper form of the lesion occurs which is associated with a prominent superficial and deep lymphoid infiltrate with prominent perivascular cuffing. In the authors' experience, however, EAC frequently lacks the classic "coat-sleeve" effect. Clinical correlation is therefore of importance in evaluating such less characteristic histologic presentations.

**Differential Diagnosis.** EAC must be differentiated from other causes of type IV hypersensitivity reactions, including those directly the result of overlying dermatophytosis, contact dermatitis, and drugs. The PAS stain is often performed, particularly because tinea corporis is a clinical possibility. The characteristic coat-sleeve nature of the inflammatory infiltrate, although not entirely specific and not consistently present, is the most helpful histologic sign in determining the correct diagnosis. The histologic findings may be identical to those of the rare condition, erythema gyratum repens, highlighting the importance of accurate correlative clinical information. Erythema gyratum repens, in contrast to EAC, is characterized by annular plaques distributed widely and forming concentric rings with a "wood-grain" pattern. This disorder affects middle-aged to elderly individuals, and is highly associated with internal malignancy.

**Treatment and Prognosis.** The treatment depends upon the cause, if one can be identified. In idiopathic lesions, topical steroids or systemic steroids may be helpful. Recurrence is common. Topical and systemic antipruritic agents are useful for pruritic lesions. The lesions commonly resolve after appropriate treatment (92).

## ECZEMATOUS STASIS DERMATITIS

**Definition.** *Stasis dermatitis* is characterized by a variety of associated epidermal alterations, ranging from atrophy to acanthosis, the latter often having a variable degree of spongiosis. This common condition is a frequent mimic of primary forms of spongiotic dermatitis.

**Clinical Features.** Lesions most often involve leg skin, especially the lower legs and ankles. They generally present as variably erythematous, scaling, and hyperpigmented plaques (fig. 2-28). The lesions are frequently biopsied, with differential clinical diagnoses that encompass melanocytic proliferative processes, pigmentary purpura, postinflammatory hyperpigmentation, poikiloderma, and superficial pigmented dysplasia or neoplasia (e.g., pigmented actinic keratosis, multicentric pigmented basal cell carcinoma). Localized stasis dermatitis is a frequent cause of confusion with a primary eczematous (spongiotic) or neoplastic process. In addition to variable epidermal atrophy and thickening, with or without evidence of vesicles or weeping, dermal vascular proliferation and dermal edema and fibrosis eventually occur. Some chronic lesions are woody hard and deeply pigmented, the latter due to hemosiderin deposition in the tissue. This pigment accounts in large part for the zones of tan-brown coloration appreciated clinically and grossly (93).

**Pathologic Findings.** Biopsy specimens of localized stasis dermatitis lesions reveal hemosiderin-laden macrophages (i.e., siderophages) about superficial dermal vessels and sometimes diffusely within the papillary dermis. The following associated features are also generally present in varying degrees: epidermal alterations, consisting of hyperkeratosis with hyperplasia and spongiosis; superficial dermal vascular ectasia and proliferation; superficial dermal edema; and mild dermal fibroplasia (fig. 2-29). As the lesions become more chronic, dermal fibrosis increases, and may extend into the deep dermis

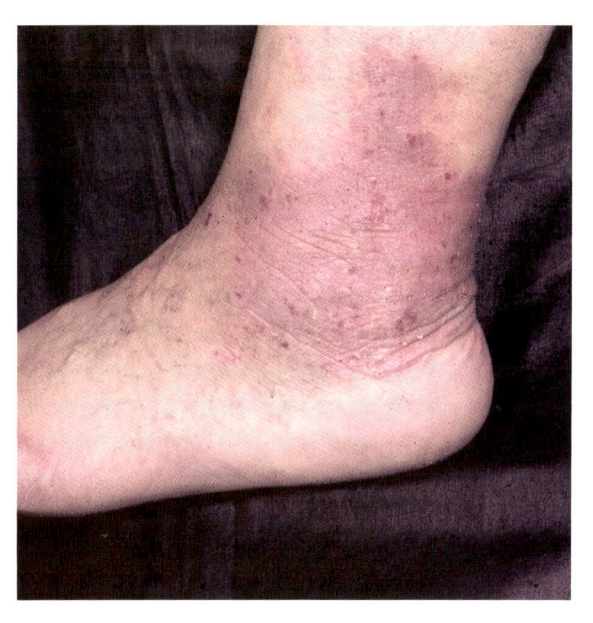

Figure 2-28
SPONGIOTIC STASIS DERMATITIS
The erythematous scaling plaque involves the skin of the distal extremity in this patient with chronic stasis change.

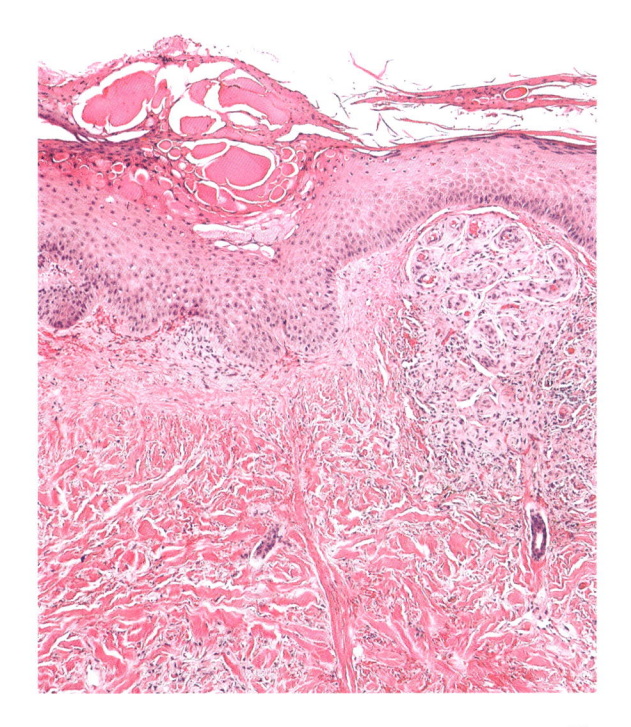

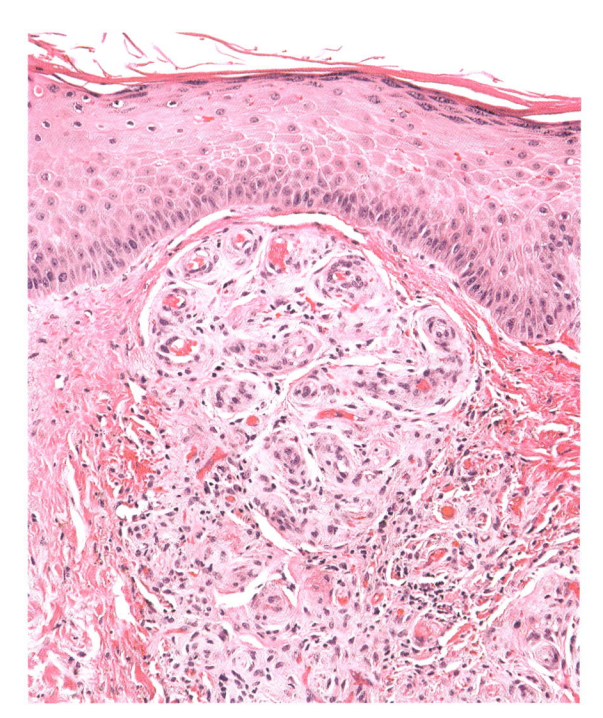

Figure 2-29
SPONGIOTIC STASIS DERMATITIS
Left: Intraepidermal vesicles are associated with characteristic vascular proliferative changes.
Right: Higher magnification shows mild diffuse spongiosis associated with characteristic vascular proliferative changes involving the superficial capillary loop.

and subcutis in severe cases. Hemosiderin accumulates, predominantly in macrophages, but is also scattered free throughout the dermis. Stasis dermatitis differs from the other common cause of hemosiderin deposition within the superficial dermis, pigmentary purpura, in that the latter has a pericapillary and often band-like lymphocytic infiltrate within dermal papillae and lacks the aforementioned findings associated with chronic stasis. Stasis dermatitis differs from allergic spongiotic dermatitis by lacking the characteristic superficial lymphocytic infiltrate often containing eosinophils and the associated formation of Langerhans cell microgranulomas in the epidermis.

**Differential Diagnosis.** The differential diagnosis includes spongiotic dermatitis with chronic excoriation, in which repeated papillary dermal hemorrhage provoked by trauma may mimic the hemosiderin deposition associated with underlying stasis. The characteristic vascular alterations of stasis dermatitis are not observed in most forms of primary spongiotic dermatitis. One complicating factor, however, is that mild stasis-like superficial vascular proliferations may occur secondarily in any chronic inflammatory lesion on the lower extremity.

**Treatment and Prognosis.** Therapy includes topical agents to minimize inflammation and scaling, as well as approaches to enhance circulation and tissue oxygenation. The wearing of pressure stockings is critical because it prevents the dilation of veins in the already compromised vasculature that with chronicity becomes surrounded by fibrosis. The persistent dilation leads to extravasation of red blood cells and release of fluid, resulting in ever-increasing edema.

## PARAPSORIASIS, INCLUDING SMALL PLAQUE AND SUPERFICIAL DIGITATE DERMATOSIS TYPES

**Definition.** *Parapsoriasis* takes different forms, one of which is an acute scaly eruption that has been designated *small plaque parapsoriasis* (SPP); its variant is *superficial digitate dermatosis*. *Guttate parapsoriasis*, a distinct, persistent, nonpruritic, recalcitrant dermatitis that is generally distributed over the trunk and proximal extremities as small, drop-like, pink-tan plaques covered by scant adherent scale, is considered in the section dealing with pityriasis lichenoides chronica. SPP, including its variant form, benign superficial digitate dermatosis, includes small oval lesions, with a fine scale occurring predominantly on the trunk and upper portion of the extremities. SPP and pityriasis rosea (PR) are differentiated primarily by their clinical features: both are low-grade subacute spongiotic dermatitides that may resemble each microscopically.

**Clinical Features.** SPP is an eruption, predominantly on the trunk, that is scaly and variably pruritic (fig. 2-30). The lesions are generally 1 to 2 cm in diameter, and often oval. There is scant superficial scale and lesions may resemble PR. This type of parapsoriasis also occurs in a digitate form, in which the lesions extend onto the trunk and sometimes the abdomen and flank. Such lesions often abut one another in parallel finger-like array, and thus have been given the name "digitate." Lesions are chronic, but do not progress to the atrophic form of large-plaque parapsoriasis or to mycosis fungoides. Like psoriasis, parapsoriasis may occur as small guttate plaques, indistinguishable from PR, that have a chronic course and may be recalcitrant to treatment. The small plaque variant of parapsoriasis is usually diagnosed when an episode of presumed PR becomes chronic and persistent without response to therapy. SPP is distinct from patch- and early plaque-stage cutaneous T-cell lymphoma, which regrettably has been referred to as parapsoriasis of the large plaque type (i.e., parapsoriasis en plaques).

**Pathologic Findings.** At scanning magnification, SPP can appear identical to PR, demonstrating mild epidermal hyperplasia and spongiosis accompanied by a superficial perivascular lymphocytic infiltrate (fig. 2-31). Upon closer inspection, foci of mound-like parakeratotic scale in a lenticular pattern are observed. In contrast to PR, the scale of guttate parapsoriasis maintains its lenticular appearance and either adheres to the epidermal surface or lifts off evenly as a single entity without the angulation characteristic of PR. PSS seldom shows prominent inflammation and does not exhibit superficial dermal hemorrhage, as may be encountered in PR. In examples of PR in which hemorrhage cannot be detected, however, biopsy specimens may closely resemble those of SPP. Overall, SPP shows a characteristic scale with rather prominent retiform hyperplasia, with a perivascular

*Inflammatory Disorders with Primary Epidermal Alterations: Spongiotic Dermatitis*

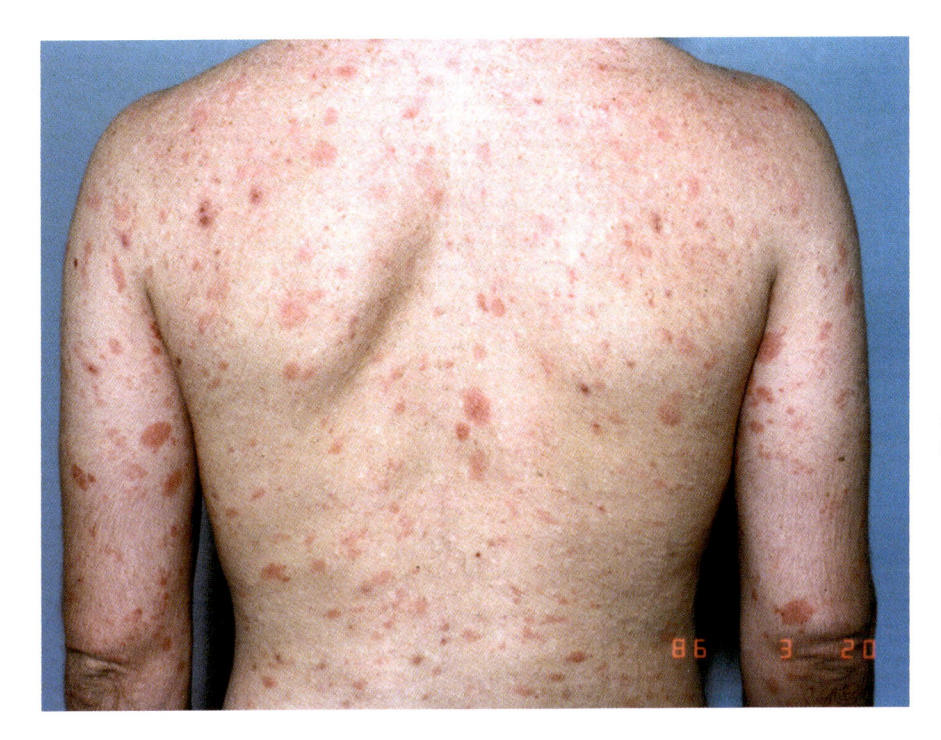

Figure 2-30

**SMALL PLAQUE PARAPSORIASIS**

Multiple erythematous scaling plaques involve the skin of the back.

Figure 2-31

**SMALL PLAQUE PARAPSORIASIS**

The changes are of a subacute low-grade spongiotic dermatitis with an associated superficial perivascular lymphocytic infiltrate. Even at this magnification, the characteristic scale pattern is evident. This pattern consists of multiple discrete mounds of parakeratotic scale. Note the mound at the far right that is evenly lifting off from the underlying epidermis.

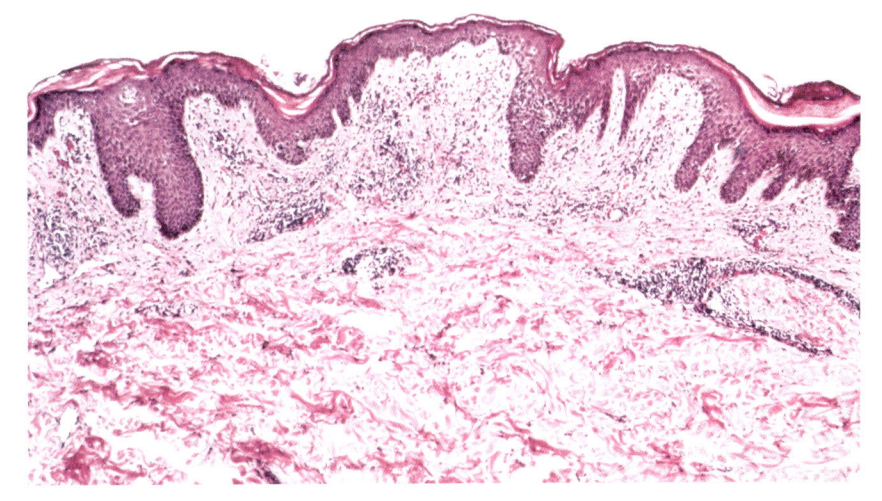

infiltrate of lymphoid cells. There may be delicate papillary dermal fibrosis scattered below the epidermal hyperplasia.

**Differential Diagnosis.** The primary differential diagnostic considerations are PR, mild nummular eczema (multifocal small plaques of spongiotic dermatitis), secondary syphilis, and tinea corporis. Ultimately, the diagnosis is a clinicopathologic one, where the typical, albeit not entirely specific and subtle, histopathology matches a clinical course involving indolent and chronic guttate patches and plaques that prove to be recalcitrant to therapy. The characteristic scale pattern of SPP and PR is frequently only focally present, and multiple levels may be required in order to segregate low-grade spongiotic dermatitis into these categories. In contrast to secondary syphilis, SPP and PR virtually never demonstrate plasma cells in their infiltrates, and affected vessels show only moderate endothelial prominence. Examples of secondary syphilis without plasma cells closely mimic SPP and PR both clinically and histologically, although such lesions generally show some degree of basal cell layer vacuolization and deeper perivascular involvement. Serologic exclusion of secondary

## Inflammatory Disorders of the Skin

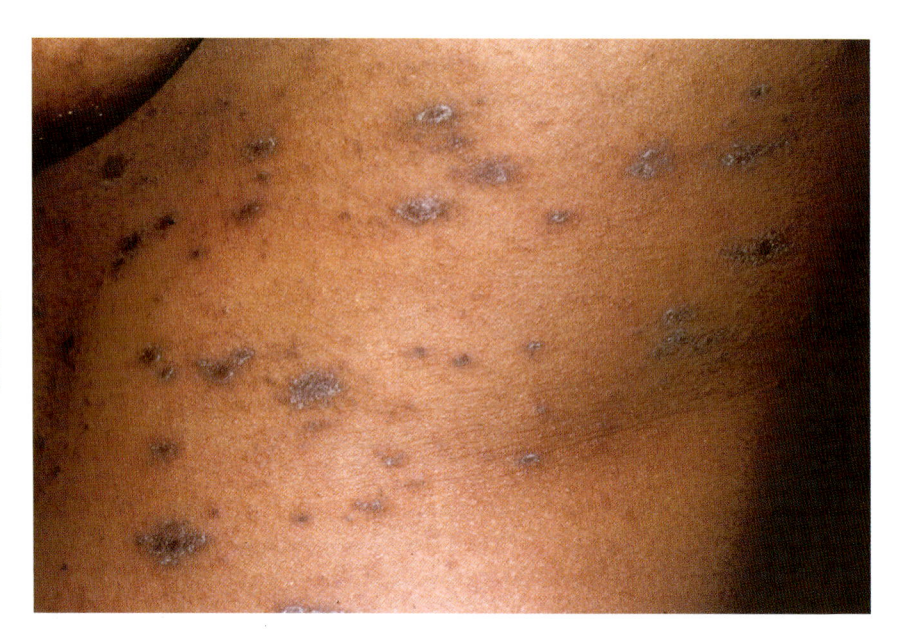

**Figure 2-32**

**PITYRIASIS ROSEA**

In this darkly pigmented individual, the multiple ovoid plaques are hyperpigmented, and have a finely adherent surface scale.

syphilis is recommended when this entity is a clinical diagnostic possibility, even when the corresponding histopathology suggests guttate SPP or PR (94).

**Treatment and Prognosis.** The treatment of SPP and its variant, superficial digitate dermatosis, involves topical steroid creams, which are helpful in some patients. Other patients respond to ultraviolet light, be it natural sunlight or broadband ultraviolet B, or even narrow band ultraviolet B and PUVA.

### PITYRIASIS ROSEA

**Definition.** *Pityriasis rosea* (PR) is a common, self-limited, sometimes epidemic, benign disorder of the skin that is preceded at times by a prodrome. The eruption of scaly oval papules on the trunk in a "fir or Christmas tree" distribution is characteristic and remission is spontaneous. The cause is unknown, although a viral etiology has been conjectured. In one study, results failed to support a causal relationship between PR and Epstein-Barr virus (EBV) or cytomegalovirus (CMV), but indicated a possible role for human herpesvirus (HHV)-6 and especially HHV-7 in a group of Turkish patients, concluding, however, that other etiologic factors may exist (95).

**Clinical Features.** PR is a common dermatitis that is mimicked clinically by secondary syphilis, guttate SPP, and nummular eczema; consequently, biopsies are frequently performed. The disorder presents with a "herald patch," a 2- to 10-cm, usually oval plaque, that is salmon to dusky pink-red in color, with a delicate scale scattered over the surface (fig. 2-32). In 7 to 10 days, multiple lesions appear, usually on the trunk and proximal extremities, but occasionally generalized. The individual lesion is oval, 1- to 2-cm, salmon colored in most Caucasians, and deeply pigmented in more heavily melanized skin. A delicate scale ("cigarette paper-like" scale) forms a collarette around the periphery of the lesion. Lesions vary in number from a few to sometimes hundreds. Typically, patches and plaques are arranged in a fir tree-like pattern on trunk skin, although some individuals present with a more acral distribution that often also involves the groin and buttocks, "inverted PR." Whereas PR resolves within months, SPP is refractory to treatment and may persist for years.

A papular variant is more common in childhood, in pregnant women, and in African Americans. An inflammatory form exhibits edematous, extremely pruritic, sometimes vesicular lesions, always surrounded by the collarettes of scale that allows for the clinical diagnosis. Some patients with papular PR are asymptomatic, but most lesions are very pruritic, with patients experiencing considerable discomfort.

**Pathologic Findings.** PR is a mild, subacute spongiotic dermatitis. In contrast to secondary syphilis, plasma cells are not observed, and en-

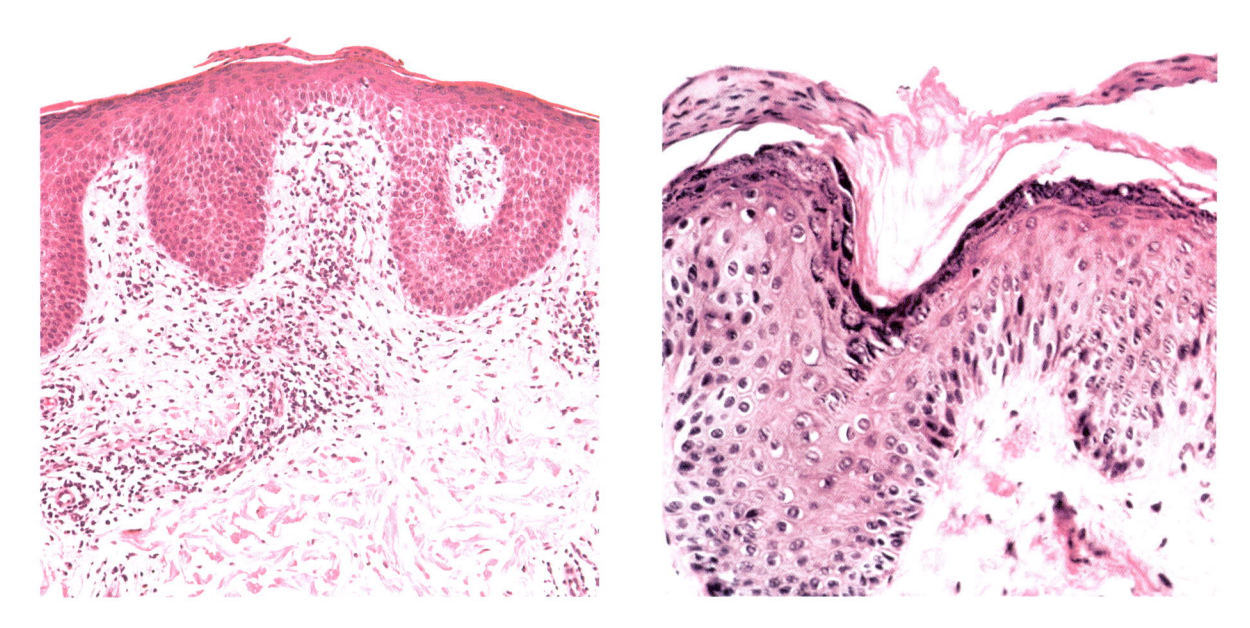

**Figure 2-33**

**PITYRIASIS ROSEA**

Left: Foci of mound-like parakeratosis are associated with a mildly spongiotic epidermis.

Right: At higher magnification, low-grade subacute spongiotic dermatitis is seen. The characteristic scale pattern consists of discrete mounds of parakeratosis. Note the mound at the far right lifting off at an angle from the underlying epidermis. Often such lesions also show foci of papillary dermal hemorrhage.

dothelial cells, although somewhat activated, seldom are so enlarged as to obstruct lumens. A characteristic finding is the presence of small foci of tightly compacted, parakeratotic scale forming mound-like configurations (fig. 2-33). Frequently, the affected scale appears to be desquamating from the underlying epidermis, and as it lifts off the surface it stays attached at one end, with a resultant angulated appearance. This scale pattern is unusual in nummular dermatitis and seborrheic dermatitis. A differential feature is the occasional presence of small foci of papillary dermal hemorrhage in PR. In contrast to early pityriasis lichenoides et varioliformis acuta, the extravasation does not extend into the epidermis but stops abruptly at the basement membrane zone. The herald patch has certain distinct histologic features. It shows a more prominent diffuse retiform epidermal hyperplasia but is surmounted by multiple typical PR-like scales. Also, there is multifocal extravasation of red blood cells. The perivascular inflammatory infiltrate is more extensive and shows intermittent exocytosis of lymphocytes, sometimes with patterned regularity, alternating with areas of extravasation.

**Differential Diagnosis.** The herald patch is often considered to be a tinea infection or nummular eczema, before the eruptive character of the disorder appears. Examination of the scrapings of the lesion with a potassium hydroxate (KOH) stain excludes tinea. The clinical course and the multiple scales and patterned exocytosis help exclude nummular eczema. Secondary syphilis must always be considered as a possibility. Involvement of the palms and soles is characteristic in the secondary manifestation of lues, and allows for diagnosis. It is advisable that any patients with PR have a serologic test for syphilis.

Lesions of PR that persist for more than 6 months are unusual and are regarded as a subset or variant of parapsoriasis, the so-called small plaque or benign superficial digitate type. A biopsy may permit differentiation. Occasionally, lesions of psoriasis and nummular eczema resemble PR, but biopsy often assists in this differential.

**Treatment and Prognosis.** Topical steroids may be helpful in resolving the lesions. The severe pruritus may respond to oral antihistamines, but at times, a brief course of oral prednisone is necessary. Often, erythemogenic doses

*Inflammatory Disorders of the Skin*

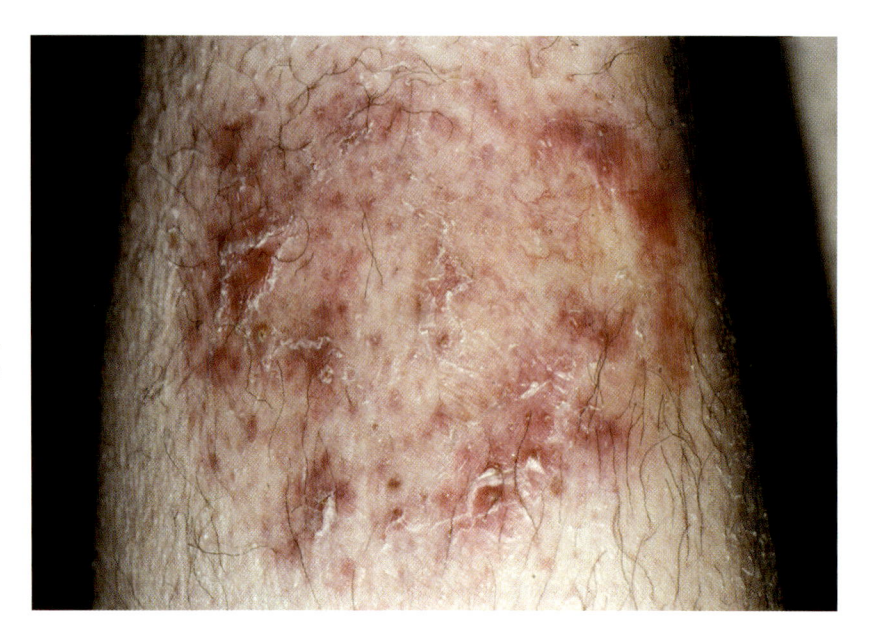

**Figure 2-34**

**SPONGIOTIC DERMATOPHYTE INFECTION**

The vaguely annular erythematous and scaling plaque involves extremity skin.

of ultraviolet B light for 5 days or direct sunlight helps to both relieve symptoms and resolve the lesions. A role for antibiotic therapy, particularly erythromycin, has been postulated.

## DERMATOPHYTOSIS

**Definition.** *Dermatophytosis* is a superficial fungal infection that mimics both the gross and histologic pathology of noninfectious spongiotic dermatitis. It should be suspected whenever a biopsy specimen of low-grade subacute dermatitis shows mild, nonspecific spongiotic changes in the absence of an obvious clinical cause. Tinea probably elicits a mild, indolent contact hypersensitivity response as a result of the incorporation of protein excretory and possibly secretory products into the stratum corneum. Hydration of scale may facilitate the detection of these potential antigens by immune skin cells, which then incite a delayed hypersensitivity reaction. Frequently hydrated intertriginous regions are particularly prone to the inflammatory sequelae of dermatophytosis.

**Clinical Features.** Lesions typically present as pink erythematous plaques, sometimes with vesicles, but with central clearing and peripheral scale (fig. 2-34).

**Pathologic Findings.** Aside from the mild subacute spongiotic dermatitis, the histologic changes in dermatophytosis may be protean (fig. 2-35). Focal parakeratotic scale alternating vertically with compacted hyperorthokeratotic scale is an important clue. This abnormality produces a sandwich-like effect within the scale and is associated with the accumulation of occasional neutrophils. Although fungi may be visible in routine preparations, variability in staining among laboratories often necessitates the use of the PAS stain for their confirmation (fig. 2-36). In such preparations, hyphal forms are present within the affected scale. Proteinaceous material and inflammatory debris may also stain with PAS; therefore, definitive criteria for hyphal morphology must be met, including branching and septation. The finding of yeast forms alone does not constitute a diagnosis of dermatophytosis.

**Differential Diagnosis.** The differential diagnosis of dermatophytosis often includes other causes of spongiotic dermatitis (contact, irritant, or atopic).

**Treatment and Prognosis.** Topical antifungal agents are generally effective. Steroid treatment may result in temporary clinical improvement, although lesions recur upon cessation due to the persistence of organisms. A major problem is the premature cessation of antifungal topical therapy based on lesion improvement alone. Lesions partially treated prior to biopsy may harbor ballooned and distorted hyphal forms or too few organisms to permit diagnosis. Therapy should be discontinued, and lesions resampled at least 2 to 3 weeks after cessation in such instances. Biopsies should only be encouraged

*Inflammatory Disorders with Primary Epidermal Alterations: Spongiotic Dermatitis*

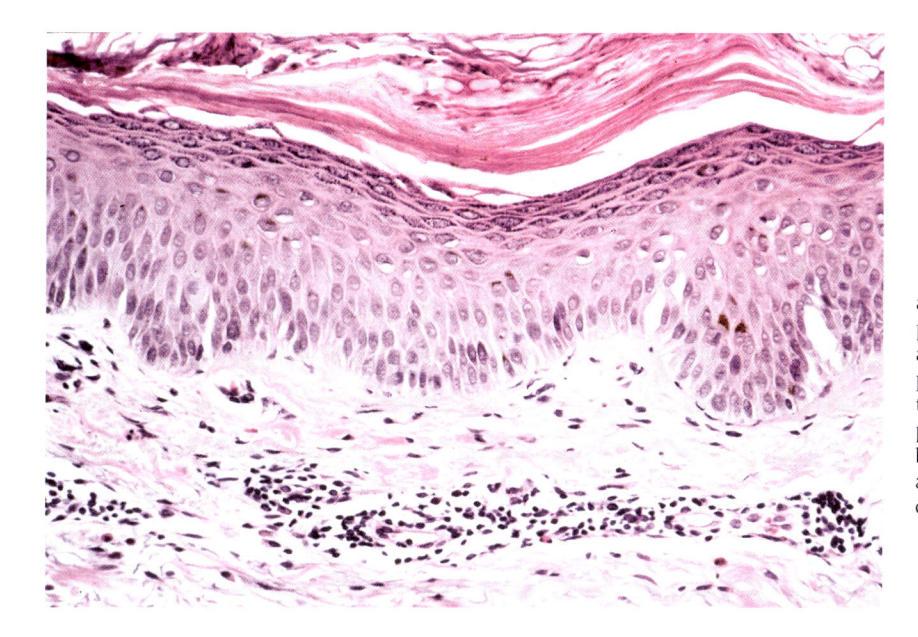

### Figure 2-35

### SUPERFICIAL DERMATOPHYTE INFECTION WITH ASSOCIATED ECZEMATOUS CHANGES

Mild acanthosis, spongiosis, and compact orthokeratotic and parakeratotic scale formation are accompanied by a superficial perivascular lymphocytic infiltrate. Unless entertained as a potential infectious process, this biopsy could easily be diagnosed as low-grade subacute spongiotic dermatitis.

### Figure 2-36

### SPONGIOTIC DERMATOPHYTE INFECTION

Periodic acid–Schiff (PAS) stains numerous hyphal organisms within the stratum corneum.

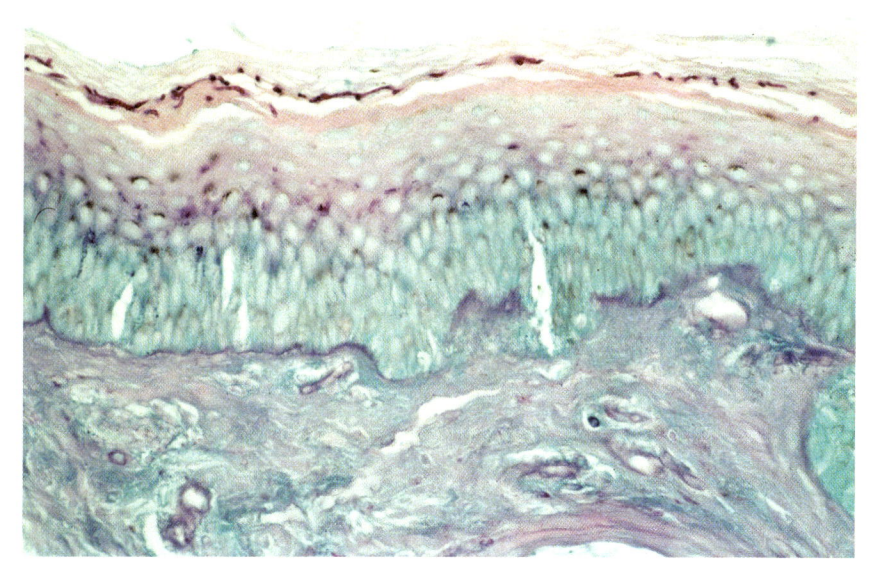

and performed if simpler and more economical approaches (e.g., KOH preparations) fail to yield definitive diagnostic information (96). Oral antifungal therapy is reserved for disseminated eruptions and hair or nail involvement.

## SCABIES

**Definition.** *Scabies* results from the superficial cutaneous infestation by the mite, *Sarcoptes scabiei*. The resultant delayed hypersensitivity reaction produces an intensely pruritic dermatitis that often shows spongiotic epidermal alterations.

**Clinical Features.** Although anyone may be infested, institutionalized individuals and children are particularly susceptible. Lesions are intensely pruritic papules to eczematous patches and plaques, and acral distribution is often observed (particularly involving the wrists and fingers). The papules may coalesce to form curvilinear lesions, termed burrows, and small pinpoint vesicles. Scraping of these burrows with a sharp blade occasionally reveals evidence of the offending organism, obviating the need for a biopsy. A form of the disorder termed *Norwegian scabies* occurs in elderly and immunocompromised

*Inflammatory Disorders of the Skin*

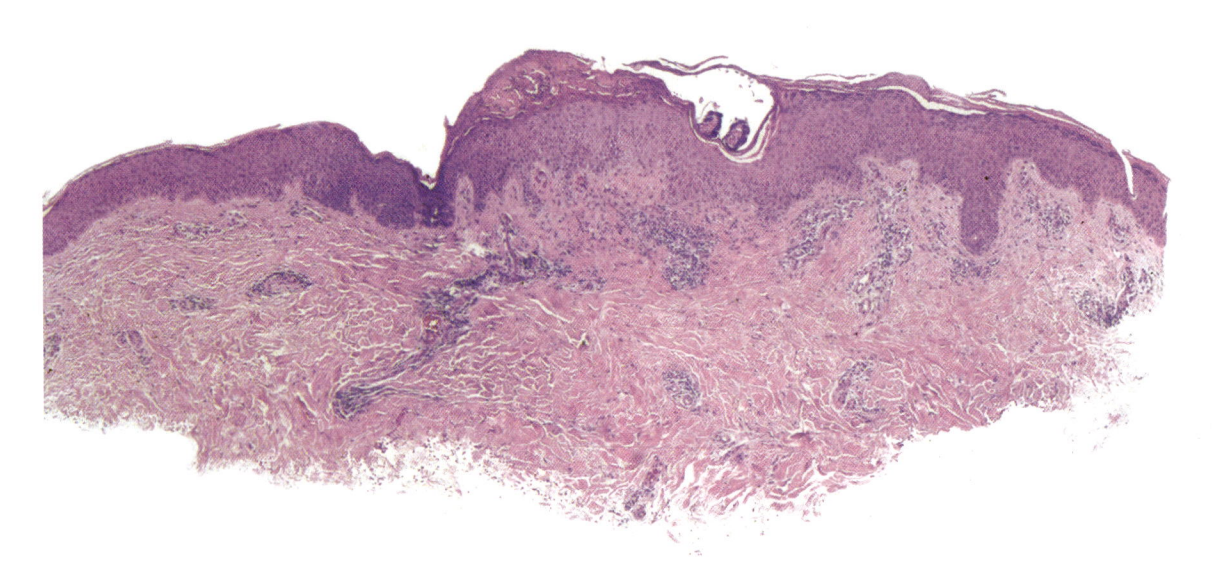

Figure 2-37

**SCABETIC SPONGIOTIC DERMATITIS**

At scanning magnification, there are irregular acanthosis, spongiosis with foci of abnormal scale formation, and a superficial perivascular inflammatory infiltrate. One small intracorneal cavity hints at the underlying cause.

Figure 2-38

**INTRACORNEAL SCABIES MITE**

In cross section, a portion of the mite is present within the intracorneal tunnel that it has formed. The surrounding epidermal layer shows acanthosis and spongiosis.

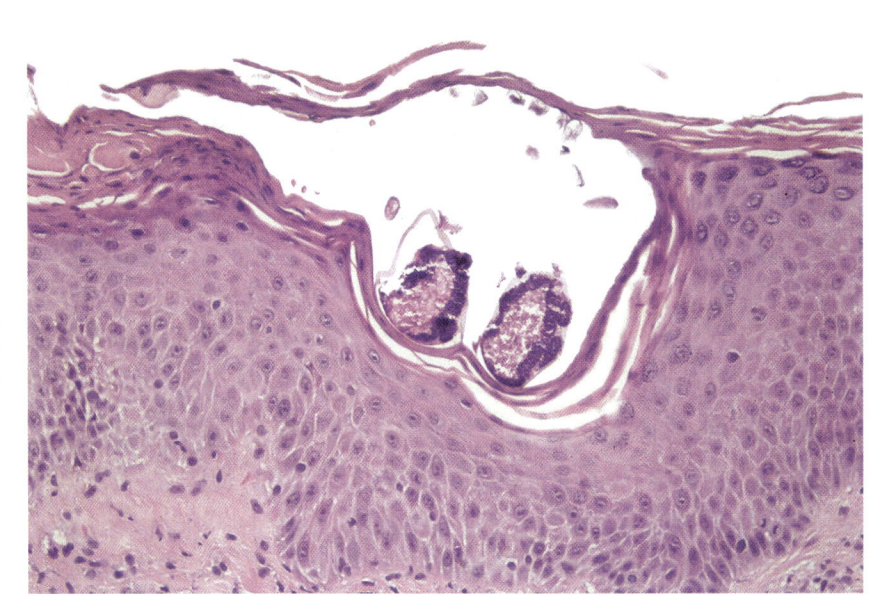

individuals and is characterized by thickened, hyperkeratotic plaques replete with organisms (97).

**Pathologic Findings.** There is acute to subacute spongiotic dermatitis associated with an underlying superficial and mid-dermal perivascular lymphocytic infiltrate, often containing numerous eosinophils (fig. 2-37). The presence of prominent retiform hyperplasia with a dense band-like infiltrate of lymphohistiocytic cells replete with eosinophils should lead to a strong suspicion of a scabetic infestation. Organisms and associated eggs or fecal material should be sought directly beneath or within the stratum corneum, although multiple levels may be required for their detection (figs. 2-38, 2-39). Occasionally, a burrow is observed as a cleft or minute space filled with inflammatory debris beneath the stratum corneum. Although these

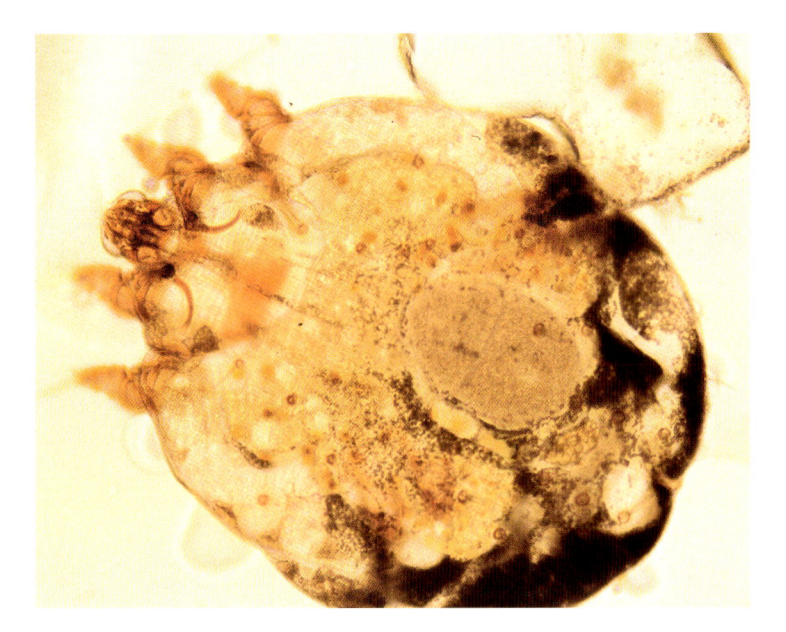

Figure 2-39

**OIL DROP PREPARATION SHOWING SCABIES MITE**

Such preparations are obtained by immersing scrapings of the clinical lesion in a drop of oil, and examining them by routine microscopy, obviating the need for a skin biopsy.

findings are nonspecific, they are suggestive and should prompt examination of multiple levels through the biopsy to attempt to document the presence of the organism. Spongiotic and inflammatory alterations continue in some patients after therapy, presumably due to the persistence of protein antigens within the scale. The Norwegian form of the disease is characterized by exuberant epidermal proliferation and enumerable organisms within the hyperkeratotic and crusted scale.

**Differential Diagnosis.** The differential diagnosis is as for other forms of spongiotic dermatitis, particularly contact dermatitis and pruritic drug eruptions. Occasionally, the urticarial/pruritic variant of pemphigoid and dermatitis herpetiformis are considered, prompted by the intense itching experienced by the patient.

**Treatment and Prognosis.** Antiscabetic topical lotions are most effective. Because the disorder is highly contagious, all household members potentially exposed must be treated, and contaminated clothing either discarded or treated in a manner to render organisms or their eggs incapable of infestation.

## PAPULAR ACRODERMATITIS OF CHILDHOOD (GIANOTTI-CROSTI SYNDROME)

**Definition.** *Papular acrodermatitis of childhood*, also termed *Gianotti-Crosti syndrome*, is a reaction to infection, most commonly viral, in children. It characteristically presents on the face and limbs and hence is designated papular acrodermatitis.

**Clinical Features.** The patient presents with a rapidly evolving eruption of papules or papulovesicles that are 2 to 3 mm in width and pink to salmon to red in color. These lesions are characteristically present on the face and the limbs, while the trunk is usually spared. The lesions are sometimes pruritic, sometimes vesicular, and usually last for no more than 2 to 3 weeks. Fever and inguinal and axillary adenopathy are common. Patients often have acute hepatitis B; however, hepatitis A, EBV, CMV, and Coxsackie virus are also associated with the disease.

**Pathologic Findings.** The findings are generally indistinguishable from those of other forms of subacute spongiotic dermatitis: focal spongiosis associated with hyperorthokeratosis and parakeratosis. There is a superficial perivascular lymphocytic infiltrate with associated eosinophils and variable papillary dermal edema. In the rare cases that we have observed, there were multiple dyskeratotic (apoptotic) cells scattered randomly throughout the affected epidermis.

**Differential Diagnosis.** The differential diagnosis includes the id reaction, airborne contact dermatitis, pityriasis lichenoides, and, at times when the papules are lichenoid, a photoallergic reaction or even lichen planus.

**Treatment and Prognosis.** The lesions are self-limited and resolve within a few weeks. If there is an associated infection, it should be treated (98).

## TOXIC SHOCK SYNDROME

**Definition.** *Toxic shock syndrome* is an uncommon and sometimes fatal disease resulting from infection with *Staphylococcus aureus*. The bacteria produce toxic shock syndrome toxin. In women, there is an approximate 4 percent fatality rate; men are only occasionally affected but have a higher rate of death in the range of 10 to 15 percent. The *S. aureus* toxins produced in women are often elaborated after prolonged use of superabsorbent vaginal tampons during menstruation.

**Clinical Features.** Originally, the etiology was the use of tampons with marked absorbency. Other causes associated with infection and the syndrome have now been described. Infections with *S. aureus* affecting the skin, either nonbroken or at the site of a surgical wound, are common causes. Entry through the nasal mucosa after packing also is associated with this disorder. Infections of soft tissue, bone, and lung with *S. aureus* have been described as causative of toxic shock syndrome.

The disorder is initially identified by fever, hypotension, and diffuse, sunburn-like erythema characterized by a superficial mixed inflammatory infiltrate containing neutrophils and eosinophils in addition to mononuclear cells. Rarely, influenza produces a disease that has features resembling Kawasaki syndrome, scarlet fever, and toxic shock syndrome.

Toxic shock syndrome has well-defined criteria. There are four major clinical features. First is the precipitous onset of fever between 102°F (38.9°C) and 104°F (40°C) or greater. Second, there is a rapid evolution of a diffuse scarlatiniform erythroderma, with prominent involvement of the palms and soles, with their subsequent desquamation. The third component is striking inflammation or erythema of the conjunctiva and the oropharynx, sometimes with ulceration. There may also be vaginal erythema and even a discharge. The fourth criterion is often striking hypotension.

Several other symptoms may present indicating involvement of different organ systems. These include vomiting or diarrhea, the gastrointestinal sign; elevation of creatine phosphokinase; a sign of musculoskeletal involvement; confusion or disorientation, a sign of nervous system involvement; evidence of hepatic dysfunction; thrombocytopenia; cardiopulmonary symptoms with electrocardiographic changes; and finally, endocrinopathic involvement with metabolic abnormalities, especially those involving calcium and phosphorus metabolism. The four major criteria plus involvement of at least three organ systems must be present to make the diagnosis.

Other dermatologic manifestations include petechiae on the extremities and marked edema of the hands and feet. Telogen effluvium and nail loss are late sequelae in about half the patients.

**Pathologic Findings.** The spongiosis is associated with dermal and epidermal neutrophil infiltration, necrotic keratinocytes, and occasional subepidermal blisters (fig. 2-40).

**Differential Diagnosis.** Another precipitous cutaneous disorder that must be differentiated from toxic shock syndrome is a drug eruption, which results in more of a maculopapular or morbilliform rash, usually with peripheral eosinophilia and without hypotension. Kawasaki syndrome usually exhibits fever lasting 10 days or longer and unilateral cervical adenopathy. Conjunctival and oral pharyngeal injection, hand and foot erythema, and even desquamation can occur in both Kawasaki and toxic shock syndromes, leading to confusion in the diagnosis.

The rash of scarlet fever has a definite prodrome, and usually spares the palms and soles early. There is a pinpoint character to the rash, which is associated with positive throat cultures and a rising antistreptolysin O (ASO) titer. The staphylococcal scalded skin syndrome exhibits diffuse erythema with tenderness, and widespread sloughing of the skin. Positive cultures can be obtained from eligible sites of infection, such as the pharynx or conjunctiva.

Viral exanthemas must be considered, but the characteristic patterns of their exanthemas, prodromes, and enanthems, with positive viral cultures, allow for correct diagnosis.

**Treatment and Prognosis.** Appropriate beta-lactamase–resistant antibiotics and protein synthesis inhibitors (i.e., clindamycin) are intravenously administered with supportive fluid therapy, and must continue well beyond the resolution of the severe symptoms because of the duration of effects of the toxin. Local treatment of known etiologic sites, such as impetigo or abscess, must be carried out. The shock syndrome

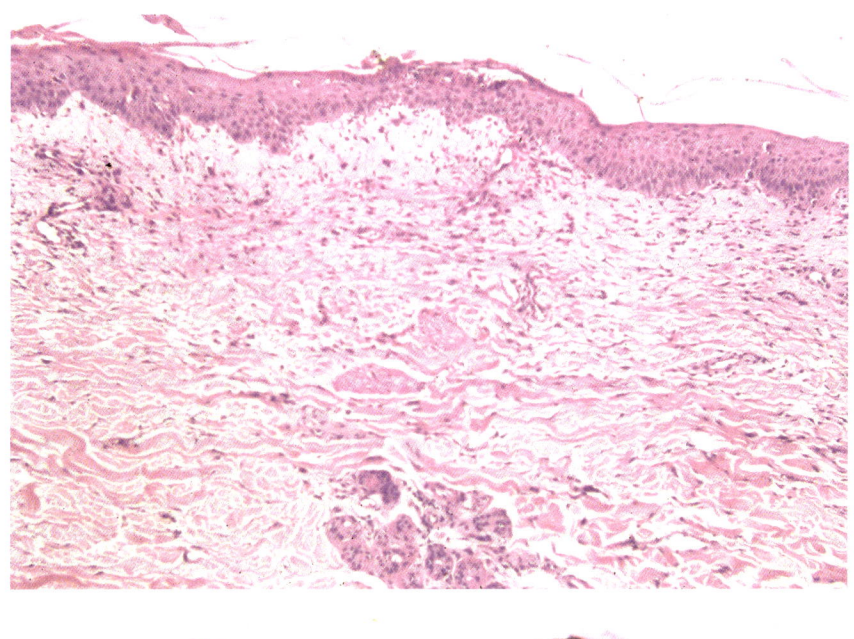

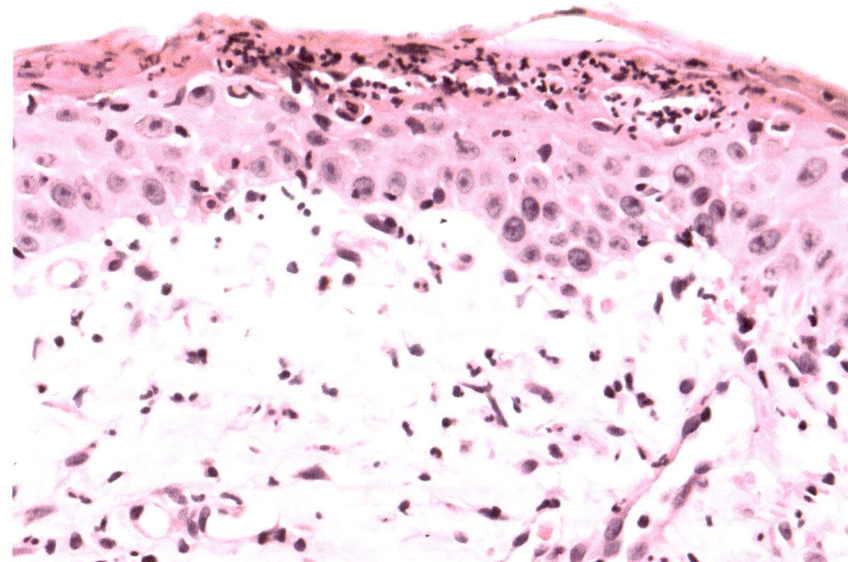

**Figure 2-40**
**TOXIC SHOCK SYNDROME**

Top: At scanning magnification, irregular acanthosis, spongiosis, abnormal scale formation, and a superficial perivascular inflammatory infiltrate with associated papillary dermal edema are seen.

Bottom: At higher magnification, there is a characteristic edematous papillary dermis containing a perivascular and interstitial mixed inflammatory infiltrate. The epidermal layer shows apoptosis as well as focal spongiosis. Neutrophils accumulate within the more superficial layers.

associated with influenza usually produces tracheitis, pharyngitis, or viral pneumonia in which the toxic shock syndrome Tox-1–producing bacteria cause superinfection, and appropriate antibiotic therapy must be instituted. Intravenous immunoglobulin and clindamycin have been used to neutralize the effect of the toxin and/or impair further toxin production (99).

## REFERENCES

1. Murphy GF. Dermatopathology: a practical guide to common disorders. Philadelphia: Saunders; 1995:3-48.
2. Murphy GF, Herzberg AJ. Atlas of dermatopathology. Philadelphia: Saunders; 1996:2-29.
3. Guitart J. Spongiotic dermatitis. In: Farmer ER, Hood AF. Pathology of the skin. New York: McGraw-Hill; 2000:152-67.
4. Ackerman AB. Histologic diagnosis of inflammatory skin disease. Philadelphia: Lea & Febiger; 1978.
5. Streilein JW, Bergstresser PR. Two antigen presentation pathways, only one of which requires Langerhans cells, lead to the induction of contact hypersensitivity. J Invest Dermatol 1983;80:302.
6. Lewis RE, Buchsbaum M, Whitaker D, Murphy GF. Intercellular adhesion molecule expression in the evolving human cutaneous delayed hypersensitivity reaction. J Invest Dermatol 1989;93:672-7.
7. Klein LM, Lavker RM, Matis WL, Murphy GF. Degranulation of human mast cells induces an endothelial antigen central to leukocyte adhesion. Proc Natl Acad Sci U S A 1989;86:8972-6.
8. Abell E. Spongiotic dermatitis. In: Farmer ER, Hood AF, eds. Pathology of the skin, Norwalk CT: Appleton & Lange; 1990:74.
9. Girolomoni G, Sebastiani S, Albanesi C, Cavani A. T-cell subpopulations in the development of atopic and contact allergy. Curr Opin Immunol 2001;13:733-7.
10. Wolf R, Wolf D. Contact dermatitis. Clin Dermatol 2000;18:661-6.
11. Traidl C, Merk HF. Cavani A, Hunzelmann N. New insights into the pathomechanisms of contact dermatitis by the use of transgenic mouse models. Skin Pharmacol Appl Skin Physiol 2000;13:300-12.
12. Xu H, Bjarnason B, Elmets CA. Sensitization versus elicitation in allergic contact dermatitis: potential differences at cellular and molecular levels. Am J Contact Dermat 2000;11:228-34.
13. Weston WL, Bruckner A. Allergic contact dermatitis. Pediatr Clin North Am 2000;47:897-907.
14. Mowad CM. Update on contact dermatitis. Adv Dermatol 1999;14:61-87.
15. Jakob T, Udey MC. Epidermal Langerhans cells: from neurons to nature's adjuvants. Adv Dermatol 1999;14:209-58.
16. Waldorf HA, Walsh LJ, Schechter NM, Murphy GF. Early cellular events in evolving cutaneous delayed hypersensitivity in humans. Am J Pathol 1991;138:477-86.
17. Dvorak HF, Mihm MC Jr, Dvorak AM. Morphology of delayed-type hypersensitivity reactions in man. J Invest Dermatol 1976;67:391-401.
17a. Petzelbauer P, Gröger M, Kunstfeld R, Petzelbauer E, Wolff K. Human delayed-type hypersensitivity reaction in a SCID mouse engrafted with human T cells and autologous skin. J Invest Dermatol 1996;107:576-81.
18. Willis I, Kligman AM. The mechanism of photoallergic contact dermatitis. J Invest Dermatol 1968;51:378-84.
19. Harber LC, Baer RL. Pathogenic mechanisms of drug-induced photosensitivity. J Invest Dermatol 1972;58:327-42.
20. Cronin E. Contact dermatitis. Edinburgh, Scotland: Churchill Livingstone; 1980.
21. Fisher AA. Contact dermatitis, 3rd ed. Philadelphia: Lea & Febiger; 1986.
22. Holdiness MR. Contact dermatitis to topical drugs for glaucoma. Am J Contact Dermat 2001;12:217-9.
23. Yu HS, Lee CH, Jee SH, Ho CK, Guo YL. Environmental and occupational skin diseases in Taiwan. J Dermatol 2001;28:628-31.
24. Kanerva L. Cross-reactions of multifunctional methacrylates and acrylates. Acta Odontol Scand 2001;59:320-9.
25. English J. Current concepts in contact dermatitis. Br J Dermatol 2001;145:527-9.
26. Merk HF, Sachs B, Baron J. The skin: target organ in immunotoxicology of small-molecular-weight compounds. Skin Pharmacol Appl Skin Physiol 2001;14:419-30.
27. Reese DJ, Reichl RB, McCollum J. Latex allergy literature review: evidence for making military treatment facilities latex safe. Mil Med 2001;166:764-70.
28. Wolf R, Wolf D, Tüzün B, Tüzün Y. Contact dermatitis to cosmetics. Clin Dermatol 2001;19:502-15.
29. Wolf R, Wolf D, Tüzün B, Tüzün Y. Soaps, shampoos, and detergents. Clin Dermatol 2001;19:393-7.
30. Jeebhay MF, Robins TG, Lehrer SB, Lopata AL. Occupational seafood allergy: a review. Occup Environ Med 2001;58:553-62.
31. Koutis D. Freeman S. Allergic contact stomatitis caused by acrylic monomer in a denture. Australas J Dermatol 2001;42:203-6.
32. Holdiness MR. Contact dermatitis from topical antiviral drugs. Contact Dermatitis 2001;44:265-9.
33. Bruckner AL, Weston WL. Beyond poison ivy: understanding allergic contact dermatitis in children. Pediatr Ann 2001;30:203-6.

34. Zhai H, Maibach HI. Skin occlusion and irritant and allergic contact dermatitis: an overview. Contact Dermatitis 2001;44:201-6.
35. Kurup VP, Fink JN. The spectrum of immunologic sensitization in latex allergy. Allergy 2001;56:2-12.
36. Huygens S, Goossens A. An update on airborne contact dermatitis. Contact Dermatitis 2001;44:1-6.
37. Scheman A. Adverse reactions to cosmetic ingredients. Dermatol Clin 2000;18:685-98.
38. Lushniak BD. Occupational skin diseases. Prim Care 2000;27:895-916.
39. Shaffer MP, Belsito DV. Allergic contact dermatitis from glutaraldehyde in health-care workers. Contact Dermatitis 2000;43:150-6.
40. Matura M, Goossens A. Contact allergy to corticosteroids. Allergy 2000;55:698-704.
41. English JS. Corticosteroid-induced contact dermatitis: a pragmatic approach. Clin Exp Dermatol 2000;25:261-4.
42. Willis CM, Stephens CJ, Wilkinson JD. Epidermal damage induced by irritants in man: a light and electron microscopy study. J Invest Dermatol 1989;93:695-9.
43. Slodownik D, Lee A, Nixon R. Irritant contact dermatitis: a review. Australas J Dermatol 2008;49:1-9.
44. Taylor RM. Histopathology of contact dermatitis. Clin Dermatol 1986;4:18-22.
45. Crotty C, Pittelkow M, Muller SA. Eosinophilic spongiosis: a clinicopathological review of seventy-one cases. J Am Acad Dermatol 1983;8:337-43.
46. Ruiz E, Deng JS, Abell EA. Eosinophilic spongiosis: a clinical, histologic, and immunopathologic study. J Am Acad Dermatol 1994;30:973-6.
47. Burkert KL, Huhn K, Menezes DW, Murphy GF. Langerhans cell microgranulomas (pseudo-Pautrier abscesses): Morphologic diversity, diagnostic implications, and pathogenetic mechanisms. J Cutan Pathol 2002;29:511-6.
48. Ackerman AB, Breza TS, Capland L. Spongiotic simulants of mycosis fungoides. Arch Dermatol 1974;109:218-20.
49. Baxevanis CN, Papadopoulos NG, Katsarou-Katsari A, Papamichail M. Regulation of allergic-specific immune responses by CD4+ CD45R+ cells in patients with allergic contact dermatitis. J Allergy Clin Immunol 1994;94:917-27.
50. Levin C, Maibach HI. An overview of the efficacy of topical corticosteroids in experimental human nickel contact dermatitis. Contact Dermatitis 2000;43:317-21.
51. Mihm MC Jr, Soter NA, Dvorak HF, Austen KF. The structure of normal skin and the morphology of atopic eczema. J Invest Dermatol 1976;67:305-12.
52. Rothke MJ, Grant-Kels JM. Atopic dermatitis; an update. J Am Acad Dermatol 1996;35:1-13.
53. Graham-Brown RA. Atopic dermatitis. Semin Dermatol 1988;7:37-42.
54. Schultz Larsen F. Atopic dermatitis. A genetic-epidermiologic study in a population-based twin sample. J Am Acad Dermatol 1993;28:719-23.
55. Krutmann J. Phototherapy for atopic dermatitis. Clin Exp Dermatol 2000;25:552-558.
56. Landow K. Hand dermatitis. The perennial scourge. Postgrad Med 1998;103:141-2, 145-8, 151-2.
57. Kutzner H, Wurzel RM, Wolff HH. Are acrosyringia involved in the pathogenesis of "dyshidrosis"? Am J Dermatopathol 1986;8:109-16.
58. Khanna M, Qasem K, Sasseville D. Allergic contact dermatitis to tea tree oil with erythema multiforme-like id reaction. Am J Contact Dermatitis 2000;11:238-42.
59. Magro CM, Crowson AN. A distinctive cutaneous reaction pattern indicative of infection by reactive arthropathy-associated microbial pathogens: the superantigen ID reaction. J Cutan Pathol 1998;25:538-44.
60. Gianni C, Betti R. Crosti C. Psoriasiform id reaction in tinea corporis. Mycoses 1996;39:307-8.
61. Rocamora V, Romani J, Puig L, de Moragas JM. Id reaction to molluscum contagiosum. Pediatr Dermatol 1996;13:349-50.
62. Derebery J, Berliner KI. Foot and ear disease—the dermatophytid reaction in otology. Laryngoscope 1996;106:181-6.
63. Jordaan HF, Schneider JW. Papular urticaria: a histopathologic study of 30 patients. Am J Dermatopathol 1997;19:119-26.
64. Shaffer B, Jacobson C, Beerman H. Histopathologic correlation of lesions of papular urticaria and positive skin test reactions to insect antigens. Arch Derm Syphilol 1954;70:437-42.
65. Stibich AS, Carbonaro PA, Schwartz RA. Insect bite reactions: an update. Dermatology 2001;202:193-7.
66. Reschly MJ, Ramos-Caro FA, Mathes BM. Multiple fire ant stings: report of 3 cases and review of the literature. Cutis 2000;66:179-82.
67. Metry DW, Hebert AA. Insect and arachnid stings, bites, infestations, and repellents. Pediatr Ann 2000;29:39-48.
68. Gilliam AC, Wood GS. Cutaneous lymphoid hyperplasias. Semin Cutan Med Surg 2000;19:133-41.
69. Schexnayder SM, Schexnayder RE. Bites, stings, and other painful things. Pediatr Ann 2000;29:354-8.
70. Kain KC. Skin lesions in returned travelers. Med Clin North Am 1999;83:1077-102.

71. King TP. Immunochemical studies of stinging insect venom allergens. Toxicon 1996;34:1455-8.
72. Graft DF. Stinging insect hypersensitivity in children. Curr Opin Pediatr 1996;8:597-600.
73. Stafford CT. Hypersensitivity to fire ant venom. Ann Allergy Asthma Immunol 1996;77:87-95.
74. Elder C, Harris J, Williams D. Allergy to bee and wasp venom. Br J Hosp Med 1996;55:349-52.
75. Fellner MJ, Prutkin L. Morbilliform eruptions caused by penicillin. A study of electron microscopy and immunologic tests. J Invest Dermatol 1970;55:390-5.
76. Shin HT, Chang MW. Drug eruptions in children. Curr Prob Pediatr 2001;31:207-34.
77. Tokura Y. Immune responses to photohaptens: implications for the mechanisms of photosensitivity to exogenous agents. J Dermatol Sci 2000;23(Suppl 1):S6-9.
78. Krutmann J. Ultraviolet A radiation-induced biological effects in human skin: relevance for photoaging and photodermatosis. J Dermatol Sci 2000;23(Suppl 1):S22-6.
79. Epstein JH. Phototoxicity and photoallergy. Semin Cutan Med Surg 1999;18:274-84.
80. Taylor CR. Photosensitivity: classification, diagnosis, and treatment. Dermatol Nurs 1998;10:323-30.
81. Tokura Y. Quinolone photoallergy: photosensitivity dermatitis induced by systemic administration of photohaptenic drugs. J Dermatol Sci 1998;18:1-10.
82. Wolf R, Oumeish OY. Photodermatoses. Clin Dermatol 1998;16:41-57.
83. Schauder S, Ippen H. Contact and photocontact sensitivity to sunscreens. Review of a 15-year experience and of the literature. Contact Dermatitis 1997;37:221-32.
84. Epstein JH. Polymorphous light eruption. Photodermatol Photoimmunol Photomed 1997;13:89-90.
85. Isaksson M, Bruze M. Photopatch testing. Clin Dermatol 1997;15:615-8.
86. Gonzalez E, Gonzalez S. Drug photosensitivity, idiopathic photodermatoses, and sunscreens. J Am Acad Dermatol 1996;35:871-85.
87. Dooms-Goossens A, Blockeel I. Allergic contact dermatitis and photoallergic contact dermatitis due to soaps and detergents. Clin Dermatol 1996;14:67-76.
88. Wrangsjo K, Ros AM. Compositae allergy. Semin Dermatol 1996;15:87-94.
89. Lovell CR. Current topics in plant dermatitis. Semin Dermatol 1996;15:113-21.
90. Farage MA, Miller KW, Berardesca E, Maibach HI. Clinical implications of aging skin: cutaneous disorders in the elderly. Am J Clin Dermatol 2009;10(2):73-86. doi: 10.2165/00128071-200910020-00001.
91. Stefanaki I, Katsambas A. Therapeutic update on seborrheic dermatitis. Skin Therapy Lett 2010;15:1-4.
92. Hsu S, Le EH, Khoshevis MR. Differential diagnosis of annular lesions. Am Fam Physician 2001;64:289-96.
93. Reinharez D. Varicose eczema. Phlebologie. 1982;35:259-72.
94. Belousova IE, Vanecek T, Samtsov AV, Michal M, Kazakov DV. A patient with clinicopathologic features of small plaque parapsoriasis presenting later with plaque-stage mycosis fungoides: report of a case and comparative retrospective study of 27 cases of "nonprogressive" small plaque parapsoriasis. J Am Acad Dermatol 2008;59:474-82.
95. Canpolat Kirac B, Adisen E, Bozdayi G, et al. The role of human herpesvirus 6, human herpesvirus 7, Epstein-Barr virus and cytomegalovirus in the aetiology of pityriasis rosea. J Eur Acad Dermatol Venereol 2009;23:16-21.
96. Kaur IP, Kakkar S. Topical delivery of antifungal agents. Expert Opin Drug Deliv 2010;7:1303-27. Epub 2010 Oct 20.
97. Walton SF. The immunology of susceptibility and resistance to scabies. Parasite Immunol 2010;32:532-40.
98. Wu CY, Huang WH. Question: Can you identify this condition? Gianotti-Crosti syndrome. Can Fam Physician 2009;55:712, 716.
99. Silversides JA, Lappin E, Ferguson AJ. Staphylococcal toxic shock syndrome: mechanisms and management. Curr Infect Dis Rep 2010;12:392-400.

# 3 ACANTHOTIC DERMATITIS (RETIFORM EPIDERMAL HYPERPLASIA)

*Psoriasiform dermatitis* is a term commonly used for inflammatory disorders that exhibit primarily epidermal hyperplasia involving acanthosis (diffuse epidermal thickening). The acanthosis is initiated by proliferation within the epidermal rete ridges (retiform hyperplasia). Psoriasis and lichen simplex chronicus are the two primary forms of dermatitis with retiform epidermal hyperplasia, which is often referred to as psoriasiform and nonpsoriasiform, respectively. The former indicates a type of epidermal hyperplasia in which the rete ridges undergo regular downward elongation such that their tips appear to approximate a straight line parallel to the overlying epidermal layer. The latter conveys a form of epidermal hyperplasia in which the rete tips extend to different depths beneath the epidermal layer.

Retiform epidermal hyperplasia is either a primary process, as in psoriasis, or an evolutionary stage in lesion progression, as in chronically rubbed or excoriated spongiotic dermatitis. Accordingly, some disorders discussed in this section are also described in different temporal stages in other chapters.

Most forms of retiform epidermal hyperplasia share the common clinical feature of abnormal scale formation overlying a variably erythematous patch, plaque, papule, or nodule. There exist important clinical differences, however, and these include the color of the scale (e.g., yellow-tan versus silvery white); the configuration of the lesion (e.g., papules versus circinate plaques); associated structures (e.g., involvement or sparing of hair follicles); and regional variations (e.g., the presence or absence of nail changes).

The immunofluorescence pattern of psoriasis consists of accumulation of immunoglobulin and complement within the parakeratotic stratum corneum. This finding is nonspecific, and may be seen in any disorder where serum collects within the uppermost epidermal layers (such as spongiotic dermatitis or impetiginization). Histochemical stains are useful in evaluating forms of acanthosis associated with dermal inflammatory infiltrates that potentially represent immune responses to infectious agents (e.g., as with blastomycosis).

Traditional animal models for acanthosis and retiform epidermal hyperplasia have relied upon the topical application of primary irritants to rodent skin. Phorbol esters, a variety of irritants, and topical retinoids are known to produce an exuberant epidermal proliferative response resulting in a form of acanthotic dermatitis (1). Because rodent skin does not exhibit rete ridges as does porcine and primate skin, the replication of lesions of lichen simplex chronicus is incomplete with respect to induction of true retiform epidermal hyperplasia and attendant vertically oriented papillary dermal fibrosis. The epidermal proliferative alterations in such models have, however, paved the way for the current understanding of stem cell populations that are likely to be stimulated in acanthotic reactions and in the wound healing response. These apoptosis-resistant cells appear to reside either in the bulge regions of hair follicles or at the tips of epidermal rete ridges (2,3). This concept has resulted in the notion that future therapeutic strategies to control the epidermal proliferative response could be directed toward molecular or genomic modification of these stem cell regions.

The "flaky skin" mouse mutation (fsn/fsn) is responsible for an autosomal recessive genetic disease with clinical and histopathologic features that resemble human psoriasis (4). Human psoriatic skin has been successfully xenografted onto immunodeficient mice, and lesions similar to human psoriasis have been induced in normal human skin xenografts from psoriatic patients by injecting their lymphocytes into the engrafted skin (5). This latter finding suggests that psoriasis is a systemic disorder in which specifically activated lymphocytes are capable of producing disease when introduced into appropriate target tissues.

**Figure 3-1**

**LICHEN SIMPLEX CHRONICUS AND PRURIGO NODULARIS**

Thickened plaques and coalescent nodules have formed in the extremities in response to chronic excoriation and trauma.

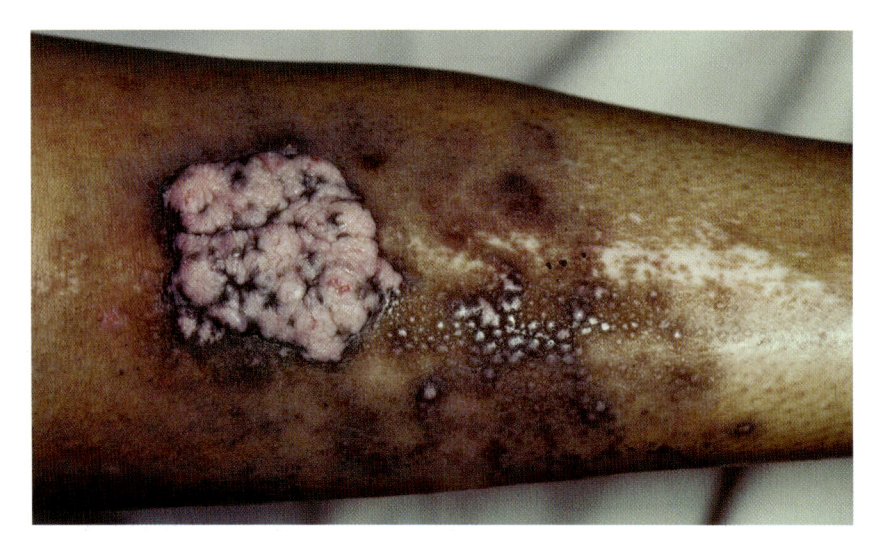

## LICHEN SIMPLEX CHRONICUS AND PRURIGO NODULARIS

**Definition.** The term *lichen simplex chronicus* implies an uncomplicated, persistent condition superficially resembling botanical lichen, a plant consisting of a fungus in close combination with certain algae which forms a scaling growth on rocks or tree trunks. In humans, lichen simplex chronicus is a disorder characterized by the development of scaling, often erythematous plaques at the site of chronic rubbing or irritation. *Prurigo nodularis* is lichen simplex chronicus that develops as scaling papules and nodules at discrete sites of persistent itching (6,7).

**Clinical Features.** Lichen simplex chronicus presents as one or more scaling, variably erythematous plaques affecting individuals of any age. Extensor surfaces that are prone to repeated trauma, sites chronically rubbed due to environmental or occupational irritation (e.g., violin player's chin), or the posterior surface of the neck where patients often scratch inadvertently are most often affected by lichen simplex chronicus (fig. 3-1). Prurigo nodularis is generally manifested by solitary or multiple papules and nodules that are firm, variably erythematous, and covered by a thick scale. In contrast to the easily abraded silvery white scale of psoriasis, both lichen simplex chronicus and prurigo nodularis are characterized by more adherent, slightly off-white to yellow scales. Postinflammatory hypopigmentation or hyperpigmentation may occur at sites of lichen simplex chronicus, particularly in individuals with increased endogenous melanization.

A traumatic cause in lichen simplex chronicus and prurigo nodularis is evidenced by the detection of recent excoriations in clinically uninvolved skin. Care must be taken not to overlook primary disorders that may give rise to lichen simplex chronicus after repeated scratching (e.g., primary contact dermatitis and atopy, scabies, dermatophytosis and other superficial fungal infections such as candidiasis, mast cell disorders, and pruritic vesiculobullous disorders such as the urticarial variant of pemphigoid or dermatitis herpetiformis). Metabolic causes of pruritus and secondary lichen simplex chronicus (e.g., renal [8] or hepatic dysfunction) should also be considered in certain patients.

**Pathologic Features.** Both lichen simplex chronicus and prurigo nodularis have similar histologic features. There is variably compact hyperorthokeratosis, hypergranulosis, focal irregularly scattered parakeratosis, and acanthosis producing irregular retiform hyperplasia in which epidermal rete ridges extend to different depths within the underlying superficial dermis (fig. 3-2, above). The affected rete ridges may have irregular shapes. The bases of the rete also vary; some have pointed tips, others have broad bases. Secondary impetiginization may be observed, with neutrophils and bacterial colonies within the thickened stratum corneum. An important and characteristic finding is the development of a peculiar type of fibrosis within elongated dermal papillae where collagen fibers are

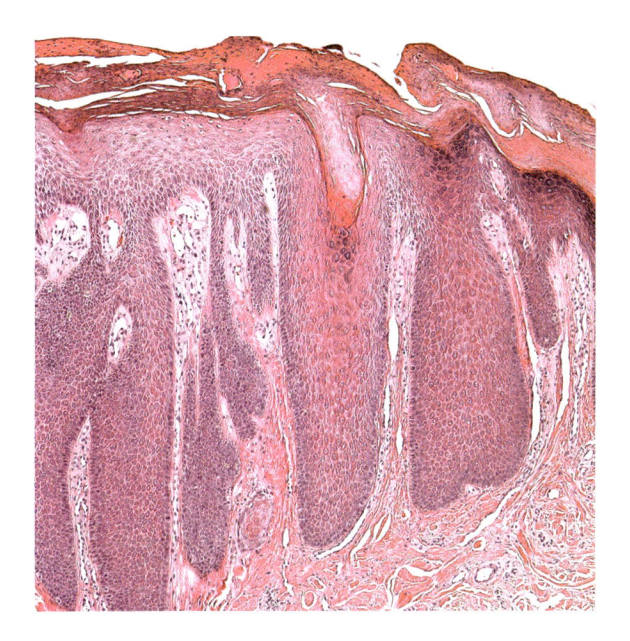

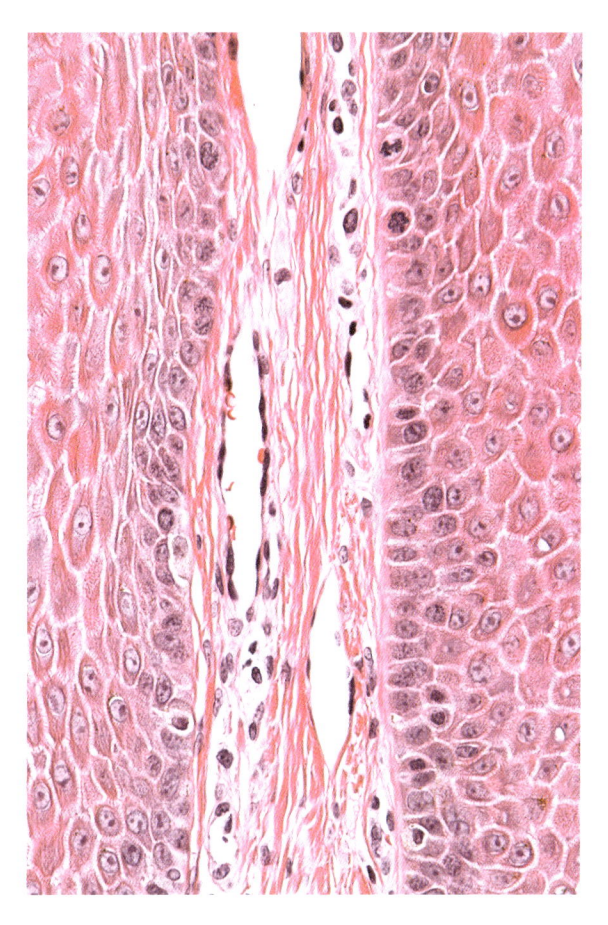

### Figure 3-2
**LICHEN SIMPLEX CHRONICUS**

Above: Marked hyperkeratosis, thickening of the stratum granulosum, irregular acanthosis with uneven elongation of rete ridges, and a sparse superficial perivascular lymphocytic infiltrate are seen at scanning magnification.

Right: At higher magnification, a characteristic finding is the linear and vertically oriented deposition of collagen (streaking) within the dermal papillae.

aligned perpendicular to the overlying epidermal layer (fig. 3-2, right) (9). Spongiosis is generally minimal. A sparse to absent mononuclear cell infiltrate is seen about vessels within the papillary dermis.

Occasionally, lichen simplex chronicus produces a verrucous architecture in which the epidermal surface is no longer relatively flat, but is in the form of irregular ridges and spires. Such variants may be particularly difficult to differentiate from chronically irritated verrucous keratoses based on histologic examination alone. As indicated above, lichen simplex chronicus and prurigo nodularis may be superimposed upon primary pruritic dermatoses, masking the latter. In the case of pruritic pemphigoid, hyperkeratotic nodules of prurigo nodularis, termed *pemphigoid nodularis*, represent a mixed variant of both disorders (10,11). Prurigo nodularis combined with atopic or contact dermatitis, cutaneous amyloid, or underlying metabolic abnormalities (e.g., renal or hepatic dysfunction) must also be considered when patients present with self-induced hyperkeratotic plaques and nodules.

*Pseudoepitheliomatous hyperplasia* is a specific type of acanthotic reaction characterized by irregular and often deeply endophytic elongation of thinned rete ridges within a chronically inflamed dermis. It lacks the highly irregular shapes of the rete and the characteristic vertically oriented fibrosis within rete ridges of lichen simplex chronicus (fig. 3-3, left). The tips of the rete have a tapered, pointed appearance, in contrast to the broader-based tips of some squamous cell carcinomas. Moreover, it is generally not the consequence of chronic rubbing, but rather the result of persistent attempts at reepithelialization at the edge of an ulcer or in association with an underlying dermal inflammatory focus (e.g., a draining fistula or sinus tract). *Syringometaplasia* is a related condition in which eccrine ductular epithelium undergoes initial hyperplasia and eventual squamous metaplasia at sites of chronic inflammation and fibrosis (fig. 3-3, right).

*Inflammatory Disorders of the Skin*

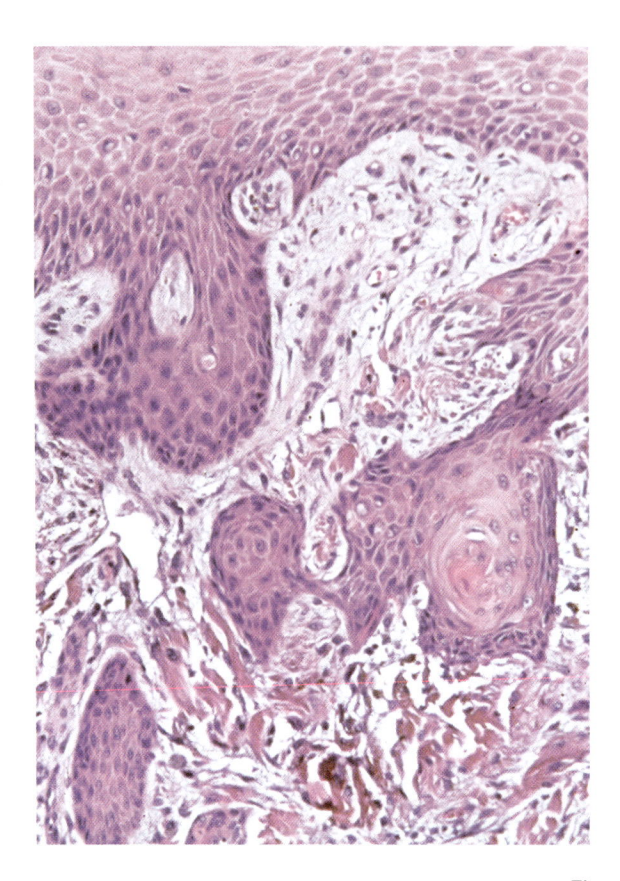

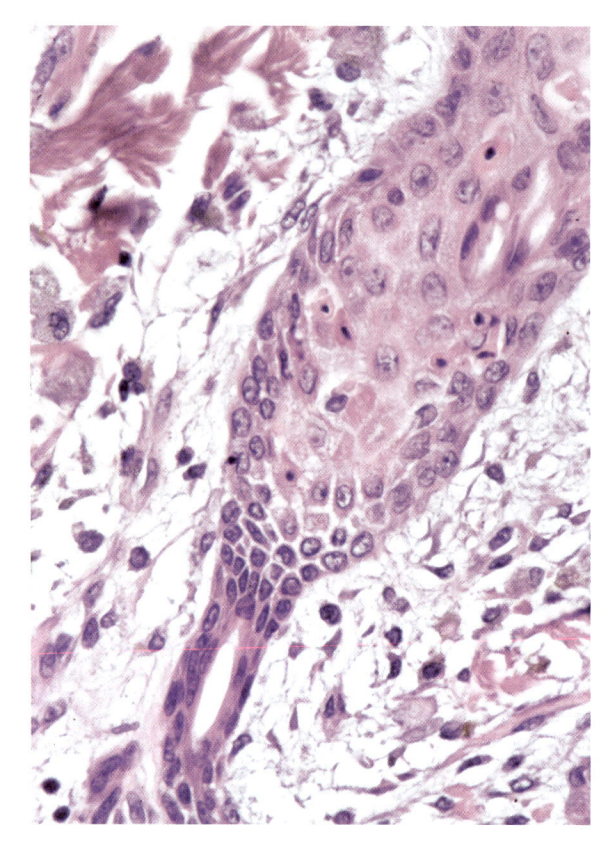

**Figure 3-3**

**PSEUDOEPITHELIOMATOUS EPIDERMAL HYPERPLASIA**

Left: In this region of scarring and chronic inflammation, there is exuberant endophytic proliferation of hyperplastic epithelium. In many areas, the diagnosis of invasive squamous cell carcinoma is suggested.

Right: Higher magnification shows areas of eccrine syringometaplasia. The endophytic squamous epithelium is surrounded by reactive stroma, with focal contiguity with a remnant of eccrine duct (lower left of field).

**Pathogenesis.** Both lichen simplex chronicus and prurigo nodularis are most commonly caused by chronic, low-grade mechanical injury and repetitive stimulation to the skin surface, as occurs with scratching or rubbing (12–14). Although such trauma has traditionally been regarded as arising from psychogenic influences (hence, the unfortunate term "neurodermatitis"), more recently, it has been acknowledged that simple somatization or neurosis is unlikely to explain many examples of this disorder. Dermal mast cells may release pruritogenic mediators, such as histamine, upon stimulation by a variety of physical factors, and thresholds for mast cell degranulation appear to differ among individuals and body sites (15). Moreover, mast cells are closely associated with unmyelinated nerve fibers which contain neuropeptides, such as substance P (16). These neuropeptides may trigger mast cell histamine release or act directly as primary pruritogenic agents. These nerves send branches into the epidermal layer (17–19) and may undergo significant proliferation at sites involved by lichen simplex chronicus and other forms of dermatitis showing retiform epidermal hyperplasia (20,21). Merkel cells occur in larger numbers in lesions of lichen simplex chronicus (22), either a secondary event, or possibly indicative of a regulatory influence over skin cell homeostasis. Other factors causing itching, such as insect bite reaction or an atopic diathesis, may represent primary stimuli for the development of prurigo nodularis and lichen simplex chronicus (23,24). Finally, dry skin in elderly patients tends to itch, providing a fertile setting for the development of the self-perpetuating "scratch-itch" cycle.

Table 3-1

DIFFERENTIAL HISTOLOGIC FEATURES OF LICHEN SIMPLEX CHRONICUS AND PSORIASIS

|  | Lichen Simplex Chronicus | Psoriasis |
|---|---|---|
| Stratum corneum | Orthokeratotic | Parakeratotic |
| Stratum granulosum | Increased | Decreased |
| Stratum spinosum | Thickened | Thickened |
| Rete extension | Irregular | Regular |
| Papillary dermal collagen | Fibrotic | Not fibrotic |
| Papillary dermal vessels | Normal | Dilated, tortuous |
| Inflammation | Neutrophils absent[a] | Neutrophils present |

[a]Unless bacterial superinfection has occurred.

How chronic and persistent mechanical irritation at the epidermal surface results in lesions of lichen simplex chronicus and prurigo nodularis is poorly understood. Chemical irritants are known to induce the production of a stimulated keratinocyte phenotype, as determined by their ability to produce cytokines and express markers of cellular activation and proliferation. Mechanical injury is likely to produce a low-grade wound healing response whereby keratinocyte stem cell populations are induced to proliferate and differentiate as a protective adaptation to insulate the traumatized site against further injury.

**Differential Diagnosis.** Lichen simplex chronicus must primarily be differentiated from psoriasis, particularly when the former has been traumatically impetiginized, resulting in accumulation of neutrophils within the stratum corneum. Table 3-1 summarizes some of the pertinent differences between lichen simplex chronicus and psoriasis.

Early psoriasis may show a somewhat irregular downward extension of epidermal rete ridges, and accordingly, this feature may not always assist in the differential diagnosis. Occasional lesions of psoriasis that are pruritic and chronically excoriated may show histologic features of both lichen simplex chronicus and psoriasis. Moreover, secondarily impetiginized lichen simplex chronicus may contain neutrophils within the uppermost epidermal layers, mimicking neutrophilic involvement in psoriasis. The absence of diffuse parakeratosis, the presence of hypergranulosis, and the finding of vertically oriented fibrosis within dermal papillae, however, should assist in the accurate recognition of superinfected lichen simplex chronicus.

Clues to an underlying cause should always be sought in biopsies of lichen simplex chronicus and prurigo nodularis. Detection of residua of arthropod body parts, eggs, or excrement within the stratum corneum should lead to diagnostic consideration of scabies, an infestation that typically leads to intense pruritus and scratching. The rare Norwegian variant of scabies is often associated with immunosuppression and results in exuberant epidermal hyperplasia replete with organisms within the thickened scale. The finding of focal spongiosis or of eosinophils admixed within the dermal inflammatory infiltrate raises the possibility of a chronic delayed hypersensitivity reaction or atopic diathesis as a cause of persistent excoriation. Eosinophils or neutrophils along the dermal-epidermal junction should draw attention to the possibility of pruritic pemphigoid or neutrophilic dermatosis variants. Finally, the mere finding of lichen simplex chronicus or prurigo nodularis in the absence of associated alterations potentially representing a cause of pruritus may not be trivial, since it could represent a manifestation of an underlying metabolic or systemic disorder that would benefit from clinical detection and treatment. Pseudoepitheliomatous hyperplasia may involve the dermis so extensively that it mimics invasive squamous cell carcinoma (24a), and is alternatively referred to as "pseudocarcinomatous epidermal hyperplasia." Syringometaplasia also may mimic invasive squamous cell carcinoma. In both pseudoepitheliomatous hyperplasia and syringometaplasia, nuclei are of a reactive phenotype, with prominent, enlarged nucleoli surrounded by a field of evenly dispersed, particulate chromatin enclosed by a thin, uniform, and smooth nuclear membrane.

### Figure 3-4
### EVOLUTIONARY STAGES OF ACANTHOTIC DERMATITIS (PSORIASIS)

The most significant changes as one progresses from normal skin (A) to early and established lesions are: initial ectasia tortuosity of capillary loops within dermal papillae (B), progressive retiform epidermal proliferation (C–E) resulting in even endophytic elongation of the rete ridges, progressive parakeratosis and scale formation (C–E), thinning of the suprapapillary plate (D,E), and progressive accumulation of neutrophils within the most epidermal layers.

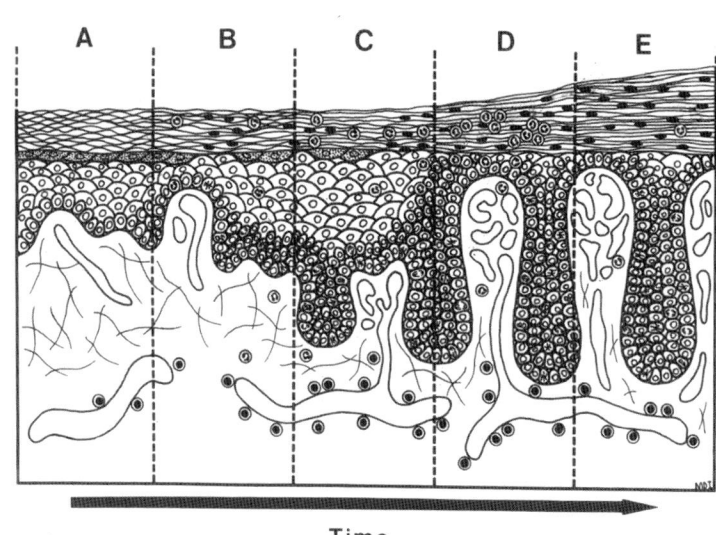

**Treatment and Prognosis.** Lichen simplex chronicus is a persistent dermatosis that is often refractory to treatment as long as chronic irritation or mechanical stimulation continues. Emollients, keratolytic agents, antipruritic preparations, and occasionally, sedation to lessen the perception of itch in established lesions are effective in certain individuals. Identification and treatment of the underlying condition that could predispose to pruritus are crucial. In particular, chronically dry skin in elderly individuals is a common cause of pruritus, and should be treated with appropriate emollients and protective agents. Ultimately, lesions should slowly regress if the irritant stimulus is completely removed, although persistent induration or nodularity may linger at sites where extensive papillary dermal fibrosis has developed.

## PSORIASIS

**Definition.** *Psoriasis* (-iasis = a condition; psor- = of itching, Greek) is a chronic and relapsing skin disease with variable clinical presentations that share the features of erythema, epidermal thickening, and scale formation. Lesions also present with pustules, which may be generalized or localized. *Psoriatic erythroderma* implies involvement of most or all of the cutaneous surface. There is often a genetic predisposition. Psoriasis may be associated with arthritis (*psoriatic arthritis*). The term "psoriasiform" refers broadly to histopathologic features of lesions in unrelated disorders that share some, but not all, of the clinical and histologic features of psoriasis that are described below. True psoriasis consists of a well-defined evolutionary sequence of histologic changes that generally enable accurate diagnosis. Figure 3-4 presents a time line for the histologic evolution of characteristic psoriasis from early to late established lesions.

The incidence of psoriasis varies. In the United States, approximately 1 percent of the population is affected, but estimates range from less than 1 percent to as high as 2.8 percent in different subgroups. Evidence for genetic susceptibility includes an increased incidence of psoriasis in relatives of patients with this disorder, offspring of a parent with psoriasis, monozygotic twins, and individuals sharing certain major histocompatibility antigens.

**Clinical Features.** In its most classic presentation, the lesions have a characteristic appearance and distribution (25). They are usually sharply demarcated and surmounted by silvery scales. The underlying skin has a homogeneous erythematous appearance. The *Auspitz sign* is a characteristic feature whereby minute bleeding points result from peeling or abrasion of the surface scale of a psoriatic plaque. The *Koebner phenomenon* (26) refers to the development of new psoriatic lesions after repeated trauma to an uninvolved area (figs. 3-5, 3-6). This is believed to be one reason why lesions tend to form on extensor surfaces prone to repetitive low-grade environmental trauma.

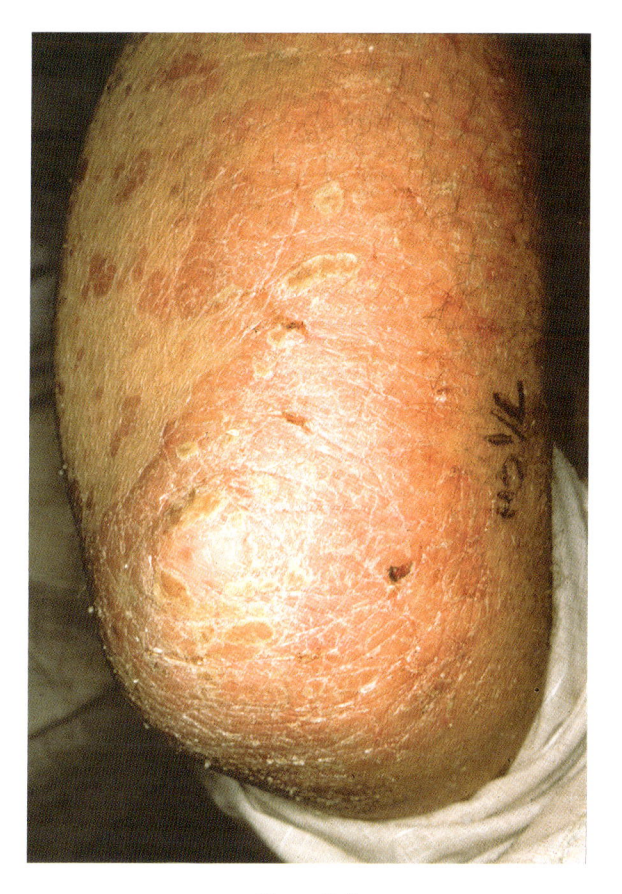

## Acanthotic Dermatitis (Retiform Epidermal Hyperplasia)

Figure 3-5
**ACTIVE PSORIASIS**
The erythematous and scaling plaque preferentially involves extensor skin of forearm and elbow. This lesion occurs at sites of potential trauma, suggesting a role for the Koebner phenomenon at such sites.

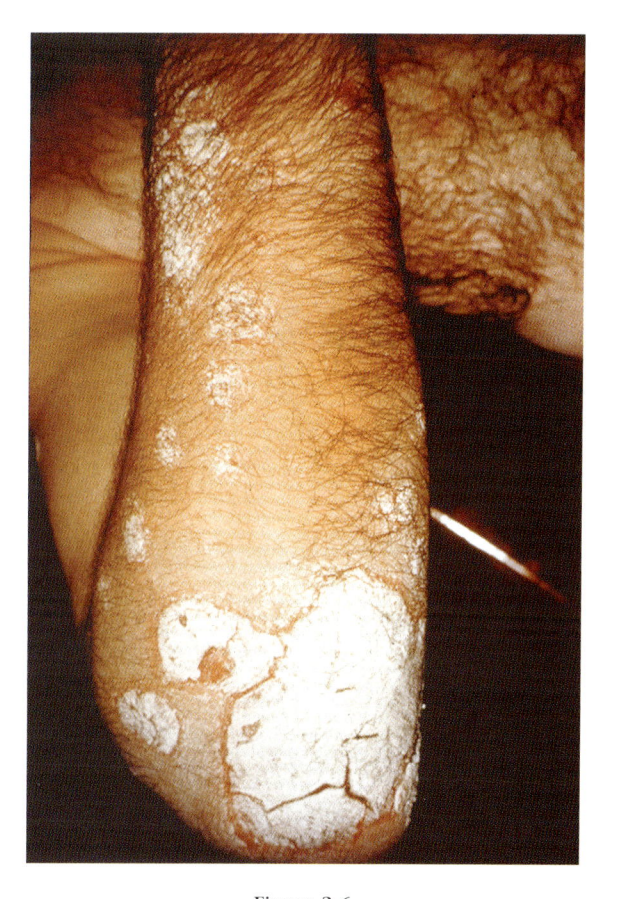

Figure 3-6
**PSORIATIC PLAQUES: ESTABLISHED CHRONIC LESIONS**
The characteristic silvery white scale covers the erythematous plaques. There is preferential involvement of elbow skin as well as skin covering other bony prominences.

Psoriasis has several clinical patterns (27). The most common and characteristic is the chronic stationary type of psoriasis, or *psoriasis vulgaris*. This is characterized by longstanding red, scaly plaques distributed on the elbows, knees, scalp, retroauricular regions, lumbar region, extensor surfaces of the arms and legs, and umbilicus. While the usual lesion is a uniform plaque, plaques may enlarge to produce a circinate or gyrate appearance. There may be central clearing, resulting in so-called *annular psoriasis*. When the disease affects intertriginous skin, there is usually minimal scaling and the erythematous plaques tend to be sharply demarcated with a glossy surface. In children and young adults, *eruptive*, or *guttate*, *psoriasis* may develop (fig. 3-7) (28), often triggered by a preceding streptococcal throat infection (29). The guttate lesions characteristically are 1.0 to 1.5 cm in diameter, and are distributed primarily over the trunk and extremities. Lesions may be surmounted by scale or even by very small pustules that are 1 to 2 mm in diameter. Early eruptive lesions of psoriasis, or certain variants throughout their evolution, may exhibit a prominent pustular component both clinically and histologically (fig. 3-8; discussed further below).

An unusual form of psoriasis is *psoriatic erythroderma* (30) in which total body psoriasis develops, with widespread involvement of the trunk, extremities, hands, feet, nails, and face. It occurs in the setting of chronic psoriasis or develops as a generalized Koebner reaction to certain treatments, such as light therapy or certain drugs (31). Involvement of the palms and soles may produce excessive buildup of keratin

*Inflammatory Disorders of the Skin*

Figure 3-7
GUTTATE PSORIASIS
Multiple erythematous lesions are covered by adherent silvery scale. Rather than forming large plaques, the individual lesions form small leaf-like and coin-like smaller plaques.

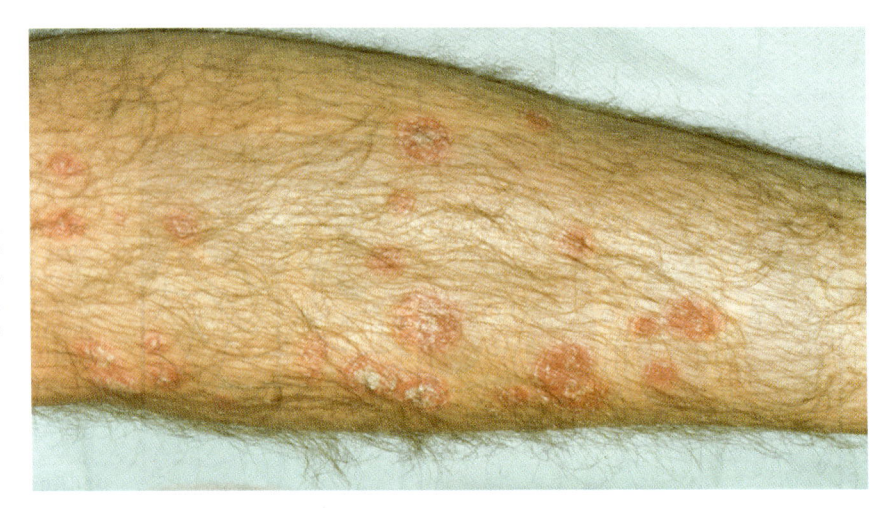

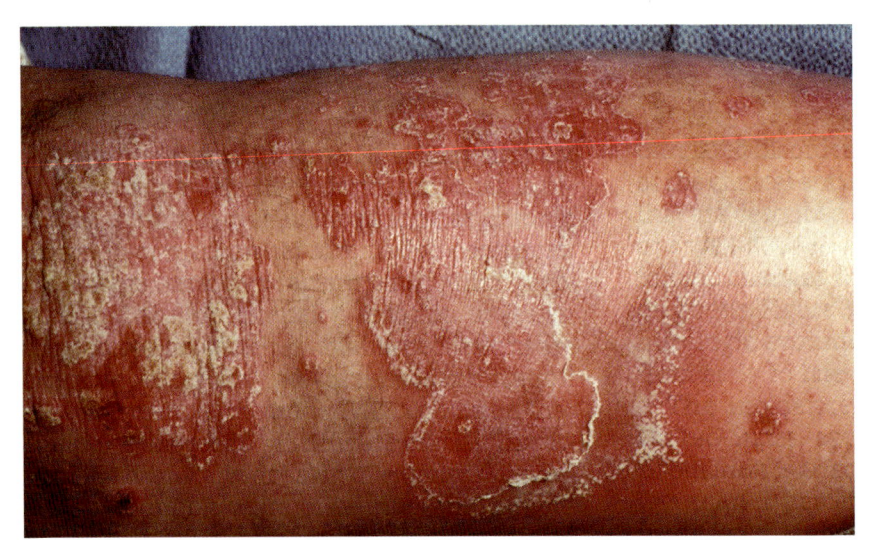

Figure 3-8
ACTIVE PSORIASIS WITH PUSTULAR COMPONENT
These erythematous and scaling plaques are studded with multiple pustules.

scale, resulting in the clinical picture of keratoderma (fig. 3-9). *Nail psoriasis* may show several characteristic alterations: pitting of the nail plate, yellow macules beneath the nail fold that extend distally toward the hyponychium (the "oil drop" change), or striking onychodystrophy with the accumulation of yellow keratinaceous debris beneath the nail (fig. 3-10). Psoriatic involvement of the distal fingers and nails is highly associated with psoriatic arthritis, which ranges from chronic, slowly progressive deformities to fulminant, mutilating disease with features that resemble rheumatoid joint disease.

The clinical differential diagnosis of psoriasis is broad (32). For the chronic plaque type, the differential includes nummular eczema, mycosis fungoides, tinea corporis, seborrheic dermatitis, pityriasis rubra pilaris, and even secondary syphilis. For guttate psoriasis, the clinical differential diagnosis includes pityriasis rosea, pityriasis lichenoides chronica, and secondary syphilis. The main differential diagnostic considerations of erythrodermic psoriasis include atopic dermatitis, drug eruption, generalized contact dermatitis, and Sézary syndrome. The differential diagnosis of psoriasis localized to the scalp and face is seborrheic dermatitis and certain chronic forms of contact allergy. Psoriasis occasionally appears as an isolated plaque on the genitalia, where the differential diagnosis includes Bowen disease, lichen planus, fixed drug eruption, or primary syphilis.

Psoriasis is one of the disorders of the skin that is occasioned by various precipitating factors. The most common of these is infection, specifically streptococcal, although other infections

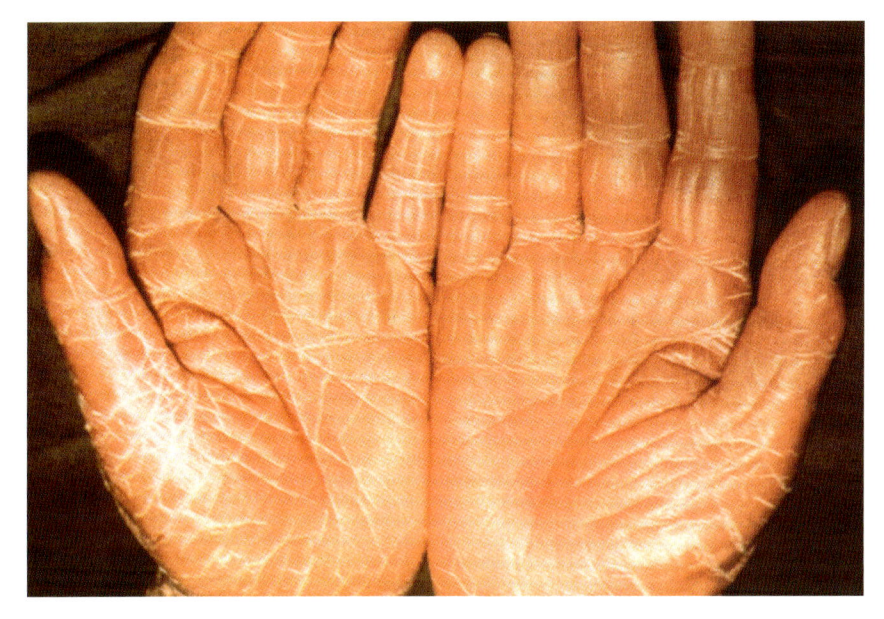

**Figure 3-9**

**PSORIASIS: PALMAR SKIN**

Thickened plaques are associated with erythema, hyperkeratosis, and accentuated skin fold markings.

cause this disorder to erupt. Drug reactions and trauma can incite the Koebner phenomenon. The drugs that are considered in the etiology include lithium, indomethacin, terfenadine, isostreptin, various nonsteroidal anti-inflammatory drugs, and certain beta-blockers.

**Pathologic Findings.** Psoriasis progresses through evolutionary stages and often has periods of exacerbation and resolution. Thus there exists a spectrum of lesions produced in the course of the disease.

The earliest change in psoriasis is focal edema of the papillary dermis, which is associated with a perivenular lymphoid infiltrate, dilatation of vessels variably containing red blood cells and neutrophils, and mild focal spongiosis of the epidermis (fig. 3-11; also see spongiotic dermatitis, chapter 2, for further discussion). This early change is rapidly followed by the migration of neutrophils into the epidermis, persistence of focal spongiosis, and formation of edema resulting in a bulbous appearance of the dermal papillae. The stratum corneum at this juncture usually shows mound-like parakeratotic scale beneath the still visible normal basket-woven orthokeratotic scale. Neutrophils may be present in this mound-like scale. Extravasation of red blood cells is often noted in the epidermis adjacent to the vessels, which now show, in addition to congestion with red blood cells, variable endothelial swelling. Mitoses may be noted in both the basilar and suprabasilar layers

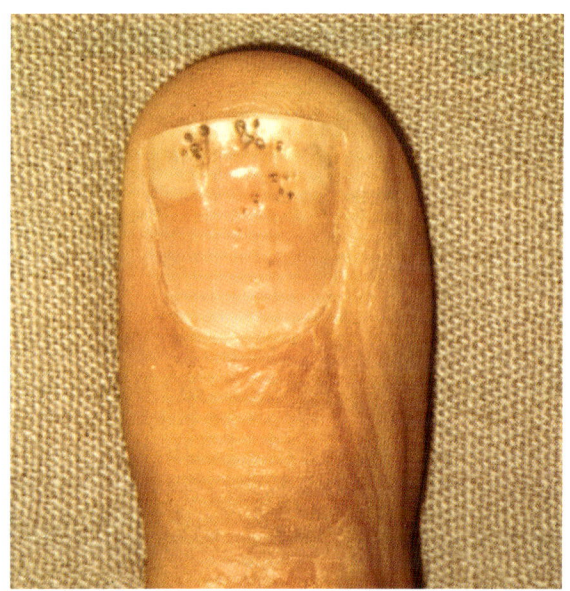

**Figure 3-10**

**PSORIASIS: NAIL INVOLVEMENT**

Multiple pits, as well as zones of thickening and yellow-white discoloration, involve the surface of the nail.

of the epidermis. The presence of mitoses in one to three layers of keratinocytes above the basal layer is very characteristic of the early guttate and early plaque stages of the disease. Other dermatoses do not exhibit this change, which is also shared by neoplastic squamous cell lesions. This type of change may be observed in all stages of guttate psoriasis, or in the earliest

**Figure 3-11**

**EARLY EVOLUTIONARY STAGE OF PSORIASIS**

There is mild acanthosis, although the typical regular elongation of rete ridges has yet to develop. An important diagnostic clue lies in the superficial blood vessels and capillaries within the dermal papillae, which already appeared dilated and tortuous.

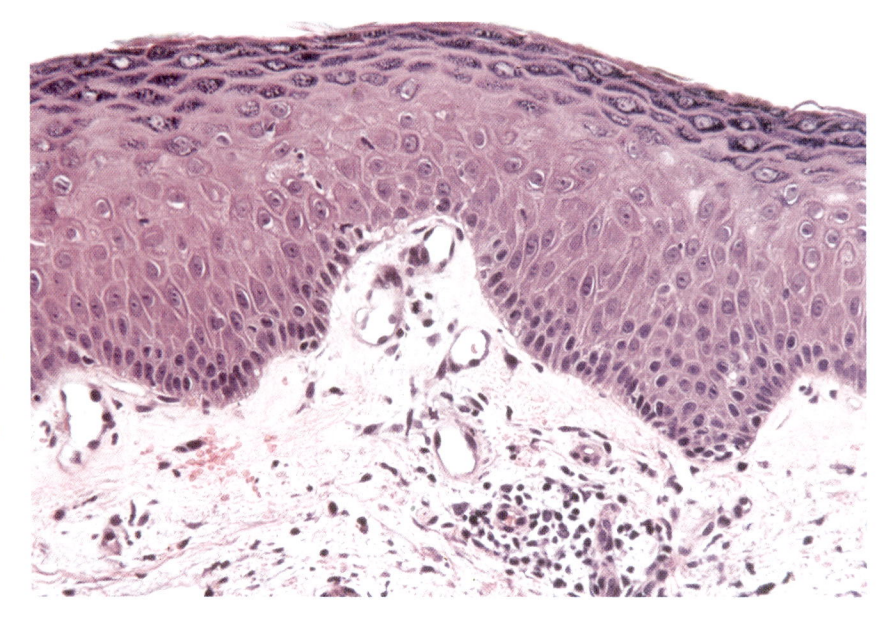

phase of the development of chronic plaque-like lesions.

The early plaque of psoriasis is characterized by well-demarcated epidermal hyperplasia with retention of the rete ridge pattern. The epidermal hyperplasia is often prominent, and the tips of the rete ridges continue to develop a bulbous or clubbed appearance. The pattern of retiform epidermal hyperplasia is striking, and one can virtually draw a straight horizontal line through the tips of the rete at scanning magnification. In addition, there are mounds of parakeratosis usually containing compressed and distorted neutrophils as well as developing regions of confluent parakeratosis. In some lesions, there may be diffuse parakeratoses at this stage. The granular cell layer is absent in the areas of parakeratosis. Intracorneal collections of neutrophils are known as *Munro microabscesses*. Their underlying precursors are small aggregates of neutrophils associated with mild spongiosis and keratinocyte degeneration within the spinous layer. These are referred to as *spongiform pustules of Kogoj*. There are often admixed lymphocytes and occasional Langerhans cells in these pustules as well, although true Langerhans cell microgranulomas tend not to form. The suprapapillary epidermal plates over the bulbous papillae are thin and exaggerate the pattern of rete hyperplasia. In the dermis, there is an often striking inflammatory infiltrate composed primarily of mononuclear cells and neutrophils. The capillaries within the dermal papillae are dilated and tortuous, and there may be hypertrophy of some of the endothelial cells. Neutrophils may migrate from the papillary dermis into the epidermis toward the mound-like parakeratotic scales and the pustules.

The established plaque of psoriasis shows again prominent and regular retiform epidermal hyperplasia (fig. 3-12). Now, however, there is prominent club-shaped thickening of the lower rete pegs, often with the appearance of prominent coalescence or bridging in histologic profiles. The bulbous dermal papillae persist, contain considerably fewer inflammatory cells, and retain prominent tortuous and ectatic vessels. Areas of parakeratosis are associated with diminution in the granular cell layer. Multiple levels often reveal areas of parakeratosis and even very small Munro microabscesses as evidence of persistent inflammatory activity in these chronic and established plaques (figs. 3-13–3-17).

The first change to occur in treated psoriasis is the reappearance of the granular cell layer in the psoriatic plaque (fig. 3-18). If the treatment has involved ultraviolet light, apoptotic or dyskeratotic cells are frequently present in the psoriatic epidermis. There is also a diminution in the inflammatory infiltrate.

Agents in topical medications, such as paraben, may elicit contact hypersensitivity in patients with psoriasis. Such lesions show a granular cell layer, focal spongiosis, and

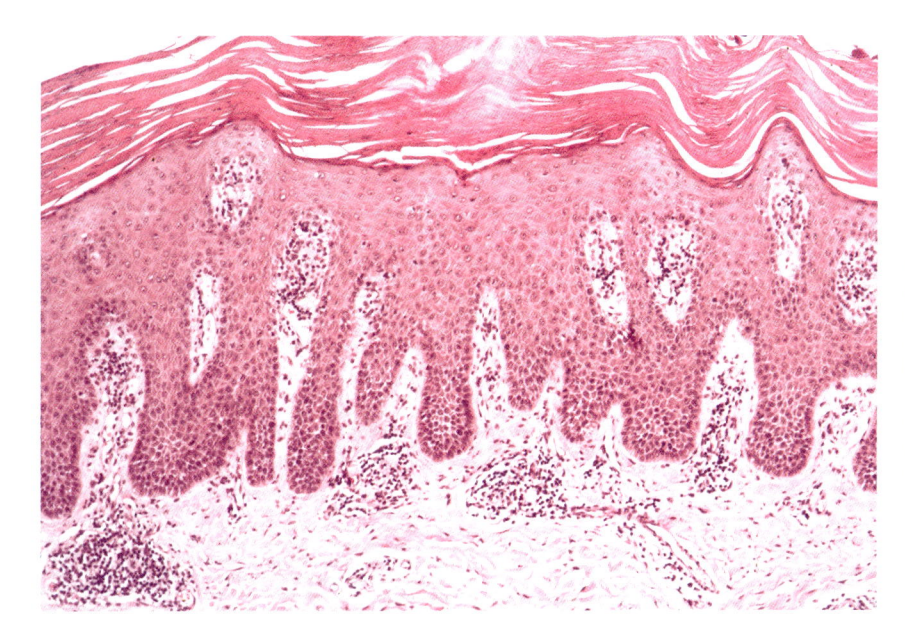

## Figure 3-12
### ESTABLISHED PSORIATIC PLAQUE
Regular acanthosis of rete ridges (retiform epidermal hyperplasia), diffuse absence of stratum granulosum, and markedly thickened scale showing foci of plate-like parakeratosis are present. There is a superficial perivascular inflammatory infiltrate composed predominantly of lymphocytes, but also with admixed neutrophils.

occasional eosinophils, but the other characteristic architectural features of psoriasis, are usually present. In resolved lesions of psoriasis, which clinically appear as either slightly erythematous and slightly scaly to normal-appearing skin, expanded and prominent dermal papillae with ectasia of vessels and deformity of rete ridges are evidence of the antecedent changes of the psoriatic lesion. Otherwise the epidermis is normal.

**Clinicopathologic Variants.** These are described at the end of the section on psoriasis.

**Pathogenesis.** Psoriasis is an example of markedly controlled and chronically localized inflammation and associated proliferation confined to the epidermis and the underlying papillary dermis. It now appears that several mechanisms play a role in lesion production. First, immunologically activated T cells and Langerhans cells are present in the epidermis and superficial dermis, implying an immune mechanism (38). Second, increased proliferation of keratinocytes suggests a role for the altered regulation of normal epidermal kinetics (39). Third, superficial dermal vessels may be abnormally stimulated, raising the possibility of endothelial pathology in lesion formation (40). Finally, genetic factors are implicated due to the heritable nature of psoriasis and its relationship to human leukocyte antigen (HLA) histocompatibility markers.

The role of immune cells in the pathogenesis of psoriasis is emphasized by experiments in

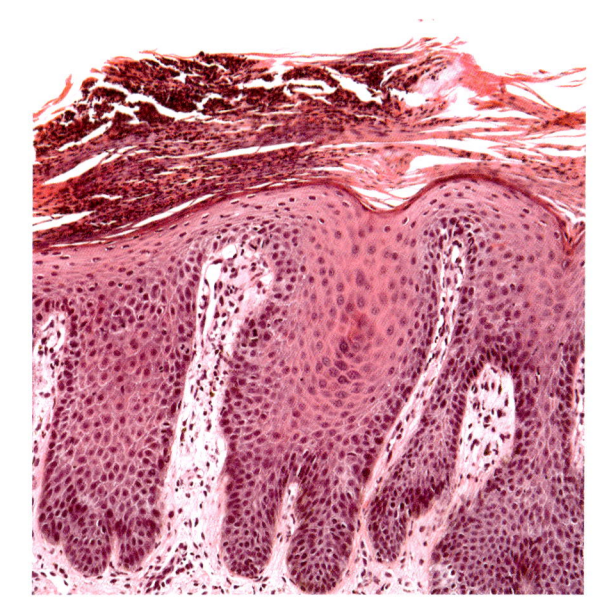

## Figure 3-13
### EARLY PSORIASIS
Note acanthosis, thinning of the stratum granulosum, and prominent ("squirting") dermal papilla containg neutrophils and erythrocytes.

which lesions are reproduced in xenografts of normal skin from psoriatics after intradermal injection of autologous lymphocytes (5). Dysregulated wound healing responses via production of nitric oxide and epidermal growth factor by Langerhans cells have been suggested as a trigger for lesion formation in predisposed individuals

*Inflammatory Disorders of the Skin*

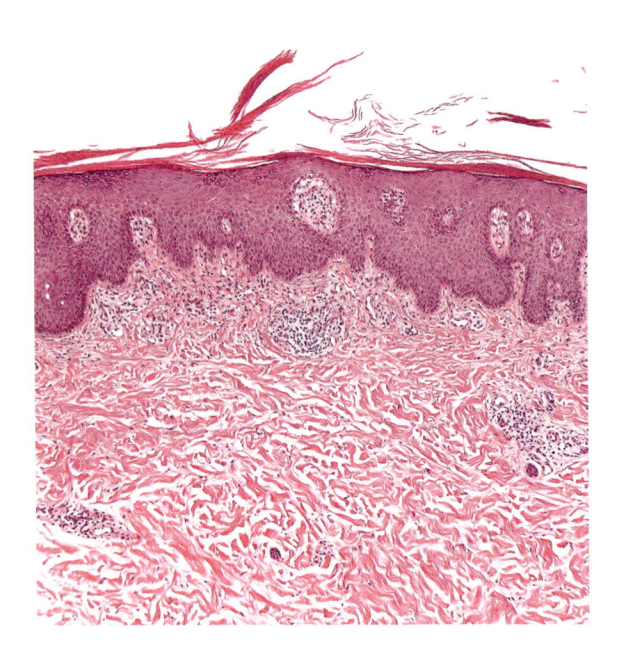

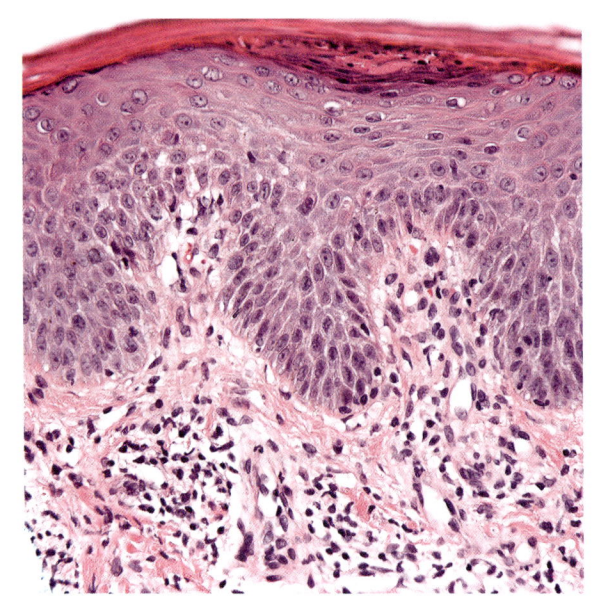

**Figure 3-14**

**GUTTATE PSORIASIS**

Left: At scanning magnification, the psoriasiform thickening of the epidermal layer is associated with forming layers of parakeratosis that focally are mound-like and "lift off" the epidermal surface.

Right: At higher magnification, parakeratosis and neutrophils are associated with a zone of hypogranulosis.

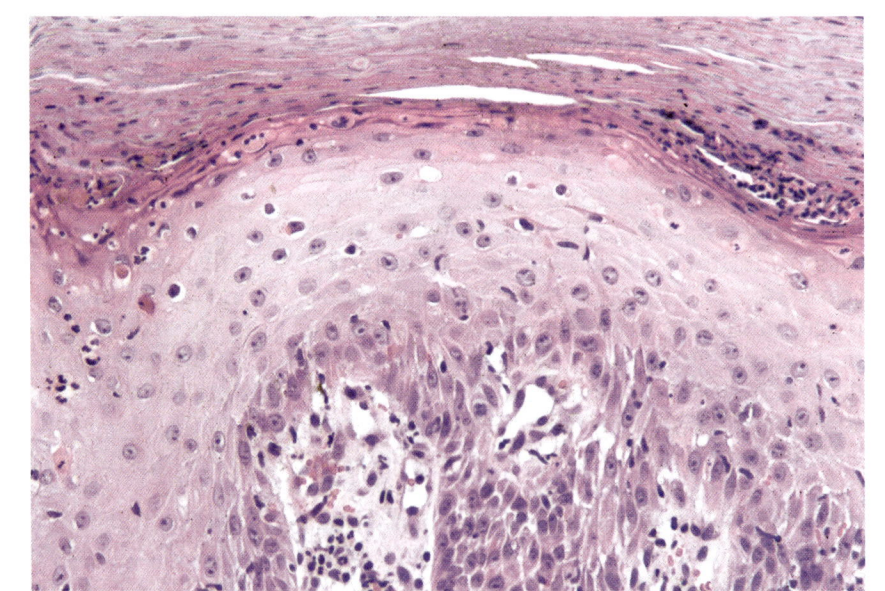

**Figure 3-15**

**ACTIVE PSORIASIS**

The dilated and ectopic vessels within dermal papillae are readily apparent, as well as the absence of stratum granulosum. Neutrophils collect within the uppermost epidermal layers and within the parakeratotic scale.

(41). Such immune factors appear to collaborate with altered epidermal proliferation, differentiation, and cytokine responsiveness to produce clinical lesions. Compelling evidence links some psoriatic flares with emotional stress, implicating immunomodulatory neuropeptides in the pathogenesis (42,43). It remains controversial, however, as to whether immune factors or epidermal proliferative defects represent the primary event in the formation of psoriatic plaques.

Genetically, psoriasis is most commonly associated with the HLA-Cw6 antigenic type (44–46). Other HLA-associated types include HLA-B13, -B17, and -Bw57. Linkage of HLA

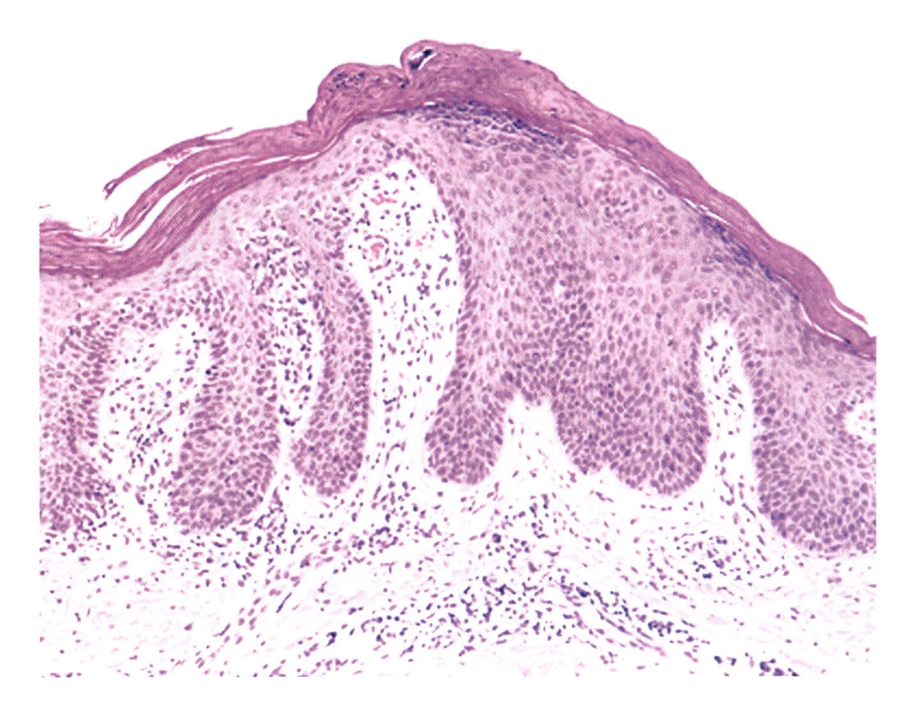

## Acanthotic Dermatitis (Retiform Epidermal Hyperplasia)

### Figure 3-16
### ESTABLISHED PLAQUE OF PSORIASIS SHOWING SCALE PATTERN

The scale is plate-like, parakeratotic, and infiltrated by neutrophils. The dermal papillae contain dilated vessels, and the suprapapillary plate is attenuated.

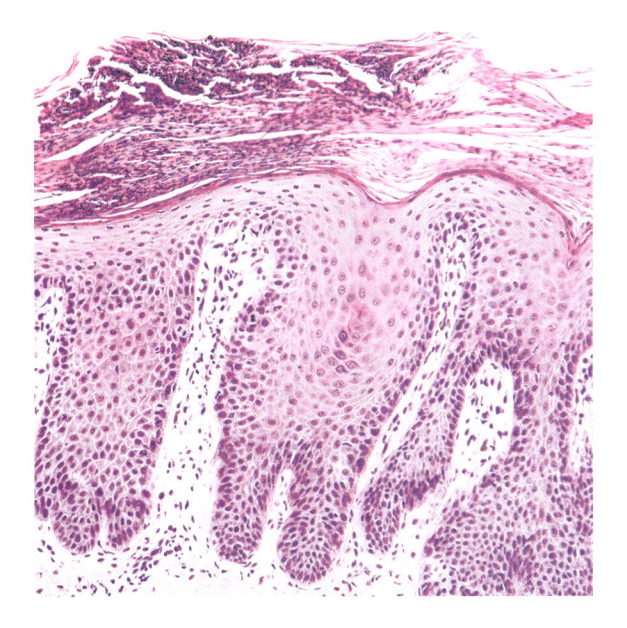

### Figure 3-17
### ESTABLISHED PSORIATIC PLAQUE

Above: Psoriatic scale of an active lesion showing marked accumulation of neutrophils in foci of parakeratosis. Also seen are absence of stratum granulosum, thinning of the suprapapillary plate, and prominent capillary loops.

Right: At higher magnification, the parakeratotic scale infiltrated by neutrophils to form Munro microabscesses, and the attenuated suprapapillary plate that separates this scale from the markedly dilated vessels within the expanded dermal papillae, are easily seen.

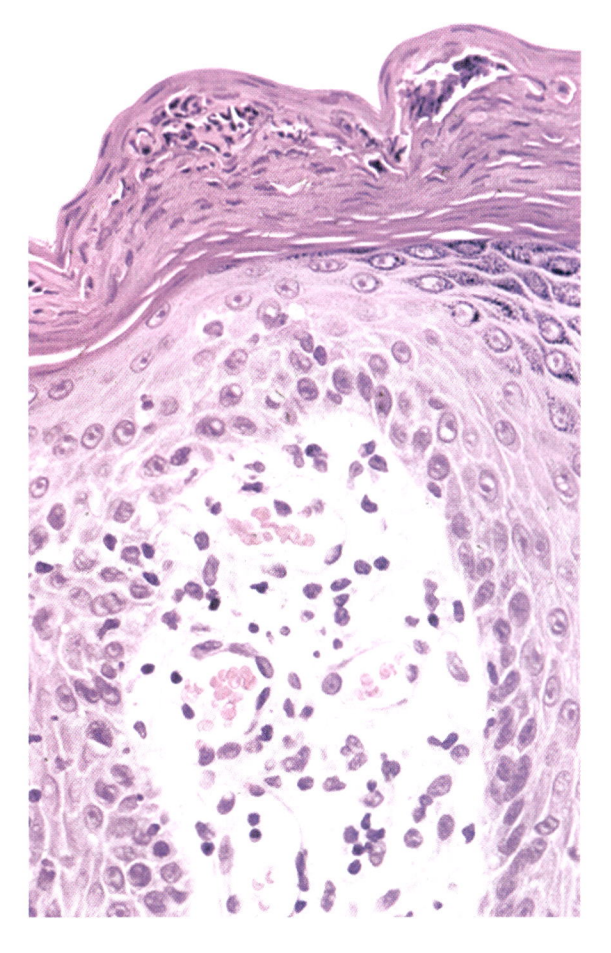

*Inflammatory Disorders of the Skin*

**Figure 3-18**
**PSORIASIS, PARTIALLY TREATED**
The stratum granulosum has begun to return in response to therapy. Scattered suprabasal mitoses (arrow) and underlying vascular changes (not represented), however, generally persist despite the confounding effect of partial treatment.

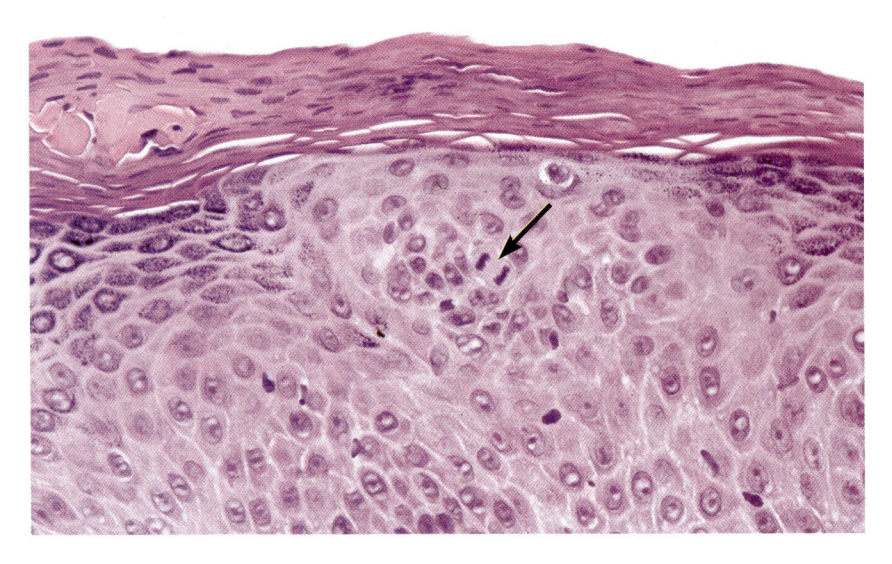

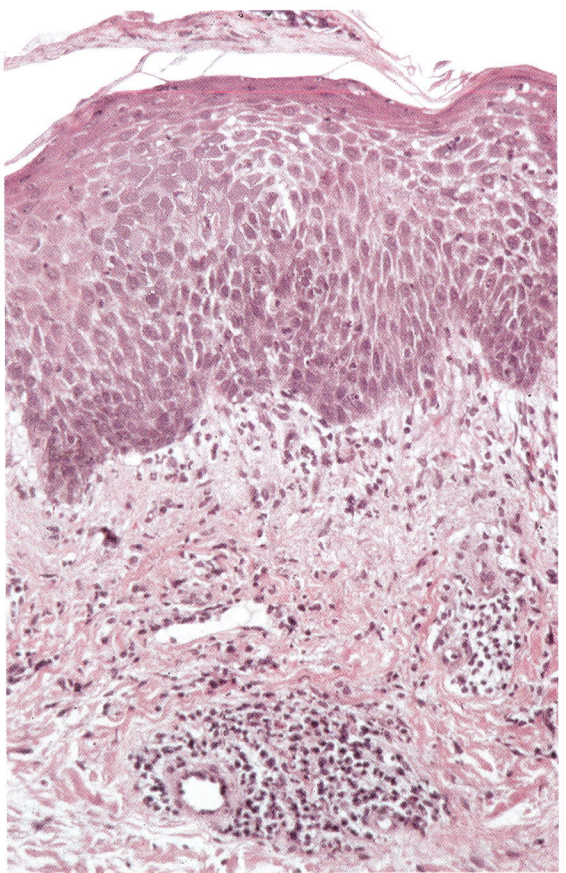

**Figure 3-19**
**PSORIASIFORM DRUG ERUPTION**
While there are parakeratosis, focal hypogranulosis, and epidermal acanthosis, the underlying perivascular lymphocytic infiltrate also contains eosinophils, an important clue to the underlying cause.

antigens with specific patterns of psoriasis has been described. Guttate psoriasis is associated with HLA-Cw6 and -B17. HLA-B13 is associated with antecedent streptococcal infections, a predisposing factor in some patients with psoriasis. HLA-B27 is associated with psoriatic arthritis.

**Differential Diagnosis.** The primary histologic differential diagnostic consideration in psoriasis is chronic eczematous dermatitis. This simulant is identified by spongiosis, the presence of an often thickened granular cell layer, presence of occasional eosinophils in the inflammatory component, and zones of parakeratosis and hyperorthokeratosis. Pustules are not present, although superinfected eczema may show subcorneal pustules as a consequence of impetiginization.

Psoriasiform drug eruptions occasionally mimic true psoriasis both clinically and histologically (fig. 3-19). The involvement of deep as well as superficial dermal vessels by the inflammatory infiltrate, the presence of occasional eosinophils, and the persistence of mild spongiosis despite chronicity separate such lesions from true psoriasis.

Lichen simplex chronicus can be differentiated from psoriasis by both epidermal and dermal alterations. There is usually quite striking dense hypergranulosis and irregular rete ridge hyperplasia rather than the regular rete ridge hyperplasia of psoriasis. Primary pustules and Munro microabscesses are not seen. Furthermore, in the dermis, there is a pattern of fibrous thickening with vertical streaking of collagen fibers as a result of repeated trauma and fibrous entrapment of the superficial venular plexus. These findings are not observed in classic psoriasis.

Pityriasis rubra pilaris shows variable psoriasiform hyperplasia, with a characteristic pattern of parakeratosis in the stratum corneum. This pattern includes vertically oriented parakeratotic scales often admixed with horizontally oriented alternating parakeratotic scales without loss of the granular cell layer. Often "shoulder parakeratosis" at the ostia of follicular epithelium is observed in pityriasis rubra pilaris. Pustular psoriasis can be differentiated on the basis of the prominent spongiform pustulation, which forms lakes of pus rather than the small pustules of Kogoj observed in classic psoriasis. Certain lesions of seborrheic dermatitis may show significant overlap with psoriasis, and accordingly the term *sebopsoriasis* has been used to denote this clinicopathologic entity.

**Treatment and Prognosis.** Psoriasis is a chronic disease that, although variably responsive to therapy, often recurs or fails to completely clear. Immunosuppressive agents, including corticosteroids and coal tar preparations, are the mainstay of topical therapy (47). In severe cases, systemic administration of methotrexate or cyclosporin A has proven effective. Complete clearing, even after treatment has ceased, is occasionally observed with PUVA (psoralen and ultraviolet light A) therapy. Topical immunomodulators are useful as steroid-sparing agents. Oral retinoids, such as acitretin, are helpful in managing extensive psoriasis, and have particularly imparted a beneficial effect in the acute treatment of erythrodermic psoriasis. Biologic therapy has been instrumental in reducing disease burden, particularly associated seronegative arthritis in the presence or absence of psoriatic skin disease.

## Reiter Disease

*Reiter disease,* a clinicopathologic variant of psoriasis, is a tripartite symptom complex that includes aseptic arthritis, enteritis, and urethritis, the latter usually caused by an infectious agent (33). Young men are commonly affected by this illness, which is episodic and often followed by recovery. In some instances, however, permanent arthritic changes result. About 50 percent of patients have cutaneous lesions. These lesions have a predilection for the palms and soles, subungual areas, and the glans penis. On the glans penis the lesion is described as *balanitis circinata,* and on the palms and soles is termed *keratoderma blennorrhagicum*. On the penises of uncircumcised men, lesions generally present in a serpiginous pattern formed by crusted erosions. In circumcised men, lesions usually are formed by an array of coalescent erythematous papules. The lesions on the palms and soles are often striking and consist of markedly hyperkeratotic excrescences. These may be associated with pustules, and the combination of pustules and hyperkeratosis is the essential component of keratoderma blennorrhagicum.

The infectious agents that have been associated with Reiter disease are usually *Chlamydia trichomonas, Ureaplasma urealyticum, Campylobacter cusidia,* and *Salmonella*. Approximately 50 percent of patients who have Reiter disease have had *Chlamydia trichomonas* cultured from their urethra. Although joint cultures are sterile for bacteria, *Chlamydia* RNA has been described in synovial specimens.

Disequilibrium in patients with Reiter disease has been found in the major histocompatability antigens, specifically HLA-B27. The arthritis of Reiter disease is similar to psoriatic arthritis clinically, and thus resembles rheumatoid joint disease. In neither case, however, is the rheumatoid factor positive.

In early lesions of keratoderma blennorrhagicum, small spongiform pustules are observed in the upper epidermis. With progression of the lesions, there is striking parakeratosis and hyperkeratosis, with a prominent admixture of neutrophils and cellular debris in the parakeratotic scale. Large spongiform pustules are associated with regular retiform epidermal hyperplasia that resembles psoriasis vulgaris. In late lesions, spongiform pustules disappear, but retiform epidermal hyperplasia resembling psoriasis persists. The changes of balanitis circinata include small spongiform pustules and Munro microabscesses in association with psoriasiform epidermal hyperplasia.

## Pustular Psoriasis

*Pustular psoriasis,* another clinicopathologic variant of psoriasis, is either generalized or diffuse, or localized (34). The generalized forms are acute generalized pustular psoriasis or the so-called Von Zumbusch type, generalized pustular psoriasis of pregnancy, so-called impetigo herpetiformis, infantile and juvenile pustular psoriasis, and the annular or circinate group of pustular psoriasis.

The cutaneous eruption of acute generalized pustular psoriasis is usually associated with a fever preceding and continuing throughout the episode, with the abrupt onset of tiny, pinpoint, 1- to 2-mm pustules that are scattered over the trunk, extremities, and palms and soles. The pustular psoriasis of pregnancy occurs during the last trimester and is usually associated with the appearance of psoriasis in flexural areas associated with a generalized pustular eruption. The annular or circinate type of psoriasis may be generalized or localized. When localized, it is difficult to differentiate from subcorneal pustular dermatosis. It consists of a circinate or annular distribution of pustules. The juvenile or infantile type is a rare form of pustular psoriasis in children that is associated often with spontaneous remission.

*Localized pustular psoriasis* may occur with established psoriasis, and is characterized by psoriatic plaques and scattered localized pustules. More commonly, however, the so-called localized acrodermatitis continuo of Hallopeau often evolves into a generalized disorder. Pustular psoriasis of the palms and soles includes the variants of *pustulosis palmaris et plantaris* and *acute palmar plantar pustulosis* or *pustular bacterid*.

*Acrodermatitis continua of Hallopeau* is a pustular eruption involving the distal portions of the hands and feet. These may be the only areas affected and may be limited to one digit. When the generalized type evolves, large areas of the skin may be involved in addition to the extremities. *Pustulosis palmaris et plantaris* is a chronic disorder affecting either the palms or soles, or both. Crops of deeply seated pustules are accompanied by erythema and prominent scaling. Early on, the lesions may resemble dyshidrotic eczema, appearing as vesicles that may become pustular. The most common sites of involvement are the thenar eminence, heels, insteps of the feet, and palms.

In the generalized forms of pustular psoriasis, pustules appear to evolve in the same manner as the classic pustule derived from the spongiform pustule of Kogoj. Such pustules are formed as a consequence of migration of neutrophils into the epidermis which come to occupy spaces produced by the degeneration of keratinocytes. These micropustules are bordered by thinned epidermal cells, which surround the former areas of keratinocyte degeneration. In pustular psoriasis, however, the pustules increase in size to form large "lakes" of subcorneal neutrophils (fig. 3-20). At the periphery of such lakes, the characteristic spongiform pustular changes typical of this disorder is observed. These changes are observed in association with exocytosis of neutrophils into the stratum corneum, where large Munro microabscesses appear. This feature is associated with loss of the granular cell layer and other changes of psoriasis described above, including elongation of the rete ridges, clubbing of the rete, and formation of bulbous dermal papillae. As pustular psoriasis resolves, changes similar to those associated with the plaques of classic, nonpustular psoriasis appear.

In the localized forms, similar histologic alterations are observed, as is the case in digital skin in acrodermatitis continua of Hallopeau. In this variant, however, the nail bed is also involved, with striking formation of pustules, epidermal hyperplasia, and mounds of parakeratosis with entrapped neutrophils. Only rarely is the nail matrix involved. In pustulosis palmaris et plantaris, a striking unilocular pustule is found in the epidermis. This pustule is usually discretely marginated at its periphery, with characteristic rounding off of keratinocytes. Careful inspection, however, generally reveals small spongiform pustules at the periphery of the lake of pus.

### Follicular Psoriasis

*Follicular psoriasis*, another variation of psoriasis, shows marked follicular plugging, often with striking regions of confluent parakeratosis that extend to the middle of the follicular ostium. This diffuse parakeratosis may be associated with pustules and Munro microabscesses. Shoulder parakeratosis at the edges of the follicular ostium is not observed. Rather, diffuse parakeratosis involving the edges and extending down along the ostium is generally encountered. There is also a mild perivenular inflammatory infiltrate.

### Erythrodermic Psoriasis

When diagnostic, *erythrodermic psoriasis* (35) is characterized by early plaques of psoriasis

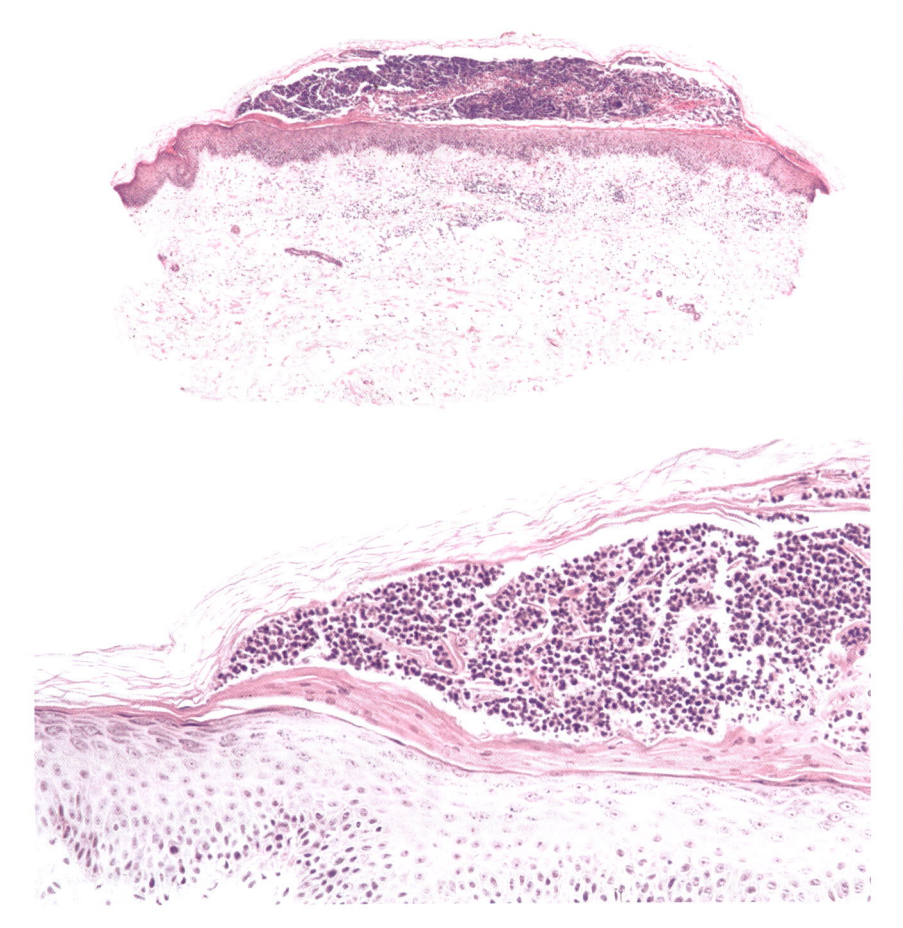

**Figure 3-20**

**PUSTULAR PSORIASIS**

Top: At scanning magnification, a prominent subcorneal pustule is seen. While the epidermis shows diffuse acanthosis, the characteristic diagnostic changes of psoriasis are lacking in this acute lesion.

Bottom: At higher magnification, the well-formed intracorneal pustule as well as the underlying epidermal acanthosis and parakeratosis are seen.

with prominent papillary dermal vascularity, focal parakeratosis, and loss of the granular cell layer. Occasionally the changes are nonspecific, however, consisting of mild epidermal hyperplasia with a slight perivenular lymphoid infiltrate. The skin of the patient should be palpated to detect any evidence of thickening. Biopsies should be obtained from such sites, which usually are representative of residual plaques of psoriasis in the erythrodermic patient. Eosinophils are observed in the infiltrate of this variant of psoriasis. The presence of eosinophils should suggest either a lesion of psoriasis with a superimposed contact dermatitis or erythrodermic drug-induced psoriasis (see below).

### Psoriasis and Acquired Immunodeficiency Syndrome (AIDS)

Patients with AIDS may develop cutaneous changes characteristic of psoriasis (36,37), with an incidence that is higher than that of the general population. Histologically, epidermal hyperplasia, bulbous dermal papillae with overlying parakeratosis, and loss of the granular cell layer occur, but there may be foci of spongiosis, apoptotic cells or necrotic keratinocytes, and plasma cells in the lymphohistiocytic infiltrate.

### PITYRIASIS RUBRA PILARIS

**Definition.** *Pityriasis rubra pilaris*, as the name implies, is a dermatitis involving perifollicular erythema and follicular hyperkeratosis (48). Upon confluence, pityriasis rubra pilaris may result in extensive involvement of the body surface by erythematous plaques.

**Clinical Features.** Pityriasis rubra pilaris affects both children and adults, and the disease is usually self-limiting. In all age groups, the lesions appear as erythematous follicular papules or large erythematous plaques containing sharply demarcated, normal-appearing islands of skin (fig. 3-21). Children may develop a form characterized primarily by erythematous and hyperkeratotic follicular papules (fig. 3-22) and

*Inflammatory Disorders of the Skin*

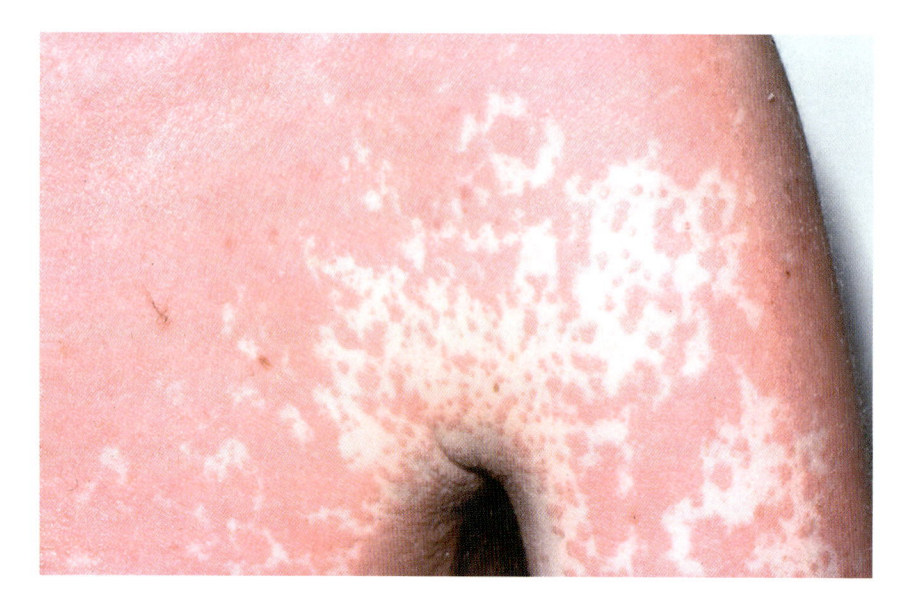

**Figure 3-21**

PITYRIASIS RUBRA PILARIS

Characteristic zones of erythema with sharply demarcated areas (islands) of sparing are typical of this disorder clinically.

**Figure 3-22**

PITYRIASIS RUBRA PILARIS: FOLLICULAR INVOLVEMENT

Multiple erythematous punctate zones represent involvement of individual follicular infundibula.

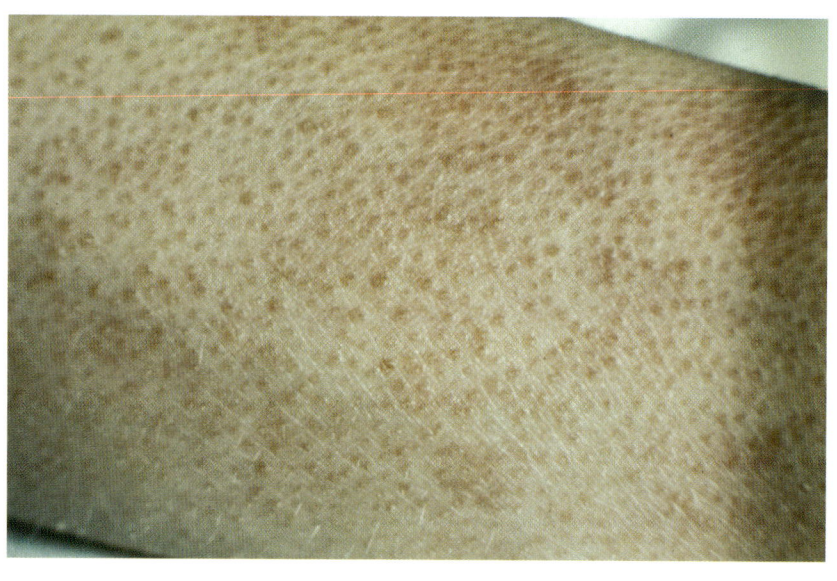

well-defined zones of erythema preferentially affecting the knees and elbows. Pityriasis rubra pilaris, along with dermatitides such as psoriasis and seborrheic dermatitis, is a cause of erythroderma in certain individuals.

**Pathologic Findings.** The histopathology of pityriasis rubra pilaris is subtle yet characteristic (49). There is slightly irregular acanthosis involving the interfollicular epidermis, with zones of parakeratosis and orthokeratosis that may initially resemble evolving psoriasis. The abnormal scale in pityriasis rubra pilaris typically shows focal parakeratosis and compact orthokeratosis that alternate with basket-weave patterns of orthokeratosis, both along a horizontal (parallel to the epidermis) and vertical (perpendicular to the epidermis) axis (fig. 3-23). Multiple biopsy levels may be necessary, however, to demonstrate these features. A superficial perivascular lymphoid infiltrate is generally present in the papillary dermis, which does not contain the dilated and tortuous capillary loops so typical of true psoriasis. Involved hair follicles show orthokeratotic plugging involving the infundibulum, and often there are discrete mound-like "shoulders" of parakeratosis at the site where the epidermis interfaces with the infundibular ostium, called "shoulder parakeratosis." A variant form which may show focal acantholysis has recently been recognized (50).

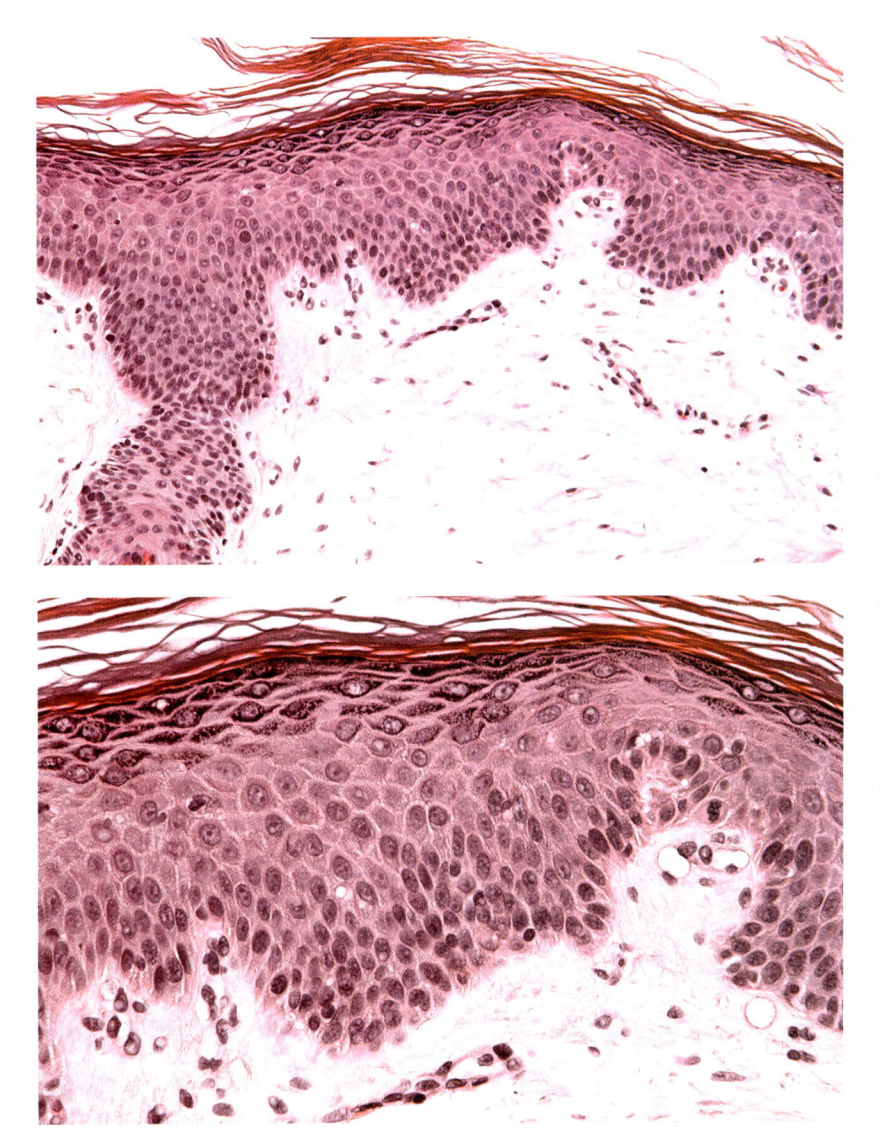

## Figure 3-23
**PITYRIASIS RUBRA PILARIS**

Top: At medium magnification, the abnormal scale shows alternating zones of parakeratosis and laminated orthokeratosis. The parakeratotic scale often is more prominent at the "shoulders" of follicular infundibula, as seen here. Note the keratotic infundibular plug as well.

Bottom: At high magnification, the zones of alternating compacted orthokeratosis are juxtaposed with regions of normal basket-weave stratum corneum.

Although the precise cause of pityriasis rubra pilaris remains to be elucidated, it appears to involve disordered and potentially aberrant epidermal differentiation. For example, lesional skin has been shown to express certain cytokeratin molecules that are not seen in normal skin (K6 and K16) (50a). A genetic diathesis may play a role in some patients, as evidenced by a familial form of the disease that is inherited in an autosomal dominant pattern (51).

**Differential Diagnosis.** The differential diagnosis of pityriasis rubra pilaris includes early or partially treated psoriasis and early primary irritant dermatitis evolving in the direction of lichen simplex chronicus. Because pityriasis rubra pilaris does not contain neutrophils or express capillary loop abnormalities within dermal papillae, distinction from psoriasis is usually not problematic. Early lichen simplex chronicus tends to show hypergranulosis and is relatively devoid of well-developed alternating regions of parakeratosis. Over time, lichen simplex chronicus is characterized by vertically oriented fibrosis within dermal papillae. These alterations are not typical of pityriasis rubra pilaris.

**Treatment and Prognosis.** As with similar forms of psoriasiform dermatitis, topical steroids have proven successful. This is most commonly observed in localized variants of the disease. If left untreated, the disorder may spontaneously clear within several years, or may persist until adolescence, in the case of certain juvenile

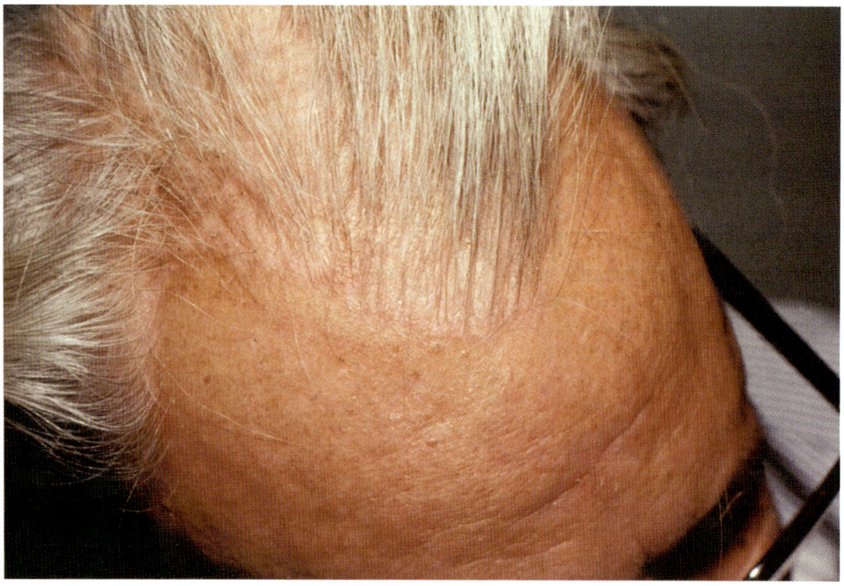

**Figure 3-24**

**SEBORRHEIC DERMATITIS**

Subtle erythema and scaling involve the skin of the scalp, particularly the hair-bearing areas.

forms of the disease. PUVA therapy is successful in some patients, as are oral retinoids. The successful use of biological therapies has also been reported, mostly as case reports (51a).

## CHRONIC SEBORRHEIC DERMATITIS

**Definition.** *Seborrheic dermatitis* is a common, poorly understood disorder resulting in erythematous patches and plaques covered by tan-yellow, oily scales. *Sebopsoriasis* (see below) is a clinical and histologic variant of seborrheic dermatitis in which lesions possess features hybrid between those of seborrheic dermatitis and psoriasis.

**Clinical Features.** Seborrheic dermatitis affects individuals of any age. In adults, the lesions generally consist of erythematous patches and plaques covered by oily yellow scales and occasionally by scale crust (fig. 3-24). Areas preferentially involved include the scalp (a common manifestation of "dandruff"), nasolabial folds, eyebrows, periauricular regions, central chest, and inguinal folds. Lesions may be asymptomatic or mildly pruritic. In infants, generalized erythema and scaling may be seen, giving rise to consideration of more potentially life-threatening conditions, such as Langerhans cell histiocytosis. In patients with AIDS, facial involvement in the nasolabial folds and cheeks may be so severe that the butterfly exanthem of lupus erythematosus may be considered clinically.

**Pathologic Findings.** The histologic findings in chronic seborrheic dermatitis are often subtle. In early lesions, there is edema within the papillary dermis associated with a variable infiltrate of lymphocytes and neutrophils about superficial dermal venules. The epidermis may show focal spongiosis associated with scattered intraepidermal neutrophils, and accordingly, this evolutionary phase can be alternatively considered under the category of spongiotic dermatitis (see chapter 2). There is generally parakeratosis, which occasionally is most prominent in the vicinity of follicular ostia. This form of shoulder parakeratosis includes also neutrophilic debris. Neutrophils thus may be found not only in the superficial dermis, but also in the epidermis and in association with parakeratotic foci within the stratum corneum.

With chronicity, acanthosis supervenes and may dominate the histologic picture (fig. 3-25). Although somewhat irregular, the acanthotic epidermis may mimic that of evolving psoriasis. This, coupled with the persistence of neutrophils in the inflammatory infiltrate and the scale of seborrheic dermatitis, may lead to diagnostic confusion. The absence of hypogranulosis, tortuous and dilated papillary dermal capillary loops, true spongiform pustules, or Munro microabscesses in seborrheic dermatitis is helpful.

**Clinicopathologic Variants.** *Sebopsoriasis.* Unlike chronic seborrheic dermatitis, sebopsoriasis may closely recapitulate the epidermal

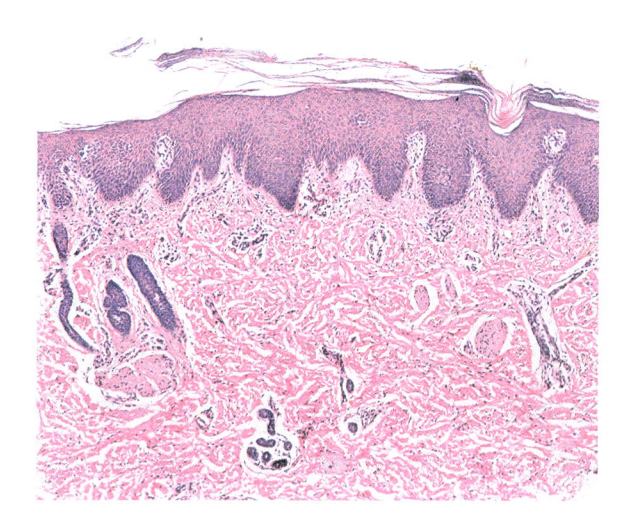

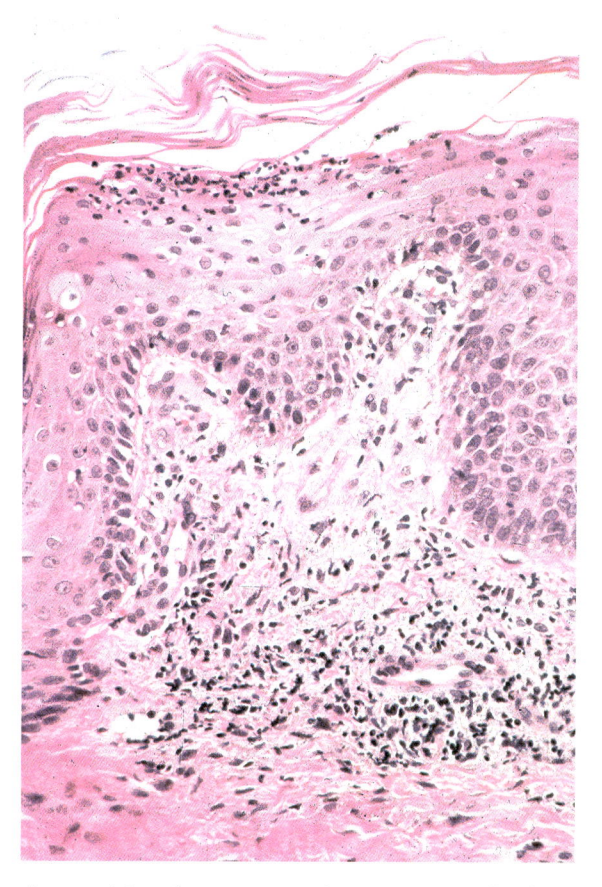

## Acanthotic Dermatitis (Retiform Epidermal Hyperplasia)

**Figure 3-25**

**SEBORRHEIC DERMATITIS**

Above: At scanning magnification, irregular epidermal hyperplasia with focal psoriasiform architecture and multiple foci of abnormal scale formation are seen. The inflammatory infiltrate is largely superficial and perivascular.

Right: At higher magnification, the dermal infiltrate consists of lymphocytes with admixed neutrophils. The epidermis shows irregular acanthosis with features that overlap with psoriasis. Occasional neutrophils are detected in the hyperkeratotic and parakeratotic scale.

architecture and inflammatory alterations observed in true psoriasis. Intracorneal neutrophilic microabscesses are generally not prominent in sebopsoriasis, however, and papillary dermal vessels are not as tortuous or ectatic. The distinction may be extremely problematic, however, both clinically and histologically. Indeed, it is possible that sebopsoriasis represents one of several true hybrid dermatoses, such as also observed in the lichen planus/lupus crossover.

*Seborrheic Dermatitis in AIDS.* Seborrheic dermatitis in AIDS patients shows more striking inflammation than in ordinary disease. Occasional plasma cells and necrotic keratinocytes within the lowermost epidermal layers are also observed, and serve as clues of potential underlying immunodeficiency.

**Pathogenesis.** The cause of seborrheic dermatitis is unknown. Although there is an association between the occurrence of seborrheic dermatitis and psoriasis in some patients, and some lesions may have ambiguous clinical and histologic features, the two disorders appear to be separate entities. Because seborrheic dermatitis often occurs in areas enriched in hair follicles, it has been posited that demodex folliculorum or common folliculotropic fungi may play a causative role. Definitive evidence for this, however, is lacking. The increased incidence and severity of seborrheic dermatitis in certain immunodeficiency states, such as AIDS, raises the possibility of immunologic dysregulation as an important contributing factor (52).

**Differential Diagnosis.** Chronic seborrheic dermatitis must be differentiated from primary spongiotic dermatitis (e.g., contact allergy) and evolving or partially treated psoriasis. Table 3-2 provides a summary of several useful findings in making these distinctions. Seborrheic dermatitis, along with pityriasis rosea, guttate parapsoriasis, and pityriasis rubra pilaris, is a condition that may show prominent mound-like parakeratosis (fig. 3-26), and care must be taken to identify other histologic differentiating features as well as obtaining clinical correlation when rendering a diagnosis of seborrheic dermatitis.

**Treatment and Prognosis.** Seborrheic dermatitis is often a life-long disorder that waxes and

*Inflammatory Disorders of the Skin*

Table 3-2

DIFFERENTIAL DIAGNOSIS OF SEBORRHEIC DERMATITIS, ALLERGIC CONTACT DERMATITIS (ACD), AND EARLY/PARTIALLY TREATED PSORIASIS

|  | Seborrheic Dermatitis | ACD | Psoriasis |
| --- | --- | --- | --- |
| Spongiosis | Minimal | Often pronounced | Minimal to none |
| Scale | Focal parakeratosis containing neutrophils | Focal parakeratosis containing serum | Diffuse parakeratosis containing neutrophils |
| Epidermotropism | Neutrophils | Lymphocytes and Langerhans cells | Neutrophils |
| Dermal infiltrate | Lymphocytes and neutrophils | Lymphocytes and often eosinophils | Primarily lymphocytes |
| Dermal vessels | Normal | Normal | Tortuous and ectatic |

Figure 3-26

CHRONIC SEBORRHEIC DERMATITIS

There is prominent acanthosis. The parakeratosis surrounding a follicular ostium is in a pattern similar to that of the shoulder parakeratosis that typifies pityriasis rubra pilaris.

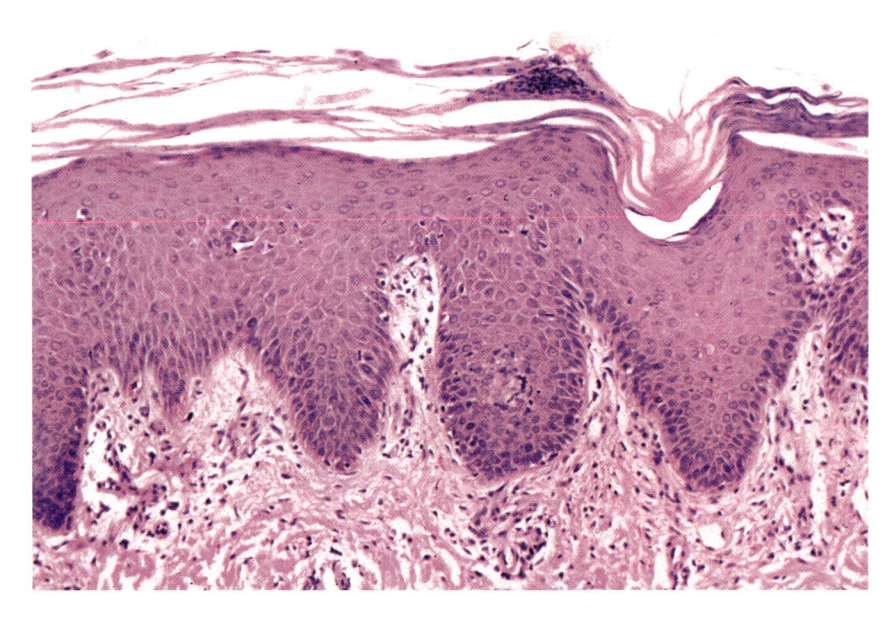

wanes. Topical steroids may be effective during flares, although these are of limited use on facial skin, where they may elicit significant atrophy as a side effect. Certain foods and drinks (alcohol) have been implicated in worsening seborrheic dermatitis, and there is at least anecdotal information that emotional stress may play a role. Ketoconazole cream is often very effective. This response lends some credence to the hypothesis that possibly demodex folliculorum and certain intrafollicular fungi may be etiopathogenic. Pruritic forms of the disease are complicated by excoriation, impetiginization, and superimposition of lichen simplex chronicus. Topical immunomodulators as well as mild topical steroids have been used for acute flares, or even for maintenance therapy, particularly for recalcitrant cases that are often confounded by immunosuppression.

## PITYRIASIS ROSEA

**Definition.** *Pityriasis rosea* is a self-limited disorder that, in its most characteristic presentation, has an evolutionary course which includes the initial appearance of a larger plaque, the so-called *herald patch*, followed by the eruption of multiple smaller oval plaques involving the trunk, neck, and upper arms. These usually last for 6 to 8 weeks.

**Clinical Features.** Pityriasis rosea occurs principally in the spring and fall, although it is occasionally observed in the winter or summer. It typically begins with an edematous scaling plaque on the trunk (the herald patch) followed in a few days to a few weeks by an eruption on the back of the neck, upper arms, and trunk, which is distributed along the lines of skin cleavage. This distribution on truncal skin results in a

## Acanthotic Dermatitis (Retiform Epidermal Hyperplasia)

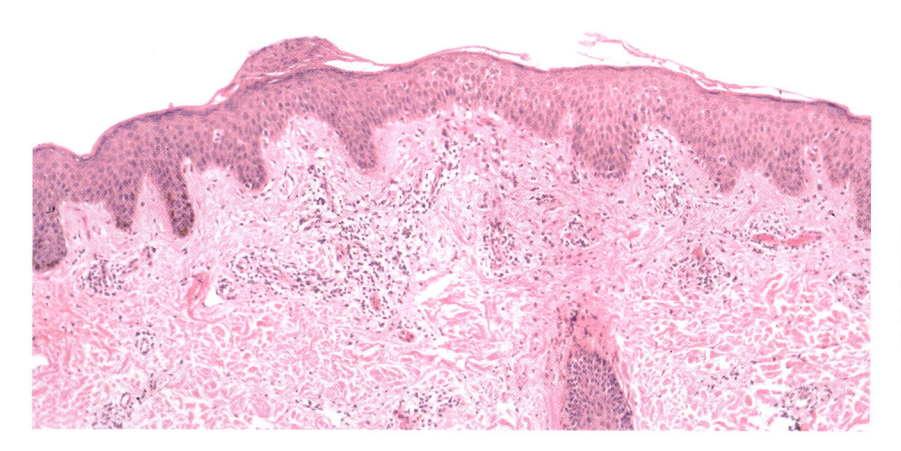

**Figure 3-27**

**PITYRIASIS ROSEA: HERALD PATCH**

At scanning magnification, there is a superficial perivascular lymphoid inflammatory infiltrate, as well as irregular acanthosis and the suggestion of discrete mounds of parakeratotic scale.

"fir tree pattern." The eruption may be associated with marked pruritus. The herald patch varies from a centimeter to several centimeters in size, is a dusky red or salmon pink, and is surmounted by fine scales. Occasionally, minute vesicles are noted on its surface. The remainder of the eruption consists of oval, salmon-pink plaques surrounded by a delicate collarette of "cigarette paper" scale. In most patients, the eruption occurs only once, and is self-limiting.

Clinical variants include *papular and inflammatory pityriasis rosea* in which lesions are markedly edematous, may show petechiae, and are surmounted by a fine scale in a peripheral or central distribution. *Vesicular pityriasis rosea* refers to an eruption in which one or more tiny vesicles surround the oval patches or plaques. *Inverse pityriasis rosea* describes an unusual presentation in which the herald patch appears in the buttock area and the eruption may be confined to the bathing trunk area. The lesion may be vesicular, urticarial, or hemorrhagic. In all of these variants, the characteristic scale is present. The urticarial form may show scattered petechiae, but the typical cigarette paper scale helps in excluding urticarial vasculitis. *Recurrent pityriasis rosea* describes multiple episodes of the disease, recurring, for example, each spring or fall.

**Pathologic Findings.** The herald patch of pityriasis rosea shows variable and occasionally striking psoriasiform epidermal hyperplasia, and accordingly pityriasis rosea is considered here in the context of acanthotic dermatitis. At scanning magnification, there is a focal, compact parakeratotic scale (fig. 3-27) that in some foci has a tendency to separate from the underlying epidermis at one end, with the other end remaining attached to the underlying superficial epidermis. This scale has a mound-like appearance and lies at an acute angle to the long axis of the epidermis. It occasionally contains small foci of serous fluid. The underlying psoriasiform epidermis shows focal intercellular edema, often directly beneath the scale, with associated exocytosis of lymphocytes. Edematous dermal papillae contain lymphocytes and extravasated erythrocytes below the basement membrane zone, although some red blood cells migrate into the epidermis (53). Exocytosis of lymphocytes is often observed and is a helpful diagnostic sign. In the dermis, there are perivenular aggregates of lymphocytes and occasionally rare eosinophils (54). Some lesions, however, show a less than specific pattern (fig. 3-28) or findings that typify a more generalized eruption (fig. 3-29). Accordingly, careful correlation with clinical parameters is recommended in diagnosing pityriasis rosea by histologic evaluation of a herald patch.

In the early lesions of the generalized eruption, there is a focal, mound-like parakeratotic scale that overlies foci of intercellular edema affecting a mildly hyperplastic epidermis (also see chapter 2 for a detailed discussion of the spongiotic presentation). A sparse, perivenular lymphocytic infiltrate is present beneath the areas of epidermal involvement, and randomly scattered red blood cells are present in the edematous papillary dermis. In the better-developed lesion, there is more marked psoriasiform epidermal hyperplasia and the scale is more prominent. The perivenular infiltrate is moderate, and extravasated red blood cells focally infiltrate the epidermis.

*Inflammatory Disorders of the Skin*

**Figure 3-28**

**PITYRIASIS ROSEA: HERALD PATCH**

Acanthosis and compacted hyperkeratotic scale produce a nonspecific pattern.

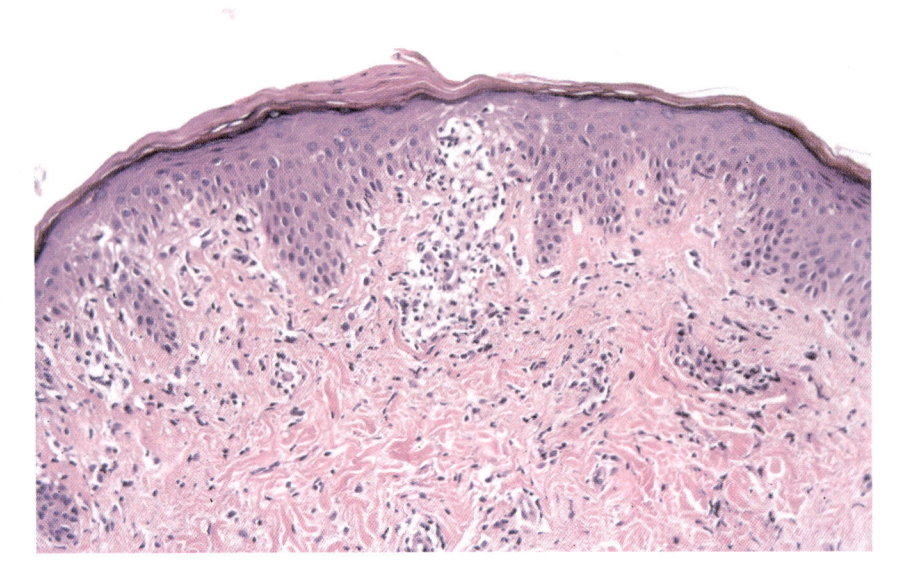

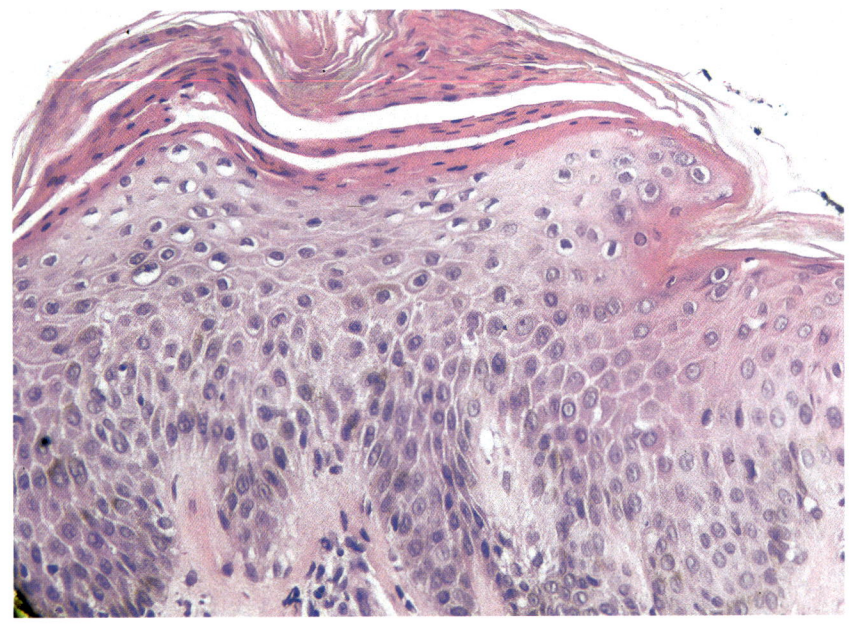

**Figure 3-29**

**PITYRIASIS ROSEA: HERALD PATCH**

The typical mound-like parakeratotic scale surmounts the zone of acanthosis.

Inflammatory pityriasis rosea has more prominent spongiosis, epidermal hyperplasia, scale-crust formation, and extravasation of red blood cells. The characteristic mound-like appearance of the parakeratotic scale persists, however, and is a clue to the diagnosis.

In the urticarial variant, there is marked papillary dermal edema. The characteristic scale pattern remains, however, and extravasated erythrocytes within the superficial epidermis is a helpful diagnostic feature. The vesicular variant shows marked intercellular edema and often prominent scale-crust formation with retention of focal mounds of tightly compacted parakeratotic scale. Inverse pityriasis rosea may show any one of the features described for the other variants, but most often resembles the inflammatory variant.

**Pathogenesis.** Pityriasis rosea often is considered to be caused by a virus, although a definite etiologic agent has not as yet been discovered. Epidemic forms of the disease among persons in barracks or dormitories support an infectious cause. An immunologic basis for the evolution of the disease also has been implicated by the finding of numerous CD4-positive helper cells in the epidermal and dermal infiltrate, along with increased numbers of CD1a-positive Langerhans cells in both the lesional epidermis and dermis (55). In foci of the epidermis infiltrated by lymphocytes, activated keratinocytes express HLA-DR (56).

**Differential Diagnosis.** The herald patch of pityriasis rosea may be confused with pityriasis lichenoides et varioliformis acuta (PLEVA), as, occasionally, may the well-developed and inflammatory generalized lesions. Pityriasis rosea is diagnosed by the characteristic "lifting off" mound-like parakeratotic scale, the confinement of the red blood cells to the edematous dermal papillae without prominent extravasation into the epidermis (this does occur but generally is subtle and focal), the absence of extensive dyskeratosis and vacuolization of the basement membrane zone, and the absence of the wedge-like pattern resulting from the deep angiocentric infiltrate often observed in PLEVA.

Small plaque parapsoriasis may resemble pityriasis rosea, but the parakeratotic scale in the former tends to remain attached to the granular cell layer or lifts off parallel to it. Also, small plaque parapsoriasis tends to lack focal spongiosis, edema within dermal papillae, and extravasation of erythrocytes into the papillary dermis (57). Early psoriasis may show focal spongiosis and parakeratosis with extravasation of red blood cells within the superficial dermis. Neutrophils are often present in the epidermis of early psoriasis, however, and the dermal papillae are bulbous and contain dilated capillary loops. Moreover, early psoriasis generally exhibits increased numbers of mitoses within the keratinocytes of the basal and suprabasal layers.

Superficial gyrate erythema may be confused with early pityriasis rosea. The former tends to show a characteristic "coat sleeve" infiltrate where lymphocytes are tightly aggregated along the walls of superficial dermal vessels. Although focal parakeratosis and spongiosis are occasionally seen in superficial gyrate erythema, superficial dermal hemorrhage is absent.

**Treatment and Prognosis.** Pityriasis rosea is generally self-limiting, with resolution within months of onset. Occasionally, topical steroid therapy hastens this process. Lesions that persist and prove refractory to topical immunosuppressive therapy should be reevaluated for a possible diagnosis of small plaque parapsoriasis. Two or three treatments on successive days with erythemogenic doses of UVB are extremely effective in some patients with severe pruritus. Oral antibiotics such as erythromycin may expedite improvement in some patients (57a).

## PSORIASIFORM STASIS DERMATITIS

**Definition.** *Stasis dermatitis* is a complication of impaired venous return or lymphatic drainage, and generally affects the lower extremities. *Acroangiodermatitis* is a form of stasis dermatitis that results in abundant proliferation of superficial dermal blood vessels and associated edema and fibrosis, resulting in a histologic picture that initially may be confused with Kaposi sarcoma. *Elephantiasis verrucosa nostra* is a chronic condition resulting from impaired drainage of fluid from the lower extremity which results in striking verrucous and nodular enlargement of the affected limb.

**Clinical Features.** Stasis dermatitis is characterized by brawny, sometimes papulonodular induration, pigmentary alterations, plaques covered with hyperkeratotic scale, and regions of atrophy. The affected extremity is generally enlarged due to accumulation of edema and extracellular matrix. Localized zones of hyperkeratosis may exist within a field of chronic stasis or in stasis associated with other forms of dermatitis, and occasionally, these are sampled to exclude keratosis, atypia, or carcinoma.

**Pathologic Findings.** Common to all forms of stasis dermatitis are the following: striking proliferation and tortuosity of superficial dermal vessels, including capillaries within dermal papillae; dermal edema and variable fibrosis; and foci of hemorrhage and hemosiderin deposition. In advanced lesions, the proliferating capillaries within each dermal papilla may resemble miniature glomeruli (fig. 3-30). The epidermis is generally covered with hyperorthokeratotic scale, and interestingly, the underlying viable epidermal layer is either atrophic or acanthotic. In the latter, there is irregular psoriasiform epidermal hyperplasia with associated zones of hypergranulosis and occasional foci of parakeratosis. In some instances, the epidermal surface is thrown up into verrucous folds, resembling the papillomatous architecture of some benign keratoses and the verrucous variant of lichen simplex chronicus.

**Figure 3-30**

**PSORIASIFORM STASIS DERMATITIS**

The irregular acanthosis overlies a fibrotic and vascularized superficial dermis typical of chronic stasis.

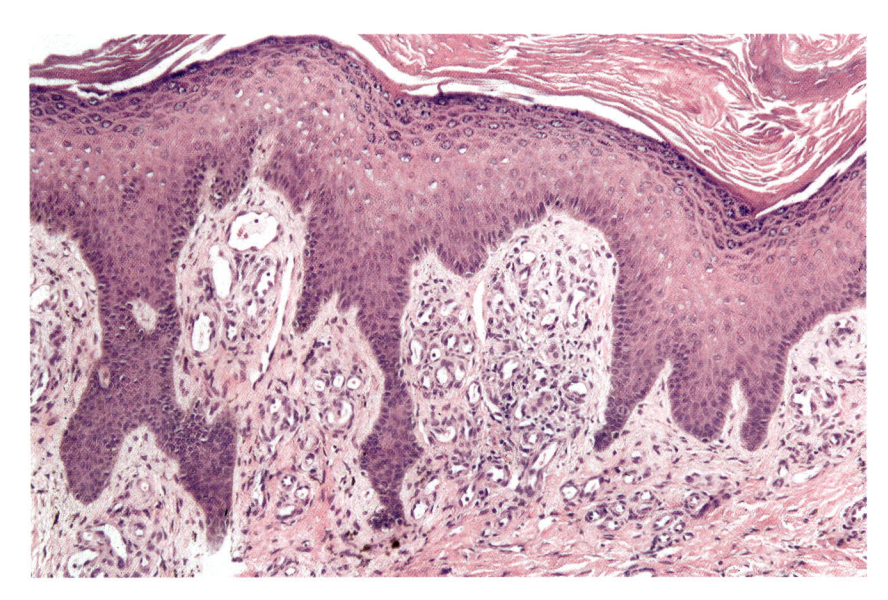

Although the epidermis is generally primarily affected in advanced stasis dermatitis, occasionally adnexal epithelia are involved. Extensive squamous eccrine metaplasia and proliferation may occur, and a syringofibroadenomatous variant resembling multiple eccrine syringofibroadenomas has been described in chronically edematous lower extremities (57b).

**Differential Diagnosis.** The primary difficulty when interpreting biopsies of psoriasiform stasis dermatitis, particularly superficial ones, is differentiating localized plaque-like disease form benign keratoses, lichen simplex chronicus, and psoriasis. Recognition of the characteristic vascular alterations of stasis helps eliminate the first two possibilities. Advanced and established psoriasis, however, may harbor capillaries within dermal papillae that are similar in architecture to those found in early stasis dermatitis. Careful examination of the epidermal layer to document diffuse parakeratosis, hypogranulosis, and the participating neutrophils is generally helpful in discriminating psoriasis of the lower extremity from psoriasiform stasis dermatitis in a superficial sample.

**Treatment and Prognosis.** Treatment, including surgical intervention to promote drainage, is generally directed at the underlying cause of the vascular stasis. Pressure dressings and leg elevation may minimize edema, but once changes are advanced, they are extremely difficult to reverse. Topical steroids may be beneficial when there is an inflammatory component, particularly in early disease. Previously, eligible patients were treated with removal of affected large veins (stripping). More recently, intravascular laser therapy has produced remarkable results.

## HYPERKERATOSIS LENTICULARIS PERSTANS (FLEGEL DISEASE)

**Definition.** *Hyperkeratosis lenticularis perstans,* also known as *Flegel disease,* is a rare disorder characterized by the development in later life of persistent hyperkeratotic papules, usually distributed on the lower extremities and dorsa of the feet (58). The disease may occur spontaneously or be associated with an autosomal dominant pattern of inheritance.

**Clinical Features.** Patients present with multiple asymptomatic, hyperkeratotic flat papules ranging from 1 to 5 mm in diameter. As mentioned above, the lower legs and dorsa of the feet tend to be preferentially involved. Traumatic stripping of the adherent surface scale may result in small bleeding points. At the perimeter of the most prominent scale, there may exist a collarette composed of more delicate scale.

**Pathologic Findings.** The histopathology of hyperkeratosis lenticularis perstans involves irregular acanthosis, hyperorthokeratosis with admixed parakeratosis, and a superficial perivascular lymphoid inflammatory infiltrate surrounding often ectatic vessels. In some lesions, the infiltrate is well demarcated and closely associated with the epidermal layer. Better-developed lesions show a characteristic

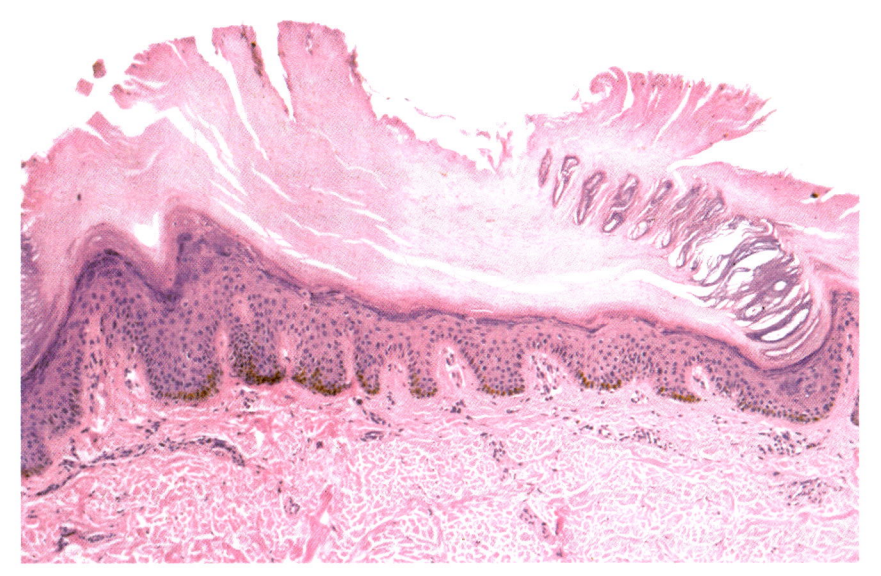

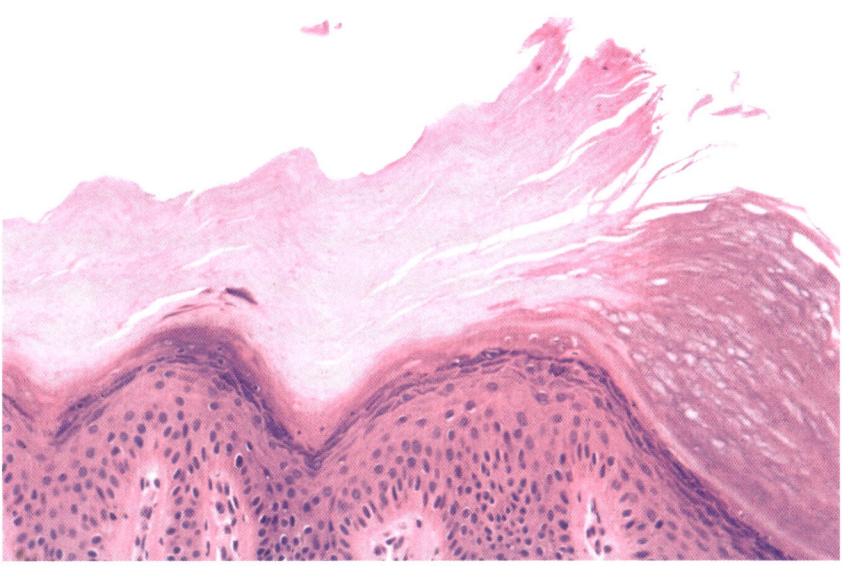

## Figure 3-31

**HYPERKERATOSIS LENTICULARIS PERSTANS**

Top: There is a zone of acanthosis surmounted by a discrete region of hyperkeratotic scale.
Bottom: At higher magnification, the abrupt demarcation of the zone of hyperkeratosis, a characteristic feature, is seen.

markedly thickened, compacted, eosinophilic scale sharply juxtaposed to adjacent stratum corneum demonstrating a normal basket-weave pattern (fig. 3-31). Occasionally, the zone of central hyperorthokeratosis originates from an epidermal layer that is slightly depressed, and the more peripheral epidermis may show a papillomatous architecture.

**Pathogenesis.** The precise cause of hyperkeratosis lenticularis perstans is unknown. Upon ultrastructural examination, occasional cases have an absence of membrane-coating granules (Odland bodies), and this may represent a primary defect. The lesions are associated with dermal inflammation, however, and thus it is unclear whether this condition represents a true dermatitis or a primary disorder of epidermal maturation.

**Differential Diagnosis.** Because the histopathology of hyperkeratosis lenticularis perstans is nonspecific, it must be differentiated from other causes of verrucous epidermal proliferation and hyperorthokeratosis, including lichen simplex chronicus and benign keratoses. Correlation of the histopathology with clinical presentation is important in formulating a correct diagnosis of this rare disorder.

**Treatment and Prognosis.** Lesions develop in older individuals, persist indefinitely, and are fairly refractory to current therapies.

## RETIFORM EPIDERMAL HYPERPLASIA INDUCED BY MYCOTIC INFECTION

**Definition.** Irregular epidermal hyperplasia with retention of the rete ridge pattern is characteristic of certain deep fungal infections affecting the skin. This hyperplasia is usually associated with intraepidermal abscesses that include neutrophils along with mononuclear cells, including multinucleated giant cells. The infecting organism is often identified within the intraepidermal abscess, as well as within granulomatous inflammatory foci in the underlying dermis. Occasionally, more superficial fungal infections are associated with retiform epidermal hyperplasia.

**Clinical Features.** Retiform epidermal hyperplasia induced by deep mycotic infection occurs in two settings. The first is a site that has been inoculated directly, and the second involves metastatic deposition of fungal elements within the skin. Primary inoculation of the skin occurs in chromomycosis and sporotrichosis, but also occurs in alternariosis, coccidiomycosis, and North American blastomycosis, with resultant deep fungal infections. It is now thought that cutaneous involvement in most cases of alternariosis, North and South American blastomycosis, and coccidioidomycosis result from secondary (metastatic) spread. Both primary and secondary forms may present as raised hyperkeratotic, sometimes verrucous plaques and pustules. The plaques tend to be well-demarcated and show a halo of surrounding erythema. Certain infections, such as North American blastomycosis, have a characteristic annular border formed by erythema and pustules surrounding a zone of central clearing. Other lesions simply are large plaques which coalesce to cover a regional area of the skin, such as in pretibial involvement by chromoblastomycosis. Inoculation sites, as may occur in coccidioidomycosis, appear as small, hyperkeratotic plaques several centimeters in diameter, studded superficially with small pustules.

**Pathologic Findings.** The characteristic histologic feature in psoriasiform deep fungal infection of the skin is hyperkeratosis associated with irregular epidermal hyperplasia (fig. 3-29). Occasionally, there is a papillary component to the hyperplastic reaction, with associated focal to diffuse parakeratosis. The rete ridges extend within the dermis to variable depths, exhibiting irregular shapes and sizes that may mimic pseudoepitheliomatous epidermal hyperplasia. This type of endophytic acanthosis may be associated with large, bulbous rete ridges formed by pale squamous cells surrounded by a distinctive basal layer. The inflammatory reaction generally consists of neutrophils, lymphocytes, histiocytes, and eosinophils, with focal intraepidermal abscesses formed by neutrophils and occasional mononuclear cells. Multinucleated giant cells are also present, and many of these contain infective organisms (fig. 3-32).

Marked retiform epidermal hyperplasia also occurs with chronic superficial infections by *Candida* and occasionally, dermatophytes. The epidermis shows irregular acanthosis and there may be parakeratosis associated with hypergranules or hypogranulosis, resembling that of psoriasis (fig. 3-33). Yeast and/or hyphal forms are generally present in association with the abnormal scale, although multiple periodic acid–Schiff (PAS) or silver stains are required for their detection. It is especially useful to search in intraepidermal and intradermal abscesses with special stains, in addition to granulomatous areas, to discover organisms.

**Differential Diagnosis.** The differential diagnosis of granulomatous dermatitis associated with an acanthotic epidermal reaction largely depends upon the identification of the offending organism by PAS or silver staining. Table 3-3 provides a summary of the salient features of most organisms that result in this form of psoriasiform dermatitis. It is also advisable to consider the possibility of superficial infection, as occasional lesions of dermatophytosis have an unusual degree of acanthosis. Superficial biopsies from immunocompromised patients may bear a striking resemblance to well-differentiated invasive squamous cell carcinoma, and yet ultimately prove to represent acanthotic changes overlying deep mycotic infection.

**Treatment and Prognosis.** Treatment is directed toward eradication of offending organisms, and may involve administration of systemic antifungal medications.

## PSORIASIFORM REACTIONS TO HALOGENS

**Definition.** Ingestion, intravenous administration, or even topical application of halogen-containing substances, usually drugs or contrast

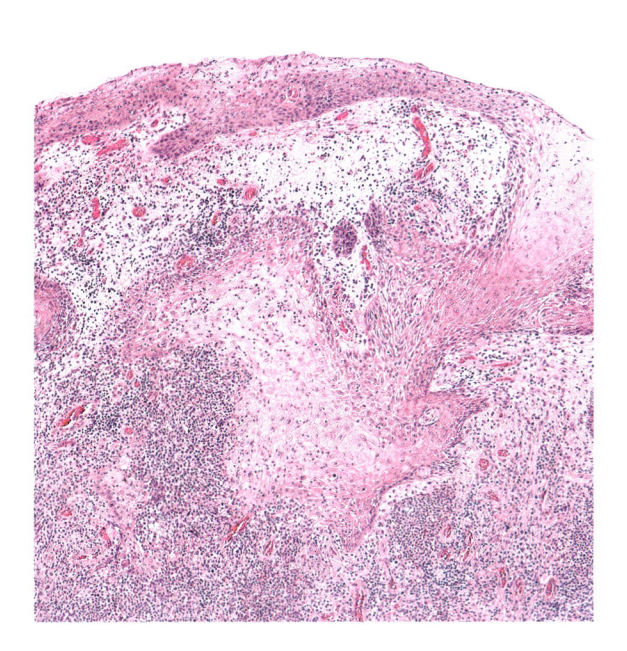

## Acanthotic Dermatitis (Retiform Epidermal Hyperplasia)

**Figure 3-32**

**PSORIASIFORM MYCOTIC INFECTION: BLASTOMYCOSIS**

Above: At scanning magnification, there is striking endophytic epidermal proliferation with a robust associated inflammatory infiltrate.

Right: The underlying dermal inflammatory infiltrate is obviously granulomatous. Blastomycosis organisms are present within the cytoplasm of multinucleated histiocytes.

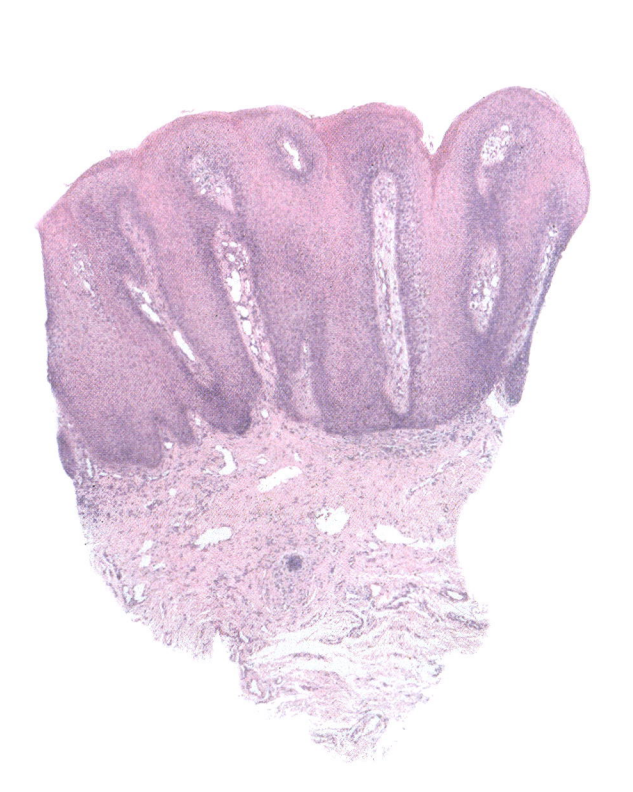

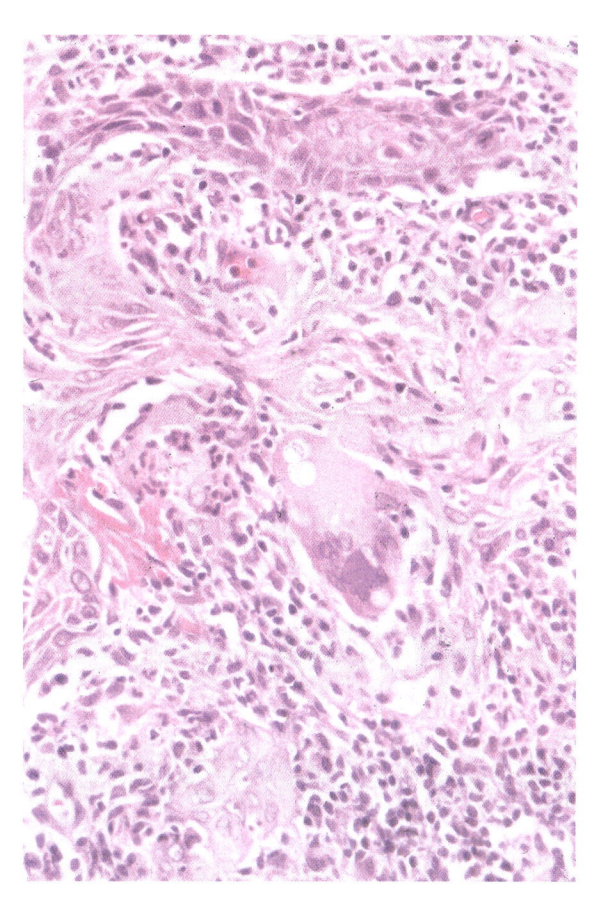

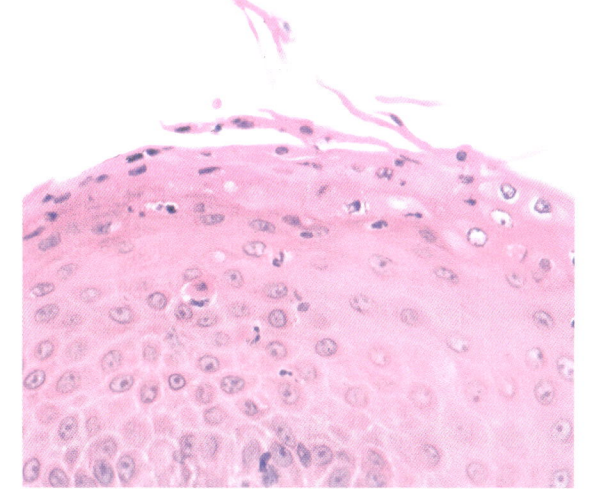

**Figure 3-33**

**PSORIASIFORM REACTION TO DERMATOPHYTE INFECTION**

Left: Regular downward acanthosis of the epithelial layer.

Above: At higher magnification, dermatophyte organisms are detected in the surface scale without the assistance of special stains.

*Inflammatory Disorders of the Skin*

Table 3-3

DEEP FUNGAL INFECTIONS ASSOCIATED WITH RETIFORM EPIDERMAL HYPERPLASIA

| Diseases | Histologic Appearance | Organism Size/Morphology |
|---|---|---|
| Alternariosis | Pseudoepitheliomatous hyperplasia, intraepidermal microabscesses, suppurative granulomatous dermal infiltrate | 5-7-µm septate hyphae with variable branching and brown pigmentation; 3-10 mm found in oval spores, often with double contours |
| North American blastomycosis | Pseudoepitheliomatous hyperplasia, intraepidermal microabscesses, suppurative/granulomatous dermal infiltrate with giant cells | 8-15-µm thick-walled spores with single broad-based buds |
| Paracoccidioidomycosis | Like North American blastomycosis | 6-20-µm spores with narrow-necked, single or multiple buds; "mariner wheels" up to 60 mm in diameter |
| Chromoblastomycosis | Like North American blastomycosis | 6-12-µm thick-walled, dark-brown spores, often in clusters; some possess cross walls |
| Coccidioidomycosis | Primary inoculation: mixed dermal infiltrate with neutrophils, lymphocytes, and occasional giant cells. Systemic: like North American blastomycosis, but granulomas may be more tuberculoid | 10-80-µm thick-walled spores with granular cytoplasm; larger spores contain endospores |
| Sporotrichosis | Cutaneous lesions: epidermal hyperplasia with intraepidermal microabscesses, suppurative granulomatous dermal infiltrate, occasional asteroid bodies. Subcutaneous nodules: central zones of neutrophils surrounded by zones of epithelioid histiocytes and lymphocytes | 4-6-µm round to oval spores; often difficult to detect in infected tissue |

media containing bromide, iodide, or fluoride, may result in a form of psoriasiform dermatitis (59). The three major classes of psoriasiform dermatitis induced by halogens are termed *iododerma*, *bromoderma*, and *fluoroderma*.

**Clinical Features.** Bromide-induced eruptions often form papillomatous plaques with a predilection for the lower extremities. Individual plaques frequently exhibit small pustules at their peripheries. Iodides, particularly those in radiographic contrast media, produce lesions on the face. These are vegetating and pustular, and may ulcerate (fig. 3-34) (60). Fluoroderma generally involves the face and neck, producing scattered papules and nodules that develop after the topical application of fluoride gel to the oral cavity.

**Pathologic Findings.** In all forms of halogen eruptions, the dermis contains a dense mixed inflammatory infiltrate composed of neutrophils, eosinophils, and mononuclear cells. Microabscesses formed by neutrophils, edema, and hemorrhage are often seen in early, active lesions. The epidermal alterations, which tend to be most pronounced in bromoderma, consist of surface papillomatosis, endophytic hyperplasia of rete ridges resulting in the appearance of pseudoepitheliomatous hyperplasia, and intraepidermal microabscesses (fig. 3-35). Occasionally, follicular infundibula appear to be preferentially involved by the acanthotic reaction. Microabscesses contain neutrophils, eosinophils, and degenerating and acantholytic keratinocytes. Ulceration with adjacent pseudoepitheliomatous hyperplasia should heighten the suspicion that iodide is the offending agent.

**Pathogenesis.** Psoriasiform halogen eruptions appear to be based upon a peculiar type of allergic response, which is initially delayed in onset. Upon readministration of the offending agent, the onset of the eruption occurs within several days, suggesting the involvement of a recall phenomenon. In vitro, lymphocytes of sensitized individuals undergo blastogenesis upon exposure to the offending agent, an observation in keeping with a delayed type hypersensitivity reaction.

**Differential Diagnosis.** Psoriasiform halogen eruptions must be differentiated from deep mycotic infections associated with epidermal hyperplasia and microabscess formation. The

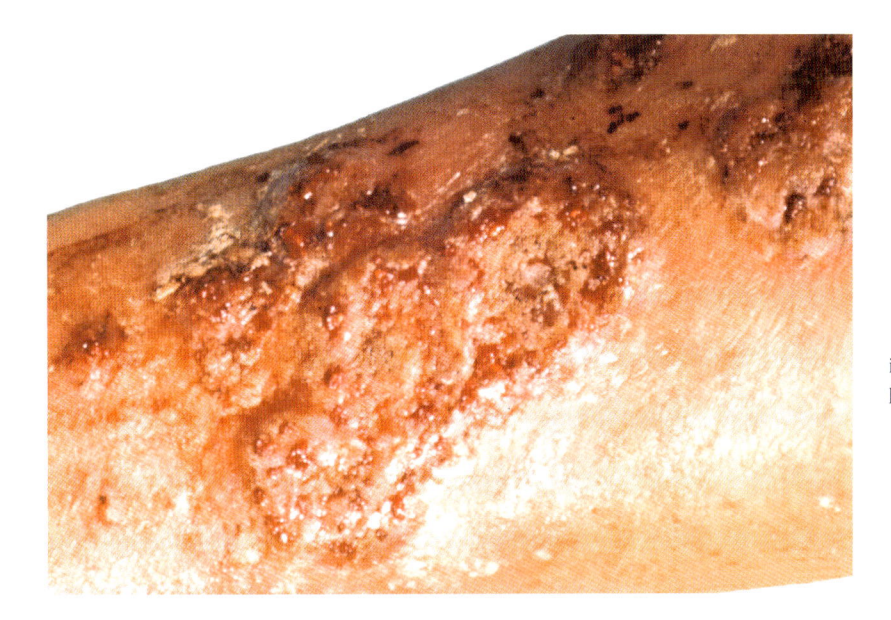

## Figure 3-34

### PSORIASIFORM REACTION TO HALOGEN: BROMODERMA

The clinical manifestations include vegetating and pustular plaques that focally ulcerate.

## Figure 3-35

### BROMODERMA

There is marked pseudocarcinomatous acanthosis of the epidermal layer. The inflammatory component within the dermis consists of a dense admixture neutrophils, eosinophils, and mononuclear cells.

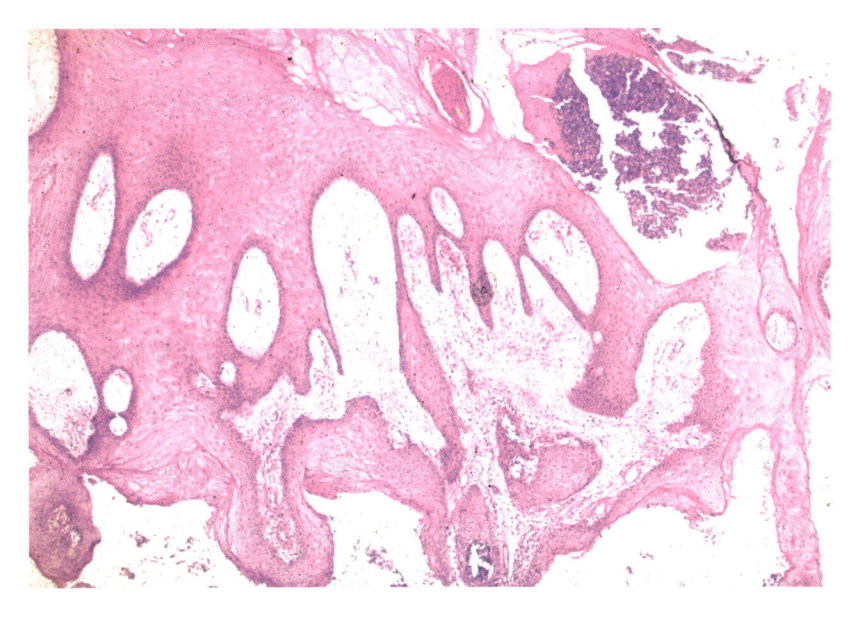

presence of numerous eosinophils in halogen eruptions, and of giant cells and organisms in cutaneous fungal infections, are the most helpful differentiating features. Pemphigus vegetans may show verrucous epidermal hyperplasia and an infiltrate containing eosinophils, but also demonstrates acantholysis that is independent of microabscesses and only rarely contains neutrophils.

**Treatment and Prognosis.** Lesions slowly resolve with avoidance of the offending agent. Re-exposure at a later date may result in a markedly accelerated and severe clinical course.

## INTERFACE DERMATITIS WITH RETIFORM EPIDERMAL HYPERPLASIA

**Definition.** This category involves disorders that are generally classified under the category of cytotoxic/lichenoid dermatitis, but which exhibit variant forms in which the acanthosis predominates over other histologic features. They thus present a hybrid of two distinct patterns. Disorders in this category include hypertrophic variants of lichen planus and lupus erythematosus, as well as certain lichenoid manifestations of treponemal infection in which psoriasiform epidermal hyperplasia typically develops (59,61). Hybrid presentations in skin should always bring to mind connective tissue diseases, certain drug reactions, certain infections, and T-cell dyscrasias.

Although the variant disorders discussed in this section share the common features of interface change and epidermal hyperplasia, their causes are different, and accordingly, are discussed individually in the chapters that deal with their more classic presentations (e.g., lupus erythematosus and lichen planus). The treponemal infections that are characterized by interface change and epidermal hyperplasia include condyloma lata, lichenoid secondary syphilis, secondary yaws, and secondary pinta. Secondary syphilis is caused by infection by *Treponema pallidum;* yaws by *T. pallidum* subspecies *pertenue;* and pinta by *T. carateum*.

**Clinical Features.** The clinical features of psoriasiform lichenoid forms of dermatitis are dominated by the formation of hyperkeratotic scale overlying what otherwise would present as erythematous plaques and nodules. In hypertrophic variants of lichen planus, individual lesions may coalesce to form scaling plaques that resemble psoriasis or lichen simplex chronicus. Hypertrophic lupus erythematosus most often manifests as scaling plaques and nodules that occasionally give rise to zones of atypical epidermal proliferation and even frank squamous cell carcinoma. Secondary syphilis often presents as brown to erythematous scaling papules and small plaques that may be serpiginous or resemble guttate forms of psoriasis or pityriasis rosea. Pitted hyperkeratotic papules involving the palms and soles (syphilis cornee), and zones occupied by confluent exophytic papules involving anogenital skin (condyloma lata) are also observed. Secondary yaws may present as circinate scaling plaques resembling dermatophytosis and condylomatous vegetations involving axillary and groin skin. Hyperkeratotic palmar and plantar lesions may be observed. Secondary pinta produces hyperkeratotic papules that typically coalesce to form psoriasiform plaques. The lichen planus-like drug reaction resembles lichen planus but is in a different distribution and has a somewhat different clinical appearance. Mycosis fungoides, as it progresses, becomes more palpable due to the deep neoplastic and dermatitic infiltrates that have supervened on the prior, predominantly epidermotropic process and may be associated with sometimes marked epidermal thickening.

**Pathologic Findings.** Hypertrophic lichen planus characteristically has features of ordinary lichen planus, namely, a band-like infiltrate of lymphocytes along the dermal-epidermal junction; vacuolization, colloid body formation, squamatization, and a "saw-tooth" configuration involving the basal cell layer and rete ridges; epidermal hyperplasia; hypergranulosis (often focal and wedge-shaped); and hyperorthokeratosis. The epidermal hyperplasia, hypergranulosis, and hyperkeratosis are often pronounced, resembling that seen in advanced lichen simplex chronicus. Indeed, hypertrophic lichen planus may be regarded as a chronic form of lichen planus in which pruritus-induced excoriation has resulted in the superimposition of lichen simplex chronicus. Hypertrophic forms of lupus erythematosus, on the other hand, are rare and distinctive. Lesions may show variable papillary dermal and deeper periadnexal lymphoid infiltrate containing occasional plasma cells, vacuolization involving the basal cell layer of the epidermis and follicular infundibula, hyperorthokeratosis involving the surface epidermis and follicular ostia, and dermal mucin deposition and vascular telangiectasia (fig. 3-36). The typical epidermal atrophy seen in classic forms of lupus erythematosus is replaced by irregular endophytic epidermal and follicular infundibular hyperplasia. In occasional patients, areas of true dysplasia and transition to invasive squamous cell carcinoma are documented.

The histopathology of all secondary forms of cutaneous treponemal infection involves variable vacuolization of the basal cell layer. In secondary syphilis, this is associated with a lichenoid papillary dermal infiltrate of lymphocytes and occasional plasma cells surrounding blood vessels lined by swollen endothelial cells. The epidermis generally shows psoriasiform hyperplasia, focal spongiosis, lymphocyte epidermotropism, surface hyperorthokeratosis and parakeratosis, and migration of neutrophils to spongiotic and parakeratotic foci (figs. 3-37, 3-38). In secondary yaws, the histopathology resembles that of psoriasiform secondary syphilis, although there is more exuberant

## Acanthotic Dermatitis (Retiform Epidermal Hyperplasia)

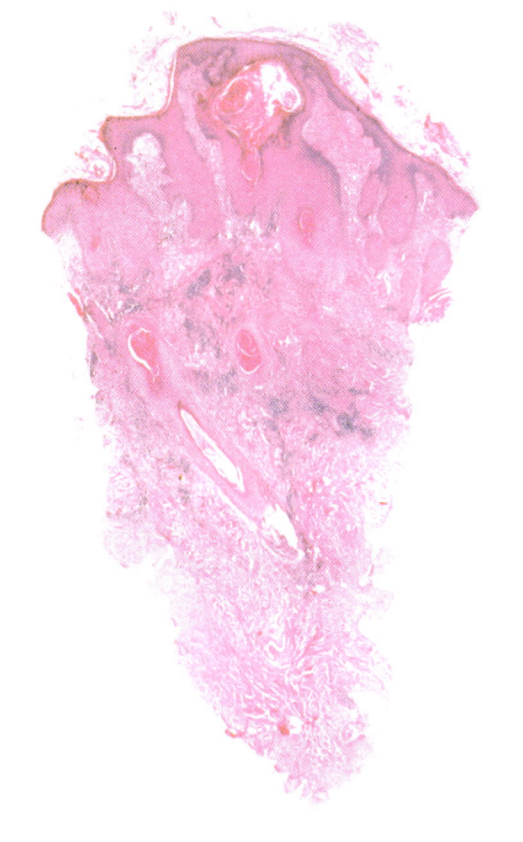

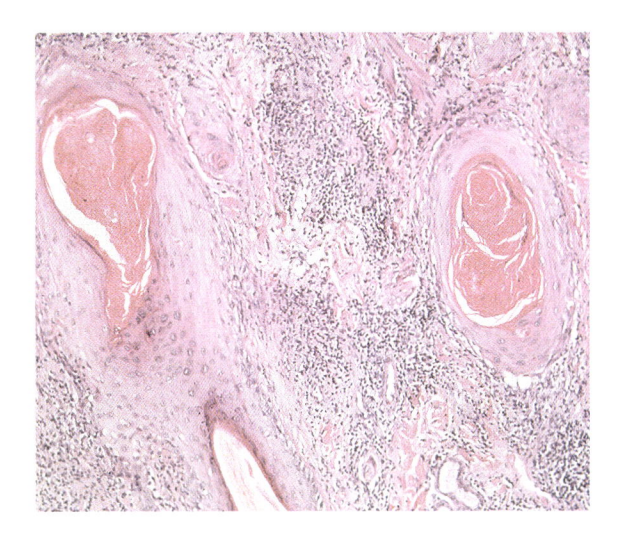

**Figure 3-36**

**PSORIASIFORM INTERFACE DERMATITIS: HYPERTROPHIC LUPUS ERYTHEMATOSUS**

Left: At scanning magnification, there is a markedly endophytic epithelial proliferation associated with a patchy perivascular and periadnexal, superficial and deep inflammatory infiltrate.

Above: At higher magnification, the markedly dilated and hyperplastic follicular infundibula are rimmed by lymphocytes with associated interface injury to the basal cell layer.

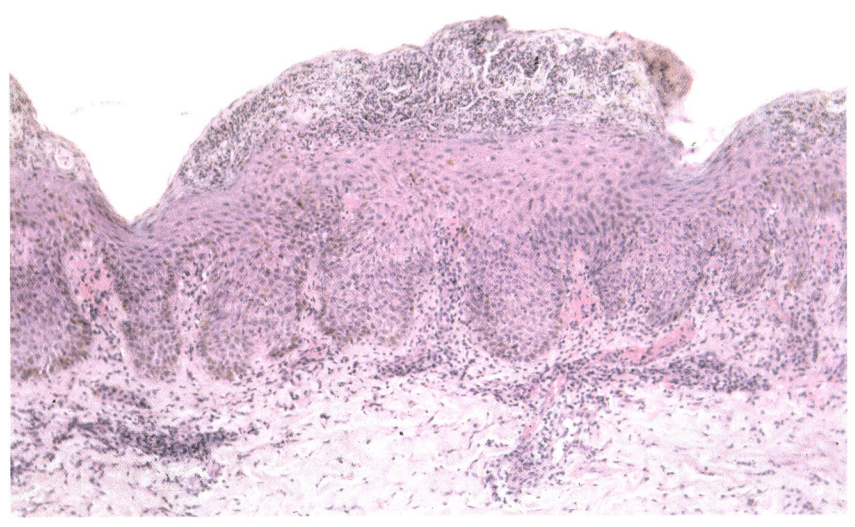

**Figure 3-37**

**PSORIASIFORM SECONDARY SYPHILIS**

Irregular acanthosis and an associated superficial dermal perivascular and papillary dermal interstitial inflammatory infiltrate are present.

epidermal hyperplasia with the formation of intraepidermal microabscesses, and the dermal inflammatory infiltrate tends to be more diffusely distributed. Secondary pinta is characterized by lesions that show epidermal hyperplasia with hypergranulosis and hyperkeratosis; focal spongiosis; basal cell layer vacuolization; a dermal infiltrate composed of lymphocytes, plasma cells, and neutrophils; and dermal vascular ectasia without significant endothelial swelling.

The condyloma lata variant of secondary syphilis shows much more epidermal thickening and hyperkeratosis (fig. 3-39), and often prominent intraepidermal microabscess formation. Unlike psoriasiform secondary syphilis, spirochetes are easily identified in lesions of

*Inflammatory Disorders of the Skin*

**Figure 3-38**

**PSORIASIFORM SECONDARY SYPHILIS**

In addition to epidermal hyperplasia, exocytotic lymphocytes and neutrophils accumulate in the orthokeratotic and parakeratotic scale. The interface inflammatory infiltrate contains both lymphocytes and plasma cells.

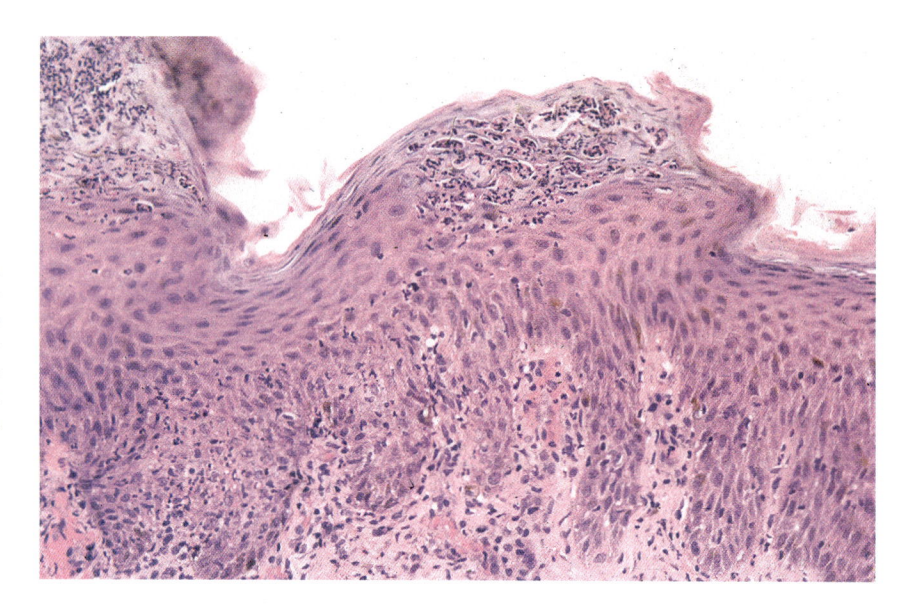

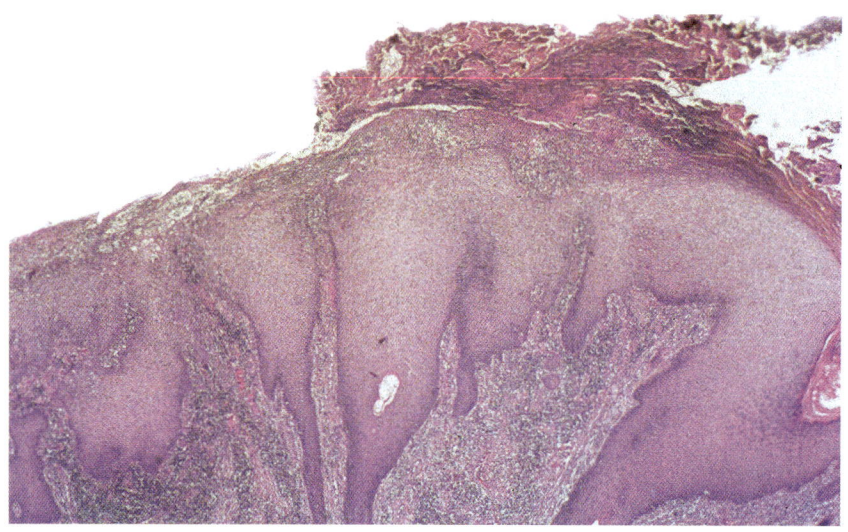

**Figure 3-39**

**PSORIASIFORM EPIDERMAL HYPERPLASIA IN CONDYLOMA LATA**

The mucosal epithelium shows markedly endophytic acanthosis surmounted by inflamed scale. The connective tissue is infiltrated by lymphocytes and plasma cells.

condyloma lata with the Warthin-Starry stain. The syphilis cornee variant of psoriasiform secondary syphilis shows acanthosis bordering a zone of focal hyperorthokeratosis and parakeratosis, which forms an invagination within the superficial epidermal layers. The underlying dermis contains a superficial perivascular lymphoplasmacytic infiltrate. Psoriasiform forms of lichen planus and lupus erythematosus are variants of primary dermatitides.

The lichen planus-like drug reaction exhibits focal parakeratosis, a variably thickened granular cell layer, and sparse interface dermatitis. In addition, there is a superficial and deep perivascular lymphoeosinophilic infiltrate.

The plaque stage of mycosis fungoides, as it progresses from patch to plaque and then to tumor, may exhibit associated psoriasiform dermatitis with a deep perivascular infiltrate.

**Differential Diagnosis.** Hypertrophic lupus erythematosus must be differentiated from hypertrophic lichen planus. The former shows dermal mucin deposition, vascular telangiectasia, and fewer colloid bodies; the latter exhibits prominent hypergranulosis and colloid body formation and seldom has a deep periadnexal inflammatory component or plasma cells within the dermal infiltrate. True psoriasis superficially resembles psoriasiform secondary syphilis. The latter, however, shows variable interface changes and does not exhibit the characteristic epidermal thinning overlying individual dermal papillae that is generally present in established lesions of psoriasis.

**Treatment and Prognosis.** Psoriasiform treponemal infections are treated with appropriate antibiotics. A variety of antiinflammatory strategies are utilized in the therapy for lupus erythematosus and lichen planus.

## PSORIASIFORM NUTRITIONAL DISORDERS

**Definition.** Nutritional disorders that are characterized by acanthosis include *pellagra (acquired vitamin B3 deficiency), chronic necrolytic migratory erythema (glucagonoma syndrome),* and *acrodermatitis enteropathica.*

**Clinical Features.** The cutaneous manifestations of pellagra are characterized by erythematous and exfoliative photodermatitis, painful genital and perineal erosions that may be induced by pressure or trauma, a seborrheic dermatitis-like facial eruption, and lip and oral mucosal involvement consisting of erythema and fissuring. In necrolytic migratory erythema due to glucagonoma, erythema, erosions, and flaccid vesicles and pustules, often with a circinate appearance, develop in a perioral, paranasal, perineal, and genital distribution (fig. 3-40). The lower legs and feet may also be involved. Acrodermatitis enteropathica occurs in infants during the first 4 to 10 weeks of life, and presents as acral and periorificial erythema, oozing, and occasional vesiculation. There also may be diffuse partial alopecia.

**Pathologic Findings.** In pellagra, the acanthosis is associated with hyperorthokeratosis, parakeratosis, and a superficial perivascular lymphocytic infiltrate. A myriad of associated findings have been described, including necrotic keratinocytes, focal loss of the stratum granulosum, and abnormal epidermal maturation. Some lesions exhibit vacuolization, cellular pallor, and apparent necrosis of the uppermost epidermal layers in a manner similar to that seen in necrolytic migratory erythema. Acanthosis, diffuse parakeratosis, and a characteristic form of hydropic clearing within the cytoplasm of the keratinocytes of the upper layers of the stratum spinosum are the most common features of both necrolytic migratory erythema and acrodermatitis enteropathica (fig. 3-41). Both also may show architectural disarray, suggesting abnormal epidermal maturation, and neutrophil infiltration into the uppermost epidermal layers, sometimes resulting in subcorneal microabscesses (62).

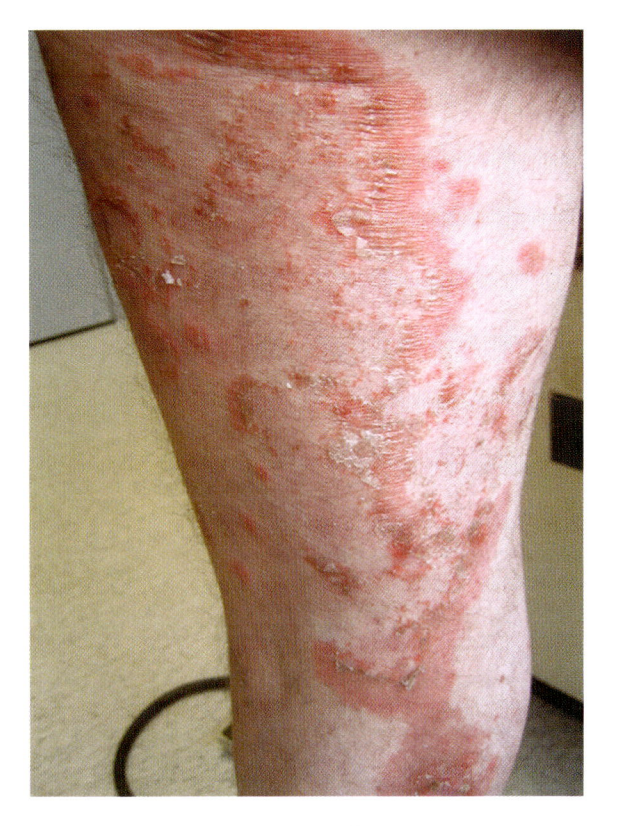

**Figure 3-40**

**NECROLYTIC MIGRATORY ERYTHEMA**

The lesion consists of a slightly circinate erythematous plaque involving the dorsum of the thigh.

**Pathogenesis.** The pathogenesis of the acantholytic response in nutritional disorders affecting the skin is poorly understood. In pellagra, kynurenic acid accumulates as a consequence of a deficiency in nicotinamide, which blocks its formation. Also urocanic acid in the epidermal layer is deficient as a result of a reduction of histidine and histidase activity. These abnormalities are believed to result in photosensitivity, which, upon chronicity, results in acanthosis. In glucagonoma, there is sustained gluconeogenesis with associated amino acid degradation, which may affect epidermal proteins. Necrolytic migratory erythema also may develop in the setting of malabsorption, where essential fatty acids, zinc, and amino acids become depleted. It has been speculated that the pathogenesis may involve a phospholipid fatty acid abnormality

*Inflammatory Disorders of the Skin*

**Figure 3-41**

NECROLYTIC MIGRATORY ERYTHEMA

Top: At scanning magnification, the characteristic pallor of the uppermost epidermal layers is visible.

Bottom: At higher magnification, the epidermis is slightly acanthotic, with characteristic pallor within the upper epidermal layers. Pallor is partially the result of hydropic clearing within the cytoplasm of the affected keratinocytes.

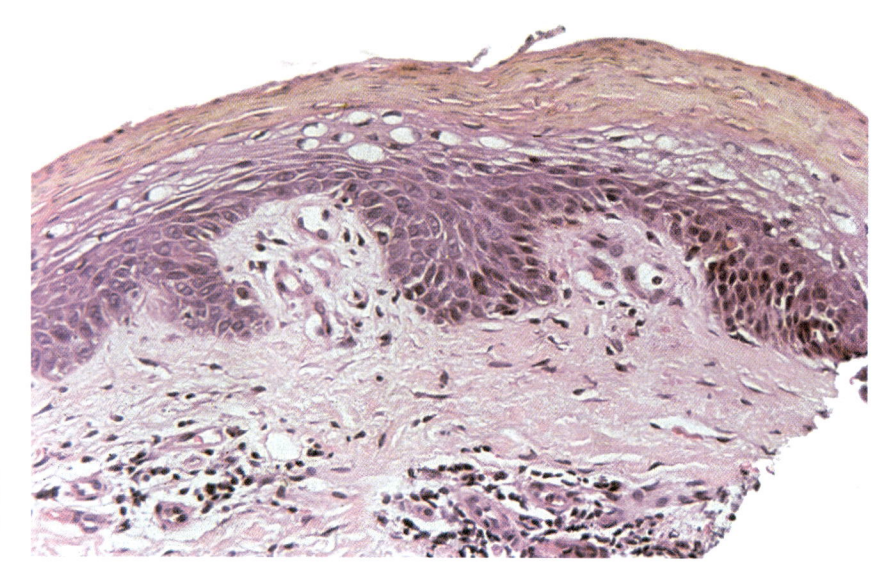

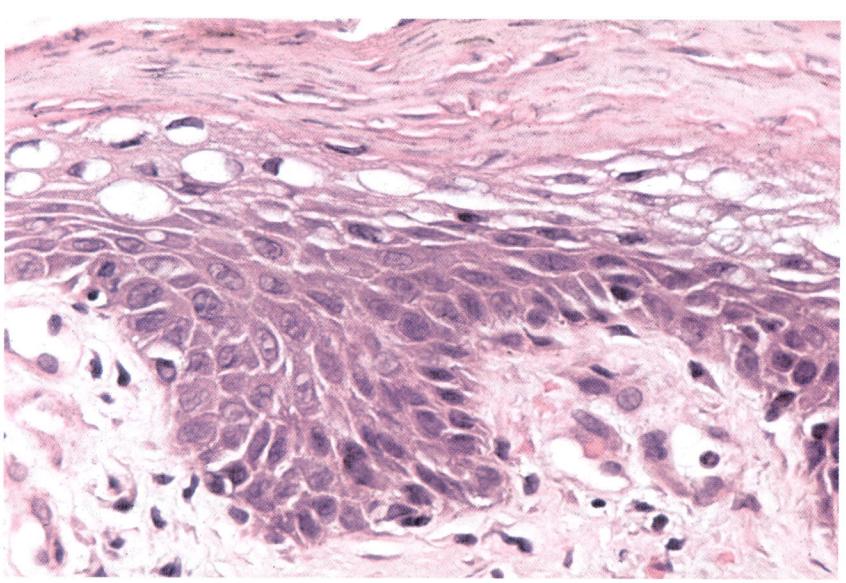

as a result of defective delta-6-desaturase enzyme, which is inhibited in the setting of zinc deficiency. A similar role for zinc has been suggested in acrodermatitis enteropathica, and oral administration of zinc sulfate leads to the reversal of this disease.

**Differential Diagnosis.** The histopathologic features of pellagra, necrolytic migratory erythema, and acrodermatitis enteropathica, although distinctive, require clinical correlation for definitive diagnosis. Such conditions—along with several other unrelated disorders and their variants (summarized in Table 3-4)—are rare, and although one must be aware of their existence, the likelihood of their encounter in routine practice is small.

**Treatment and Prognosis.** These nutritional disorders respond to correction of the underlying deficiency either by supplementation or by treatment of the underlying condition (e.g., as in glucagonoma).

Table 3-4

RARE DISORDERS ASSOCIATED WITH EPIDERMAL HYPERPLASIA

| Disorder | Clinical Characteristics | Histology |
|---|---|---|
| Psoriasiform cutaneous T-cell lymphoma (CTCL) | Verrucous, erythematous plaques | Pautrier microabscesses |
| Verrucous incontinentia pigmenti | Linear verrucous plaques following erythema and bullae; X-linked dominant inheritance | Verrucous acanthosis with whirling zones of dyskeratosis, persistent eosinophils |
| Acrodermatitis enteropathica | Zinc deficiency; hair loss, gastrointestinal complaints, bullous to verrucous skin lesions in infancy | Verrucous acanthosis with dyskeratotic epidermal cells, perivascular lymphocytes |
| Pellagra | Niacin deficiency; erythema, vesicles, and thickened plaques in photodistribution | Psoriasiform acanthosis, confluent parakeratosis, pallor to superficial keratinocytes |
| Necrolytic migratory erythema | Weight loss, diabetes mellitus, anemia, and vesicular to psoriasiform skin lesions (glucagonoma syndrome) | Psoriasiform acanthosis, pyknosis, pallor, and necrosis of keratinocytes in uppermost epidermis |
| Lamellar ichthyosis | Ichthyosiform scales at birth, flexural skin may be more severely affected | Normal or thickened granular layer, compact lamellar hyperorthokeratosis |
| Psoriasiform (hypertrophic) lupus erythematosus | Verrucous plaques in patients with chronic cutaneous lupus erythematosus | Hyperkeratosis, acanthosis, pseudo-epitheliomatous hyperplasia associated with interface dermatitis |

## REFERENCES

1. Ha HY, Kim Y, Ryoo ZY, Kim TY. Inhibition of the TPA-induced cutaneous inflammation and hyperplasia by EC-SOD. Biochem Biophys Res Commun 2006;348:450-8.
2. Zhan Q, Signoretti S, Whitaker-Menezes D, Friedman TM, Korngold R, Murphy GF. Cytokeratin15-positive basal epithelial cells targeted in graft-versus-host disease express a constitutive antiapoptotic phenotype. J Invest Dermatol 2007;127:106-15.
3. Cotsarelis G. Epithelial stem cells: a folliculocentric view. J Invest Dermatol 2006;126:1459-68.
4. Conrad C, Nestle FO. Animal models of psoriasis and psoriatic arthritis: an update. Curr Rheumatol Rep 2006;8:342-7.
5. Boyman O, Hefti HP, Conrad C, Nickoloff BJ, Suter M, Nestle FO. Spontaneous development of psoriasis in a new animal model shows an essential role for resident T cells and tumor necrosis factor-alpha. J Exp Med 2004;199:731-6.
6. Lee MR, Shumack S. Prurigo nodularis: a review. Australas J Dermatol 2005;46:211-8.
7. Dunford J, Crutchfield CE. Prurigo nodularis. Dermatol Nurs 2003;15:444.
8. Dyachenko P, Shustak A, Rozenman D. Hemodialysis-related pruritus and associated cutaneous manifestations. Int J Dermatol 2006;45:664-7.
9. Frithz A, Lagerholm B. Lichen simplex chronicus Vidal: comparative submicroscopic aspects of acanthotic disorders. Acta Derm Venereol 1977;57:103-11.
10. Tashiro H, Arai H, Hashimoto T, Takezaki S, Kawana S. Pemphigoid nodularis: two case studies and analysis of autoantibodies before and after the development of generalized blistering. J Nippon Med Sch 2005;72:60-5.
11. McGinness JL, Bivens MM, Greer KE, Patterson JW, Saulsbury FT. Immune dysregulation, polyendocrinopathy, enteropathy, X-linked syndrome (IPEX) associated with pemphigoid nodularis: a case report and review of the literature. J Am Acad Dermatol 2006;55:143-8.
12. Bernardin RM, Altman CE, Meffert JJ. What is your diagnosis? Lichen simplex chronicus. Cutis 2006;78:96, 101-2.
13. Kuwahara RB, Skinner RB Jr. An itch that must be scratched. Am Fam Physician 2006;73:299-300.
14. Chey WY, Kim KL, Yoo TY, Lee AY. Allergic contact dermatitis from hair dye and development of lichen simplex chronicus. Contact Dermatitis 2004;51:5-8.
15. Wallengren J. Neuroanatomy and neurophysiology of itch. Dermatol Ther 2005;18:292-303.

16. Nakamura M, Toyoda M, Morohashi M. Pruritogenic mediators in psoriasis vulgaris: comparative evaluation of itch-associated cutaneous factors. Br J Dermatol 2003;149:718-30.
17. Torii H, Tamaki K, Granstein RD. The effect of neuropeptides/hormones on Langerhans cells. J Dermatol Sci 1998;20:21-8.
18. Asahina A, Hosoi J, Grabbe S, Granstein RD. Modulation of Langerhans cell function by epidermal nerves. J Allergy Clin Immunol 1995;96:1178-82.
19. Hosoi J, Murphy GF, Egan CL, et al. Regulation of Langerhans cell function by nerves containing calcitonin gene-related peptide. Nature 1993;363:159-63.
20. Doyle JA, Connolly SM, Hunziker N, Winkelmann RK. Prurigo nodularis: a reappraisal of the clinical and histologic features. J Cutan Pathol 1979;6:392-403.
21. Abadia Molina F, Burrows NP, Jones RR, Terenghi G, Polak JM. Increased sensory neuropeptides in nodular prurigo: a quantitative immunohistochemical analysis. Br J Dermatol 1992;127:344-51.
22. Nahass GT, Penneys NS. Merkel cells and prurigo nodularis. J Am Acad Dermatol 1994;31:86-8.
23. Lynch PJ. Lichen simplex chronicus (atopic/neurodermatitis) of the anogenital region. Dermatol Ther 2004;17:8-19.
24. Rowland Payne CM, Wilkinson JD, McKee PH, Jurecka W, Black MM. Nodular prurigo—a clinicopathological study of 46 patients. Br J Dermatol 1985;113:431-9.
24a. Murphy GF, Elder D. Non-melanocytic tumors of the skin. AFIP Atlas of Tumor Pathology, 3rd Series, Fascicle 1. Washington DC: American Registry of Pathology; 1991.
25. Gottlieb AB, Mease PJ, Mark Jackson J, et al. Clinical characteristics of psoriatic arthritis and psoriasis in dermatologists' offices. J Dermatolog Treat 2006;17:279-87.
26. Weiss G, Shemer A, Trau H. The Koebner phenomenon: review of the literature. J Eur Acad Dermatol Venereol 2002;16:241-8.
27. Aslanian FM, Lisboa FF, Iwamoto A, Carneiro SC. Clinical and epidemiological evaluation of psoriasis: clinical variants and articular manifestations. J Eur Acad Dermatol Venereol 2005;19:141-2.
28. Guldbakke KK, Khachemoune A. Guttate psoriasis. Dermatol Nurs 2006;18:369.
29. Zhao G, Feng X, Na A, et al. Acute guttate psoriasis patients have positive streptococcus hemolyticus throat cultures and elevated antistreptococcal M6 protein titers. J Dermatol 2005;32:91-6.
30. Rongioletti F, Borenstein M, Kirsner R, Kerdel F. Erythrodermic, recalcitrant psoriasis: clinical resolution with infliximab. J Dermatolog Treat 2003;14:222-5.
31. O'Brien M, Koo J. The mechanism of lithium and beta-blocking agents in inducing and exacerbating psoriasis. J Drugs Dermatol 2006;5:426-32.
32. Smith CH, Barker JN. Psoriasis and its management. BMJ 2006;19;333:380-4.
33. Alebiosu CO, Raimi TH, Badru AI, Amore OO, Ogunkoya JO, Odusan O. Reiters syndrome - a case report and review of literature. Afr Health Sci 2004;4:136-8.
34. Iizuka H, Takahashi H, Ishida-Yamamoto A. Pathophysiology of generalized pustular psoriasis. Arch Dermatol Res 2003;295(Suppl 1):S55-59.
35. Rym BM, Mourad M, Bechir Z, et al. Erythroderma in adults: a report of 80 cases. Int J Dermatol 2005;44:731-5.
36. Namazi MR. Paradoxical exacerbation of psoriasis in AIDS: proposed explanations including the potential roles of substance P and gram-negative bacteria. Autoimmunity 2004;37:67-71.
37. Utikal J, Beck E, Dippel E, Klemke CD, Goerdt S. Reiter's syndrome-like pattern in AIDS-associated psoriasiform dermatitis. J Eur Acad Dermatol Venereol 2003;17:114-6.
38. Nickoloff BJ, Nestle FO. Recent insights into the immunopathogenesis of psoriasis provide new therapeutic opportunities. J Clin Invest 2004;113:1664-75.
39. Cribier B. Psoriasis under the microscope. J Eur Acad Dermatol Venereol 2006;20(Suppl 2):3-9.
40. Petzelbauer P, Pober JS, Keh A, Braverman IM. Inducibility and expression of microvascular endothelial adhesion molecules in lesional, perilesional, and uninvolved skin of psoriatic patients. J Invest Dermatol 1994;103:300-5.
41. Gokhale NR, Belgaumkar VA, Pandit DP, Deshpande S, Damle DK. A study of serum nitric oxide levels in psoriasis. Indian J Dermatol Venereol Leprol 2005;71:175-8.
42. Saraceno R, Kleyn CE, Terenghi G, Griffiths CE. The role of neuropeptides in psoriasis. Br J Dermatol 2006;155:876-82.
43. Zegarska B, Lelinska A, Tyrakowski T. Clinical and experimental aspects of cutaneous neurogenic inflammation. Pharmacol Rep 2006;58:13-21.
44. Biral AC, Magalhaes RF, Wastowski IJ, et al. Association of HLA-A, -B, -C genes and TNF microsatellite polymorphism with psoriasis vulgaris: a study of genetic risk in Brazilian patients. Eur J Dermatol 2006;16:523-9.
45. Paladini F, Taccari E, Fiorillo MT, et al. Distribution of HLA-B27 subtypes in Sardinia and continental Italy and their association with spondylarthropathies. Arthritis Rheum 2005;52:3319-21.

46. Korendowych E, McHugh N. Genetic factors in psoriatic arthritis. Curr Rheumatol Rep 2005;7:306-12.
47. Ortonne JP. A paradigm for the systemic treatment of plaque psoriasis. J Eur Acad Dermatol Venereol 2006;20(Suppl 2):77-9.
48. Pincus DJ. Pityriasis rubra pilaris: a clinical review. Dermatol Nurs. 2005;17:448-51.
49. White KL. Pityriasis rubra pilaris. Dermatol Online J 2003;9:6.
50. Howe K, Foresman P, Griffin T, Johnson W. Pityriasis rubra pilaris with acantholysis. J Cutan Pathol 1996;23:270-4.
50a. Vanderhooft SL, Francis JS, Holbrook KA, Dale BA, Fleckman P. Familial pityriasis rubra pilaris. Arch Dermatol 1995;131:448-53
51. Sehgal VN, Jain S, Kumar S, Bhattacharya SN, Sardana K, Bajaj P. Familial pityriasis rubra pilaris (adult classic-I): a report of three cases in a single family. Skinmed 2002;1:161-4.
51a. Garcovich S, Di Giampetruzzi AR, Antonelli G, Garcovich A, Didona B. Treatment of refractory adult-onset pityriasis rubra pilaris with TNF-alpha antogonists: a case series. J Eur Acad Dermatol Venereol 2010;8:881-4.
52. Rigopoulos D, Paparizos V, Katsambas A. Cutaneous markers of HIV infection. Clin Dermatol 2004;22:487-98.
53. Chuh A, Lee A, Zawar V, Sciallis G, Kempf W. Pityriasis rosea—an update. Indian J Dermatol Venereol Leprol 2005;71:311-5.
54. Panizzon R, Bloch PH. Histopathology of pityriasis rosea Gibert. Qualitative and quantitative light-microscopic study of 62 biopsies of 40 patients. Dermatologica 1982;165:551-8.
55. Sugiura H, Miyauchi H, Uehara M. Evolutionary changes of immunohistological characteristics of secondary lesions in pityriasis rosea. Arch Dermatol Res 1988;280:405-10.
56. Aiba S, Tagami H. HLA-DR antigen expression on the keratinocyte surface in dermatoses characterized by lymphocytic exocytosis (e.g. pityriasis rosea). Br J Dermatol 1984;111:285-94.
57. Bowers S, Warshaw EM. Pityriasis lichenoides and its subtypes. J Am Acad Dermatol 2006;55: 557-72.
57a. Sharma PK, Yadav TP, Gautam RK, Taneja N, Satyanarayana L. Erythromycin in pityriasis rosea: a double-blind, placebo-controlled clinical trial. J Am Acad Dermatol 2000;42(Pt 1):241-4.
57b. Tey HL, Tan SH. Reactive eccrine syringofibroadenomatosis associated with venous stasis and plaque psoriasis. Acta Derm Venereol 2008; 88:82-4.
58. Ando K, Hattori H, Yamauchi Y. Histopathological differences between early and old lesions of hyperkeratosis lenticularis perstans (Flegel's disease). Am J Dermatopathol 2006;28:122-6.
59. Welsh JP, Skvarka CB, Allen HB. A novel visual clue for the diagnosis of hypertrophic lichen planus. Arch Dermatol 2006;142:954.
60. Alagheband M, Engineer L. Lithium and halogenoderma. Arch Dermatol 2000;136:126-7.
61. Daldon PE, Macedo de Souza E, Cintra ML. Hypertrophic lupus erythematosus: a clinicopathological study of 14 cases. J Cutan Pathol 2003;30:443-8.
62. Bolotin D, Racz MI, Petronic-Rosic V, Sethi A. Acquired combined nutritional deficiency presenting as psoriasiform dermatitis. J Am Acad Dermatol. 2010 Apr;62(4):715-8.

# 4  PRIMARY ACANTHOLYTIC DERMATITIS

The disorders considered here are dermatoses in which acantholysis is the predominant histologic finding. Acantholysis indicates the loss of normal intercellular adhesive interactions among epidermal keratinocytes, resulting in cleft and blister formation. Unlike blisters formed by spongiosis, where keratinocytes are literally torn apart due to the forces of intercellular edema, acantholytic blisters are associated with often viable cells that are present as free, "rounded up" cells within the blister cavity or blister edge. In some lesions, acantholysis is associated with necrosis or dyskeratosis. Dyskeratosis is a much abused term. Here it is used to indicate faulty or premature keratinization, manifested by cytoplasmic hypereosinophilia and nuclear alterations. It does not necessarily suggest necrosis, although some dyskeratotic cells may be rapidly approaching premature programmed cell death (apoptosis). While it is arguable as to whether conditions mediated by focal acantholytic dyskeratosis should be grouped as inflammatory or noninflammatory disorders, the persistent tendency for them to have dermal lymphocytic infiltrates often containing eosinophils is the rationale for their inclusion here. Acantholysis associated with keratinocyte necrosis is exemplified by infection by herpesvirus. Cytopathologic alterations of other, less frequently encountered, viruses are beyond the scope of the present discussion, and are considered in Fascicles dealing with infectious diseases or tumor-like epidermal proliferations.

## PATHOGENESIS

*Pemphigus* refers to a group of autoimmune blistering diseases involving the skin and mucous membranes. There are several clinical variants, all of which have circulating antibodies against epithelial intercellular substance (1). All have in common the histologic findings of intraepithelial acantholysis and deposition of immunoglobulins in the intercellular spaces. Immunoelectron microscopy reveals immunoglobulin deposition on the cell surface of keratinocytes without extension into the cytoplasm of cells. The antigenic binding site of pemphigus vulgaris antibodies is a 130-kD glycoprotein (i.e., the pemphigus vulgaris complex), where desmoglein 3 is linked to plakoglobin, an 85-kD protein found in both adherens junctions and desmosomes (1a). In pemphigus foliaceus, or superficial pemphigus, the antigen complex is desmoglein 1, a 160-kD desmosomal core glycoprotein that is linked to plakoglobin (2). Direct immunofluorescence shows intercellular deposition of immunoglobulin (Ig) G and C3 indistinguishable from that of pemphigus vulgaris. Frequently, however, the staining is predominantly in the superficial epidermal layers. Brazilian pemphigus foliaceus, or fogo selvagem, which is endemic in rural South America, is clinically and pathologically indistinguishable from other cases of pemphigus foliaceus (3). These patients also have autoantibodies that bind to the same desmoglein 1 protein.

The cause of acantholytic/dyskeratotic disorders of skin is not as yet fully elucidated, although defective synthesis or aberrant proteolytic degradation of desmosomal components is suspected. Virally induced acantholysis is thought to represent a manifestation of early cytopathic alteration, a hypothesis that is supported by the association between acantholysis and necrosis in herpetic blisters.

## SPECIAL DIAGNOSTIC STUDIES

All the pemphigus variants have circulating antibodies against epithelial intercellular substances (4,5). Pemphigus vulgaris, the most common of the subgroups, shows intercellular deposition of IgG in nearly 100 percent of patients with active disease. The immunoreactant deposition is in a fine, uniform, fish-net or honeycomb pattern. A similar pattern is reproduced in monkey esophagus when patient serum is evaluated by indirect immunofluorescence. C3 may be detected alone or in addition to IgG in up to 50 percent of cases. However, intercellular complement binding without IgG has been reported in normal skin as well. IgA and IgM are seen in addition to IgG in approximately 30 to 50 percent of cases.

As stated, direct immunofluorescence of pemphigus foliaceus shows intercellular deposition of IgG and C3 indistinguishable from that of pemphigus vulgaris. Frequently, however, the staining is predominantly in the superficial epidermal layers. In Senear-Usher syndrome, or pemphigus erythematosus, patients develop scaly, erythematous lesions in a photodistributed pattern. The results of direct immunofluorescence are similar to those of pemphigus vulgaris and pemphigus foliaceus, but additionally, there is granular deposition of IgG and C3 at the dermal-epidermal junction, such as is seen in a positive lupus band test. These immunoreactants have been demonstrated on facial lesions and sun-exposed skin. Although coexistent systemic lupus erythematosus and pemphigus have been reported, patients with Senear-Usher syndrome generally do not develop systemic lupus with visceral organ involvement. Positive antinuclear antibodies (ANAs) are present in approximately 30 percent of these patients. These ANAs may produce a false-negative indirect immunofluorescence result for circulating pemphigus antibodies due to an interference phenomenon termed the prozone effect.

Pemphigus vegetans occurs in two clinical subtypes: the Neumann type, which has a more aggressive course, and the Hallopeau type, which tends to be less severe. Histopathology shows pseudoepitheliomatous hyperplasia, intraepidermal abscesses of eosinophils, and suprabasal acantholysis. Immunofluorescence, however, is indistinguishable from that of pemphigus vulgaris.

Pemphigus herpetiformis shows intercellular deposition of IgG and C3 similar to pemphigus vegetans on direct immunofluorescence. A recently described entity characterized by circulating or in vivo bound IgA antibodies to intercellular substance has been termed IgA pemphigus, intraepidermal neutrophilic IgA dermatosis, or intercellular IgA vesiculopustular dermatosis (IAVPD). Immunopathology reveals deposition of IgA in a pattern similar to that of pemphigus; however, recent immunoblot analysis suggests that IAVPD is a different entity than pemphigus.

Immunofluorescence is generally negative or nonspecific for other forms of acantholytic dermatitis, and the diagnosis generally depends on the interpretation of conventionally stained sections. In the case of early herpesvirus infections, immunohistochemical probes for detection of herpes simplex virus (HSV) are available.

Animal models for the reproduction of immunologically mediated acantholytic disorders have traditionally relied upon the passive transfer of human autoantibodies into rodents, resulting in variable blister formation. More recently, human skin xenografted onto genetically immunocompromised mice has served as a suitable substrate for the reproduction of lesions like pemphigus upon administration of autoantibody-producing leukocytes from patients. Evidence of the functional significance of target molecules has been demonstrated using mice whose relevant genes for these structural proteins have been deleted. Desmoglein 3 knockout mice develop a pemphigus-like epithelial pathology (6–8). An inbred canine model has also been described for the study of Hailey-Hailey disease (9). Animal models also exist for the study of herpesvirus infection, particularly with regard to the phenomenon of photoactivation.

## PEMPHIGUS GROUP

**Definition.** *Pemphigus vulgaris* (PV) is a blistering disorder characterized by bullous lesions that are flaccid and break easily in the skin, and mucosal lesions that are painful and in many are the presenting sign of the disease (10). Before the onset of corticosteroid therapy, this form of pemphigus was usually fatal, with patients dying from protein loss and sepsis. PV affects men and women with equal frequency. The median age is 50 years. It is more common in Jewish persons and persons of Mediterranean descent.

The *foliaceus variant of pemphigus* (PF) is characterized by crusted lesions often in a seborrheic distribution. Lesions tend not to involve the mucosae, and follow a less aggressive course with less mortality. The disorder most commonly occurs in middle to late life. PF also has a more localized form, *pemphigus erythematosus,* and an endemic form in Brazil, known as *fogo selvagem*; this usually occurs in younger patients, even in childhood.

**Clinical Features.** PV most often begins as a persistent, painful oral erosion or multiple erosions. In some patients, these lesions are the only sign of the disease for several months. The discomfort caused by the disease may impair the patient's ability to eat and drink. We have the clinical dictum that a persistent, painful erosion of more than two months' duration should be biopsied not only to rule out a malignancy but also to exclude pemphigus. The lesions begin as blisters but are rarely observed as such, because they rapidly break down. The erosions may appear anywhere in the buccal mucosa and may affect the pharynx or even the larynx. Other mucosal areas may be affected, including the conjunctiva, anus, and genitalia.

The cutaneous manifestation of PV is a flaccid blister, sometimes referred to as a "droopy drawers" blister, that can occur anywhere on the skin surface including the scalp. A weeping scalp lesion always suggests the consideration of pemphigus. The lesion may arise on normal-appearing skin or on an inflamed base (fig. 4-1). Because the blisters are fragile, they rapidly break down and lead to erosions that are painful (fig. 4-2). A characteristic response of the skin to shearing trauma, with the formation of a blister, has been designated the *Nikolsky sign*. A similar phenomenon can be elicited by the application of lateral trauma to a blister. This sign is not specific for pemphigus and is seen in other bullous disorders.

Some patients exhibit a striking response to the formation of erosions, with granulation tissue and vegetations, especially in intertriginous areas. When this response is the only manifestation of the disease, it has been designated *pemphigus vegetans of Hallopeau* (11). Another variant, *pemphigus vegetans of Neumann*, begins with vegetations but goes on to the development of the typical erosive lesions of pemphigus vulgaris. Patients with the Hallopeau variant, before current therapies were available, had a less serious prognosis than those with the Neumann variant, who had a high mortality rate.

*Neonatal pemphigus* (12) is an acquired variant occurring in children of mothers with PV. It varies greatly in extent and severity, with most extreme cases of disseminated blisters and erosions associated with stillbirth. This disease is self-remitting and should not be confused with the occurrence of pemphigus in childhood.

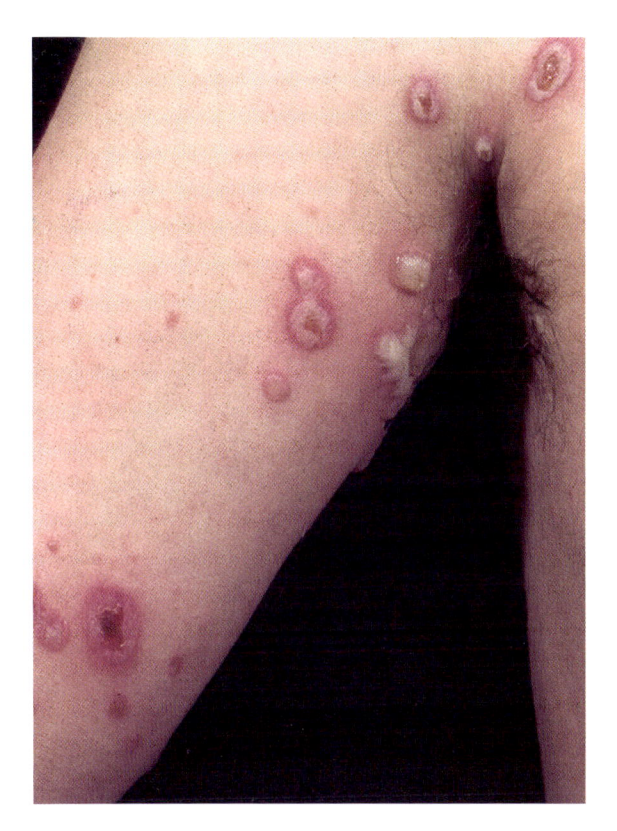

Figure 4-1
PEMPHIGUS VULGARIS: LOCALIZED
Central erosions are rimmed by discrete zones of erythema. Intact blisters are also evident.

Although the primary lesion of PF is a small blister, it is almost never observed (fig. 4-3). Rather, it quickly breaks down and leads to a scaling, crusted lesion on an erythematous base. Frequently, at the periphery of the lesion, which can exhibit a quite hyperkeratotic surface, a small vesicle is seen. PF lesions usually measure a few centimeters and have a round, oval, or irregular shape. The distribution is often in the so-called seborrheic areas of the body, including face, scalp, and trunk. Although the disorder is usually localized for some time in most patients, it can become rapidly progressive and even lead to an exfoliative erythroderma. The lesions are induced or exacerbated by exposure to light or heat. Infection with *Candida* can also induce a localized lesion. PF does not generally involve the mucosa and thus differs significantly from PV.

One form of this disease occurs endemically in Brazil, mainly along the riverbeds of the interior. The disease follows the distribution

*Inflammatory Disorders of the Skin*

Figure 4-2
**PEMPHIGUS VULGARIS**
The axilla is extensively involved by erosions representing sites of previous evanescent bullae.

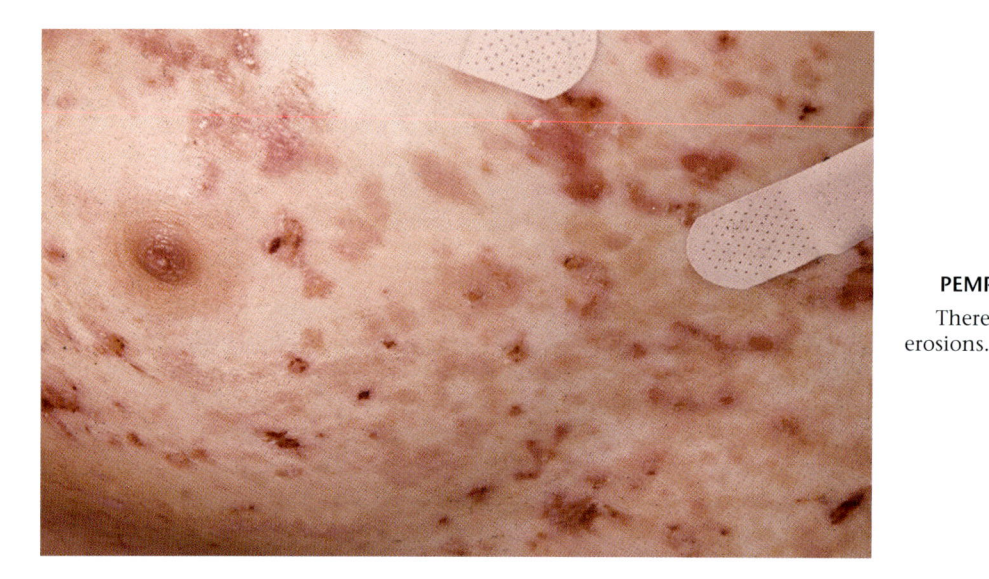

Figure 4-3
**PEMPHIGUS FOLIACEUS**
There are multiple superficial erosions.

of the black fly, *Simulium pruinosum*. Family members are often affected, but there is no know predilection for the disease. Clinically, the lesions resemble PF, but they have more symptomatology, including marked burning. There is a more obvious relationship to sun exacerbation in these patients.

Another form of PF is *pemphigus erythematosus* (13), or *Senear-Usher syndrome*, which describes crusted lesions localized to the malar region and other sites affected by seborrhea. These patients sometimes show the serologic changes of lupus erythematosus, but the two diseases do not usually overlap. Pemphigus erythematosus can lead to a generalized eruption following its initial localized form.

**Pathologic Findings.** Histologically, the common denominator of the pemphigus group of disorders is acantholysis. This term implies dissolution, or lysis, of the intercellular adhesion sites within a squamous epithelial surface. Acantholytic cells that are no longer attached to other epithelial cells lose their polyhedral shape and characteristically become rounded. In PV and pemphigus vegetans, acantholysis selectively involves the layer of cells immediately above the basal cell layer (figs. 4-4–4-7). This pathologic change correlates with the deposition of circulating autoantibodies to the intercellular spaces, specifically in association with the intercellular junctions (fig. 4-8; also see below). The vegetans variant also shows

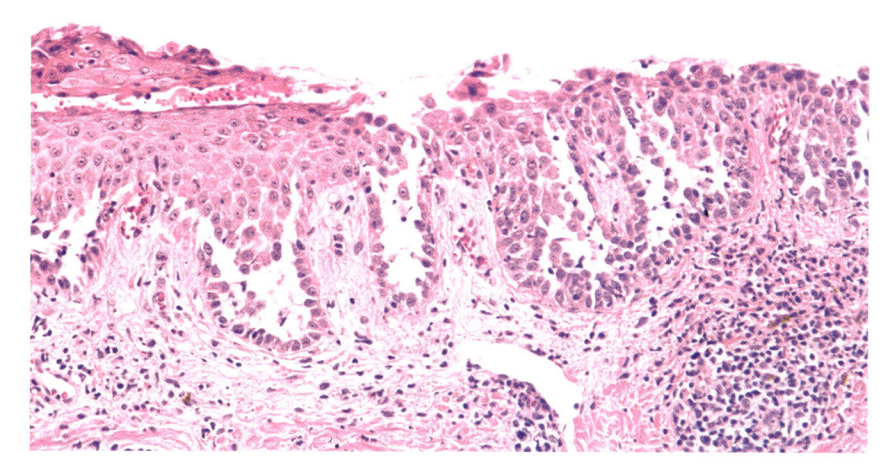

**Figure 4-4**

**PEMPHIGUS VULGARIS**

A suprabasal blister forms as a result of keratinocyte acantholysis.

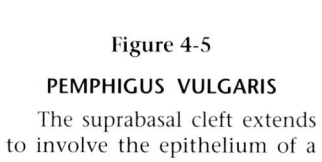

**Figure 4-5**

**PEMPHIGUS VULGARIS**

The suprabasal cleft extends to involve the epithelium of a hair follicle.

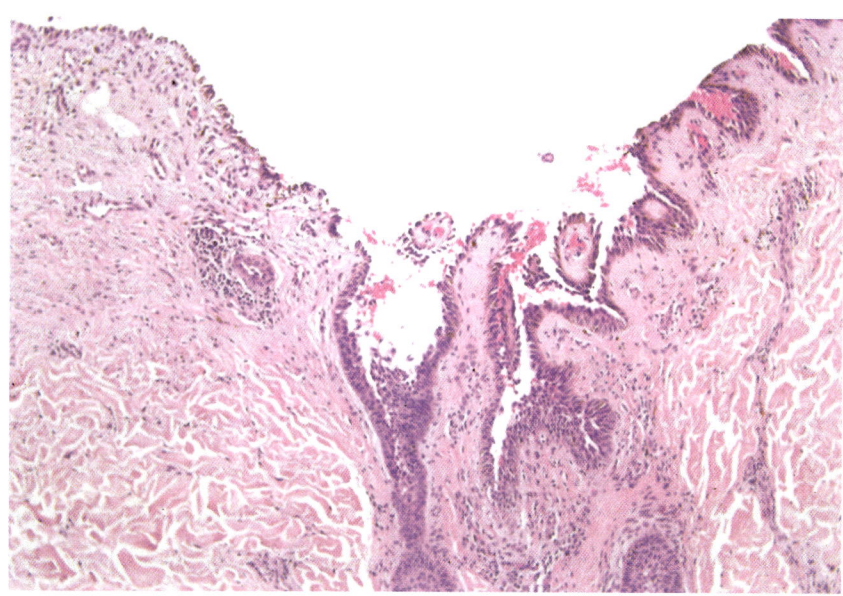

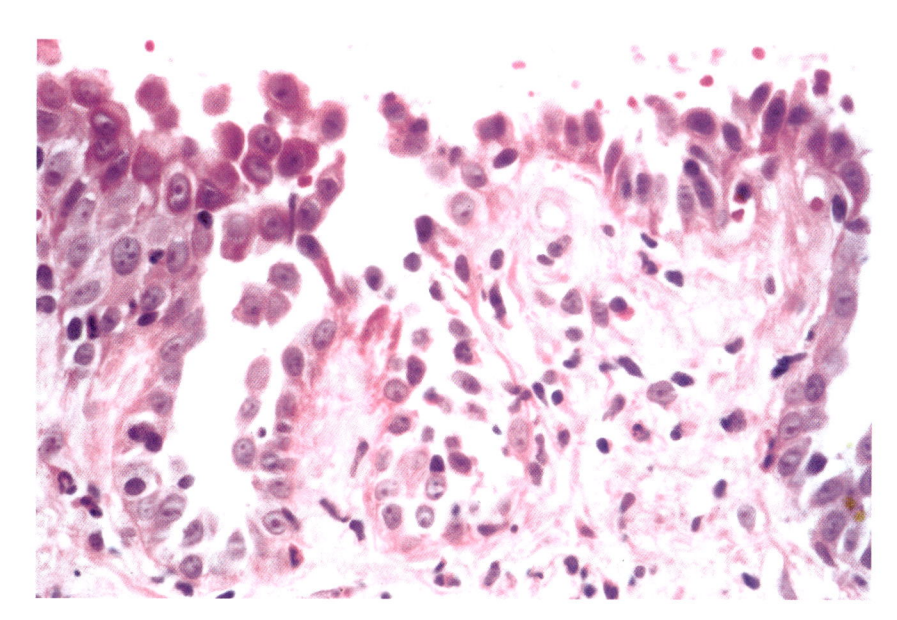

**Figure 4-6**

**PEMPHIGUS VULGARIS: BLISTER BASE**

At high magnification, the intact basal cells demonstrate the characteristic "tombstone" appearance.

*Inflammatory Disorders of the Skin*

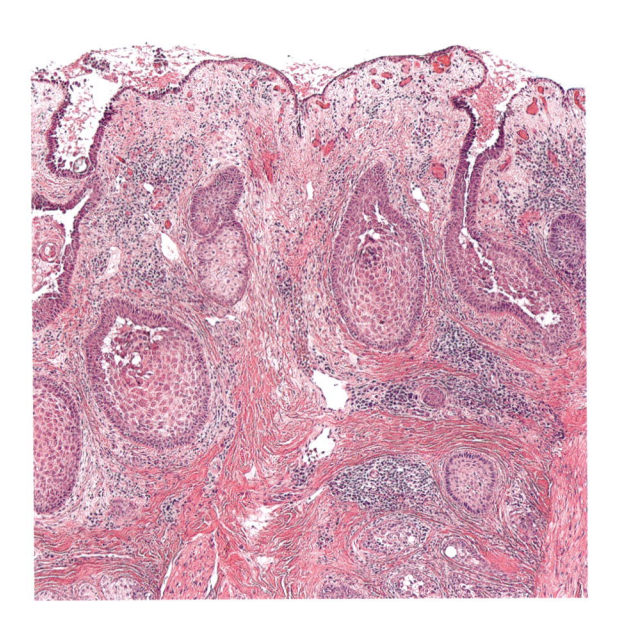

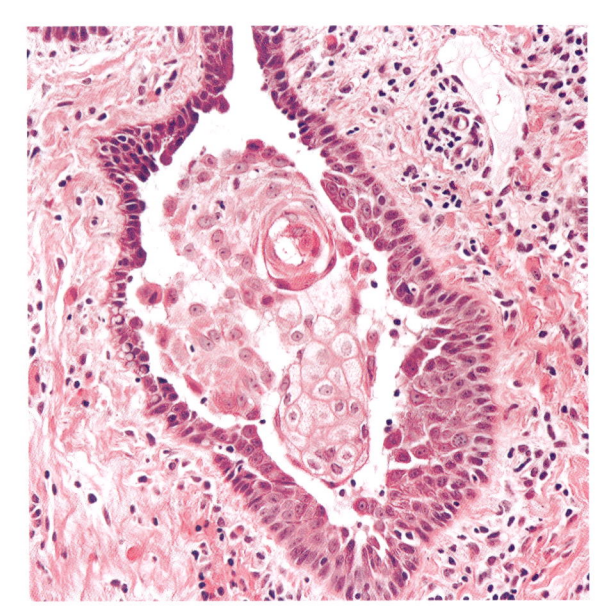

Figure 4-7

**PEMPHIGUS VULGARIS**

Left: Scanning magnification of follicular involvement. Only the basal layer of the epidermis is present, and acantholytic alterations extend deeply into most hair follicles.

Right: High magnification of acantholytic changes shows involvement of the pilosebaceous unit.

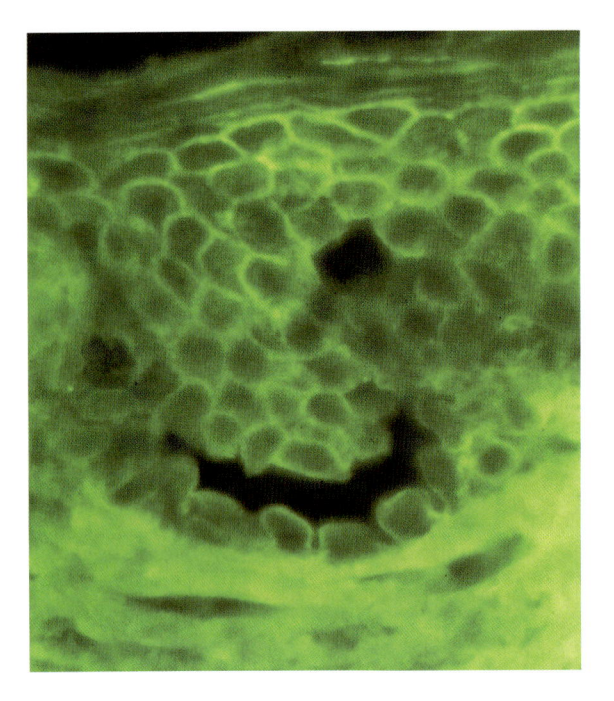

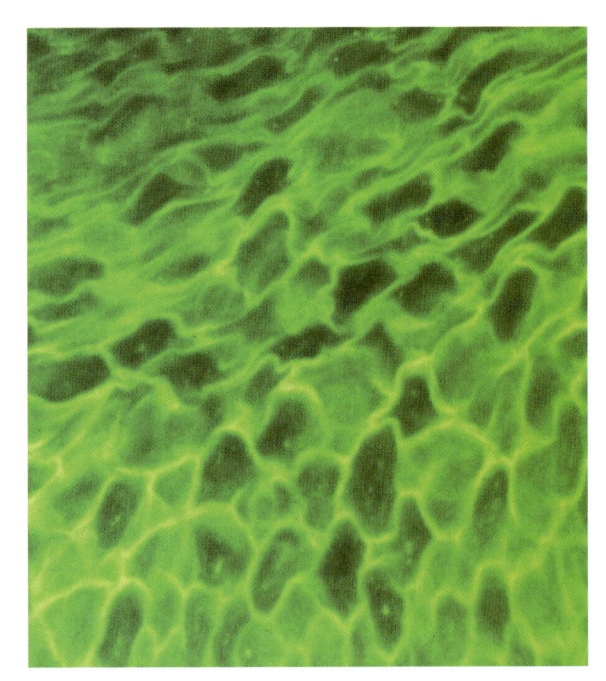

Figure 4-8

**PEMPHIGUS VULGARIS**

Left: By direct immunofluorescence, this lesion shows the typical intercellular pattern of immunoglobulin (Ig) G deposition. A suprabasal acantholytic cleft in an early formative stage is seen.

Right: Indirect immunofluorescence shows IgG directed against desmoglein 3 of the keratinocyte desmosomal complexes in monkey esophagus incubated with patient serum. The "fish net" pattern is characteristic.

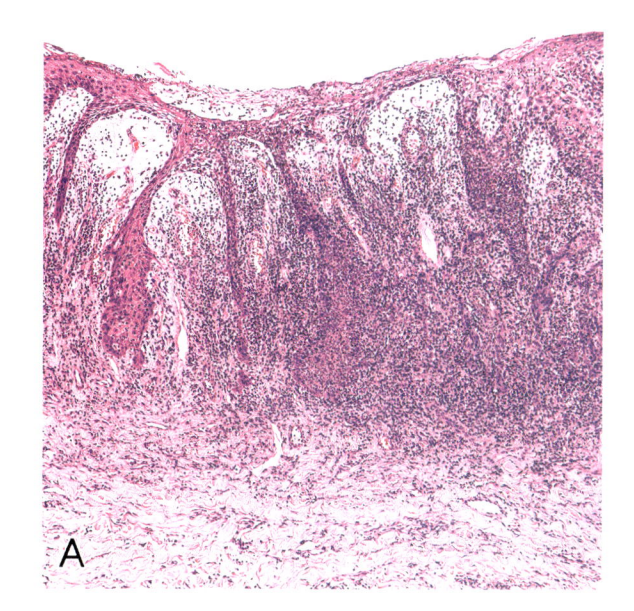

#### Figure 4-9
#### PEMPHIGUS VEGETANS
A: At low magnification, there is endophytic epidermal proliferation and a striking inflammatory infiltrate.
B: High magnification of the endophytic component of pemphigus vegetans shows intraepithelial microabscesses.
C: Endophytic epithelial proliferation is characterized by destructive microabscess formation and a marked surrounding inflammatory response.

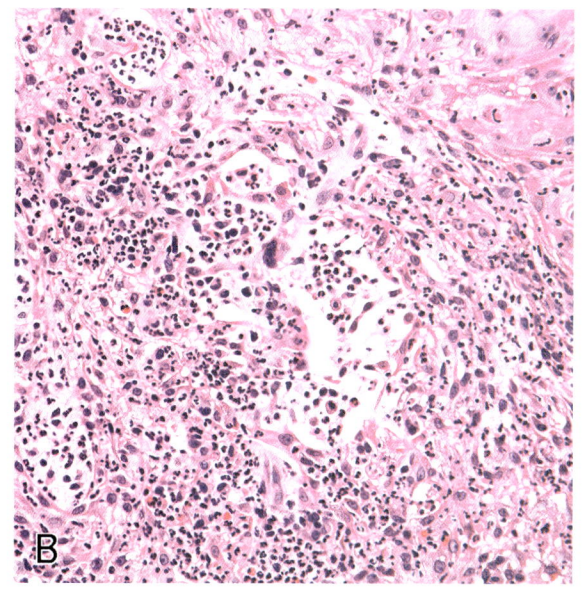

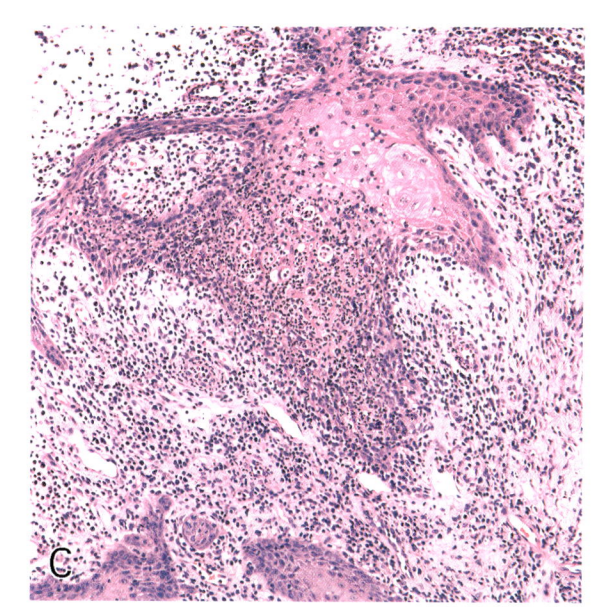

considerable epidermal hyperplasia as well as intraepidermal microabscesses (fig. 4-9). In PF, a blister forms by similar mechanisms, but unlike PV, it selectively involves the superficial epidermis at the level of the stratum granulosum (figs. 4-10–4-12). Variable superficial dermal infiltration by lymphocytes, histiocytes, and eosinophils accompanies all forms of pemphigus.

Sera from patients with PV contain antibodies of the IgG type, which react with the intercellular cement substance of skin and mucous membranes. This phenomenon is the basis for direct and indirect diagnostic immunofluorescence testing of skin and serum, respectively (fig. 4-8). Lesional skin shows a net-like pattern of intercellular IgG deposition localized to sites of developed or incipient acantholysis.

**Clinicopathologic Variants.** *Pemphigus as a reaction to drugs.* Two drugs, penicillamine (14) and captopril, are associated with symptoms and signs of pemphigus, more commonly of the foliaceus type. These drugs have sulfhydryl residues that reduce disulfide bonds and directly cause acantholysis.

*Paraneoplastic Pemphigus.* This eruption consists of oral erosions and a complex skin erup-

*Inflammatory Disorders of the Skin*

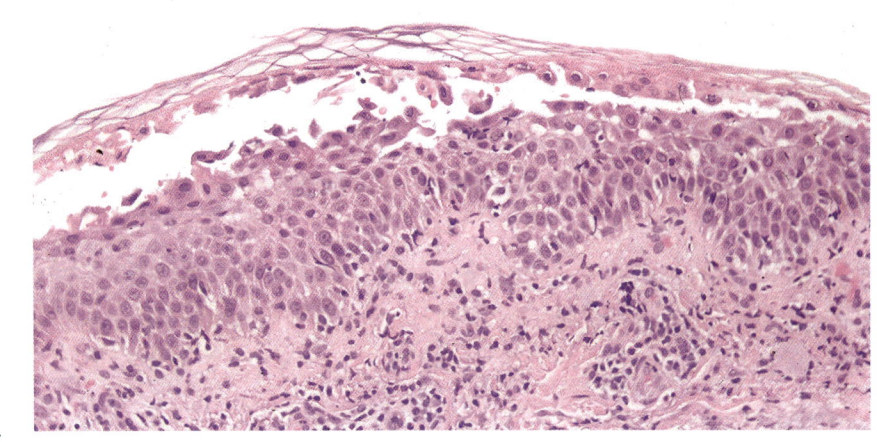

**Figure 4-10**

**PEMPHIGUS FOLIACEUS**

Top: At scanning magnification, the stratum corneum appears to be separating from the underlying epidermis, producing a cleft that at first may be overlooked as artifact.

Bottom: At higher magnification, individual acantholytic cells derived from the subcorneal layer are evident.

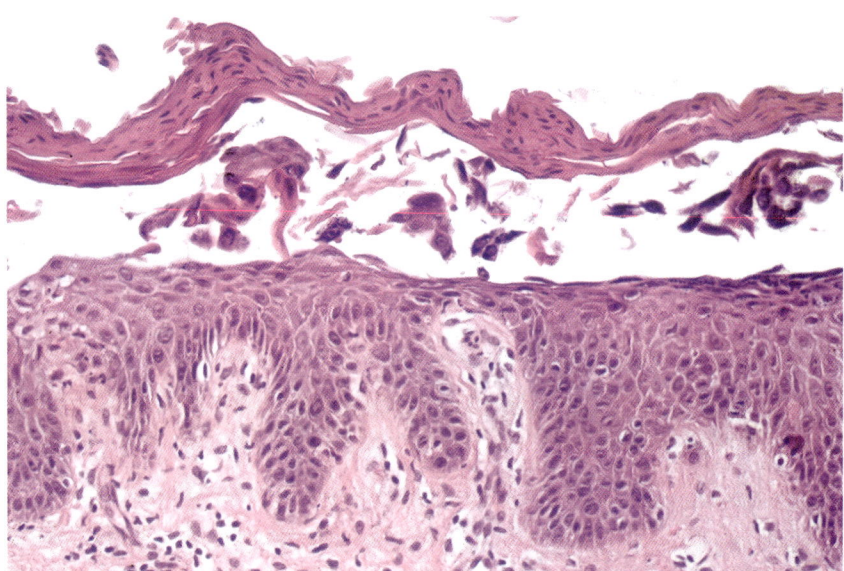

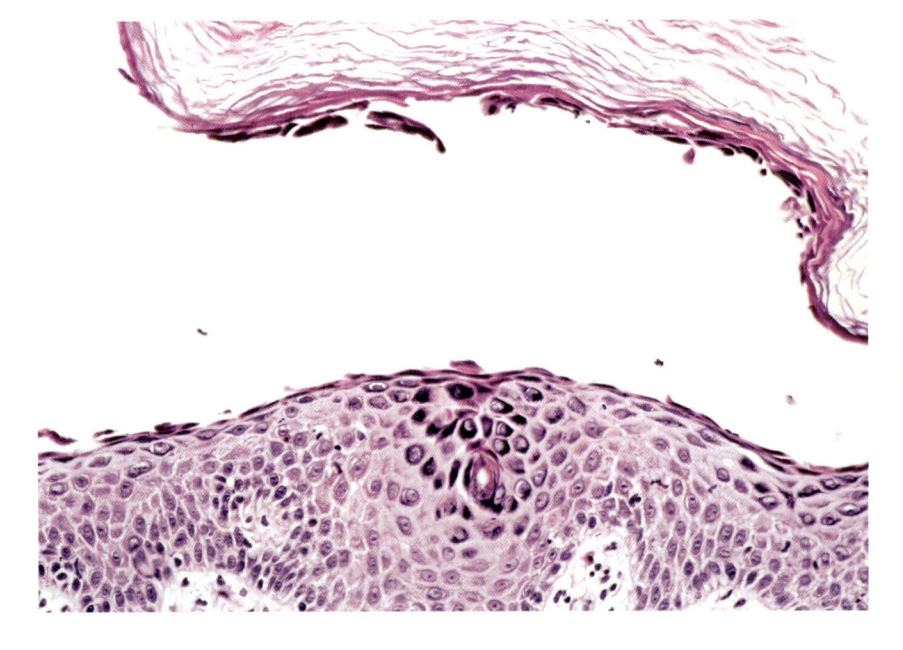

**Figure 4-11**

**PEMPHIGUS FOLIACEUS**

A subcorneal blister shows rare acantholytic stratum granulosum cells. Identification of this subtle feature is important for diagnosis.

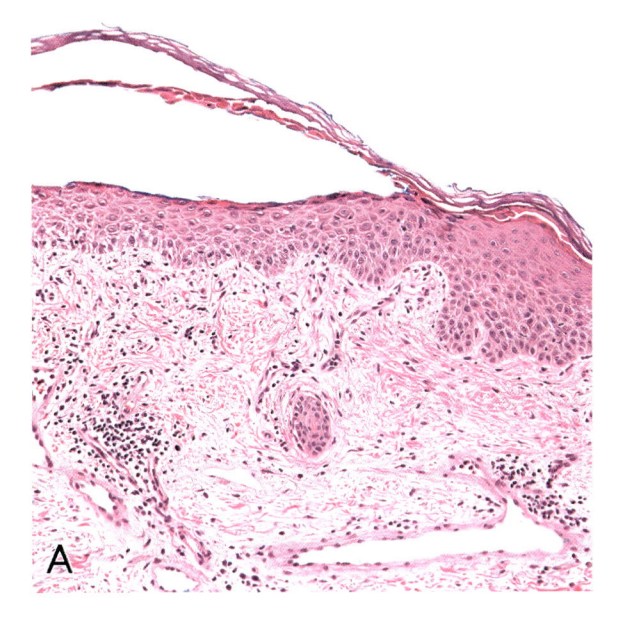

### Figure 4-12
### PEMPHIGUS FOLIACEUS

A: At scanning magnification, the stratum corneum is lifting off of the superficial epidermis as a result of subtle acantholysis at the level of the stratum granulosum.

B: Higher magnification shows superficial acantholytic cells present at the forming blister edge.

C: Subtle acantholysis involves the most superficial layers of the follicular infundibulum.

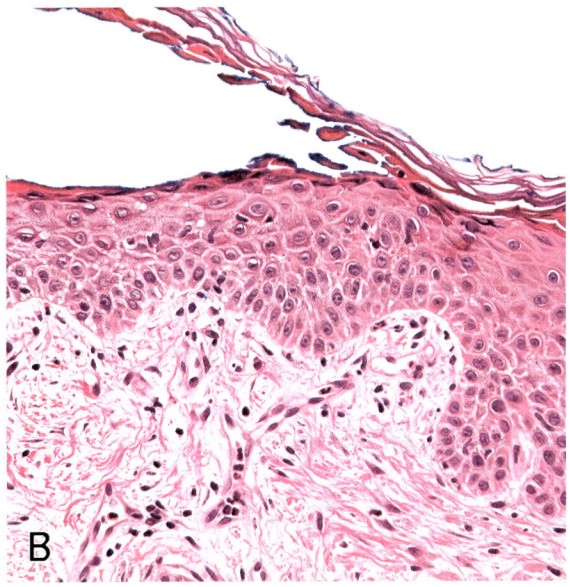

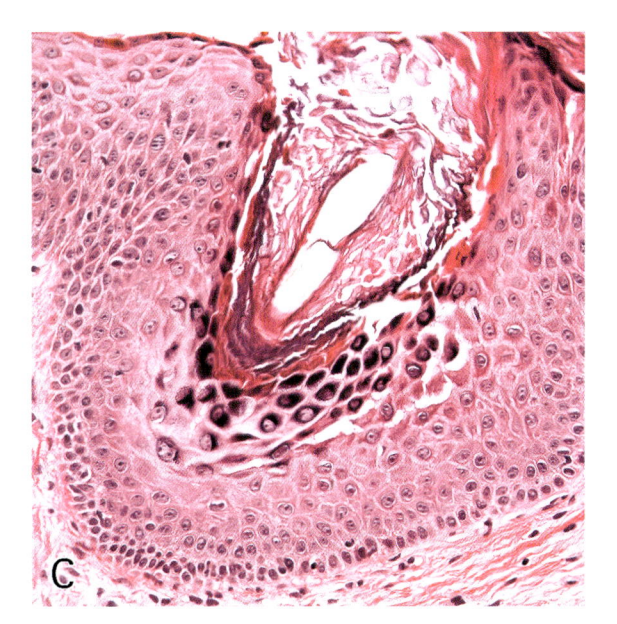

tion that includes erythematous plaques, blisters, and erythema multiforme-like lesions. It principally occurs in association with lymphoproliferative disorders and thymoma (15). Histologically, paraneoplastic pemphigus often shows an interface dermatitis which may be associated with necrosis of keratinocytes in the lower epidermis, in addition to acantholysis (fig. 4-13).

Patients present with a variety of lesions in the skin. Some resemble erythema multiforme, others subacute lupus erythematosus, others are eczematous, and all result in blistering. Erosions commonly follow. Oral lesions are the second manifestation of the disease and are associated with erosions. The patients respond to treatment of the underlying disorder.

*IgA Pemphigus.* This pustulovesicular disorder is one of the causes of intraepidermal neutrophils and is often classified with the neutrophilic type of dermatoses (16). The lesions of IgA pemphigus comprise a strikingly pruritic, vesicular and pustular rash that occurs predominantly in mid-life and the elderly, with the main age of onset in the sixth to seventh decades. The clinical findings are a crossover between subcorneal pustulosis and PF. Thus there are small vesicles and blisters

## Inflammatory Disorders of the Skin

**Figure 4-13**

**PARANEOPLASTIC PEMPHIGUS**

A: Lymphocyte-mediated interface change and suprabasal acantholysis are present.
B: There is prominent zone of suprabasal acantholysis.
C: High magnification demonstrates combined interface and acantholytic changes.

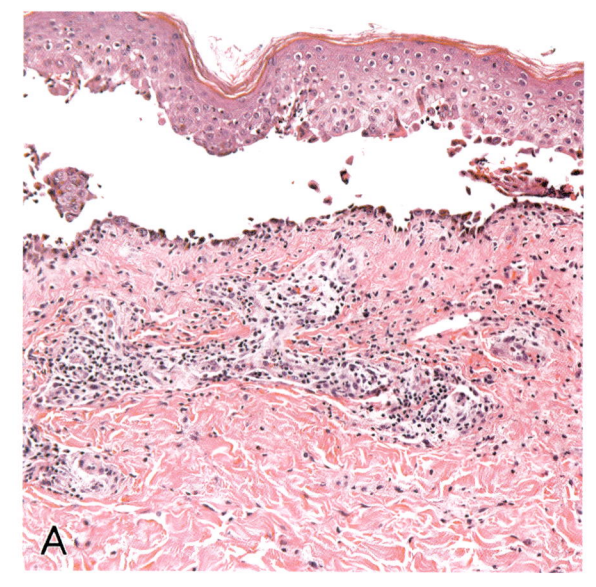

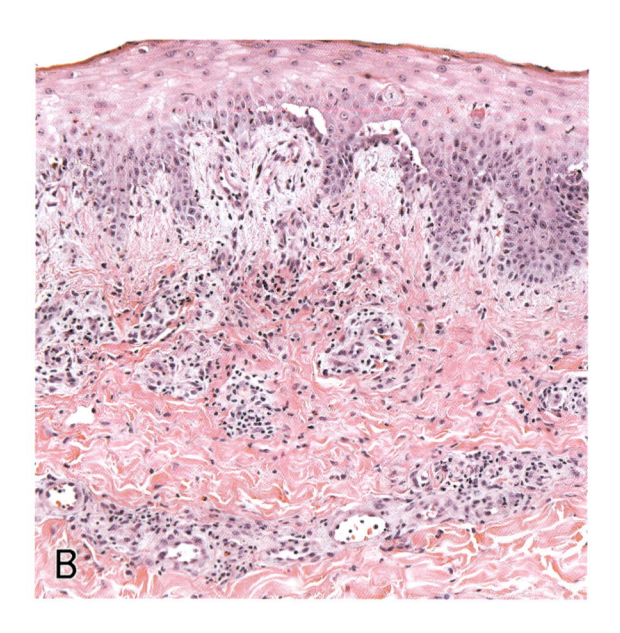

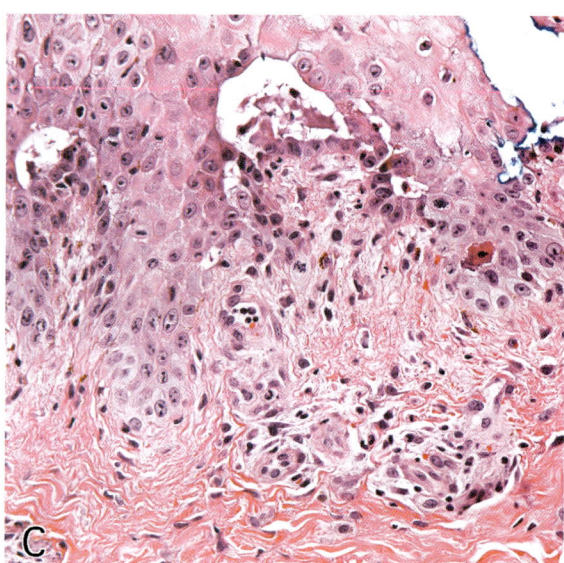

that can rupture and give rise to crusted areas or there are pustules or an admixture of pustules, bullae, and flaccid vesicles. The patients either have a subcorneal pustular type of lesion or an intraepidermal pustular disorder. There is often an annular arrangement to these lesions.

The differential diagnosis includes the subcorneal pustular dermatosis of Sneddon-Wilkinson. Pustular psoriasis, impetigo, and the pemphigus group of disorders (PV and PF) must likewise be distinguished. Immunofluorescence findings are very helpful in making the appropriate diagnosis.

**Treatment and Prognosis.** The first line of defense for pemphigus lesions, which has resulted in a markedly improved prognosis, is glucocorticoid therapy. The initial dose of therapy is very high in order to suppress the disease. The dosage is tapered as the disease clears. Because these high dosages may result in complications, including diabetes, infection, and gastrointestinal ulceration and bleeding, other modalities of therapy have been sought. In order to avoid these complications, immunosuppressive agents such as mycophenolate mofetil, azathioprine, intravenous immunoglobulin, and rituximab have been added to the therapeutic armamentarium with great success. Other agents have been used, including dapsone, cyclosporine,

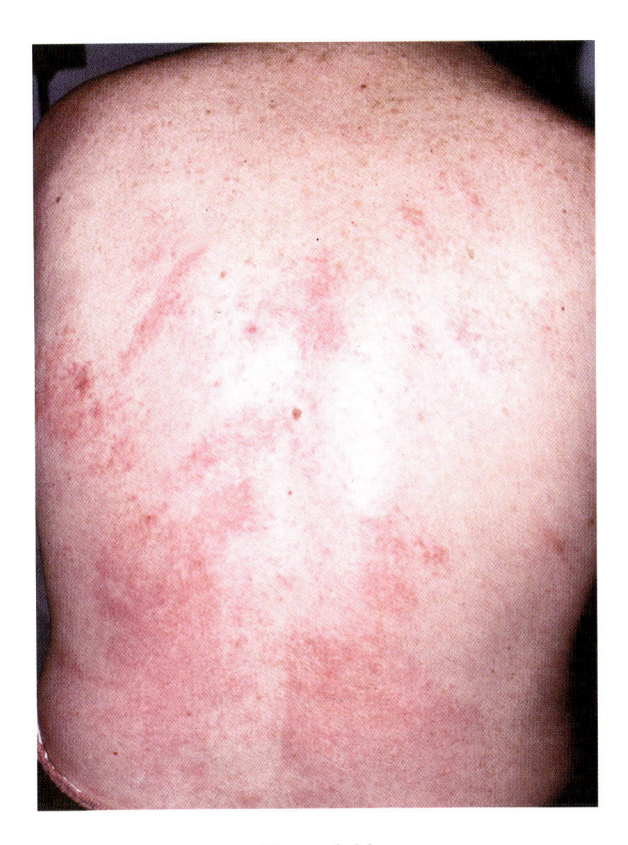

**Figure 4-14**
**GROVER DISEASE**
There are multiple erythematous, hyperkeratotic papules focally coalescing into plaques on the truncal skin.

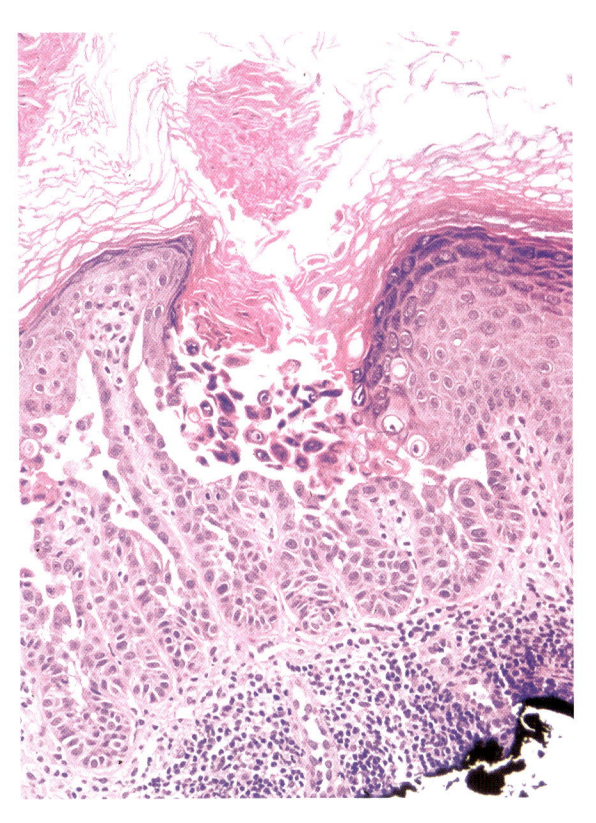

**Figure 4-15**
**GROVER DISEASE**
There is a discrete zone of suprabasal acantholysis, dyskeratosis, and hyperkeratosis.

cyclophosphamide, and even plasmapheresis with variable success. Most clinicians use a combination of corticosteroid therapy with immunosuppressive agents. Mortality has been greatly reduced, as have complications. Many lesions of the IgA variant pemphigus respond to sulfone therapy. Topical steroid therapy combined with topical antibiotics is successful for some patients with crusted lesions.

## GROVER DISEASE (TRANSIENT ACANTHOLYTIC DERMATOSIS)

**Definition.** *Grover disease*, or *transient acantholytic dermatosis* (TAD), is a self-limited disorder that occurs principally on the trunk as crops of pruritic papulovesicles. The etiology is unknown (16,17). The characteristic histopathology involves focal acantholysis and dyskeratosis. Like cornoid lamella formation and epidermolytic hyperkeratosis, focal acantholytic dyskeratosis may indicate either a specific disorder or a secondary alteration in epidermal maturation. Therefore, clinical parameters are important for accurate histologic interpretation.

**Clinical Features.** The abrupt onset of pruritus heralds the first manifestation of Grover disease, which consists of crops of papules and papulovesicles (fig. 4-14). They occur principally on the trunk of men, although women are affected as well. Precipitating factors are excessive sun exposure, fever, and sometimes, excessive exercise or sweating due to occlusion clothing. The papules are 3 to 5 mm, with a slight scale, but may show some vesiculation. The vesiculated lesions become eroded and result finally in scaly papules. The lesions tend to affect central areas of the trunk. The disorder, while designated transient, sometimes persists for years, although there is an acute and transient form.

**Pathologic Findings.** Grover disease demonstrates zones of hyperorthokeratosis associated with focal acantholytic dyskeratosis, a reaction

## Inflammatory Disorders of the Skin

**Figure 4-16**

**GROVER DISEASE**

Top: The pemphigus vulgaris-like pattern shows prominent suprabasal acantholysis involving a small and discrete zone of the epidermis. This early lesion shows only slight hyperkeratosis and minimal dyskeratosis.

Bottom: This superficial histologic variant shows primarily subcorneal acantholysis and dyskeratosis with associated hyperkeratosis.

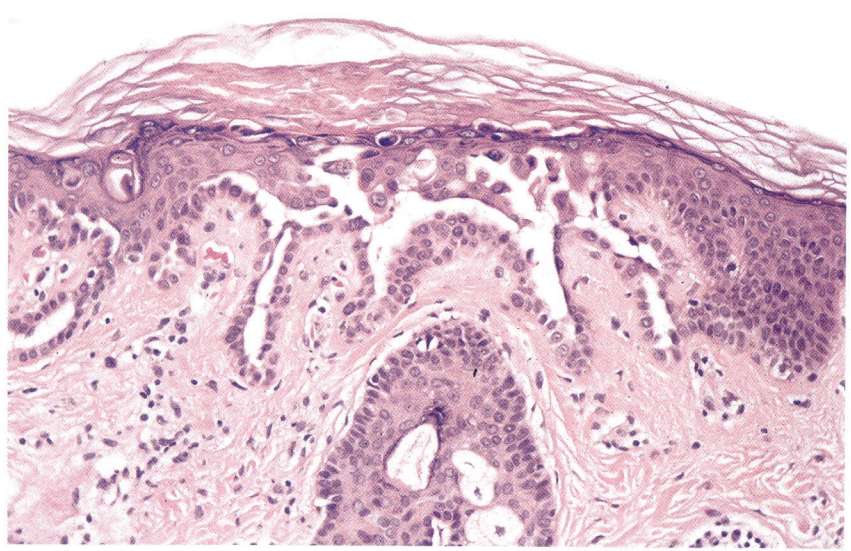

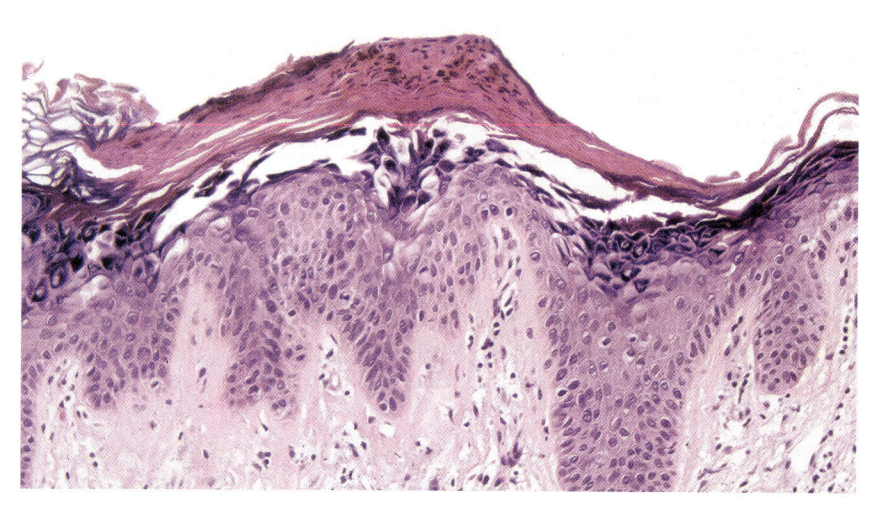

pattern consisting of suprabasal acantholysis and dyskeratosis of the sloughed acantholytic keratinocytes (figs. 4-15–4-17). This is in contradistinction to PV and Hailey-Hailey disease, which show suprabasal and full-thickness acantholysis, respectively, without dyskeratosis. This is an important distinction because some lesions of Darier disease clinically mimic vesiculobullous disease. The suprabasal acantholysis seen in most forms of Grover disease leaves an intact basal cell layer overlying dermal papillae and predominantly involves the cells of the lower stratum spinosum. The dyskeratosis typically occurs along a continuum, defined at one extreme by large, round acantholytic cells showing early nuclear degeneration in the form of chromatin clumping, perinuclear clear zones (i.e., halos), and slight cytoplasmic eosinophilia; the other extreme of the continuum is defined by small, millet seed–shaped acantholytic cells characterized by compact, pyknotic nuclei and dense, eosinophilic cytoplasm. The larger cells are commonly referred to as *corps ronds* and the smaller ones as *corps grains*.

Several histologic variants exist, based on superficial mimicry with spongiotic dermatitis, PV, Hailey-Hailey disease, and Darier disease. These variants only indicate that occasional lesions show associated intercellular edema, full-thickness acantholysis, or less conspicuous dyskeratosis, and do not represent true clinicopathologic or biologically significant variants.

**Differential Diagnosis.** Darier disease is the principal entity in the differential diagnosis of Grover disease, and can be differentiated both on its clinical extent and histopathology. Insect bite

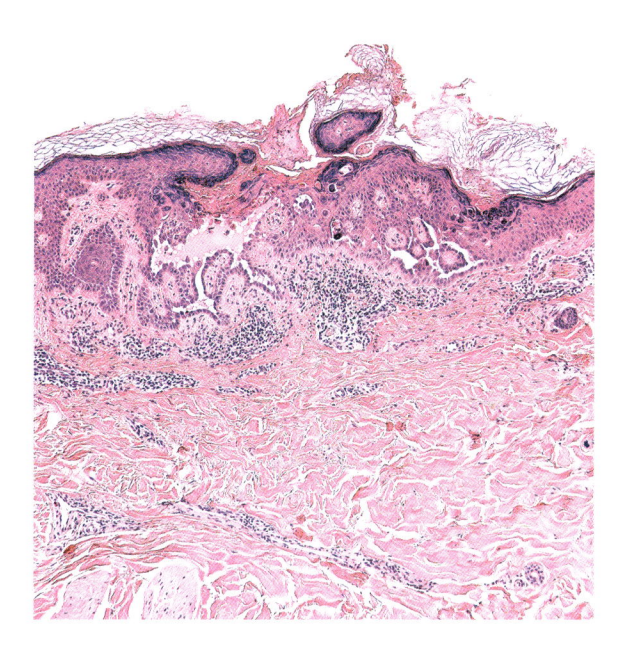

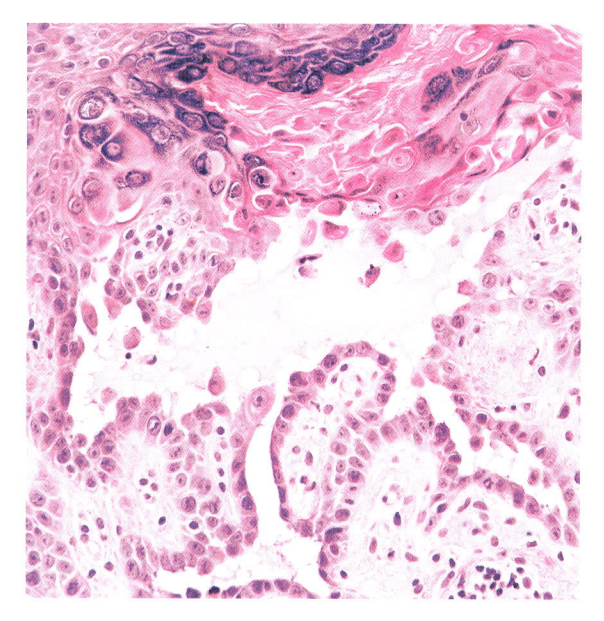

**Figure 4-17**

**GROVER DISEASE**

Left: There is discrete and focal suprabasal acantholysis associated with altered scale formation and a superficial perivascular inflammatory infiltrate.

Right: Unlike pemphigus vulgaris, the suprabasal acantholysis is associated with premature keratinization (dyskeratosis) of the acantholytic cells.

reactions, herpetic infestations, and dermatitis herpetiformis can also resemble Grover disease. Drug reactions and different infectious folliculitides must be considered as well.

Darier disease shows verrucous epidermal hyperplasia associated with focal to diffuse, well-formed acantholytic dyskeratosis; Grover disease simply demonstrates minute skip areas of focal acantholytic dyskeratosis within an otherwise unremarkable epidermal layer. Often, a nonspecific superficial perivascular inflammatory infiltrate containing mononuclear cells and eosinophils is present in Grover disease. The acantholysis of Grover disease is not always as discrete and localized within the lowermost epidermal layers as that seen in Darier disease. Certain biopsy specimens may show acantholysis at all levels of the epidermis in Grover disease, whereas others demonstrate only superficial epidermal acantholysis reminiscent of that seen in PF, bullous impetigo, and staphylococcal scalded skin syndrome. Other examples may resemble suprabasal spongiosis more than true acantholysis. All forms, however, show at least minute foci of hyperkeratosis and acantholysis at scanning magnification that usually correlate with a clinical history of pruritic hyperkeratotic papules of recent onset in older individuals.

**Treatment and Prognosis.** Topical corticosteroids, especially under wrap, are useful. In some severely affected patients, oral administration of corticosteroids and dapsone has resulted in remission but does not completely eradicate the disease. UVB and PUVA therapy have also been used.

## DARIER DISEASE (KERATOSIS FOLLICULARIS)

**Definition.** Typical patients with *Darier disease* inherit the disorder in an autosomal dominant pattern. Darier disease and Grover disease, two unrelated disorders, share in common the occurrence of multiple zones of focal acantholytic dyskeratosis. This shared feature is not diagnostically trivial, and confusion may result because large lesions of Grover disease may histologically mimic small papules of Darier disease.

**Clinical Features.** The eruption of Darier disease (18,19), which is persistent and slowly progressive, consists of multiple hyperkeratotic and crusted papules that coalesce to form verrucous plaques, often with a seborrheic distribution (fig.

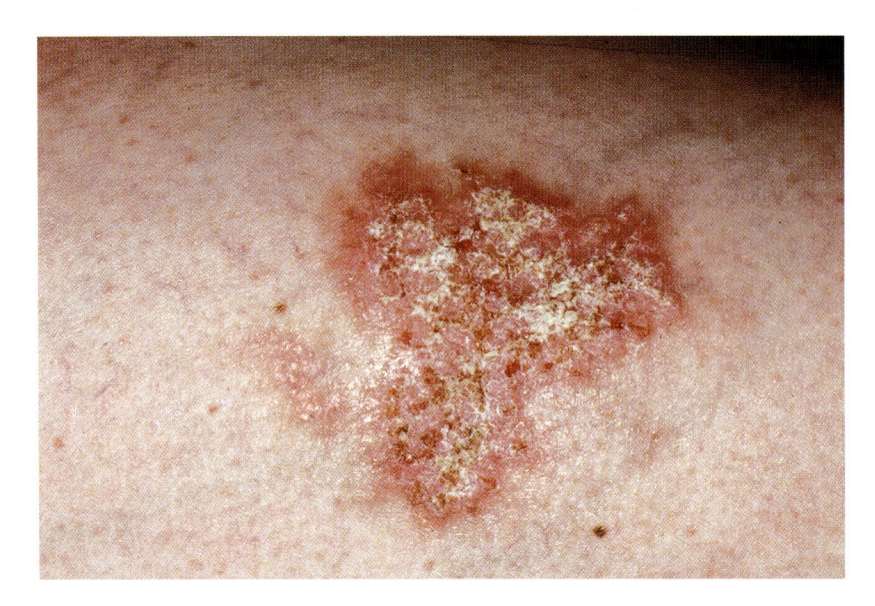

**Figure 4-18**

**DARIER DISEASE**

The well-defined erythematous plaque is surmounted by prominent scale.

4-18). Individual papules may show a follicular distribution (hence the alternative term, keratosis follicularis), although oral mucosal involvement has also been documented. Several clinical variants have been described: a hyperkeratotic form, which preferentially involves intertriginous skin; a vesiculobullous type; and a linear or systematized variant that probably represents epidermal nevi predominated by the reaction pattern of focal acantholytic dyskeratosis.

**Pathologic Findings.** The same basic histologic reaction pattern of focal acantholytic dyskeratosis seen in Grover disease is observed in the lesions of Darier disease (fig. 4-19). In Darier disease, however, the lesion is more organized and better developed. In the stratum corneum there is abundant dyskeratosis, beneath which are the very small "millet seed-like" cells. These may be focally attached to the stratum corneum or lie in the cavity between the stratum corneum and the basal keratinocytes that form the base of the apparent blister. Along the sides near the surface of this cavity are the large, round dyskeratotic cells that have been described as the corps ronds. The mixed features of spongiosis and irregular dyskeratosis at all levels that characterize Grover disease are not present. Individual lesions of Darier disease are much larger than those of Grover disease, showing verrucous epidermal proliferation and occasionally involving follicular infundibula. A variant of Darier disease presents with proliferative hyperkeratotic nodules, *hypertrophic Darier disease*. There are exuberant areas of epidermal hyperplasia that involve the follicles, toward the base of which the characteristic picture of Darier disease can be found.

**Differential Diagnosis.** Another form of inherited acantholytic dermatosis is Hailey-Hailey disease, also known as benign familial pemphigus. Inherited as an autosomal dominant trait, the rarely encountered Hailey-Hailey disease differs from Darier disease in that typical lesions present as recurrent vesicles on an erythematous base, often forming circinate configurations affecting intertriginous skin. Histologically, these lesions do not show acantholytic clefts confined to a suprabasal plane, as is the case in Darier disease, but rather show suprabasal acantholysis affecting all epidermal layers to form a "dilapidated brick wall" appearance.

**Treatment and Prognosis.** Treatment is difficult, since the basic defect is genetic. Topical tretinoin and systemic retinoids may result in improvement, although lesions may worsen with cessation of therapy. It is important to minimize the complications of bacterial impetiginization with antibiotics.

## BENIGN FAMILIAL "PEMPHIGUS" (HAILEY-HAILEY DISEASE)

**Definition.** Just as epidermolysis bullosa acquisita is not a true form of epidermolysis bullosa, so too *benign familial pemphigus* is pathogenetically unrelated to the immunologically mediated acantholytic disorder, pemphigus. *Hailey-Hailey disease* is inherited as an autosomal

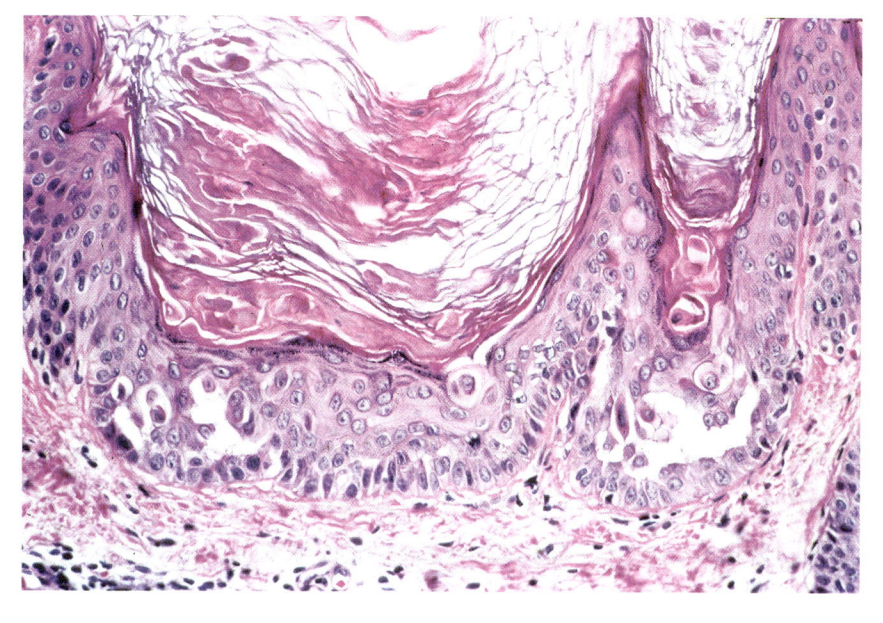

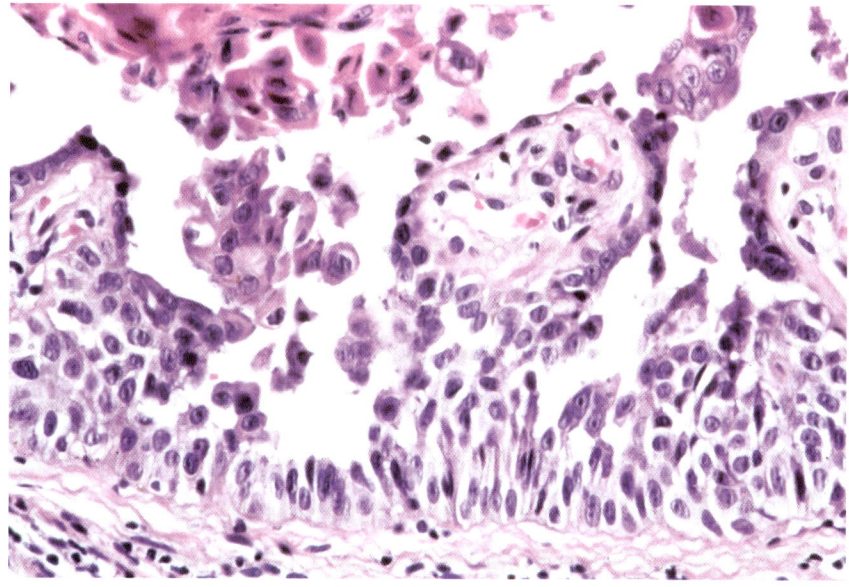

**Figure 4-19**

**DARIER DISEASE**

Top: The suprabasal acantholysis, dyskeratosis, and overlying hyperkeratosis show significant overlap with the changes of Grover disease.

Bottom: At higher magnification, a hallmark of this condition is dyskeratosis affecting the acantholytic cells, producing characteristic corps ronds and corps grains.

dominant condition with variable penetrance (20–22). This rare condition is believed to represent a defect in epidermal differentiation affecting cell-cell adhesion and resulting in erosions that are often provoked at sites of environmental trauma or irritation.

**Clinical Features.** Lesions usually are first noted in late adolescence and consist initially of confluent vesicles at sites of friction and moisture, particularly involving intertriginous skin, such as axillae and inguinal and perianal regions (fig. 4-20). Soon lesions become erythematous and often pruritic ovoid to circinate patches and plaques with prominent fissures. The surfaces are often oozing, with formation of malodorous scale-crust and minute vegetations.

**Pathologic Findings.** The hallmark of Hailey-Hailey disease is acantholysis that at least focally involves all or most of the epidermal layer, producing a "dilapidated brick wall" appearance (figs. 4-21, 4-22). Rare dyskeratotic cells are seen, but not in the number typical of Grover or Darier disease. Mixed inflammation is observed in the underlying dermis, and focal acanthosis and surface impetiginization are common findings.

*Inflammatory Disorders of the Skin*

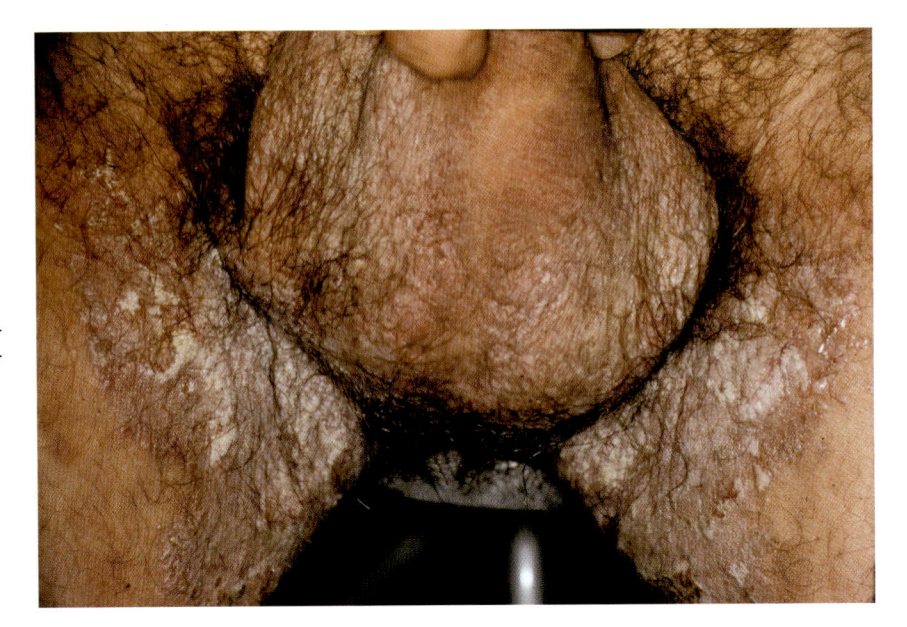

**Figure 4-20**

**HAILEY-HAILEY DISEASE**

The moist, macerated, hyperkeratotic plaques affect the intertriginous skin.

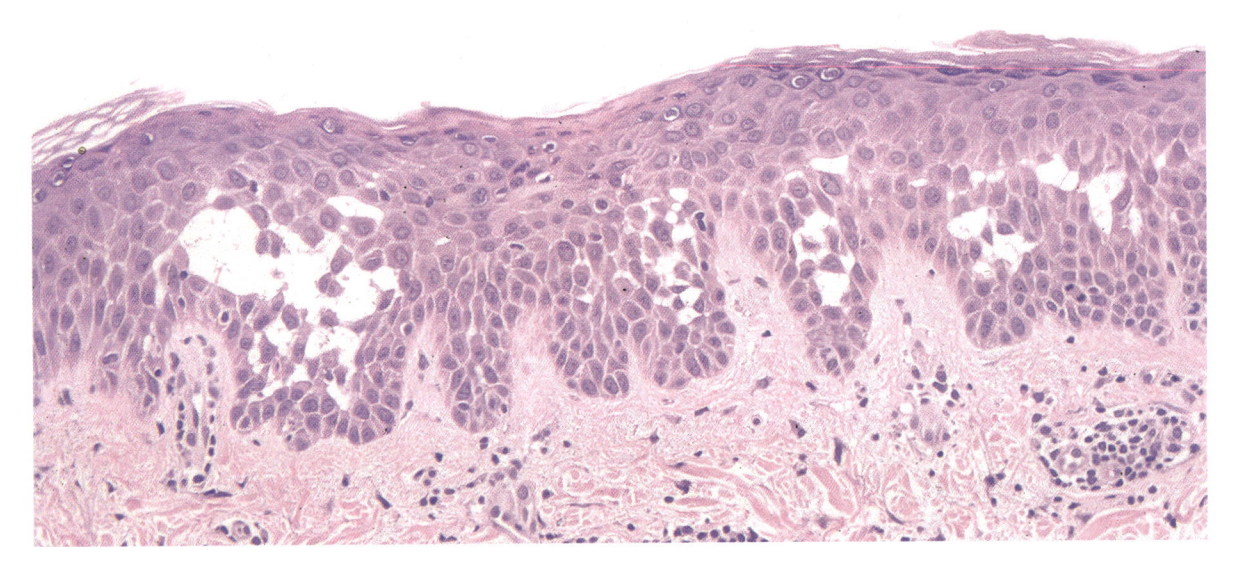

**Figure 4-21**

**HAILEY-HAILEY DISEASE**

Multiple foci of epidermal acantholysis involve various epidermal levels, producing the "dilapidated brick wall" architecture that is characteristic of this condition.

**Differential Diagnosis.** The finding of full-thickness acantholysis with minimal dyskeratosis is characteristic of this condition and is not observed in other acantholytic dermatoses, save for very focal involvement in the Hailey-Hailey variant of Grover disease. Occasionally in pemphigus, there are mixed features of the vulgaris and foliaceus variants, and rare transitional zones may resemble Hailey-Hailey disease. Virally induced acantholysis related to herpes is associated with cytopathic alterations not seen in the affected keratinocytes of Hailey-Hailey disease.

**Treatment and Prognosis.** Topical steroids and antibiotics, and avoidance of precipitating environmental factors (heat, friction), have been effective in more localized and less severe forms of the disease. Systemic administration

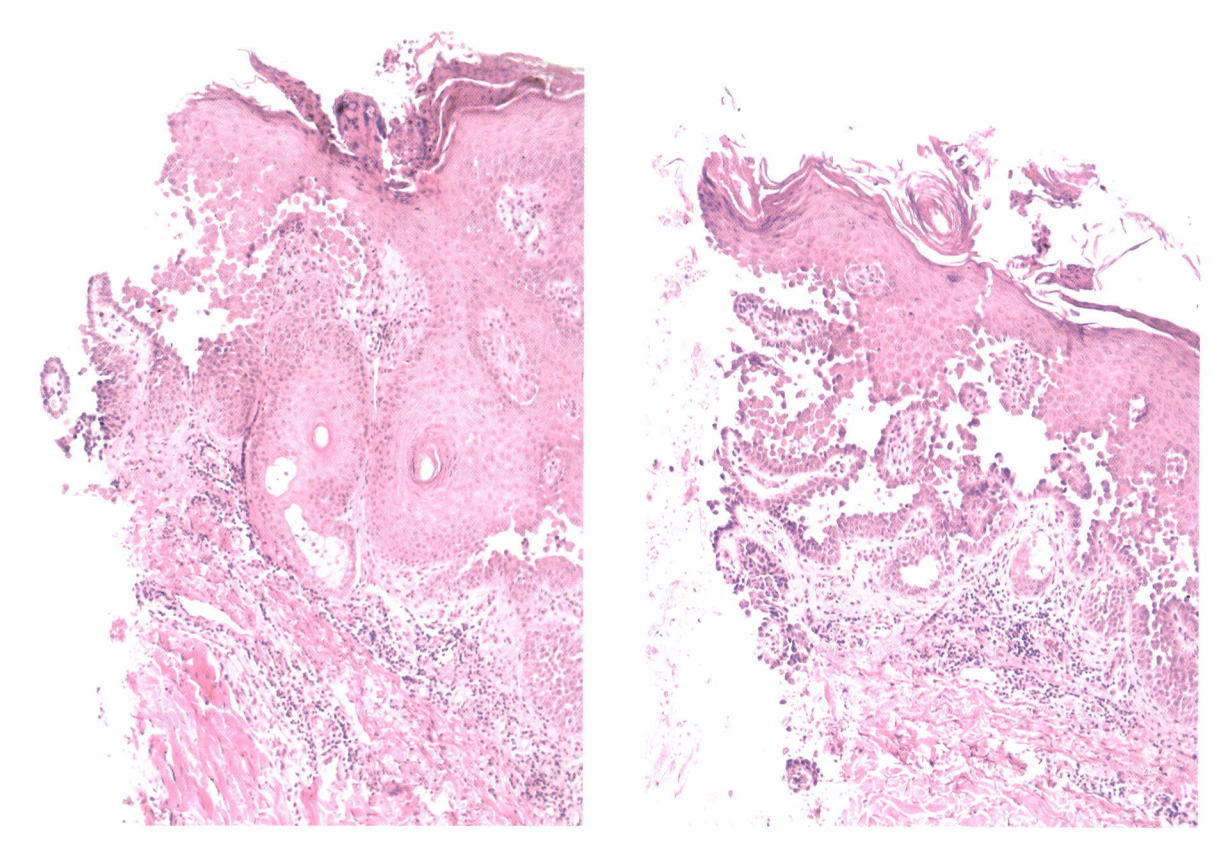

**Figure 4-22**

**HAILEY-HAILEY DISEASE**

Left: This biopsy site exhibits reactive acanthosis in addition to foci of acantholysis.
Right: The acantholysis is primarily suprabasal, producing the false impression of pemphigus vulgaris. In other regions, however, the acantholysis was more haphazard, involving all levels of the epidermis.

of retinoids, glucocorticoids, and antibiotics (if impetiginized) may be helpful during flares.

## HERPETIC BLISTERS

**Definition.** Members of the *herpesvirus* family typically induce cytopathic alterations in infected keratinocytes, leading to the formation of inflammatory acantholytic intraepidermal blisters.

**Clinical Features.** The most commonly encountered vesicular eruption resulting from viral infection is that of herpes simplex virus (23–25). Both the simplex and zoster variants produce grouped erythematous papules that rapidly develop central vesiculation ("dew drops on rose petals"), although the latter occurs along a dermatomal distribution. Early vesicular lesions may be mistaken for other forms of vesicular dermatitis (e.g., acute spongiotic dermatitis, dermatitis herpetiformis). Older lesions may become superinfected, resulting in grouped pustules (fig. 4-23).

A variant of herpes simplex affects only the follicles and presents as a cluster of inflamed follicular-based papules that are extremely pruritic. A variant of herpes zoster that affects the first branch of the trigeminal nerve results in herpes zoster ophthalmicus, a condition that may produce blindness as a result of corneal involvement. While almost always unilateral, there are rare cases that are bilateral. Two other variants of herpes simplex are auricular herpes, which is spread through the ear canal and can result in herpetic encephalitis, and herpes gladiatorum, which is usually contracted by athletes, especially wrestlers, on any part of the exposed body. The mode of transmission is from herpes labialis, communicated either by direct skin

*Inflammatory Disorders of the Skin*

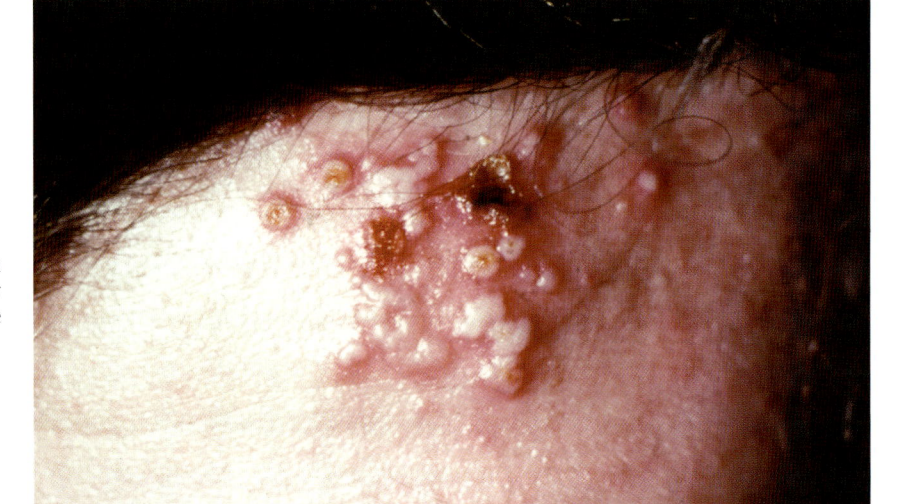

**Figure 4-23**

**HERPES BLISTERS**

These grouped, herpetiform lesions have undergone secondary superinfection, resulting in the formation of pustules.

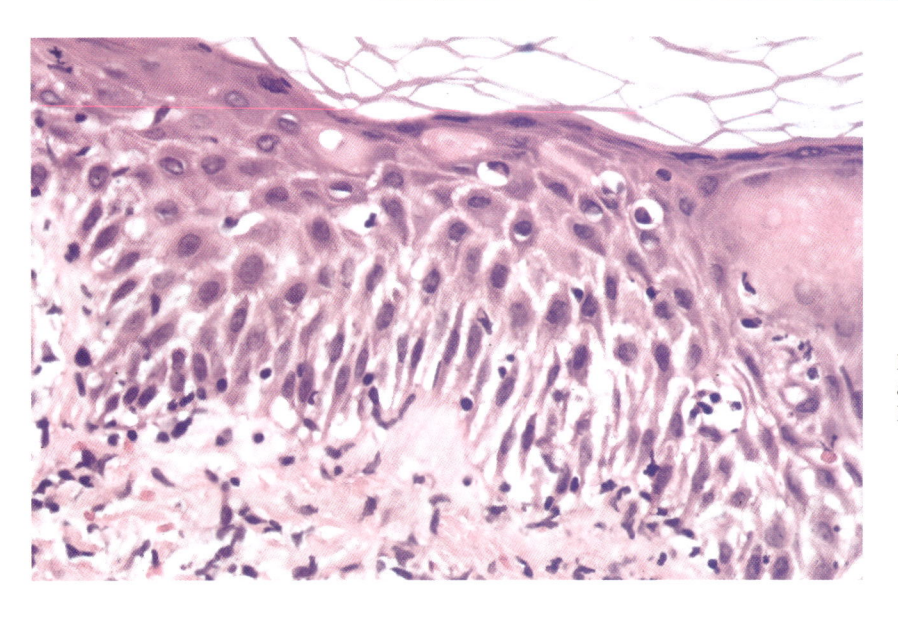

**Figure 4-24**

**EARLY CYTOPATHIC ALTERATIONS OF HERPES/VARICELLA**

Maturation disorder and early hydropic changes affect the keratinocytes. Specific alterations, however, are not as yet evident.

contact or as a result of viral shedding onto surfaces such as the wrestler's mat.

**Pathologic Findings.** Acute early lesions of herpesvirus infection may show only a mixed superficial and periadnexal inflammatory infiltrate predominated by neutrophils and lymphocytes, associated with disordered overlying epidermal maturation and slight cytoplasmic ballooning (figs. 4-24, 4-25). Clues to the diagnosis are the presence of the mixed neutrophilic and lymphocytic (i.e., "dirty") infiltrate with debris and associated subtle epidermal changes. These changes may take the form of cytoplasmic pallor and disordered maturation, both nonspecific findings. In the earliest lesions, there are multiple, small bluish dots along the nuclear membrane. These structures have been designated as nucleolini, or Cowdry B bodies, as they were described after the Cowdry A bodies discussed below. Eventually, an intraepidermal acantholytic blister forms, which is easily detected at scanning magnification (figs. 4-26, 4-27).

Although acantholytic cells are present within the blister fluid, dyskeratotic cells are not. The acantholysis is not exclusively between the basal cell layer and suprabasal cells, as is the case in PV. At least some of the acantholytic cells are multinucleated, a characteristic cytopathic change of herpesvirus which correlates with the presence of intranuclear inclusions

*Primary Acantholytic Dermatitis*

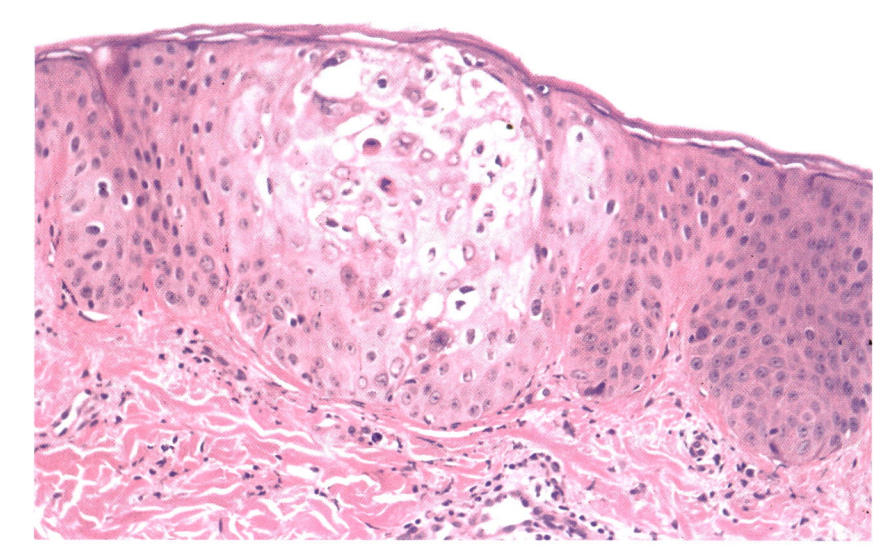

**Figure 4-25**

**VARICELLA: EARLY LESION**

A focus of ballooning degeneration of keratinocytes shows evidence of early cellular necrosis.

**Figure 4-26**

**VARICELLA: INTERMEDIATE LESION**

A vesicle has developed as a consequence of acantholysis and necrosis of infected keratinocytes. Occasional multinucleated keratinocytes containing nuclei with viral cytopathic changes are seen (arrow). A developing dermal inflammatory response is also evident.

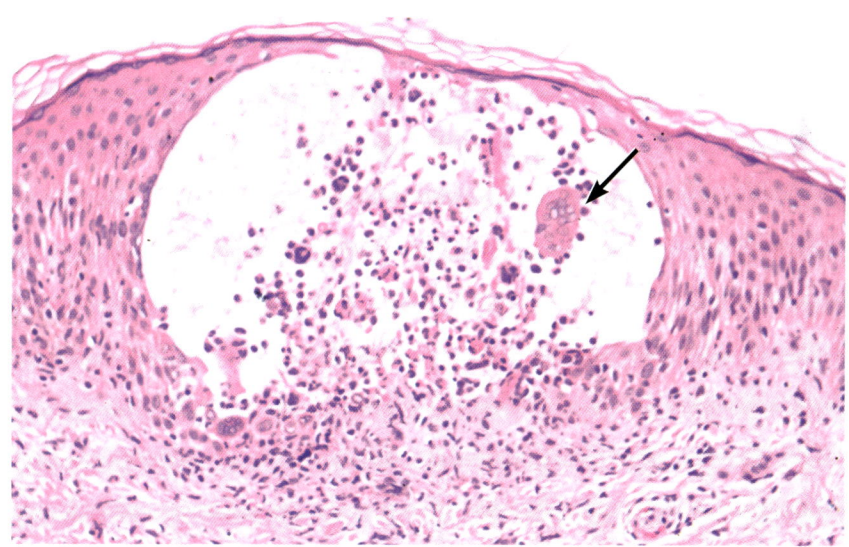

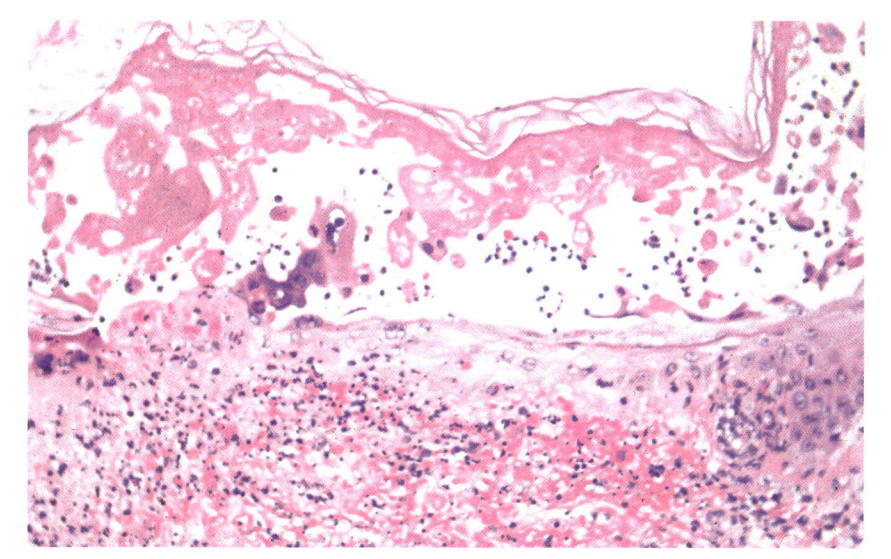

**Figure 4-27**

**VARICELLA: LATE LESION**

Most of the involved epidermal cells have undergone necrosis, and nuclei are indistinct. At this juncture, careful scrutiny and multiple levels may be required to delineate diagnostic viral cytopathic changes.

131

**Figure 4-28**

**VARICELLA ZOSTER**

A: At scanning magnification, there is an acantholytic intraepidermal vesicle with an associated superficial and deep inflammatory infiltrate.

B: Higher magnification shows variably necrotic and focally multinucleated acantholytic cells.

C: Characteristic multinucleation and nuclear cytopathic changes are present in both necrotic and viable infected acantholytic cells

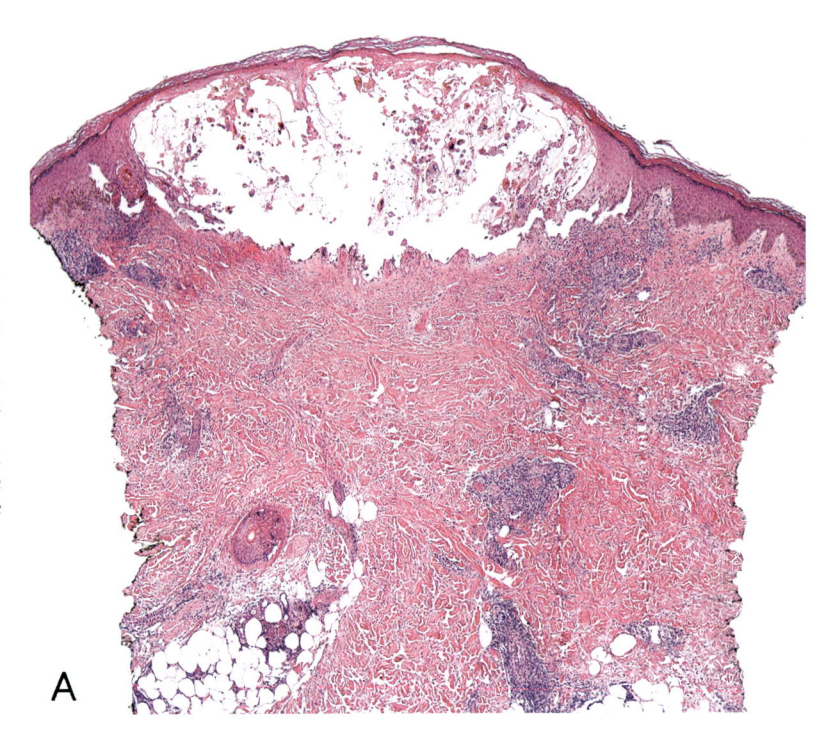

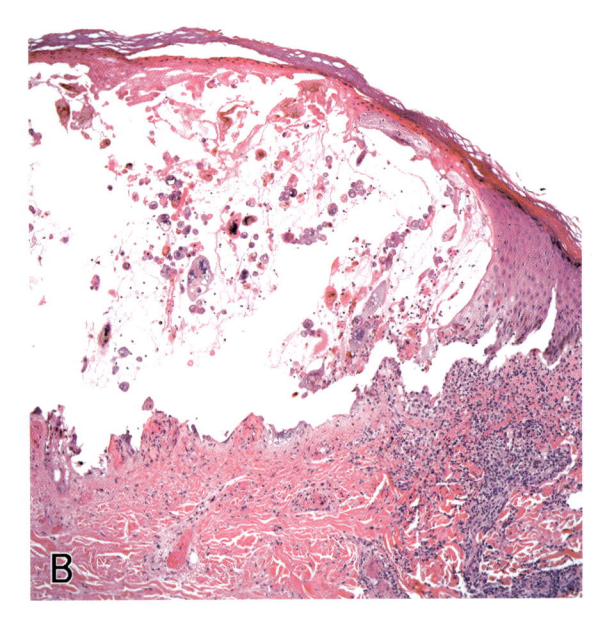

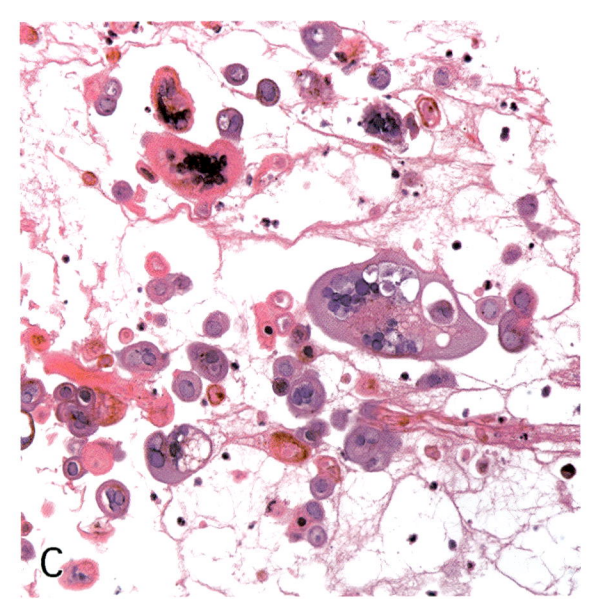

(fig. 4-28). Such cells may also be observed in Tzanck stains of blister contents prior to biopsy (fig. 4-29). The individual, densely basophilic nuclei filled with virus within the multinucleated cells mold to one another, an additional feature of diagnostic significance. There is clearing of the nuclear chromatin as the virus passes into the cytoplasm. The residual is an eosinophilic body lying in a halo formed by the nuclear membrane. This eosinophilic structure is considered characteristic and is described as a Cowdry A body. These virally infected acantholytic cells may account for only a minority of the cells within the blister cavity and therefore are easy to overlook (figs. 4-27–4-29).

Varicella zoster has epidermal changes identical to those described for herpes simplex infection, as does the exanthem of chickenpox.

*Primary Acantholytic Dermatitis*

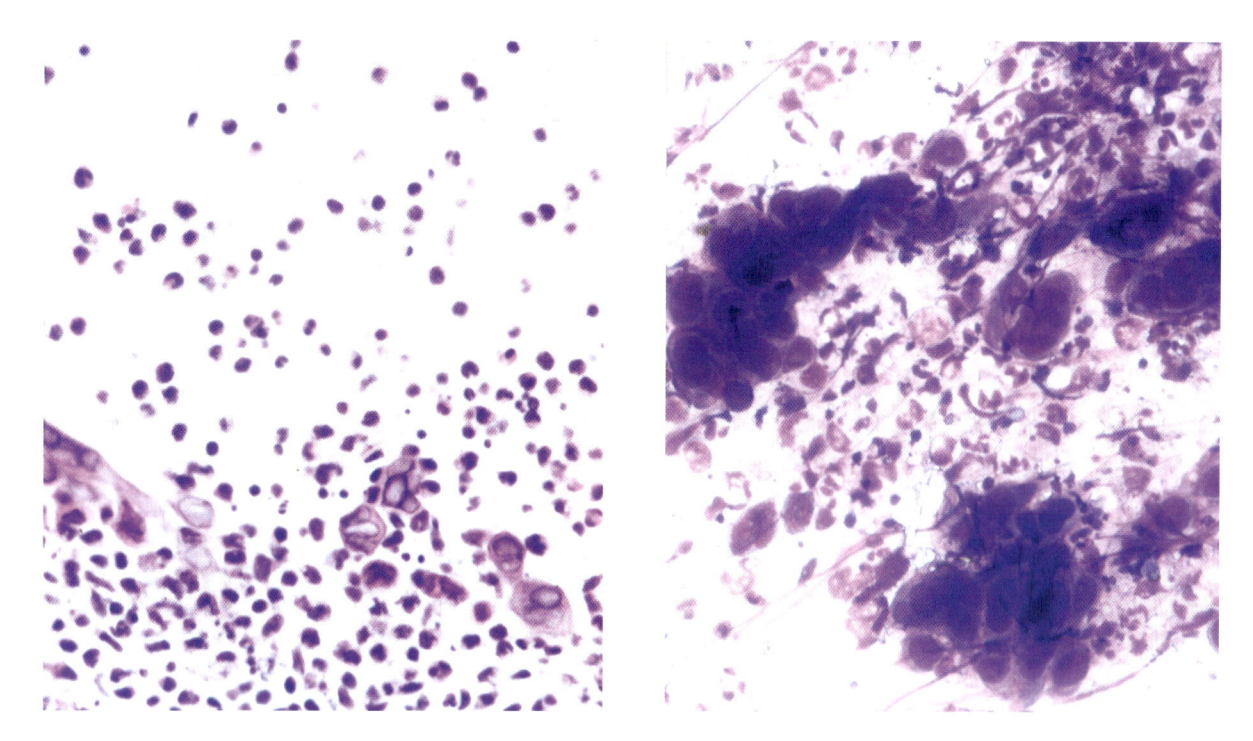

Figure 4-29

SUPERINFECTED (BACTERIAL) HERPETIC VESICLE

Left: Neutrophils and residual multinucleated acantholytic cells infiltrate the lower portion of the field. These cells still demonstrate sufficient viral cytopathic alterations for a definitive diagnosis.
Right: The contents of a vesiculopustule show occasional multinucleated cells suggestive of herpetic infection (Tzanck stain).

Varicella zoster, however, often shows associated vasculitis within the superficial dermis, whereas herpes simplex does not. This vasculitis consists of a perivascular infiltrate of neutrophils and mononuclear cells with associated nuclear dust formation, fibrinoid necrosis of vessels walls, and perivascular hemorrhage (fig. 4-30). It is indistinguishable from necrotizing cutaneous vasculitis. Herpesvirus infections at times preferentially involve the hair follicle (figs. 4-31, 4-32). Therefore, follicular epithelium should also be carefully scrutinized for evidence of viral changes, particularly in biopsy specimens of vesicular dermatoses from facial or scalp skin. Rarely, preferential eccrine involvement is seen, and it too may be difficult to detect, requiring multiple levels to insure representative sampling of the eccrine apparatus.

The immune response may provide a helpful clue to the diagnosis of herpes infection. The presence of an interface dermatitis involving the epidermis and hair follicle, with associated sebaceous gland necrosis, occurs in some cases

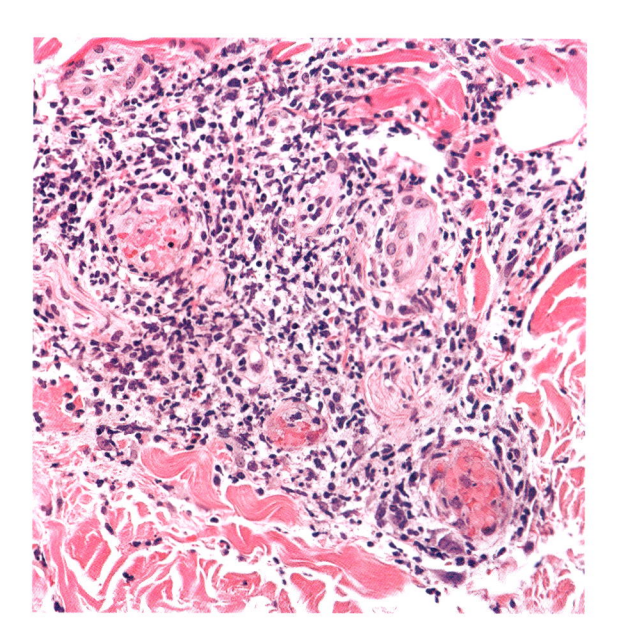

Figure 4-30

VASCULAR ALTERATIONS IN VARICELLA ZOSTER

There is thrombotic and necrotizing vasculitis associated with a mixed inflammatory infiltrate.

## Inflammatory Disorders of the Skin

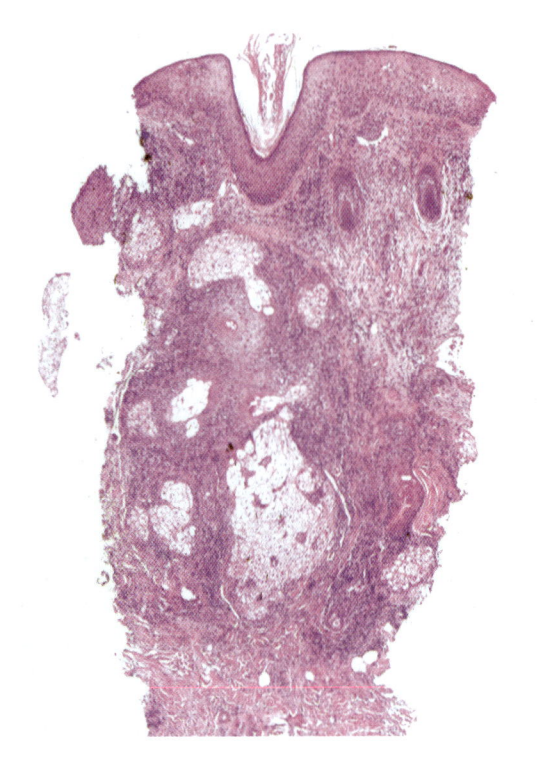

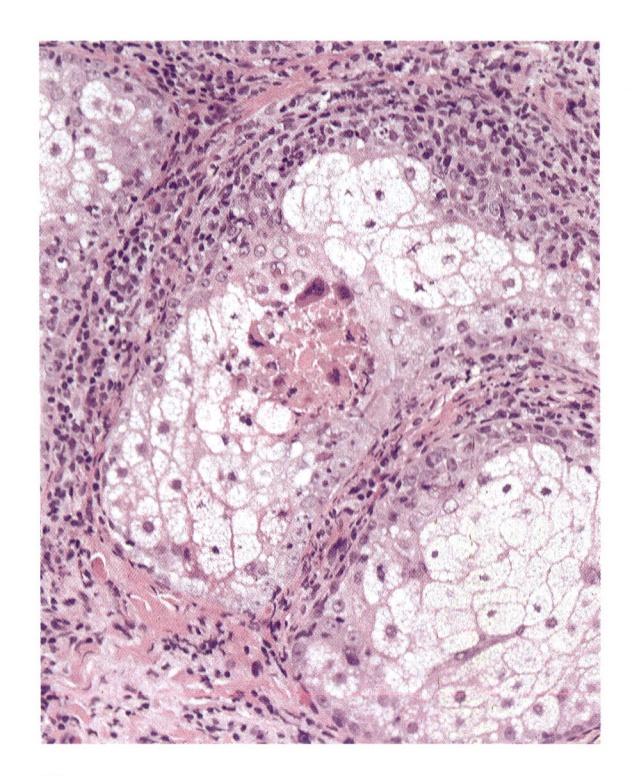

**Figure 4-31**

**HERPETIC FOLLICULITIS**

Left: On scanning magnification, the pathology may appear to represent primary inflammatory folliculitis.
Right: At higher magnification, careful search reveals a central cluster of degenerating follicular epithelial cells exhibiting viral cytopathic changes.

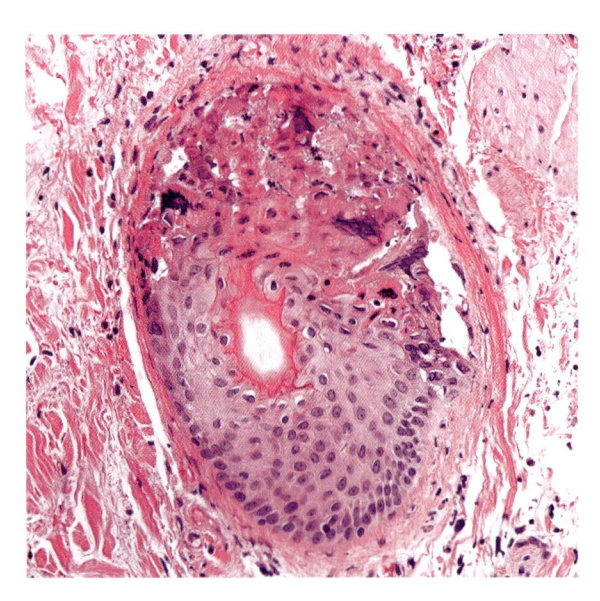

**Figure 4-32**

**FOLLICULAR INVOLVEMENT IN VARICELLA ZOSTER**

The zonal necrosis and incipient acantholysis are associated with subtle viral cytopathic change and focal multinucleation.

of herpes simplex. Often the infiltrate is mixed, containing an admixture predominantly of lymphocytes and neutrophils, with associated nuclear debris.

**Differential Diagnosis.** Because the viral cytopathic changes of herpes are so characteristic, few conditions enter into the differential diagnosis. Early lesions without significant vesiculation may mimic toxic epidermal alterations due to drugs (e.g., chemotherapeutic agents). Swelling of keratinocytes in the uppermost stratum spinosum and stratum granulosum has been suggested to represent a clue to early herpetic involvement (see fig. 4-25). Immunohistochemical stains for HSV I and II are used in equivocal cases (fig. 4-33).

**Treatment and Prognosis.** Topical and systemic antiviral agents (Acyclovir) are effective both for treatment and prophylaxis.

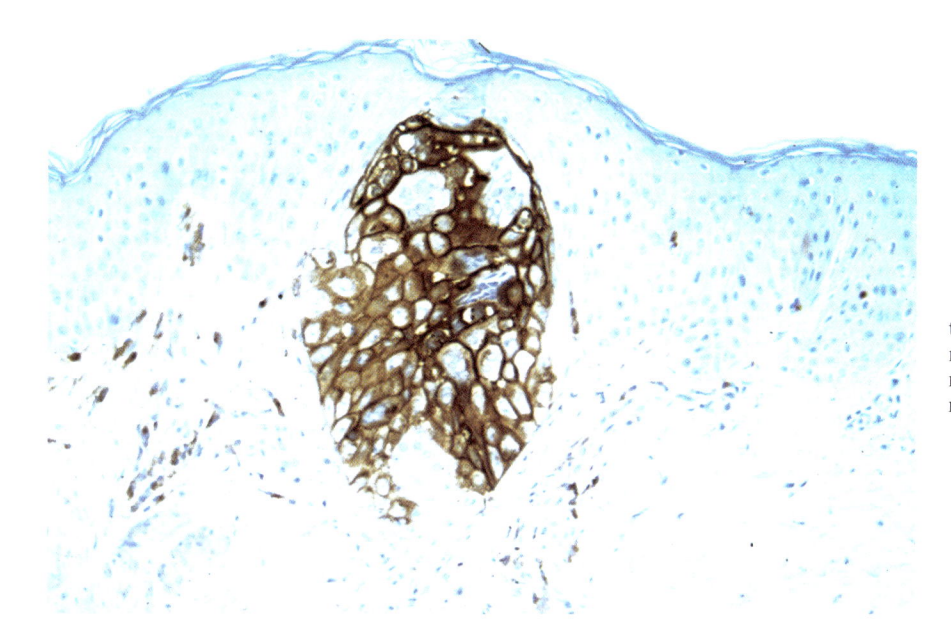

**Figure 4-33**

**EARLY VARICELLA**

Immunohistochemistry to varicella envelope protein reveals a discrete region of reactivity, facilitating the diagnosis of early disease.

## REFERENCES

1. Tron F, Gilbert D, Joly P, et al. Immunogenetics of pemphigus: an update. Autoimmunity 2006;39:531-9.
1a. Roh JY, Stanley JR. Plakoglobin binding by human Dsg3 (pemphigus vulgaris antigen) in keratinocytes requires the cadherin-like intracytoplasmic segment. J Invest Dermatol 1995;104:720-4.
2. Gniadecki R. Desmoglein autoimmunity in the pathogenesis of pemphigus. Autoimmunity 2006;39:541-7.
3. Empinotti JC, Aoki V, Filgueira A, et al. Clinical and serological follow-up studies of endemic pemphigus foliaceus (fogo selvagem) in Western Parana, Brazil (2001-2002). Br J Dermatol 2006;155:446-50.
4. Balighi K, Taheri A, Mansoori P, Chams C. Value of direct immunofluorescence in predicting remission in pemphigus vulgaris. Int J Dermatol 2006;45:1308-11.
5. McCuin JB, Hanlon T, Mutasim DF. Autoimmune bullous diseases: diagnosis and management. Dermatol Nurs 2006;18:20-25.
6. Kurzen H, Brenner S. Significance of autoimmunity to non-desmoglein targets in pemphigus. Autoimmunity 2006;39:549-56.
7. Aoki-Ota M, Tsunoda K, Ota T, et al. A mouse model of pemphigus vulgaris by adoptive transfer of naive splenocytes from desmoglein 3 knockout mice. Br J Dermatol 2004;151:346-54.
8. Hanakawa Y, Matsuyoshi N, Stanley JR. Expression of desmoglein 1 compensates for genetic loss of desmoglein 3 in keratinocyte adhesion. J Invest Dermatol 2002;119:27-31.
9. Sueki H, Shanley K, Goldschmidt MH, Lazarus GS, Murphy GF. Dominantly inherited epidermal acantholysis in dogs, simulating human benign familial chronic pemphigus (Hailey-Hailey disease). Br J Dermatol 1997;136:190-6.
10. Stanley JR, Amagai M. Pemphigus, bullous impetigo, and the staphylococcal scalded-skin syndrome. N Engl J Med 2006;26;355:1800-10.
11. de Almeida HL Jr, Neugebauer MG, Guarenti IM, Aoki V. Pemphigus vegetans associated with verrucous lesions: expanding a phenotype. Clinics (Sao Paulo) 2006;61:279-82.
12. Bonifazi E, Milioto M, Trashlieva V, Ferrante MR, Mazzotta F, Coviello C. Neonatal pemphigus vulgaris passively transmitted from a clinically asymptomatic mother. J Am Acad Dermatol 2006;55:S113-4.

13. Malik M, Ahmed AR. Dual diagnosis of pemphigus vulgaris and connective tissue disease. J Am Acad Dermatol 2006;55:699-704.
14. Brenner S, Ruocco V. D-penicillamine-induced pemphigus foliaceus with autoantibodies to desmoglein-1. J Am Acad Dermatol 1998;39:137-8.
15. Billet SE, Grando SA, Pittelkow MR. Paraneoplastic autoimmune multiorgan syndrome: Review of the literature and support for a cytotoxic role in pathogenesis. Autoimmunity 2006;39:617-30.
16. Kowalewski C, Hashimoto T, Amagai M, Jablonska S, Mackiewicz W, Wozniak K. IgA/IgG pemphigus: a new atypical subset of pemphigus? Acta Derm Venereol 2006;86:357-8.
17. Quirk CJ, Heenan PJ. Grover's disease: 34 years on. Australas J Dermatol 2004;45:83-6.
18. Reinstein E, Shoenfeld Y. Darier's disease. Isr Med Assoc J 2006;8:588.
19. Sehgal VN, Srivastava G. Darier's (Darier-White) disease/keratosis follicularis. Int J Dermatol 2005;44:184-92.
20. McKibben J, Smalling C. Hailey-Hailey. Skinmed 2006;5:250-2.
21. Chave TA, Milligan A. Acute generalized Hailey-Hailey disease. Clin Exp Dermatol 2002;27:290-2.
22. McGrath JA. Hereditary diseases of desmosomes. J Dermatol Sci 1999;20:85-91.
23. Knight J. An introduction to the herpes viruses. Dent Assist 2006;75:20-3.
24. Boer A, Herder N, Blodorn-Schlicht N, Steinkraus V, Falk TM. Refining criteria for diagnosis of cutaneous infections caused by herpes viruses through correlation of morphology with molecular pathology. Indian J Dermatol Venereol Leprol 2006;72:270-5.
25. Tan HH, Goh CL. Viral infections affecting the skin in organ transplant recipients: epidemiology and current management strategies. Am J Clin Dermatol 2006;7:13-29.

# 5 NONACANTHOLYTIC VESICULOBULLOUS AND VESICULOPUSTULAR DERMATITIS

## GENERAL CONSIDERATIONS

One of the most important and misunderstood areas of dermatopathology is vesiculobullous disease (1–4). This divergent group of disorders may be life-threatening, and accurate diagnosis and implementation of correct therapy may have profound therapeutic implications. The ability to make an accurate diagnosis, however, is often confounded by the histologic subtleties inherent in the stage of lesion evolution, the slight nuances in architecture and inflammatory cytology that separate certain disorders, and the plethora of divergent stimuli that eventuate in the common intraepidermal or subepidermal blister (e.g., antibody attack, cellular attack, ischemia, or viral cytopathologic changes).

The nomenclature of blistering diseases is simple. The term "vesicle," from the Latin word *vesicula*, meaning small blister, generally implies lesions ranging up to 1 cm in diameter. The term "bulla," from the Latin word *bulla*, meaning bubble-like, connotes a large blister. Blisters form from spongiosis, reticular degeneration, vacuolar degeneration, acantholysis, and lysis of the dermal matrix (i.e., dermolysis).

This chapter concentrates on those nonacantholytic disorders that commonly manifest as blisters at the most classic stage of their clinical evolution. Diseases that may form blisters but are better known for changes inherent in nonvesicular stages (e.g., erythema multiforme) or disorders that occasionally, but not ordinarily, give rise to blisters and erosions (e.g., lupus erythematosus, fixed drug eruption, lichen sclerosus) are discussed in other chapters. Occasional lesions that form blisters may also, but not invariably, show acantholytic cells (e.g., staphylococcal scalded skin syndrome, IgA pemphigus), and these are discussed here to emphasize that they must be recognized independent of acantholytic alterations.

Appreciation of the gross pathology of blistering diseases is of critical importance when evaluating a skin biopsy specimen. Early blisters may not appear as such, and the accompanying history may describe urticaria, erythema, induration, or simply pruritic normal-appearing skin. Some blisters are so fulminant and rapid that the predominant lesion is a shallow erosion. Later in the course of blistering disease, lesions may be appreciated primarily as pustules (due to superinfection), eschars, or zones of re-epithelialization. It is imperative to ascertain the type of lesion that was biopsied when evaluating the possibility of a blistering disorder. Ideally, a recent, fluid-filled blister is sampled; however, biopsy of the midportion of the lesion jeopardizes dermal-epidermal integrity and minimizes the possibility of gaining insight into the evolutionary histology of the process. Samples should ideally be obtained from the blister edge, with no more than two thirds of the biopsy diameter representing the blister and at least one third representing the presumably intact perilesional skin. Often, the clinically normal skin is inflamed, and early blister formation is seen. Biopsy specimens obtained in this manner generally include a spectrum of histologic changes ranging from the early stages of the blister formation at one edge or in the middle, and frank vesicle formation at the other edge. Specimens for direct immunofluorescence examination should be transported in appropriate medium.

Regardless of whether a blister arises as a result of spongiosis, cell injury or death, or defective cell-matrix interactions, the common denominator is a fluid-filled cavity within the epidermis or superficial dermis (fig. 5-1). Most acute blisters contain a proteinaceous serum transudate, and therefore are filled with homogenous pink material; traumatized blisters contain numerous erythrocytes; and superinfected blisters are infiltrated by neutrophils and may mimic primary neutrophilic and pustular dermatoses. The early stages of blister formation,

*Inflammatory Disorders of the Skin*

**Figure 5-1**

**PROTOTYPICAL CUTANEOUS BLISTER**

A small vesiculopustule on the back, with the pus accumulating at the base of the blister due to gravity.

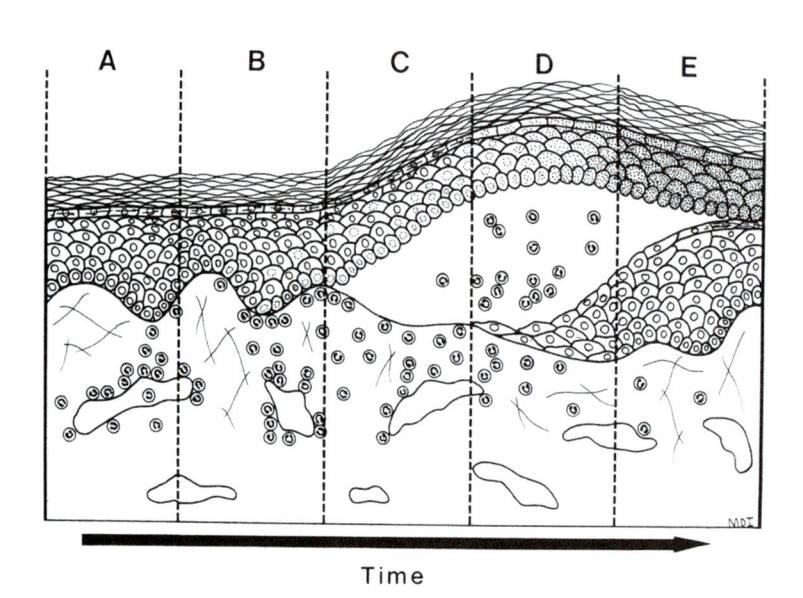

**Figure 5-2**

**SEQUENTIAL EVOLUTION OF SUBEPIDERMAL BLISTER**

The earliest phase (A) shows nonspecific dermal inflammation. Early injury to the basal cell zone (B) is followed by the formation of a subepidermal, fluid-filled cavity (C). D and E depict later phases, where re-epithelialization partially to completely covers the blister base, potentially leading to diagnostic confusion as to the primary plane of blister formation.

however, are generally more subtle. Because most vesiculobullous disorders are inflammatory, there is usually an early superficial perivascular infiltrate, occasionally with leukocytes in association with epidermal cells, in a pattern that may be helpful diagnostically (e.g., degranulating eosinophils along the dermal-epidermal interface in early bullous pemphigoid). Subtle early cellular alterations also may be helpful in discerning the cause of the blister.

Whereas the early evolutionary phases of blisters provide important diagnostic clues, the late stages are usually confusing and problematic (fig. 5-2). Dermatitis herpetiformis, for example, which during the active stages is predominated by neutrophils, may contain eosinophils in later stages, resulting in confusion with active bullous pemphigoid. Resolving lesions of the subepidermal blistering disorder bullous pemphigoid, on the other hand, may show significant re-epithelialization along the blister base, giving the false impression in some samples that the blister cavity is really intraepidermal. Precise understanding of the evolutionary patterns of

Table 5-1

ANTIBODIES IN BULLOUS DISEASE

| Bullous Disorder | Epitope | Size |
| --- | --- | --- |
| Bullous pemphigoid | BPAg1 | 230 kD |
|  | BPAg2 (NC16A domain) | 180 kD |
| Cicatricial pemphigoid | BPAg2 (distal C-terminal) | 180 kD |
| (Ocular) | β-4-integrin |  |
| (Malignancy-associated) | Laminin 5 (epilligrin) | Heterotrimer |
| Epidermolysis bullosa aquisita | Type VII collagen | 290 kD |
| Linear IgA | Part of PBAg2 (LAD-1) | 97 kD |
| Chronic bullous disease of childhood | Part of PBAg2 | 97 kD |
| Dermatitis herpetiformis | Transglutaminase 3 | 77 kD |
| Bullous lupus erythematosus | NC1 region of collagen type VII | 145 kD, 290 kD |

how blisters form and heal is integral to accurate histologic interpretation. Close clinicopathologic correlation is required in the evaluation of most forms of vesiculobullous dermatitis.

## PATHOGENESIS

Blistering disorders of skin are often, although not exclusively, autoimmune phenomena where antibodies form aberrantly to structural proteins integral to dermal-epidermal stability (Table 5-1). The bullous pemphigoid antigen is a group of glycoproteins produced by keratinocytes; it is a constituent of normal squamous epithelium. The antigen is composed of a major 230-kD antigen (BPAg1) and a minor 180-kD protein (BPAg2-NC16A domain). Sera from patients with both localized and generalized bullous pemphigoid have antibodies that immunoprecipitate the 230-kD antigen. Electron microscopy shows disintegration of the basement membrane and fragmentation of anchoring fibrils, anchoring filaments, and hemidesmosomes. Neutrophil elastase and matrix metalloproteinase-9 cleave the 180-kD protein in vitro. Immune reactants are localized to the upper lamina lucida by immunoelectron microscopy.

In patients with cicatricial pemphigoid, antibodies against BPAg2 (distal C-terminal domain) are present in mucosal and cutaneous lesions. Patients with primary ocular disease have antibodies against β-4-integrin. Rarely, when cicatricial pemphigoid is associated with malignancy, antibodies against laminin 5 (epiligrin) are detected. Laminin 5 (α3β3γ2) is a heterotrimeric adhesion molecule that is associated with anchoring filaments in the lamina lucida. Other targets, including a 168-kD antigen expressed in buccal mucosa and a 45-kD antigen in ocular disease, await confirmation.

The epidermolysis bullosa acquisita (EBA) antigen is a large glycoprotein in the lamina densa that develops at 8 to 10 weeks of gestation. Two bands are identified by polyacrylamide gel electrophoresis (PAGE) in sera of patients with EBA: the major band is a 290-kD protein of type VII collagen, and the 145-kD band is the noncollagenous C-terminal glycoprotein domain of the type VII collagen.

In linear immunoglobulin (Ig)A bullous dermatosis, immunoelectron microscopy has localized immune deposits to the lamina lucida, sublamina densa, or both. PAGE of the serum of patients with linear IgA disease identifies a 97-kD band in both dermal and epidermal skin extracts; this antigen may be produced and secreted by fibroblasts and subsequently binds to the lamina lucida. This 97-kD protein is part of BPAg2. The serum of these patients may contain circulating IgA antibasement membrane zone antibodies. IgA antiendomysial antibodies, which are seen in dermatitis herpetiformis, are absent.

The immunopathogenesis of dermatitis herpetiformis involves the production of IgA antibodies to connective tissue components of the gastrointestinal tract (i.e., antiendomysial antibodies). These antibodies occur in 70 to 80 percent of patients with dermatitis herpetiformis and in a somewhat lower percentage of patients with celiac disease. They have also been detected in other enteropathies. Antibodies against transglutaminase 3 are produced. Patients with dermatitis herpetiformis or celiac disease also have antigliadin and antigluten antibodies of the IgA subclass, which cross-react with reticulin fibers. This latter phenomenon may be responsible for the deposition of IgA on the tips of dermal papillae, where reticulin fibers are concentrated.

The immunopathology of bullous lupus erythematosus involves autoantibodies to type VII collagen. These autoantibodies recognize epitopes within the noncollagenous (NC1) region of type VII collagen. That region is composed of fibronectin type III homology units that may contribute to intermolecular cross-linking and the basement membrane adhesion functions of type VII collagen.

The immunopathology of staphylococcal scalded skin syndrome involves exfoliative toxin A, with the structure of a serine proteinase, produced by *Staphylococcus aureus* group 2 phage type 71. This molecule cleaves desmoglein 1, resulting in a proteolytic attack on this keratinocyte adhesion molecule that is most concentrated just below the stratum corneum (4a).

## SPECIAL DIAGNOSTIC STUDIES

Direct and indirect immunofluorescence studies are the adjunctive mainstays for the diagnosis of vesiculobullous conditions of the skin. In pemphigoid, for example, direct immunofluorescence of skin biopsy specimens reveals strong, continuous, linear deposition of complement at the dermal-epidermal junction in nearly 100 percent of patients. It is of critical importance to recognize and differentiate the linear pattern from the granular staining seen in lupus erythematosus. Linear staining often has an undulant, glassy quality that has been likened to ribbon candy. IgG is the most common immunoglobulin seen in pemphigoid, occurring in 45 to 90 percent of patients. IgM and IgA are present in 25 to 30 percent of patients and are usually of lesser intensity. IgD and IgE are rare. The intensity of C3 staining is greater than that of IgG or other immunoglobulins, a feature that is helpful in excluding EBA from the differential diagnosis. Indirect immunofluorescence using the patient's serum produces a linear basement membrane pattern of reactivity in appropriate substrates, such as monkey esophagus, and decorates substrates that have been split via salt solutions at the dermal-epidermal junction along the epidermal portion, which contains the lamina lucida–associated bullous pemphigoid antigen. False-negative immunofluorescence in patients with bullous pemphigoid may occur in biopsy specimens from the lower extremities, and biopsy specimens from flexural sites may produce the most accurate results. Biopsy specimens of blistered skin or old lesions that have begun to re-epithelialize may yield discontinuous staining or negative results because the basement membrane has been destroyed. A biopsy adjacent to a new blister is optimal. Specimens from patients in remission or on corticosteroid or other immunosuppressive therapy also may fail to show deposition of immunoreactants.

Herpes gestationis, a rare vesiculobullous disorder that occurs in pregnant women and during the puerperium, may produce a histologic and direct immunofluorescence picture that is indistinguishable from pemphigoid. Therefore, this diagnosis is made largely on clinical parameters. Perilesional skin most commonly reveals C3 and other complement components in linear array along the dermal-epidermal junction. Immune deposits may be present in the walls of cutaneous vessels. Linear C3 is a consistent finding; linear IgG, usually of lesser intensity, is present in 30 to 50 percent of patients. Similar direct immunofluorescence findings are seen in the neonates of affected mothers, regardless of whether or not the infant has clinical lesions. Immunoelectron microscopy reveals C3 deposition within the lamina lucida, as observed in patients with pemphigoid. IgG is also located in the lamina lucida, but it is concentrated near the dermal side of the basal cell plasma membrane and in association with hemidesmosomes. In most cases, indirect immunofluorescence fails to identify antibasement membrane zone antibodies in the serum of herpes gestationis patients, probably because the concentration of circulating autoantibody is below the level of sensitivity of the technique. Sera from affected individuals contain a substance that is capable of fixing C3 to the basement membrane zone of normal human skin. This antibody is identified as the HG factor (herpes gestationis), which is a complement-fixing factor also present in cord serum from infants of affected patients.

In cicatricial pemphigoid, also known as benign mucosal pemphigoid, patients develop subepidermal blisters on mucosal surfaces, predominantly the oral and conjunctival skin. Skin lesions are present in 10 to 30 percent of patients. The Brunsting-Perry type of cicatricial pemphigoid is characterized by localized, scarring lesions, frequently on the scalp, without mucosal involvement. On direct immunofluorescence, these changes are similar to those seen in bullous pemphigoid: linear, ribbon-like deposition of C3 at the dermal-epidermal junction. IgG is the most common of the immunoglobulins detected in addition to C3. Immunoelectron microcopy has localized the immune reactants to the lower portion of the lamina lucida.

EBA is an acquired, adult-onset bullous disease characterized by skin fragility, trauma-induced blisters, healing with scars and milia, and possible scarring alopecia and oral dystrophy. Typical blisters are noninflammatory clinically and show an acral distribution. Some EBA patients present with widespread inflammatory disease resembling bullous pemphigoid. Oral involvement is seen in 30 to 50 percent of these patients. Direct immunofluorescence of perilesional skin reveals a broad, homogeneous, linear band of IgG and C3 at the basement membrane zone in nearly all cases. IgA, IgM, C1q, C4, factor B, and properidin are present in a much lower frequency. IgG is the most intense immunoreactant, and generally, all four subclasses of IgG are found in patients with EBA. IgG deposits are detected in the oral and esophageal mucosa of patients who do not have mucosal disease clinically. Immunopathologically, EBA may be difficult to differentiate from bullous pemphigoid, cicatricial pemphigoid, and herpes gestationis. The presence of linear IgG deposition that is stronger in intensity than the deposition of C3 favors a diagnosis of EBA. Definitive diagnosis, however, frequently requires immunoelectron microscopy or indirect immunofluorescence using sodium split skin specimens, in which the serum autoantibody localizes the dermal portion of the split skin. Ultrastructural analysis reveals a band of amorphous material beneath the lamina densa, corresponding to the accumulation of immunoglobulins and complement. Direct immunoelectron microscopy also reveals corresponding immune complexes below the lamina densa.

Dermatitis herpetiformis is an autoimmune blistering disease that produces intensely pruritic, grouped, erythematous papulovesicles on skin, particularly overlying extensor surfaces. Accordingly, the clinical differential diagnosis ranges from contact allergy and drug eruptions to the urticarial and pruritic forms of pemphigoid. Direct immunofluorescence is generally confirmatory, revealing granular deposits of IgA, with or without fibrin, within dermal papillae. Early lesions show fine, barely perceptible strands of fluorescence for IgA at the tips of dermal papillae. Late lesions show granular reactivity evenly distributed along the dermal-epidermal junction in a pattern that mimics a positive lupus band test. In such instances, however, the predominant immunoglobulin subclass is consistently IgA. Positive direct immunofluorescence results are observed in 85 to 90 percent of patients affected with dermatitis herpetiformis, although step sections through biopsy specimens may be required to increase yield due to the focality of the deposits. False-negative results occur when a biopsy specimen includes predominantly lesional tissue and insufficient quantities of perilesional skin. Perilesional skin or even normal buttock skin may disclose IgA deposits even in patients undergoing clinical remission.

Linear IgA bullous dermatosis is a pruritic skin disease that frequently presents with vesicles and bullae in clusters. Because of histologic similarities, the differential diagnosis usually includes dermatitis herpetiformis. By definition, direct immunofluorescence reveals linear deposition of IgA in the basement membrane zone. C3 and IgG may also be present, but generally stain with less intensity. If the staining intensity of C3 is stronger than IgA, a diagnosis of bullous pemphigoid should be considered. Immunoelectron microscopy has localized these deposits to the lamina lucida, sublamina densa, or both. PAGE of the sera of patients with linear IgA disease identifies a 97-kD band in both dermal and epidermal skin extracts; it is suggested that this antigen is produced and secreted by fibroblasts and subsequently binds to the lamina lucida. The sera of these patients may contain circulating IgA antibasement membrane zone antibodies. IgA antiendomysial antibodies, which are seen in dermatitis herpetiformis, are absent.

The immunofluorescence pattern in bullous lupus erythematosus shows linear deposition of predominantly IgG along the dermal-epidermal interface. This is in contradistinction to a classic lupus band test, where the deposits are granular, and is similar to the pattern of deposition in EBA.

## ANIMAL MODELS

Passive transfer of bullous pemphigoid antisera using rodent models has contributed significantly to the elucidation of the pathogenesis and target molecules in this disorder (5–8). Passive transfer of anti-BP180 produces findings similar to those of human bullous pemphigoid in a murine model of the disease. Recently, a humanized murine model, in which BP180 murine protein was replaced by the human analogue, closely recapitulated human disease. The role of mast cells, neutrophils, proteinases, and complement activation can be fully studied in this model (9,10). Similar findings have been noted in models for herpes gestationis. Canine models of cicatricial pemphigoid are available, although epitopes may be different than those seen in human disease (11). By immunizing mice with autologous type VII collagen, blistering disease akin to EBA is produced (12).

## BULLOUS PEMPHIGOID

**Definition.** *Bullous pemphigoid* is a disease usually of late life that presents with widespread, tense, subepidermal blisters that usually spare the mucosa (13–15). The disease affects both sexes equally and shows no racial or ethnic predilection. The disorder is mediated by autoimmune, complement-fixing antibodies directed against basement membrane antigens, the demonstration of which by immunofluorescence is used in diagnosis.

*Cicatricial pemphigoid* is a variant that affects predominantly mucosa but also skin. It is a chronic, recurrent and persistent disease with striking sequelae due to scarring. The mouth and eyes are most commonly affected. This disorder usually occurs in middle to late life and affects females twice as often as males. It also has an immunopathologic basis, which allows for diagnosis by immunofluorescence.

**Clinical Features.** Bullous pemphigoid is characterized by subepidermal bullae and a chronic, self-limited course (fig. 5-3). Although rare among dermatitides, this disorder is more common than pemphigus (see chapter 4) or dermatitis herpetiformis. In many immunofluorescence laboratories, bullous pemphigoid accounts for more than 40 percent of all specimens of blistering diseases received for diagnostic evaluation. Bullous pemphigoid usually occurs after the age of 60 years and is rare before the age of 40 years (13). The lesions occur anywhere on the skin, but there is a predilection for the lower abdomen, groin, inner aspects of the thighs, and flexor surfaces of the forearms. In one third of patients, the mouth is involved, but these lesions are small, heal quickly, and are much less significant than the oral lesions of pemphigus. The development of typical lesions of bullous pemphigoid may be heralded by one or more areas of localized pruritus. These lesions are often urticarial, and in some patients, urticarial lesions may predominate or persist in the absence of overt blisters. Cicatricial pemphigoid is an erosive, scarring variant with a predilection for involvement of conjunctival and mucosal epithelium (16).

The individual cutaneous lesion of bullous pemphigoid is a tense, often clear-filled, blister on normal skin or, at times, on an inflamed base. The lesion may be hemorrhagic. Some patients present with an urticarial phase while others, an eczematous phase. Many bullae may arise in the urticarial or eczematous plaques, and these patients have marked pruritus. The urticarial lesions sometimes have an arcuate appearance, with blisters occurring at the periphery. In some patients, there are numerous serpiginous plaques surmounted by blisters, admixed with widely scattered blisters on both erythematous and normal skin.

A variant of bullous pemphigoid, designated *localized type,* can persist and recur, usually on the lower legs, for years. The disease may progress to generalized bullous pemphigoid.

Bullous pemphigoid can occur in association with lichen planus, and patients have lesions that simultaneously resemble both disorders. This occurrence is termed *lichen planus pemphigoides.* When the bullae of lichen planus pemphigoides occur in a lesion of lichen planus, there are the classic morphologic changes of lichen planus in the overlying epidermis. Other

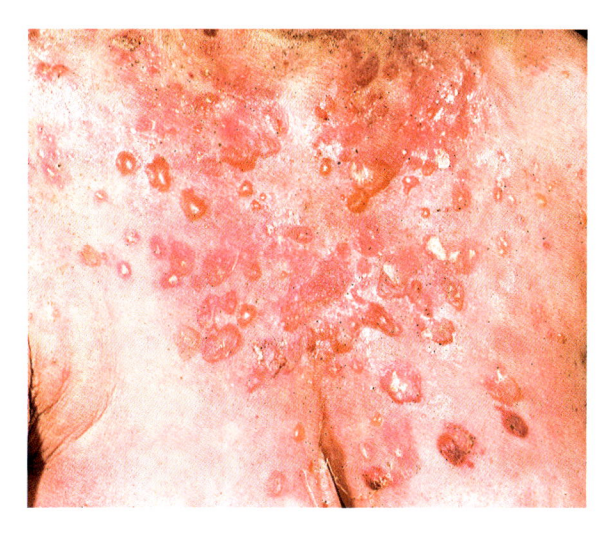

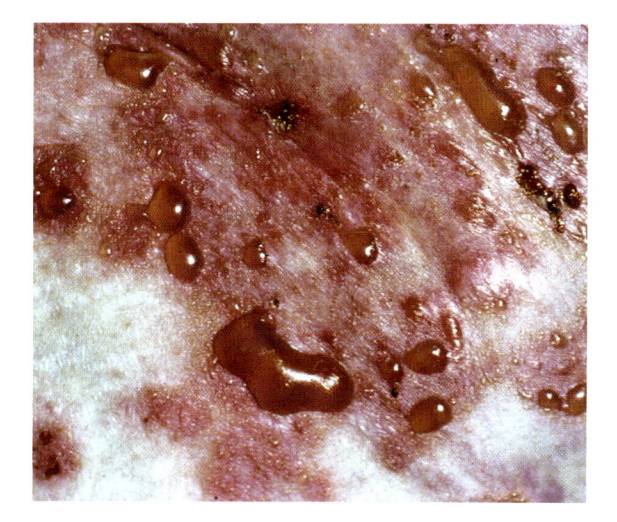

**Figure 5-3**
**BULLOUS PEMPHIGOID**
Left: Multiple clear blisters on both inflamed and noninflamed backgrounds characterize bullous pemphigoid. Eroded lesions form crusts. The trunk and extremities are typical sites.
Right: Tense clear blisters of skin surmount an erythematous patch on an urticarial to eczematous base.

bullous lesions in these patients have the typical features of bullous pemphigoid. This feature, along with the absence of spongiosis and acantholysis, allows for separation of lichen planus pemphigoides from paraneoplastic pemphigus, where the interface and acantholytic alterations develop in the same lesion. Thus, in lichen planus pemphigoides, lesions with bulla formation and those with lichenoid interface changes are separate, whereas in paraneoplastic pemphigus, the intraepidermal sites of blister formation are directly associated with the interface changes in a single biopsy. In those rare lesions where lichen planus in lichen planus pemphigoides has sufficient interface injury to form a bulla, there is overlying hypergranulosis and hyperkeratosis, and adjacent saw-tooth architecture to the chronically injured rete ridges (fig. 5-4), in contrast to the less characteristic interface alteration seen in paraneoplastic pemphigus.

Bullous pemphigoid was considered for years to be associated with systemic malignancy. It is now believed that there is no association and that the initial studies reflected a coincidence of increased incidence of the two diseases in the elderly population. Bullous pemphigoid can be precipitated by ultraviolet (UV) light, both by UVB and by UVA and psoralens.

The usual presentation of cicatricial pemphigoid is erosive lesions of either the conjunctiva, oral mucosa, or both. Lesions first appear as bullae but quickly become eroded. The gingival erosions are usually painful and, when extensive, have been labeled clinically as one of the causes of desquamative gingivitis. Other bullous diseases present with this painful erosive clinical appearance. In cicatricial pemphigoid, erosions of the palate and buccal mucosa are usually present. Involvement of the eye begins as nonspecific conjunctivitis affecting one or both eyes, and only rarely do vesicles form. The inflammation gradually gives way to scarring, which can progress to ankyloblepharon, that is, a destructive obliteration of the conjunctiva. The lacrimal ducts become scarred and tearing is impaired. Corneal abrasions from distorted eyelid hairs, along with the scarring, lead to blindness.

The distribution of lesions of cicatricial pemphigoid includes other mucosal sites such as the nasopharynx, esophagus, larynx, and anogenital mucous membranes. The resultant scarring can lead to many complications associated with obstruction of vital organs and functions. Hoarseness is usually the earliest sign of tracheal lesions. The skin is involved in 25 to 30 percent of cases, and the eruption may be scarring or nonscarring.

*Inflammatory Disorders of the Skin*

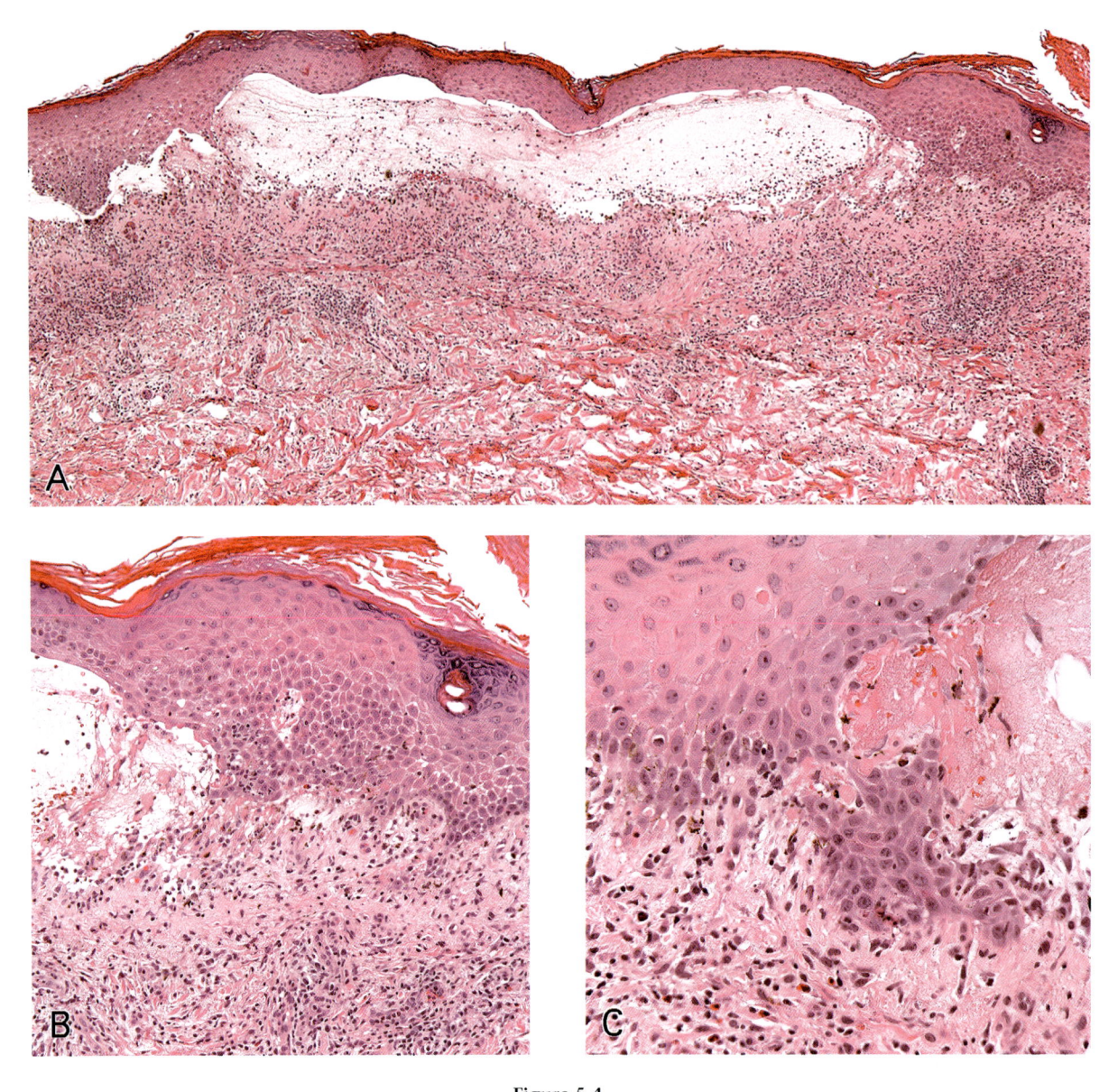

**Figure 5-4**

**LICHEN PLANUS PEMPHIGOIDES**

A: Scanning magnification shows inflammatory subepidermal blister formation.

B: High magnification of the blister edge. There is a lymphocytic infiltrate with eosinophils associated with lichen planus-like interface change.

C: The colloid/apoptotic bodies are associated with a superficial lymphocytic infiltrate containing eosinophils.

The former occurs in the head and neck region usually and presents as a blister that is tense and inflamed. In one variant, known as *Brunsting-Perry type,* the lesions scar and are recurrent in the head and neck region but without mucosal involvement. Nonscarring lesions usually present on a red or urticarial base as blisters that resolve gradually without scar.

**Pathologic Findings.** At scanning magnification, bullous pemphigoid is easily recognized as a subepidermal, inflammatory blistering disorder. Early changes, often appreciated at the blister edge, consist of vacuolization at the dermal-epidermal junction and small collections of degranulating eosinophils and mast cells within the most superficial stratum

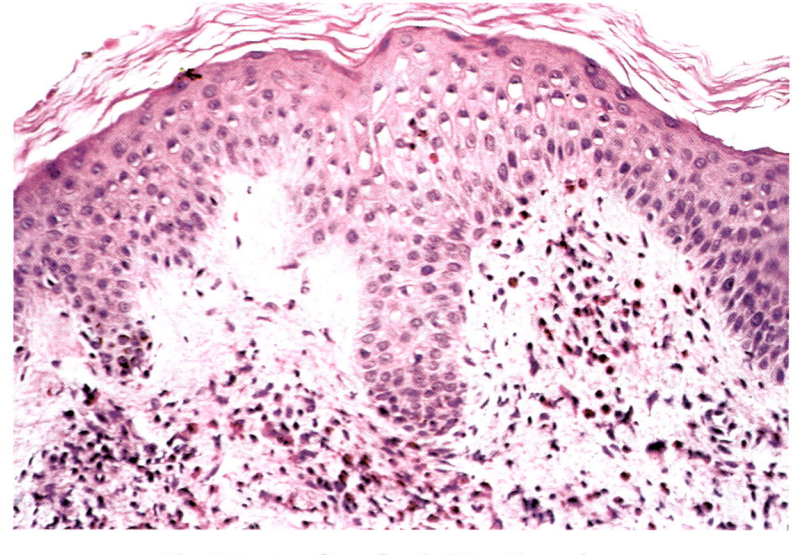

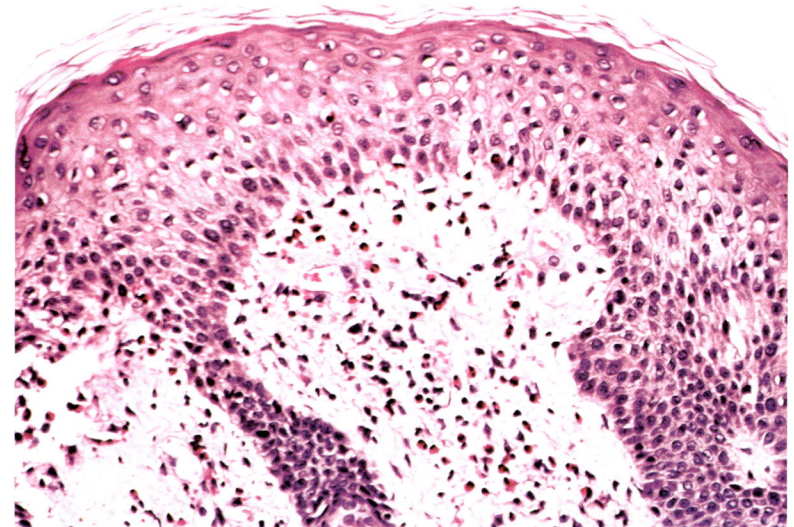

### Figure 5-5
### BULLOUS PEMPHIGOID

Top: The presence of eosinophils scattered along the dermal-epidermal junction, with basal cell layer vacuolization, is a typical finding in bullous pemphigoid. Eosinophils in the uppermost portion of the edematous papillary dermis are also typical.

Bottom: Degranulation of eosinophils leads to basal cell necrosis and vacuolization, formation of small clefts via coalescence, and early bulla formation.

of the papillary dermis, directly beneath the basement membrane zone (fig. 5-5). Vacuoles within basal keratinocytes coalesce to form a subepidermal bulla (fig. 5-6); within and below the bulla, there is an infiltrate of eosinophils, mast cells, lymphocytes, histiocytes, and rare neutrophils (fig. 5-7). Pulses of eosinophils in regions of spongiosis may occur (i.e., eosinophilic spongiosis). Epidermal regeneration, or re-epithelialization of the blister base, begins within 2 days of blister formation at the edges of the bulla and gradually extends centripetally toward the center of the bulla. Acantholysis is not observed, and neutrophilic papillary dermal microabscesses, a requisite feature for the diagnosis of dermatitis herpetiformis, are never seen. In urticarial lesions, the dermal infiltrate may predominate, with the epidermis showing only subtle basal layer vacuolization.

Immunoelectron microscopy reveals that the bullous pemphigoid antigen to which these immune reactants bind is associated with the lamina lucida of the basement membrane and is present in the portion of basal keratinocyte cytoplasm that apposes the basement membrane. Circulating antibody directed against the dermal-epidermal junction is detected in 70 percent of patients. A proposed sequence of events in the pathogenesis of bullous pemphigoid is the deposition of immunoglobulin and complement at the dermal-epidermal junction, followed by degranulation of mast

*Inflammatory Disorders of the Skin*

**Figure 5-6**

**BULLOUS PEMPHIGOID**

At the edge of a forming subepidermal blister is a subepidermal cleft with normal epidermis, except for prominent basal cells with slightly ragged borders. This is characteristic of bullous pemphigoid, as are the edematous papillae jutting into the bullae cavity. Inflammatory cells are along the dermal-epidermal junction and there is a perivascular lymphoeosinophilic infiltrate.

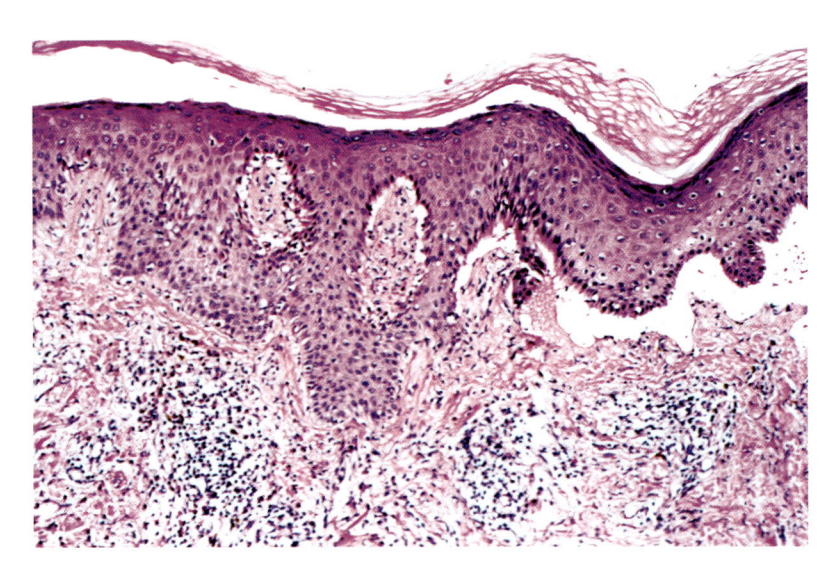

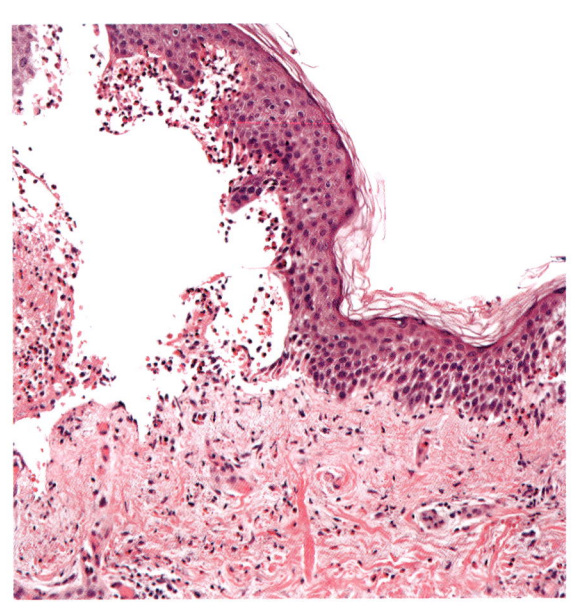

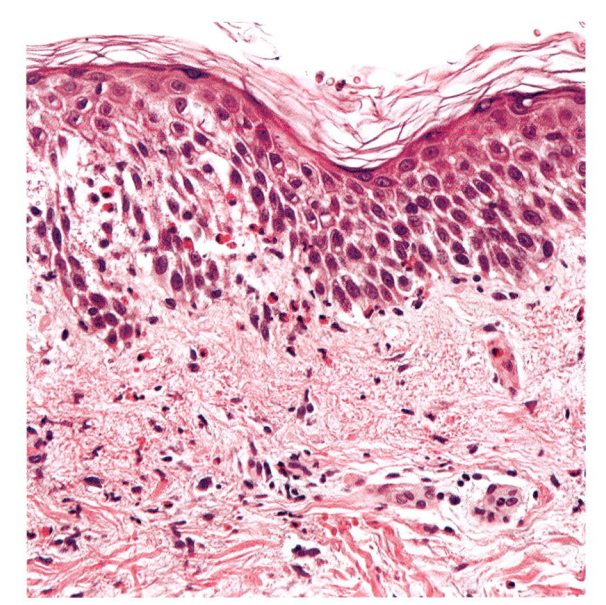

**Figure 5-7**

**BULLOUS PEMPHIGOID**

Left: On the right side of the blister edge, numerous eosinophils are observed directly beneath the epidermal layer, a characteristic finding.

Right: Eosinophils are present both beneath and within the epidermal layer in this higher magnification of the epidermis bordering the forming blister.

cells, resulting in eosinophil recruitment and degranulation. The proteolytic enzymes released by eosinophils damage the basement membrane zone, with subsequent blister formation.

**Differential Diagnosis.** Bullous pemphigoid must be differentiated clinically from pemphigus vulgaris, which is associated with scalp and persistent oral involvement. Pemphigus, but not pemphigoid, shows a Nikolsky sign. Erythema multiforme can sometimes resemble bullous pemphigoid but shows target lesions and may have oral and conjunctival involvement. EBA exhibits a characteristic clinical sign of blistering with milia formation following trauma. Porphyria cutanea tarda has a characteristic distribution and other signs such as hypertrichosis.

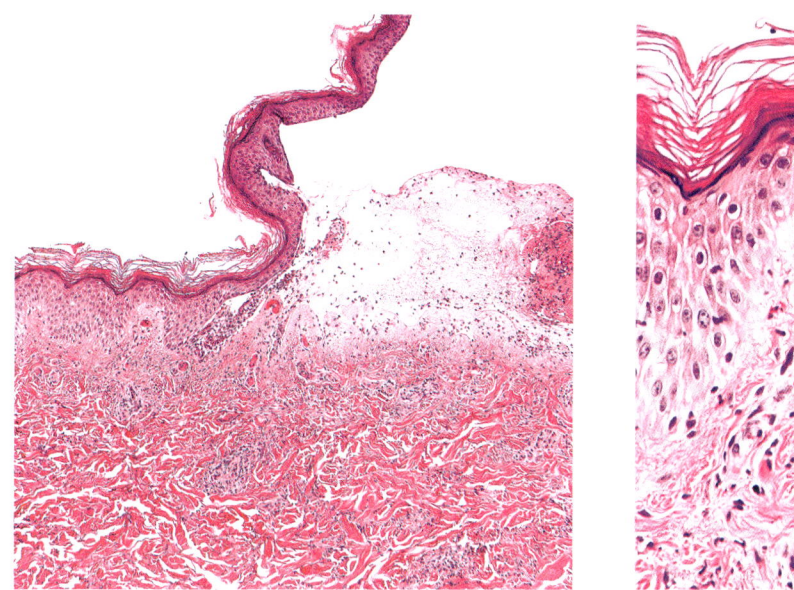

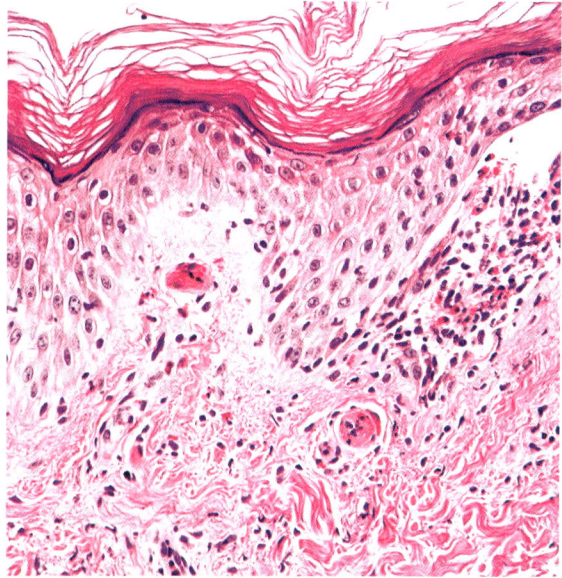

**Figure 5-8**

**BULLOUS PEMPHIGOID-LIKE DRUG ERUPTION**

Left: There is a subepidermal blister associated with a mixed superficial infiltrate containing eosinophils.
Right: Higher magnification shows degranulating eosinophils, many associated with a focally vacuolated epidermal layer, at the edge of the forming blister.

There are a number of disorders that may mimic bullous pemphigoid histologically. These include herpes gestationis, EBA, insect-bite reactions, drug eruptions (fig. 5-8), old lesions of dermatitis herpetiformis, and rarely, certain stages of drug-induced erythema multiforme. Direct immunofluorescence of a perilesional specimen, including the edge of lesional skin, is generally recommended as a confirmatory test when bullous pemphigoid is suspected by conventional histology (fig. 5-9). As stated previously, immunofluorescence microscopy discloses deposition of C3, usually with IgG, in a linear pattern at the dermal-epidermal junction. C3 usually predominates over IgG in intensity.

**Treatment and Prognosis.** The advent of corticosteroid therapy has resulted in impressive control of widespread disease with orally administered therapy (17–20). Because the disease occurs predominantly in the elderly, the course of systemically administered prednisone is as brief as possible, or if prolonged, is given every other day to avoid complications. Unlike patients with pemphigus, patients with pemphigoid may show increased mortality when systemic immunosuppressants are used (20a).

Thus, a strict and careful topical regime with corticosteroids and immunomodulators is often the best first step. Following this, treatment with oral nicotinamide and tetracycline may obviate the need for systemic corticosteroids and their side effects. Immunosuppressive therapy with agents such as mycophenolate, cyclosporine, and azathioprine reduces the need for higher doses of corticosteroids (21). Localized disease can be treated by topical steroid application, often with great success (22–24). The eruption may be self-limited and spontaneously remit within 1 to 2 years, or it can persist and recur for months to years, with individual lesions lasting for many years. Patients have a good prognosis, but in the elderly, it has proven fatal, especially in debilitated persons.

The basic treatment modalities for cicatricial pemphigoid are systemic therapy with dapsone or prednisone and immunosuppressive therapy. Treatment is directed at the control of mucosal scarring. For early conjunctival involvement, dapsone is used. For progressive involvement with scarring, the immunosuppressive drugs, such as mycophenolate, cyclophosphamide, or azathioprine, are used. For those who present

### Figure 5-9
**BULLOUS PEMPHIGOID**

Direct immunofluorescence shows linear deposition of IgG (60 to 80 percent) and complement (100 percent) along the dermal-epidermal junction, a characteristic finding in bullous pemphigoid. Indirect immunofluorescence studies reveal positivity in 75 to 80 percent of cases.

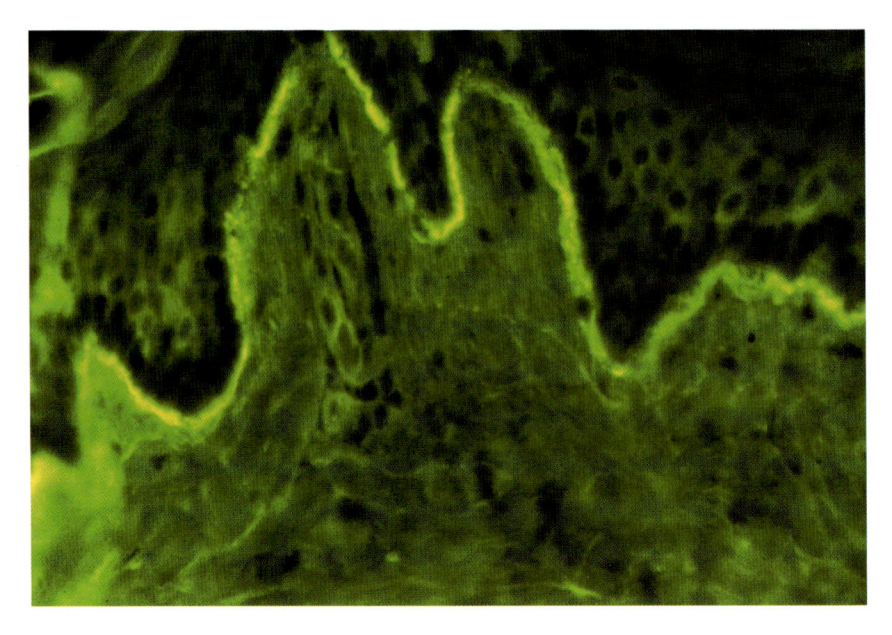

with advanced or rapidly progressive disease, and for those with esophageal, anal, or laryngeal lesions, intravenous gammaglobulin and/or rituximab may be necessary. The results of therapy are variable. Etanercept and infliximab have been used for cicatricial pemphigoid. Delay in systemic therapy portends a poor prognosis, particularly if the cornea scars.

## HERPES GESTATIONIS

**Definition.** *Herpes gestationis* is one of the group of dermatoses that occur in pregnancy, as well as the postpartum period (25–33). It appears to represent an autoimmune disease characterized by a complement-fixing IgG.

**Clinical Features.** The eruption occurs in the fourth to seventh month of pregnancy, rarely earlier in pregnancy, and in the postpartum period (25,26). Although herpes gestationis may not necessarily recur in subsequent pregnancies, it is sometimes exacerbated by the use of contraceptive, estrogen, or progesterone medications. It is present in all races.

The eruption is severely pruritic and begins mainly on the central and lateral aspects of the trunk and on the abdomen. The rest of the body may be involved, including extremities and even the palms and soles. The lesions vary from papules to urticarial papules and plaques, and are often surmounted by blisters that are tense but can break down and become eroded (fig. 5-10). Unlike bullous pemphigoid or erythema multiforme, it is less likely to affect the mucous membranes. The hair and nails are also spared.

**Pathologic Findings.** There are subtle yet important differences between the histology of herpes gestationis and bullous pemphigoid. Both are subepidermal blistering disorders. In herpes gestationis, however, there is often marked papillary dermal edema which expands dermal papillae and which, in tangential section, appears as intraepidermal vesicles (figs. 5-11, 5-12). The epidermis may show focal spongiosis and infiltration of eosinophils (i.e., eosinophilic spongiosis). While bullous pemphigoid is associated with vacuolization of the basal cell layer, herpes gestationis often demonstrates dyskeratosis and colloid body formation, similar to that seen in lichen planus. Herpes gestationis must be differentiated from pruritic urticarial papules and plaques of pregnancy (PUPPP). PUPPP, an itchy papular eruption, generally does not vesiculate, shows no evidence of cytolytic or dyskeratotic injury along the dermal-epidermal junction, and is negative by routine direct immunofluorescence testing. Immunofluorescence testing of lesional or nonlesional skin in herpes gestationis reveals findings identical to those of bullous pemphigoid (fig. 5-13). It has been hypothesized that herpes gestationis is a hormonally modulated autoimmune disease directed against chorioallantoic and trophoblastic (paternally derived) antigens that cross-react with basement membrane zone antigens. Circulating antibasement membrane zone antibodies are less frequently detected in herpes gestationis than in bullous pemphigoid.

**Differential Diagnosis.** The principal entity in the differential diagnosis is PUPPP, which also occurs toward the end of pregnancy. The lesions of PUPPP are not vesicular, however, and they do not have positive immunofluorescence, a helpful diagnostic finding. Also, they do not characteristically occur in the postpartum period. Other bullous disorders, such as bullous pemphigoid, erythema multiforme, or bullous drug reactions, must be considered.

**Treatment and Prognosis.** Because the eruption occurs late in pregnancy, oral corticosteroids are tolerated with fewer side effects. Low doses may lead to remission of the lesions (34). Occasionally, only topical corticosteroids are necessary in addition to antihistamines.

## EPIDERMOLYSIS BULLOSA ACQUISITA, INFLAMMATORY VARIANT

**Definition.** *Epidermolysis bullosa acquisita* (EBA) is a chronic, subepidermal blistering disease that resembles hereditary epidermolysis bullosa of the dystrophic type in that blisters are associated with increased skin fragility (35). Healing likewise occurs with scarring and milia. An underlying immunopathologic mechanism derives from the patient's autoimmunity to type VII collagen fibers. The disease occurs in adult life without gender predilection (35); children are rarely affected (36–38). Patients seem to have a genetic predisposition to other autoimmune diseases. Human leukocyte antigen (HLA)-DR2 haplotype expression is found, especially in patients who also have bullous systemic lupus

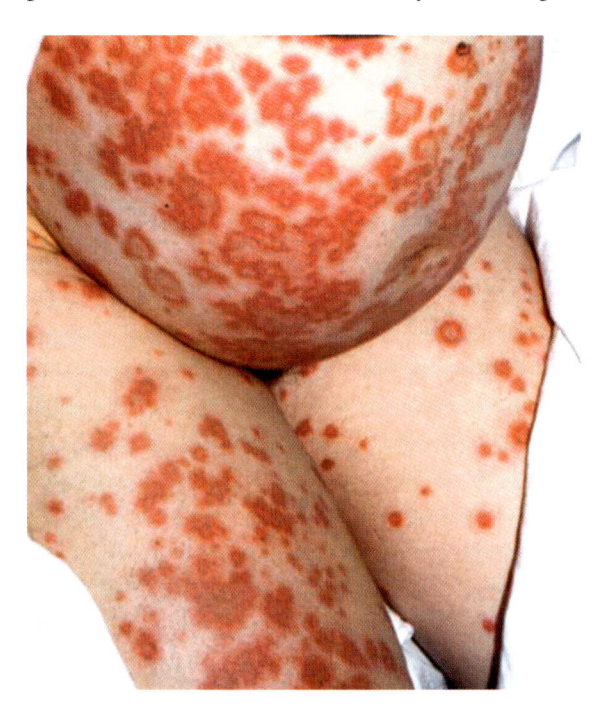

Figure 5-10

**HERPES GESTATIONIS**

The lesions are polymorphic, ranging from urticarial, erythematous papules and plaques, to more polycyclic regions. Early vesiculation was also present.

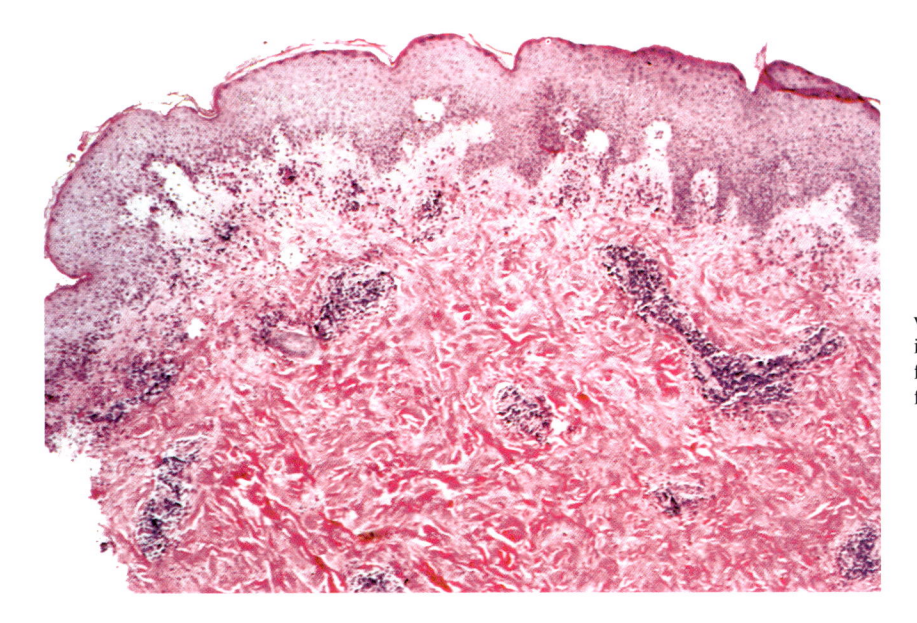

Figure 5-11

**HERPES GESTATIONIS**

There is a superficial perivascular and papillary dermal inflammatory infiltrate. The findings at scanning magnification are nonspecific.

## Inflammatory Disorders of the Skin

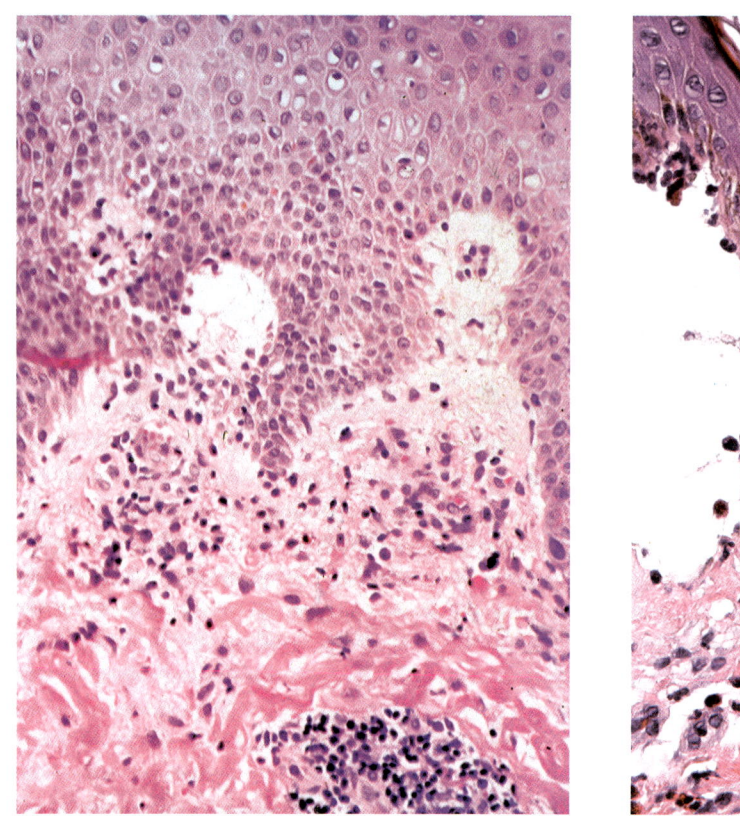

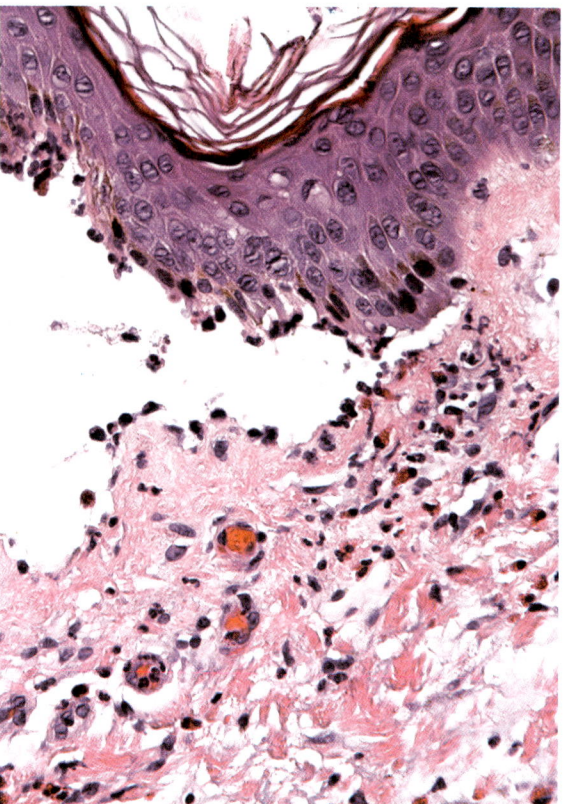

**Figure 5-12**

**HERPES GESTATIONIS**

Left: High magnification shows marked papillary dermal edema with lymphocytes and eosinophils in the dermis and along the dermal-epidermal junction. Eosinophilic spongiosis may be observed.

Right: A subepidermal blister ensues with numerous associated eosinophils.

**Figure 5-13**

**HERPES GESTATIONIS**

Direct immunofluorescence of perilesional skin in herpes gestationis demonstrates linear C3 in virtually all cases and IgG in a third of patients.

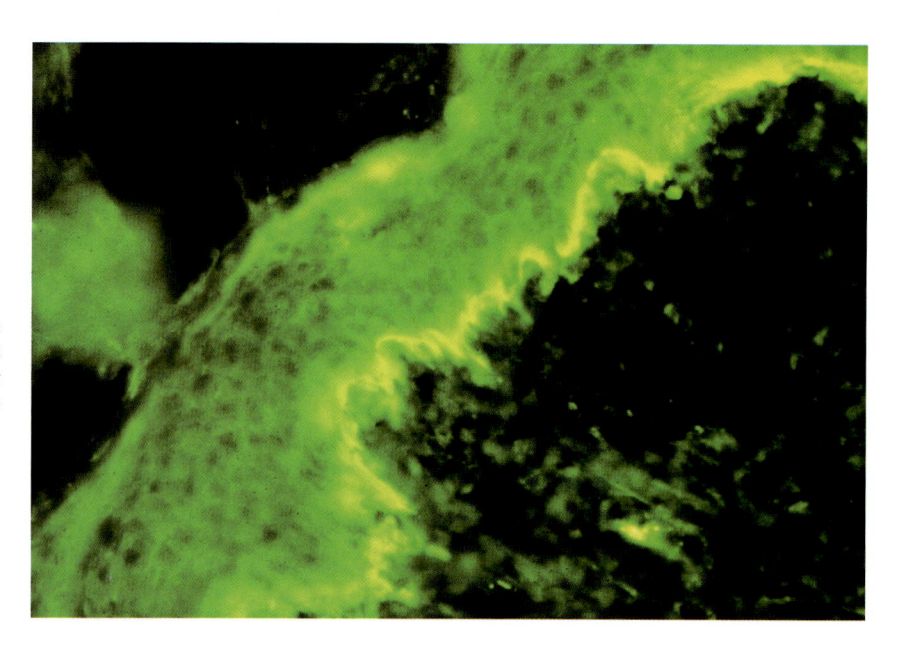

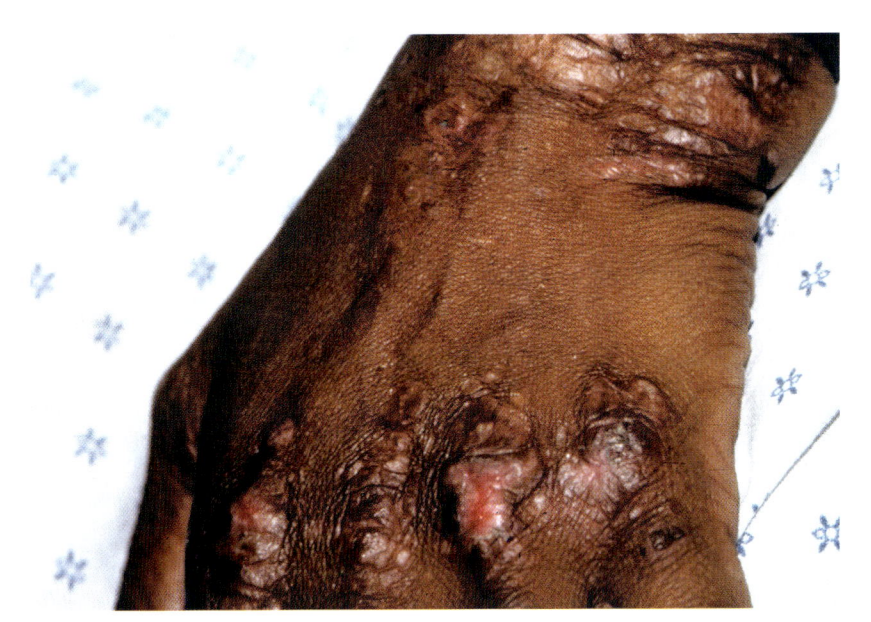

**Figure 5-14**

**EPIDERMOLYSIS BULLOSA ACQUISITA**

Acral blisters that lead to scarring and milia formation on a noninflammatory base are characteristic. In this form, alopecia and nail dystrophy also occur.

erythematosus. Black patients with this haplotype have a higher relative risk of developing EBA than Caucasians.

**Clinical Features.** There are two clinical presentations in patients with this disorder. The first and classic is as a noninflammatory blistering eruption on the extremities that heals with scarring and the formation of milia (fig. 5-14). The presentation may be mild and resemble porphyria cutanea tarda, or severe and resemble the recessive form of hereditary epidermolysis bullosa dystrophica. There is increased skin fragility and the blisters are thus localized to sites of trauma. Intact blisters, which may be hemorrhagic, may be very tense but are present on a noninflamed base. Erosions lead to crusting and eventual scarring with milia formation. Blisters may appear on previously unaffected skin or on scarred areas. Other clinical and laboratory features of porphyria cutanea tarda are missing and allow for distinction from that entity.

The second manifestation of EBA, which occurs in as many as half the patients, resembles bullous pemphigoid. It presents as a generalized inflammatory dermatosis in which tense blisters surmount a reddened or urticarial base. Like bullous pemphigoid, the lesions affect the trunk and flexural areas, begin as plaque-like urticarial lesions, and may not scar, although, over the course of repeated bouts, the lesions become less inflamed and may scar. Mucosal involvement occurs in both types and in rare cases may be the only manifestation of the disease, resembling cicatricial pemphigoid.

EBA has been anecdotally associated with a variety of disorders including autoimmune diseases, endocrinopathies, and neoplasms. Significant association, however, only occurs with systemic lupus erythematosus and inflammatory bowel disease.

**Pathologic Findings.** The histology may be identical to that of bullous pemphigoid (fig. 5-15), although there are usually more neutrophils than in pemphigoid, with both neutrophils and eosinophils at the dermal-epidermal junction. Direct immunofluorescence, although often negative, may show a linear pattern for IgG that predominates over that of C3. Indirect immunofluorescence of split skin preparations, immunocytochemical mapping of basement membrane zone components of lesional skin, or immunoelectron microscopy of lesional skin may be required to definitively differentiate EBA from bullous pemphigoid.

**Differential Diagnosis.** The characteristic scarring helps to differentiate the disease from bullous pemphigoid or erythema multiforme. At times, biopsy is required to differentiate cicatricial pemphigoid from EBA. Porphyria cutanea tarda is also associated with milia formation and scarring, but has other symptoms and signs, including differences in immunofluorescence.

**Treatment and Prognosis.** The treatment of this disease poses a great problem to clinicians

*Inflammatory Disorders of the Skin*

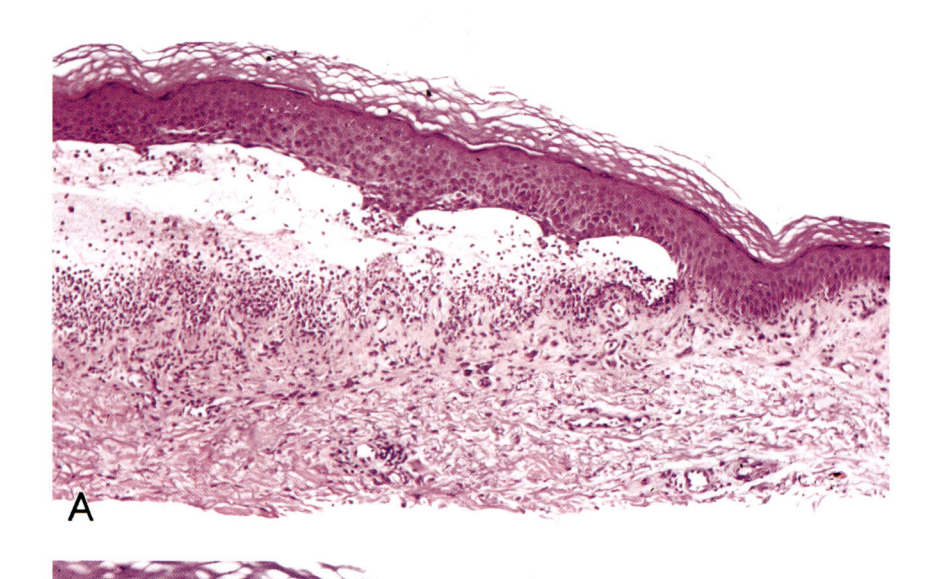

**Figure 5-15**

**EPIDERMOLYSIS BULLOSA ACQUISITA**

A: Subepidermal bulla shows lymphocytes and neutrophils in a papillary dermal and perivascular array.

B: There is prominent edema with minimal inflammation. This form of EBA, the bullous pemphigoid-like form, is associated with a striking number of neutrophils and lymphocytes with rare eosinophils admixed.

C: At higher magnification, the inflammatory component is better seen.

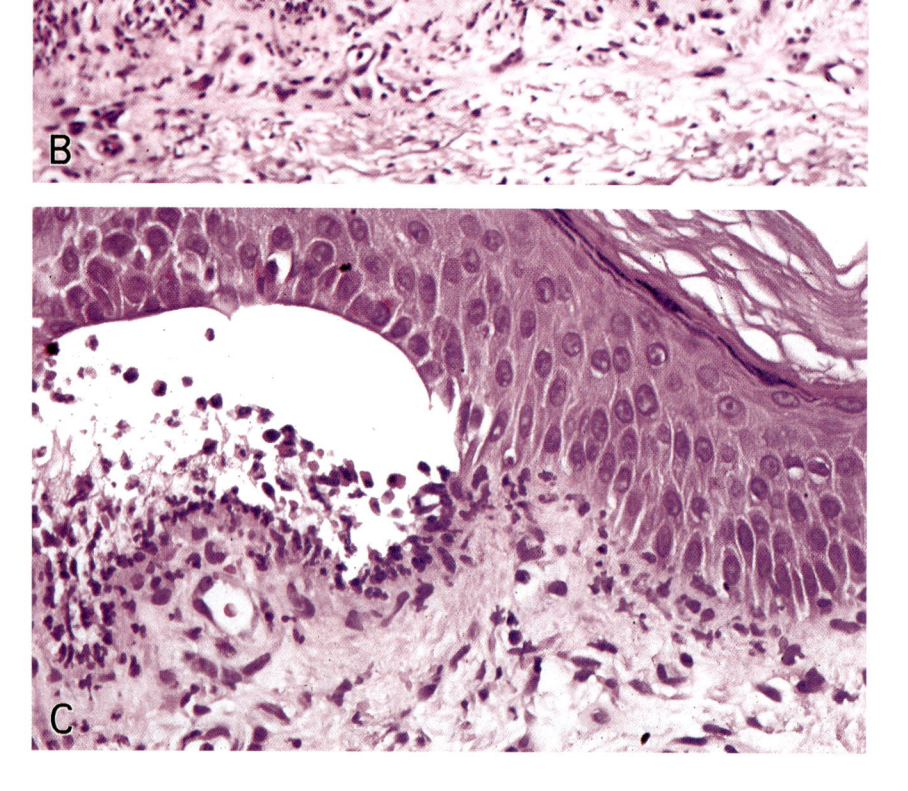

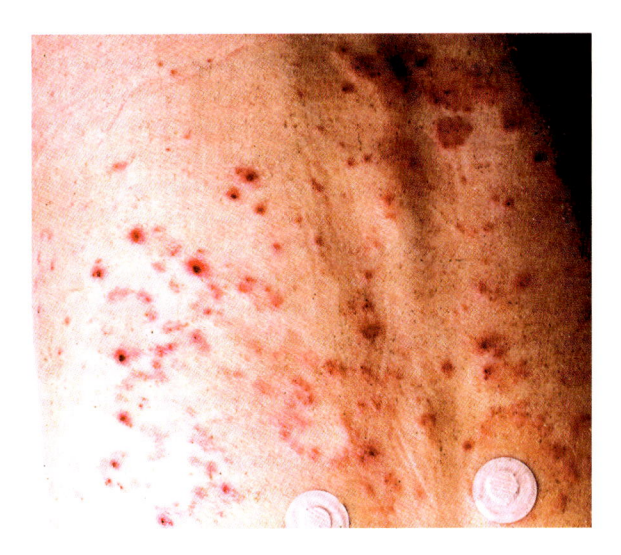

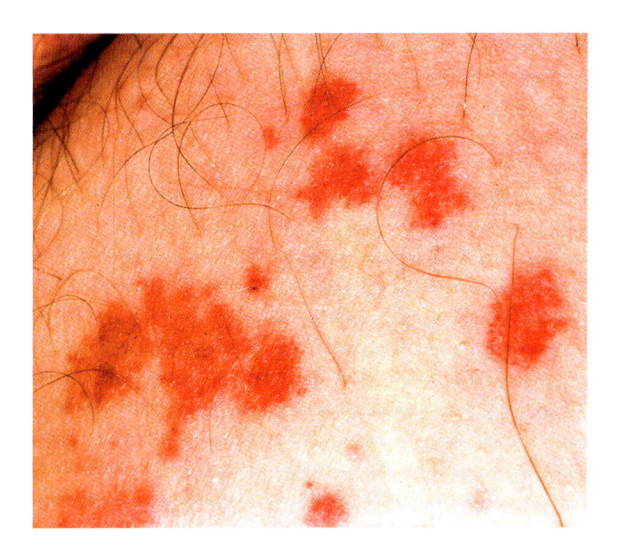

## Figure 5-16
### DERMATITIS HERPETIFORMIS

Left: Symmetrical grouped vesicles on an erythematous base are characteristic of dermatitis herpetiformis. Lesions are extremely pruritic.

Right: Grouped erythematous vesicles of dermatitis herpetiformis.

(39–47). The usual treatments, such as systemic steroids, methotrexate, and azathioprine, to which other bullous diseases respond, are generally not effective, except for partially treating the inflammatory form of the disease. In patients with a prominent neutrophilic component, some response with dapsone has been reported (44,45). There has been success with high doses of cyclosporine (46); however, the toxicity of the drug limits its use. Intravenous gammaglobulin has been used with variable results. Rituximab and extracorporeal photopheresis have been attempted in recalcitrant cases. Wound infections must be prevented at affected sites.

## DERMATITIS HERPETIFORMIS

**Definition.** *Dermatitis herpetiformis* is a chronic, extremely pruritic eruption composed of both papules and vesicles, with a characteristic distribution on extensor surfaces (48–52). The rash is often symmetrical, for example, on buttocks, both elbows, and both scapulae. Occurring at any age, the disorder most commonly presents in the second to the fourth decades. Patients often have associated gluten-sensitive enteropathy and exhibit granular deposits of IgA in a characteristic distribution in their skin (53–55), evidence of the autoimmune nature of the disease and a useful finding for the immunofluorescence diagnosis of dermatitis herpetiformis. Also, these patients express the HLA-B8 and Dr3 haplotypes as do other patients with autoimmune disorders.

**Clinical Features.** The onset of this disorder is usually heralded by itching, burning, or stinging in involved sites 8 to 12 hours before the appearance of the most characteristic lesion: a papule that rapidly becomes vesicular (48). At times, urticarial plaques appear. The blisters average less than 5 mm and thus are true vesicles. Because of their striking pruritus they are excoriated; hence, the lesions may all consist of erythematous erosions. The term herpetiform derives from the clustering of the papules and vesicles on an erythematous base (fig. 5-16). The lesions often appear symmetrically on the scapulae, buttocks, sacrum, elbows, knees, and scalp. The face may be affected. When lesions occur on the palms and soles, they are hemorrhagic. Because lesions are grouped or localized and pruritic, the clinical differential diagnosis includes insect-bite reaction, scabies, contact dermatitis, and the pruritic variant of bullous pemphigoid. Mucosal involvement is uncommon. Patients often relate the onset of their disease or exacerbations to iodide-containing foods, such as seafood, and to the consumption of gluten-containing products.

## Inflammatory Disorders of the Skin

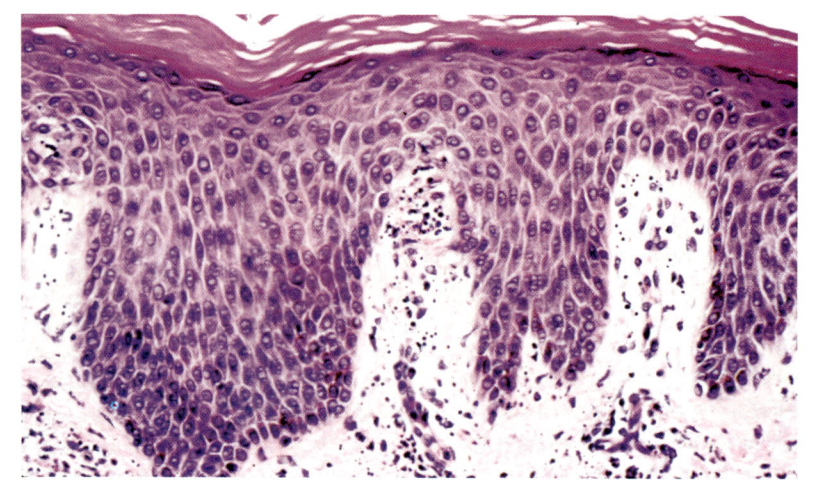

**Figure 5-17**

**DERMATITIS HERPETIFORMIS**

Top: Neutrophils at the tips of the dermal papillae forming incipient papillary microabscesses are characteristic of early dermatitis herpetiformis.

Bottom: A more advanced lesion shows well-developed microabscesses at the tips of dermal papillae.

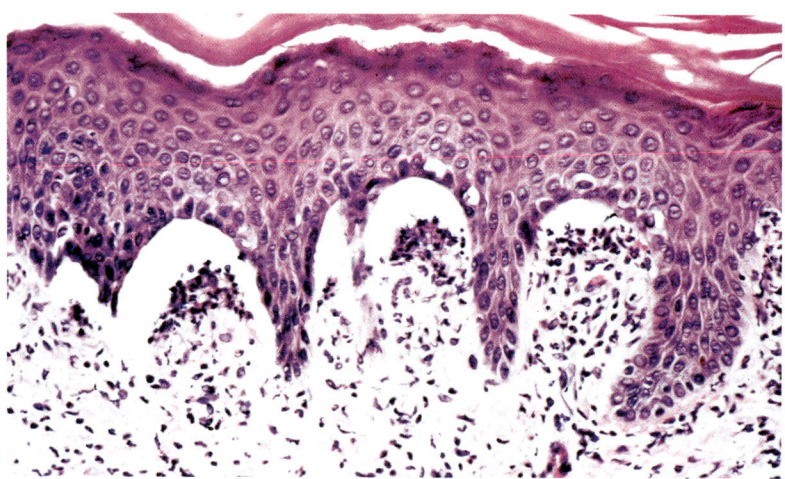

The relationship of dermatitis herpetiformis to gluten appears to be an intrinsic pathogenetic one. It is likely that all patients with this eruption have the abnormality, no matter whether or not clinically apparent. Many asymptomatic patients, when given large doses of gluten-containing foods, such as wheat, rye, or oats, demonstrate sprue-like symptoms.

**Pathologic Findings.** Scanning magnification reveals a forming or established subepidermal blister associated with concentrations of neutrophils within the tips of dermal papillae. Early changes include deposition of fibrin in dermal papillae, nuclear dust (i.e., fragments) beneath a vacuolated basal cell layer overlying the dermal papillae, and the notable absence of spongiosis or eosinophils (figs. 5-17, 5-18). Importantly, neutrophils are not concentrated at rete tips, a common site of inflammatory involvement in linear IgA disease (discussed later).

Old lesions may show influx of eosinophils, re-epithelialization, and impetiginization, which may confuse the diagnostic picture. Direct immunofluorescence reveals predominantly IgA and fibrin in a granular array in the tips of dermal papillae (fig. 5-19)

**Differential Diagnosis.** Linear IgA dermatitis can exhibit similar findings clinically but also involves the palms and soles; it additionally has larger vesicles. The severe pruritus helps to differentiate dermatitis herpetiformis from other bullous disorders. Histologically, it is unusual to find papillary dermal microabscesses in other disorders, although they occur, rarely, in necrotizing cutaneous vasculitis.

**Treatment and Prognosis.** Initiating a gluten-free diet is the first therapeutic step. Patients rapidly respond to dapsone and sulfapyridine (56). Ingestion of the medication results in rapid diminution of symptoms, in many cases

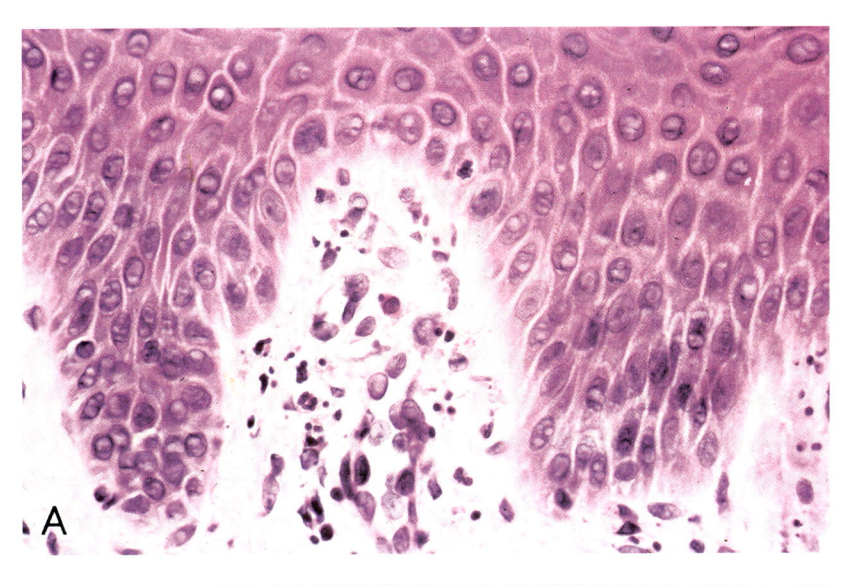

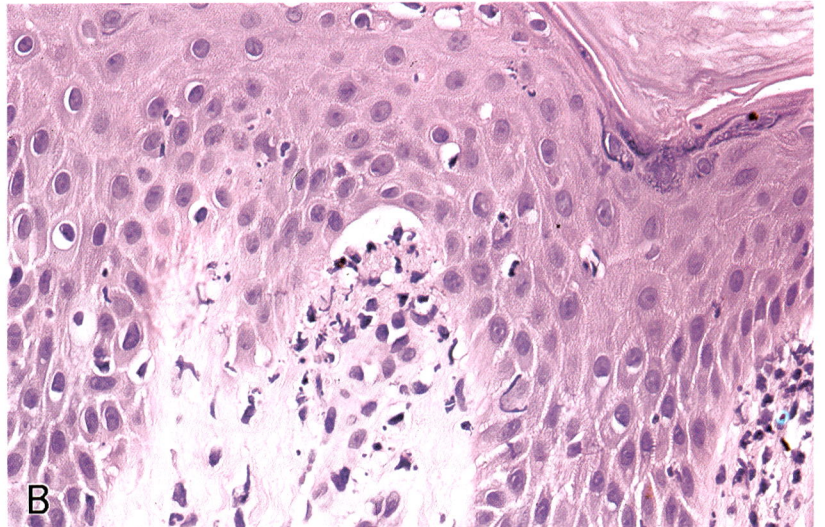

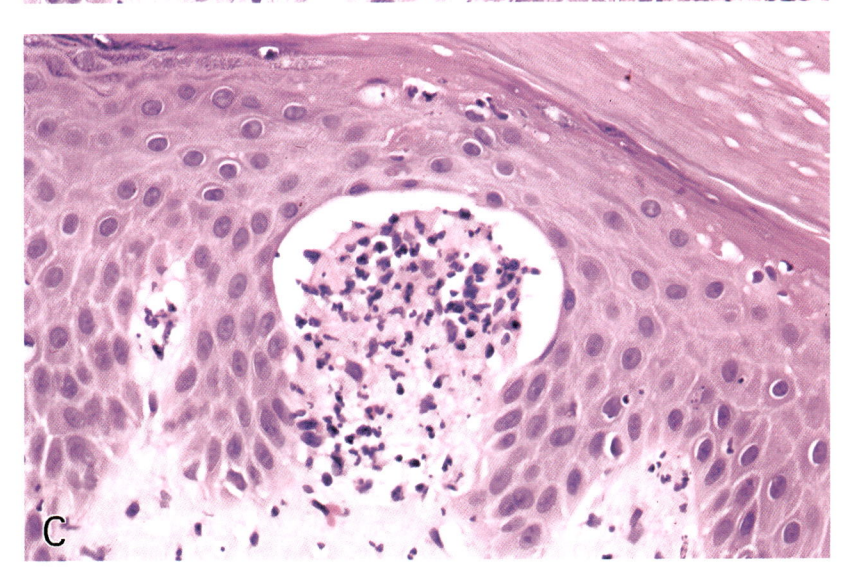

### Figure 5-18
### DERMATITIS HERPETIFORMIS

A-C: Progressive accumulation of neutrophils, at first with nuclear debris, leads to focal separation of the epidermis, and finally clefting in dermatitis herpetiformis. As the neutrophils increase, rare admixed eosinophils are seen as well as apoptotic keratinocytes. Degradation of laminin and type IV collagen by neutrophilic enzymes leads to bulla formation due to coalescence of the suprapapillary clefts.

## Inflammatory Disorders of the Skin

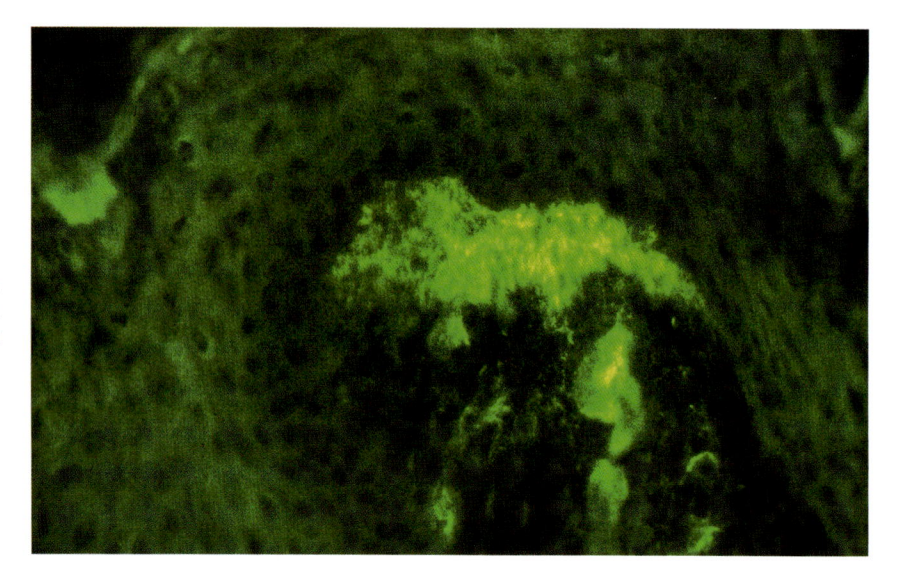

Figure 5-19

**DERMATITIS HERPETIFORMIS**
Granular and thready deposits of IgA at the tip of a dermal papilla are revealed by direct immunofluorescence.

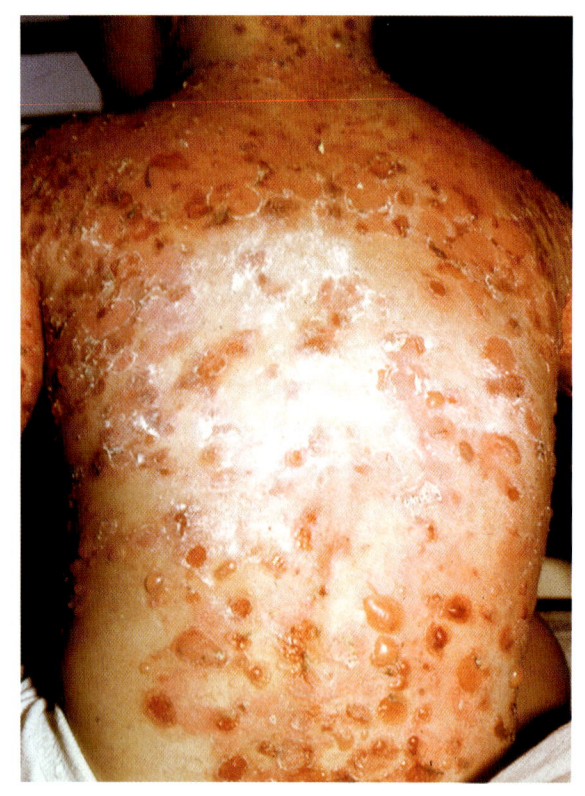

Figure 5-20

**LINEAR IgA DERMATOSIS/ BULLOUS DISEASE OF CHILDHOOD**

This disorder presents in adults with papulovesicles that are less pruritic and less symmetrical than in dermatitis herpetiformis and often involve the palms and soles. Oral and ocular lesions are found in 50 percent of patients. In the childhood form of linear IgA disease, the lesions form in a linear array as a "string of pearls" and begin in the genital area or buttocks.

within a few hours. In other cases, improvement is more gradual. Discontinuance of the drugs is usually followed by exacerbation of the eruption. The response to these drugs is so effective that it may be used as an aid in diagnosis. Colchicine may also be helpful. Systemic immunosuppression is rarely needed, but if so, prednisone, mycophenolate, azathioprine, and cyclosporine are used.

### BULLOUS DISEASE OF CHILDHOOD

**Definition.** The chronic *bullous disease of childhood* is an acquired disorder that occurs in young children and is distinguished from other disorders by the presence of a linear band of IgA at the dermal-epidermal junction, as detected by immunofluorescence.

**Clinical Features.** The lesions occur usually before the age of 10 years and there is equal distribution among male and female children. It has been determined that the condition is associated with the HLA-B8 haplotype. The lesions usually appear on normal skin, or on skin that is slightly erythematous, as large, tense bullae (fig. 5-20). They often occur in the diaper area and concentrate on the lower abdomen, the perineum, and the lower extremities; the genitalia are often affected. Perioral lesions also occur. The lesions are often annular or irregular in shape and have blisters at the periphery. The appearance of new blisters at the site of previous crusted lesions is characteristic, and the result is known as "the rosette affect."

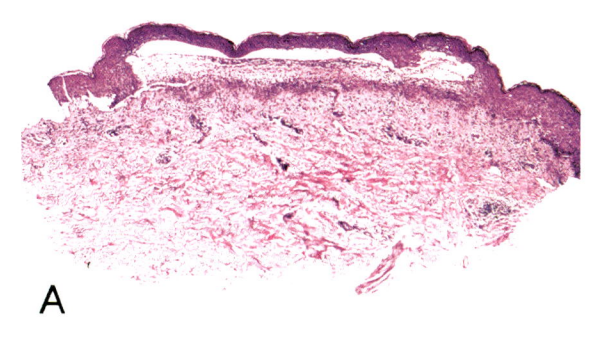

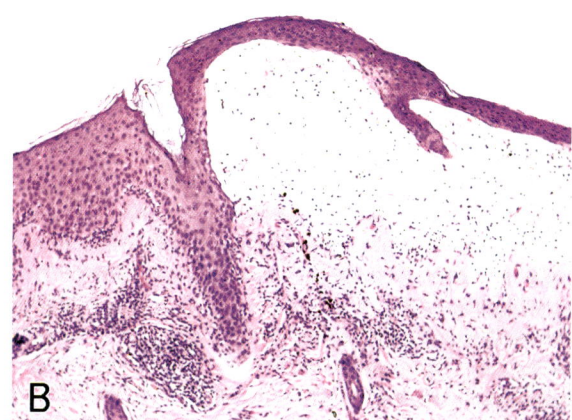

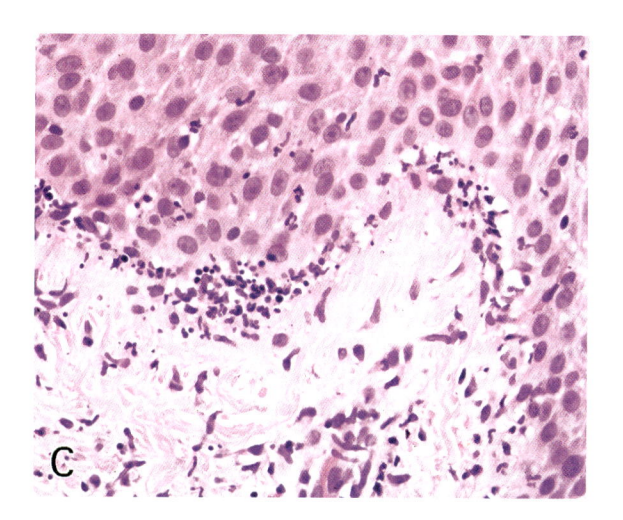

### Figure 5-21
### LINEAR IgA DERMATOSIS/ BULLOUS DISEASE OF CHILDHOOD

A: A characteristic subepidermal bulla is present. Biopsies must be taken from the edge of the lesion to reveal the diagnostic features.
B: Higher-magnification view of blister edge.
C: Neutrophils line up along the entire dermal-epidermal junction. Involvement of the tips of the rete ridges helps to distinguish the lesion from dermatitis herpetiformis.

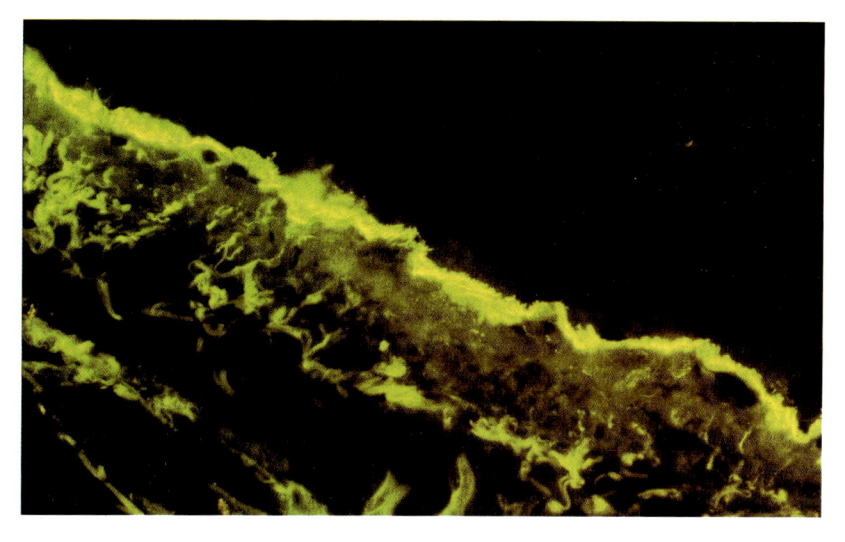

### Figure 5-22
### LINEAR IgA DERMATOSIS/ BULLOUS DISEASE OF CHILDHOOD

Direct immunofluorescence shows the deposition of IgA in a linear array, characteristic of this disorder.

**Pathologic Findings.** Although the histologic appearance superficially mimics dermatitis herpetiformis, important differences exist (fig. 5-21). Most critical of these is the localization of neutrophils evenly and linearly along the dermal-epidermal interface to include the tips of the rete ridges. Confirmation of the diagnosis requires direct immunofluorescence, which shows a linear pattern of IgA deposition along the dermal-epidermal interface in contrast to the localized granular IgA deposits in dermatitis herpetiformis (fig. 5-22).

**Differential Diagnosis.** These lesions must be distinguished from childhood bullous pemphigoid or dermatitis herpetiformis. Immunofluorescence allows for the correct diagnosis.

**Treatment and Prognosis.** Fortunately, most children will exhibit spontaneous remission after about the second year of life. Almost all cases remit before puberty. Even if the disease lasts into early adult life, the lesions become much less severe. Patients have been treated with dapsone and sulfapyridine. Usually they respond well; if not, they may respond to oral steroids or mycophenolate mofetil.

## LINEAR IgA DISEASE

**Definition.** *Linear IgA disease* is an uncommon blistering disease representing the adult form of the disorder associated with linear IgA deposition along the dermal-epidermal junction (57–59). It clinically shares features with EBA, bullous pemphigoid, and dermatitis herpetiformis. While the childhood disease occurs in those under 10 years of age, this form occurs in later life, most commonly in the fourth decade.

**Clinical Features.** Lesions vary from grouped pruritic papules, to papulovesicles in an arcuate array, to large bullae over the trunk and extremities. When grouped, the lesions often are present along the extensor surfaces; otherwise, they are mainly truncal. An unusual feature of the disorder is the presence of urticarial lesions on the palms and soles. Mucosal involvement is common, sometimes affecting two thirds of the patients with shallow oral ulcers. The disorder has been associated with certain drugs, including vancomycin and lithium, among others (60–62). There is no convincing evidence of a gluten-associated enteropathy. The lesions also have been associated with underlying lymphoproliferative disorders and other malignant tumors.

**Pathologic Findings.** The lesions initially are associated with a perivenular lymphoid infiltrate, occasionally admixed with eosinophils. As the lesions evolve, neutrophils migrate and are dispersed along the dermal-epidermal junction in a scattered array, but notably involving the tips of the rete ridges. A subepidermal blister ensues, with neutrophils and occasional admixed eosinophils in the blister cavity. In some cases, eosinophils and lymphocytes are present at the dermal-epidermal junction. The initial separation occurs either within the lamina lucida or below the lamina densa.

**Differential Diagnosis.** The clinical differential diagnosis includes dermatitis herpetiformis, bullous pemphigoid, cicatricial pemphigoid, and even EBA. The presence of an annular array of blisters is often helpful, as is the involvement of the palms and soles with urticaria. The final diagnostic resolution lies in appropriately performed immunofluorescence with the detection of linear IgA along the dermal-epidermal junction in the absence of IgG and in most cases, the third component of complement.

The histologic differential diagnosis includes bullous lupus erythematosus and rarely, herpes gestationis with neutrophils. In both of these disorders, neutrophils and debris are scattered along the dermal-epidermal junction.

**Treatment and Prognosis.** The lesions usually respond to sulfapyridine or dapsone (63,64). In some patients, oral corticosteroids are administered to inhibit blistering. The disease usually responds to elimination of a causative drug or associated underlying systemic disorder, although not in all cases remits. Dicloxacillin and colchicine are also accepted treatments. Only rarely is further immunosuppression needed.

## BULLOUS LESIONS OF INTERFACE DERMATITIS

These disorders include *erythema multiforme, toxic epidermal necrolysis, bullous lupus erythematosus, bullous/erosive lichen planus, bullous lichen sclerosus,* and *bullous fixed drug eruption* (65–75). Figures 5-23 through 5-27 illustrate various disorders that share the potential for bullous lesions to evolve from lymphocyte-mediated interface dermatitis. Just as vascular ischemia may produce blisters, so too may interface dermatitis. Interface dermatitis generally results only in a band-like lymphocytic infiltrate along the dermal-epidermal interface and chronic alterations to basal cells (i.e., dyskeratosis, squamatization) that do not eventuate in dermal-epidermal separation. This implies that neutrophils and eosinophils may be far more potent than lymphocytes in producing the degree of acute epidermal injury that results in the formation of a subepidermal vesicle. In rare instances, interface dermatitis mediated by lymphocytes produces erosive and bullous

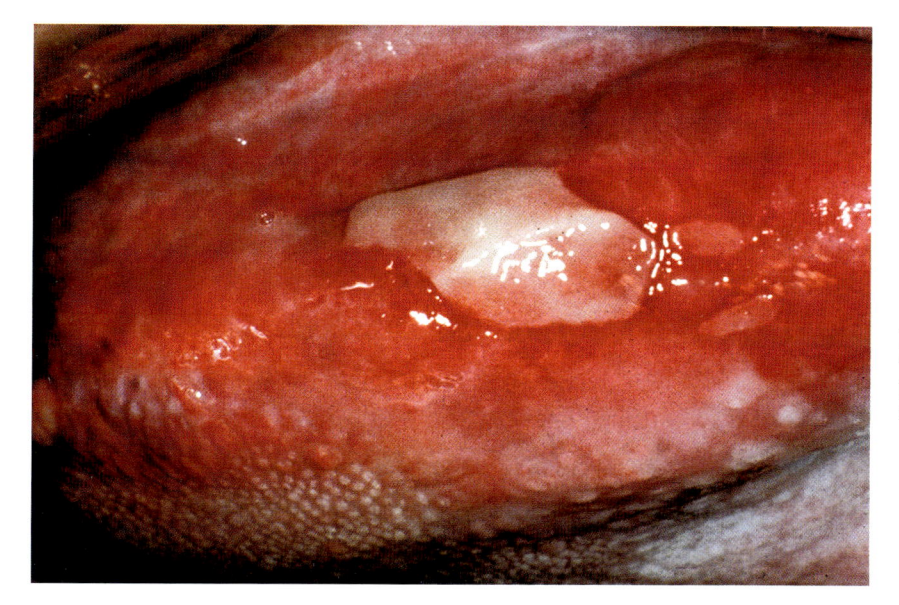

### Figure 5-23
### BULLOUS LICHEN PLANUS: ORAL LESION
The lesion presents as white patches in the mucosa, often associated with a reticulated pattern referred to as Wickham striae.

### Figure 5-24
### BULLOUS LICHEN PLANUS
There is a subepidermal bulla, the roof of which is formed by an epidermis with rete ridges in a sawtooth–like appearance. A dense band-like infiltrate of lymphocytes, here associated with fibrovascular proliferation, is also apparent.

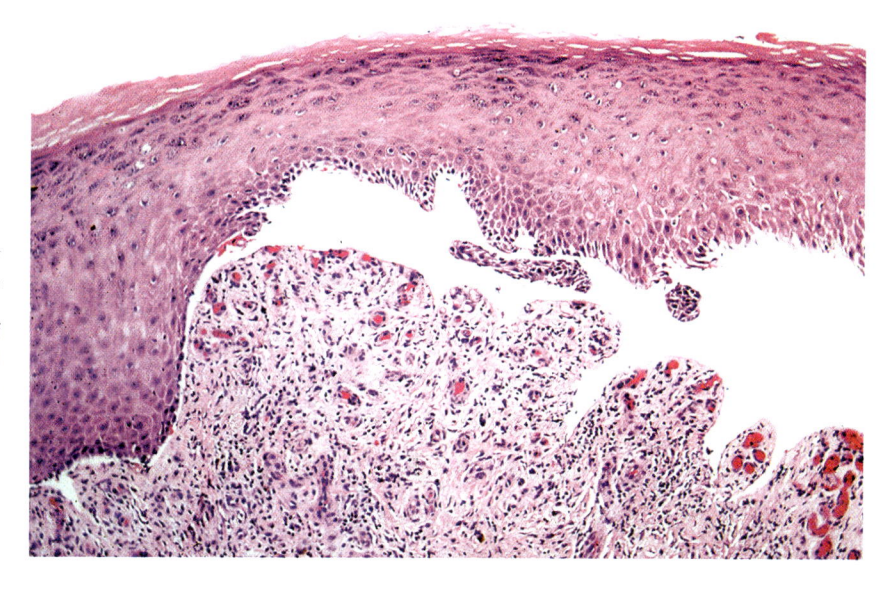

lesions resulting from destruction of the basal cell layer and basement membrane zone. The more common disorders that produce such alterations include erythema multiforme, lichen planus, and fixed drug eruption. *Pityriasis lichenoides et varioliformis acuta* may also result in bullous lesions due to lymphocyte-mediated dermal-epidermal separation. Bullous lupus erythematosus involves an admixture of neutrophils and lymphocytes along the basement membrane zone of a forming dermal-epidermal separation. Such lesions mimic linear IgA disease, and direct immunofluorescence to exclude linear IgA deposits is helpful.

## STAPHYLOCOCCAL SCALDED-SKIN SYNDROME (RITTER DISEASE)

**Definition.** *Staphylococcal scalded-skin syndrome* (SSSS), or *Ritter disease*, is an acute desquamation of the skin that follows erythema and tenderness subsequent to an acute bacterial infection (76). This disorder is due to *Staphylococcus aureus* which produces epidermolysin as an exotoxin (77,78). The condition is associated with subtle cleft formation beneath the stratum corneum that may, but is not invariably associated with obvious acantholysis, and therefore the condition is discussed in this chapter. Although listed here as a nonacantholytic blistering disorder, it must

*Inflammatory Disorders of the Skin*

**Figure 5-25**

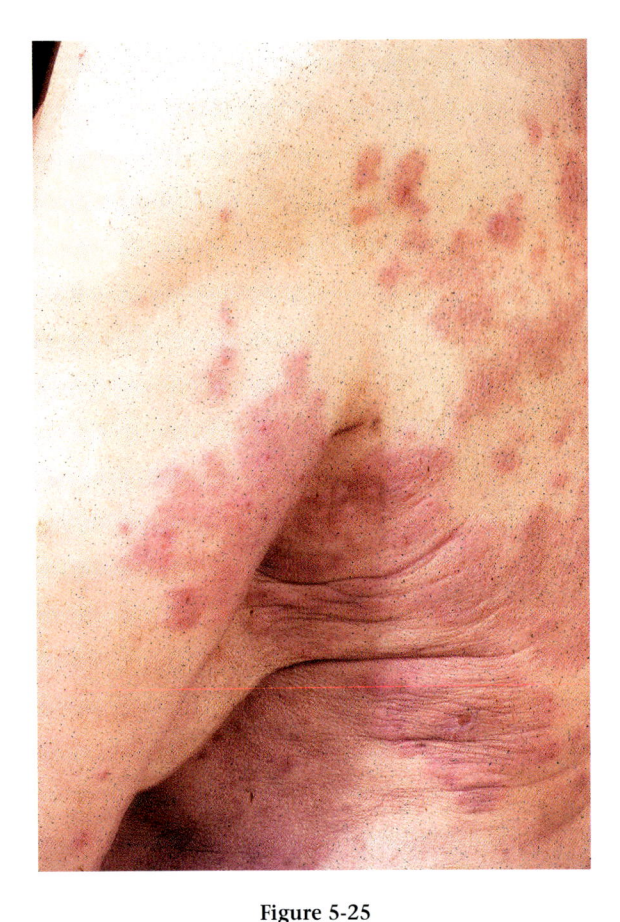

**ERYTHEMA MULTIFORME**

There are multiple coalescent plaques, many with central regions showing dusky erythema and correlating with the characteristic "targetoid" pattern.

be remembered that the target epitope that is compromised by the epidermolysin is analogous to the desmoglein affected in pemphigus foliaceus (79). SSSS occurs in nursery epidemics.

**Clinical Features.** Children usually 2 to 30 days of age exhibit an abrupt onset of generalized erythema (76). Within 24 hours this is followed by bullae formation; exfoliation of large sheets of skin follows within the first 2 days (fig. 5-28). The lesions occur around the head and neck, buttocks, groin, and axillae as well as the periumbilical area of the abdomen. The diagnosis is made by histopathology. Cultures of the skin are taken at the perianal area and groin. Antistaphylococcal antibiotics are administered with appropriate fluid and electrolyte replacement. These children should be treated as patients with second degree burns and need immediate therapy. The disease also occurs in adults, particularly the immunosuppressed or those with renal insufficiency, probably due to decreased excretion of toxin.

**Pathologic Findings.** The histology shows subtle foci of cleft formation within the superficial stratum spinosum and stratum granulosum (figs. 5-29, 5-31) (80). Occasionally, multiple levels are required to detect the characteristic alterations. Acantholytic cells may or may not be prominent, as emphasized by the placement of this condition in this section. Unlike the subcorneal separation of bullous impetigo, there are few inflammatory cells, and bacteria are not observed by Gram stain.

**Figure 5-26**

**ERYTHEMA MULTIFORME**

Biopsy of an early lesion reveals a normal stratum corneum. The characteristic vacuolization of the dermal-epidermal junction is associated with lymphocyte tagging that results in interface dermatitis. Occasionally, apoptotic cells in the epidermis may be noted. A perivascular lymphoid infiltrate is characteristic.

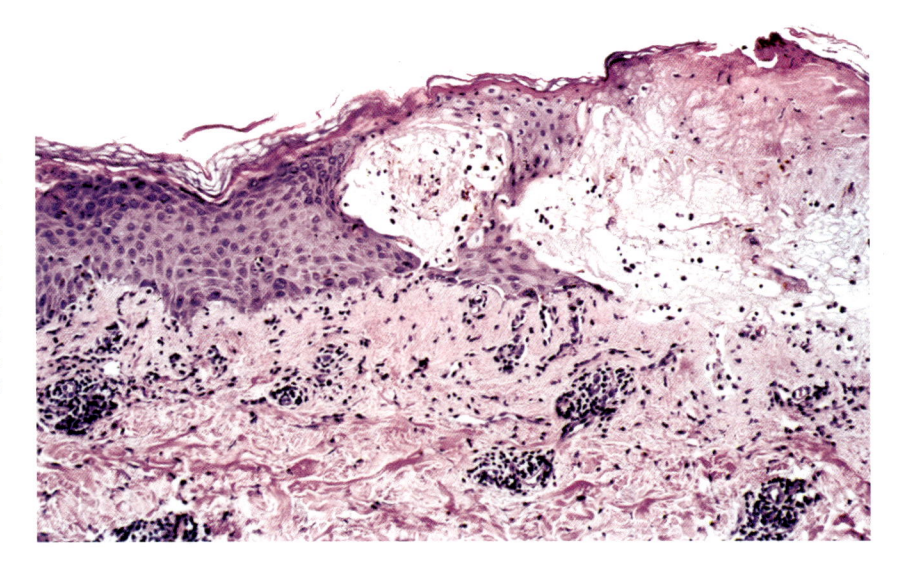

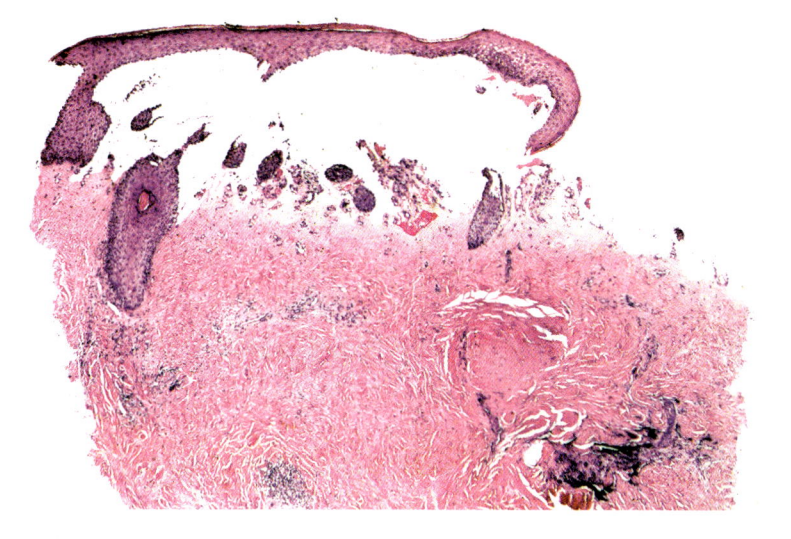

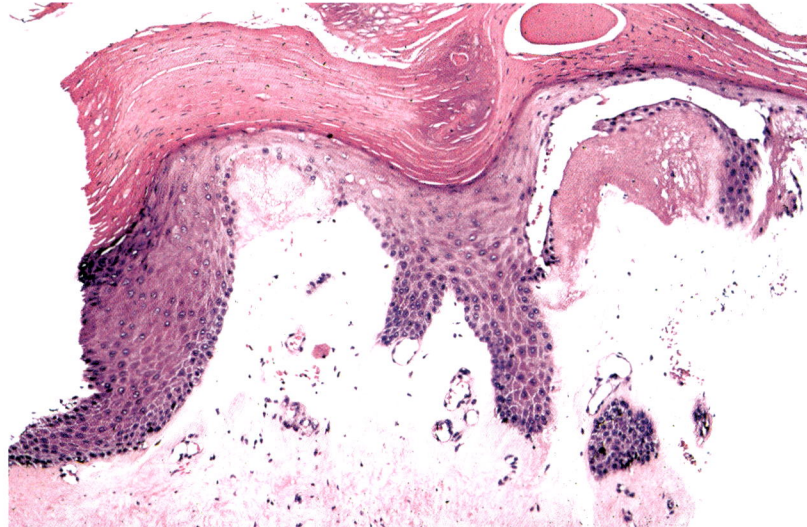

## Figure 5-27

**BULLOUS LICHEN SCLEROSUS**

Top: A subepidermal bulla is shearing away from the structures below that are left in the hyalinized dermis.

Bottom: The hyalinized tissue with ectatic vessels lies at the base of the bulla, which exhibits hemorrhage and fibrin deposition.

## Figure 5-28

**STAPHYLOCOCCAL SCALDED SKIN SYNDROME (SSSS)**

There is diffuse shedding of skin without evidence of inflammation. Sometimes a whole cast of an extremity can be removed due to sloughing of the superficial skin layers.

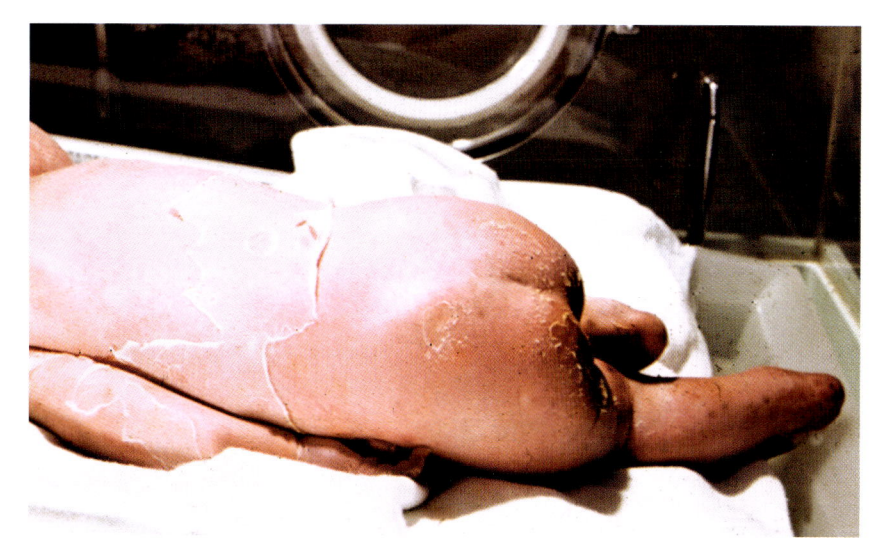

*Inflammatory Disorders of the Skin*

**Figure 5-29**

**EARLY LESION OF SSSS**

Top: At low magnification, the findings are extraordinarily subtle and may appear nonspecific.

Bottom: At higher magnification, the stratum corneum "lifts off" the underlying keratinocytes due to the epidermolysin produced by the staphylococcal organism. Dermal edema, and scattered lymphocytes and neutrophils, are present. In the process of lysis, a few parakeratotic cells are shed. When one produces a "jelly roll" rotating an applicator stick to wind shedding skin, only stratum corneum and a rare parakeratotic or acantholytic cell are noted on histologic exam.

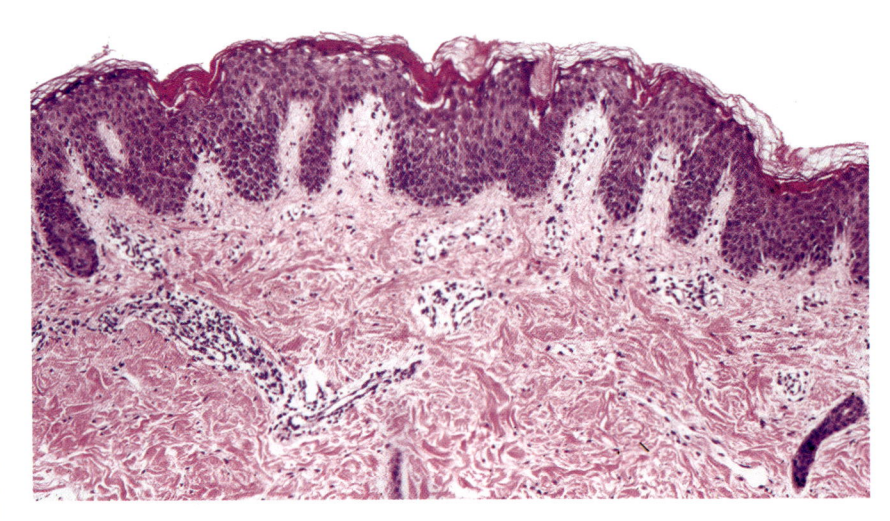

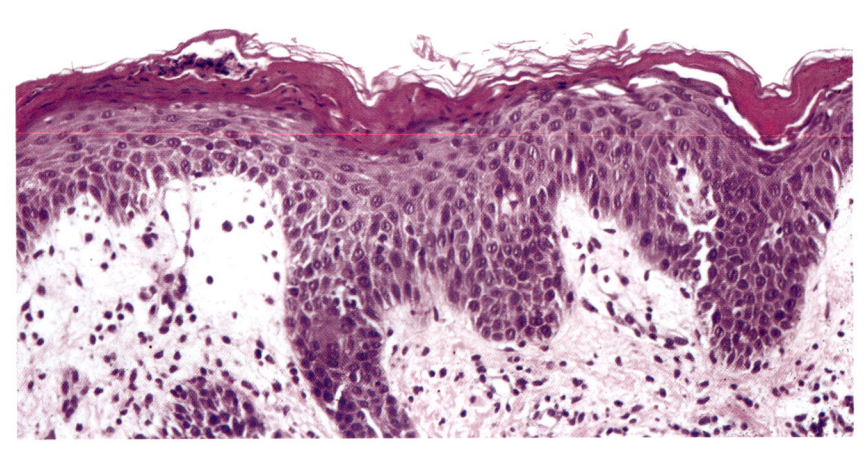

**Differential Diagnosis.** Toxic shock syndrome and toxic epidermolysis need to be considered in the clinical differential diagnosis. These lesions are rare in the neonatal period, however. Systemic mastocytosis with accompanying erythroderma may be confused with this disorder but the skin biopsy is negative.

**Treatment and Prognosis.** Cultures should be taken from the skin, nasopharynx, and genital area and groin (81,82). The organism is thus identified. Supportive skin care follows proper antibiosis.

## INFLAMMATORY VESICULOBULLOUS LESIONS DUE TO ISCHEMIA

### Bullous Manifestations of Primary Vasculopathic Injury

Blister formation may result from ischemic insult to the superficial dermis and, more commonly, to the epidermis. Injury to large vessels, which potentially may not be included in the biopsy specimen, results in noninflammatory cytolytic injury to the basal cell layer, leading to sites of dermal-epidermal separation. *Bullous vasculitis* is one of the more common forms of ischemic bullae formation. In this condition, clinical bullae result from necrotizing vasculitis, and involve leukocytoclasis, fibrinoid necrosis, and intraluminal thrombus formation, presumably leading to nutrient deficiency and hypoxia to the overlying epidermal layer (fig. 5-31).

### Bullae Due to Physical Agents

Blisters and bullae occur in response to physical agents (heat, pressure, friction). *Friction blisters* occur at sites of repeated trauma in which there is a shearing motion. These blisters are usually superficial and heal rapidly if abraded.

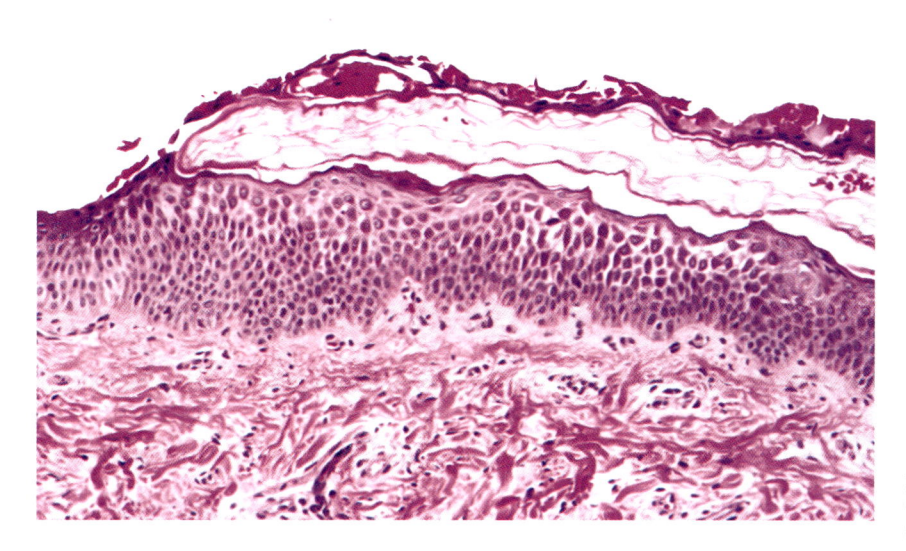

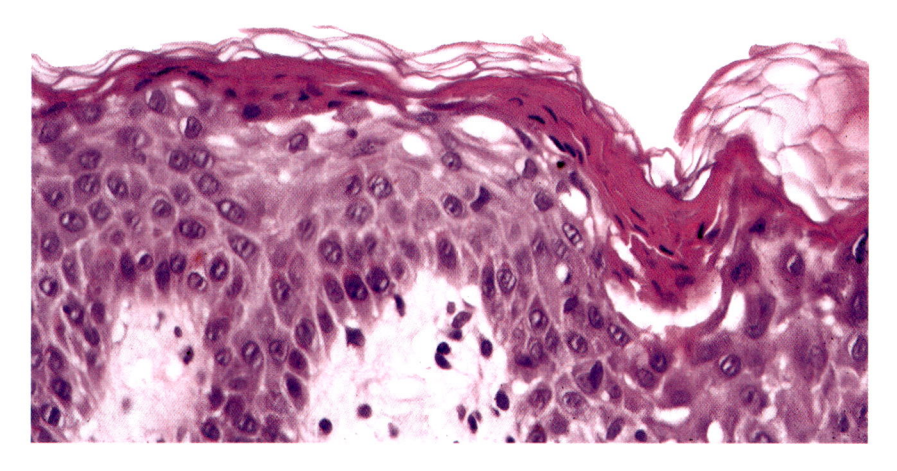

**Figure 5-30**

**OLDER LESION OF SSSS**

Top: The residue of the previous superficial blister is evidenced by a thin zone representing the blister roof, which adheres to the underlying normal stratum corneum.

Bottom: Higher-magnification view.

*Pressure bullae,* or so-called *coma bullae,* are associated with subepidermal blisters that appear at sites of prolonged application of pressure. Thus, for example, a person in a coma who lies on their forehead may have a coma bulla on the forehead or on the hip or at whichever point of pressure is the most sustained during the episode of unconsciousness (figs. 5-32, 3-33). While originally these blisters were thought to be due to barbiturate intoxication, it is now clear that they are due to pressure because they result in subepidermal blisters that are identifiable at the pressure sites. Necrosis of adnexal epithelium, in particular, the eccrine apparatus, is typical of coma blisters. Inflammation, if present, is secondary to the necrosis.

Blisters due to heat vary according to the degree of *thermal injury* that occurs. First-degree burns are superficial and result in simple desquamation. Second-degree burns cause a cleft in the epidermis itself, and similar features are also caused by severe cold injury. Severe burns are also associated with subepidermal blister formation and erosions, as are severe cold-induced injuries. These result in ulcers as they break down.

Generally, biopsy of blisters secondary to trauma reveals only an intraepidermal, subepidermal, or subcorneal vesicle without evidence of active acantholysis or spongiosis. Inflammation is minimal. The blister cavity contains serum and erythrocytes undergoing cytolysis and coagulation necrosis. When due to pressure, as with coma blisters, there is extensive necrosis of the eccrine glands and even of adjacent vessels. Thermal burns (i.e., infrared) and ultraviolet light B–induced injury (i.e., sunburn) usually produce subepidermal blisters as a result of individual cell or widespread keratinocyte necrosis.

*Inflammatory Disorders of the Skin*

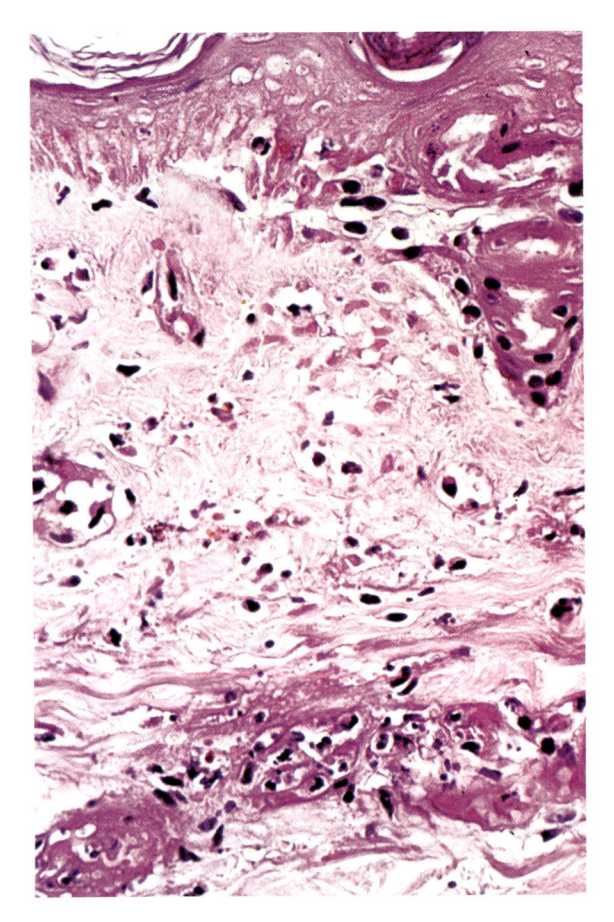

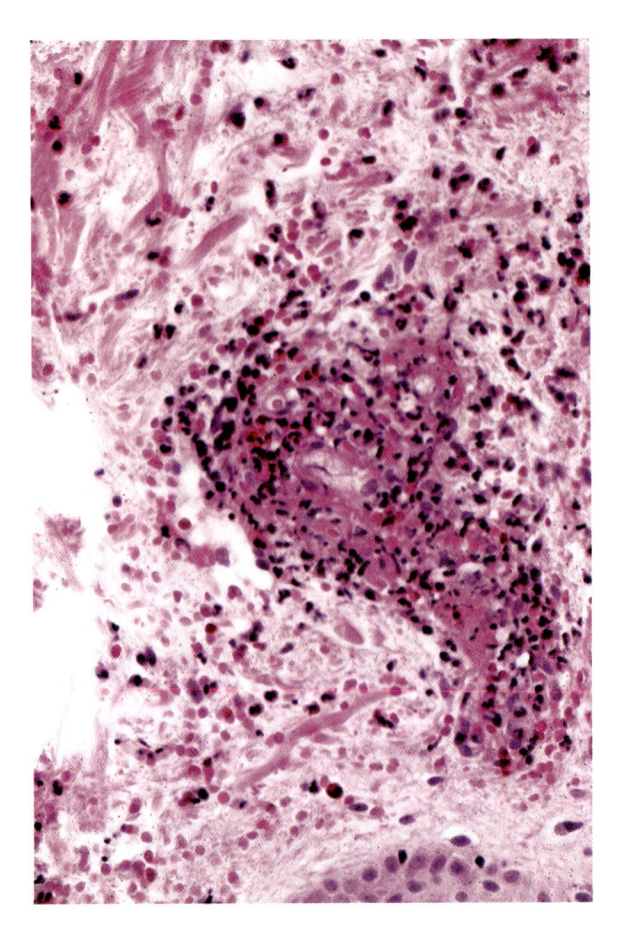

**Figure 5-31**

**NECROTIZING VASCULITIS**

Left: The roof of the blister associated with necrotizing vasculitis is usually necrotic. There is necrosis of the acrosyringium and underlying vasculitis.

Right: Classic necrotizing vasculitis involves a dermal vessel. There is marked fibrinoid necrosis; neutrophils infiltrate the wall of vessels with associated nuclear debris and hemorrhage.

**Figure 5-32**

**PRESSURE BLISTER**

The lesions develop at sites of continuous pressure applied for a prolonged period of time.

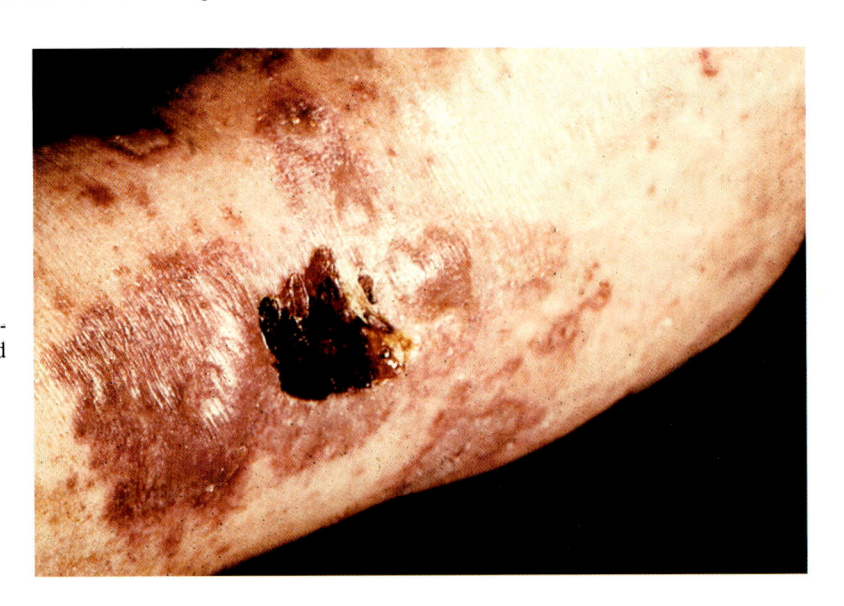

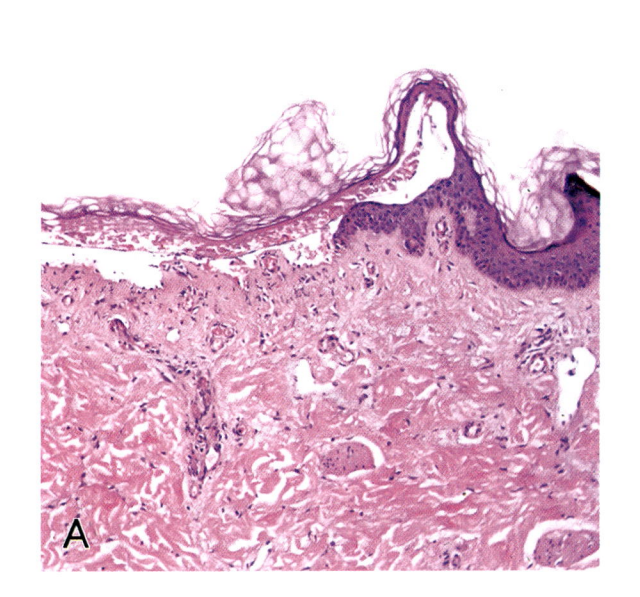

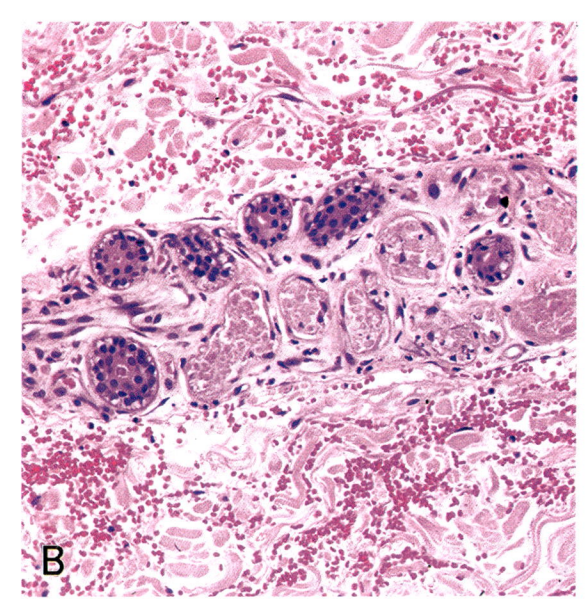

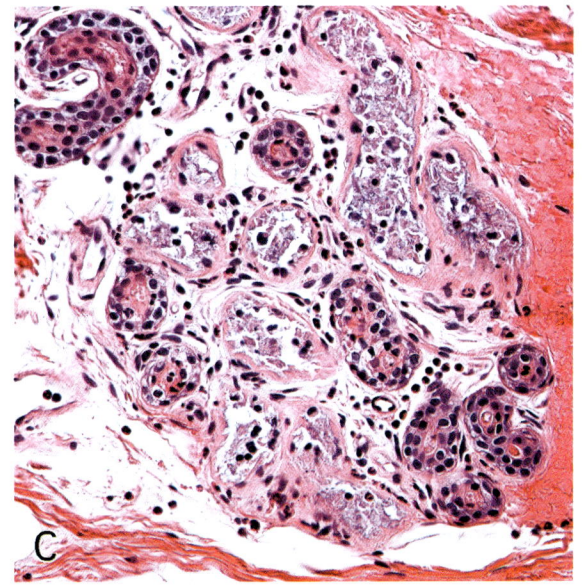

**Figure 5-33**

**PRESSURE (COMA) BULLA**

A: The lesion shows epidermal necrosis and necrosis of underlying dermal vessels with minimal inflammation.

B: Necrosis of an eccrine gland due to ischemia induced by pressure is a characteristic finding of pressure bullae.

C: The eccrine coil shows characteristic early necrosis at higher magnification.

Inflammation may be minimal in comparison to the extent of epidermal injury. First-degree thermal burns differ from sunburn by showing necrosis of the more superficial epidermal layers; sunburn shows individual cell necrosis (i.e., sunburn cells) in the basal cell layer. Second-degree thermal burns are characterized by full-thickness epidermal necrosis, usually dermal-epidermal separation and blister formation, and sometimes superficial dermal necrosis; adnexa, however, remain viable. Third-degree thermal burns involve adnexal necrosis as well as extensive dermal necrosis. Moreover, third-degree burns characteristically show neutrophilic infiltration of the subcutaneous fat. It is important for the dermatopathologist to make these distinctions, because the presence of third-degree changes mandates skin grafting.

*Freeze injury* to viable skin produces diffuse nuclear and cytoplasmic shrinkage and distortion similar to that observed in routinely stained frozen sections. In addition, there may be widespread vascular thrombosis and subepidermal blister formation, which are probably the result of both direct epidermal injury and vascular ischemia. During the winter months in colder

## Inflammatory Disorders of the Skin

**Figure 5-34**

**DERMAL-EPIDERMAL SEPARATION MIMICKING BLISTER AT SITE OF SCAR FORMATION**

The impaired dermal-epidermal adhesion promotes the formation of either true friction blisters or blister-like separation artifact upon biopsy and tissue processing.

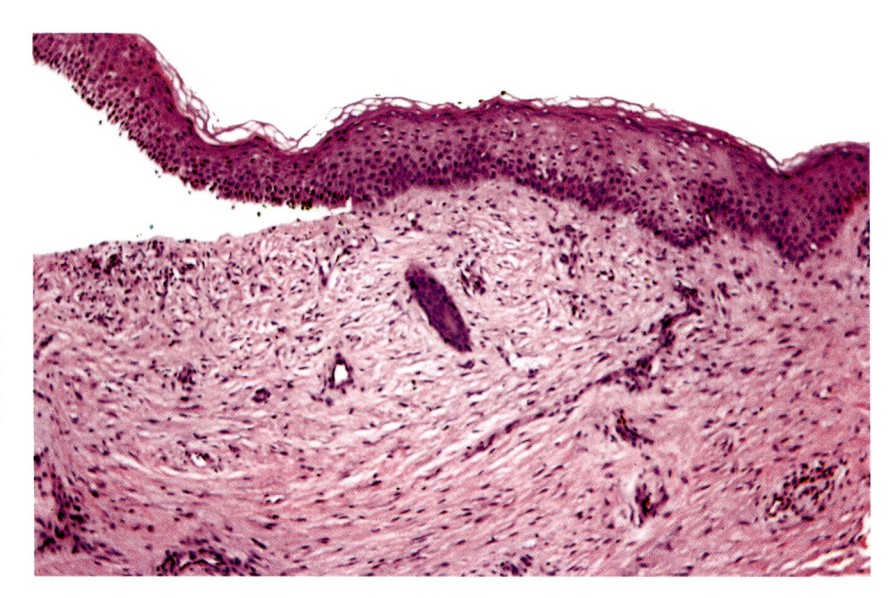

climates, freezing artifact may be seen in formalin-fixed tissue after transportation in fixative that was not pretreated with an antifreeze reagent. Individual cells in fixed frozen tissue undergo striking ballooning artifact, which may render accurate interpretation impossible.

*Electrical injury* may produce dermal-epidermal separation as a result of direct epithelial necrosis. This is characterized by nuclear thinning, elongation, and alignment of each nucleus in parallel to the next diffusely throughout the specimen. Similar alterations are routinely encountered at the edges of biopsy specimens exposed to electrocautery.

The differential diagnosis depends upon the history, the site of involvement, and the nature of the blister, be it superficial or through the midepidermis or as a cause of subepidermal bullous disease. Most of these types of blisters respond to local care, but the offending physical agent must be removed. Any chronic condition that impairs the integrity of dermal-epidermal adhesion, including dermal fibrosis and epidermal atrophy, lowers the threshold for the formation of blisters as a result of acute physical injury (fig. 5-34).

### SUBCORNEAL PUSTULAR DERMATOSIS (SNEDDON-WILKINSON DISEASE)

**Definition.** *Subcorneal pustular dermatosis (SPD)*, also referred to as *Sneddon-Wilkinson disease*, is a chronic dermatitis characterized by aggregated pustules, often arranged in serpiginous arrays, most often involving abdominal skin and the skin of the axillary and inguinal folds (83,84). Early pustules contain both clear serum and neutrophils, and pus may segregate within the lower half of larger pustules. This unusual recurrent and chronic pustular eruption occurs in women more often than men and in Caucasians more commonly than in other racial groups. SPD is associated with monoclonal gammopathy, most commonly IgA paraproteinemia, and with the eventual development of IgA myeloma. While immunofluorescence testing has led to some evidence that IgA or other intraepidermal immunoglobulins have a role in the disorder, those cases have been documented as IgA pemphigus. In general, the term SPD is used in those patients with suggestive pathology but with negative immunofluorescence studies.

**Clinical Features.** The characteristic lesion begins as a vesicle that quickly becomes pustular and flaccid, and rapidly occurs in crops in otherwise normal skin (fig. 5-35) (85). The patient has no systemic symptoms associated with an infectious process. At times, itching or burning herald the onset of the eruption. As the lesions coalesce, they form groups in an arcuate or figurate array. As the lesions resolve, they become scaly but tend to spread peripherally, adding to the unusual shapes associated with SPD. The axillae, groin, trunk, and especially submammary areas are common sites of often symmetrical involvement. Scalp, face, and other mucosae are spared, but the palms and soles are

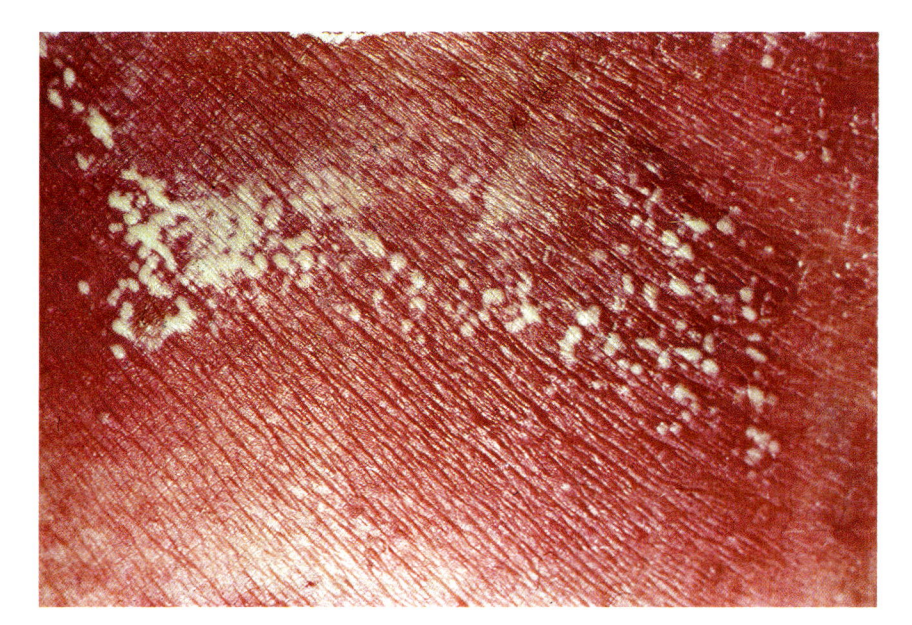

**Figure 5-35**

**SUBCORNEAL PUSTULAR DERMATOSIS**

The trunk, flexural areas, and groin are affected. The lesion often forms in a serpiginous or grouped pattern. Some cases have been associated with IgA gammopathy and myeloma.

occasionally affected. The crops of eruptions are separated by a few weeks to months. Culture of the pustules shows no bacterial growth.

**Pathologic Findings.** Scanning magnification reveals a well-formed, subcorneal pustule filled with mature neutrophils and admixed serum (fig. 5-36). Adjacent to the blister, there may be spongiosis, and in advanced lesions, secondary acantholysis. There is a variable underlying dermal infiltrate composed of lymphocytes, neutrophils, and occasional eosinophils.

**Differential Diagnosis.** The differential diagnosis includes many pustular eruptions. First, the abrupt presentation of the lesions, especially in intertriginous areas, most resembles impetigo contagiosa, but the subsequent distribution, the absence of systemic symptoms and of bacteria in the pustules, and the failure of response to antibacterial therapy eliminate this diagnostic possibility. The arcuate shape of the lesions resembles dermatitis herpetiformis. The highly pruritic nature of dermatitis herpetiformis, the distribution of the eruption, and the histopathologic and immunofluorescence examination all allow for differentiation. Pemphigus foliaceus with impetiginization resembles SPD but the course of the disorder and the histopathologic and immunofluorescence findings aid in differentiation. Acute pustular psoriasis of the von Zumbusch type is differentiated by the systemic symptoms and widespread nature of the psoriatic eruption. Acute generalized pustulosis shows prominent distribution on the distal extremities and is associated with necrotizing vasculitis. Differentiation of lesions of SPD from those of bullous impetigo may be difficult by histology alone. Impetigo may show bacteria by special stains, but this is variable, and culture is a more sensitive means of detecting organisms. Correlation with the clinical setting in which the lesions arose (e.g., facial vesiculopustules in a child versus serpiginous truncal pustules in an adult) generally assists in the correct diagnosis. Acute generalized exanthematous pustulosis (AGEP), a form of pustular drug eruption, may show many features of SPD; however, lesions of AGEP generally contain eosinophils and show a temporal relationship to drug ingestion, such as amoxicillin (86).

**Treatment and Prognosis.** Dapsone usually controls the eruption. Sometimes the severe acute eruptions require systemic steroids or phototherapy (PUVA [psoralen with UVA]). Sulfapyridine is also effective in some patients. Interestingly, prednisone is usually ineffective. Case reports exist of the use of minocycline, tetracycline, adalimumab, infliximab, and mycophenolate for treatment.

## IgA PEMPHIGUS

**Definition.** The pustulovesicular disorder, *IgA pemphigus*, is one of the causes of intraepidermal neutrophils and is often classified as a neutrophilic type of dermatosis (87–90).

*Inflammatory Disorders of the Skin*

**Figure 5-36**

**SUBCORNEAL PUSTULAR DERMATOSIS**

Top: The pustule in early lesions is classically subcorneal, with the normal stratum corneum above the lesion. Neutrophils are scattered in the superficial dermis.

Bottom: There is no spongiform pustule formation, a distinguishing feature of pustular psoriasis. A rare acantholytic cell, resulting from neutrophilic enzyme digestion of intercellular substances, may be noted.

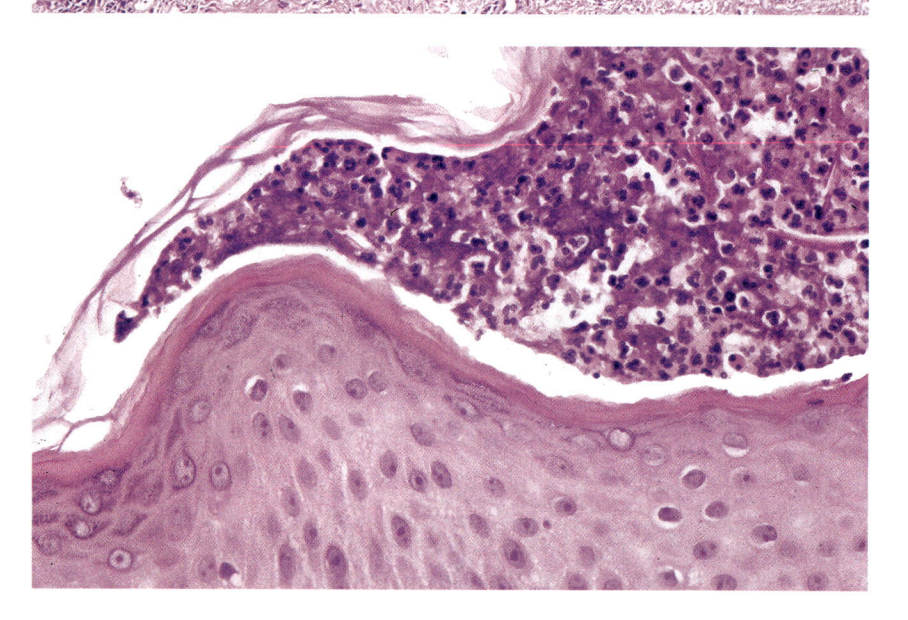

**Clinical Features.** IgA pemphigus is a strikingly pruritic, vesicular and pustular rash that occurs predominantly in mid-life and the elderly, with the main age of onset in the sixth to seventh decade. The clinical findings are a crossover between subcorneal pustular dermatosis and pemphigus foliaceus. Thus, there are small vesicles and blisters that can rupture and give rise to crusted areas or there may be pustules or an admixture of pustules, bullae, and flaccid vesicles. The patients either have a subcorneal pustular type of lesion or an intraepidermal pustular disorder. There is often an annular arrangement to these lesions.

**Pathologic Findings.** Subcorneal vesiculopustules may be the dominant finding, or in some cases, acantholytic intraepidermal vesiculopustules are seen (enzymatic acantholysis may develop in any intraepidermal neutrophilic infiltrate, and thus need not imply a primary event). In some patients, direct immunofluorescence reveals IgA deposition in the uppermost epidermal layers in a cell-membrane, pemphigus-like pattern (91). These antibodies are believed to bind to the desmocollin component of desmosomes.

**Differential Diagnosis.** The differential diagnosis includes SPD. Pustular psoriasis, impetigo, and the pemphigus group of disorders (pemphigus vulgaris and pemphigus foliaceus) must likewise be distinguished. Immunofluorescence findings are very helpful in making the appropriate diagnosis.

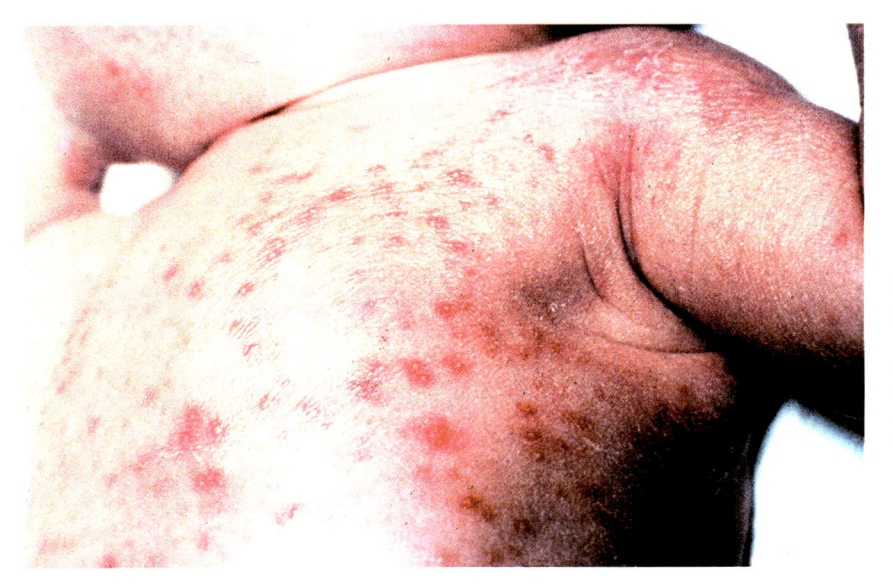

**Figure 5-37**

**ERYTHEMA TOXICUM NEONATORUM**

The lesions occur in about half of full-term infants as a patchy erythema with papules and pustules. Lesions appear in the first 2 days of life, are asymptomatic, affect pressure areas, and disappear in a few days.

**Treatment and Prognosis.** Many lesions respond to sulfone therapy. Topical steroid therapy with topical antibiosis is successful in some of the crusted lesions. In patients with a more pemphigus vulgaris-like disorder, oral corticosteroids and oral retinoids are effective.

## PUSTULAR ERUPTIONS OF INFANCY

### Erythema Toxicum Neonatorum

**Definition.** *Erythema toxicum neonatorum* is a transient exanthem that occurs in approximately 50 percent of term infants (92). This disorder is less common in premature infants and its cause is unknown.

**Clinical Features.** Poorly defined and blotchy erythematous macules of 2 to 3 cm in diameter, are surmounted by a small 2 to 4 mm central vesicle or pustule (fig. 5-37). The lesions are usually not present at birth but occur within the first 24 to 48 hours. They occur principally on the trunk but also on the face and the upper portions of the extremities. The palms and soles are characteristically spared.

Generally, there is eosinophilia within the peripheral blood. An easy way to establish the diagnosis is by scraping a pustular lesion and examining a smear of the exudate, which is dominated by eosinophils.

**Pathologic Findings.** Biopsy specimens reveal different alterations depending on the stage of lesional evolution (93). Early lesions show only a perifollicular lymphocytic and eosinophilic infiltrate, often centered about hair follicles. With time, eosinophils progressively migrate into follicular epithelium, where small follicular infundibular abscesses form (fig. 5-38). Although incontinentia pigmenti also produces subcorneal eosinophilic pustules, this lesion is invariably interfollicular rather than follicular.

**Differential Diagnosis.** The differential diagnosis includes transient neonatal pustular melanosis, which is differentiated by simply smearing the vesicle and finding neutrophils rather than eosinophils, the characteristic finding in erythema toxicum neonatorum. Some bacterial infections and candida mimic erythema toxicum and cultures of the lesions help to rule these out.

**Treatment and Prognosis.** The lesions resolve spontaneously.

### Transient Neonatal Pustular Melanosis

**Definition.** *Transient neonatal pustular melanosis* is a neonatal blotchy erythema that is quite transient as the name implies, and leaves residual pigmentation with clearing. It is more common among African-American newborns. The disorder results from obstruction of the pilosebaceous orifices of the skin, but the cause for this is unknown.

**Clinical Features.** This congenital type of erythema is present as vesicles, pustules, or ruptured vesicles or pustules, with a collarette of scale around the pustular area. There may be pigmented macules present at birth but they definitely

*Inflammatory Disorders of the Skin*

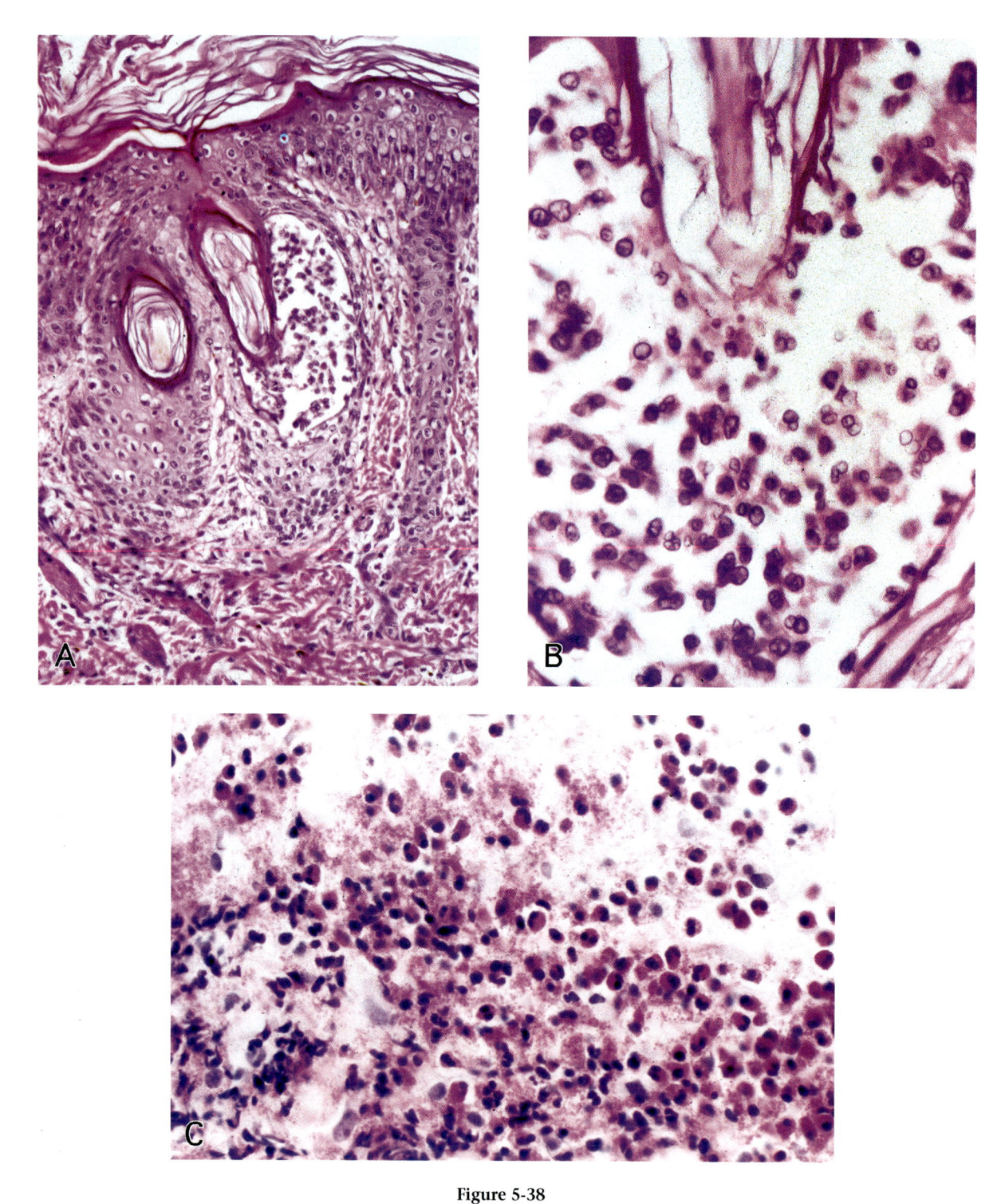

**Figure 5-38**

**ERYTHEMA TOXICUM NEONATORUM**

A: The follicle is the affected structure in which eosinophils aggregate. There is dermal edema with occasional dermal eosinophils in a perivascular distribution.

B: Numerous eosinophils affect the follicle and overlying epidermis, eventually forming a subcorneal eosinophilic pustule with rare neutrophils.

C: A smear of the follicle reveals numerous eosinophils.

develop with evolution to pustules or vesicles. These lesions occur on the trunk and proximal extremities but spare the palms and soles.

**Pathologic Findings.** Macular lesions show basal cell layer hyperpigmentation. Pustules are observed beneath the stratum corneum as well as within the epidermis. They are composed primarily of neutrophils, with a minor component of eosinophils, and may contain partially degraded remnants of hair shafts. A mixed dermal inflammatory infiltrate may be present about the pustular focus (94).

**Differential Diagnosis.** The differential diagnosis includes miliaria, which usually exhibits small foci of erythema of 1 or 2 mm as opposed to the larger 2 to 3 cm of erythema seen in erythema toxicum and transient neonatal pustular dermatosis. Erythema toxicum shows no bacteria but numerous eosinophils, whereas neutrophils are seen in neonatal pustular dermatosis. Cultures rule out infection with *Candida* or bacteria.

**Treatment and Prognosis.** The lesions spontaneously resolve. The residual pigmentation also gradually resolves.

### Acropustulosis of Infancy

**Definition.** *Acropustulosis* is an eruption of infancy that occurs most commonly on palms and soles. African-American children are most frequently affected.

**Clinical Features.** The lesions begin as small, 1- to 2-mm, extremely pruritic pustules on the palms and soles and then extend to the dorsa of the hands and feet. Occasionally, lesions extend onto the wrists, ankles, and buttocks. The lesions last 1 or 2 weeks, but may recur periodically for 2 to 4 weeks. Onset is at birth and during the first 2 years of life. The disorder usually spontaneously remits in the first 3 to 5 years of life. The pustules are sterile.

**Pathologic Findings.** Micropustules composed primarily of neutrophils are present within the epidermis and beneath the stratum corneum. The superficial dermis shows edema and a sparse mixed perivascular inflammatory infiltrate.

**Differential Diagnosis.** The most important entity in differential diagnosis is pustular superinfected scabies. The predominance of the lesions in the interdigital folds favors a diagnosis of scabies. Impetigo shows larger pustules that are not as pruritic, and bacterial smears offer the correct diagnosis. Dyshidrotic eczema can occur in children but is usually vesicular.

**Treatment and Prognosis.** Topical steroids are useful in some children, but in others, the disorder must run its course. Dapsone has been used in difficult cases. Topical pramoxine and oral antihistamines provide a valuable adjunct to therapy (95).

### INTESTINAL BYPASS SYNDROME

The appearance of asymmetrical polyarteritis, tenosynovitis, sterile skin pustules, thrombophlebitis, ulcerations of the mucosae, and vasculitis in the retina has been noted as a complication of *intestinal bypass surgery* for morbid obesity. Because this disorder is characterized by both blistering lesions and vasculitis, it is more specifically discussed in chapter 11.

A variety of changes are described, with epidermal hyperplasia, subcorneal and intracorneal vesiculopustule formation, and vascular injury with immune complex deposition representing the dominant findings. In some cases, there is pustular vasculitis.

### IMPETIGO

**Definition.** *Impetigo* is a common superficial infection of the skin, generally caused by staphylococci and streptococci. Impetigo is most often seen in infants, young children, and adults in poor health. Cultures most frequently grow coagulase-positive *Staphylococcus*, group A β-hemolytic *Streptococcus*, or both. Nephritogenic strains of *Streptococcus* cause impetigo, particularly in tropical areas and in the southern United States.

**Clinical Features.** Impetigo usually involves exposed skin, particularly that of the face and hands. Initially, it is an erythematous macule, but multiple small pustules rapidly supervene. As pustules break, shallow erosions form and are covered with drying serum, which gives the characteristic clinical appearance of honey-colored crust (fig. 5-39). If the crust is not removed, new lesions form about the periphery, and extensive epidermal damage may ensue. Clinical variants of impetigo include *impetigo contagiosa*, an epidemic form of this disorder affecting preschool children, and *bullous impetigo*, characterized by rapidly progressive vesicles and bullae that may be confused with SSSS.

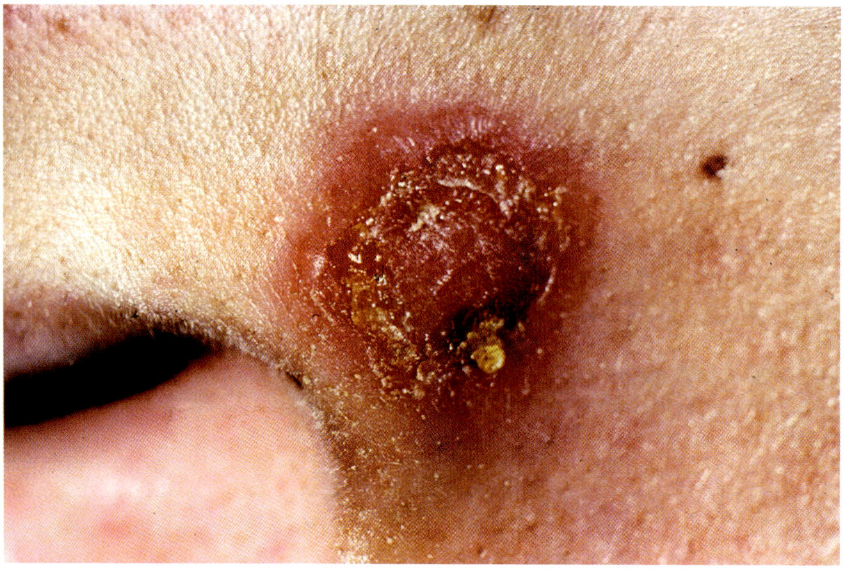

**Figure 5-39**

**IMPETIGO**

The erythematous plaque is covered with the characteristic honey-colored scale-crust.

**Pathologic Findings.** The characteristic microscopic feature of impetigo is accumulation of neutrophils within and beneath the stratum corneum, often with the formation of a subcorneal pustule (fig. 5-40). Special stains reveal the presence of bacteria in these foci. Nonspecific, reactive epidermal alterations and superficial dermal inflammation accompany these findings. The rupture of pustules results in superficial layering of serum, neutrophils, and cellular debris to form the characteristic clinical crust. Bullous forms of impetigo are characterized by a blister with secondary acantholysis at or directly beneath the granular cell layer. Bullae are fluid filled, and neutrophils are frequently scarce.

**Differential Diagnosis.** Bullous impetigo is differentiated from SSSS, which produces similar epidermal changes as a result of the distant release of the phage group II staphylococcal toxin, exfoliatin, by the demonstration of bacteria in lesions by culture. Also, bullous impetigo, but not SSSS, shows inflammatory infiltration of the superficial dermis that underlies the forming blister.

These findings are of significance only in the context of the gross pathology. For example, such histologic findings, along with the demonstration of bacteria by special stains or culture, result in a diagnosis when the biopsy specimen is obtained from a crusted or pustular lesion in a child. In adults, however, impetiginization may be a secondary phenomenon, as is frequently the case in actinic keratosis.

**Treatment and Prognosis.** Systemic or topical antibiotics based on culture sensitivity are most effective (96).

## PUSTULAR CANDIDIASIS

**Definition.** Acute mucocutaneous *pustular candidiasis* is caused by *Candida albicans,* a dimorphous fungus producing both yeast and filamentous growth in the superficial epidermal layers. It is a benign, self-limited disease that occurs as a result of immunosuppression, changes in the topical cutaneous environment (e.g., excessive sweating), and overgrowth of this commensal organism in the setting of systemic antibiotic therapy.

**Clinical Features.** Intertriginous areas, oral cavity, paronychial skin, and vulva are preferentially affected. Generalized neonatal and congenital forms exist in which infection is acquired via passage through the birth canal or as a result of ascending intrauterine spread. Clinical lesions consist of beefy red plaques covered by small pustules (fig. 5-41).

**Pathologic Findings.** The multiple foci of neutrophilic infiltration of the stratum corneum are best appreciated at scanning magnification. Well-formed foci are represented by subcorneal pustules, often associated with foci of neutrophilic infiltration and spongiosis involving the upper stratum spinosum (i.e., spongiform pustules similar to those observed in psoriasis) (fig. 5-42). Mycelia and spores are detected by

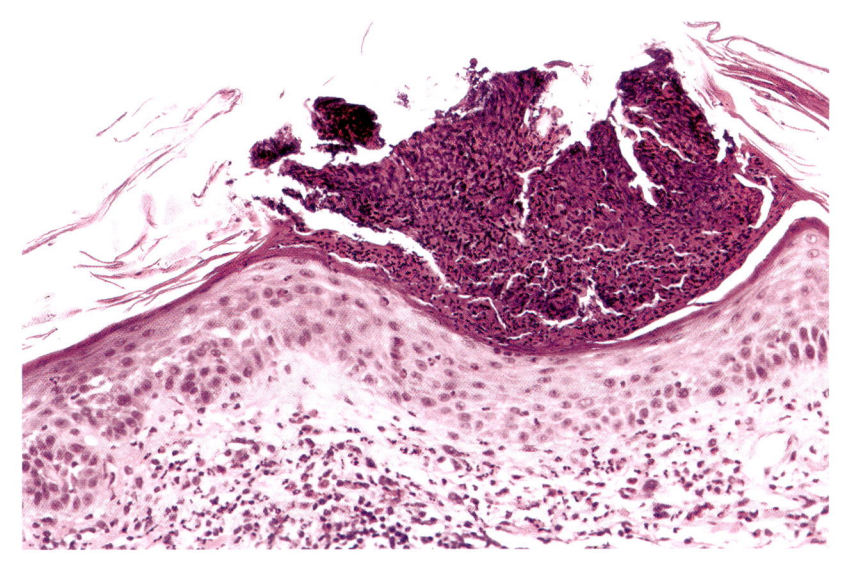

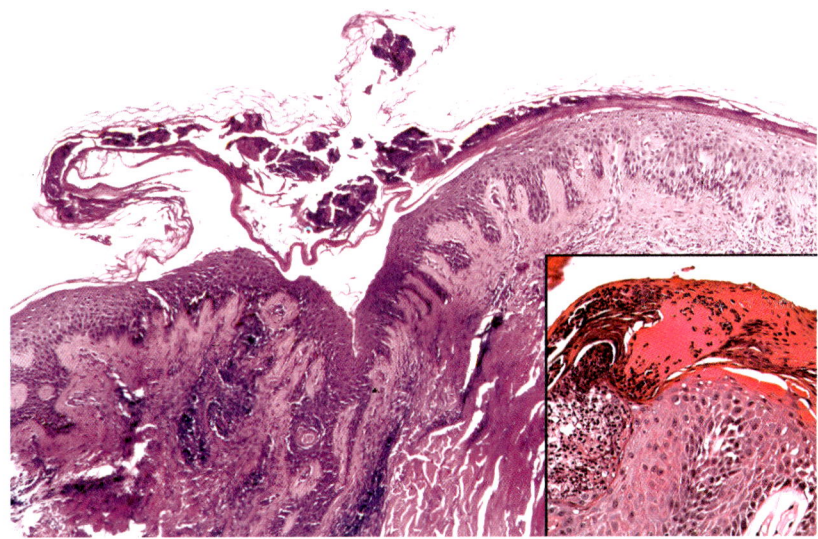

### Figure 5-40

**IMPETIGO**

Top: The scale-crust is composed of aggregated neutrophils and desiccated serum. Associated bacterial colonies are within the stratum corneum.

Bottom: In addition to accumulation of neutrophils and bacteria in the superficial scale, there is a forming subcorneal vesicle as a result of superficial secondary acantholysis. The inset shows "scale crust," with neutrophilic infiltration and associated bacteria.

periodic acid–Schiff (PAS) stain in the affected stratum corneum, although they are also often apparent in routinely stained sections (fig. 5-43). Mycelia are pseudoseptate and branch; spores are ovoid and range between 2 and 5 µm in diameter. Invasion of the epidermal layer by organisms raises the possibility of chronic mucocutaneous candidiasis, a form of infection associated with defective cell-mediated immunity.

**Differential Diagnosis.** Generally, bacterial infection and sterile pustules associated with primary forms of pustular dermatitis must be excluded by appropriate stains. Rarely, dermatophytosis also shows pustule formation within the stratum corneum.

**Treatment and Prognosis.** Topical anticandidal agents are useful for localized disease; systemic antifungal therapy is indicated in the setting of tissue invasion or immunosuppression (97).

## PUSTULAR VASCULITIS

**Definition.** *Pustular vasculitis* describes a reaction pattern in which there are pustules associated with necrotizing vasculitis. The pustules have follicular prominence and are surrounded by hemorrhage.

**Clinical Features.** Pustular vasculitis presents as multiple pustules and petechiae scattered over the extremities and occasionally onto the trunk.

*Inflammatory Disorders of the Skin*

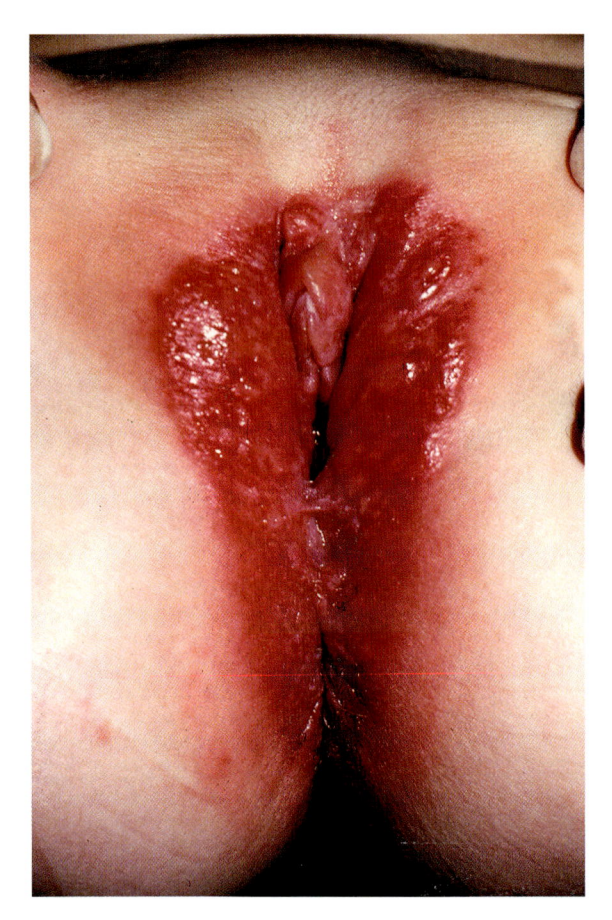

**Figure 5-41**

**CUTANEOUS CANDIDIASIS**

A beefy red patch or plaque studded with pustules is often along the advancing edge.

There are areas of focal hemorrhage in the skin, which are sometimes purpura-like and associated with pustulation superficially. Follicular prominence of the pustules is often observed.

**Pathologic Findings.** In addition to the findings of necrotizing cutaneous vasculitis, there is microabscess formation within the superficial epidermis or within the follicular infundibular epithelium. Fibrin thrombi may be present in vessel lumens. In some patients, the vessel involvement resembles that of Sweet syndrome, with prominent endothelial swelling. There is also a perivenular infiltrate of lymphocytes, eosinophils, and neutrophils with debris. If the cause is sepsis, organisms may be demonstrated within neutrophils (e.g., as in the pustular vasculitic lesions of meningococcemia and gonococcemia). Polymerase chain reaction (PCR) and immunoperoxidase techniques reveal bacterial remnants in the affected vessels or in associated inflammatory cells.

**Differential Diagnosis.** Pustular vasculitis includes a broad differential diagnosis, including IgA vasculitis. Patients who present with IgA vasculitis may have an antecedent infection. Streptococcal pharyngitis frequently precedes the eruption of so-called Henoch-Schönlein purpura; however, other infectious disorders give rise to a pustular IgA-related vasculitis, including *Mycoplasma pneumoniae*, other streptococcal infections, and hepatitis A and C, among others. Other disorders that give rise to IgA-related pustular vasculitis are noninfectious IgA vasculitis, Sjögren syndrome (especially associated with the presence of anti-Ro antibodies), IgA paraproteinemia, inflammatory bowel disease, and underlying neoplasia of other types. Behçet disease, Reiter disease, and reactions to drugs including carbamazepine are also considered. Finally, the intestinal bypass syndrome, or so-called bowel arthritis dermatosis syndrome, and septic vasculitis can cause pustular vasculitis.

**Treatment and Prognosis.** Treatment of the underlying disorder resolves the lesion (98).

## VESICULOPUSTULAR ERUPTION OF HEPATOBILIARY DISEASE

**Definition.** One of the clues to the diagnosis of *hepatobiliary disease* is a neutrophilic dermatosis-like lesion that rapidly erupts and can be widespread (99). The disorder is considered by some to represent a vesiculopustular variant of pyoderma gangrenosum.

**Clinical Features.** Patients with hepatobiliary disease of various causes, including hepatitis B, hepatitis C, and sclerosing cholangitis, among others, can present with a pustular eruption affecting the trunk, upper arms, and upper extremities, or a folliculitis that goes on to focal ulceration. The superficial lesions break down and lead to erosions. The follicular lesion may result in multiple ulcers. These changes sometimes are a clue to the diagnosis. The lesions may also occur in association with inflammatory bowel disease.

**Pathologic Findings.** There is a subepidermal blister containing serum and aggregated neutrophils (fig. 5-44), marked papillary dermal

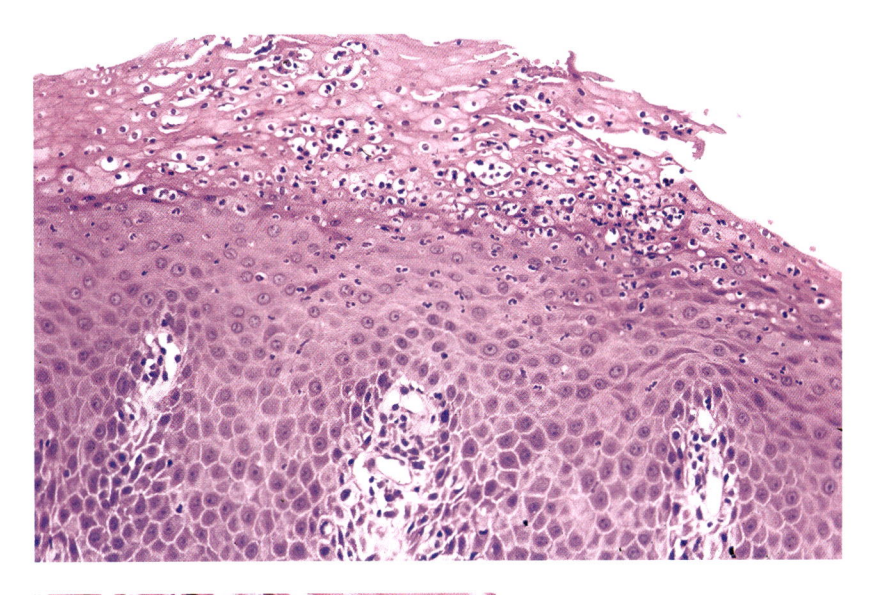

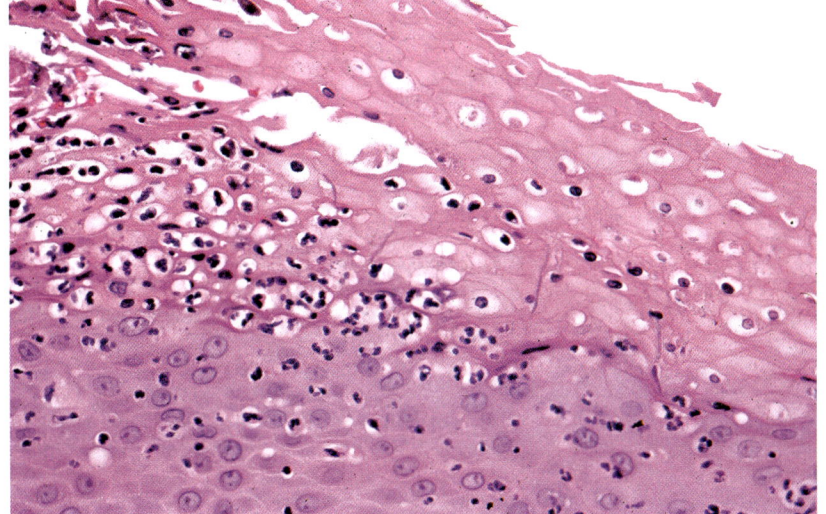

## Nonacantholytic Vesiculobullous and Vesiculopustular Dermatitis

**Figure 5-42**

**CUTANEOUS CANDIDIASIS**

Top: All spongiform pustules in vulvar biopsies must be stained with periodic acid–Schiff (PAS) to demonstrate possible organisms.

Bottom: Higher-magnification view.

**Figure 5-43**

**CUTANEOUS CANDIDIASIS**

Pseudohyphae of *Candida* are seen on hematoxylin and eosin (H&E)-stained sections. Confirmation with a PAS stain is recommended.

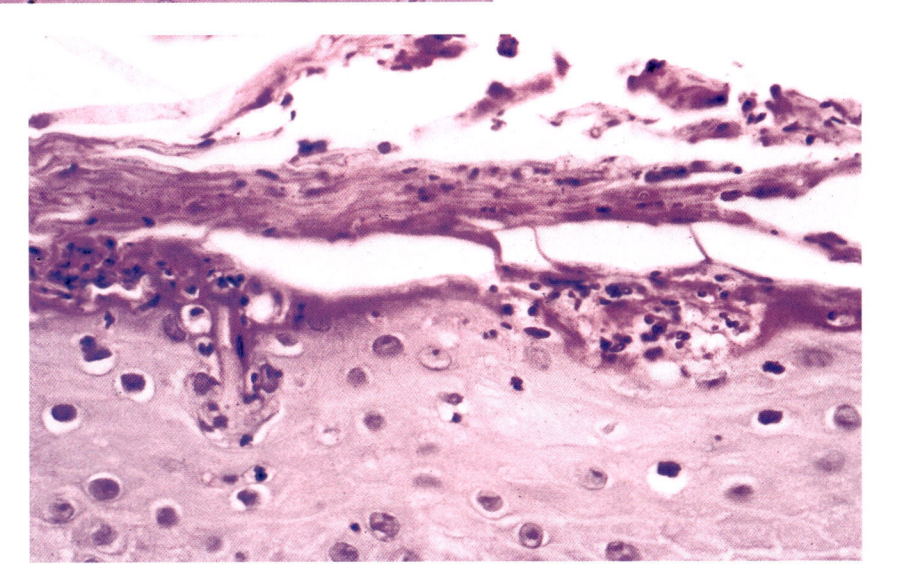

*Inflammatory Disorders of the Skin*

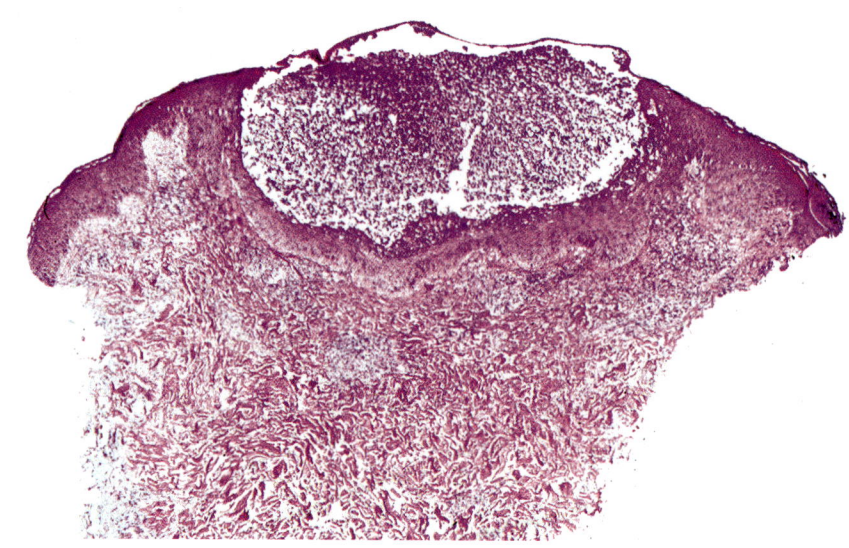

**Figure 5-44**

**PUSTULAR ERUPTION OF HEPATOBILIARY DISEASE**

Top: A prominent intraepidermal pustule is apparent at scanning magnification.
Bottom: Higher-magnification view.

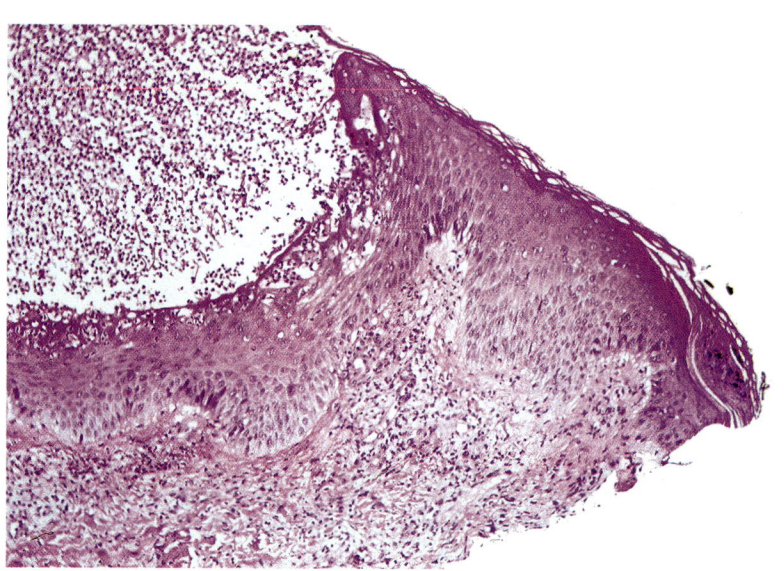

edema, and prominent, often folliculocentric formation of nuclear dust. There is also an associated perivascular lymphocytic inflammatory component without evidence of significant vascular injury.

**Differential Diagnosis.** SPD must be considered in the differential diagnosis, as should pyoderma gangrenosum. When the lesions are nodular, neutrophilic eccrine hidradenitis is also a possibility.

**Treatment and Prognosis.** The treatment of the underlying disorder results in regression of the eruption.

# REFERENCES

1. Kolanko E, Bickle K, Keehn C, Glass LF. Subepidermal blistering disorders: a clinical and histopathologic review. Semin Cutan Med Surg 2004;23:10-8.
2. Yeh SW, Ahmed B, Sami N, Razzaque Ahmed A. Blistering disorders: diagnosis and treatment. Dermatol Ther 2003;16:214-23.
3. Mutasim DF. Autoimmune bullous dermatoses in the elderly: diagnosis and management. Drugs Aging 2003;20:663-81.
4. Verdolini R, Cerio R. Autoimmune subepidermal bullous skin diseases: the impact of recent findings for the dermatopathologist. Virchows Arch 2003;443:184-93.
4a. Stanley JR, Amagai M. Pemphigus, bullous impetigo, and the staphylococcal scalded-skin syndrome. N Eng J Med 2006;355:1800-10.
5. Liu Z. Bullous pemphigoid: using animal models to study the immunopathology. J Investig Dermatol Symp Proc 2004;9:41-6.
6. Olivry T, Jackson HA. Diagnosing new autoimmune blistering skin diseases of dogs and cats. Clin Tech Small Anim Pract 2001;16:225-9.
7. Zone JJ, Egan CA, Taylor TB, Meyer LJ. IgA autoimmune disorders: development of a passive transfer mouse model. J Investig Dermatol Symp Proc 2004;9:47-51.
8. Kalaher KM, Scott DW. Subcorneal pustular dermatosis in dogs and in human beings: comparative aspects. J Am Acad Dermatol 1990;22(Pt 1):1023-8.
9. Heimbach L, Li N, Diaz A, Liu Z. Experimental animal models of bullous pemphigoid. G Ital Dermatol Vener 2009:144:423-31.
10. Liu Z, Diaz L, Swartz S. Molecular mapping of a pathogenically relevant BP180 epitope associated with experimentally induced murine bullous pemphigoid. J. Immunol 1996:155:5449-54.
11. Olivry T, Dunston SM, Schachter M, et al. A spontaneous canine model of mucosal membrane (cicatricial) pemphigoid, an autoimmune blistering disease affecting mucosae and mucocutaneous junctions. J Autoimmun 2001:16:411-21.
12. Sitaru C. Experimental models of epidermolysis bullosa acquisita. Exp Dermatol 2007:16:520-31.
13. Walsh SR, Hogg D, Mydlarski PR. Bullous pemphigoid: from bench to bedside. Drugs 2005;65:905-26.
14. Cecchi R, Paoli S, Giomi A. Peristomal bullous pemphigoid. J Eur Acad Dermatol Venereol 2004;18:515-6.
15. Liu Z, Diaz LA. Bullous pemphigoid: end of the century overview. J Dermatol 2001;28:647-650.
16. Fleming TE, Korman NJ. Cicatricial pemphigoid. J Am Acad Dermatol 2000;43:571-91.
17. Swerlick RA, Korman NJ. Bullous pemphigoid: what is the prognosis? J Invest Dermatol 2004;122:XVII-XVIII.
18. Fontaine J, Joly P, Roujeau JC. Treatment of bullous pemphigoid. J Dermatol 2003;30:83-90.
19. Khumalo NP, Murrell DF, Wojnarowska F, Kirtschig G. A systematic review of treatments for bullous pemphigoid. Arch Dermatol 2002;138:385-9.
20. Cooper SM, Wojnarowska F. Treatments of choice for bullous pemphigoid. Skin Therapy Lett 2002;7:4-6.
21. Kirtschig G, Khumalo NP. Management of bullous pemphigoid: recommendations for immunomodulatory treatments. Am J Clin Dermatol 2004;5:319-26.
22. Stockman A, Beele H, Vanderhaeghen Y, Naeyaert JM. Topical class I corticosteroids in 10 patients with bullous pemphigoid: correlation of the outcome with the severity degree of the disease and review of the literature. J Eur Acad Dermatol Venereol 2004;18:164-68.
23. Khumalo N, Kirtschig G, Middleton P, Hollis S, Wojnarowska F, Murrell D. Interventions for bullous pemphigoid. Cochrane Database Syst Rev 2003;:CD002292.
24. Claudy A. Evaluation of the safety and efficacy of a potent topical cortico-steroid in the treatment of bullous pemphigoid. Clin Dermatol 2001;19:778-80.
25. Lin MS, Arteaga LA, Diaz LA. Herpes gestationis. Clin Dermatol 2001;19:697-702.
26. Shornick JK. Dermatoses of pregnancy. Semin Cutan Med Surg 1998;17:172-81.
27. Kroumpouzos G, Cohen LM. Specific dermatoses of pregnancy: an evidence-based systematic review. Am J Obstet Gynecol 2003;188:1083-92.
28. Weisshaar E, Witteler R, Diepgen TL, Luger TA, Stander S. [Pruritus in pregnancy. A frequent diagnostic and therapeutic challenge.] Hautarzt 2005;56:48-57. [German]
29. Shornick JK. Herpes gestationis. Dermatol Clin 1993;11:527-33.
30. Morrison LH, Anhalt GJ. Herpes gestationis. J Autoimmun 1991;4:37-45.
31. Yancey KB. Herpes gestationis. Dermatol Clin 1990;8:727-35.
32. Engineer L, Bhol K, Ahmed AR. Pemphigoid gestationis: a review. Am J Obstet Gynecol 2000;183:483-91.

33. Wever S, Burger M, Langfritz K, et al. [Herpes gestationis. Clinical spectrum and diagnostic possibilities.] Hautarzt 1995;46:158-64. [German]
34. Jenkins RE, Hern S, Black MM. Clinical features and management of 87 patients with pemphigoid gestationis. Clin Exp Dermatol 1999;24:255-9.
35. Hallel-Halevy D, Nadelman C, Chen M, Woodley DT. Epidermolysis bullosa acquisita: update and review. Clin Dermatol 2001;19:712-8.
36. Trigo-Guzman FX, Conti A, Aoki V, et al. Epidermolysis bullosa acquisita in childhood. J Dermatol 2003;30:226-9.
37. Wu JJ, Wagner AM. Epidermolysis bullosa acquisita in an 8-year-old girl. Pediatr Dermatol 2002;19:368-71.
38. Schmidt E, Hopfner B, Chen M, et al. Childhood epidermolysis bullosa acquisita: a novel variant with reactivity to all three structural domains of type VII collagen. Br J Dermatol 2002;147:592-7.
39. Kirtschig G, Murrell D, Wojnarowska F, Khumalo N. Interventions for mucous membrane pemphigoid and epidermolysis bullosa acquisita. Cochrane Database Syst Rev 2003;:CD004056.
40. Engineer L, Ahmed AR. Emerging treatment for epidermolysis bullosa acquisita. J Am Acad Dermatol 2001;44:818-28.
41. Arora KP, Sachdeva B, Singh N, Bhattacharya SN. Remission of recalcitrant epidermolysis bullosa acquisita (EBA) with colchicine monotherapy. J Dermatol 2005;32:114-9.
42. Abecassis S, Joly P, Genereau T, et al. Superpotent topical steroid therapy for epidermolysis bullosa acquisita. Dermatology 2004;209:164-6.
43. Gourgiotou K, Exadaktylou D, Aroni K, et al. Epidermolysis bullosa acquisita: treatment with intravenous immunoglobulins. J Eur Acad Dermatol Venereol 2002;16:77-80.
44. Hughes AP, Callen JP. Epidermolysis bullosa acquisita responsive to dapsone therapy. J Cutan Med Surg 2001;5:397-9.
45. Miyake H, Morishima Y, Komai R, Hashimoto T, Kishimoto S. Epidermolysis bullosa acquisita: correlation of IgE levels with disease activity under successful betamethasone/dapsone combination therapy. Acta Derm Venereol 2001;81:429.
46. Maize JC Jr, Cohen JB. Cyclosporine controls epidermolysis bullosa acquisita co-occurring with acquired factor VIII deficiency. Int J Dermatol 2005;44:692-4.
47. Feliciani C, Tulli A. Topical cyclosporin in the treatment of dermatologic diseases. Int J Immunopathol Pharmacol 2002;15:89-93.
48. Nicolas ME, Krause PK, Gibson LE, Murray JA. Dermatitis herpetiformis. Int J Dermatol 2003;42:588-600.
49. Kárpáti S. Dermatitis herpetiformis: close to unravelling a disease. J Dermatol Sci 2004;34:83-90.
50. Collin P, Reunala T. Recognition and management of the cutaneous manifestations of celiac disease: a guide for dermatologists. Am J Clin Dermatol 2003;4:13-20.
51. Fry L. Dermatitis herpetiformis: problems, progress and prospects. Eur J Dermatol 2002;12:523-31.
52. Reunala TL. Dermatitis herpetiformis. Clin Dermatol 2001;19:728-36.
53. Zone JJ. Skin manifestations of celiac disease. Gastroenterology 2005;128:S87-91.
54. Oxentenko AS, Murray JA. Celiac disease and dermatitis herpetiformis: the spectrum of gluten-sensitive enteropathy. Int J Dermatol 2003;42:585-7.
55. Collin P, Kaukinen K, Maki M. Clinical features of celiac disease today. Dig Dis 1999;17:100-6.
56. Paniker U, Levine N. Dapsone and sulfapyridine. Dermatol Clin 2001;19:79-86.
57. Zone JJ. Clinical spectrum, pathogenesis and treatment of linear IgA bullous dermatosis. J Dermatol 2001;28:651-3.
58. Guide SV, Marinkovich MP. Linear IgA bullous dermatosis. Clin Dermatol 2001;19:719-27.
59. Egan CA, Zone JJ. Linear IgA bullous dermatosis. Int J Dermatol 1999;38:818-27.
60. Waldman MA, Black DR, Callen JP. Vancomycin-induced linear IgA bullous disease presenting as toxic epidermal necrolysis. Clin Exp Dermatol 2004;29:633-6.
61. Neughebauer BI, Negron G, Pelton S, Plunkett RW, Beutner EH, Magnussen R. Bullous skin disease: an unusual allergic reaction to vancomycin. Am J Med Sci 2002;323:273-8.
62. Klein PA, Callen JP. Drug-induced linear IgA bullous dermatosis after vancomycin discontinuance in a patient with renal insufficiency. J Am Acad Dermatol 2000;42:316-23.
63. Cooper SM, Powell J, Wojnarowska F. Linear IgA disease: successful treatment with erythromycin. Clin Exp Dermatol 2002;27:677-9.
64. Korman NJ. New and emerging therapies in the treatment of blistering diseases. Dermatol Clin 2000;18:127-37.
65. Letko E, Papaliodis DN, Papaliodis GN, Daoud YJ, Ahmed AR, Foster CS. Stevens-Johnson syndrome and toxic epidermal necrolysis: a review of the literature. Ann Allergy Asthma Immunol 2005;94:419-36.
66. Williams PM, Conklin RJ. Erythema multiforme: a review and contrast from Stevens-Johnson syndrome/toxic epidermal necrolysis. Dent Clin North Am 2005;49:67-76.
67. Fritsch PO, Sidoroff A. Drug-induced Stevens-Johnson syndrome/toxic epidermal necrolysis. Am J Clin Dermatol 2000;1:349-60.

68. Ringheanu M, Laude TA. Toxic epidermal necrolysis in children—an update. Clin Pediatr (Phila) 2000;39:687-94.
69. Wolkenstein P, Revuz J. Toxic epidermal necrolysis. Dermatol Clin 2000;18:485-95.
70. Rogers RS 3rd, Eisen D. Erosive oral lichen planus with genital lesions: the vulvovaginal-gingival syndrome and the peno-gingival syndrome. Dermatol Clin 2003;21:91-8.
71. Rencic A, Goyal S, Mofid M, Wigley F, Nousari HC. Bullous lesions in scleroderma. Int J Dermatol 2002;41:335-9.
72. Yesudian PD, Sugunendran H, Bates CM, O'Mahony C. Lichen sclerosus. Int J STD AIDS 2005;16:465-73.
73. Funaro D. Lichen sclerosus: a review and practical approach. Dermatol Ther 2004;17:28-37.
74. Yawalkar N. Drug-induced exanthems. Toxicology 2005;209:131-4.
75. Pichler WJ, Yawalkar N, Britschgi M, et al. Cellular and molecular pathophysiology of cutaneous drug reactions. Am J Clin Dermatol 2002;3:229-38.
76. Patel GK, Finlay AY. Staphylococcal scalded skin syndrome: diagnosis and management. Am J Clin Dermatol 2003;4:165-75.
77. Hanakawa Y, Stanley JR. Mechanisms of blister formation by staphylococcal toxins. J Biochem 2004;136:747-50.
78. Ladhani S. Understanding the mechanism of action of the exfoliative toxins of Staphylococcus aureus. FEMS Immunol Med Microbiol 2003;39:181-9.
79. Stanley JR, Amagai M. Pemphigus, bullous impetigo, and the staphylococcal scalded-skin syndrome. N Engl J Med 2006;355:1800-1810.
80. Dobson CM, King CM. Adult staphylococcal scalded skin syndrome: histological pitfalls and new diagnostic perspectives. Br J Dermatol 2003;148:1068-9.
81. Patel GK. Treatment of staphylococcal scalded skin syndrome. Expert Rev Anti Infect Ther 2004;2:575-87.
82. Johnston GA. Treatment of bullous impetigo and the staphylococcal scalded skin syndrome in infants. Expert Rev Anti Infect Ther 2004;2:439-46.
83. Reed J, Wilkinson J. Subcorneal pustular dermatosis. Clin Dermatol 2000;18:301-13.
84. Sneddon IB, Wilkinson DS. Subcorneal pustular dermatosis. Br J Dermatol 1979;100:61-8.
85. Lutz ME, Daoud MS, McEvoy MT, Gibson LE. Subcorneal pustular dermatosis: a clinical study of ten patients. Cutis 1998;61:203-8.
86. Fairris GM, Ashworth J, Cotterill JA. A dermatosis associated with bacterial overgrowth in jejunal diverticula. Br J Dermatol 1985:112:709-13.
87. Robinson ND, Hashimoto T, Amagai M, Chan LS. The new pemphigus variants. J Am Acad Dermatol 1999;40:649-71.
88. Hashimoto T, Yasumoto S, Nagata Y, Okamoto T, Fujita S. Clinical, histopathological and immunological distinction in two cases of IgA pemphigus. Clin Exp Dermatol 2002;27:636-40.
89. Niimi Y, Kawana S, Kusunoki T. IgA pemphigus: a case report and its characteristic clinical features compared with subcorneal pustular dermatosis. J Am Acad Dermatol 2000;43:546-9.
90. Harman KE, Holmes G, Bhogal BS, McFadden J, Black MM. Intercellular IgA dermatosis (IgA pemphigus)—two cases illustrating the clinical heterogeneity of this disorder. Clin Exp Dermatol 1999;24:464-6.
91. Hashimoto T. Immunopathology of IgA pemphigus. Clin Dermatol 2001;19:683-9.
92. Liu C, Feng J, Qu R, et al. Epidemiologic study of the predisposing factors in erythema toxicum neonatorum. Dermatology 2005;210:269-72.
93. Marchini G, Ulfgren AK, Lore K, Stabi B, Berggren V, Lonne-Rahm S. Erythema toxicum neonatorum: an immunohistochemical analysis. Pediatr Dermatol 2001;18:177-87.
94. O'Connor NR, McLaughlin MR, Ham P. Newborn skin: Part I. Common rashes. Am Fam Physician 2008;77:47-52.
95. Mengesha YM, Bennett ML. Pustular skin disorders: diagnosis and treatment. Am J Clin Dermatol 2002;3:389-400.
96. Bernard P. Management of common bacterial infections of the skin. Curr Opin Infect Dis 2008;21:122-8.
97. Wilkerson A, Smoller B. The pustular disorders. Semin Cutan Med Surg 2004;23:29-38.
98. Del Pozo J, Sacristán F, Martínez W, Paradela S, Fernández-Jorge B, Fonseca E. Neutrophilic dermatosis of the hands: presentation of eight cases and review of the literature. J Dermatol 2007;34:243-7.
99. Magro CM, Crowson AN. A distinctive vesiculopustular eruption associated with hepatobiliary disease. Int J Dermatol 1997;36:837-44.

# 6  INTERFACE DERMATITIS (ACUTE CYTOTOXIC DERMATITIS)

## GENERAL CONSIDERATIONS

There are only a finite number of reaction patterns that occur in human skin consequent to the infiltration by reactive T lymphocytes. One pattern involves intercellular epidermal edema, or spongiosis. Spongiosis occurs when antigen-specific T cells generally of the helper subtype infiltrate at sites of antigen challenge. Other subtypes of effector lymphocytes produce different alterations within the epidermal layer. For example, experimentally, when autosensitized cytotoxic T cells enter the skin, the pattern consistently involves degeneration and death of keratinocytes (i.e., cytotoxicity), particularly those of the lower epidermal layers. Acute cytotoxicity may take the form of basal cell layer vacuolization, an accelerated rate of programmed cell death (i.e., apoptosis), or direct cell-cell killing via effector-target cell apposition (i.e., satellitosis). This tends to obscure the dermal-epidermal interface, and hence, the application of the term *interface dermatitis*.

For purposes of this Fascicle, the acute forms of cytotoxic dermatitis are considered separately from the more chronic forms, which are often alternatively termed *lichenoid dermatitis* due to their presentation as scaling elevated plaques that mimic lichens that grow on the surfaces of rocks and tree trunks. Some acute forms of cytotoxic dermatitis evolve over time to more chronic, lichenoid lesions, and therefore, the separation between these two categories is not always absolute. Figure 6-1 provides a conceptual schema of the temporal evolution of acute cytotoxic dermatitis to more chronic forms.

## PATHOGENESIS

The underlying causes of most forms of acute cytotoxic dermatitis are protean, although it is generally assumed that autoantigens within the epidermal layer provoke an autoimmune reaction directed against keratinocytes. In other settings, such as erythema multiforme, infectious agents and ingested drugs are likely to alter epidermal antigens in a manner that provokes reactivity of an otherwise normal T-cell axis. In situations such as acute graft-versus-host disease, provocative histocompatibility differences are implicated, although the precise identity and tissue distribution of the primary target molecules remain to be elucidated.

The clinical appearance of cytotoxic dermatitis is different in the acute and chronic forms (Table 6-1). Because early lesions often involve abrupt destruction of the basal cell layer, there may be blister formation or erosion of the epidermal surface. Accordingly, acute forms of cytotoxic dermatitis are considered in the clinical differential diagnosis of primary vesiculobullous disorders of the skin, as well as some acute vesicular lesions of spongiotic dermatitis. Certain chronic forms of cytotoxic dermatitis produce lichenoid plaques as a result of inflammation and associated epidermal hyperplasia, and therefore, may be confused with forms of psoriasiform dermatitis. Other types of chronic cytotoxic dermatitis result in epidermal atrophy, vascular ectasia, and loss of melanin pigment into the underlying dermis and therefore may be confused with variants of cutaneous T-cell lymphoma, superficial basal cell carcinomas, or even primary abnormalities of skin pigmentation.

## PATHOLOGY

The generic forms of cytotoxic dermatitis share the following common features: 1) a superficial perivascular and interstitial papillary dermal infiltrate; 2) apposition of lymphocytes along a focally damaged basal cell layer characterized by either vacuolization, dyskeratosis, or squamatization; 3) epidermotropic migration of lymphocytes associated with necrosis/apoptosis of epidermal cells in direct contact; and 4) epidermal pigment incontinence and dermal fibrosis or basement membrane thickening with chronicity. Early in the course of the disease,

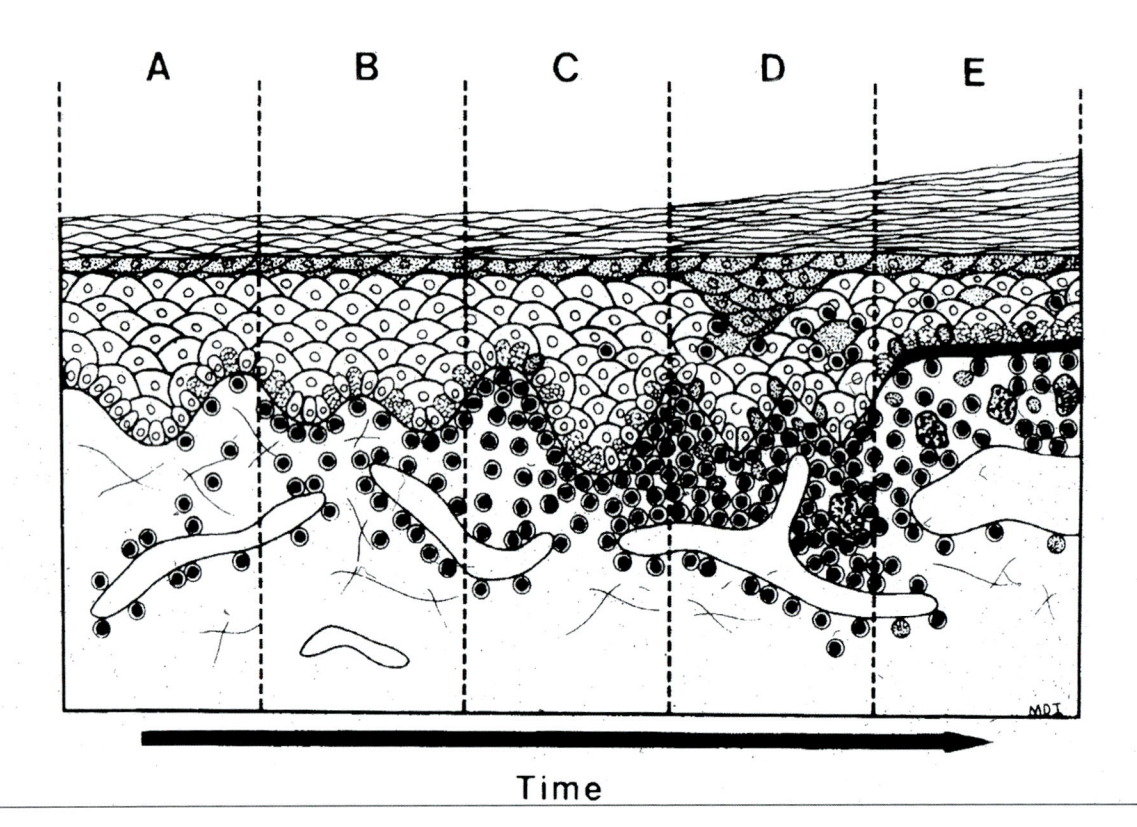

*Inflammatory Disorders of the Skin*

#### Figure 6-1
#### TEMPORAL EVOLUTION OF CYTOTOXIC DERMATITIS

Acute cytotoxic dermatitis begins as a perivascular accumulation of lymphocytes associated with a gradual accumulation of lymphocytes along the dermal-epidermal interface (A,B). Over time, the lymphocytes that accumulate along the dermal-epidermal interface produce a "tagging" pattern and become progressively associated with evidence of injury to the basal cell layer. As lymphocytes migrate into the epidermal layer (C,D), apoptotic cells become surrounded by lymphocytes, a phenomenon known as satellitosis. With chronicity, the epidermis undergoes reactive change, resulting either in epidermal hyperplasia (D) or atrophy (E). These epidermal changes are associated with transition from the tagging lymphocytic infiltrate to a more band-like or lichenoid pattern of lymphoid infiltration, heralding the onset of the subacute to chronic stage of cytotoxic dermatitis known as lichenoid dermatitis.

Table 6-1

**CLINICAL APPEARANCE OF VARIOUS FORMS OF CYTOTOXIC DERMATITIS**

| Gross Pathology | Histology | Representative Disorder |
| --- | --- | --- |
| Urticarial | Dermal edema, angiocentric lymphocytic infiltrate with mild basal cell layer injury | Erythema multiforme, early |
| Vesiculobullous | Marked basal cell layer injury | Erythema multiforme, advanced |
| Erythematous plaque | Marked dermal inflammation, focal epidermal injury | Fixed drug eruption, active |
| Pigmented macule | Dermal melanin incontinence | Fixed drug eruption, inactive |
| Hyperkeratotic plaque | Epidermal hyperplasia with hyperkeratosis, focal basal layer injury | Lichen planus |
| Erosion | Epidermal slough after diffuse, severe basal layer injury | Toxic epidermal necrolysis |
| Translucent, scaling plaque with telangiectasia | Epidermal atrophy, hyperkeratosis, vessel ectasia | Lupus erythematosus (discussed in chapter 7 given its predominant reaction pattern) |

only a sparse superficial, dermal perivascular lymphocytic infiltrate, with hints of lymphoid migration into the papillary dermis, is seen. Somewhat later, lymphocytes become aligned along the dermal-epidermal interface in association with subtle evidence of basal cell layer destruction. This tagging of lymphocytes is typical of the early stages of erythema multiforme, although it may be encountered in acute and subacute forms of lupus erythematosus. Generally, the stratum corneum maintains a basket-weave configuration at this juncture, because adequate time has not elapsed for transmission of evidence of full-thickness epidermal injury.

## SPECIAL DIAGNOSTIC STUDIES

In special situations, immunofluorescence or immunohistochemical examination is useful. For example, apoptotic cells may be documented by their tendency to take up immunoglobulin (Ig)M, as evidenced by direct immunofluorescence testing, or their reactivity in the terminal deoxynucleotidyl transferase (TdT)-mediated nick end labeling (TUNEL) assay. In most situations, however, careful correlation of clinical information with conventional histologic findings is the mainstay of diagnosis.

## ANIMAL MODELS

Probably the best animal model for the study of acute cytotoxicity is that of murine acute graft-versus-host disease (GVHD) (1). In this model, allostimulated donor effector cells home to skin (and other target organs) where they become associated with cellular targets, inducing apoptotic injury. This model has permitted elegant sequential analysis of lesion formation, and has provided significant insights into the coordinated cellular and molecular events responsible for lesion formation and resolution.

Recently, the acute GVHD model, in conjunction with correlative studies in human skin, has suggested that discrete subpopulations of basal epithelial cells may be selectively vulnerable to acute cytotoxic injury (2). Whether this phenomenon is more generalizable to forms of cytotoxic dermatitis other than GVHD remains to be determined. Nonetheless, at least in acute GVHD, the pattern of early injury to subpopulations of basal epithelial cells is considered of some diagnostic importance.

## ERYTHEMA MULTIFORME GROUP

**Definition.** *Erythema multiforme* is an uncommon but not rare, self-limiting disorder that is an acute cytotoxic manifestation of cell-mediated hypersensitivity that is often provoked by certain infections and drugs (3,4). Unlike contact allergy, which is a form of spongiotic dermatitis, erythema multiforme is a prototype of an acute cytotoxic reaction pattern. This disorder affects individuals of any age. It is associated with the following conditions: 1) infections such as herpes simplex, mycoplasma, histoplasmosis, coccidioidomycosis, typhoid, and leprosy: 2) administration of certain drugs, such as sulfonamides, penicillin, barbiturates, salicylates, hydantoins, and antimalarials; 3) malignancy (i.e., carcinomas and lymphomas); and 4) collagen-vascular (i.e., connective tissue) diseases, such as lupus erythematosus, dermatomyositis, and polyarteritis nodosa.

There are two forms of erythema multiforme, the so called minor and major types, the most severe of which is the *Stevens-Johnson syndrome*. *Toxic epidermal necrolysis* is thought to be related to the major form, representing the most extreme manifestation, because many cases begin with target lesions that are characteristic of erythema multiforme.

Erythema multiforme and toxic epidermal necrolysis describe basic underlying reaction patterns of the skin that are thought to share an underlying etiology, namely, a hypersensitivity reaction that expresses itself as a combination of a dermal process and a keratinocytic-cytotoxic process. The two forms of erythema multiforme are self-limited and have a variable picture of involvement. Toxic epidermal necrolysis is a severe disorder usually caused by drugs. There is widespread involvement of skin, and even at times internal organs, with frequent associated mortality.

**Clinical Features.** Clinically, affected individuals present with an array of "multiform" lesions, including macules, papules, vesicles, and bullae, as well as the characteristic target lesion, consisting of a red macule or papule with a pale, vesicular or eroded center (fig. 6-2). Lesions may be widely distributed, and symmetric involvement of the extremities is frequent. An extensive and symptomatic febrile form of the disease, which is more common in children,

*Inflammatory Disorders of the Skin*

**Figure 6-2**

**ERYTHEMA MULTIFORME**

Numerous erythematous plaques, many with central regions of dusky pallor rimmed by more intense erythema, form on the palm. Some of these central areas represent early blister formation. This is the characteristic targetoid appearance of erythema multiforme.

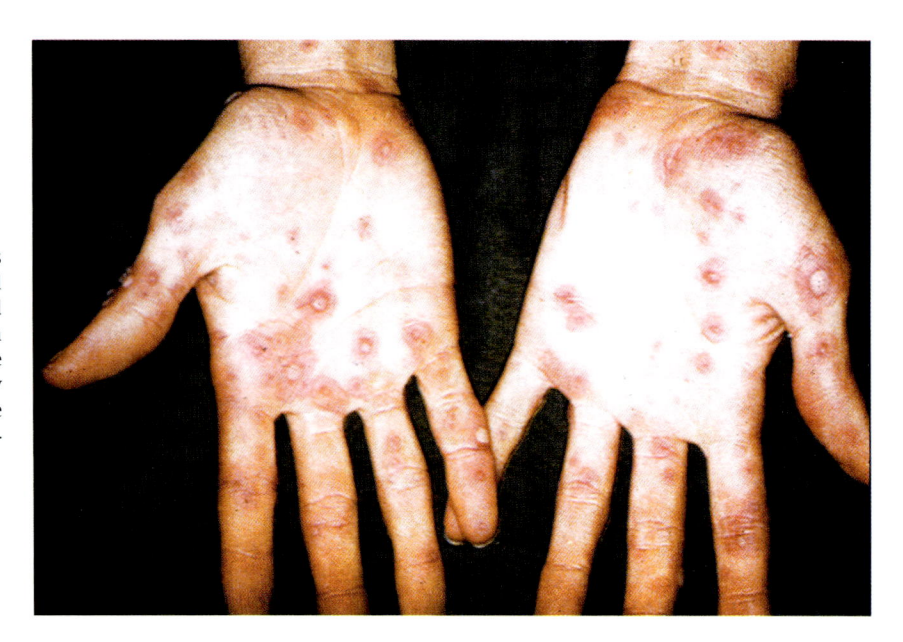

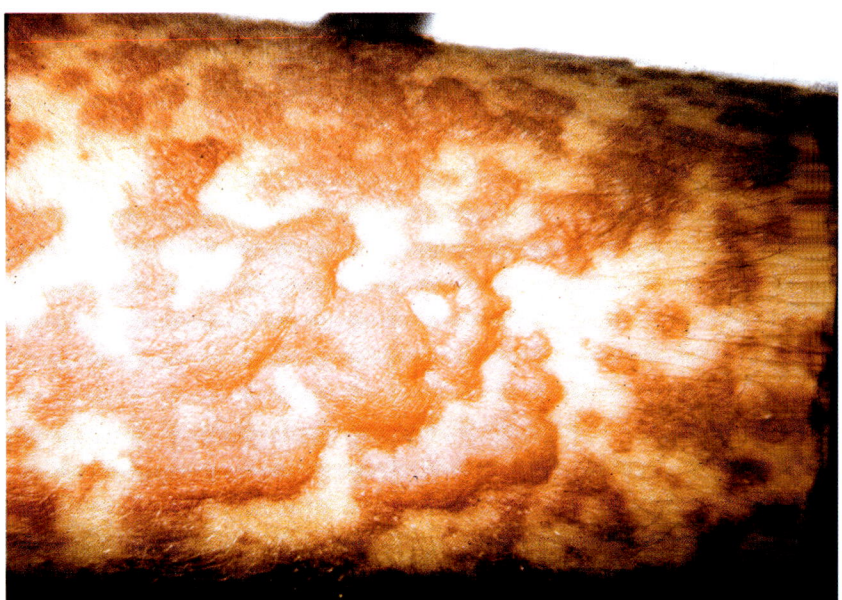

**Figure 6-3**

**STEVENS-JOHNSON SYNDROME**

Multiple, coalescent, focally bullous lesions are present. Not shown is involvement of the squamous mucosae.

is the Stevens-Johnson syndrome (fig. 6-3). In this disorder, erosions and hemorrhagic crusts involve the lips and oral mucosa. In addition, the conjunctiva, urethra, and anogenital regions may be involved. Life-threatening sepsis may result from infection of involved areas. Toxic epidermal necrolysis is characterized by diffuse necrosis and sloughing of cutaneous and mucosal epithelial surfaces, including oropharynx, esophagus, and even bronchial epithelium. This produces clinical manifestations similar to those of extensive thermal burns.

*Erythema Multiforme, Minor.* This self-limited and recurrent disorder is usually caused by herpes simplex viral infection. Prodromal symptoms are minimal or absent. The lesions are fixed plaques, characteristically distributed symmetrically and limited to acral sites. The characteristic target lesion has a dusky center with an erythematous rim. Mucosae are usually not involved in this variant and there are few constitutional symptoms and no internal organ involvement. The self-limited eruption lasts 1 to 3 weeks. There are usually no complications, no associated mortality, and the lesions heal without scarring.

*Erythema Multiforme, Major.* This acute and also self-limited form of the disease is almost invariably caused by drugs, and thus may be recurrent or episodic depending on the causative agent (5). In this more severe form of the disease a prodrome is present that often includes malaise. The lesions are distributed in acral areas but may affect central areas as well, especially the face. They consist of fixed plaques with a target-like appearance, but in addition, blisters are common. Mucosae are also affected, resulting in erosions and ulcers of the mouth, conjunctiva, and genitalia. Internal organs are occasionally involved. Constitutional symptoms lasting 3 to 4 weeks may be severe during the course of this reaction. In contrast to the minor form, complications are common and include superinfection of affected sites with associated pneumonia, local cutaneous infections, septicemia, and even in severe cases, heart and kidney failure with resultant mortality (up to 15 percent of cases). Lesions, especially of mucosae, may heal with scarring.

**Pathologic Findings.** Although the end result is a blister resulting from lymphocyte-mediated epidermal injury (fig. 6-4), the earliest phases of erythema multiforme are characterized by alignment or tagging of lymphocytes along a focally vacuolated dermal-epidermal interface (figs. 6-5–6-7). At this juncture, there is an associated superficial, perivascular lymphocytic infiltrate, often containing eosinophils,

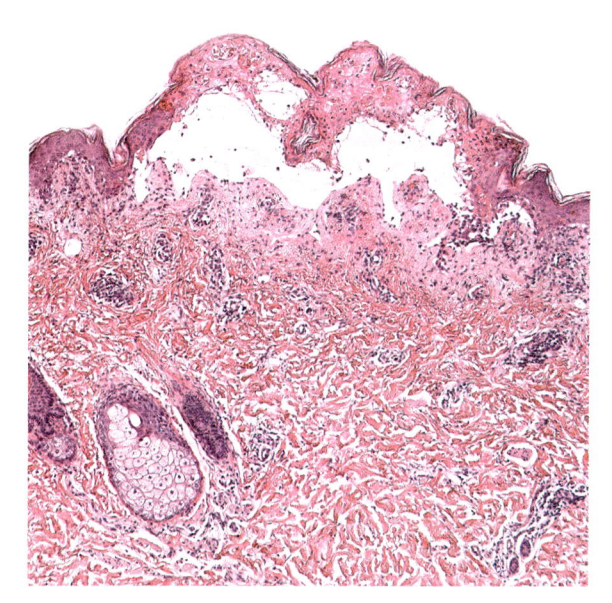

Figure 6-4

ERYTHEMA MULTIFORME

Left: The subepidermal blister has a largely necrotic roof, although the adjacent epidermis is viable with interface changes, all contributing to the targetoid clinical appearance.

Below: This lesion was initially a subepidermal blister. Now, the blister roof is largely necrotic, and the blister base is lined by a thin layer of re-epithelialization. Even at scanning magnification, the superficial perivascular lymphoid infiltrate and the tagging lymphocytes along the blister edge (right) are readily appreciated.

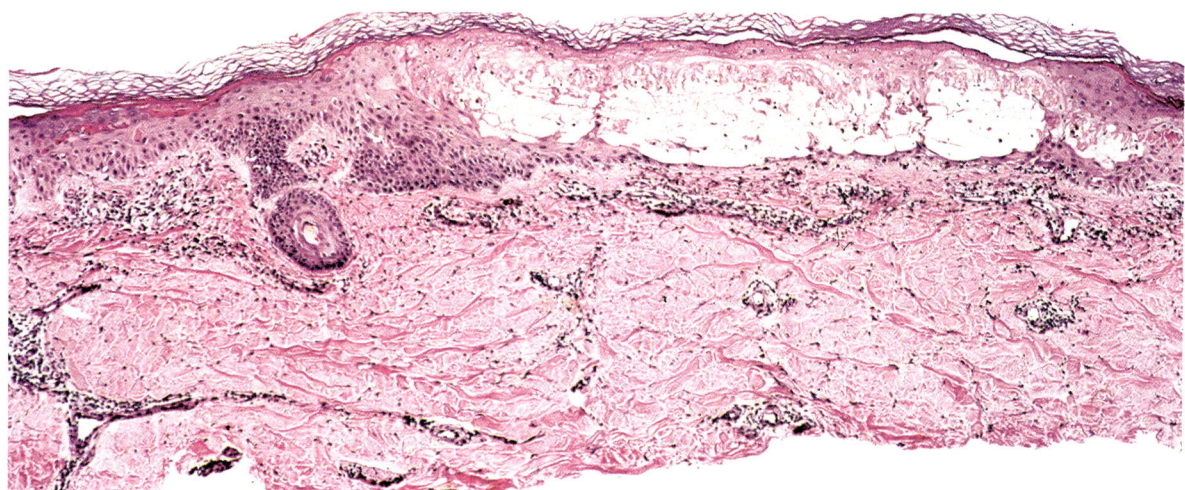

*Inflammatory Disorders of the Skin*

**Figure 6-5**

**ERYTHEMA MULTIFORME: EARLY LESION**

At high magnification, early tagging of lymphocytes is clearly seen along a focally vacuolated dermal-epidermal interface.

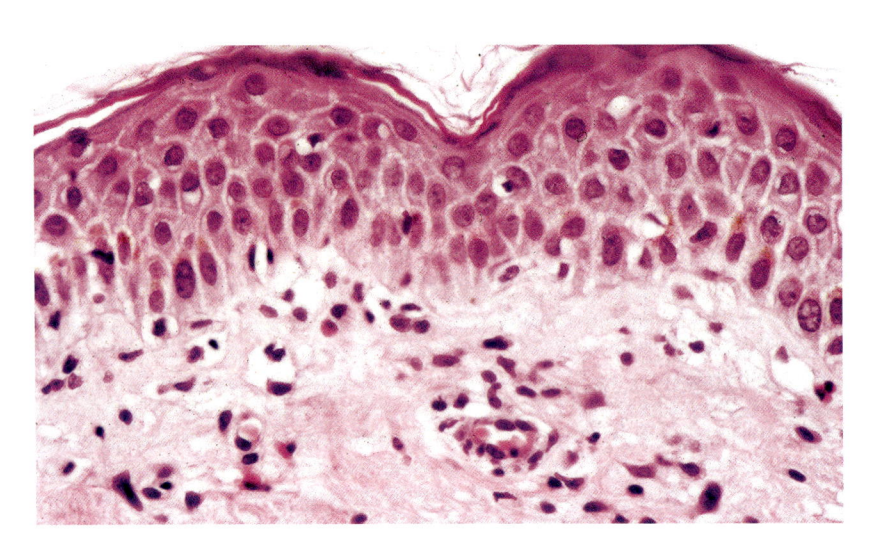

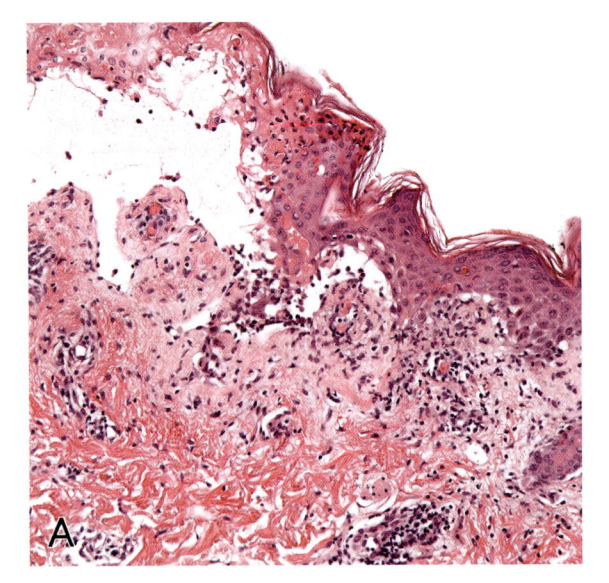

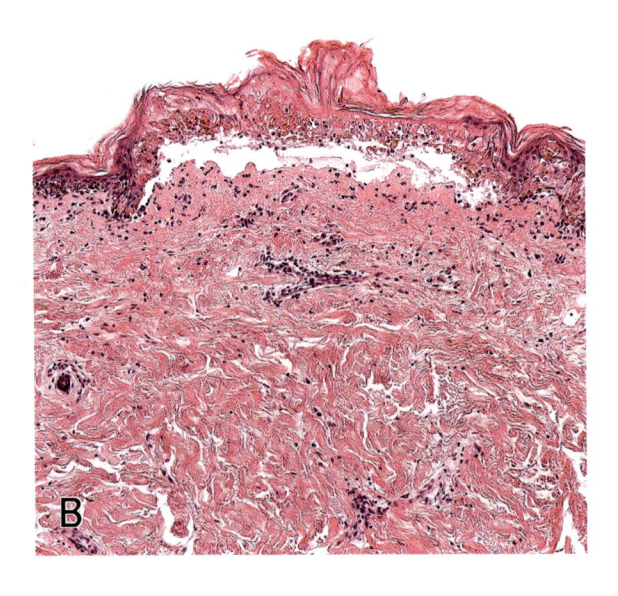

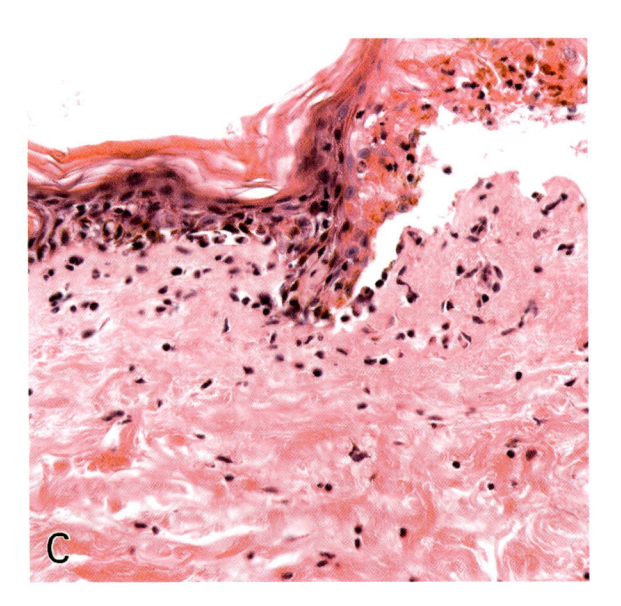

**Figure 6-6**

**ERYTHEMA MULTIFORME**

A: From right to left, there is lymphocyte-mediated interface dermatitis, leading to apoptosis and subepidermal blister formation.

B: The early blister shows central necrosis of the roof; subtle lymphocyte-mediated interface changes are present at the perimeter.

C: High magnification of the blister edge shows the lymphocyte tagging along the dermal-epidermal junction and the abrupt plane of subepidermal separation.

## Interface Dermatitis (Acute Cytotoxic Dermatitis)

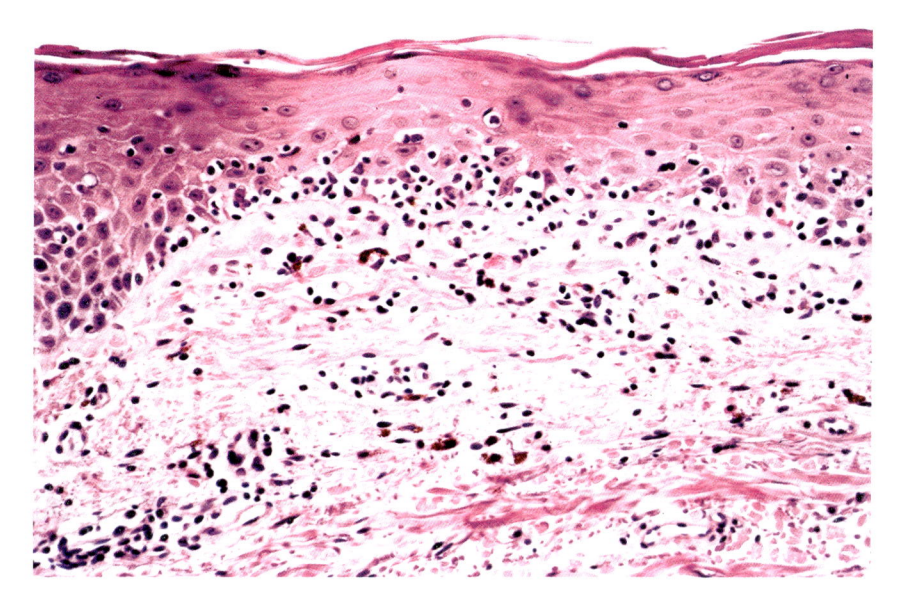

**Figure 6-7**

**ERYTHEMA MULTIFORME: ACTIVE EDGE OF LESION**

There is marked tagging of lymphocytes along the dermal-epidermal junction, with focal migration of lymphocytes into the epidermal layer. In many areas, lymphocytes begin to surround target keratinocytes in the process of early satellitosis. The papillary dermis is also infiltrated by lymphocytes and shows moderate edema.

**Figure 6-8**

**ERYTHEMA MULTIFORME: CENTRAL LESION ZONE**

The area of pallor comprises the central zone of the target lesion. It is composed of a zone of full-thickness epidermal necrosis forming the blister roof. The base is beginning to be recovered by the process of re-epithelialization. Subepidermal blisters with re-epithelialization occasionally mimic intraepidermal blisters. Therefore, careful evaluation of the blister edge where the dermal-epidermal junction remains intact is important in arriving at a correct diagnosis in such instances.

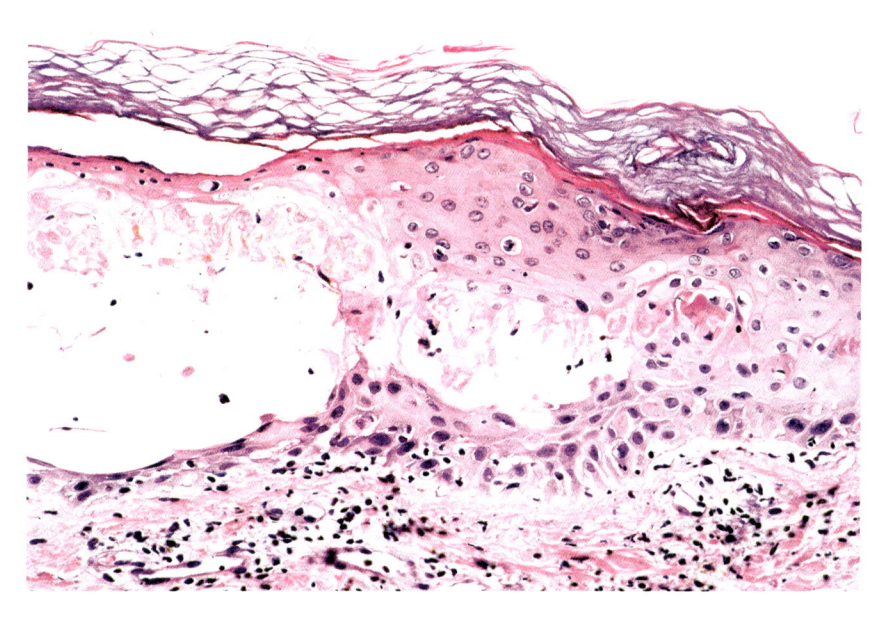

and papillary dermal edema. As lymphocytes migrate into the epidermis, they provoke single cell and focally clustered epidermal necrosis. With progressive accumulation of lymphocytes along a damaged dermal-epidermal interface, subepidermal blisters eventually form. The roof of the blister often shows extensive necrosis, and in healing lesions, the roof may cover a blister base lined with a new, re-epithelializing layer of flattened keratinocytes (fig. 6-8).

Some observers have categorized erythema multiforme as a type of lymphocytic vasculitis. Although the degree of vascular injury is not like that observed in necrotizing cutaneous vasculitis mediated by neutrophils, there is endothelial enlargement, subtle degenerative alterations, and perivascular hemorrhage in erythema multiforme. These features may be useful in diagnosing early lesions, when predominantly dermal alterations are present.

**Differential Diagnosis.** The minor form, with well-developed symmetrical target lesions, is quite destructive in terms of the extent of epidermal injury. Because some lesions appear edematous, both clinically and in terms of the predominance of dermal inflammatory

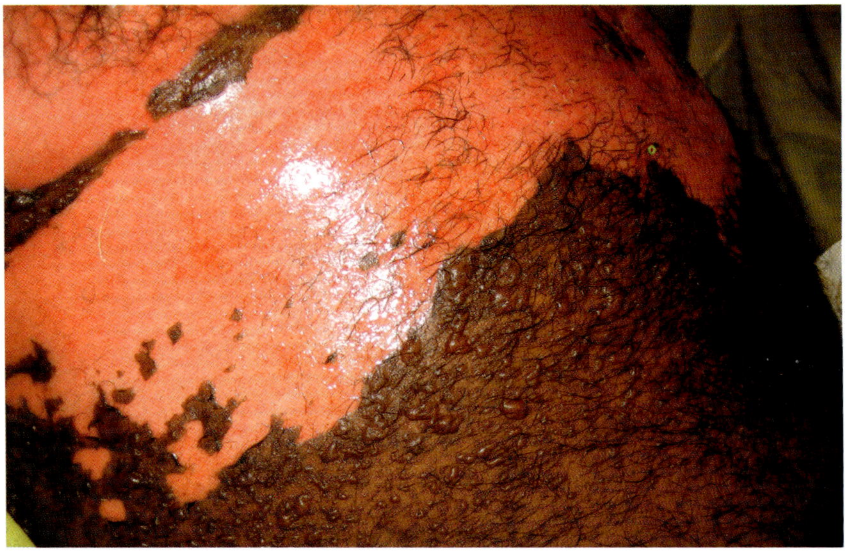

*Inflammatory Disorders of the Skin*

**Figure 6-9**

**TOXIC EPIDERMAL NECROLYSIS**

Thirty-six hours after admission, the epidermis is significantly denuded. The adjacent intact skin shows multiple foci of noninflammatory vesicle and bulla formation.

alterations, urticaria must be excluded. Also, other bullous diseases must be considered. The differential considerations for the stomatitis of erythema multiforme include herpes or aphthae. In severe erythema multiforme, the differential diagnosis includes bullous fixed drug reactions, other autoimmune bullous disorders, and severe GVHD. Exfoliative dermatitis and generalized fixed drug eruptions must also be excluded.

Erythema multiforme must be differentiated from acute GVHD in the post-transplant setting, and based on histopathology alone, this may not be possible. Viral exanthems produce superficial dermal perivascular lymphoid infiltrates with associated microvascular injury, although the characteristic interface alterations are generally lacking. Active lesions of fixed drug eruptions generally show associated melanin pigment incontinence, although any form of acute interface dermatitis may mimic this finding in the skin, especially in those individuals with prominent constitutive melanin pigmentation.

**Treatment and Prognosis.** Treatment is primarily directed against the underlying cause and local control of infection and tissue destruction. For the herpes-related diseases, antiviral therapy is helpful. For mild cases of erythema multiforme, it is useful to take antihistamines orally and to apply corticosteroids topically. For severe cases, oral corticosteroids and intravenous (IV) immunoglobulins are effective. If there is secondary infection, antibiotics are necessary. Soaks, debridement, and topical antibiotics are useful.

## TOXIC EPIDERMAL NECROLYSIS

**Definition.** *Toxic epidermal necrolysis* is an acute and explosive, yet self-limited disorder that may be episodic and is most commonly caused by drugs (6–9). The reaction leads to extensive sloughing of the skin and can lead to death from complications of fluid and electrolyte imbalance as well as infection.

**Clinical Features.** This disease affects both sexes and occurs at any age. A brief prodrome with some malaise and tenderness of the skin precedes the appearance of target lesions, progressing to a morbilliform rash with confluence to diffuse erythema. The target lesions may appear on the extremities, but the erythema appears on the face and trunk, and spreads. The lesions progress from red macules and target-like lesions to diffuse erythema with sloughing of the epidermis (fig. 6-9). The mucosae are frequently involved, resulting in serious morbidity with sloughing even of the conjunctiva. Healing, particularly of mucosal lesions, can lead to severe scarring with conjunctival symblepharon and vaginal synechiae. Internal organ involvement may occur and includes sloughing of the gastrointestinal tract, acute tubular necrosis, and upper respiratory erosion. There may be secondary infections of the eroded skin with septicemia. Cardiac and renal failure may ensue with mortality as high as 50 percent of the patients. The lesions progress for up to 4 days and then there is gradual recovery unless

*Interface Dermatitis (Acute Cytotoxic Dermatitis)*

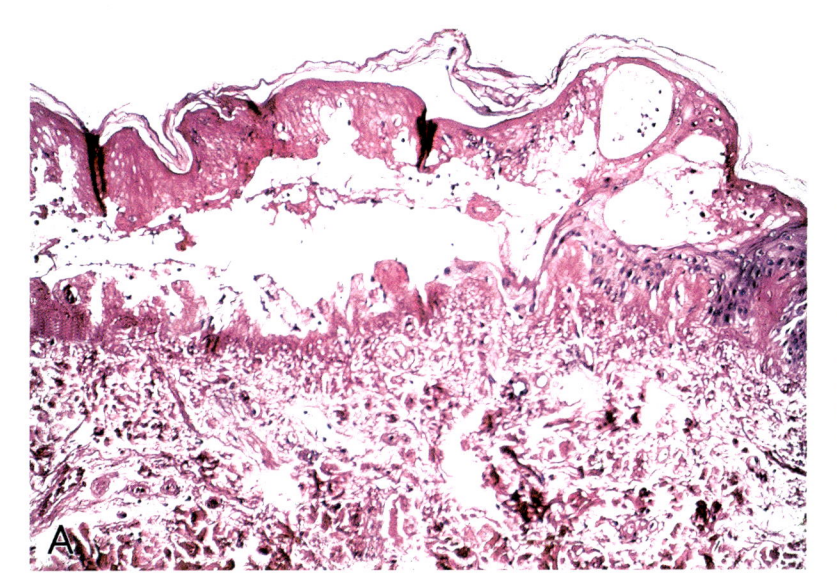

Figure 6-10

**TOXIC EPIDERMAL NECROLYSIS**

A: Subepidermal blister formation with full-thickness necrosis of the blister roof. The paucity of associated lymphoid inflammatory infiltration within the underlying dermis is characteristic.

B: In this early lesion, an exceedingly sparse lymphoid interface component is already associated with striking basal layer injury and incipient full-thickness epidermal necrosis.

C: This acute lesion already shows an extensively necrotic blister roof.

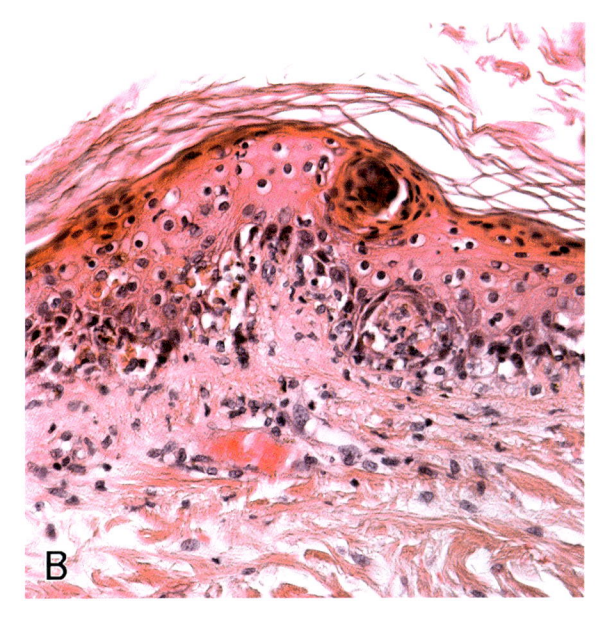

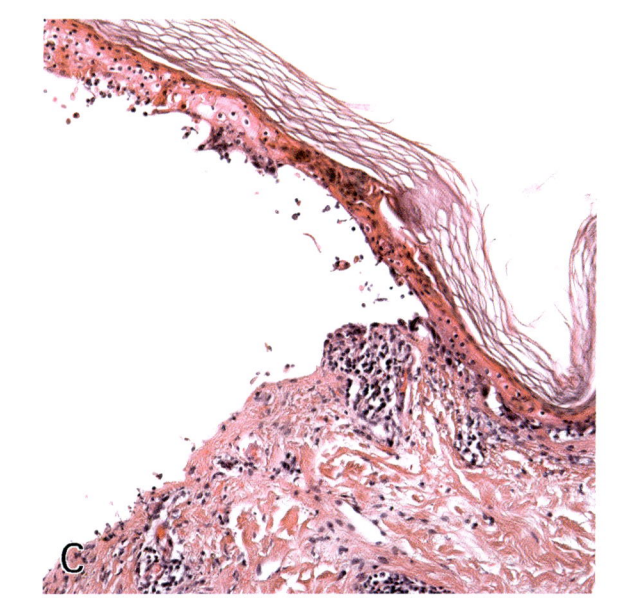

secondary complications develop. If the causative agent is not eliminated, toxic epidermal necrolysis may persist or recur.

**Pathologic Findings.** Toxic epidermal necrolysis is noted for extensive epidermal injury in the face of few effector lymphocytes (fig. 6-10). Accordingly, there is often a sparse, even inconspicuous, superficial dermal interstitial and perivascular lymphoid inflammatory infiltrate associated with zonal to confluent epidermal necrosis and focal sloughing as a result of dermal-epidermal separation. Rare admixed eosinophils may be present. Adnexal necrosis may be observed.

**Differential Diagnosis.** The differential diagnosis is diverse and highly dependent on the stage of lesion evolution. The early morbilliform rash must be differentiated from a viral exanthem or a phototoxic eruption. Toxic shock syndrome and acute GVHD must be considered. Thermal burns can appear indistinguishable. In fully developed lesions, toxic epidermal necrolysis and staphylococcal scalded skin syndrome (SSSS) are clinically similar. A diagnostic approach to separating toxic epidermal necrolysis from SSSS is the "jelly roll" technique (fig. 6-11) where a sloughed blister roof is rolled and sectioned, often by cryostat, to determine the

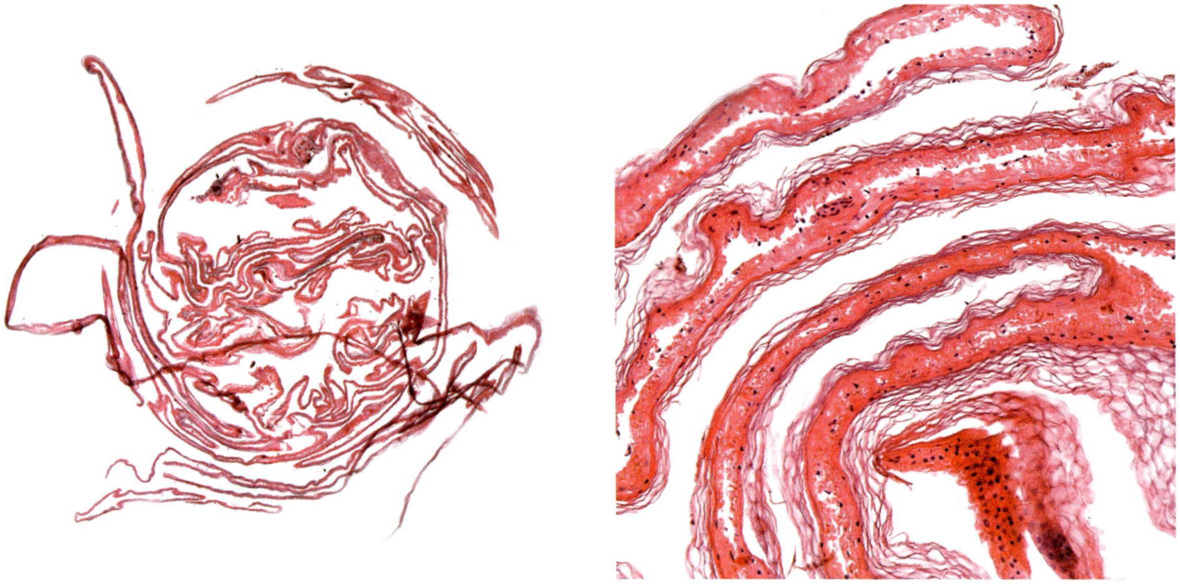

*Inflammatory Disorders of the Skin*

Figure 6-11

**TOXIC EPIDERMAL NECROLYSIS: "JELLY ROLL"**
Left: Low magnification.
Right: The epidermal layer is intact and shows full-thickness necrosis

plane of epidermal separation (subepidermal in toxic epidermal necrolysis, subcorneal in SSSS). Exfoliative erythroderma and phototoxic eruptions must be ruled out.

**Treatment.** The treatment is best carried out in a burn unit if possible (10–13). The offending agent must be withdrawn. Intravenous (IV) fluids, antibiotics, and IV immunoglobulins (Ig) are effective (14–17). Early use of systemic corticosteroids and/or IVIg is beneficial. Local burn care and local antisepsis are necessary. Care is aimed at supportive measures. Several prognostic scales, such as SCORTEN, help estimate morbidity and mortality.

## ACUTE GRAFT-VERSUS-HOST DISEASE

**Definition.** *Acute graft-versus-host disease (GVHD) is an immunologically mediated reaction of immunocompetent donor cells to host tissues due to histoincompatibility* (18–23). While acute GVHD generally develops subsequent to allogenic bone marrow transplantation (60 to 80 percent of cases), it also occurs after simple transfusion of nonirradiated blood products or as a consequence of "passenger leukocytes" after solid organ transplantation. The reaction occurs in acute, subacute, and chronic phases. A milder form occurs with autologous bone marrow transplantation. Similar reactions may also occur in immunosuppressed patients and in maternal-fetal transfer in the course of immunodeficiency disease.

The disorder presents as an inflammatory response which is mounted by the incompatible immunocompetent donor cells specifically against certain organs of the host, principally the liver, the gastrointestinal tract, and the skin. The greater the histoincompatibility of the donor and recipient match, the greater the severity of the disease.

**Clinical Features.** Very early, there is a maculopapular eruption on the trunk, hands, and feet, especially the palms and soles (fig. 6-12), with pain or discomfort. It is initially subtle and occurs generally in the first 3 months after bone marrow transplantation. The general rule that acute GVHD develops "within the first 100 days after bone marrow transplantation" varies, especially since immunosuppressive manipulation and donor lymphocyte infusions may modify the conventional time course of disease initiation and evolution. As the symptoms become more marked, the mild discomfort of pruritus leads to pain. In this phase, there may

## Interface Dermatitis (Acute Cytotoxic Dermatitis)

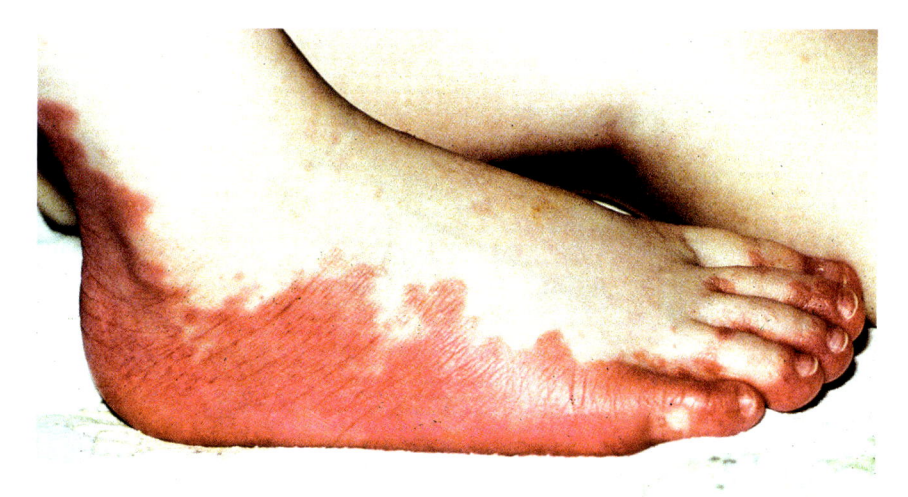

**Figure 6-12**

**ACUTE GRAFT-VERSUS-HOST DISEASE (GVHD)**

The characteristic erythema involves the sole of the foot and palm. Patients frequently have a maculopapular exanthem that may mimic a viral or drug rash.

be systemic signs and symptoms as well. If the initial eruption resolves spontaneously or is controlled by treatment, there is subsequent cutaneous desquamation and mild postinflammatory pigmentation. If the lesions progress, they become more generalized, more intense, and confluent, and lead to erythroderma, finally resulting in a toxic epidermal necrolysis–like picture. Occasionally, bullae occur, especially over areas of trauma. Localized bullae can lead to more generalized changes. The oral mucosa may be involved with lichenoid lesions or even erosive stomatitis. In severe cases, there is an oral and ocular sicca syndrome. Generalized symptoms include fever, nausea, vomiting, right upper quadrant pain and tenderness, diffuse abdominal pain, and diarrhea. Liver abnormalities are associated with abdominal pain and cramping, and with the development of dark urine.

The clinical staging of acute GVHD of the skin is as follows: stage 1, an erythematous maculopapular eruption involving less than 25 percent of the body surface; stage 2, an erythematous maculopapular eruption evolving 25 to 50 percent of the body surface; stage 3, generalized erythroderma; and stage 4, bullae formation.

**Pathologic Findings.** Histologically, a helpful diagnostic feature of GVHD is the presence of significant epidermal injury (i.e., basal cell layer vacuolization and single cell death) that is out of proportion to a relatively sparse superficial dermal perivascular lymphocytic infiltrate (fig. 6-13). A characteristic finding is satellitosis, a reaction pattern whereby a dying keratinocyte, commonly referred to as an apoptotic cell, is surrounded by several lymphocytes in direct apposition (fig. 6-13C). Apoptotic cells may be confirmed in acute GVHD using the TUNEL method, which permits detection of the laddered DNA fragments that typically are produced as a result of endonuclease activity (fig. 6-14). Although originally described in experimental acute GVHD, satellitosis is not entirely specific and also may be observed in other forms of cytotoxic dermatitis, such as lichen planus and erythema multiforme. Because the term apoptosis, when rigidly defined, implies programmed cell death, it remains to be determined whether many of the dying cells in certain forms of cytotoxic dermatitis other than acute GVHD represent true apoptotic cells.

Other features that may be seen in acute GVHD include increased mitotic activity and abnormal or disordered epidermal maturation. These may also be related to the "toxic" effects of the conditioning regimen and the influence on cell proliferation/maturation inherent in the early soluble (cytokine-mediated) phase of the disease that precedes effector cell infiltration of target tissues.

**Differential Diagnosis.** Early acute GVHD may have extraordinarily subtle findings, necessitating serial biopsies at 7- to 10-day intervals to assess disease progression, which generally occurs with this disorder, as opposed to viral exanthems. Very early lesions may show lymphoid infiltration and basal layer injury that preferentially affect the tips of epidermal rete

*Inflammatory Disorders of the Skin*

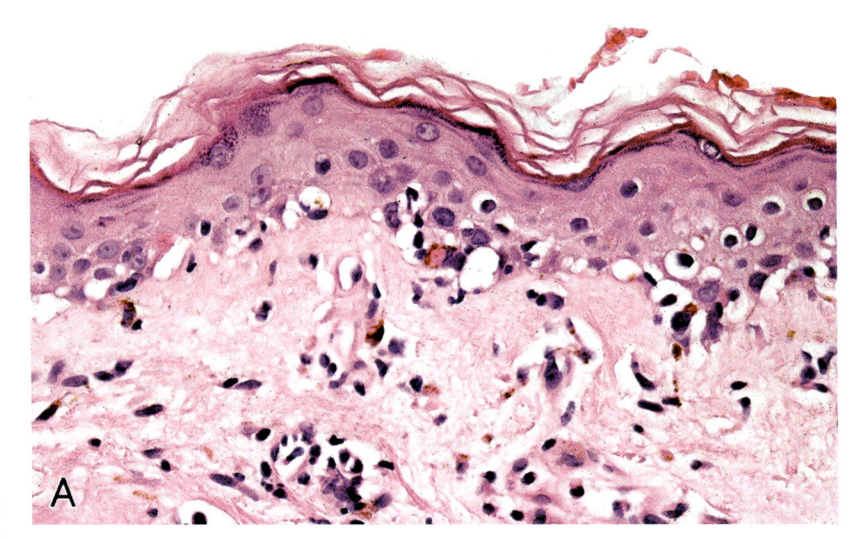

### Figure 6-13
### ACUTE GRAFT-VERSUS-HOST DISEASE: EARLY LESION

A: Although there is a paucity of infiltrating lymphocytes, there is striking vacuolization of the basal cell layer with occasional apoptotic cells. Lymphocytes are present both above the superficial postcapillary venules as well as singly along the dermal-epidermal interface. The stratum corneum shows a normal basket-weave pattern, indicative of the acute nature of this cytotoxic insult.

B: At higher magnification, in addition to showing apoptotic cells associated with lymphocytes (middle of field), the epidermis also shows "maturation disarray," a finding probably attributable to the effects of the conditioning regimen as well as the circulating "cytokine storm" that accompanies the early stages of GVHD.

C: Lymphocytes are infiltrating the dermal-epidermal interface as well as within the epidermal layer. The lymphocytes are associated with apoptotic target cells, and occasional cells show the characteristic satellitosis pattern (arrow). The epidermal layer is mildly hyperplastic at this point.

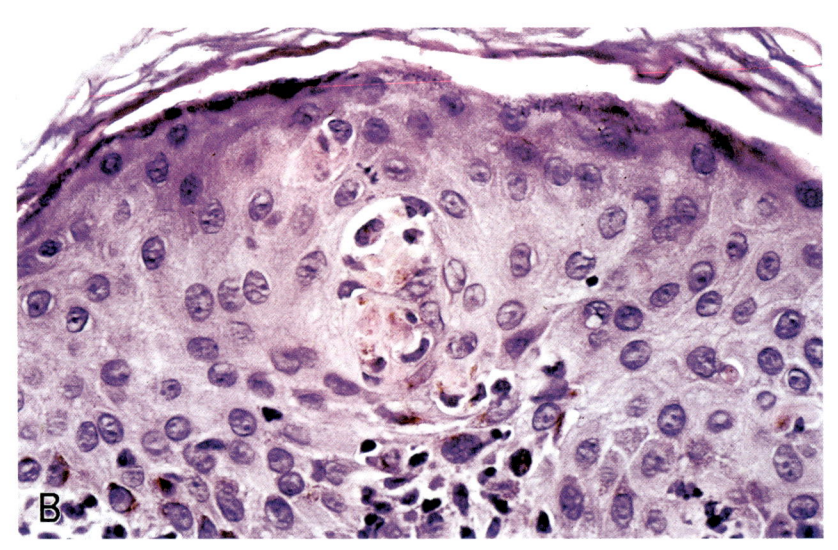

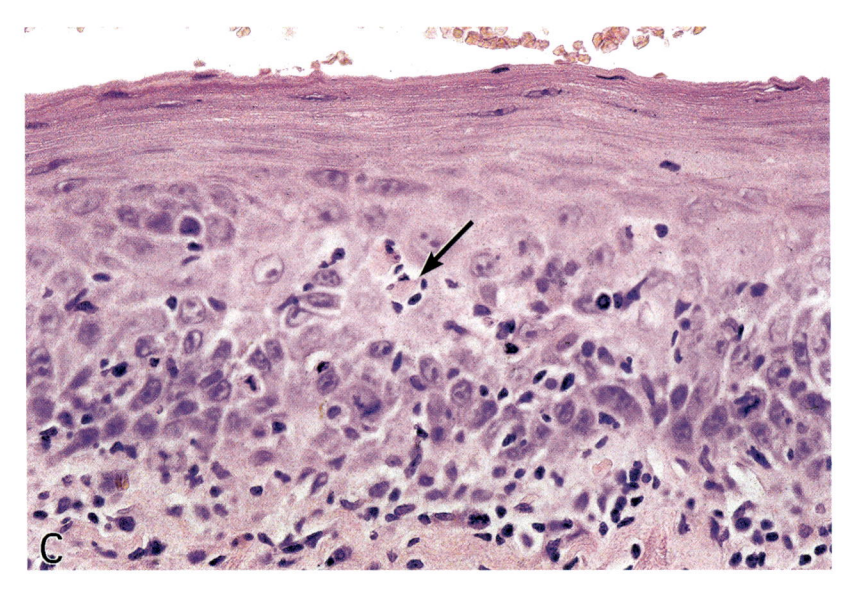

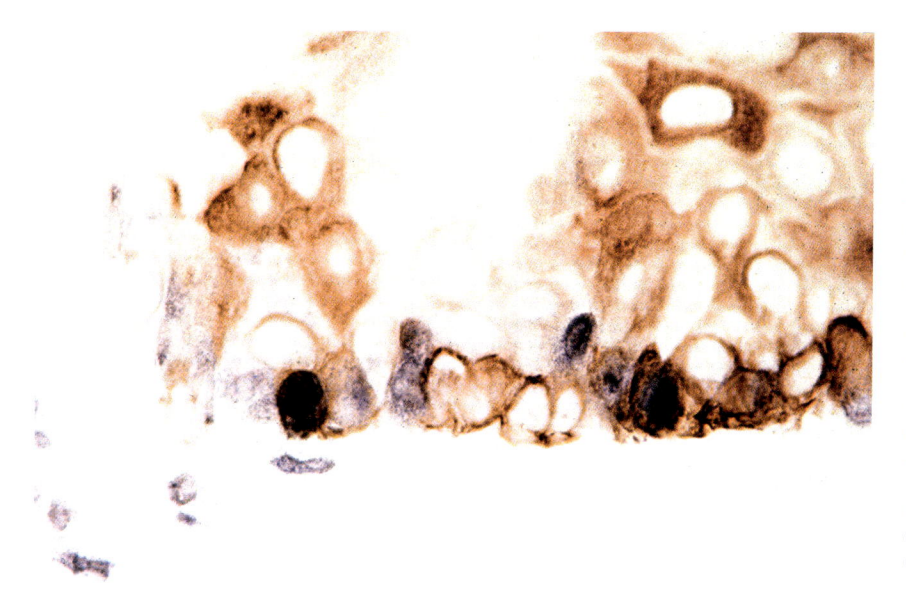

### Figure 6-14

**TUNEL IMMUNOSTAINING OF APOPTOTIC CELLS**

The presence of cytotoxic cytokines (TNFα [tumor necrosis factor alpha]) as well as alloreactive T cells in acute GVHD results in apoptosis that preferentially affects the basal cell layer (here experimentally reproduced and indicated as the dark blue to purple zone of staining). Apoptosis in GVHD may preferentially involve basal cells of the tips of the rete ridges and the bulge regions of hair follicles. (Brown staining indicates background cytokeratins within target cells.)

ridges (fig. 6-15), although the diagnostic specificity and potential utility of this finding are yet to be established. One helpful site to examine at early time points (e.g., 2 to 3 weeks after transplantation or transfusion) is the bulge region of the infundibulum of hair follicles, which in both experimental and human disease has been shown to be a very early site of target cell injury (fig. 6-16) (23a). In some cases, the eccrine duct exhibits the changes of satellitosis and infiltration by lymphoid cells (fig. 6-17). Severe and widespread acute GVHD may occasionally produce such extensive epidermal injury that it is essentially indistinguishable from toxic epidermal necrolysis by histopathology alone (fig. 6-17). Chronic GVHD may histologically resemble lichen planus or scleroderma.

The most difficult and common entity in the differential diagnosis is an exanthematous drug reaction. Viral exanthems are also confused with this disorder. Usually, drug reactions respond with withdrawal of the drug, or if there is continuation of the drug, they persist but don't evolve; viral exanthems are self-limited. For this reason, biopsies at different intervals to chart the evolution of GVHD are useful and recommended. One helpful feature in differentiating between acute GVHD and cytotoxic drug eruption is the presence of easily identified eosinophils, which favors the latter.

Toxic epidermal necrolysis or erythroderma due to other causes is considered in the differential diagnosis, emphasizing the importance of clinicopathologic correlation and documentation of extracutaneous involvement in the diagnosis of acute GVHD. The so-called rash of lymphocyte recovery also develops in the post-transplant period and may be a manifestation of extrathymic (intracutaneous) T-cell

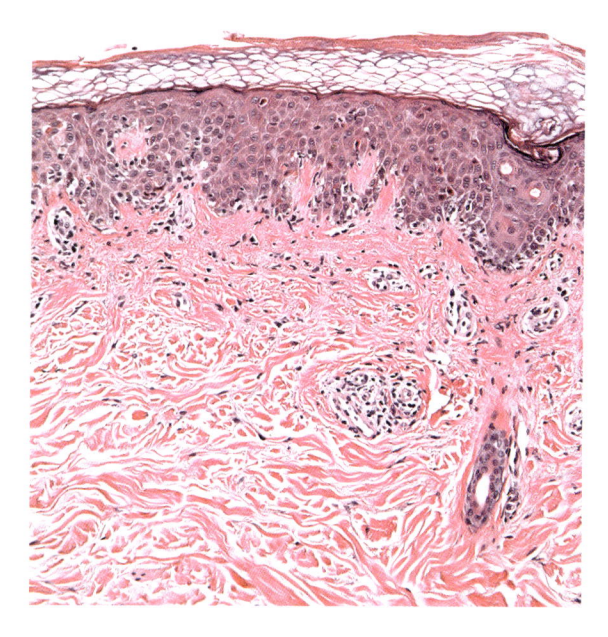

### Figure 6-15

**ACUTE GRAFT-VERSUS-HOST DISEASE**

There is an exceedingly sparse superficial lymphocytic infiltrate associated with mild interface changes that are more prominent in rete tips of this early lesion.

*Inflammatory Disorders of the Skin*

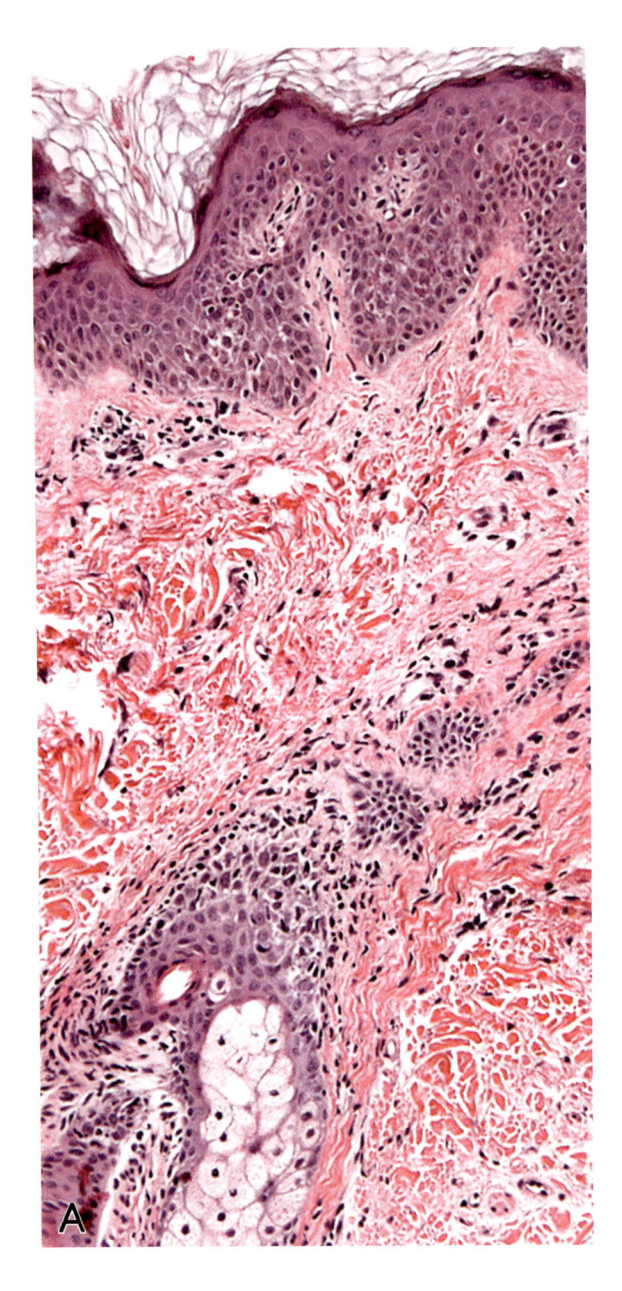

**Figure 6-16**

**ACUTE FOLLICULAR GVHD**

A: This 53-year-old male had chronic myelogenous leukemia. Eight days after allogeneic stem cell transplantation, he presented with a maculopapular rash. The inflammatory changes are restricted to the hair follicle.

B: At higher magnification, there is lymphocyte-mediated interface change, selectively involving the bulge region of the hair follicle.

C: The infiltrating lymphocytes surround target cells destined for apoptotic injury.

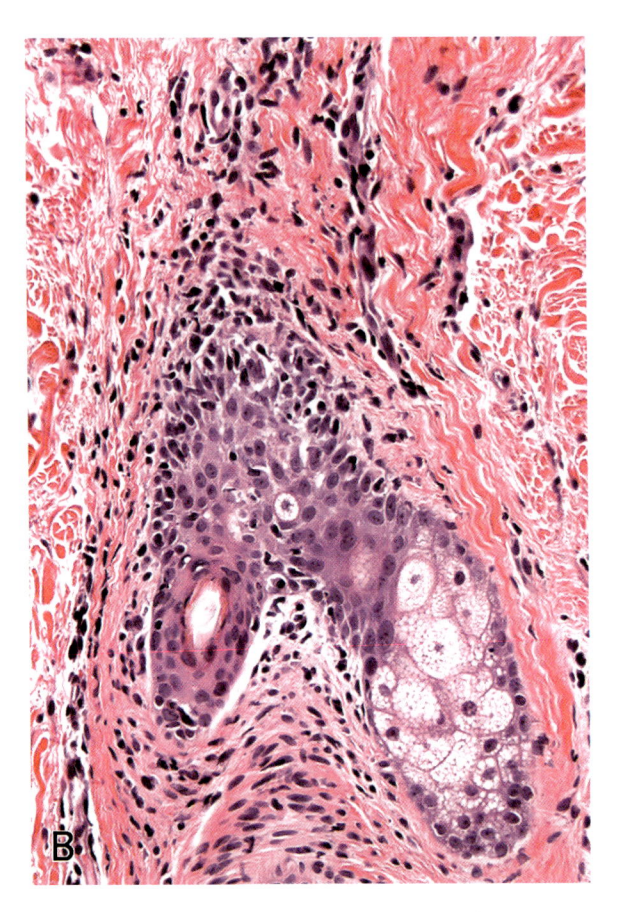

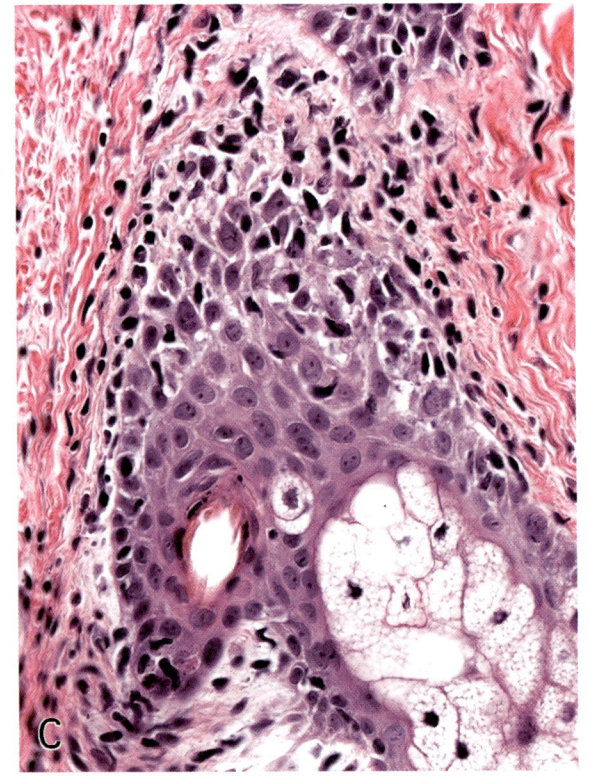

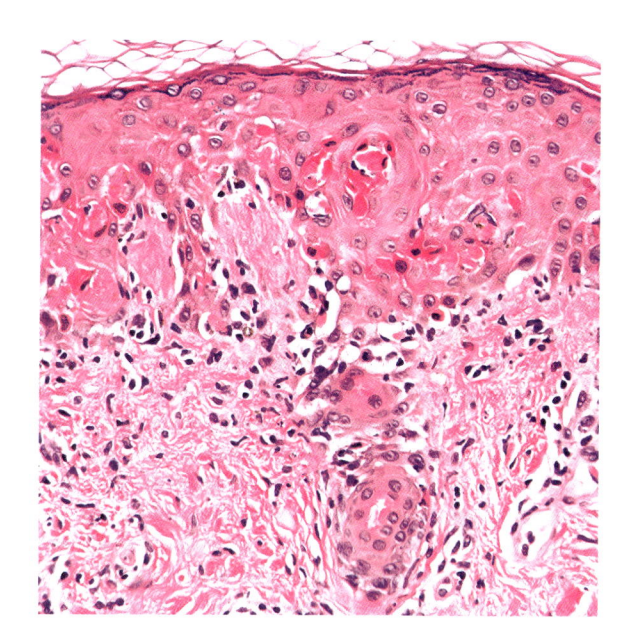

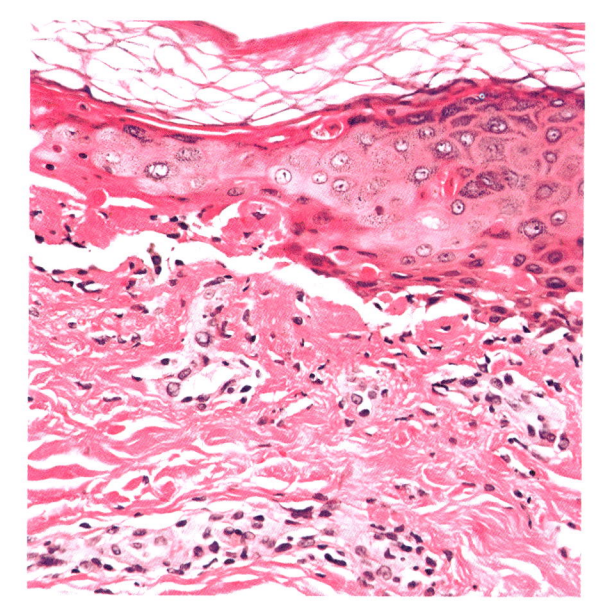

**Figure 6-17**

**ACUTE GRAFT-VERSUS-HOST DISEASE**

Left: High magnification of an advanced lesion shows extensive apoptotic injury, a sparse lymphoid component, and characteristic involvement of the superficial eccrine duct.

Right: Incipient subepidermal blister formation in the setting of relatively few effector lymphocytes. Lesions of this severity may resemble toxic epidermal necrolysis.

maturation. Although histologically subtle (as are many examples of early acute GVHD), the rash of lymphocyte recovery does not exhibit prominent satellitosis, in our experience, and trafficking lymphocytes presumably have an immature immunophenotype. Exclusion of liver and gastrointestinal involvement assists in considering the myriad other mimics of acute GVHD that may develop in the post-transplant period. Acute systemic lupus erythematosus occasionally resembles acute GVHD, and although its development after allogeneic stem cell or bone marrow transplantation would be unusual, dermatitic conditions potentially may be transferred from donor to host via cells in the inoculum.

**Treatment and Prognosis.** Usually, acute GVHD requires oral steroid therapy (24–28). In very severe cases, especially with gastrointestinal or liver involvement, cyclosporine, methotrexate, mycophenolate, or advanced immunosuppressant medications such as tacrolimus and sirulimus, are added to the regimen. Topical steroids in the form of potent glucocorticoids give only symptomatic relief for milder cases. PUVA (psoralen ultraviolet light A) therapy is used for subacute to chronic cases. Extracorporeal photopheresis has shown some benefit as well, particularly as a steroid-sparing or-reducing agent.

## PITYRIASIS LICHENOIDES ET VARIOLIFORMIS ACUTA

**Definition.** *Pityriasis lichenoides et varioliformis acuta* (PLEVA) is a disorder of unknown etiology that clinically presents with crops of lesions that are papular but that show striking variation and morphology (29–33). These include macules, papules, vesicles, pustules, and crusts in the acute form of this disorder and scaly reddish brown papules in the chronic form. In the acute form, it is characteristic to have lesions at different stages of development. It has been known by a variety of names including *Mucha-Habermann disease*, and the guttate, or chronic, form has been called *guttate parapsoriasis of Juliusberg*.

**Clinical Features.** PLEVA occurs most commonly in adolescents and young adults and is more common in males than in females. The etiology of the disorder is unknown. These

*Inflammatory Disorders of the Skin*

**Figure 6-18**

**PITYRIASIS LICHENOIDES ET VARIOLIFORMIS ACUTA (PLEVA)**

The lesions are dome-shaped and erythematous, and form characteristic "juicy red papules." The clinical differential diagnosis of such clustered papules includes insect bites.

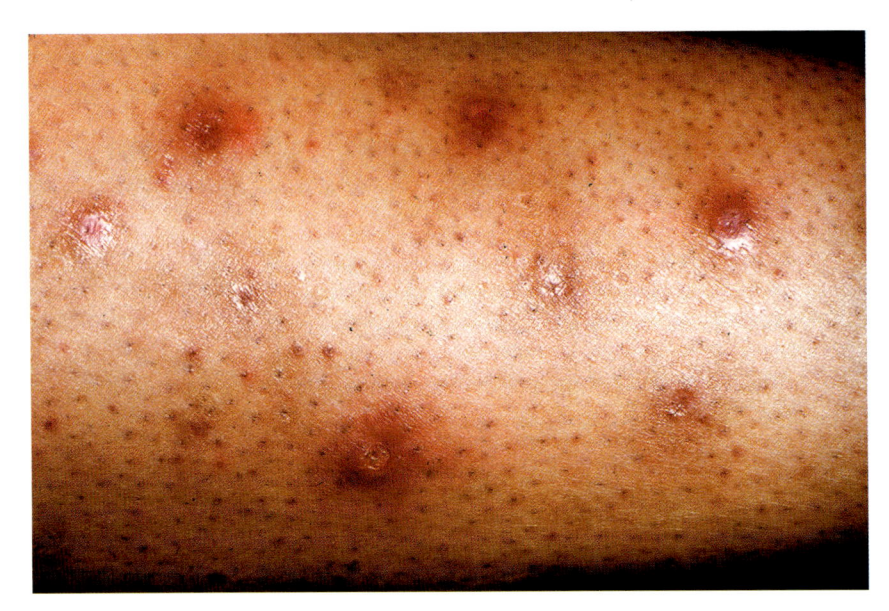

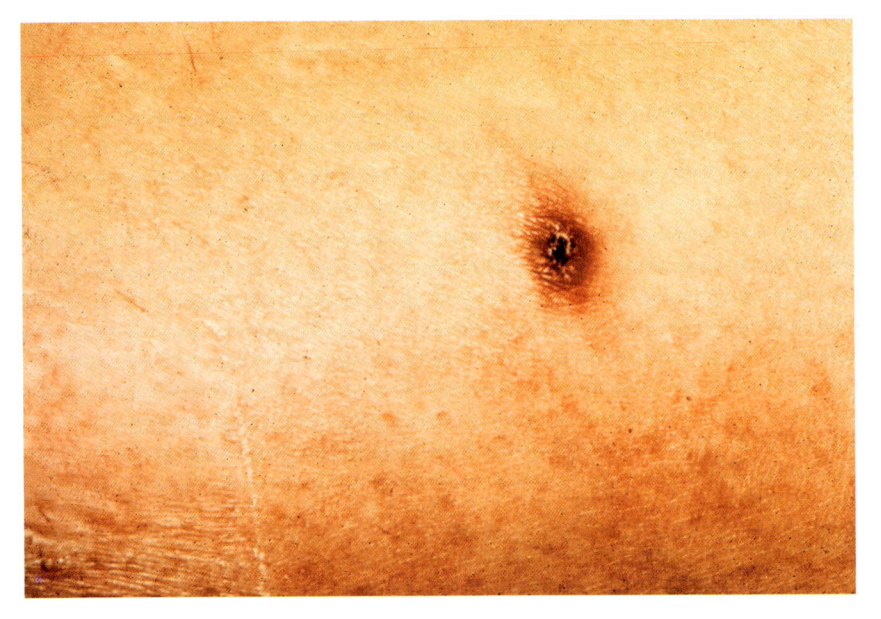

**Figure 6-19**

**PITYRIASIS LICHENOIDES ET VARIOLIFORMIS ACUTA**

The erythema is red-brown, and a central scab-like region is apparent in this older lesion.

lesions occur as crops (fig. 6-18). Patients who have an acute onset sometimes have associated fever, malaise, and headaches. Cutaneous lesions do not cause symptoms but may be pruritic or produce a sensation of discomfort upon touching. The skin lesions are randomly distributed on the trunk and upper extremities or on the proximal portions of the upper and lower extremities. The lesions begin as papules that develop into vesicles; these break down and become ulcerated papules with crusts. Crusted lesions mimic those of variola infection, hence the name varioliformis (fig. 6-19). In the acute form, there are lesions in various stages of development. The chronic form of this disorder, which is sometimes referred to as *pityriasis lichenoides chronica* and which may be the presenting form, usually consists of reddish brown papules with a central, very tightly adherent scale. When the lesions resolve, they may leave depressed or elevated white scars, or hypopigmented or hyperpigmented macules. Occasionally, the genitalia and rarely, the oral mucosa, are affected.

**Pathologic Findings.** At scanning magnification, the inflammatory infiltrate in PLEVA shows a superficial and deep angiocentric pattern as well as a cytotoxic (i.e., interface) pattern of infiltration along the dermal-epidermal junction (fig. 6-20). At higher magnification, the interface portion of the infiltrate is associated with basal cell layer vacuolization and epidermotropism with associated satellitosis (fig. 6-21). Often, single cell and zonal necroses involving clusters of keratinocytes independent of infiltrating lymphocytes are observed. The stratum corneum may show foci of parakeratosis infiltrated by neutrophils (fig. 6-22). In the early lesion, perivascular extravasation of erythrocytes is frequently present about superficial vessels, an indicator that in addition to erythema multiforme, PLEVA may represent yet another example of lymphocytic vasculitis (fig. 6-23). Indeed, in rare cases more overt vasculitic injury may be seen in PLEVA. The erythrocytes extend into the epidermis, even up to the stratum corneum, across a broad zone of the affected area, a helpful diagnostic sign. Pityriasis lichenoides chronica has many of the features of PLEVA, but the dermal infiltrate spares the deep vessels. Also, there is a prominent parakeratotic scale. There may be dermal pigment incontinence and sometimes mild papillary dermal fibrosis.

**Differential Diagnosis.** The primary differential diagnosis includes lichenoid insect bite reaction and lymphomatoid papulosis, both of which PLEVA resembles clinically (Table 6-2). Insect bite reactions may have vasculitic components with hemorrhage, basal cell layer vacuolization, and a superficial and deep perivascular polymorphous and highly activated inflammatory infiltrate that includes eosinophils in many cases. The zonal epidermal necrosis and

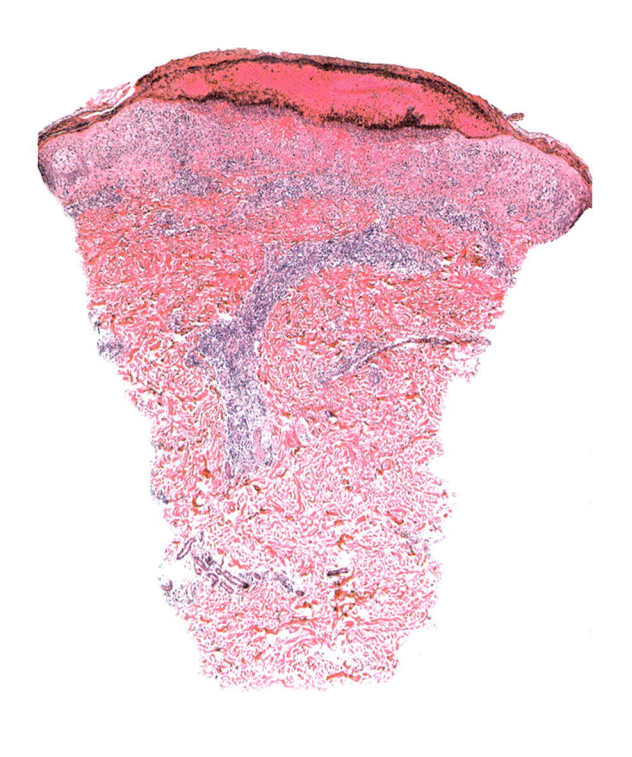

Figure 6-20

**PITYRIASIS LICHENOIDES ET VARIOLIFORMIS ACUTA**

The lesion is characterized by a superficial and deep perivascular lymphocytic infiltrate, as well as interface dermatitis with lymphocytes accumulating along the dermal-epidermal junction. Epidermal breakdown is centrally present.

Table 6-2

**DIFFERENTIAL DIAGNOSTIC FEATURES OF PITYRIASIS LICHENOIDES ET VARIOLIFORMIS ACUTA**

|  | PLEVA[a] | PLC | Lymphomatoid Papulosis | Insect Bite Reaction |
|---|---|---|---|---|
| Infiltrate |  |  |  |  |
| Depth | Superficial and deep | Superficial | Superficial and deep | Superficial and deep |
| Location | Angiocentric and interface | Angiocentric and lichenoid | Angiocentric and interstitial | Angiocentric, interstitial, and interface/lichenoid |
| Composition | Lymphocytes | Lymphocytes | Lymphocytes and atypical Reed-Sternberg–like cells | Lymphocytes and eosinophils |
| Spongiosis | Absent | Absent | Absent | Often present |
| Apoptosis | Present | Present | Absent | Often absent |
| Vascular injury | Variable | Absent | Prominent | Variable |

[a]PLEVA = pityriasis lichenoides et varioliformis acuta; PLC = pityriasis lichenoides chronica.

*Inflammatory Disorders of the Skin*

**Figure 6-21**

**PITYRIASIS LICHENOIDES ET VARIOLIFORMIS ACUTA**

Top: In an early lesion, there is a brisk infiltrate of lymphocytes along a vacuolated dermal-epidermal interface. The stratum corneum shows a basket-weave pattern, indicating the acute nature of the cytotoxic insult.

Bottom: High magnification shows a brisk lymphocytic infiltrate along the dermal-epidermal junction, obvious vacuolization of the basal cell layer, and zones of superficial epidermal hemorrhage with focal extravasation of erythrocytes into the epidermal layer.

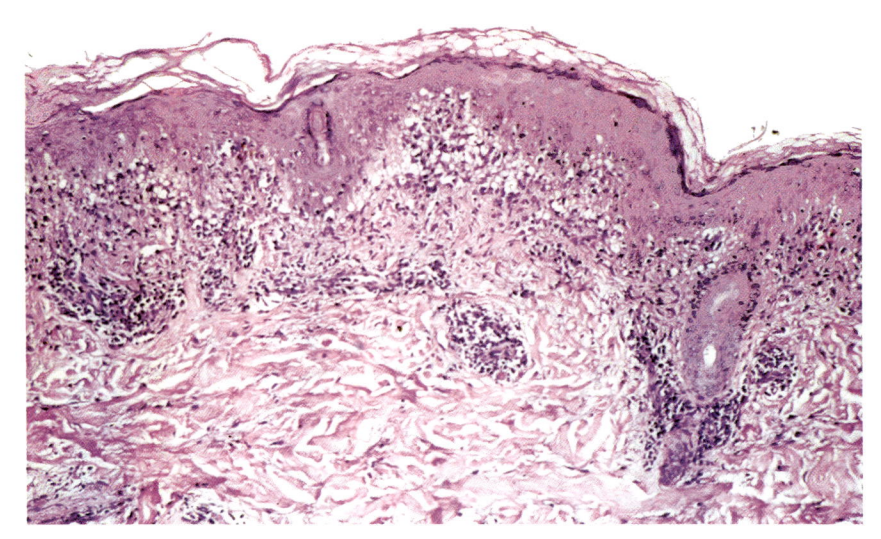

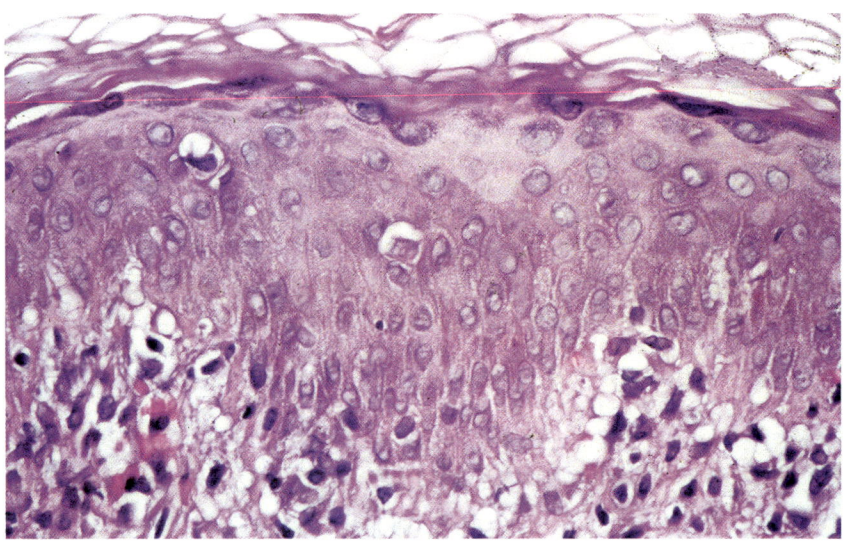

parakeratosis infiltrated by neutrophils typical of PLEVA, as well as the intraepidermal extravasated red blood cells, are generally absent in insect bites. Moreover, the latter often show foci of interstitial dermal infiltration by histiocytes (often resembling granuloma annulare in these regions) and eosinophils. Pityriasis lichenoides chronica involves a superficial perivascular lymphocytic infiltrate, and the epidermal alterations are generally less pronounced than in PLEVA. Signs of chronicity include pigment incontinence and subtle fibrosis within the papillary dermis, neither of which is prominent in PLEVA.

Lymphomatoid papulosis describes a generally asymptomatic disorder in which recurrent crops of lesions occur and heal spontaneously (34). Because a minority of cases eventuate in lymphoma or represent indolent forms of T-cell lymphoproliferative disease from the outset, differentiation from PLEVA is an important distinction. Lymphomatoid papulosis occurs any time in life, from childhood to old age, but most often in mid-life. Both sexes are affected equally and the exact etiology of the disorder is not completely understood. The lesions are papulonodules that are similar to, but larger than, those of PLEVA, approximately 5 to 10 mm in diameter. They are initially erythematous and edematous. Clinically, PLEVA may resemble lymphomatoid papulosis, but usually the lesions of PLEVA are smaller. Lymphomatoid papulosis and PLEVA also differ histologically. The former often ulcerates and may develop a central black crust. There is usually a polymorphous

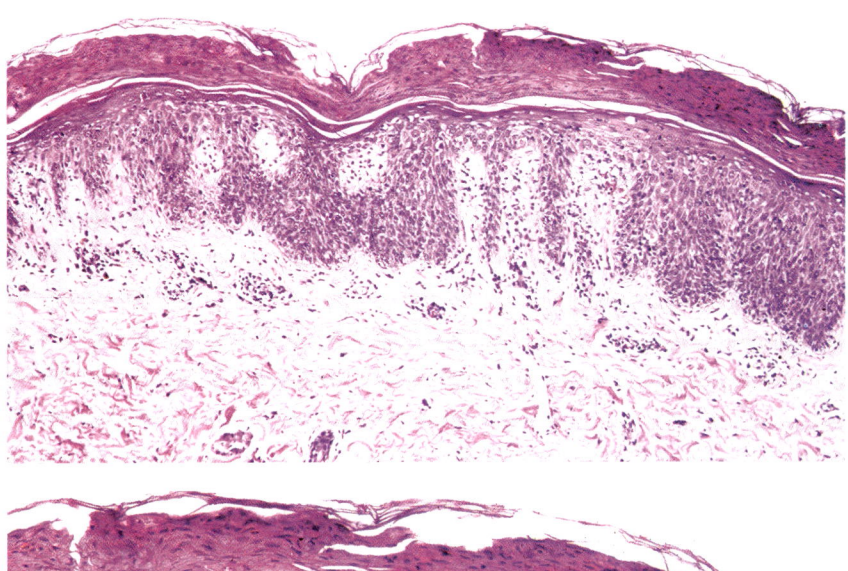

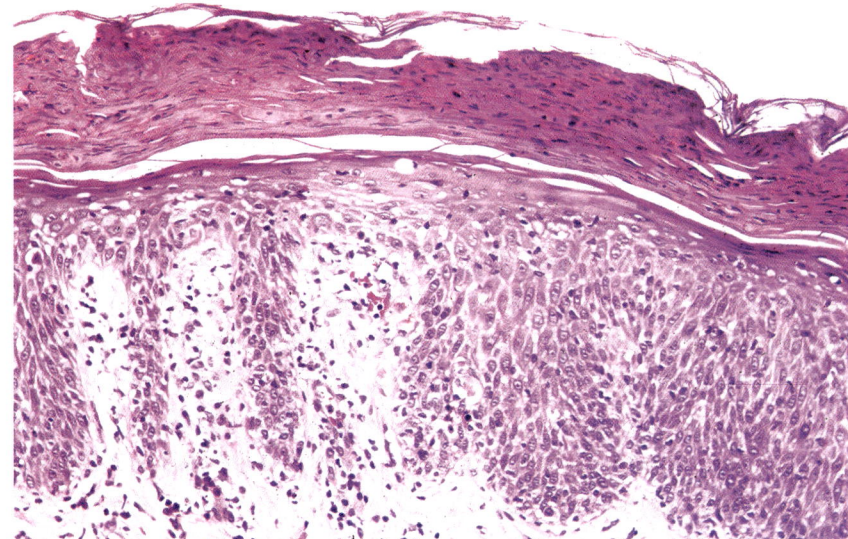

*Interface Dermatitis (Acute Cytotoxic Dermatitis)*

**Figure 6-22**

**PITYRIASIS LICHENOIDES ET VARIOLIFORMIS ACUTA**

Top: In a more advanced lesion, in addition to the acute interface changes, there is prominent parakeratosis infiltrated by neutrophils.

Bottom: At higher magnification, the characteristic epidermal changes of advanced PLEVA are apparent, namely, parakeratosis, infiltration by neutrophils, cells undergoing apoptosis, basal layer vacuolization, interface lymphocytic infiltrate with foci of epidermotropism of lymphocytes, and foci of papillary dermal hemorrhage.

**Figure 6-23**

**LYMPHOCYTIC VASCULITIS IN PLEVA**

The superficial and deep perivascular lymphocytic infiltrates of this disorder are characteristically associated with intense infiltration of venular walls by activated lymphocytes, with associated endothelial degeneration. This "lymphocytic vasculitis" is a helpful diagnostic marker of this condition.

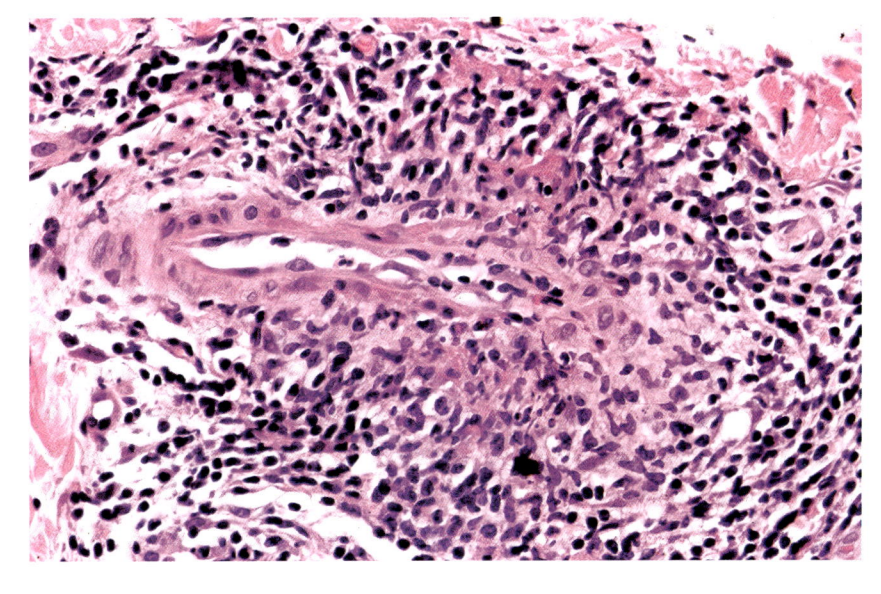

clinical appearance because as early lesions are occurring, others are maturing, and some are spontaneously resolving. Most lesions last only a few weeks, but the eruption may be chronic and recurrent over years; patients go through periods free of lesions during the course of the illness. This disorder has been associated in 10 to 20 percent of patients with an underlying lymphoma, especially mycosis fungoides, CD30-positive large cell anaplastic lymphoma, and Hodgkin disease.

Histologically, lymphomatoid papulosis occurs in several variants, all of which involve considerably more lymphoid atypia than seen in PLEVA. Lymphomatoid papulosis is a disorder that is most appropriately classified as a primary cutaneous CD30-positive T-cell lymphoproliferative disorder, and as such, is not described here in further detail (see World Health Organization [WHO] classification [35]).

**Treatment and Prognosis.** The lesions of PLEVA may heal spontaneously, sometimes with scarring, after a single episode, or multiple relapses may occur over a period of weeks. In some instances, the lesions persist as pityriasis lichenoides chronica. There is no satisfactory therapy for these lesions. Some patients respond to topical steroid preparations (36). In certain cases, oral erythromycin and tetracycline may result in healing of the disorder. Ultraviolet light therapy (UVB and PUVA) and methotrexate have been successful in some patients (37).

## ACUTE CYTOTOXIC GENERALIZED DRUG ERUPTION

**Definition.** *Drug-induced cytotoxic reactions* are adverse reactions to ingested pharmacologic agents that result in features resembling erythema multiforme (38). The reader is referred to the discussion of erythema multiforme for additional clinical and pathologic features.

**Clinical Features.** The clinical features are those of an erythema multiforme-like reaction, but the cutaneous eruption is more generalized and extensive. Iris and target-like patterns are seen, but often without the discrete lesional formation that is associated with the characteristic erythema multiforme associated with herpes infection or as a postherpetic phenomenon. Drug-induced cytotoxic reactions occur in the same distribution, however, and can lead to a Stevens-Johnson–like reaction and toxic epidermal necrolysis. The drugs that are most commonly implicated include sulfonamides and penicillin among the antibiotics, barbiturates, and phenytoin. Phenylbutazone and allopurinol are also associated with this eruption. Carbamazepine, piroxicam, chlormezanone, amithiozone, and some of the more complex sulfa derivatives including dapsone, as well as a variety of other antibiotics, including the cephalosporins, vancomycin, rifampin, and fenbufen, have likewise been associated. Rarely, some of the nonsteroidal, antiinflammatory drugs such as ibuprofen have resulted in this reaction.

**Pathologic Findings.** Cytotoxic drug eruptions are characterized by an interface and a superficial and at least mid-dermal (often deep dermal) angiocentric lymphoid inflammatory infiltrate; they thus represent a hybrid pattern of reactions. The angiocentric component generally contains eosinophils, a characteristic finding of drug eruptions (fig. 6-24). Unlike lichenoid insect-bite reactions, however, interstitial eosinophils are not prominent. The interface lymphoid component is associated with variable basal cell layer vacuolization, and may resemble the changes of erythema multiforme or acute active fixed drug eruption. Focal spongiosis is also occasionally present, emphasizing the characteristic feature of hybrid or mixed immune patterns (e.g., conventional spongiotic delayed hypersensitivity and cytotoxic immune reaction).

**Differential Diagnosis.** The differential diagnosis includes all of the drug-related causes of the erythema multiforme/Stevens-Johnson syndrome/toxic epidermal necrolysis. Bullous pemphigoid must be considered as well if bullous lesions are present. Linear IgA bullous dermatoses simulate some of these reactions.

**Treatment and Prognosis.** The withdrawal of the offending agent is paramount to recovery. Care must be taken to choose a drug that does not cross-react with the inciting agent. For severe cases, the use of oral prednisone may be necessary. Topical measures, such as soaks and corticosteroids, may be helpful.

## FIXED DRUG ERUPTION (ACTIVE PHASE)

**Definition.** A *fixed drug eruption* is both clinically and histologically distinctive (39–41). As the name implies, the lesion occurs repeatedly at

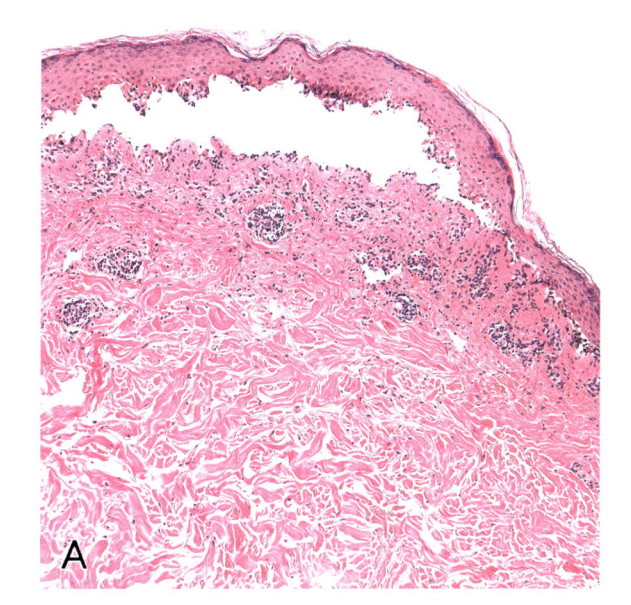

*Interface Dermatitis (Acute Cytotoxic Dermatitis)*

Figure 6-24

**CYTOTOXIC DRUG ERUPTION**

A: There is a subepidermal blister associated with a superficial epidermal lymphoid infiltrate.

B: At higher magnification, the skin adjacent to the blister shows a lymphoid infiltrate with occasional admixed eosinophils and prominent basal layer apoptosis.

C: Oil immersion magnification of effector-target interactions in cytotoxic drug eruption. Lymphocytes and eosinophils are in direct apposition to target keratinocytes undergoing apoptotic changes.

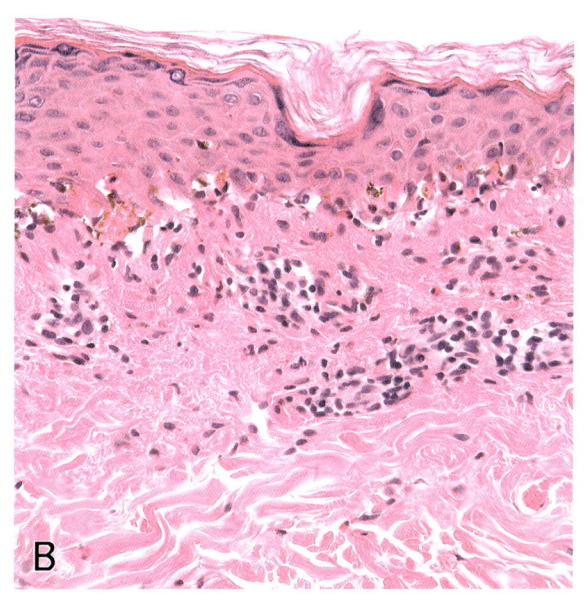

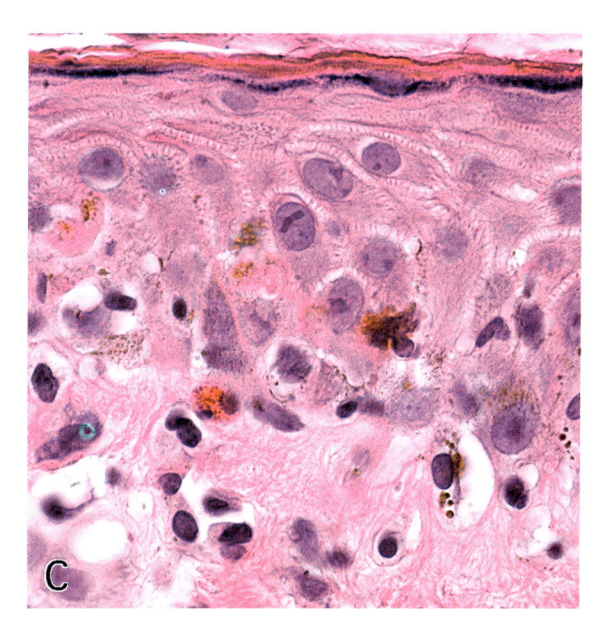

the same site after drug ingestion. Common offenders include trimethoprim-sulfamethoxazole, aspirin, tetracycline, phenolphthalein, phenylbutazone, and an extensive list of other pharmaceutical agents, including oral contraceptives.

**Clinical Features.** In the early phases, patients present with a pruritic, sometimes vesicular, plaque or multiple plaques, associated with a history of recurrence following the ingestion of a specific drug. In chronic cases, the patient has a pigmented lesion and the nature of the drug reaction is not apparent until a careful history is obtained of symptoms at the site that are intermittent and can be linked to an ingestant. The first reports of this by Bourns and Brocq described lesions due to antipyrine; in one report, the patient presented with multiple lesions (over 100) that were diagnosed as erythema multiforme originally (41a,41b).

The earliest lesion is an erythematous plaque that shows vesicles or even bullae, or may be eroded. Sometimes it is only a pruritic red raised area. This usually occurs within hours after the ingestion of a drug in a previously sensitive person. After the subsidence of the erythema of the initial lesion, the macule becomes progressively

*Inflammatory Disorders of the Skin*

**Figure 6-25**

**FIXED DRUG ERUPTION**

The solitary erythematous plaque has a characteristic hyperpigmented central zone, correlating with repeated cytotoxic insults to this site and resulting in melanin pigment incontinence.

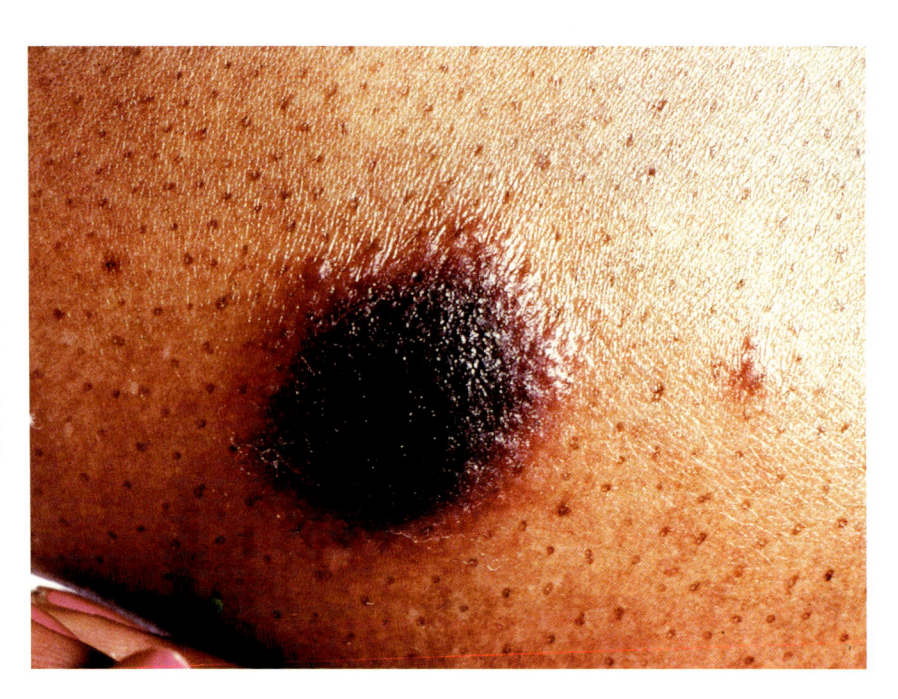

pigmented with each recurrent episode (fig. 6-25). The size of the lesion varies from a few millimeters to up to 20 cm in greatest diameter. Lesions are usually eroded and painful, especially those in genital and mucosal sites. They occur anywhere on the skin or mucosae, but the genitalia are preferentially involved; however, they have been noted in the conjunctiva, oral pharynx, vulva, and even vagina.

The offending drugs are many and include most commonly antimicrobial agents, especially sulfonamides; many antiinflammatory agents, including especially phenylbutazone and phenacetin; and various neuropsychiatric agents including fiorinal, quinine, and phenolphthalein. The reaction is also induced by additive coloring agents in food: the yellow dye in certain liquors, the phenolphthalein in maraschino cherries, and the quinine in tonic water are agents that elicit the reaction primarily or as a cross-reaction to another drug.

**Pathologic Findings.** Histologically, there is an interface (i.e., acute cytotoxic) pattern of lymphocytic infiltration within the papillary dermis, along with a superficial and at least mid-dermal perivascular lymphocytic infiltrate (fig. 6-26). Occasional eosinophils and activated histiocytes are admixed within the infiltrate. At higher magnification, lymphocytes are seen along a vacuolated dermal-epidermal junction, which may show colloid body (apoptotic keratinocyte) formation. Lymphocytes also migrate into the epidermis, where they are associated with dead and dying keratinocytes, a finding similar to that seen in erythema multiforme but different and distinctive in that there are clusters of such cells in the mid-epidermis in fixed drug eruption. The etiology of this phenomenon is unclear but may be related to antigen presentation by Langerhans cells (41c). In active as well as inactive lesions, there is often striking incontinence of melanin pigment within the underlying papillary dermis (figs. 6-27, 6-28).

**Differential Diagnosis.** Any cytotoxic dermatitis may result in marked papillary dermal deposition of melanin pigment in constitutively deeply pigmented skin; therefore, the finding of pigment incontinence need not indicate repeated insult or chronicity. The primary differential concern is interface dermatitis occurring in racial groups where papillary dermal melanophages may acutely mimic the characteristic pigment incontinence that develops only after repeated flares of the fixed drug eruption. This emphasizes the importance of basic clinical information, including gender, age, site, and constitutive degree of epidermal pigmentation, when assessing biopsies of inflammatory skin disease. Other diagnostic considerations include an early lichen planus–like reaction with

*Interface Dermatitis (Acute Cytotoxic Dermatitis)*

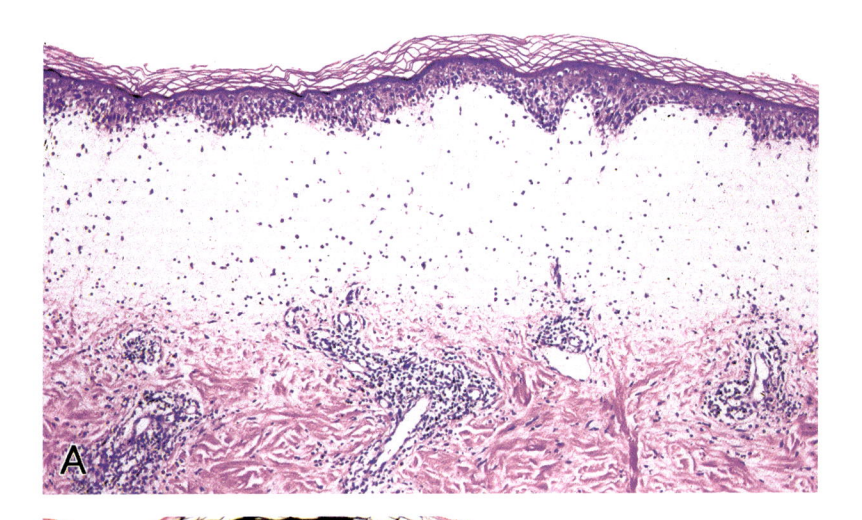

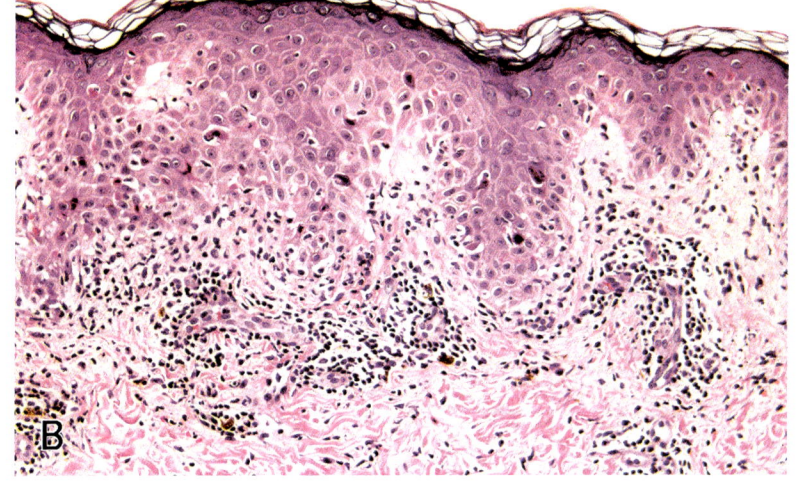

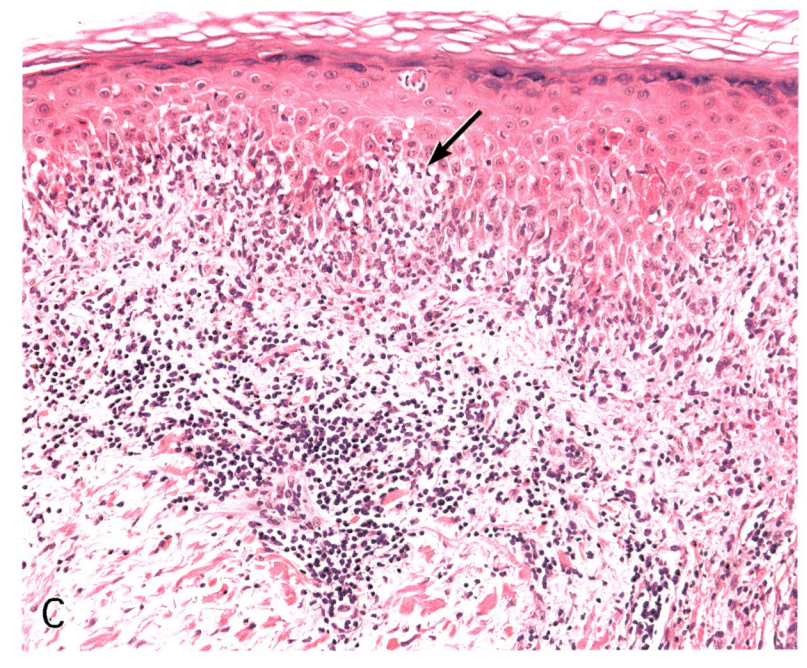

**Figure 6-26**

**FIXED DRUG ERUPTION**

A: The unremarkable epidermis, replete with a normal basket-weave stratum corneum, surmounts a zone of marked papillary dermal edema in an early stage lesion. The underlying perivascular inflammatory infiltrate and the tagging pattern of lymphocytes along the dermal-epidermal junction are seen.

B: Lymphocytes infiltrate the dermal-epidermal junction, with focal migration of lymphocytes into the epidermal layer in a more advanced lesion. The basal layer is vacuolated, and numerous apoptotic cells, some in clusters, are present within the epidermis.

C: There is a prominent superficial lymphocytic infiltrate with scattered eosinophils, brisk interface change, and clusters of apoptotic cells (arrow) within the affected epidermis.

## Inflammatory Disorders of the Skin

**Figure 6-27**

**FIXED DRUG ERUPTION: PIGMENT INCONTINENCE**

This active lesion, characterized by an interface of lymphocytes with attendant injury to the epidermal layer, is also associated with an accumulation of melanophages within the papillary dermis, evidence of previous cytotoxic insult to the basal cell layer at this site.

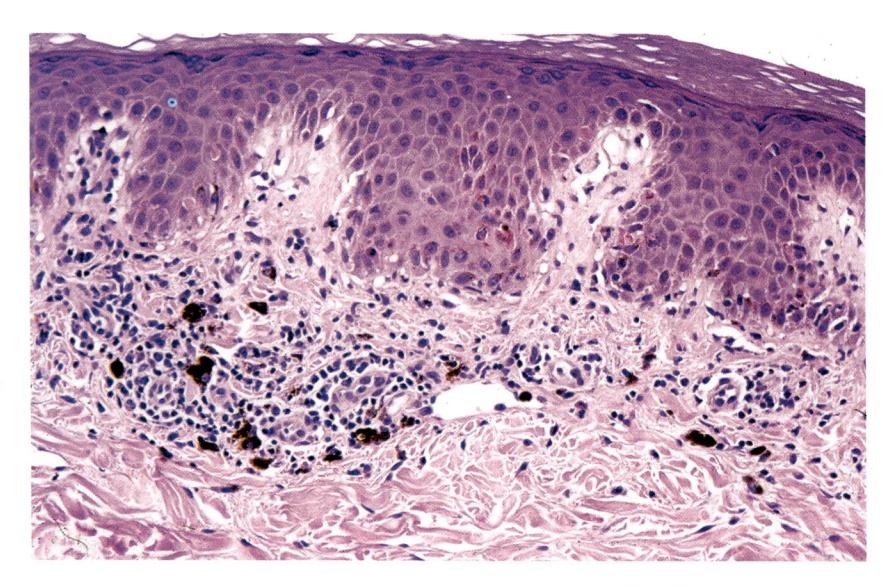

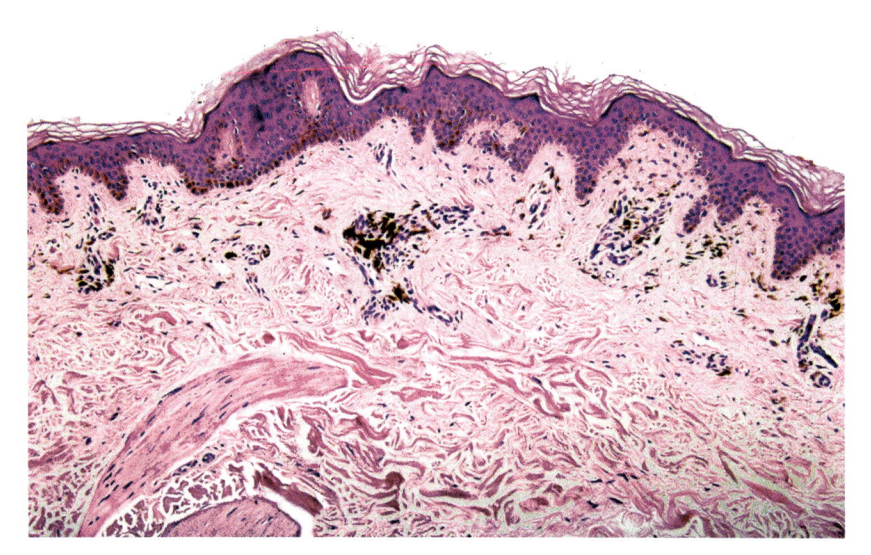

**Figure 6-28**

**FIXED DRUG ERUPTION: INACTIVE**

Evidence of active interface dermatitis is absent. Residual melanin pigment incontinence is present within the papillary dermis (postinflammatory hyperpigmentation).

pigment incontinence, a regressed pigmented lesion, and entities such as "ashy dermatosis" (erythema dyschromicum perstans), which can be eliminated by clinical correlation. Sometimes, only a careful history and documentation that the same sites become symptomatic at every episode result in the correct diagnosis.

**Treatment and Prognosis.** While topical antiinflammatory agents may be helpful in active stages, the primary goal of treatment is the identification and avoidance of offending agents. Topical measures for acute lesions include soaks and local corticosteroids. Doxepin may help with symptoms. Local depigmentary agents such as hydroquinone are useful for chronic lesions. Fixed drug eruptions result from a plethora of agents, including those not generally perceived as drugs and therefore not elicited in a patient history (e.g., aspirin, oral contraceptives). Moreover, in some patients it is possible that endogenous factors play a role. We have observed one patient, for example, who developed a fixed drug eruption coincident with each flare of multiple sclerosis.

## INTERFACE DERMATITIS OF HUMAN IMMUNODEFICIENCY VIRUS

**Definition.** Patients infected with *human immunodeficiency virus* (HIV) or who present with acquired immunodeficiency syndrome (AIDS) or AIDS-related complex (ARC) may develop generalized maculopapular exanthems that

## Interface Dermatitis (Acute Cytotoxic Dermatitis)

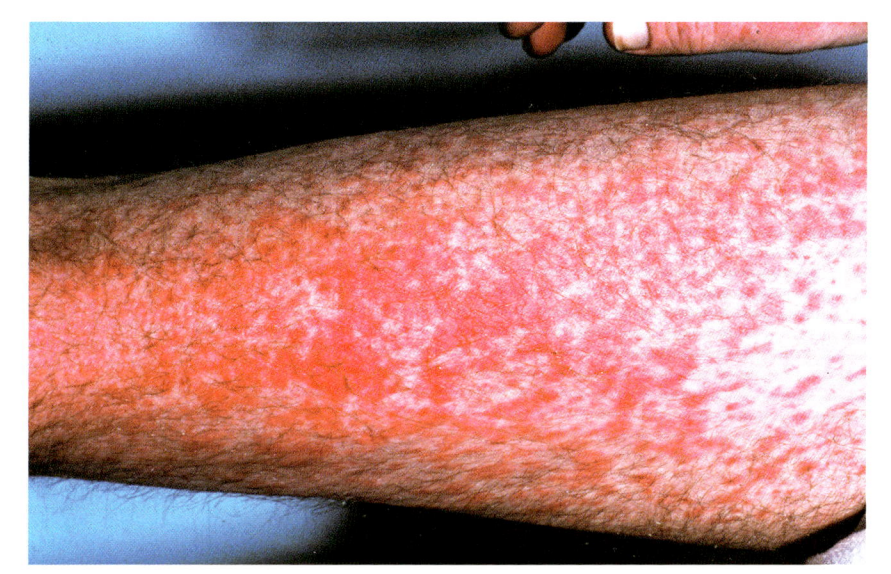

**Figure 6-29**

**LICHENOID ERUPTION IN ACQUIRED IMMUNODEFICIENCY SYNDROME (AIDS)**

The maculopapular exanthem gives rise to differential diagnostic possibilities of a viral rash or drug eruption.

resemble morbilliform drug eruptions and viral exanthems (42,43). Unlike drug eruptions or viral rashes occurring in immunologically intact individuals, these lesions closely resemble the alterations characteristic of acute GVHD. Interestingly, there are a number of immunologic similarities between bone marrow recipients experiencing acute GVHD and patients with AIDS. A similar eruption has been described in simian immunodeficiency virus (SIV)-infected macaques, indicating that not all such eruptions are superficial drug eruptions in immunocompromised individuals (43a). In this experimental model, cytotoxic T cells appear to be targeting epidermal Langerhans cells, which become infected with the retrovirus.

**Clinical Features.** Patients generally present with nonspecific morbilliform eruptions resembling drug-related exanthems. The papules are widespread over the trunk and extremities (fig. 6-29). They wax and wane. The lesions are characteristic in their presentation as being an eruptive type of flat-topped papular exanthem.

**Pathologic Findings.** Histologically, there is a sparse papillary dermal infiltrate of lymphocytes and occasionally rare plasma cells associated with often marked basal cell layer vacuolization and keratinocyte necrosis (fig. 6-30). Satellitosis, in which epidermotropic lymphocytes surround dead and dying keratinocytes, is frequently encountered. The epidermal layer may show focal parakeratosis and evidence of disordered maturation (i.e., irregularity in maturation from the vertically oriented cells of the stratum basalis to the horizontally oriented cells of the uppermost stratum corneum).

**Differential Diagnosis.** The differential diagnosis of interface dermatitis of AIDS includes secondary syphilis, drug eruption, viral exanthem, erythema multiforme, and acute GVHD, especially if the patient has received nonirradiated blood products within 100 days of onset. Lesional skin biopsies in GVHD generally do not contain plasma cells, and occlusive endothelial activation as seen in secondary syphilis is not typical of the lichenoid dermatitis of AIDS. This latter condition may be difficult to differentiate from syphilis, however, particularly because AIDS patients may have seronegative syphilis. Although certain drug eruptions have an interface pattern, they generally contain eosinophils, a finding not observed in interface dermatitis of AIDS. Nonspecific viral exanthems often show a sparse superficial perivascular lymphocytic infiltrate with foci of perivascular hemorrhage, and usually no cytotoxic alterations within the epidermal layer. The targetoid lesions of erythema multiforme are not seen in interface dermatitis of AIDS.

Biopsy specimens of dermatitis from patients with known or suspected immunodeficiency may harbor other alterations indicative of contemporaneous infection or infestation within epidermal and dermal components. For example, infection with cytomegalovirus or atypical mycobacteria may superimpose unrelated cutaneous pathology in skin lesions (fig. 6-31).

## Inflammatory Disorders of the Skin

**Figure 6-30**

**INTERFACE ERUPTION IN AIDS**

The interface change resembles acute GVHD or erythema multiforme, although other alterations, such as parakeratosis and acanthosis, may be observed.

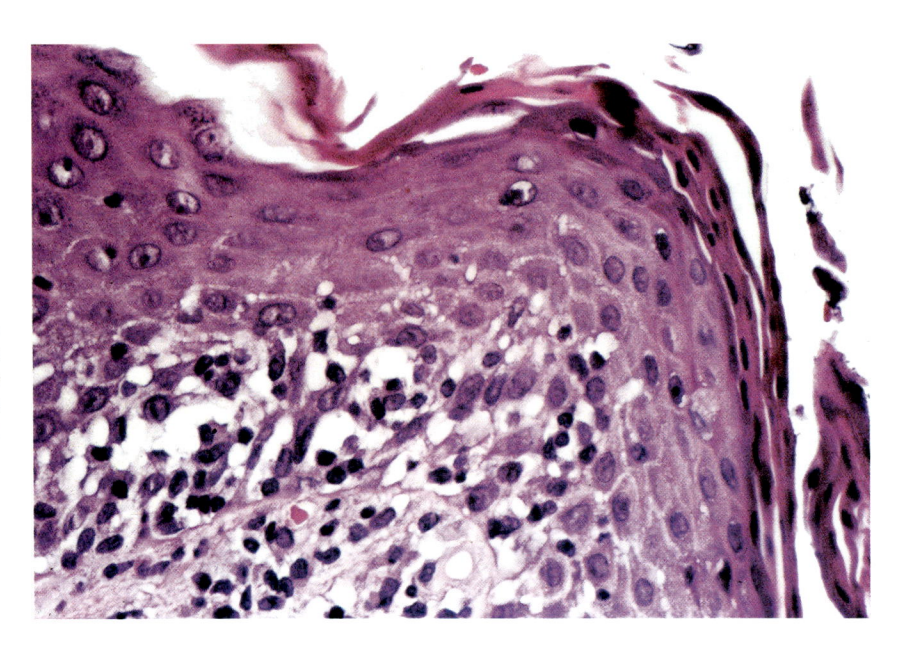

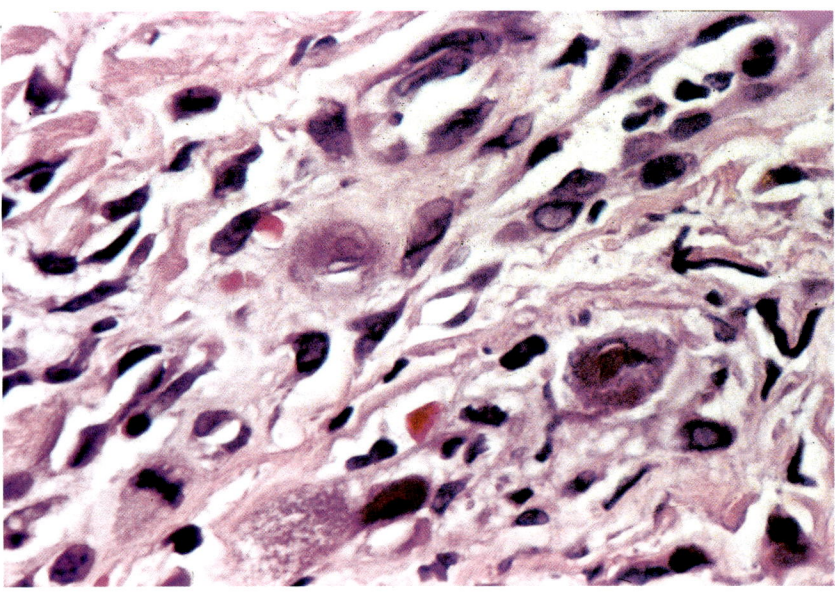

**Figure 6-31**

**INTERFACE ERUPTION IN AIDS**

The inflammatory component should be inspected closely for evidence of associated pathology or infection. In this case, inclusions of cytomegalovirus are observed in occasional dermal cells.

**Treatment and Prognosis.** The rash is generally self-limiting. Its significance resides in its potential biological relationship to cytotoxic attack against HIV-infected cells, and the potential for HIV infection to initially present as a cytotoxic skin rash.

### PARANEOPLASTIC PEMPHIGUS

**Definition.** *Paraneoplastic pemphigus* consists of oral erosions and a complex skin eruption that includes erythematous plaques, blisters, and erythema multiforme–like lesions. It is associated with lymphoproliferative disorders and thymoma (44–49).

**Clinical Features.** Patients present with a variety of skin lesions. Some of them resemble erythema multiforme, others subacute lupus erythematosus, others eczematous conditions, all of which finally result in blistering and erosions. Oral lesions, often eroded, are the second manifestation of the disease (fig. 6-32).

**Pathologic Findings.** An erythema multiforme–like acute interface dermatitis is combined with features of pemphigus vulgaris.

*Interface Dermatitis (Acute Cytotoxic Dermatitis)*

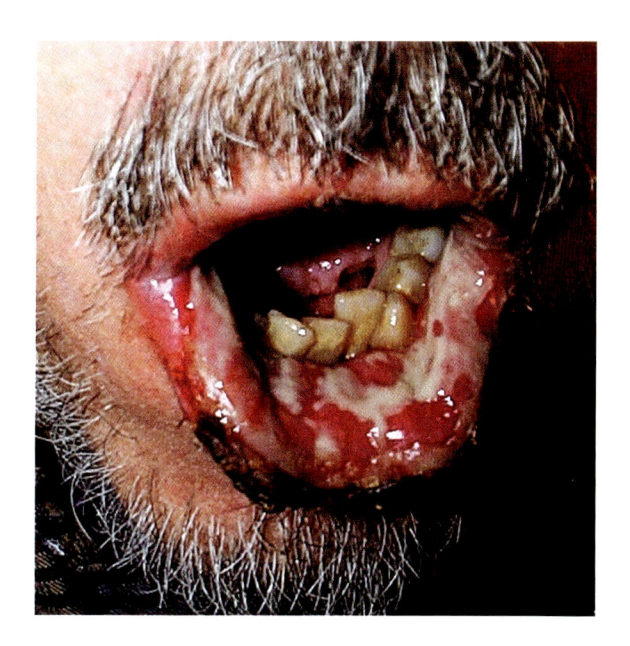

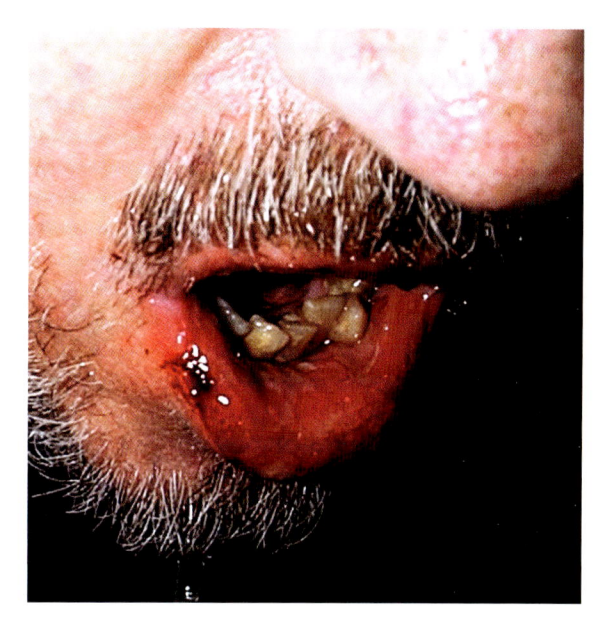

Figure 6-32

PARANEOPLASTIC PEMPHIGUS

Left: The epithelium and mucosa of the lip show multiple erosions and areas of leukoplakia associated with necrotic blister roofs.

Right: In the healing phase, there is some degree of re-epithelialization, although scabbed erosions persist focally.

Accordingly, there is basal cell layer vacuolization, keratinocyte apoptosis, acantholysis, and exocytosis of lymphocytes within the lowermost epidermal layers (fig. 6-33). Direct immunofluorescence shows a pemphigus-like pattern of intercellular deposition of IgG and C3, as well as granular deposition of these immune reactants along the dermal-epidermal interface. Serum characteristically reacts by indirect immunofluorescence to both stratified squamous epithelial substrates (e.g., monkey esophagus) and nonstratified epithelium (rodent urinary bladder). This indicates reactivity to intracytoplasmic desmoplakins, which are expressed by both stratified and nonstratified epithelial surfaces, in contradistinction to desmosomal proteins (desmogleins), which are the targets of classic pemphigus and are expressed only by stratified squamous epithelium.

**Differential Diagnosis.** The unique combination of histologic and immunologic features limits the differential diagnosis. Diagnostic difficulty is generally related only to problems in the sampling of lesions, or lack of knowledge concerning this rare but important form of interface dermatitis.

**Treatment and Prognosis.** The patients may respond to treatment of the underlying disorder, which includes lymphoma, leukemia, certain sarcomas, breast cancer, thymoma, and Castleman disease (50). Most commonly, the disease course is independent of the associated malignancy. The patient may enter oncologic remission, but continue to suffer from paraneoplastic pemphigus, which is now considered to be a paraneoplastic autoimmune multiorgan syndrome (PAMS). Stomatitis tends to be the most recalcitrant symptom. Patients are treated with systemic corticosteroids, methotrexate, and advanced immunosuppressants such as tacrolimus. Wound care and dental care are paramount. The development of bronchiolitis obliterans–like lung disease often imparts a poor prognosis. Only a few patients have survived a year following the onset of lung disease, which often necessitates severely immunosuppressive regimens with agents such as rituximab, alemtuzumab, or daclizumab.

*Inflammatory Disorders of the Skin*

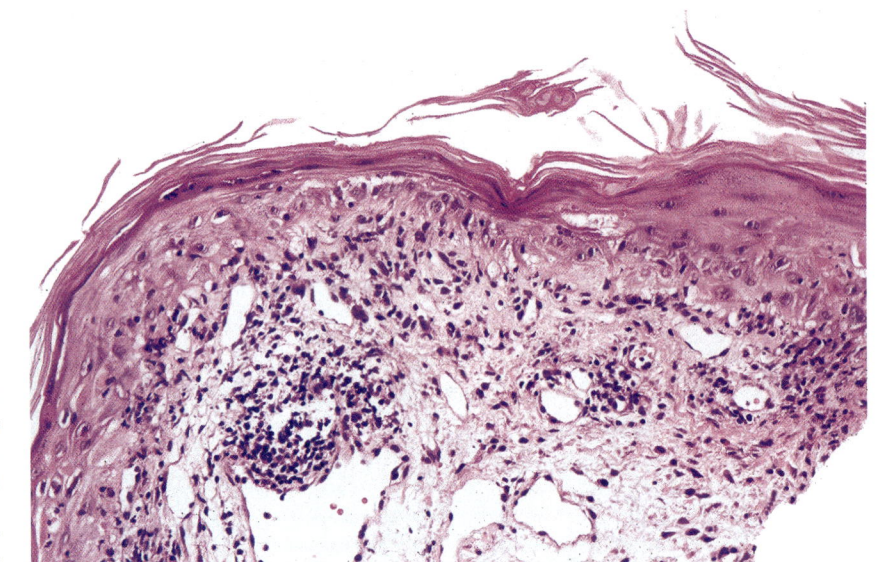

**Figure 6-33**

**PARANEOPLASTIC PEMPHIGUS**

Top: The interface infiltrate of lymphocytes along the dermal-epidermal junction is associated with epidermal alterations, including the formation of cleft-like spaces due to acantholysis-like alterations.

Bottom: High magnification shows the accumulation of lymphocytes along a vacuolated dermal-epidermal interface. The underlying epidermis shows foci of spongiosis. Pigment incontinence is observed within the underlying papillary dermis.

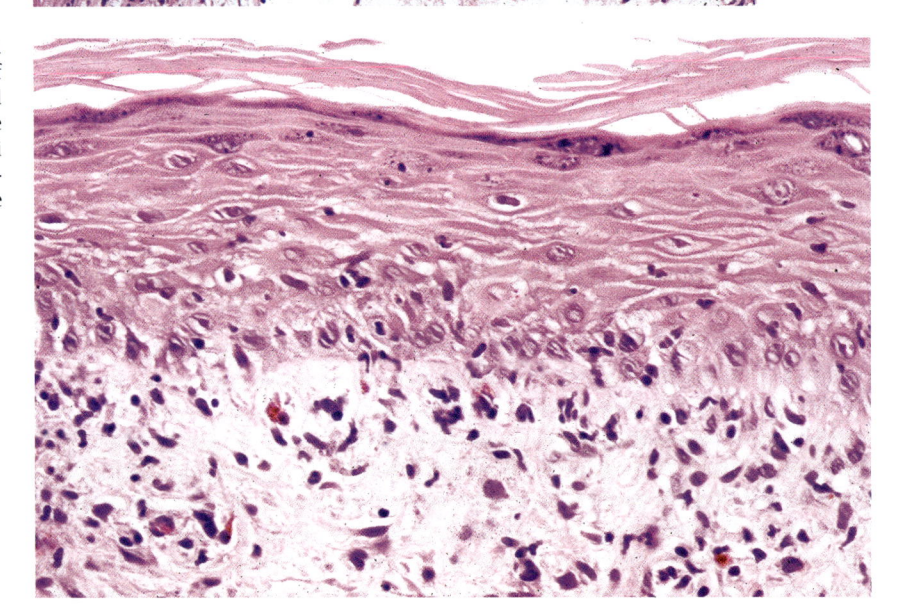

## REFERENCES

1. Yada S, Takamura N, Inagaki-Ohara K, et al. The role of p53 and Fas in a model of acute murine graft-versus-host disease. J Immunol 2005;174:1291-7.
2. Murphy GF, Korngold R. Significance of selectively targeted apoptotic rete cells in graft-versus-host disease. Biol Blood Marrow Transplant 2004;10:357-65.
3. Williams PM, Conklin RJ. Erythema multiforme: a review and contrast from Stevens-Johnson syndrome/toxic epidermal necrolysis. Dent Clin North Am 2005;49:67-76.
4. Ramrakha-Jones VS, Tillman D. Erythema multiforme and erythema nodosum. Practitioner 2001;245:940-1.

5. Micali G, Linthicum K, Han N, West DP. Increased risk of erythema multiforme major with combination anticonvulsant and radiation therapies. Pharmacotherapy 1999;19:223-7.
6. Letko E, Papaliodis DN, Papaliodis GN, Daoud YJ, Ahmed AR, Foster CS. Stevens-Johnson syndrome and toxic epidermal necrolysis: a review of the literature. Ann Allergy Asthma Immunol 2005;94:419-36.
7. Prendiville J. Stevens-Johnson syndrome and toxic epidermal necrolysis. Adv Dermatol 2002;18:151-73.
8. Fritsch PO, Sidoroff A. Drug-induced Stevens-Johnson syndrome/toxic epidermal necrolysis. Am J Clin Dermatol 2000;1:349-60.
9. Wolkenstein P, Revuz J. Toxic epidermal necrolysis. Dermatol Clin. 2000 Jul;18:485-95.
10. Wolf R, Ruocco V, Jablonska S. Treatment of toxic epidermal necrolysis syndrome with "disease-modifying" drugs: the controversy goes on. Clin Dermatol 2004;22:267-9.
11. Majumdar S, Mockenhaupt M, Roujeau J, Townshend A. Interventions for toxic epidermal necrolysis. Cochrane Database Syst Rev 2002: CD001435.
12. Ghislain PD, Roujeau JC. Treatment of severe drug reactions: Stevens-Johnson syndrome, toxic epidermal necrolysis and hypersensitivity syndrome. Dermatol Online J 2002;8:5.
13. Stern RS. Improving the outcome of patients with toxic epidermal necrolysis and Stevens-Johnson syndrome. Arch Dermatol 2000;136:410-1.
14. Ruetter A, Luger TA. Efficacy and safety of intravenous immunoglobulin for immune-mediated skin disease: current view. Am J Clin Dermatol 2004;5:153-60.
15. Metry DW, Jung P, Levy ML. Use of intravenous immunoglobulin in children with Stevens-Johnson syndrome and toxic epidermal necrolysis: seven cases and review of the literature. Pediatrics 2003;112(Pt 1):1430-6.
16. Bachot N, Roujeau JC. Intravenous immunoglobulins in the treatment of severe drug eruptions. Curr Opin Allergy Clin Immunol 2003;3:269-74.
17. Rutter A, Luger TA. Intravenous immunoglobulin: an emerging treatment for immune-mediated skin diseases. Curr Opin Investig Drugs 2002;3:713-9.
18. Mielcarek M, Storb R. Graft-vs-host disease after non-myeloablative hematopoietic cell transplantation. Leuk Lymphoma 2005;46:1251-60.
19. Vargas-Diez E, Garcia-Diez A, Marin A, Fernandez-Herrera J. Life-threatening graft-vs-host disease. Clin Dermatol 2005;23:285-300.
20. Jaksch M, Mattsson J. The pathophysiology of acute graft-versus-host disease. Scand J Immunol 2005;61:398-409.
21. Couriel D, Caldera H, Champlin R, Komanduri K. Acute graft-versus-host disease: pathophysiology, clinical manifestations, and management. Cancer 2004;101:1936-46.
22. Davies JK, Lowdell MW. New advances in acute graft-versus-host disease prophylaxis. Transfus Med 2003;13:387-97.
23. Ferrara JL, Cooke KR, Teshima T. The pathophysiology of acute graft-versus-host disease. Int J Hematol 2003;78:181-7.
23a. Murphy GF, Lavker RM, Whitaker D, Korngold R. Cytotoxic folliculitis in GVHD. Evidence of follicular stem cell injury and recovery. J Cutan Pathol 1991;18:309-14.
24. Penas PF, Fernandez-Herrera J, Garcia-Diez A. Dermatologic treatment of cutaneous graft versus host disease. Am J Clin Dermatol 2004;5:403-16.
25. Devetten MP, Vose JM. Graft-versus-host disease: how to translate new insights into new therapeutic strategies. Biol Blood Marrow Transplant 2004;10:815-25.
26. Zeiser R, Marks R, Bertz H, Finke J. Immunopathogenesis of acute graft-versus-host disease: implications for novel preventive and therapeutic strategies. Ann Hematol 2004;83:551-65.
27. Antin JH, Chen AR, Couriel DR, Ho VT, Nash RA, Weisdorf D. Novel approaches to the therapy of steroid-resistant acute graft-versus-host disease. Biol Blood Marrow Transplant 2004;10:655-68.
28. Bacigalupo A, Palandri F. Management of acute graft versus host disease (GvHD). Hematol J 2004;5:189-96.
29. Kempf W, Kutzner H, Kettelhack N, Palmedo G, Burg G. Paraneoplastic pityriasis lichenoides in cutaneous lymphoma: case report and review of the literature on paraneoplastic reactions of the skin in lymphoma and leukaemia. Br J Dermatol 2005;152:1327-31.
30. Tsianakas A, Hoeger PH. Transition of pityriasis lichenoides et varioliformis acuta to febrile ulceronecrotic Mucha-Habermann disease is associated with elevated serum tumour necrosis factor-alpha. Br J Dermatol 2005;152:794-9.
31. Ito N, Ohshima A, Hashizume H, Takigawa M, Tokura Y. Febrile ulceronecrotic Mucha-Habermann's disease managed with methylprednisolone semipulse and subsequent methotrexate therapies. J Am Acad Dermatol 2003;49:1142-8.
32. Yang CC, Lee JY, Chen W. Febrile ulceronecrotic Mucha-Habermann disease with extensive skin necrosis in intertriginous areas. Eur J Dermatol 2003;13:493-6.

33. Rivera R, Ortiz P, Rodriguez-Peralto JL, Vanaclocha F, Iglesias L. Febrile ulceronecrotic pityriasis lichenoides et varioliformis acuta with atypical cells. Int J Dermatol 2003;42:26-8.
34. Van Neer FJ, Toonstra J, Van Voorst Vader PC, Willemze R, Van Vloten WA. Lymphomatoid papulosis in children: a study of 10 children registered by the Dutch Cutaneous Lymphoma Working Group. Br J Dermatol 2001;144:351-4.
35. Willemze R, Jaffe ES, Burg G, et al. WHO-EORTC classification for cutaneous lymphomas. Blood 2005;105:3768-3785.
36. Simon D, Boudny C, Nievergelt H, Simon HU, Braathen LR. Successful treatment of pityriasis lichenoides with topical tacrolimus. Br J Dermatol 2004;150:1033-5.
37. Gardlo K, Mahnke N, Megahed M, Ruzicka T, Neumann NJ. [PUVA therapy of severe-course pityriasis lichenoides et varioliformis acuta.] Hautarzt 2003;54:984-5. [German]
38. Roujeau JC. Clinical heterogeneity of drug hypersensitivity. Toxicology. 2005;209:123-9.
39. Izumi A, Katsumi S, Kobayashi N, Niizeki H, Asada H, Miyagawa S. Bucillamine-induced toxic epidermal necrolysis and fixed drug eruption. J Dermatol 2005;32:397-401.
40. Shiohara T, Mizukawa Y, Teraki Y. Pathophysiology of fixed drug eruption: the role of skin-resident T cells. Curr Opin Allergy Clin Immunol 2002;2:317-23.
41. Lee AY. Fixed drug eruptions. Incidence, recognition, and avoidance. Am J Clin Dermatol 2000;1:277-85.
41a. Bourns DC. Unusual effects of antipyrine. Br Med J 1889;2:218-20.
41b. Brocq L. Eruption érythemato-pigmentée fixe due a l'antipyrine. Ann Dermatol Syphiligr (Paris) 1894;5:308-13.
43c. Murphy GF, Guillén FJ, Flynn TC. Cytotoxic T lymphocytes and phenotypically abnormal epidermal dendritic cells in fixed cutaneous eruptions. Hum Pathol 1985;16:1264-71.
42. Rico MJ, Kory WP, Gould EW, Penneys NS. Interface dermatitis in patients with the acquired immunodeficiency syndrome. J Am Acad Dermatol 1987;16:1209-18.
43. Lapins J, Lindback S, Lidbrink P, Biberfeld P, Emtestam L, Gaines H. Mucocutaneous manifestations in 22 consecutive cases of primary HIV-1 infection. Br J Dermatol 1996;134:257-61.
43a. Ringler DJ, Hancock WW, King NW, et al. Immunophenotypic characterization of the cutaneous exanthem of SIV-infected rhesus monkeys. Apposition of degenerative Langerhans cells and cytotoxic lymphocytes during the development of acquired immunodeficiency syndrome. Am J Pathol 1987;126:199-207.
44. Stone SP, Buescher LS. Life-threatening paraneoplastic cutaneous syndromes. Clin Dermatol 2005;23:301-6.
45. Coelho S, Reis JP, Tellechea O, Figueiredo A, Black M. Paraneoplastic pemphigus with clinical features of lichen planus associated with low-grade B cell lymphoma. Int J Dermatol 2005;44:366-71.
46. Wade MS, Black MM. Paraneoplastic pemphigus: a brief update. Australas J Dermatol 2005;46:1-8.
47. Anhalt GJ. Paraneoplastic pemphigus. J Investig Dermatol Symp Proc 2004;9:29-33.
48. Hashimoto T. Immunopathology of paraneoplastic pemphigus. Clin Dermatol 2001;19:675-82.
49. Kimyai-Asadi A, Jih MH. Paraneoplastic pemphigus. Int J Dermatol 2001;40:367-72.
50. Allen CM, Camisa C. Paraneoplastic pemphigus: a review of the literature. Oral Dis 2000;6:208-14.
51. Heizmann M, Itin P, Wernli M, Borradori L, Bargetzi MJ. Successful treatment of paraneoplastic pemphigus in follicular NHL with rituximab: report of a case and review of treatment for paraneoplastic pemphigus in NHL and CLL. Am J Hematol 2001;66:142-4.

# 7  LICHENOID DERMATITIS (SUBACUTE TO CHRONIC CYTOTOXIC DERMATITIS)

## GENERAL CONSIDERATIONS

Chronic cytotoxicity is manifested by abnormal keratinization (i.e., dyskeratosis), cell death with mummification of cytoplasmic contents (i.e., colloid body formation), and altered cellular maturation for a specific epidermal stratum (i.e., squamatization of the basal cell layer). These chronic alterations, usually concentrated at the dermal-epidermal junction, and associated with epidermal changes and hyperkeratosis, produce scaling papules and plaques that have been compared to the lichen that grows on the surface of tree trunks, and hence the term, *lichenoid dermatitis,* for this group of disorders (1–3).

## PATHOGENESIS

As with acute cytotoxic dermatitis, the underlying causes of most forms of chronic cytotoxic dermatitis are protean, although it is generally assumed that autoantigens within the epidermal layer provoke an autoimmune reaction directed against keratinocytes. In connective tissue disorders such as lupus erythematosus, the primary abnormality appears to reside in the effector pathway, with immune recognition and attack directed against epitopes that normally are exempt from host surveillance. In situations such as lichen planus, it is unclear whether target or effector pathways are the primary stimulants for lesion formation.

With the chronicity of cytotoxic epidermal injury, there may be progressive squamatization and dyskeratosis of the basal cell layer, apoptosis, melanin pigment incontinence, epidermotropism of lymphocytes with apposition to degenerating keratinocytes (when lymphocytes surround a target keratinocyte, a phenomenon termed satellitosis), and abnormalities of the stratum corneum (hyperkeratosis and/or parakeratosis). In certain lesions, the dermal-epidermal interface is so compromised that microscopic zones of cleft-like separation or even clinical bullae are formed.

## SPECIAL DIAGNOSTIC STUDIES

Special diagnostic studies for subacute to chronic forms of cytotoxic dermatitis generally involve direct immunofluorescence. For example, lichen planus usually shows nonspecific yet characteristic reactivity for immunoglobulins (particularly immunoglobulin [Ig]M) within apoptotic bodies at the dermal-epidermal interface and within the superficial dermis (Civatte bodies). Lupus erythematosus is characterized by a positive band test along the dermal-epidermal interface (see below), although both false positives and false negatives exist, and serologic evaluation is often required for assessment of systemic disease. Histochemical stains for spirochetes (e.g., Warthin-Starry stain) are often obtained for the assessment of lichenoid secondary syphilis, although unlike the primary chancre, organisms are generally not detected at this stage.

## ANIMAL MODELS

Potentially the most informative and relevant model for lichenoid dermatitis, as well as a variety of other human skin disorders, involves human skin xenografted to the backs of genetically immunocompromised mice (SCID mice). Intradermal injection of heterologous human peripheral blood mononuclear cells results in allostimulation in situ, and eventual development of an eruption that shows striking similarities to epidermal-type chronic graft-versus-host disease (GVHD) and lichen planus (4). This model indicates that lichenoid tissue pathology may be duplicated by allostimulation directed against skin antigens, and further supports the autoimmune nature of many forms of naturally occurring disease.

## LICHEN PLANUS

**Definition.** *Lichen planus* is a form of chronic cytotoxic dermatitis that classically consists of pruritic, pink to purple, polygonal papules (5,6).

**Clinical Features.** This uncommon disorder affecting middle-aged adults presents as crops

# Inflammatory Disorders of the Skin

**Figure 7-1**

**LICHEN PLANUS**

There are numerous flat, pruritic papules which form hyperkeratotic plaques. In this case, marked associated hyperpigmentation has resulted from chronic pigment incontinence, a consequence of the degree constitutive melanization in this patient.

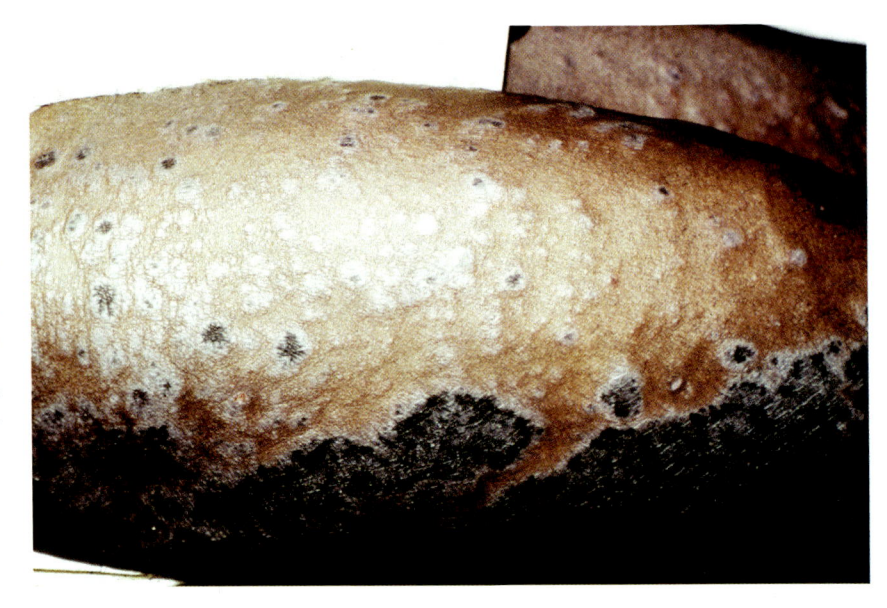

of flat-topped papules, often arranged in linear configuration, presumably elicited at sites of trauma (i.e., Koebner phenomenon). The surface of an individual lesion shows delicate white lines known as Wickham striae. These correlate with hyperplastic rete ridges, which intimately interdigitate with dermal papillae replete with lymphocytes. Coalescence of individual papules may result in plaques that mimic psoriasis or other forms of chronic dermatitis (fig. 7-1). Lesions involving the buccal mucosa or genital skin may be painful and a source of significant morbidity (7–13). Nail involvement also occurs (14–16). The course varies from short to chronic, although most cases resolve within 12 months.

The pathogenesis of lichen planus remains obscure. Leading hypotheses implicate cell-mediated autoimmune mechanisms directed against keratinocytes. The fact that chronic epidermal injury in the lichenoid variants of GVHD may be indistinguishable histologically from ordinary lichen planus supports this hypothesis. An association with human leukocyte antigen (HLA) class II DR1 has been established (16a).

Lichen planus–like drug eruptions occur commonly; therefore, the clinical differential diagnosis must also include iatrogenic causes. Offending agents include beta blockers, methyldopa, penicillamine, quinidine, nonsteroidal antiinflammatory drugs (NSAIDs), angiotensin-converting enzyme (ACE) inhibitors, sulfonylurea agents, carbamazepine, gold, lithium, and quinine. Many of these drugs result in immune dysregulation that leads to the development of an abnormal immune response. Lichen planus also develops in association with liver disease, especially with hepatitis C virus, and lesions may wax and wane during treatment for the underlying hepatic disease (17–19). Most patients with lichen planus, however, do not have detectable liver abnormalities or evidence of viral hepatitis.

**Pathologic Findings.** The histologic features vary with the site of involvement (skin, mucosa, nail bed), although there are changes common to all affected sites. At scanning magnification, the histologic alterations of lichen planus are characteristic (fig. 7-2). There is epidermal hyperplasia with hyperkeratosis and acanthosis associated with a dermal-epidermal junction that resembles the teeth of a saw rather than the normally smooth, undulant interface between rete ridges and dermal papillae (fig. 7-3). In early lesions, the band-like lymphoid infiltrate and the epidermal proliferative changes may dominate the picture (fig. 7-4). At higher magnification, the basal cell layer shows variable vacuolization, apoptosis, and prominent squamatization, with a lymphocytic infiltrate that is intimately associated with these epidermal alterations (figs. 7-5, 7-6), often producing the phenomenon of satellitosis, as described in chapter 6 for acute GVHD (fig. 7-7). As a result of chronic injury to the basal cell layer, microscopic clefts along

*Lichenoid Dermatitis (Subacute to Chronic Cytotoxic Dermatitis)*

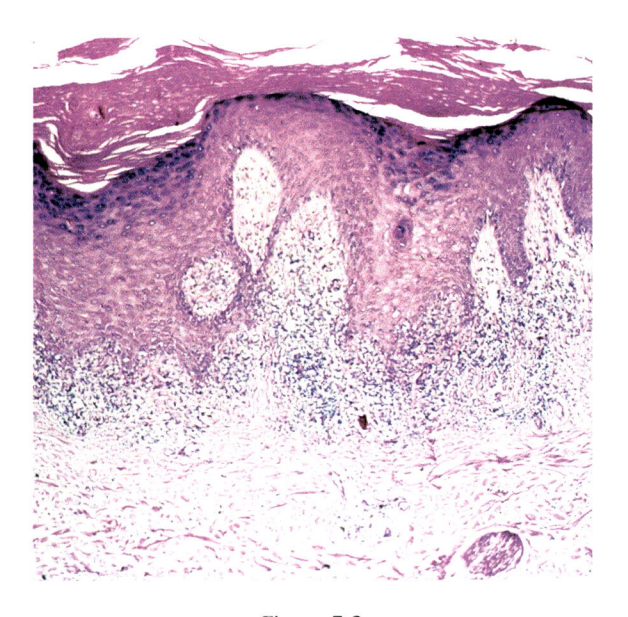

**Figure 7-2**
**LICHEN PLANUS**
At scanning magnification, there is a band-like infiltrate of lymphocytes within the papillary dermis. The dermal-epidermal interface is obscured by chronic changes, producing a "saw tooth" architecture to the rete ridges. The epidermal layer is acanthotic, and shows wedge-like zones of hypergranulosis and diffuse hyperkeratosis.

**Figure 7-3**
**LICHEN PLANUS**
At high magnification, the characteristically pointed rete ridge with evidence of apoptosis is typical of the "saw tooth" architecture of this disease.

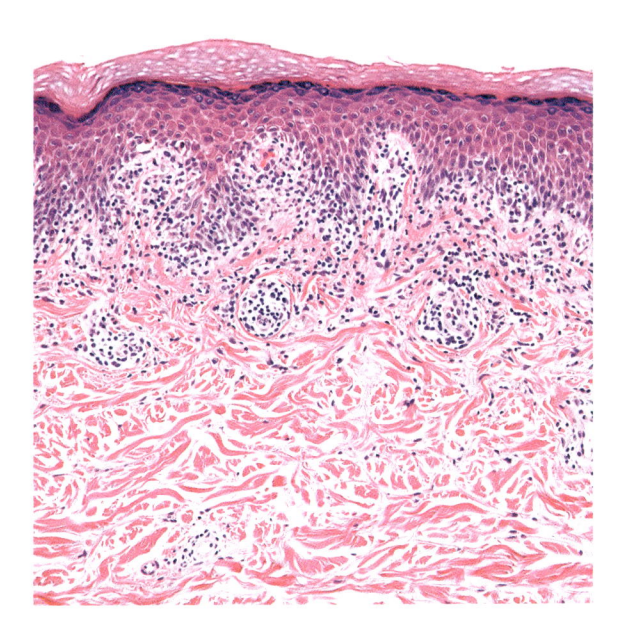

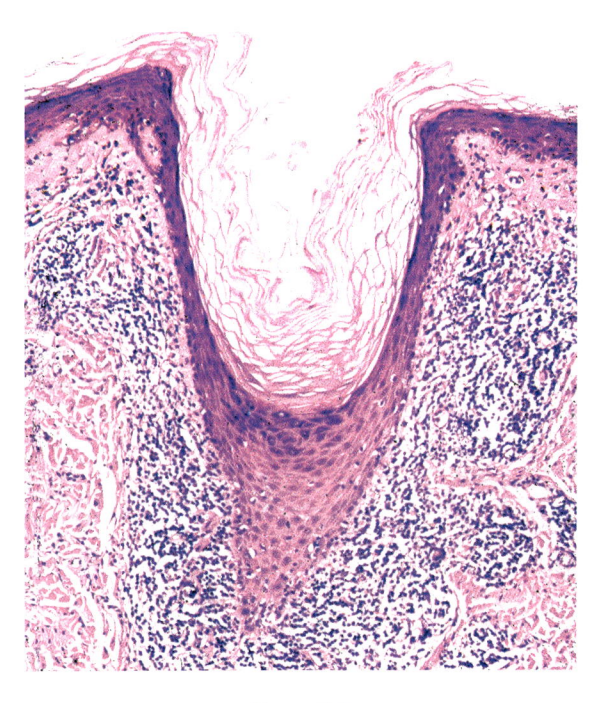

**Figure 7-4**
**LICHEN PLANUS: EARLY LESION**
The lichenoid infiltrate is associated with early basal layer injury. The epidermal proliferative changes consist of hyperkeratosis, hypergranulosis, and acanthosis.

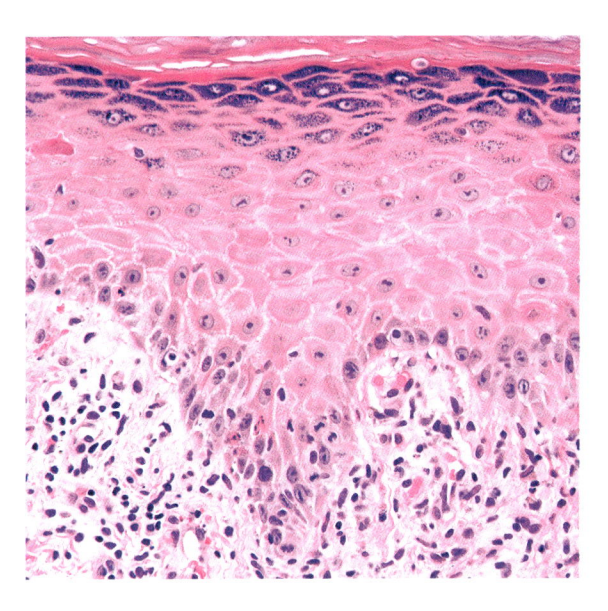

**Figure 7-5**
**LICHEN PLANUS: FOLLICULAR INFUNDIBULAR INVOLVEMENT**
The band-like infiltrate of lymphocytes involves the infundibulum. The infundibular epithelium shows hypergranulosis and hyperkeratosis, and the basal layer is squamatized, indicative of chronic interface injury.

213

*Inflammatory Disorders of the Skin*

**Figure 7-6**

**LICHEN PLANUS: FULLY DEVELOPED LESION**

Top: A pronounced band-like infiltrate of lymphocytes is within the papillary dermis. The indistinct dermal-epidermal interface is a consequence of the chronic injury to and infiltration of the lowermost epidermal layers.

Bottom: At higher magnification, there is marked basal cell layer vacuolization as well as migration of lymphocytes into the lowermost epidermal layers, where they surround target keratinocytes destined to undergo apoptotic injury (a pattern called satellitosis.)

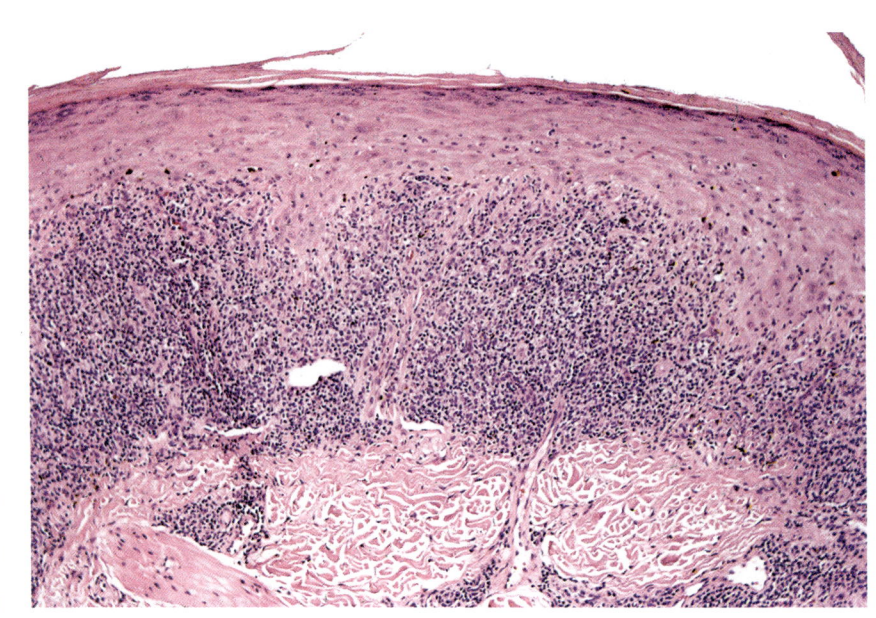

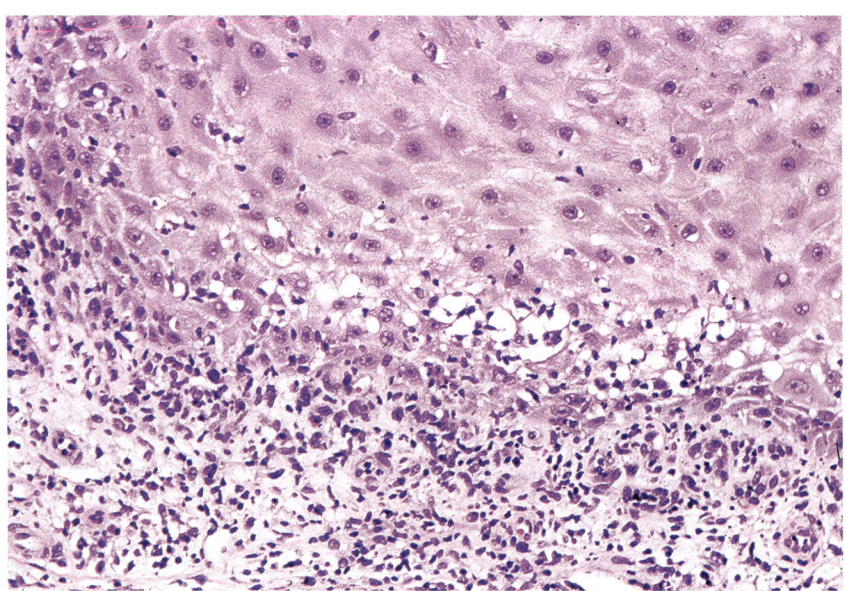

the dermal-epidermal junction (so-called Max-Joseph spaces) may develop (fig. 7-8, top). With chronicity and resolution, the infiltrate becomes less pronounced, and the papillary dermis may acquire deposits of thickened collagen bundles (fig. 7-8, bottom). The mid- and lower epidermis, as well as the papillary dermis, may contain individual and clustered apoptotic cells. These presumed residua of cytotoxic attack are the colloid, or Civatte, bodies that contain immunoglobulin (Ig)M on inspection by direct immunofluorescence and that undergo amyloid transformation over time (fig. 7-9).

Variants include *atrophic lichen planus* (fig. 7-10) and *hypertrophic lichen planus*, the latter characterized clinically by thick hyperkeratotic plaques, often on the anterior leg, and marked histologically by acanthosis, pseudocarcinomatous hyperplasia, and hyperkeratosis (figs. 7-11–7-13).

Lichen planus may preferentially involves follicular infundibular epithelium or interfollicular epithelium in a diffuse manner, leading to localized follicular papules or clinical erythroderma, respectively (fig. 7-5). The former condition, known as *lichen planopilaris*, is characterized by

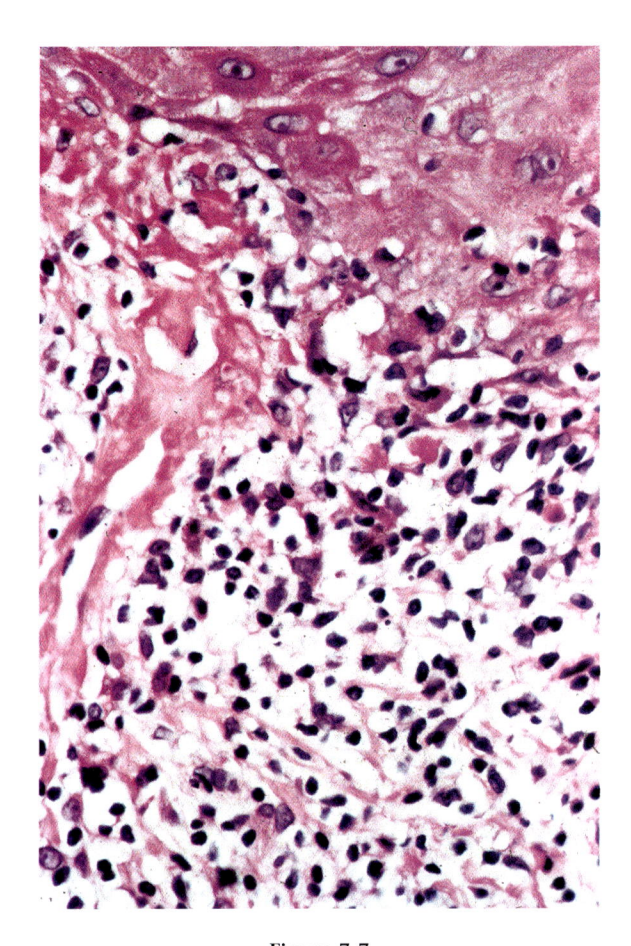

### Figure 7-7
**LICHEN PLANUS: DERMAL-EPIDERMAL INTERFACE**
Apoptotic target cells are surrounded by lymphocytes (satellitosis).

peri-infundibular lymphocytic infiltrates, which induce in the infundibular epithelium many of the same alterations produced in the interfollicular epithelium in ordinary lichen planus. These alterations include follicular infundibular acanthosis, hypergranulosis, hyperkeratosis, basal cell layer dyskeratosis, vacuolar change, and squamatization. There may be traces of inactive or chronic interfollicular lichen planus in such samples (fig. 7-14), although the dominant histologic alterations are lichenoid type that involve follicular infundibula (figs. 7-15, 7-16). In *erythrodermic lichen planus*, most of the epidermal surface is involved, including the superficial portions of the hair follicle. Lichen planus also affects the nails, producing characteristic clinical alterations and histologic changes in the nail bed and matrix, which

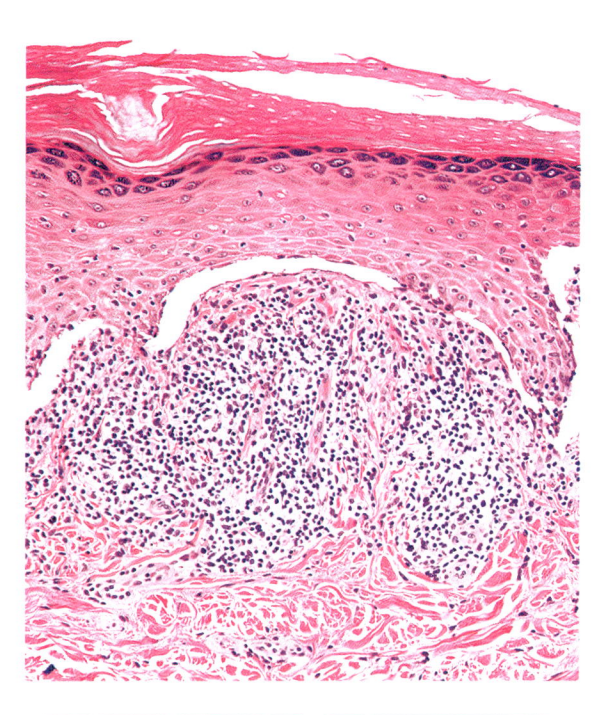

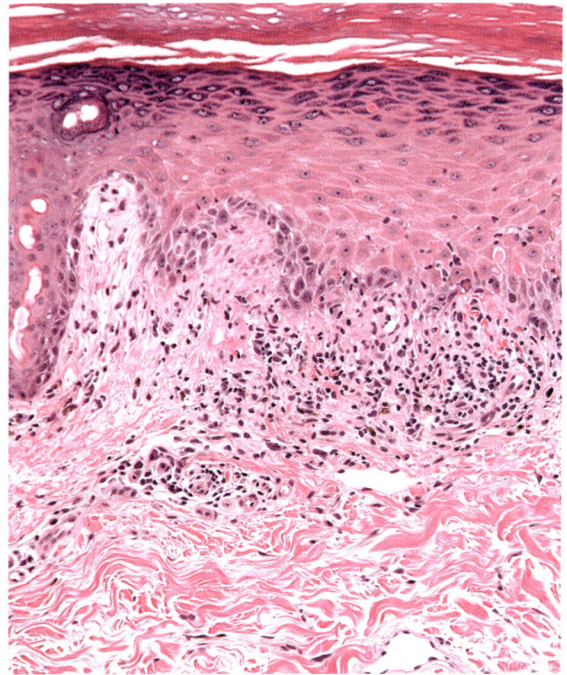

### Figure 7-8
**LICHEN PLANUS: ADVANCED LESION**
Top: The band-like lichenoid lymphocytic infiltrate is associated with subepidermal clefts (Max-Joseph spaces).
Bottom: At intermediate magnification, this older lesion shows established hypergranulosis, saw tooth rete ridge architecture, and papillary dermal fibrosis associated with a persistent lymphocytic infiltrate.

## Inflammatory Disorders of the Skin

**Figure 7-9**

**LICHEN PLANUS: DIRECT IMMUNOFLUORESCENCE FOR IgM**

Direct immunofluorescence shows "colloid bodies," rounded structures along the dermal-epidermal interface that stain strongly for IgM and that represent apoptotic target cells. Although not entirely specific, this is a characteristic immunofluorescence pattern in lichen planus.

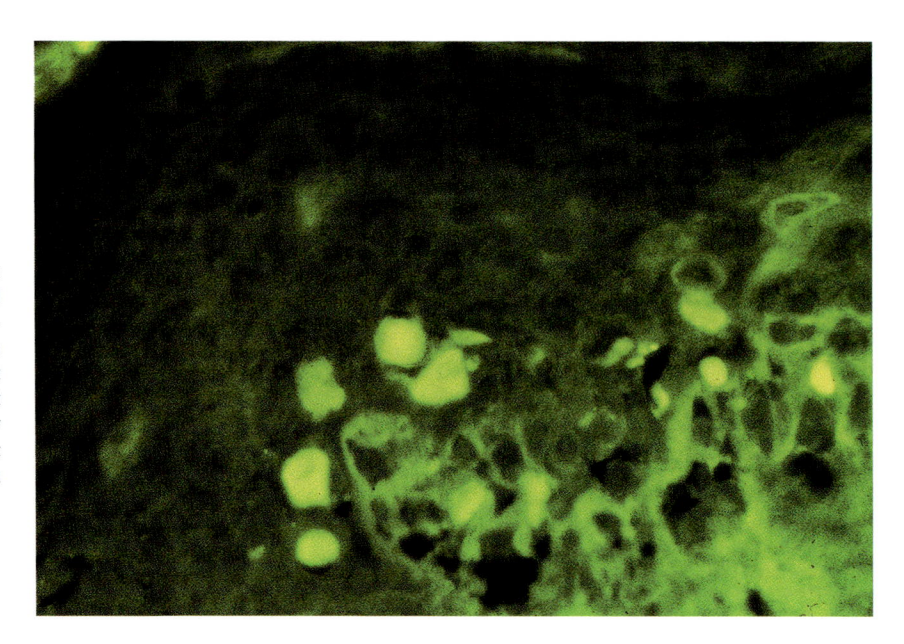

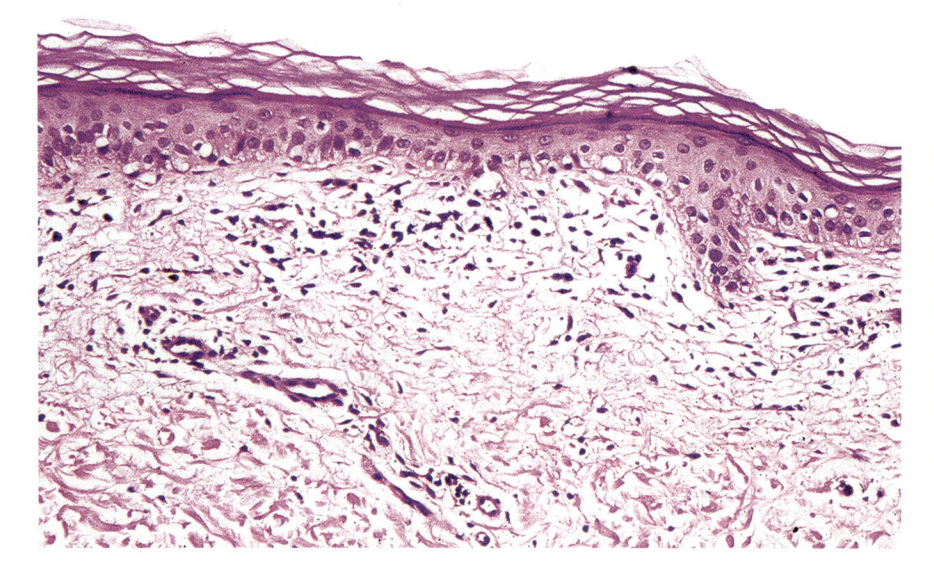

**Figure 7-10**

**LICHEN PLANUS: ATROPHIC VARIANT**

Occasionally, lichen planus produces atrophy of the epidermal layer with loss of rete ridges. There is a sparse band-like infiltrate of lymphocytes in the papillary dermis and subtle hyperkeratosis. Such lesions must be differentiated from other subacute to chronic forms of interface dermatitis that produce atrophy, such as lupus erythematosus or lupus-lichen planus crossover syndromes.

sometimes occur independent of skin lesions (figs. 7-17, 7-18). *Bullous/erosive lichen planus* is often encountered in squamous mucosae where epithelial blistering and sloughing develop as a result of coalescence of cytotoxic injury to basal keratinocytes (fig. 7-19). In general, mucous membrane (both bullous and nonbullous) involvement and nail bed involvement by lichen planus show less pronounced hypergranulosis and hyperkeratosis, and the extent of basal layer injury is often subtle; any degree of stratum granulosum or stratum corneum formation involving oral mucosa should be regarded as abnormal (figs. 7-17–7-21). At times there is only a band-like infiltrate below the altered epithelium, without evidence of characteristic basal cell changes. In our opinion, only lesions with epithelial changes should be diagnosed as consistent with lichen planus. Therapeutically recalcitrant genital lesions produce subtle histologic findings, particularly when they have been partially modified by treatment.

*Lichenoid Dermatitis (Subacute to Chronic Cytotoxic Dermatitis)*

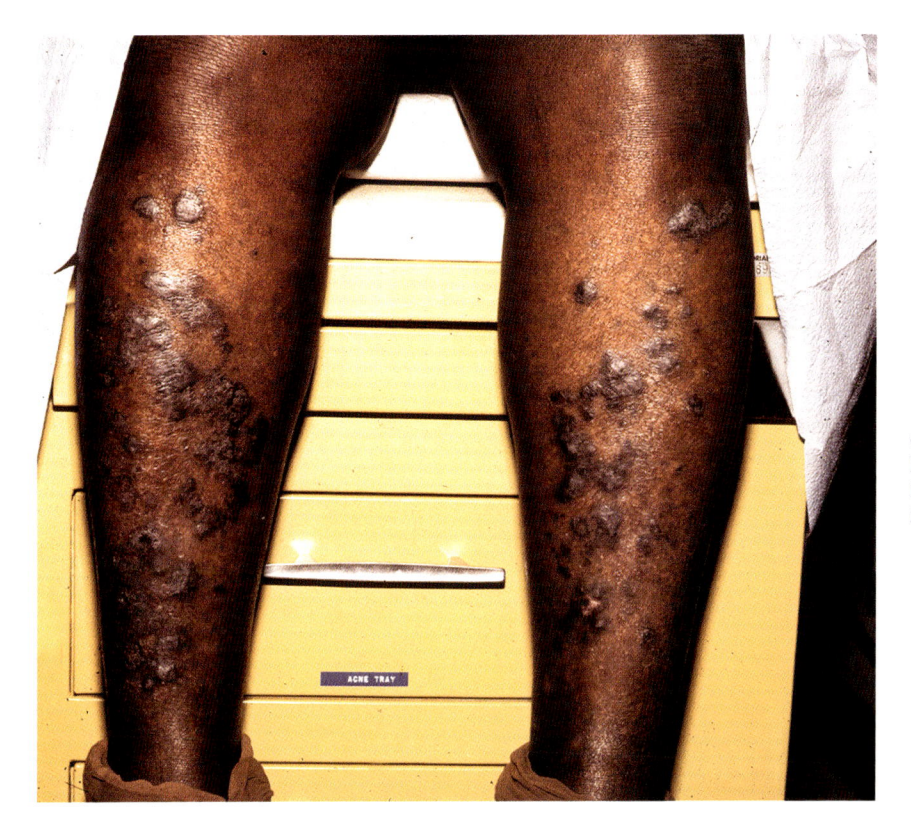

**Figure 7-11**

**LICHEN PLANUS: HYPERTROPHIC VARIANT**

Numerous papules coalescence and form plaques on the lower extremities. There is striking hyperpigmentation as well as increased surface scale.

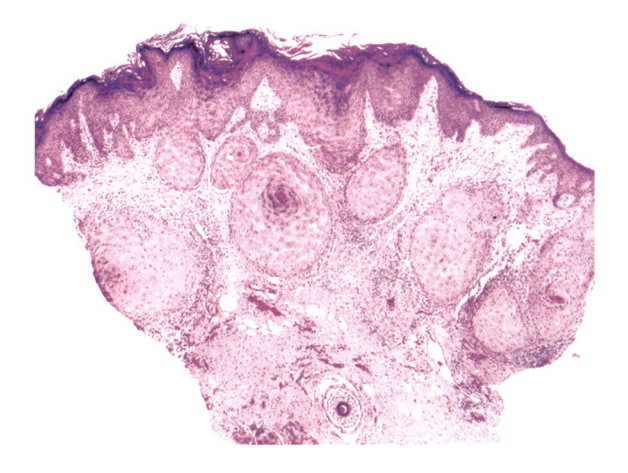

**Figure 7-12**

**LICHEN PLANUS: HYPERTROPHIC VARIANT**

Above: Multiple endophytic lobules of hyperplastic epithelium extend in a pseudoinvasive pattern into the inflamed dermis.

Right: At higher magnification, there is hyperkeratosis and wedge-shaped hypergranulosis in addition to the endophytic acanthosis extending into the superficial dermal layer.

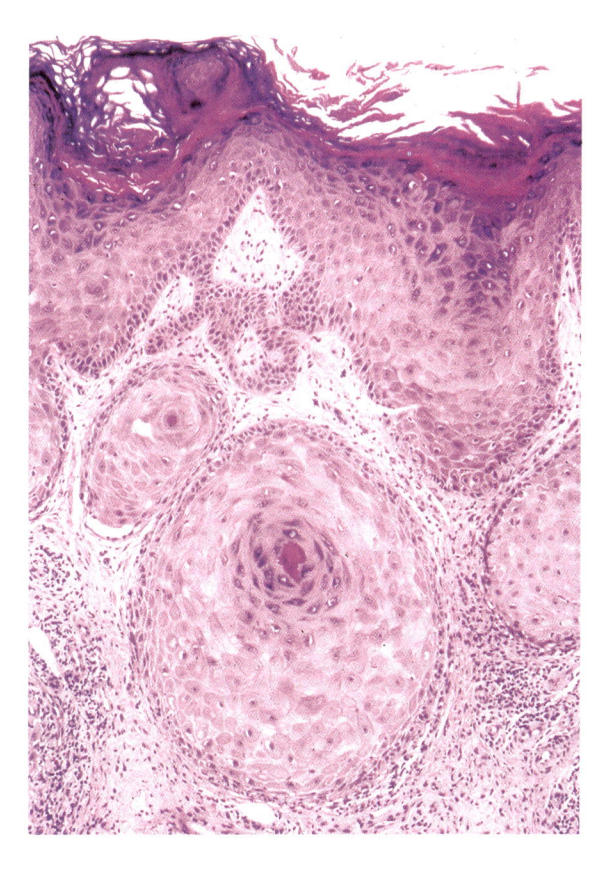

*Inflammatory Disorders of the Skin*

**Figure 7-13**

**LICHEN PLANUS: HYPERTROPHIC VARIANT**

Endophytic zones of hyperplastic epithelium are surrounded by a band of lymphocytes with evidence of chronic interface injury, features typical of more commonly encountered variants of lichen planus.

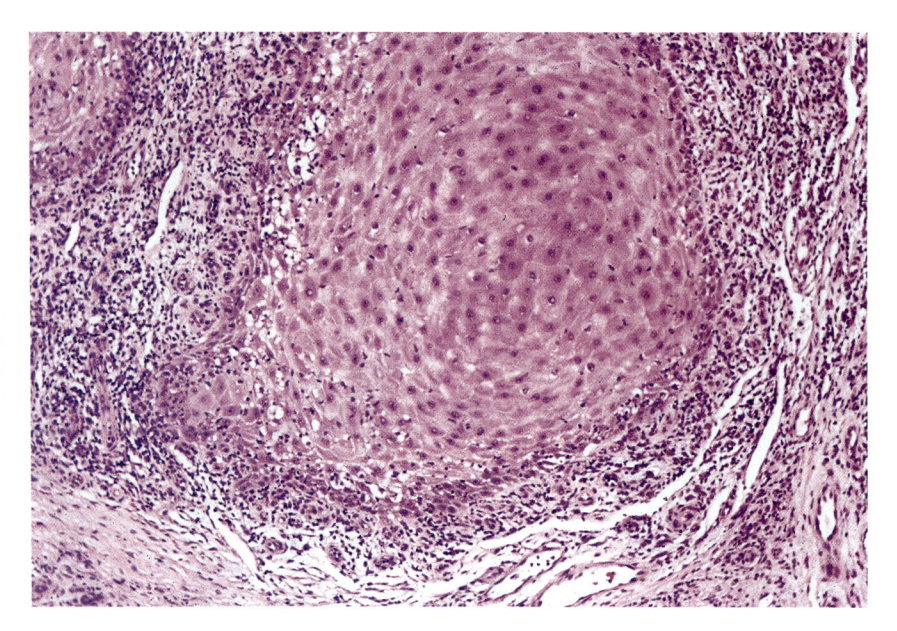

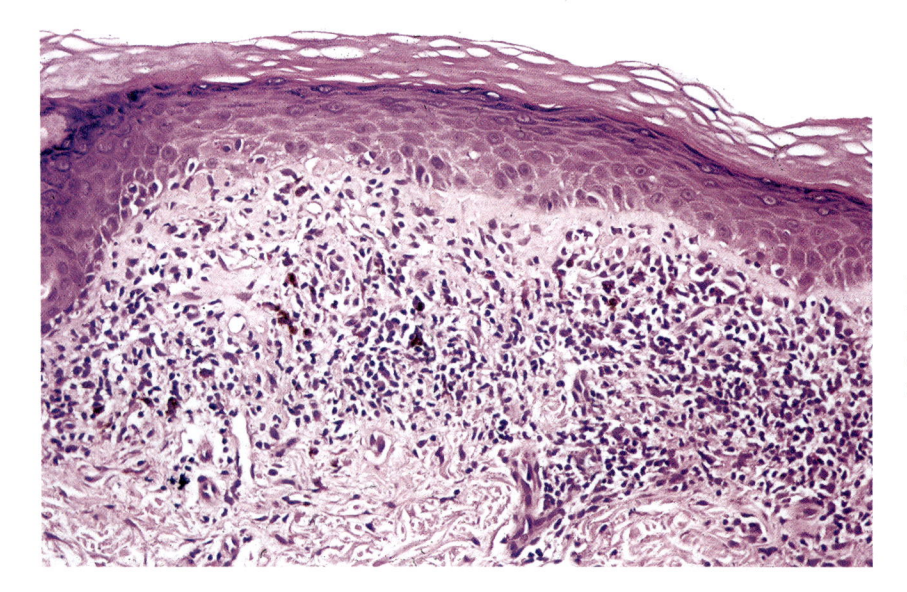

**Figure 7-14**

**LICHEN PLANUS: OLDER LESION**

With chronicity, the band-like infiltrate of lymphocytes within the papillary dermis becomes less prominent. Variable degrees of fibrosis and pigment incontinence supervene.

**Differential Diagnosis.** The histologic differential diagnosis of lichen planus includes lichen planus–like drug eruption, benign lichen planus–like keratoses, lichenoid actinic keratosis, lichenoid secondary syphilis, lichenoid GVHD, and rarely lichenoid contact hypersensitivity (particularly when affecting oral mucosa) reactions.

**Treatment and Prognosis.** Lesions may persist for many months, but spontaneously regress within one to several years in most individuals. The association of chronic oral lesions with the development of dysplasia and carcinoma is controversial (20,21).

There are a variety of therapies for lichen planus, although existing data for cutaneous involvement remain too preliminary for formulation of general recommendations (22–24). High-potency topical or intralesional corticosteroids are most effective for the treatment of oral lesions (25,26). Immunomodulators, such as pimecrolimus, have been used. Topical cyclosporine has shown variable success in steroid unresponsive cases (27,28). Retinoids, which have complex effects, have been used with positive results in certain individuals, and other forms of immunomodulatory therapy

*Lichenoid Dermatitis (Subacute to Chronic Cytotoxic Dermatitis)*

have also shown encouraging responses in some cases (29–34). Antimalarials such as hydroxychloroquine may also have a therapeutic effect. Phototherapy, both ultraviolet (UV)B and UVA, has been used successfully.

## LICHEN NITIDUS

**Definition.** *Lichen nitidus* is an idiopathic cutaneous disorder characterized by the formation of multiple, small, asymptomatic papules (35,36).

**Clinical Features.** Multiple, often grouped, nonfollicular, asymptomatic, flesh-colored papules are present (fig. 7-22). Unlike lichen planus, the lesions are small (1 to 3 mm), do not coalesce, and do not itch. The skin of the upper extremities, abdomen, and penis is most frequently involved.

**Pathologic Findings.** There is a rounded aggregate of mononuclear cells within the superficial dermis, beneath a thinned epidermal layer, often surrounded by a peripheral epithelial collarette (fig. 7-23). The overlying stratum corneum may show parakeratosis, and the basal cell layer overlying the inflammatory infiltrate may be vacuolated or squamatized. Occasional colloid bodies, as seen in lichen planus, are observed at the dermal-epidermal interface. At higher magnification, the inflammatory dermal component is predominantly composed of histiocytes admixed with lymphocytes (figs. 7-24, 7-25); the histiocytic component is often characterized by epithelioid

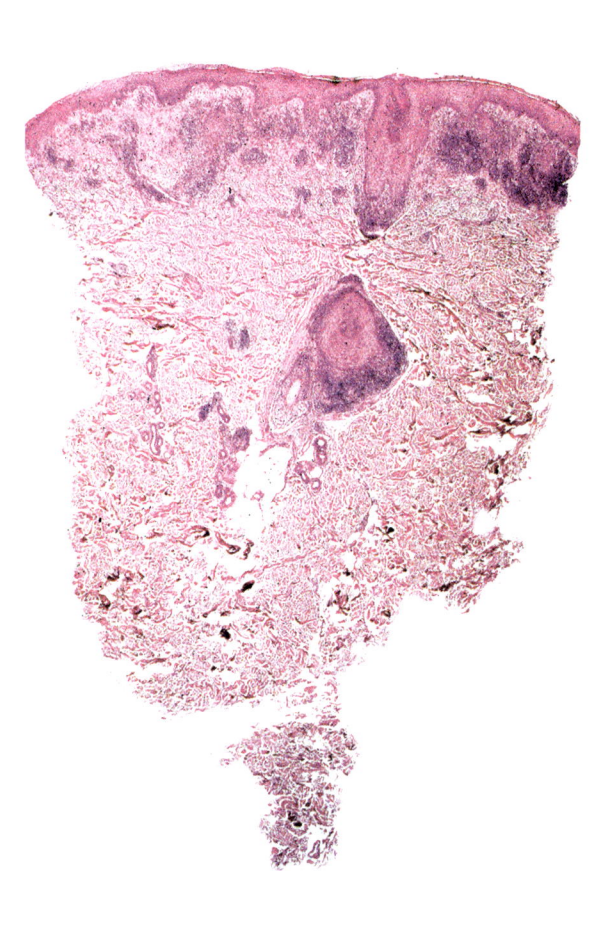

Figure 7-15

**LICHEN PLANUS: FOLLICULAR INVOLVEMENT**
The distorted, tangentially sectioned hair follicle is rimmed by lymphocytes within the mid-dermis.

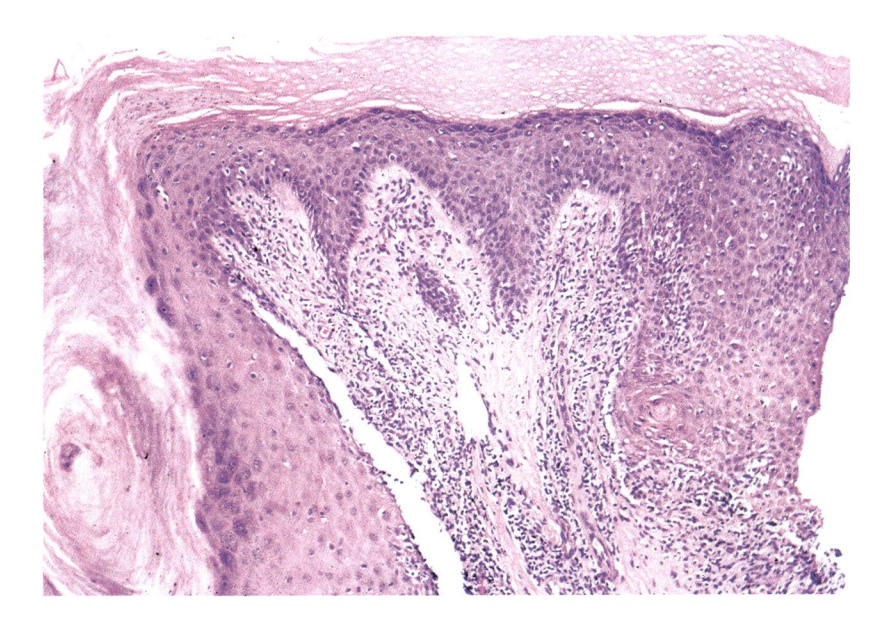

Figure 7-16

**LICHEN PLANUS: PREFERENTIAL FOLLICULAR INVOLVEMENT**

In addition to the epidermal changes typical of lichen planus, marked acanthosis, hypergranulosis, and hyperkeratosis of the follicular infundibulum are present. A cleft-like space has formed, separating a band-like infiltrate of perifollicular lymphocytes and the damaged basal cell layer of the involved follicular infundibulum. Preferential involvement of hair follicles in lichen planus, without significant epidermal involvement and often with associated hair loss, is termed lichen planopillaris.

*Inflammatory Disorders of the Skin*

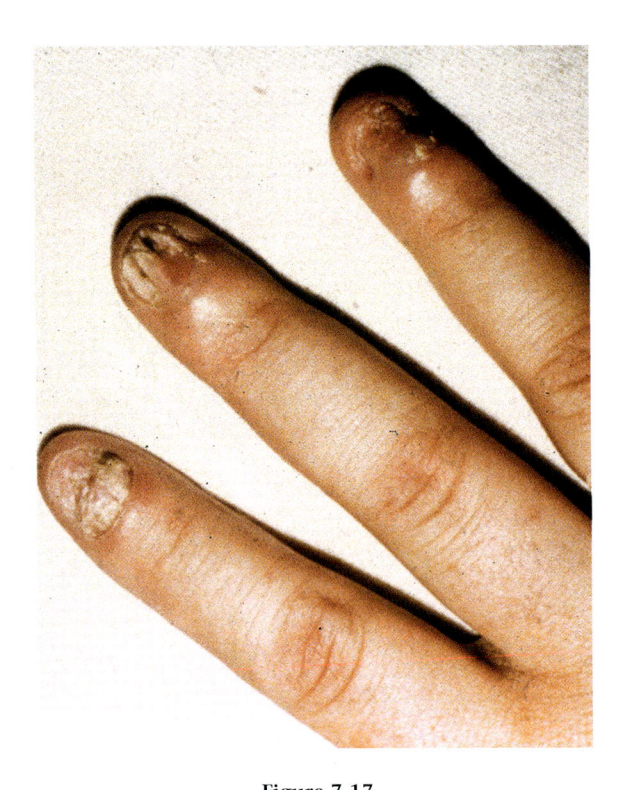

**Figure 7-17**
**LICHEN PLANUS OF THE NAIL**
Marked dystrophy of the nail plate and pterygium formation are present.

**Figure 7-18**
**LICHEN PLANUS OF THE NAIL**
A biopsy of the nail bed indicates focal separation of the bed epithelium from the dermis and an inflammatory infiltrate composed of lymphocytes. The separation is the consequence of chronic lymphocyte-mediated cytotoxicity directed against the lowermost epithelial layers of the nail bed.

mononuclear cells with larger, paler nuclei and abundant pink cytoplasm. Occasional multinucleated giant cells are seen. Focal neutrophils are sometimes admixed with the mononuclear inflammatory cells.

**Differential Diagnosis.** Early (small) lesions of lichen planus are mediated primarily by lymphocytes, not histiocytes, and a collarette is not observed. There is a greater ratio between the depth of the inflammatory infiltrate and its width in lichen nitidus than in early lesions of lichen planus (Table 7-1). Lichen striatus is often characterized by epidermal spongiosis in addition to focal lichenoid changes, and shows a deeper dermal infiltrate, usually involving sweat glands or hair follicles.

**Treatment and Prognosis.** The course and treatment are similar to those for lichen planus (see above) (37). In addition, laser therapy may be helpful for resistant cases. Occasionally, the disease is simply followed clinically without treatment, particularly in children.

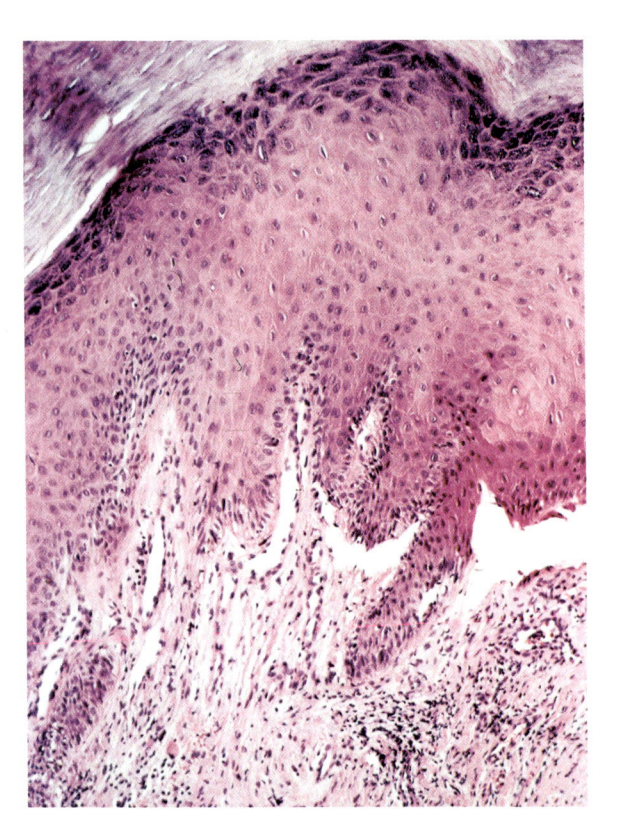

## LICHEN STRIATUS

**Definition.** *Lichen striatus* is an uncommon disorder that is often seen in children but also occurs in adults. It is characterized by minute scaling papules that occur along Blaschko lines, which define regions of melanocyte embryologic migration (38–41).

**Clinical Features.** The lesions involve the extremities, trunk, or neck, and present as contiguous or interrupted bands formed by small, variably scaling, erythematous papules. The linear band can extend from the thigh to the lower leg. The face is rarely involved. Mild pruritus may be present. Postinflammatory changes, including hypopigmentation in darkly pigmented individuals, occur. Although lesions are generally solitary and unilateral, bilateral involvement is occasionally seen.

**Pathologic Findings.** The histologic findings are variable, and both interface alterations and spongiosis replete with Langerhans cell microgranuloma formation (so-called pseudo-Pautrier abscess) may be seen. The interface alterations are mediated primarily by lymphocytes and may resemble lichen planus, with basal cell layer vacuolization, dyskeratosis, and pigment incontinence (fig. 7-26). A characteristic feature is focal involvement by the lichenoid infiltrate of the deep portion of the hair follicle, and at times, the eccrine gland. The lymphohistiocytes are mainly perivascular within the superficial dermis of some. The involvement of the eccrine gland can be quite diffuse and is then designated as *lymphocytic hidradenitis*.

**Differential Diagnosis.** The differential diagnosis includes other forms of lichenoid dermatitis, which are generally excluded by the clinical features. Inflammatory linear verrucous epidermal nevus (ILVEN), a persistent, linear, intensely pruritic erythematous plaque, probably representing an inflamed epidermal hamartoma, has a similar clinical and histologic picture. ILVEN generally shows more epidermal hyperplasia than lichen striatus, with zones of alternating parakeratosis/hypogranulosis and hyperkeratosis/hypergranulosis. Moreover, lesions of ILVEN tend to be more persistent and

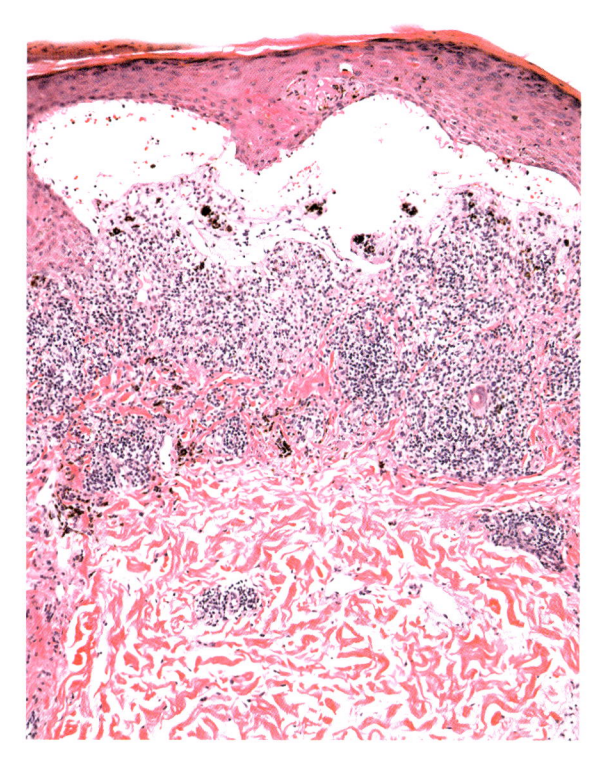

Figure 7-19
**LICHEN PLANUS: BULLOUS VARIANT**
A subepidermal vesicle is associated with a brisk lichenoid lymphocytic infiltrate and overlying epidermal changes characteristic of lichen planus.

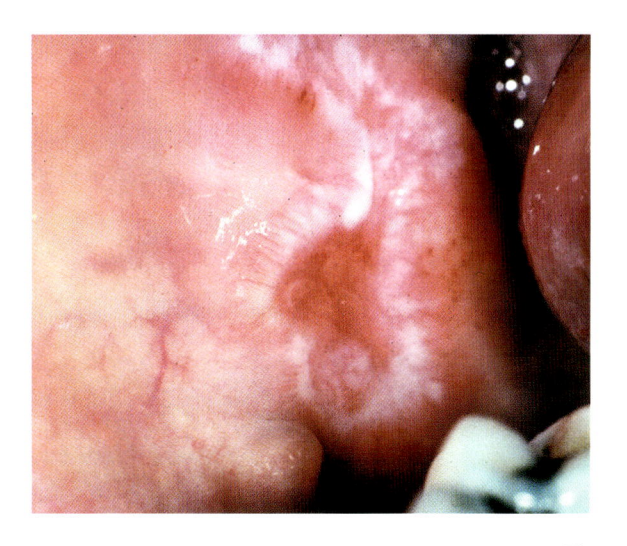

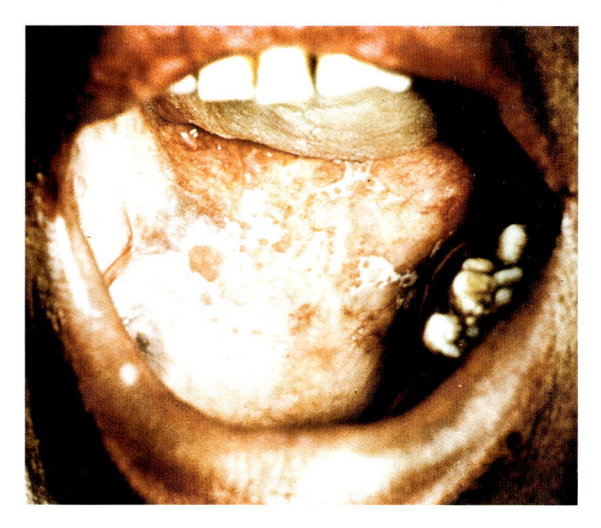

Figure 7-20
**LICHEN PLANUS: ORAL MUCOSA**
Left: In the buccal mucosa, the central atrophic zone is surrounded by radiating linear and reticular striae (Wickham striae).
Right: In a more advanced lesion, there are numerous regions of leukoplakia.

*Inflammatory Disorders of the Skin*

Table 7-1
DIFFERENTIAL DIAGNOSIS OF LICHEN NITIDUS AND LICHEN PLANUS

|  | Lichen Nitidus | Lichen Planus |
|---|---|---|
| Size | 0.1 – 0.3 cm | 0.5 – 1.0 cm |
| Pruritus | Usually absent | Usually present |
| Coalescence | Unusual | Frequently occurs |
| Collarette | Present | Absent |
| Epidermal hyperplasia | Absent | Present |
| Epidermal atrophy | Present | Usually absent |
| Parakeratosis | Present | Absent |
| Lymphocytes | Minor population | Predominant population |
| Histiocytes | Predominant population | Minor population |

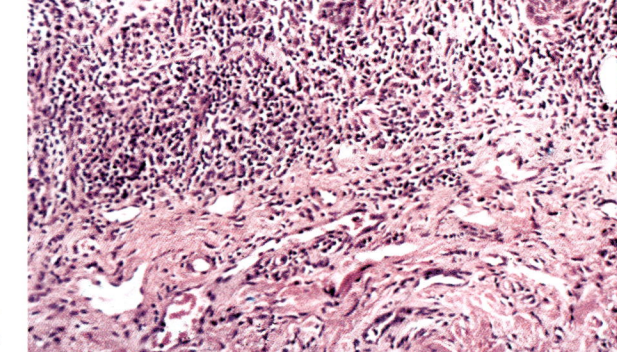

Figure 7-21

LICHEN PLANUS: ORAL MUCOSA

Top: The characteristic band-like lymphocytic infiltrate is directly beneath the acanthotic mucosal epithelial layer. In oral lichen planus, the typical sawtooth architecture of the dermal-epithelial junction and associated colloid body formation are less apparent than in the cutaneous form.

Bottom: The intraepithelial lymphocytes, disruption of the basal cells, and formation of apoptotic target cells help in formulating a more definitive diagnosis.

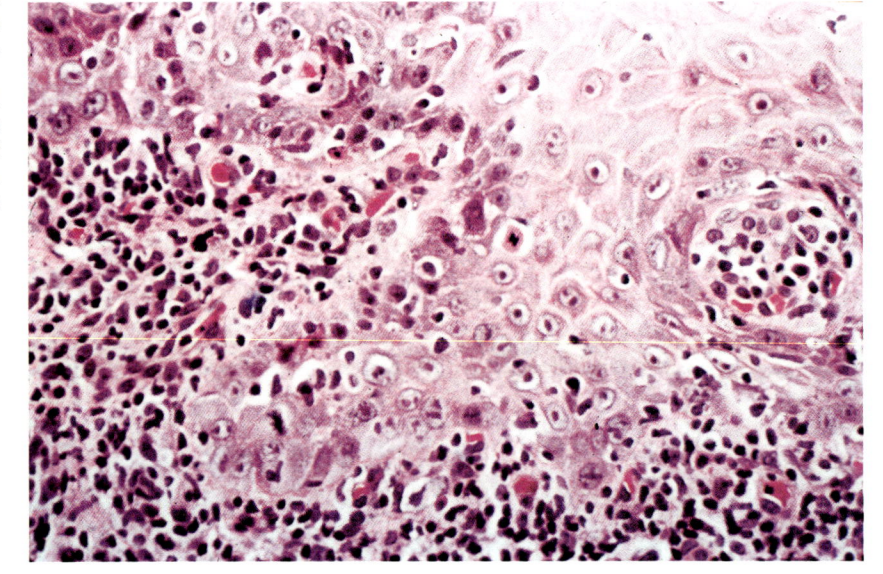

*Lichenoid Dermatitis (Subacute to Chronic Cytotoxic Dermatitis)*

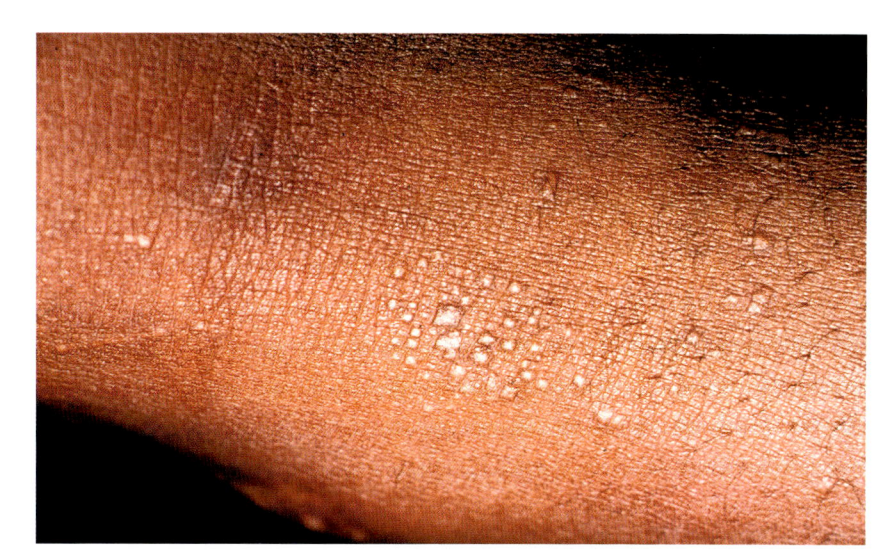

Figure 7-22
**LICHEN NITIDUS**
The multiple nonfollicular papules, like those of lichen planus, are flat-topped, although they are generally smaller.

Figure 7-23
**LICHEN NITIDUS**
There is a discrete aggregate of lymphocytes and histiocytes forming a band within the superficial dermis. The epidermis partially encloses this inflammatory aggregate in a characteristic "ball-in-claw" configuration.

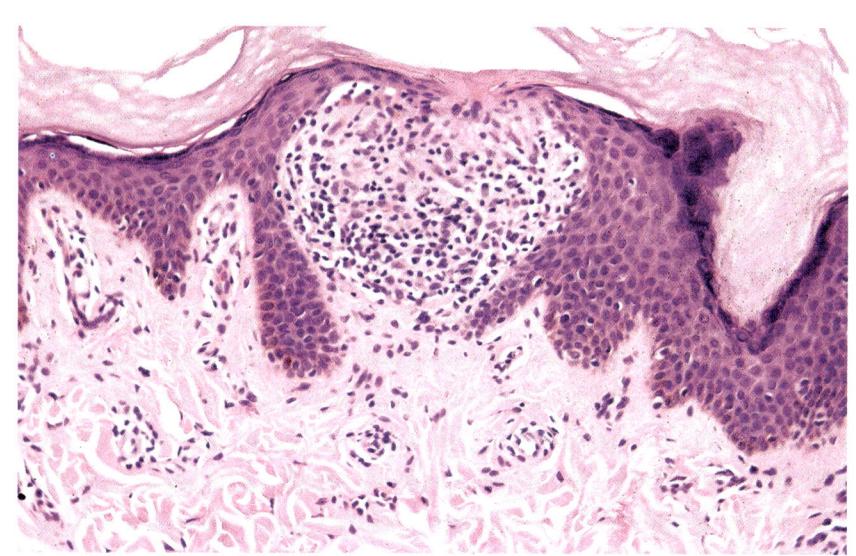

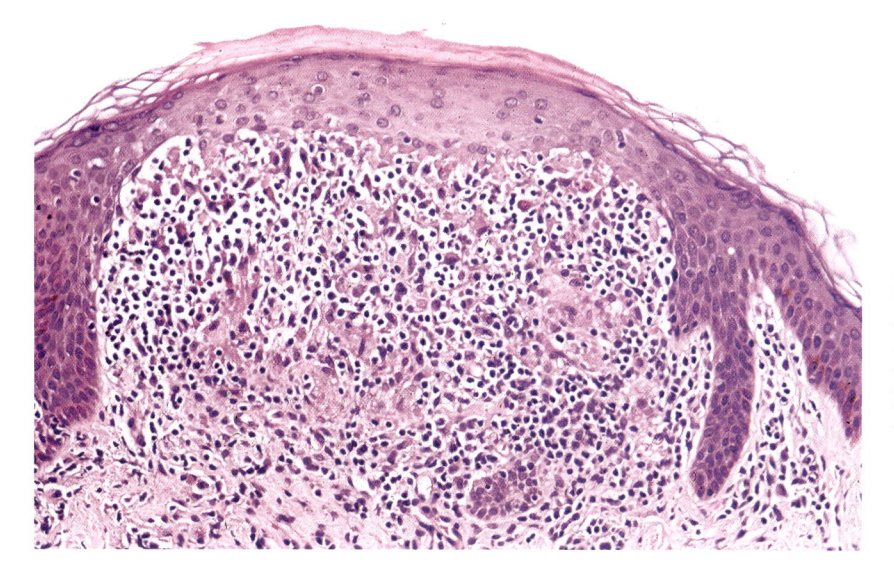

Figure 7-24
**LICHEN NITIDUS**
Higher magnification of figure 7-23 shows that the inflammatory infiltrate consists of a mixture of lymphocytes and larger histiocytes, many with pale visible cytoplasm. Squamatization and vacuolization of the basal cell layer are seen, consistent with chronic interface injury.

*Inflammatory Disorders of the Skin*

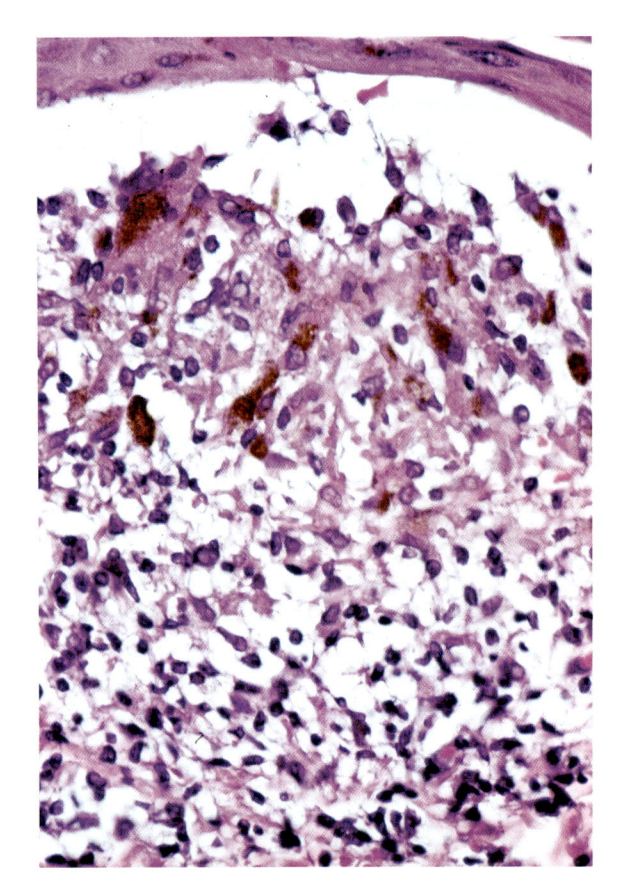

**Figure 7-25**

**LICHEN NITIDUS: INFLAMMATORY COMPONENT**

The infiltrate is composed predominantly of histiocytic cells, with admixed lymphocytes. The cleft is separating the inflammatory infiltrate from the attenuated overlying epidermis, testimony to the chronic injury to the basal cell layer typical of this disorder.

| Table 7-2 |
| :---: |
| **SOME DISORDERS SHOWING PSEUDO-PAUTRIER ABSCESS FORMATION (LANGERHANS CELL MICROGRANULOMAS)** |
| Lichen striatus |
| Inflammatory pityriasis rosea |
| Dyshidrotic eczema |
| Contact dermatitis |
| Letterer-Siwe disease |

pruritic than lichen striatus. A broad differential diagnosis is summarized in Table 7-2.

**Treatment and Prognosis.** The lesions may spontaneously regress over time, hastened by the application of topical corticosteroids.

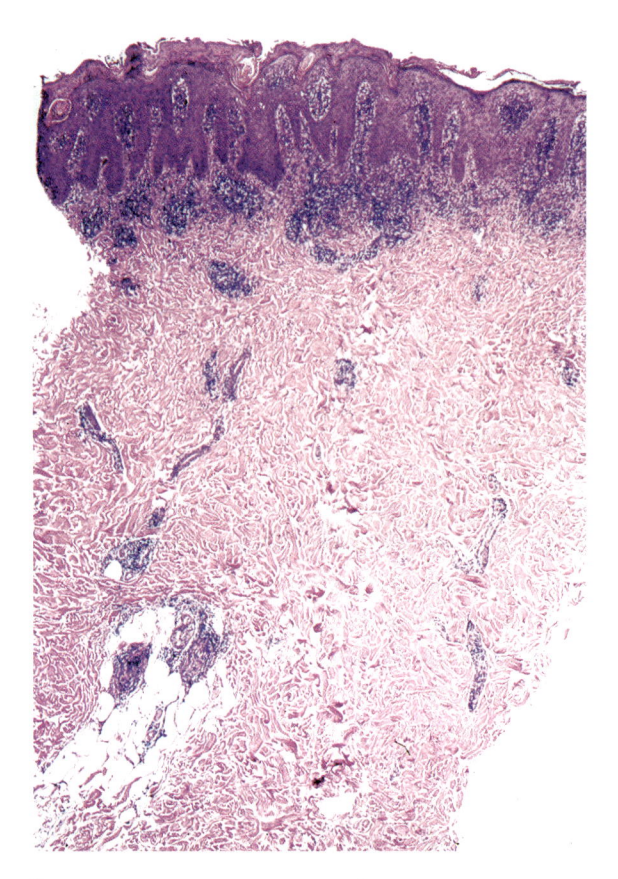

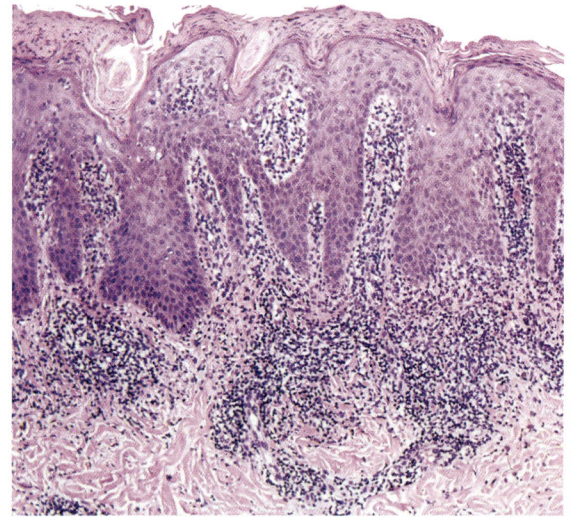

**Figure 7-26**

**LICHEN STRIATUS**

Top: There is a band-like infiltrate of lymphocytes within the superficial dermis, resembling the pattern seen in lichen planus.

Bottom: At intermediate magnification, in addition to the band-like infiltrate, there is variable injury to the epidermal layer and evidence of chronicity (acanthosis and increased scale formation).

*Lichenoid Dermatitis (Subacute to Chronic Cytotoxic Dermatitis)*

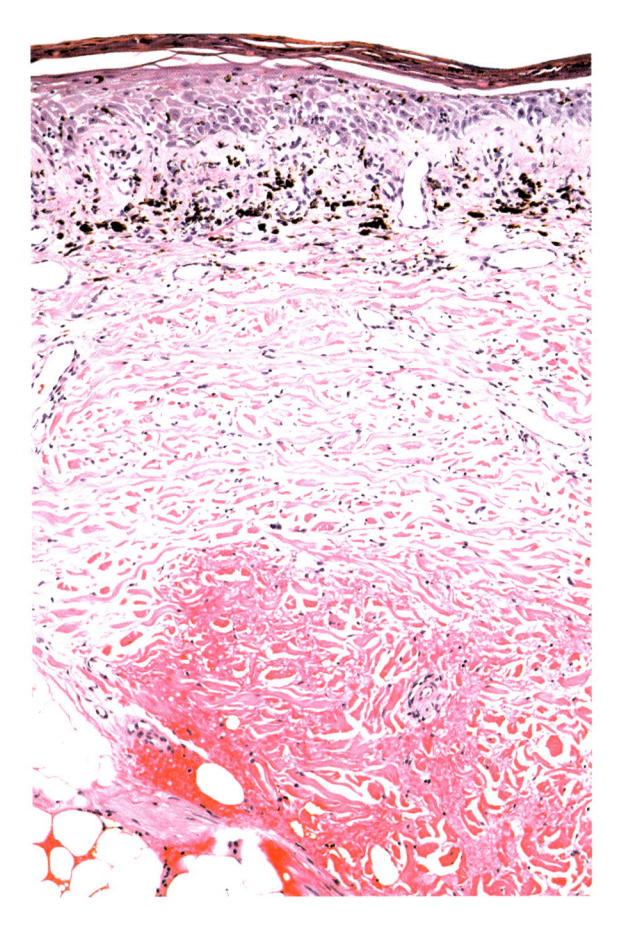

Figure 7-27

**GRAFT-VERSUS-HOST DISEASE: LICHENOID (EPIDERMAL) TYPE**

This lesion shows a band-like lichenoid infiltrate of lymphocytes and melanophages; note coexistence of early underlying sclerodermoid changes.

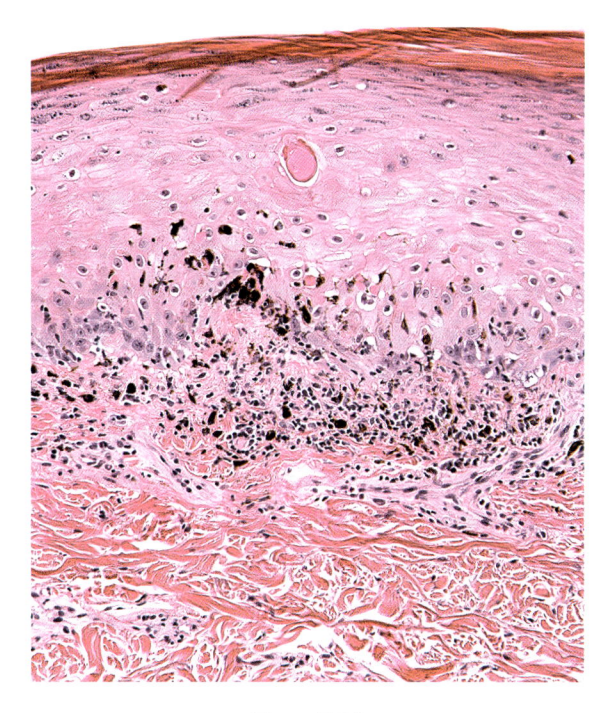

Figure 7-28

**CHRONIC GRAFT-VERSUS-HOST DISEASE: LICHENOID VARIANT**

The lichen planus-like alterations consist of hyperkeratosis, hypergranulosis, and a chronic lichenoid superficial dermal lymphoid infiltrate with associated basal layer injury and pigment incontinence.

## CHRONIC GRAFT-VERSUS-HOST DISEASE (EPIDERMAL TYPE)

**Definition.** *Chronic graft-versus-host disease* (GVHD) generally develops after the first 100 days after allogeneic bone marrow transplantation (stem cell) (42–45). Like acute GVHD, it also occurs after transplantation of nonirradiated blood products. There are two predominant forms: the *epidermal type*, which resembles lichen planus, and the *dermal type*, which resembles scleroderma.

**Clinical Features.** Patients with lichen planus–like disease develop variably pruritic lichenoid papules in a generalized distribution. The differential diagnosis ranges from drug eruption to opportunistic infection (46).

**Pathologic Findings.** The pathology is very similar, and at times essentially identical, to that of lichen planus. Clues to the diagnosis include maturation disarray of the epidermis, follicle, and eccrine duct, and scattered apoptotic cells in the stratum spinosum (figs. 7-27, 7-28). Occasional lesions have associated papillary dermal fibrosis and focal lymphocytic permeation of the reticular dermis, which may herald evolution to deeper dermal sclerosis of the sclerodermoid variant (fig. 7-29).

**Differential Diagnosis.** Lichenoid immune responses due to drugs generally contain eosinophils, which are rare in both acute and chronic epidermal forms of GVHD.

**Treatment and Prognosis.** Systemic steroids are the drugs of choice. Treatment is generally aggressive, in an effort to prevent the eventual sequelae of dermal sclerosis, which may follow

*Inflammatory Disorders of the Skin*

**Figure 7-29**

**GRAFT-VERSUS-HOST DISEASE: CHRONIC EPIDERMAL TYPE**

The lichenoid lymphocytic infiltrate within the papillary dermis has dissipated, leaving fibrosis and pigment incontinence. Such lesions may be harbingers of more sclerodermoid disease.

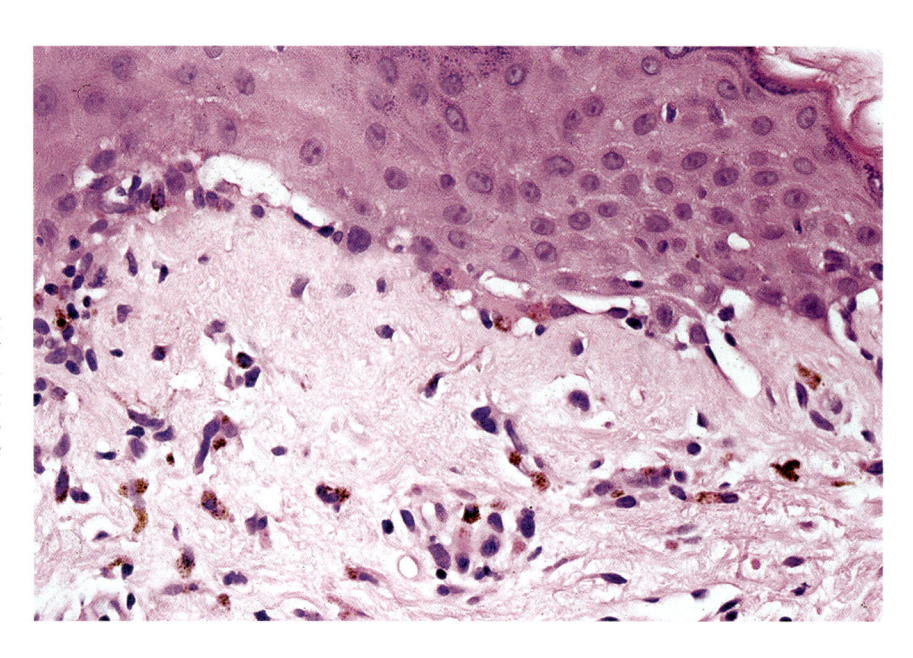

**Figure 7-30**

**DISCOID LUPUS ERYTHEMATOSUS**

These coalescent discoid plaques show erythema, central atrophy, scale formation, and peripheral hyperpigmentation as a consequence as chronic basal cell layer destruction.

the lichenoid presentation in certain individuals. Systemic immunosuppressants, phototherapy, and extracorporeal photopheresis have also been used. Mycophenolate, tacrolimus, and rituximab are helpful in steroid-refractory cases.

## LUPUS ERYTHEMATOSUS

**Definition.** The cutaneous manifestations of *lupus erythematosus* are many and varied. They include: 1) *classic discoid lupus erythematosus*; 2) *acute* and *subacute* forms of *lupus erythematosus*, characterized by subtle histologic changes; 3) *bullous lupus erythematosus*, typified by accumulation of neutrophils along the dermal-epidermal interface; 4) predominantly deep dermal and subcutaneous forms of lupus, including *lupus profundus* and *lupus panniculitis*; and 5) *necrotizing vasculitic lesions* (47–52). In addition, the malar erythema of systemic lupus erythematosus is a distinctive clinical lesion but generally is not characterized by specific diagnostic findings in biopsy specimens.

**Clinical Features.** The discoid plaques of lupus erythematosus, which predominate in disease localized to the skin but also occur with systemic disease, are well-circumscribed lesions characterized by erythema, telangiectasia, epidermal atrophy with occasional slight scale, and variability in pigmentation (fig. 7-30). The lesions may contain patulous follicular infundibula filled with cornified plugs. Discoid plaques are asymptomatic and preferentially affect the scalp, face, upper trunk, and upper extremities. Scalp lesions are frequently associated with alopecia, and therefore must be considered in the differential diagnosis of inflammatory alopecia. The acute lesions of

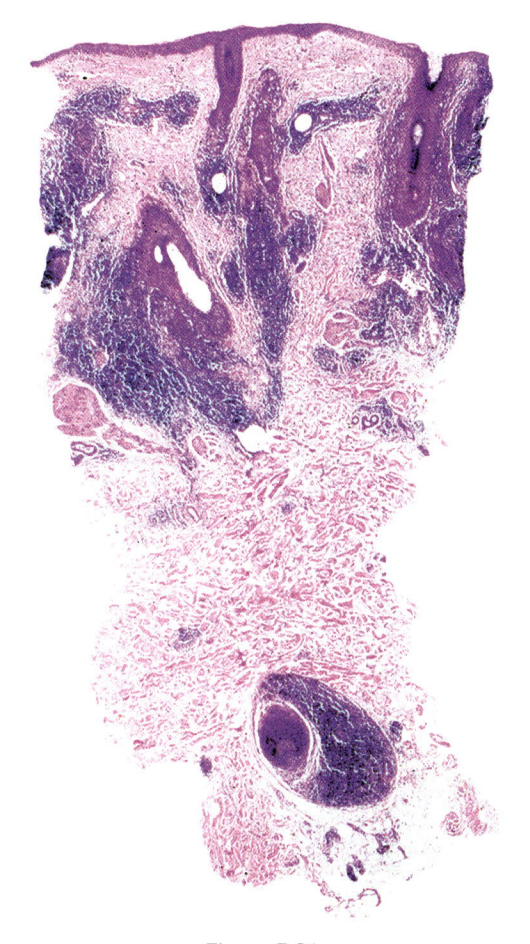

**Figure 7-31**
**DISCOID LUPUS ERYTHEMATOSUS**
There is a patchy perifollicular and perineurovascular infiltrate of inflammatory cells within the superficial and deep dermis.

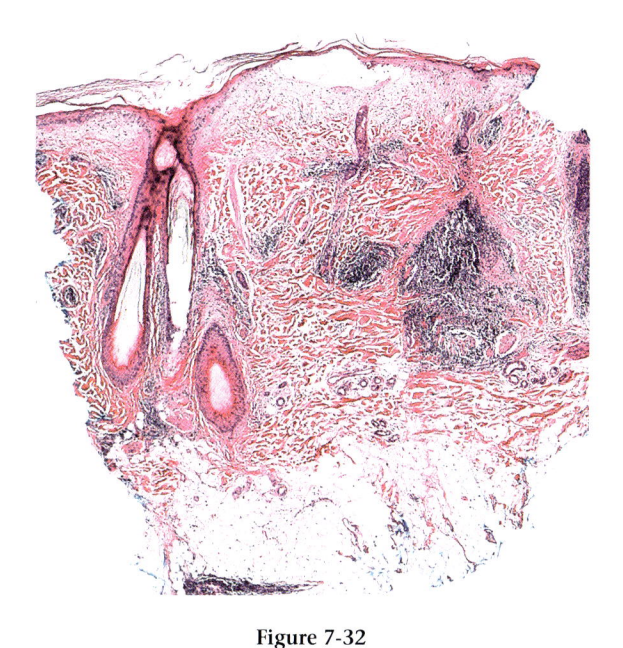

**Figure 7-32**
**DISCOID LUPUS ERYTHEMATOSUS WITH ALOPECIA: ACTIVE LESION**
Epidermal atrophy, prominent perifollicular inflammation, scarring with diminished hair density, and active telogen involution are seen.

lupus erythematosus present as a malar flush with erythema and slight scaling. They also occur as multiple erythematous papules, with slight scale confined to light-exposed areas.

Subacute lupus erythematosus presents as plaques that are often annular. They have a dusky erythematous appearance and tend to occur on light-exposed areas. The plaques may resemble psoriasis or even lichen planus, with a reddish-blue color surmounted by a delicate scale. Focal atrophy is characteristic.

**Pathologic Findings.** The histologic alterations of discoid lupus erythematosus and its variants are characteristic. At scanning magnification, there is diffuse epidermal atrophy with loss of rete ridges. Appendages are either diminished due to local destruction, or atrophic, with thinned epithelium forming follicular infundibula (figs. 7-31–7-33). The surface scale is composed of increased amounts of compacted orthokeratin, which also plugs ectatic follicles (fig. 7-34). The inflammatory infiltrate is perivascular and periadnexal (including eccrine coils), and involves the superficial and deep dermis. In some cases there is a variably dense lichenoid infiltrate along the dermal-epidermal interface, which shows coarse vacuolization of the stratum basalis (figs. 7-35, 7-36).

The periodic acid–Schiff (PAS) stain highlights the variable thickening of the basement membrane (fig. 7-37). Occasional apoptotic cells, sites of satellitosis, and superficial dermal colloid bodies are observed. Direct immunofluorescence generally demonstrates a continuous granular band of immunoglobulin and complement in the region of the affected basement membrane (fig. 7-38). A helpful diagnostic feature is the presence of diffuse mucin deposition within the superficial and deep dermis, recognized as finely granular strands of pale, gray-blue material dispersed within the slightly

*Inflammatory Disorders of the Skin*

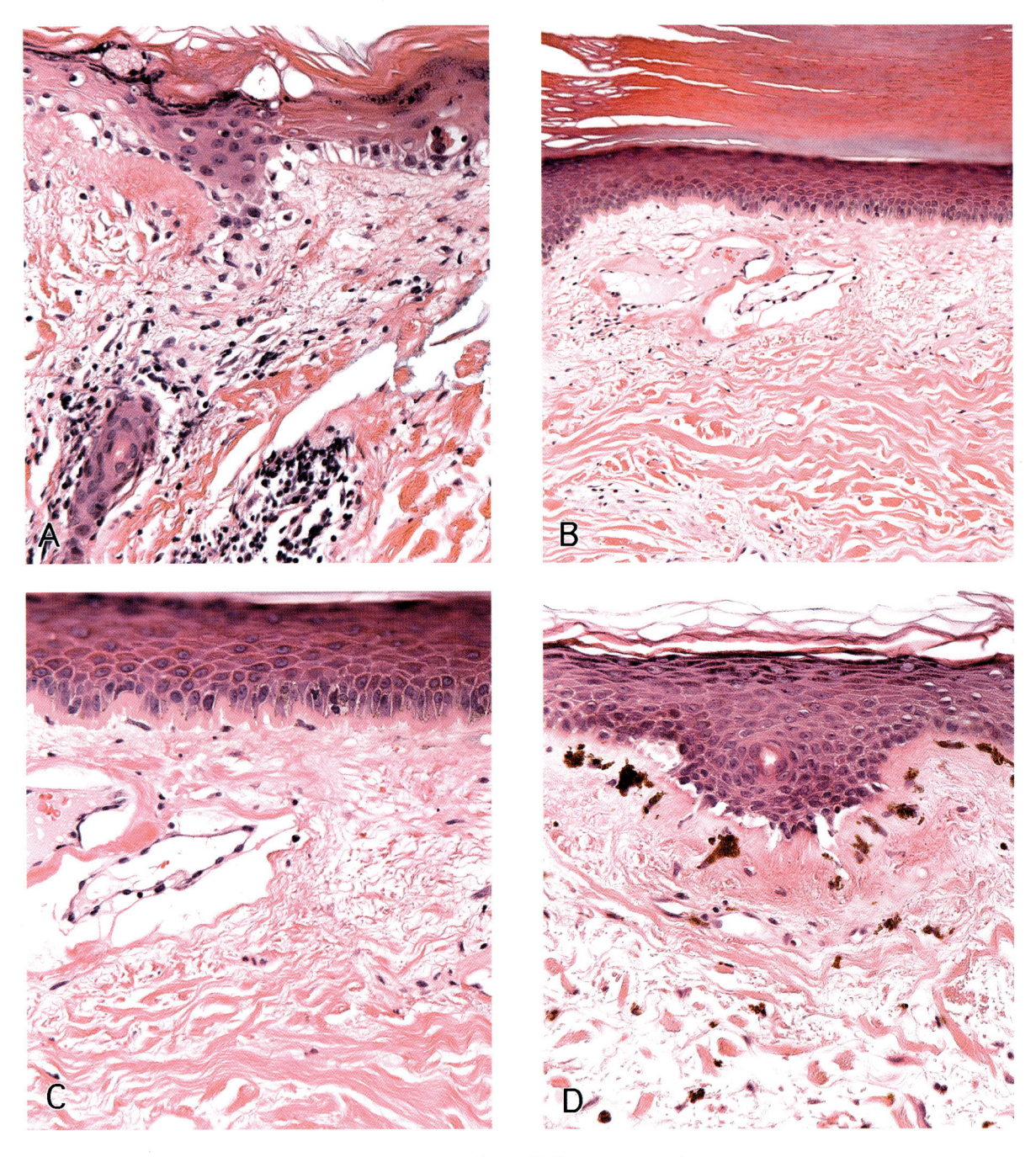

**Figure 7-33**

**DISCOID LUPUS ERYTHEMATOSUS**

A: In this active lesion, prominent basal layer vacuolization, focal apoptosis, epidermal thinning, and hyperkeratosis are present as well as eccrine duct involvement and dermal mucin deposition.

B: In this inactive lesion, hyperkeratosis is associated with epidermal atrophy and a virtually nonexistent inflammatory component.

C: In this higher magnification of the inactive lesion seen in B, in addition to epidermal atrophy, there are visibly thickened basement membrane and prominent and ectatic superficial blood vessels.

D: Inactive lesion, with persistent basement membrane thickening and pigment incontinence indicative of a previous lichenoid component.

*Lichenoid Dermatitis (Subacute to Chronic Cytotoxic Dermatitis)*

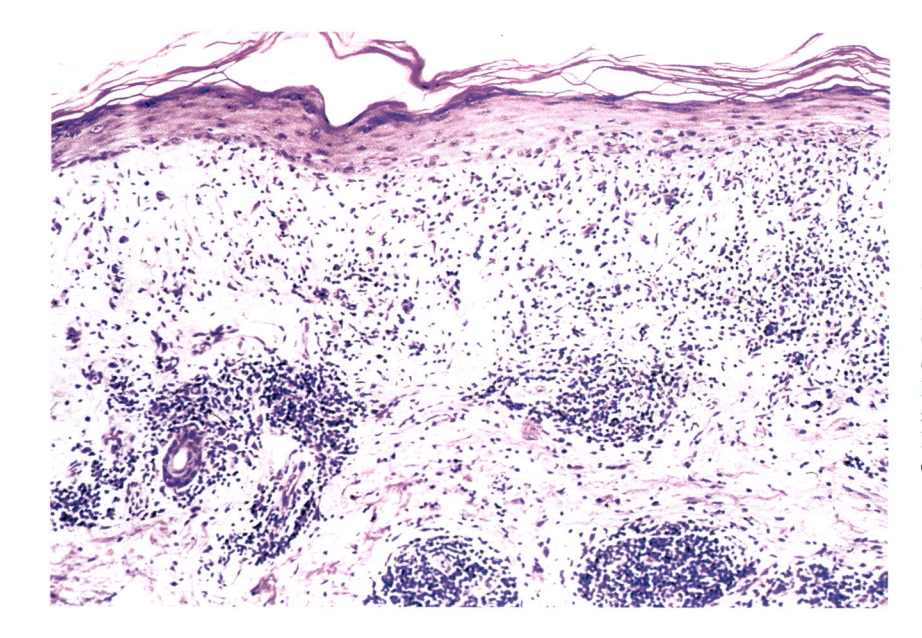

Figure 7-34

LUPUS ERYTHEMATOSUS

The superficial dermis shows a perivascular and papillary dermal interstitial lymphoid inflammatory infiltrate. The epidermis is atrophic and depleted of rete ridges, and lymphocytes are in direct apposition to a vacuolated basal cell layer. A hyperkeratotic scale is evident.

Figure 7-35

LUPUS ERYTHEMATOSUS: EARLY LESION

At high magnification, a cell-poor lymphocytic infiltrate is seen along the dermal-epidermal junction. The basal layer shows vacuolization and apoptosis; at this early juncture, the stratum corneum shows a normal basket-weave architecture, and basement membrane thickening would be inapparent by PAS staining.

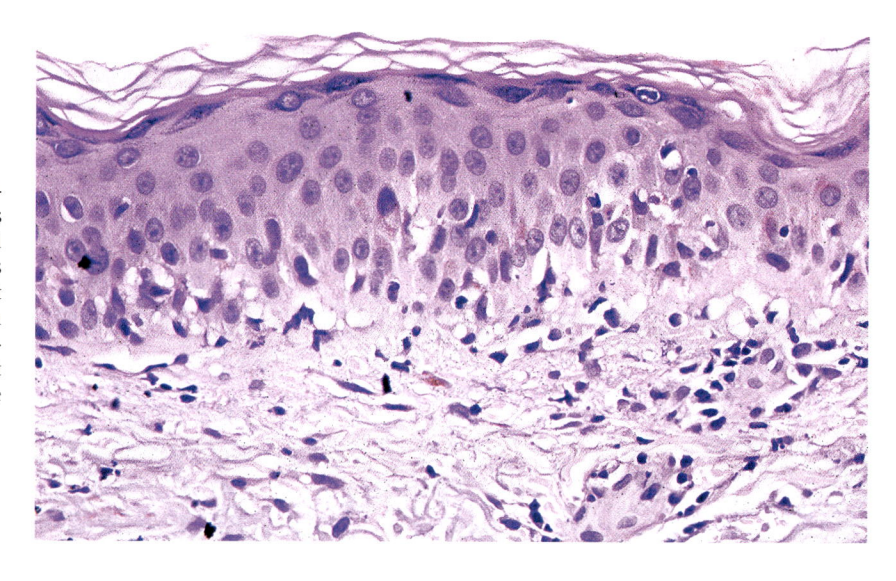

widened spaces separating collagen bundles (fig. 7-39). The use of a combined Alcian blue-PAS stain permits visualization of dermal mucin and the widened basement membrane in a single section (fig. 7-40).

The early lesions of lupus erythematosus exhibit focal hyperkeratosis overlying an atrophic epidermis, with vacuolation of the basal layer. Along the dermal-epidermal junction, granular debris, fragments of nuclei, and scattered neutrophils and occasional lymphocytes are observed. In a markedly pale dermis, ectasia of vessels is present. The pallor is shown, in part, to be mucin by stains for acid mucopolysaccharides, such as Alcian blue, ph 2.4 or colloidal iron stains. Mucicarmine, the stain for neutral mucopolysaccharides, is negative.

Subacute lupus erythematosus has distinctive histologic features. The epidermis may show focal mild retiform or psoriasiform hyperplasia surmounted by a parakeratotic scale. Infundibular hyperkeratosis is present. Focal atrophy affects limited areas of the epidermis. There is mild interface dermatitis, with vacuolation of the dermal-epidermal junction. Some lesions have a prominent lichenoid infiltrate and

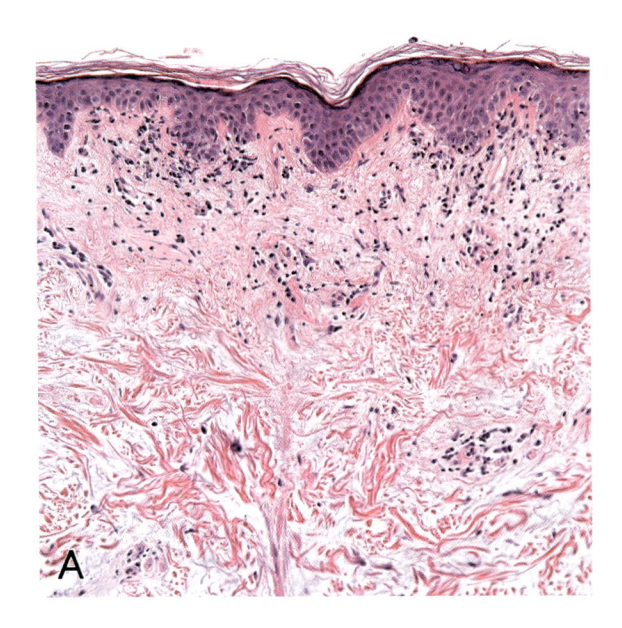

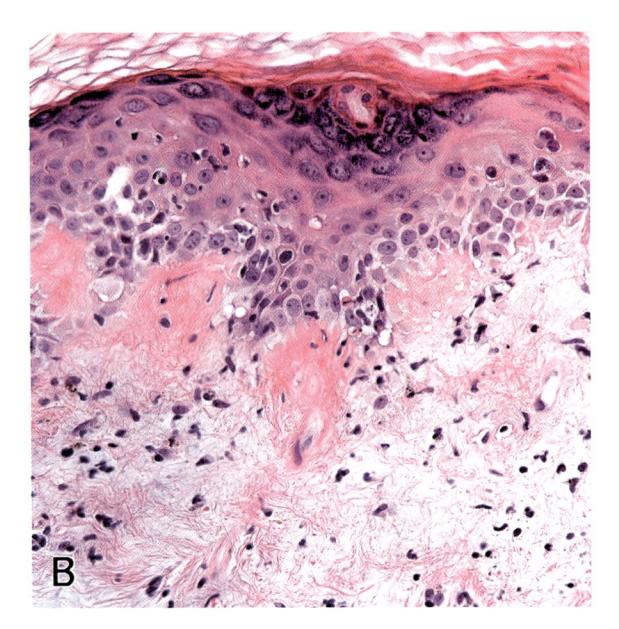

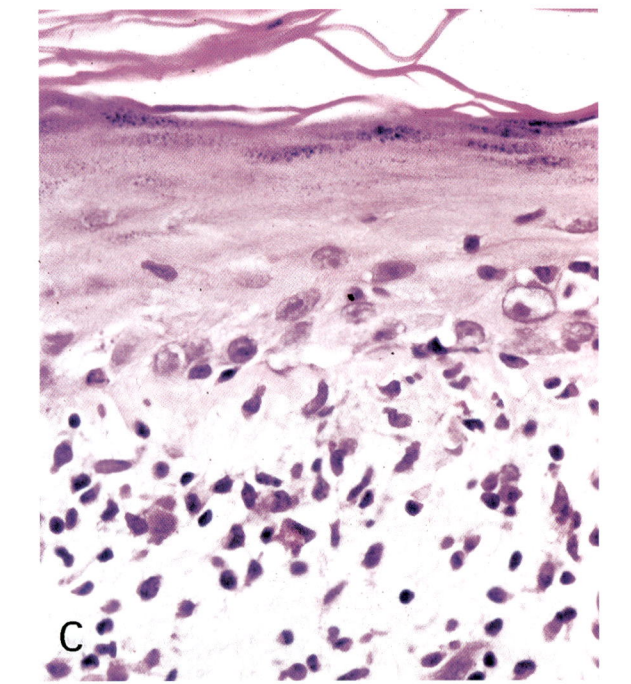

**Figure 7-36**

**SYSTEMIC LUPUS ERYTHERMATOUS**

A: At intermediate magnification, the lymphocyte-mediated interface injury is significantly more subtle than in discoid lupus. There is prominent dermal mucin deposition.

B: Lymphocyte-mediated interface injury is associated with basement membrane zone thickening and dermal mucinosis.

C: A more striking lymphocytic infiltrate within the papillary dermis is associated with vacuolization and apoptosis of the basal cell layer. The atrophic epidermis shows increased scale formation.

resemble lichen planus; others show psoriasiform change and a prominent band-like infiltrate, and represent hybrid dermatitis, that is, one showing more than one of the characteristic patterns of inflammatory reactions in the skin. A perivenular and periappendageal infiltrate is present but diminishes in intensity from the superficial to the deep dermis.

Certain lesions of lupus erythematosus show a predominance of dermal alterations and only minor or subtle changes affecting the overlying epidermis. For diagnostic purposes, such lesions are referred to as *lupus erythematosus of predominantly dermal type (lupus profundus* or *lupus tumidus)*. Lupus erythematosus of the face may show predominantly follicular involvement. Acute, subacute, and bullous variants of lupus are characterized by subtle interface changes, often without significant atrophy. A clue to the diagnosis of bullous lupus is the presence

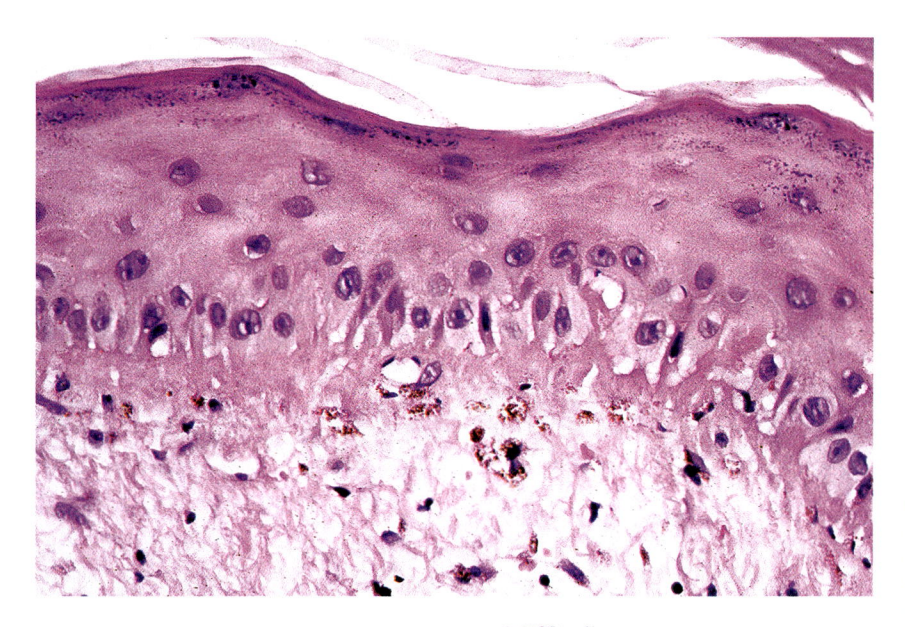

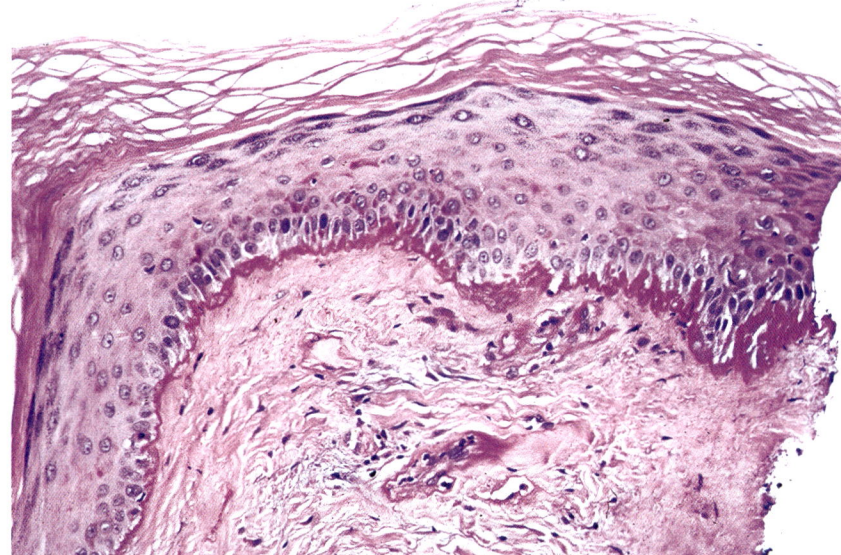

**Figure 7-37**

**DISCOID LUPUS ERYTHEMATOSUS**

Top: Advanced changes along the dermal-epidermal interface are seen. Apparent thickening of the basement membrane zone (routinely stained section) and associated melanin pigment incontinence are present.

Bottom: The thickened basement membrane zone is confirmed with a periodic acid–Schiff (PAS) stain to be consistent with the type of chronic injury to the dermal-epidermal interface observed in discoid lupus erythematosus.

of neutrophils along the dermal-epidermal junction, a feature that may cause confusion with linear IgA disease. A rare and fascinating histologic variant of lupus erythematosus produces hypertrophic lesions exhibiting verrucous epidermal hyperplasia in the presence of cytotoxic alterations along the dermal-epidermal interface (fig. 7-41).

**Special Diagnostic Studies.** The cutaneous lesions of lupus erythematosus span a spectrum of disease: discoid (chronic cutaneous) lupus, subacute cutaneous lupus, and acute lupus (usually systemic). Most patients have photodistribution of skin lesions and frequently have circulating antinuclear antibodies. Lesional skin biopsy specimens reveal granular deposition of immunoreactants at the basement membrane zone; demonstration of these immunoglobulins by immunofluorescence constitutes a positive lupus erythematosus band test (fig. 7-38).

Immunofluorescence findings, especially in lesions of recent onset, may be negative or, in some chronic lesions, show the presence of multiple immunoglobulins and complement. The finding of granular IgG, IgA, and IgM in a single biopsy specimen is highly suggestive of lupus. Both IgG and IgM are the most significant and frequent immunoglobulins deposited. Although

*Inflammatory Disorders of the Skin*

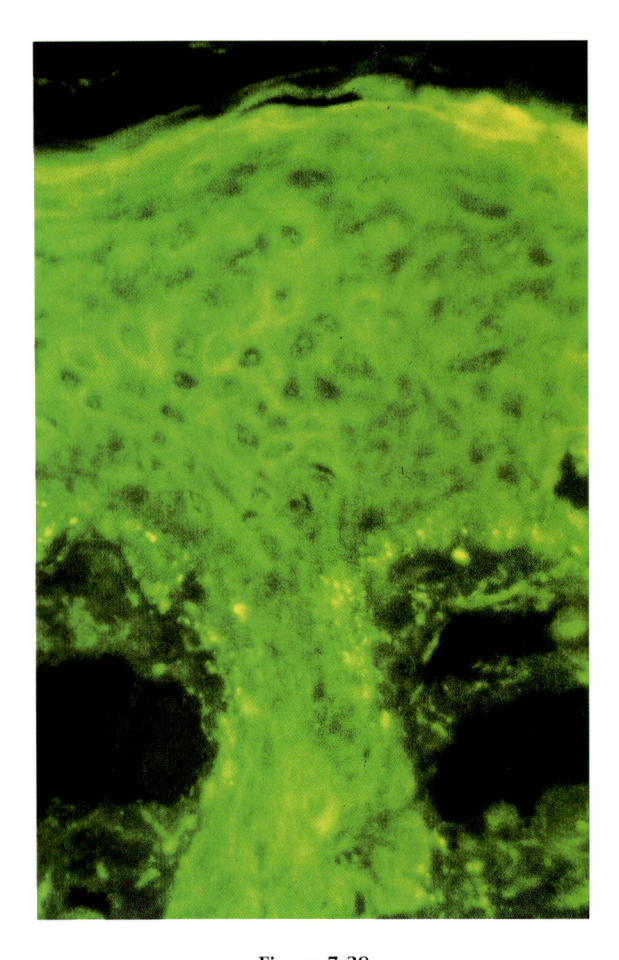

**Figure 7-38**
**LUPUS ERYTHEMATOSUS**

Direct immunofluorescence highlights this "positive lupus band test," which shows granular deposits of IgG along the dermal-epidermal interface. The presence of continuous granular deposits of immunoglobulin and/or complement is typical although not entirely specific for lupus erythematosus.

frequently only one immunoglobulin is seen in an early, evolving lupus lesion, the presence of only one immunoglobulin is also a nonspecific finding, especially in sun-exposed skin. There are a number of reasons for false-positive band tests: the more common relate to frequently encountered forms of dermatitis, such as rosacea, or simply are the result of chronic sun exposure of facial skin. The requirement of a strong continuous band of immune reactant deposition, in a pattern where fine granularity, coarse granularity, or thready or stippled fluorescence predominates, assists in differentiating a true-positive band test from apparent bands resulting

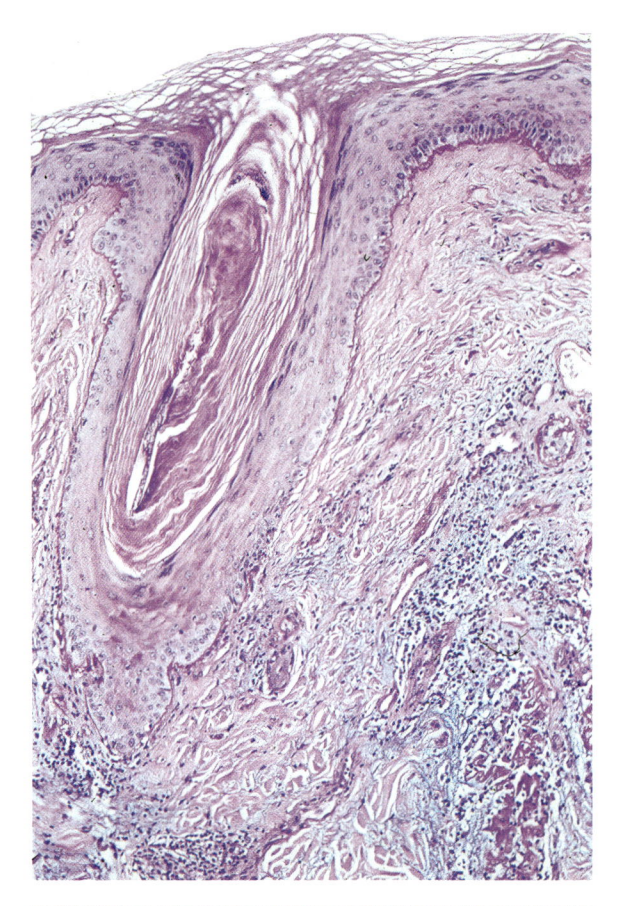

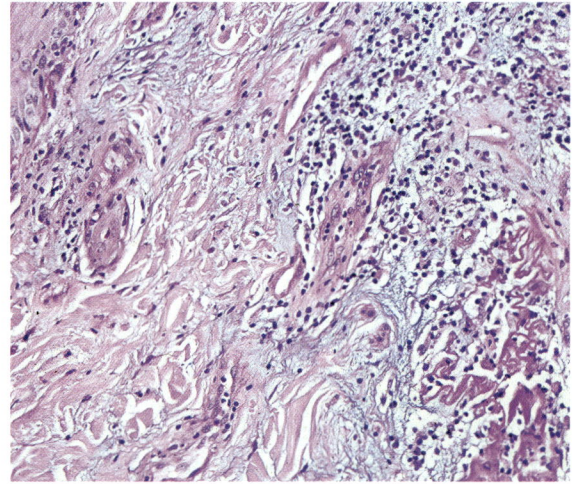

**Figure 7-39**
**DISCOID LUPUS ERYTHEMATOSUS**

Top: The follicular infundibulum is characteristically dilated and plugged by cornified material. The infundibular wall is atrophic, and a band of lymphocytes is present within the perifollicular adventitia.

Bottom: At higher magnification, a portion of a hair follicle is seen in the upper left. The adjacent dermis shows a patchy lymphoid infiltrate and increased deposition of mucin.

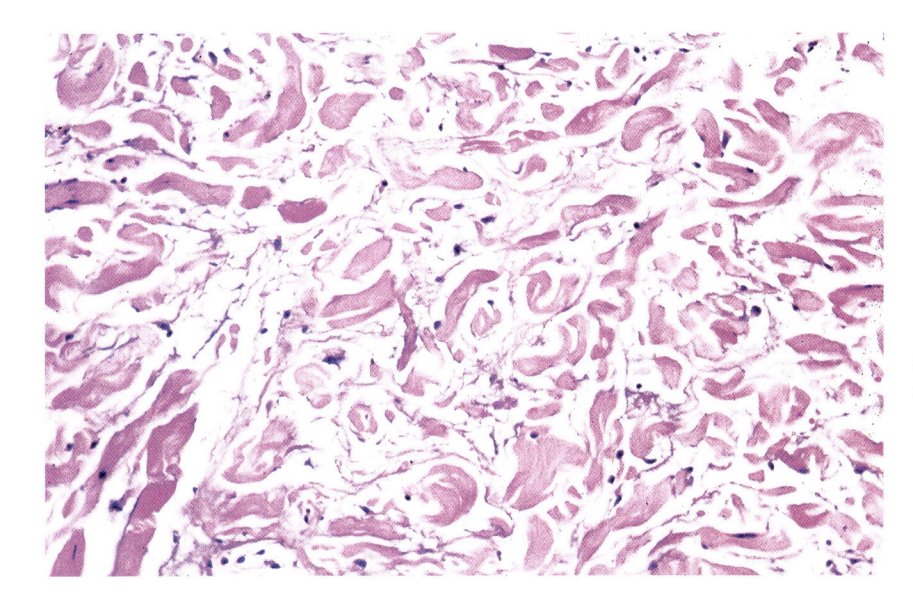

### Figure 7-40
### DISCOID LUPUS ERYTHEMATOSUS

The deposition of mucin is diffuse between the bundles of reticular dermal collagen.

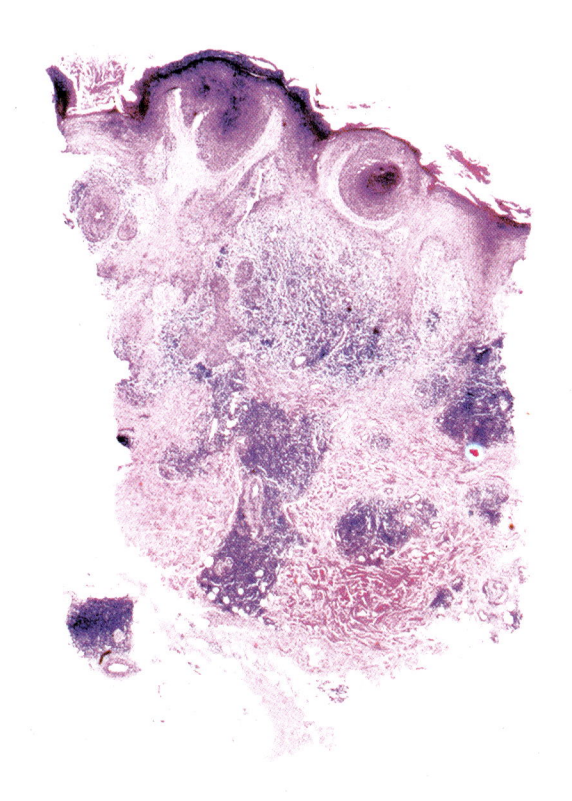

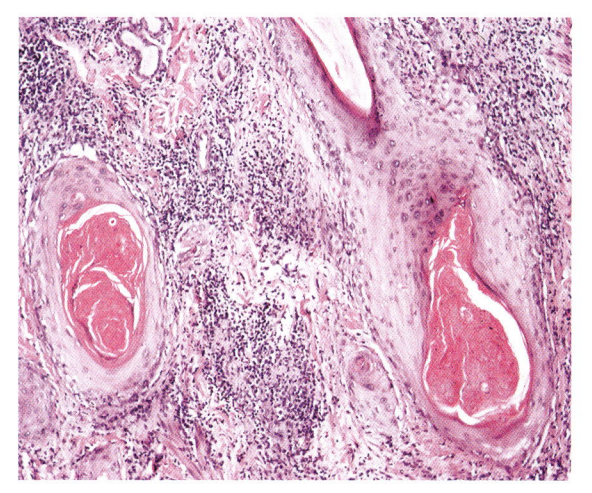

### Figure 7-41
### LUPUS ERYTHEMATOSUS: VERRUCOUS VARIANT

Left: There is a patchy lymphoid infiltrate within the superficial dermis as well as in the subcutaneous fat at scanning magnification. The epidermis and follicular infundibular epithelium appear markedly hyperplastic.

Above: At higher magnification, the epidermal layer is thrown into exophytic and endophytic undulations formed by hyperplastic epidermis and infundibular epithelium. Infundibular keratotic plugs are prominent. The brisk interface lymphocytic infiltrate is associated with variable basal cell layer destruction.

from nonspecific accretion of immune reactants along the basement membrane zone.

The presence or absence of immunoglobulins in lupus depends on several factors: 1) the type of skin lesion (acute, subacute, and chronic); 2) duration of the lesion; 3) site of biopsy; and 4) previous or concurrent administration of topical or systemic therapy. The overall prevalence of a positive lupus band test is approximately 50 to 90 percent (91 percent in patients with active disease and 33 percent in those with inactive disease). New lesions are frequently

Table 7-3

DIFFERENTIAL DIAGNOSIS OF POLYMORPHOUS LIGHT ERUPTION AND CUTANEOUS LUPUS ERYTHEMATOSUS

|  | Polymorphous Light Eruption | Cutaneous Lupus Erythematosus |
|---|---|---|
| Epidermal atrophy | Absent | Present |
| Basement membrane thickening | Absent | Present |
| Degree of deep infiltrate | Grades off | Prominent |
| Adnexal involvement | Absent | Present |
| Dermal mucinosis | Minimal | Present |

negative, whereas lesions present for more than 3 months are likely to be positive. The presence of a positive lupus band test in clinically normal, non–sun-exposed skin is strongly suggestive of systemic disease.

Granular deposits along the dermal-epidermal junction are localized, by electron microscopy, in the dermal aspect of the basal lamina, with extension into the papillary dermis. Similar deposits involve the basement membrane zone of follicular infundibula and are occasionally seen in the walls of small dermal venules.

A unique immunofluorescence staining pattern is seen in patients with subacute cutaneous lupus. This pattern consists of a particulate deposition within the lower epidermis and upper papillary dermis in both lesional and nonlesional skin. It is due to anti-Ro and anti-La antibodies reacting with these antigens or other antigens unregulated in the keratinocytes in this variant of lupus erythematosus. A similar pattern occurs in human skin grafted onto immunosuppressed mice that have been infused with anti-Ro/SSA autoantibodies (53).

**Differential Diagnosis.** Dermatomyositis may be indistinguishable histologically from lupus erythematosus, particularly the subacute variant. The destruction of endothelial cells by the circulating antiendothelial cell antibodies present in dermatomyositis, with resultant denuded and occasionally dilated superficial vessels, is not seen in lupus. Immunofluorescence, serologic, and clinical findings are critical for differentiating the cutaneous lesions of these two disorders. Occasionally, polymorphous light eruptions mimic lupus erythematosus, particularly the forms that show primarily dermal involvement (Table 7-3).

**Treatment and Prognosis.** Lupus erythematosus is a chronic, potentially progressive disease. In its purely cutaneous form, topical and sometimes systemic steroids may control lesions. Hydroxychloroquine is also an effective drug (54). In systemic disease, potent immunosuppression may be required to prevent the potentially devastating systemic complications that may result in failure of vital organs. Choices include mycophenolate, azathioprine, and cyclosporine, among others. The use of antitumor necrosis factor therapy can be plagued by a rash, similar to innate lupus, and can often induce a lupus-like systemic syndrome.

## DERMATOMYOSITIS

**Definition.** *Dermatomyositis* is a lymphocyte-mediated autoimmune disease affecting primarily skin and muscle (55–66).

**Clinical Features.** Proximal muscle weakness is the primary presenting sign of the disease, which is termed *polymyositis* when only muscle is involved. Skin manifestations include periorbital violaceous discoloration predominately affecting the upper eyelids (heliotrope eyes) and a maculopapular, scaling eruption affecting the face, neck, dorsal surfaces of the arms and legs, as well as knuckles (figs. 7-42, 7-43), elbows, and knees (Gottron papules). Periungual erythema as well as zones of epidermal atrophy, telangiectasia, and hypopigmentation and hyperpigmentation (poikiloderma) are observed (the latter potentially causing confusion with lupus erythematosus).

**Pathologic Findings.** The diagnosis often requires muscle biopsy, skin biopsy, and correlation with clinical features. Muscle biopsy reveals degenerative alterations in myocytes associated with infiltration and apposition of lymphocytes. Skin biopsy typically shows subtle but distinct findings of mild hyperkeratosis with profound epidermal atrophy and vacuolization of the

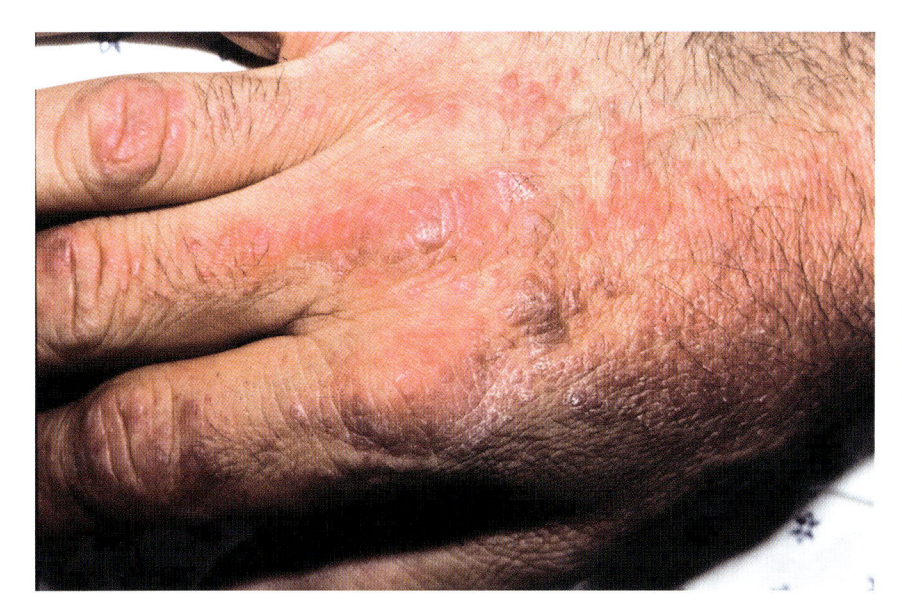

*Lichenoid Dermatitis (Subacute to Chronic Cytotoxic Dermatitis)*

**Figure 7-42**

**DERMATOMYOSITIS**

There is an erythematosus maculopapular eruption involving the dorsal skin of the hand, with some accentuation of skin involving the knuckles.

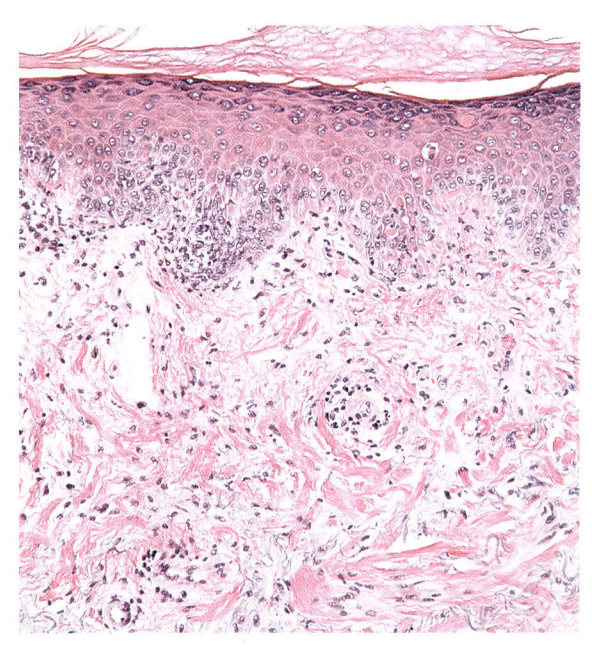

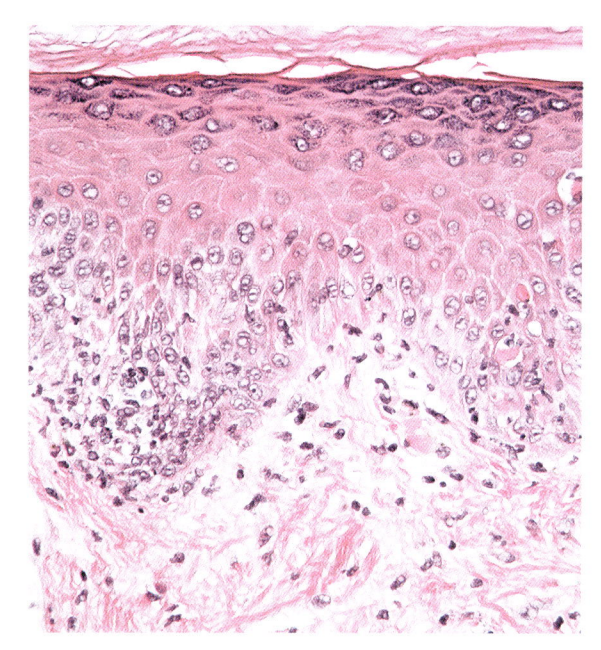

**Figure 7-43**

**GOTTRON PAPULE**

Left: The sparse lymphocytic inflammatory infiltration is associated with basal layer injury and suprabasal apoptosis at this acral site.

Right: Higher magnification shows lymphocyte-associated apoptosis favoring the rete ridge.

dermal-epidermal junction (figs. 7-44–7-46). The papillary and upper reticular dermis exhibit dilated vessels in which there are diminished endothelial cells or a vascular basement membrane zone seemingly denuded of endothelium. Careful inspection reveals clumped small aggregates of pale gray collagen, which are areas of destroyed, collapsed vessels. These changes are mediated by the presence of antiendothelial cell antibodies that result in complement fixation and destruction caused by the membrane attack complex. Immunofluorescence-labeled

*Inflammatory Disorders of the Skin*

**Figure 7-44**

**DERMATOMYOSITIS**

Top: There is a sparse inflammatory infiltrate accentuating the superficial dermal vessels. The infiltrate is inconspicuous at this magnification within the papillary dermis.

Bottom: At higher magnification, the perivascular lymphocytic component as well as the papillary dermal lichenoid component are better appreciated. Lymphocytes have migrated focally along the dermal-epidermal interface in association with a basal layer showing degenerative alterations. This pattern is similar to that seen in early or subacute lupus erythematosus and erythema multiforme.

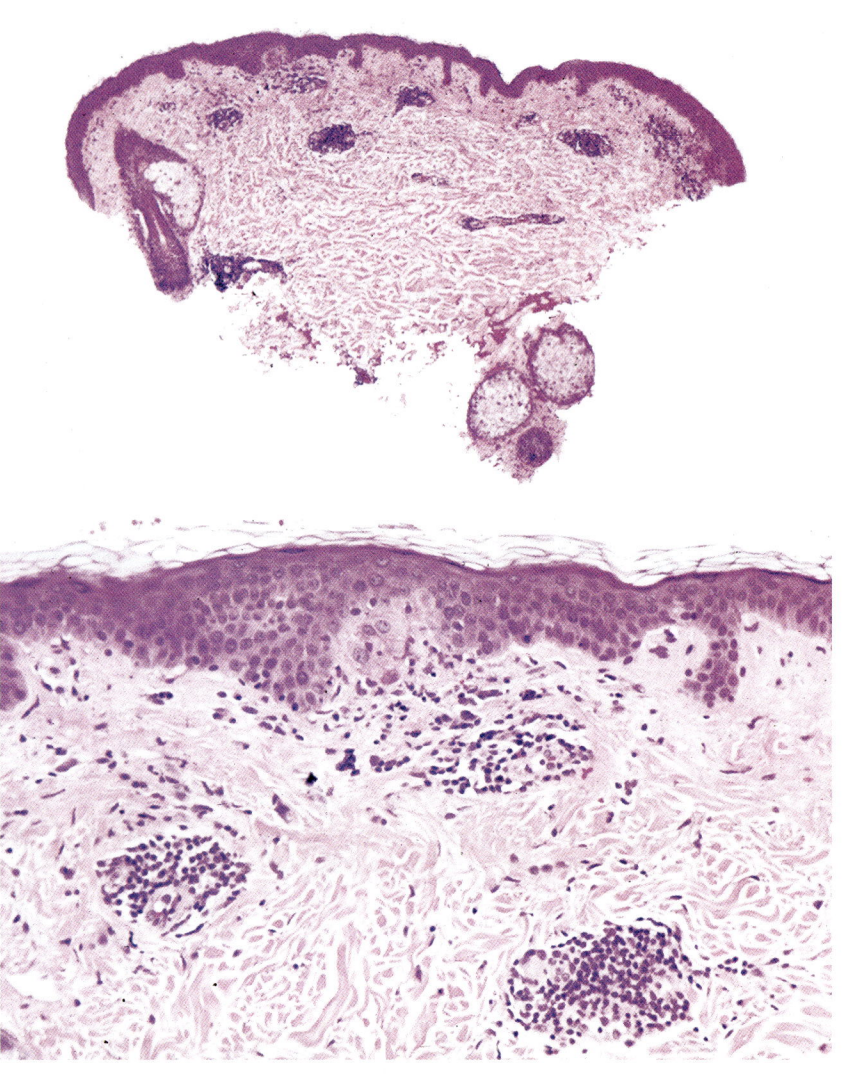

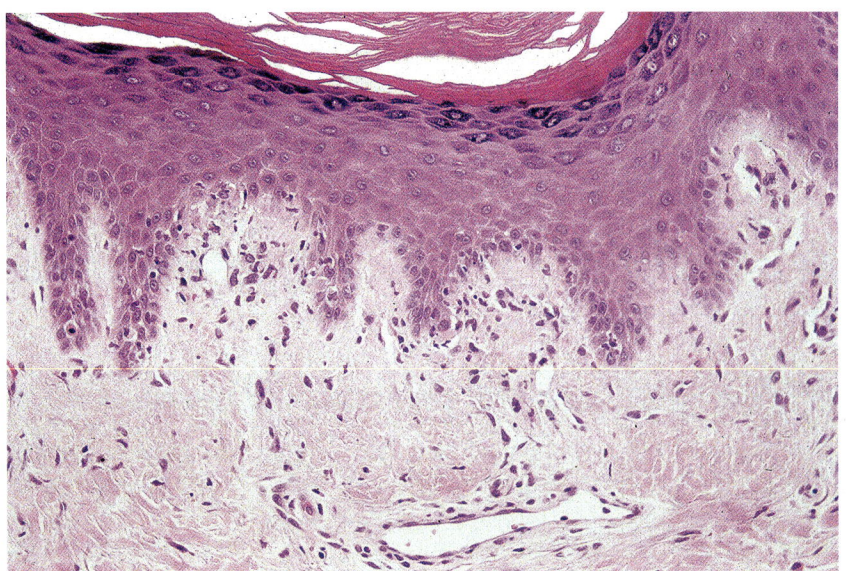

**Figure 7-45**

**DERMATOMYOSITIS**

The infiltrate of lymphocytes along the dermal-epidermal junction is sparse. Foci of apoptosis associated with lymphoid exocytosis, and mild acanthosis and hyperkeratosis of the epidermal layer, are present.

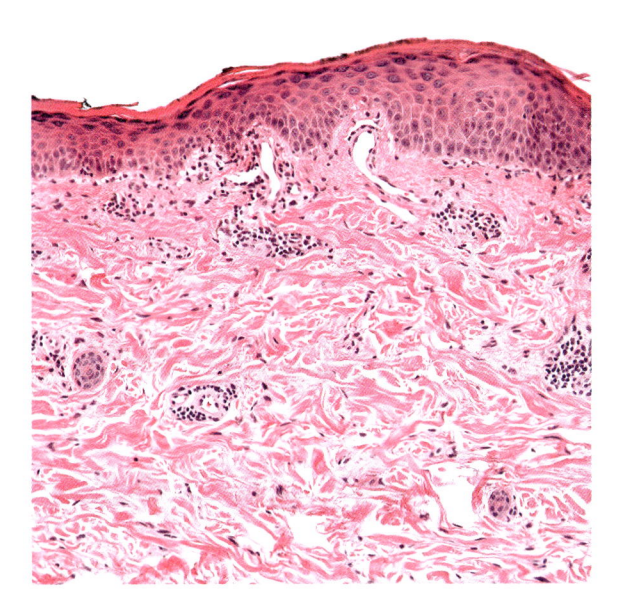

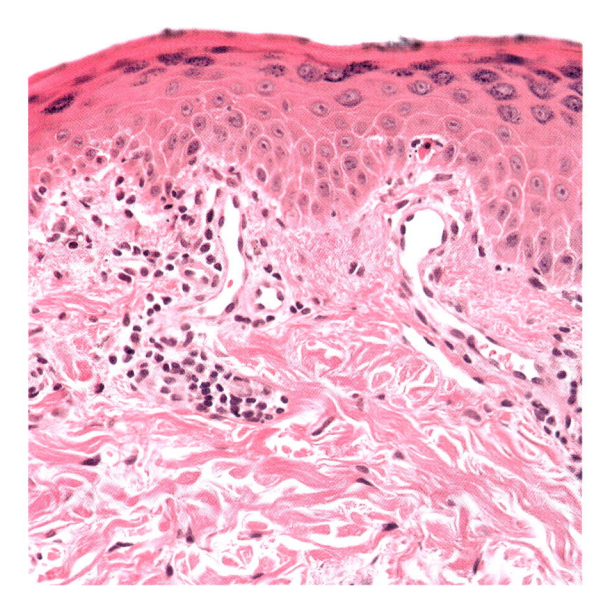

**Figure 7-46**

**DERMATOMYOSITIS**

Left: The inflammatory infiltrate is sparse and the interface changes subtle. Prominent superficial vessels are a clue to the diagnosis.

Right: At high magnification, a sparse superficial lymphocytic infiltrate, basal layer apoptosis, and prominent superficial capillary loops are seen.

antibodies against C5-9 decorate the basement membrane zone of the affected vessels as well as the collapsed vessels. In the dermis, there is a sparse, often focal, papillary dermal perivenular lymphoid infiltrate with zones of interface alteration resulting in basal cell layer vacuolization. The papillary dermis exhibits pallor due to mild dermal mucin deposition. Periadnexal lymphoid infiltration, as is observed in lupus erythematosus, is absent.

**Differential Diagnosis.** The primary entity in the differential diagnosis is the early, mild, and subacute lesion of lupus erythematosus. In addition to the differential features noted above, lesions of dermatomyositis generally fail to show a positive granular band of immunoglobulin and complement along the dermal-epidermal junction upon direct immunofluorescence testing. Evidence of the membrane attack complex, C5-9, in the areas of the upper dermis that are the sites of destroyed vessels, is helpful in distinguishing dermatomyositis from lupus erythematosus.

**Treatment and Prognosis.** The disease is chronic, although symptoms may wax and wane (67). Systemic corticosteroids may be effective in controlling symptoms, signs, and progression of this disorder (68,69). The disease may be recalcitrant to steroids, and cyclosporine, mycophenolate, azathioprine, and intravenous immunoglobulin may be necessary to control symptoms. Antitumor necrosis factor therapy is used in difficult cases (69a).

## PITYRIASIS LICHENOIDES CHRONICA

*Pityriasis lichenoides chronica* is considered a superficial variant or chronic superficial manifestation of pityriasis lichenoides et varioliformis acuta (PLEVA), and its comparative histologic features are discussed under that entity (70).

## LICHENOID IMMUNE RESPONSES

**Definition.** *Lichenoid immune response* is a diverse array of reaction patterns provoked by systemic (drug) or locally injected (insect bite) antigens (70). In many instances, the offending agent cannot be definitively identified. Other reactions include vasculitic, urticarial, spongiotic, acanthotic, and even panniculitic lesions. Lichenoid immune responses are common, and must be differentiated from primary forms of lichenoid dermatitis. Occasionally, photo-induced

*Inflammatory Disorders of the Skin*

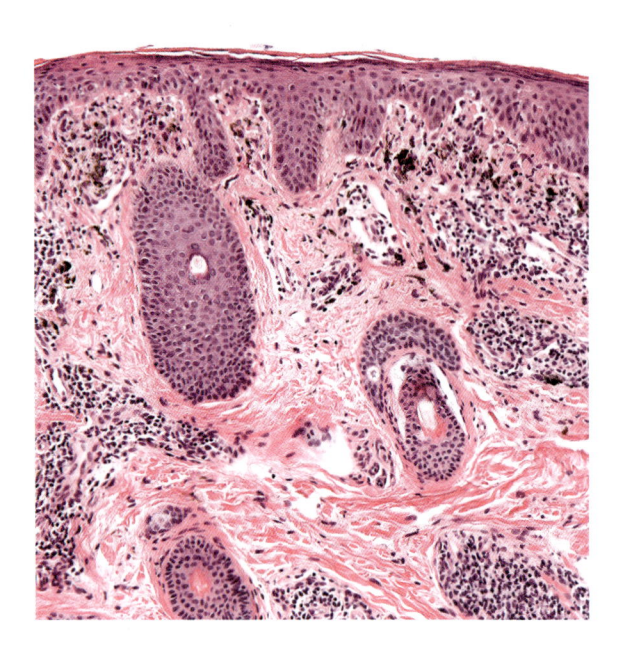

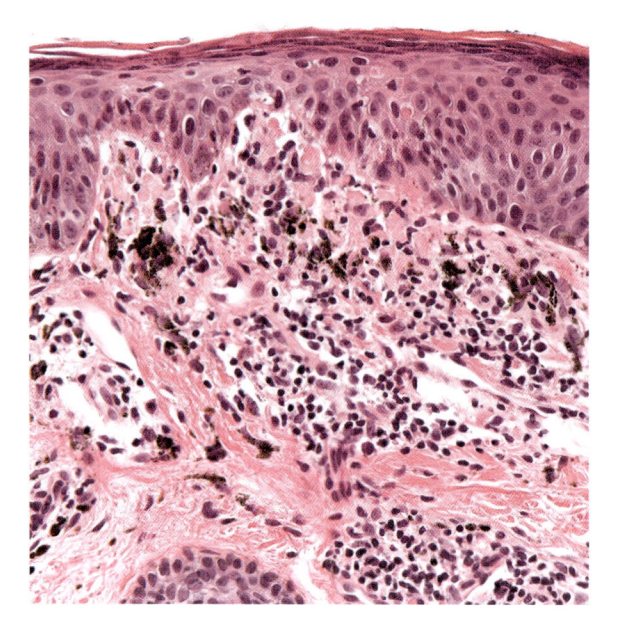

**Figure 7-47**

**LICHENOID FACIAL DERMATITIS**

Left: This presumed drug eruption shows both a lichenoid and superficial and deep perivascular inflammatory component.
Right: There is prominent apoptosis with colloid body formation and pigment incontinence.

reactions to contact sensitizers show a lichenoid reaction pattern.

**Clinical Features.** *Lichenoid drug eruptions* generally present as multiple, generalized erythematous papules within several days after drug ingestion. *Lichenoid insect bite reactions* tend to be localized to the site of the insect bite, but in extreme cases, appear generalized. More often, however, there are one to multiple erythematous papules, frequently in a linear distribution, potentially leading to confusion with Koebnerization, or with coalescence to form a linear plaque (e.g., as with lichen striatus).

A unique group of hypersensitivity responses is caused by viral and certain bacterial infections. The principle viral agents include Epstein-Barr virus, parvovirus B19, hepatitis B and C, and human immunodeficiency virus (HIV). Bacteria that contain superantigens also cause these reactions, as do some spirochetal infections. The clinical lesions may be lichenoid, or sometimes erythema multiforme–like or urticarial.

**Pathologic Findings.** Lichenoid hypersensitivity reactions due to drugs and insect bites are distinctive in being mediated by eosinophils as well as lymphocytes. Plasma cells may also be seen. The epidermal changes, however, resemble other forms of chronic cytotoxic dermatitis, with variable acanthosis, basal cell layer vacuolization, squamatization, apoptosis, colloid body formation, and pigment incontinence within the superficial dermis (fig. 7-47). There is variable hyperkeratosis, but unlike classic lichen planus, there may also be parakeratosis. The inflammatory infiltrates tend to be superficial and deep, with more prominent perivascular components than in other forms of lichenoid dermatitis. In insect bite reactions, there may also be an interstitial component, where lymphocytes, eosinophils, and histiocytes infiltrate among reticular dermal collagen bundles in a pattern similar to that seen in the early evolutionary phases of palisaded granulomatous dermatitis. In some instances, lichenoid immune responses to injected agents (e.g., tattoo pigments) are diagnosed by detecting the offending agent in the biopsy specimen (fig. 7-48).

**Differential Diagnosis.** The primary entity in the differential diagnosis is lichen planus. The presence of eosinophils, a deep component

*Lichenoid Dermatitis (Subacute to Chronic Cytotoxic Dermatitis)*

to the infiltrate, or parakeratosis is helpful in excluding this possibility. An interstitial component and vascular injury favor a lichenoid insect bite reaction over a lichenoid drug eruption.

**Treatment and Prognosis.** The lesions are self-limited with cessation and avoidance of the antigenic stimulus. In extremely acute lesions, the application of cool soaks or even ice packs is helpful. Topical corticosteroids provide relief in severe cases. In patients with a generalized eruption and marked pruritus, a brief course of oral steroids is effective.

## SECONDARY SYPHILIS

**Definition.** *Syphilis* affects skin in three phases: 1) primary chancre; 2) secondary lesions; and 3) tertiary granulomatous (gummatous) lesions (72–76). Secondary lesions are most commonly lichenoid, although striking acanthosis (condyloma lata), ulceration, pustulation, and selective follicular destruction (luetic alopecia) are rarely encountered (76,77). Thus, secondary syphilis is recognized both clinically and histologically as the mimic of a number of unrelated conditions (78).

**Clinical Features.** Secondary syphilis frequently presents as small, erythematous to red-brown plaques that resemble pityriasis rosea or small plaque parapsoriasis. There may be lichenoid or psoriasiform lesions; the latter are often referred to as *rupial secondary syphilis*. Involvement of the palms, soles (fig. 7-49), and mucosal surfaces should alert the clinician to the possibility of secondary syphilis (79). The eruption usually follows the appearance of the primary lesion by weeks to, rarely, months. In some cases, the eruption appears while the

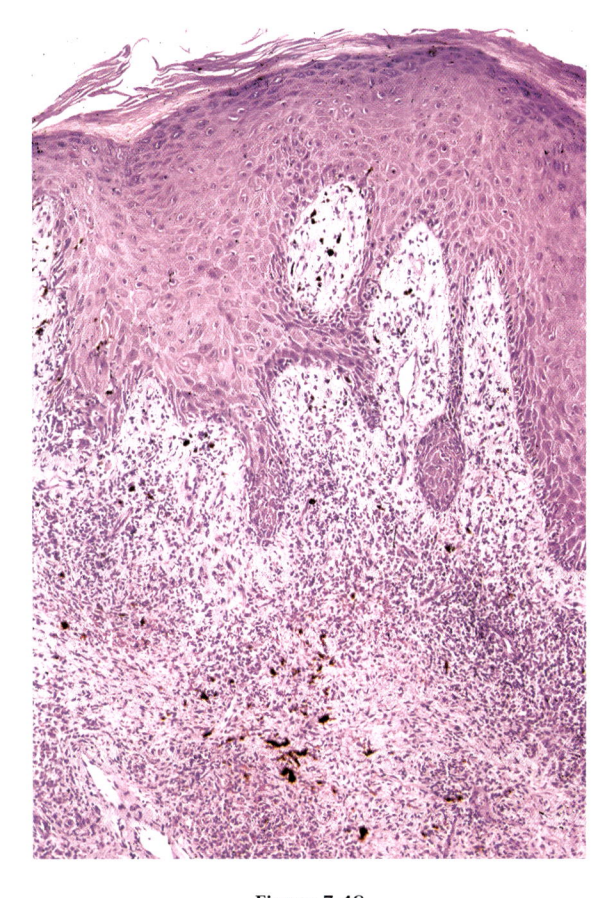

Figure 7-48

**LICHENOID REACTION PATTERN**

A patchy band-like infiltrate of lymphocytes is present along the dermal-epidermal interface of a variably hyperplastic epidermis. There are foci of subacute to chronic interface alteration. The red pigment embedded within the superficial reticular dermis is evidence of a lichenoid dermatitic response to tattoo pigment. Lichenoid reaction patterns are also seen as a consequence of insect bites or drug eruptions.

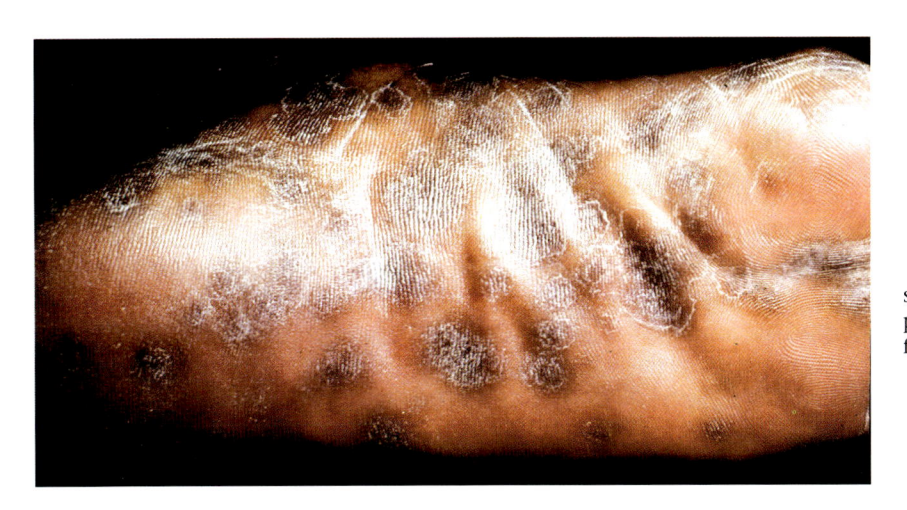

Figure 7-49

**LICHENOID SECONDARY SYPHILIS**

There are hyperpigmented scaling plaques on the sole. The patient had serologically confirmed secondary syphilis.

*Inflammatory Disorders of the Skin*

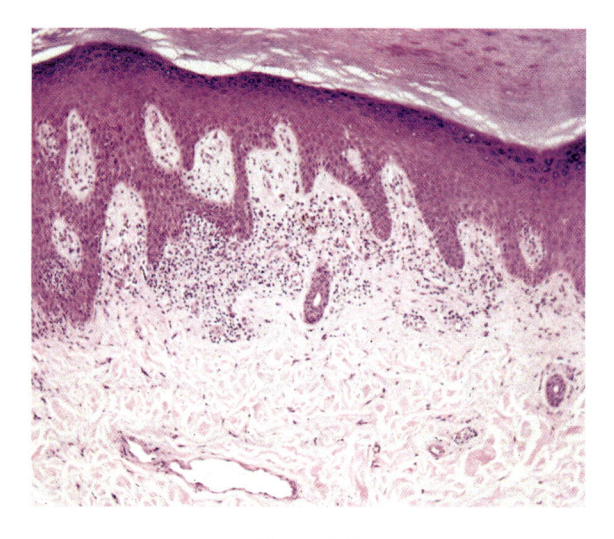

Figure 7-50

**SECONDARY SYPHILIS: EARLY LESION**

Above: There is a patchy lichenoid infiltrate of lymphocytes within the superficial dermis associated with variable epidermal hyperplasia.

Right: At higher magnification, the patchy lymphoid infiltrate is associated with vacuolization and apoptosis of the basal cell layer. Even at this magnification, occasional plasma cells are seen.

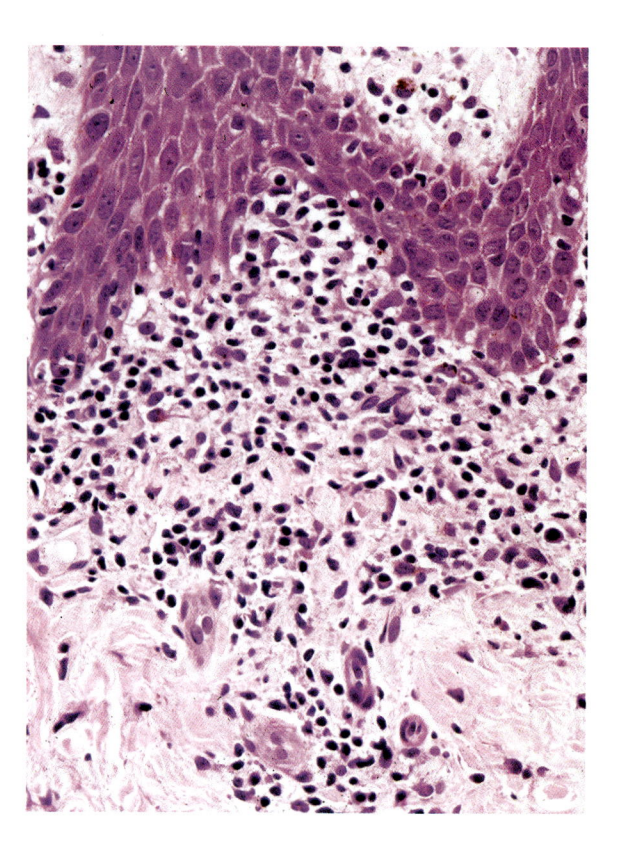

Figure 7-51

**LICHENOID SECONDARY SYPHILIS: ADVANCED LESION**

In addition to a band-like infiltrate of lymphocytes within the superficial dermis, there is a perivascular component extending into the mid to deep reticular dermis.

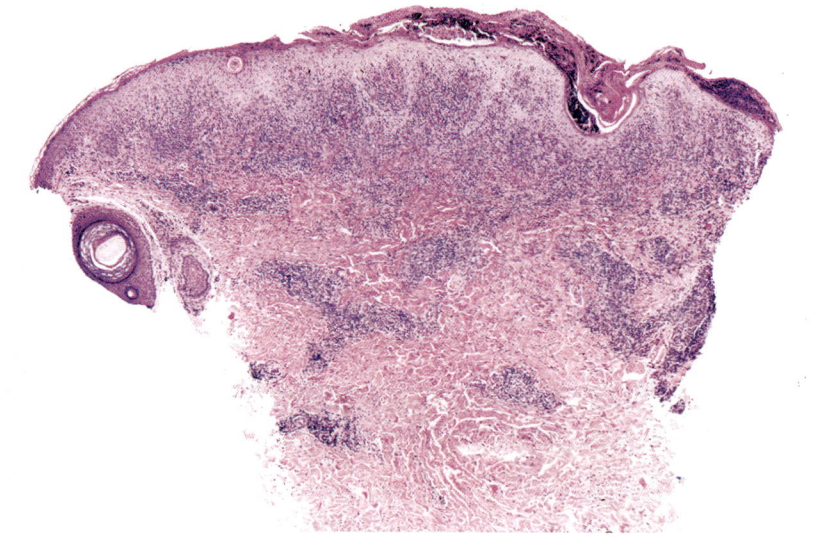

primary lesions are still visible. In some individuals a late secondary eruption occurs; often, these patients have been inadequately treated.

**Pathologic Findings.** Lichenoid secondary syphilis demonstrates a band-like infiltrate of lymphocytes and histiocytes within the papillary dermis and a deep underlying angiocentric component (figs. 7-50–7-53). There is a variable degree of injury to the basal cell layer and vacuolation of the dermal-epidermal junction. The epidermis is usually not acanthotic with a jagged dermal-epidermal interface, as is seen in lichen planus; rather, the epidermal rete may be lost and the epidermal layer thinned, or the rete may demonstrate psoriasiform hyperplasia, with thickening of the epidermal layer, the

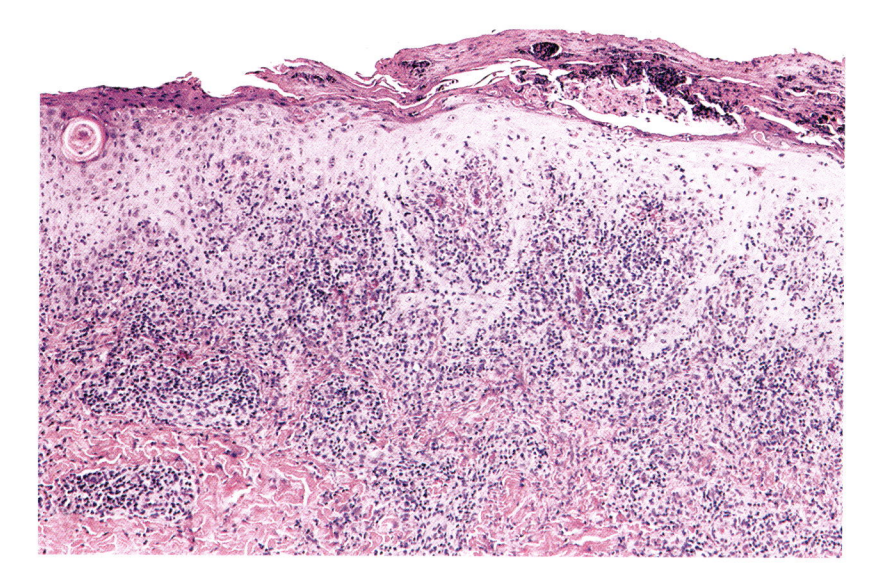

*Lichenoid Dermatitis (Subacute to Chronic Cytotoxic Dermatitis)*

**Figure 7-52**

**LICHENOID SECONDARY SYPHILIS: ADVANCED LESION**

The band-like infiltrate of lymphocytes and plasma cells obscures the dermal-epidermal interface. There is basal cell layer destruction as well as variable acanthosis and parakeratosis within the epidermis.

**Figure 7-53**

**LICHENOID SECONDARY SYPHILIS**

Foci of granulomatous inflammation are seen within the lichenoid component of the lesion.

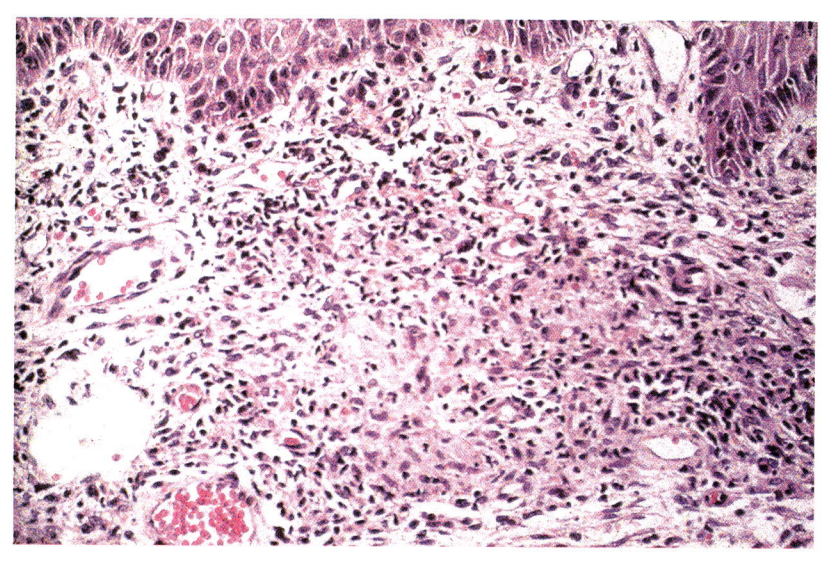

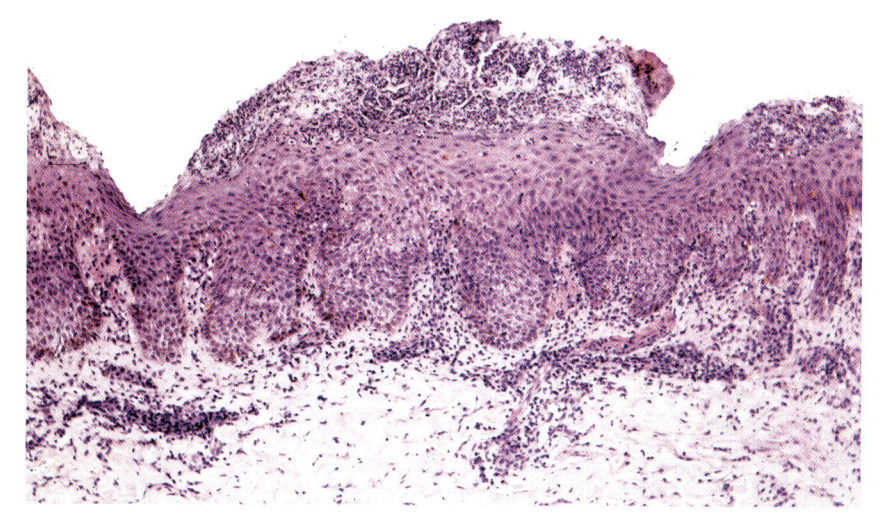

**Figure 7-54**

**LICHENOID SECONDARY SYPHILIS: RUPIAL VARIANT**

In addition to a perivascular and lichenoid infiltrate of lymphocytes and plasma cells, there is psoriasiform epidermal hyperplasia with overlying parakeratosis infiltrated by neutrophils.

*Inflammatory Disorders of the Skin*

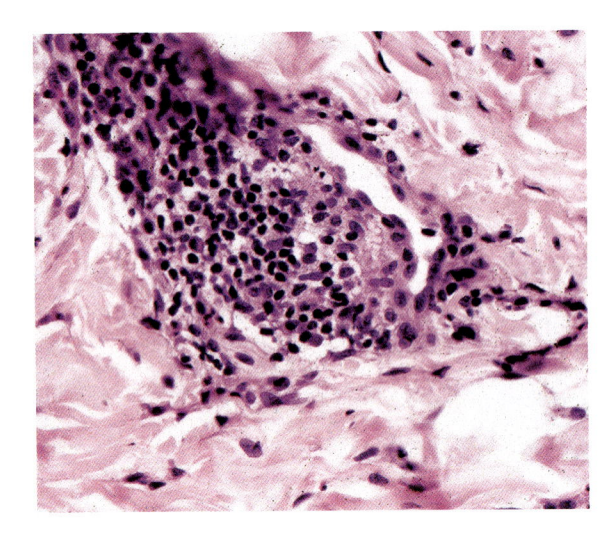

**Figure 7-55**

**DERMAL COMPONENT OF LICHENOID SECONDARY SYPHILIS: RUPIAL VARIANT**

Above: There is a perivascular cuff of lymphocytes and plasma cells, with intense permeation of the vessel wall. The endothelial cells are bulging and activated.

Right: There are activated lymphocytes and numerous plasma cells associated with vessels showing marked endothelial prominence and focal obliterative luminal changes.

rupial variant (figs. 7-54, 7-55). A low-power clue to the diagnosis is the presence of a lichenoid and deep infiltrate, with prominent perivascular and perifollicular involvement and focal cellular debris around affected areas. Another clue is the presence of unusual numbers of activated histiocytes, often associated with vague foci of granuloma formation. Most helpful are numerous plasma cells in the infiltrate. Remarkable and often occlusive endothelial swelling is usually present (figs. 7-55, 7-56). At times, the degree of endothelial swelling is so pronounced that vascular lumens are no longer detectable.

Silver stains (i.e., Warthin-Starry or Dieterle) may show thin, spiraling spirochetes in the dermal infiltrate and within the epidermal layer or follicular structures (fig. 7-57). Special stains are often negative, with the exception of the hyperplastic neutrophil-rich variant of secondary syphilis that affects mucosal surfaces, *condyloma lata*.

**Differential Diagnosis.** The presence of plasma cells in an inflammatory infiltrate, particularly when not involving mucosa or paramucosa, should always suggest syphilis.

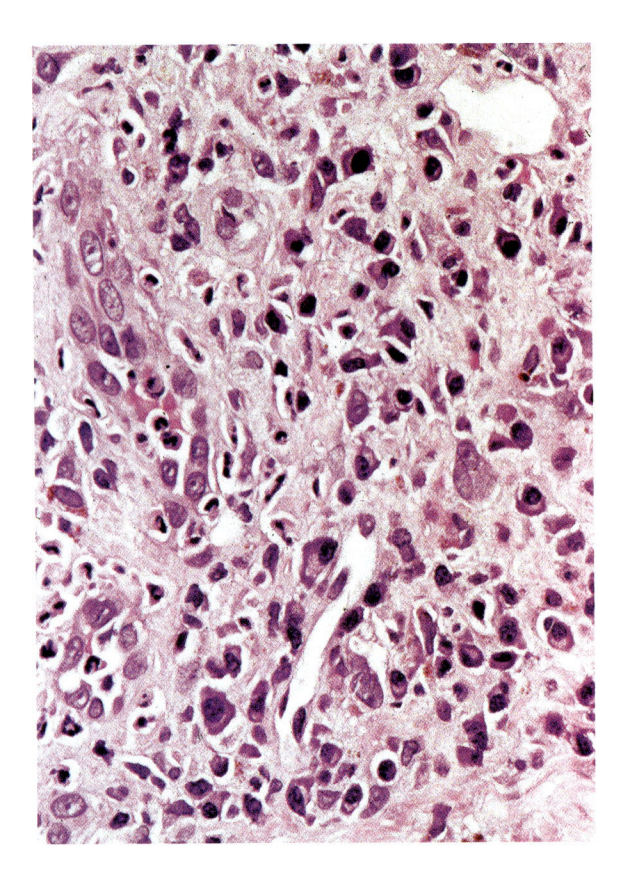

The nodular drug reaction that may occur in hypersensitivity reactions to phenytoin or other agents is rich in eosinophils in addition to lymphocytes and plasma cells, but there is massive endothelial cell hypertrophy. Psoriasiform dermatitis associated with HIV infection may have prominent plasma cells, and appropriate serologic tests must be performed to rule out syphilis. In the setting of lichenoid dermatitis that contains plasma cells, vague granulomatous foci, or marked occlusive endothelial activation, or that presents clinically as nonlichenoid dermatitis (e.g., pityriasis rosea, small plaque parapsoriasis, or guttate psoriasis), appropriate serologic testing should be performed to rule out syphilis. Special stains should also be obtained, because seronegative lesions may occur in the setting of immunodeficiency or false-negative serologies may occur for other reasons.

**Treatment and Prognosis.** Systemic antibiotics are usually curative (80–85). Untreated disease may progress to tertiary lesions after many years, with systemic (central nervous system and cardiovascular), as well as cutaneous, implications (86,87).

*Lichenoid Dermatitis (Subacute to Chronic Cytotoxic Dermatitis)*

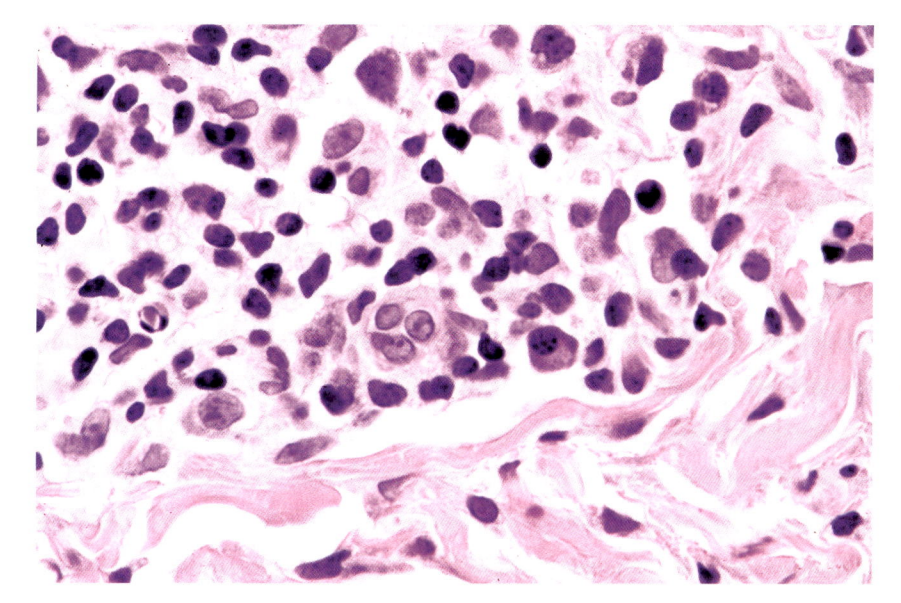

**Figure 7-56**

**LICHENOID SECONDARY SYPHILIS: PLASMA CELL COMPONENT**

Vessels are not discernable because of the endothelial swelling, which has produced obliterative luminal changes.

**Figure 7-57**

**LICHENOID SECONDARY SYPHILIS**

The Dieterle stain highlights numerous slender spiraling organisms (enclosed and in inset) within connective tissue and within the epidermal layer. Many cases are negative, however, and serologic confirmation often is more sensitive than tissue stains in establishing a definitive diagnosis.

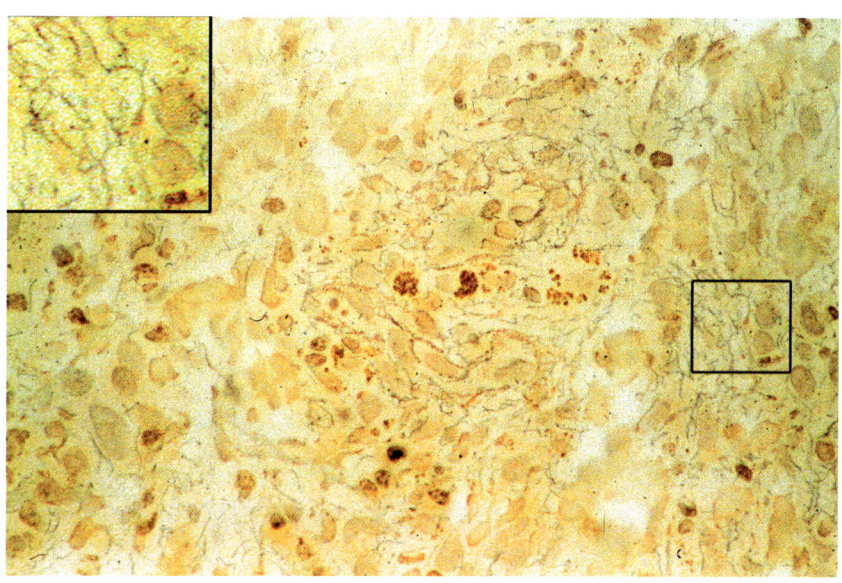

## LICHEN SCLEROSUS (EARLY/INFLAMMATORY STAGE)

**Definition.** *Lichen sclerosus* most commonly presents as a whitish, atrophic, chronic dermatitis that involves the genitalia and occasionally the nongenital skin (88–91). While the chronic lesions are classic, and often deforming in genital areas, the earliest lesions are more difficult to appreciate since they are often erythematous (92).

**Clinical Features.** Focal areas of erythema with itching and sometimes burning, especially in the vulvovaginal and perianal areas as well as in the prepuce of boys and men, should suggest lichen sclerosus in an early inflammatory phase (fig. 7-58). The erythematous plaques show, at times, evidence of sclerosis, which presents as thickening of the affected area. There may be variable hypopigmentation, although very early lesions do not show pigmentary change. A biopsy is generally necessary for diagnosis.

**Pathologic Findings.** The earliest phases of lichen sclerosus involve accumulation of lymphocytes and occasionally plasma cells about superficial dermal vessels as well as within the superficial dermal interstitium (fig. 7-59). This characteristic pattern of papillary dermal interstitial lymphoid

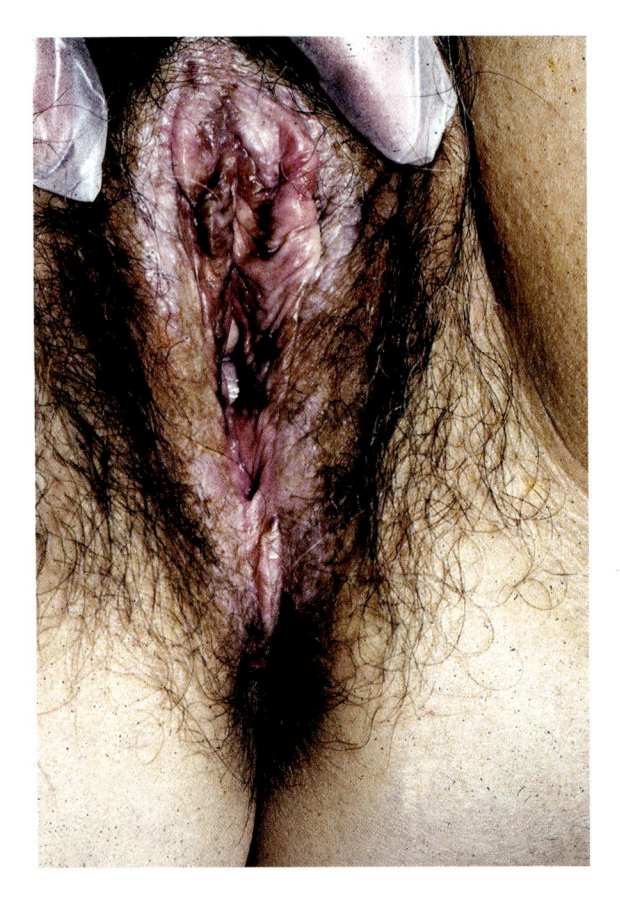

## Inflammatory Disorders of the Skin

infiltration is associated with foci of early basal cell layer vacuolization, pigment incontinence, and, at first, subtle fibrosis manifested by the formation of coarse collagen fibers. The fibers are irregularly distributed in the edematous inflamed areas, parallel to the long axis of the epidermis. Over time, these alterations within the extracellular matrix dominate the histologic picture, with characteristic pale pink, hyalinized sclerosis within the superficial dermis associated with vascular ectasia and pigment incontinence (fig. 7-60). While residual lymphocytes may persist in low numbers, the impression at this stage is generally not of active interface dermatitis, although in some lesions, epidermal atrophy is a sequela to previous chronic interface injury. Late lesions may show patulous follicular orifices plugged with infundibular keratin.

**Differential Diagnosis.** Most of the lesions that cause lichenoid dermatitis are in the differential diagnosis, but especially lichen planus involving the genitalia or the nongenital skin. Lichen simplex chronicus, chronic cutaneous lupus erythematosus, and early inflammatory vitiligo must be considered clinically. Intraepithelial neoplasia and extramammary Paget disease may also be in the differential diagnosis.

**Treatment and Prognosis.** Topical corticosteroids and immunomodulators are useful for early lesions (93,94). Some respond to hydroxychloroquine given for a brief period. Imiquimod has been shown to be helpful in early cases

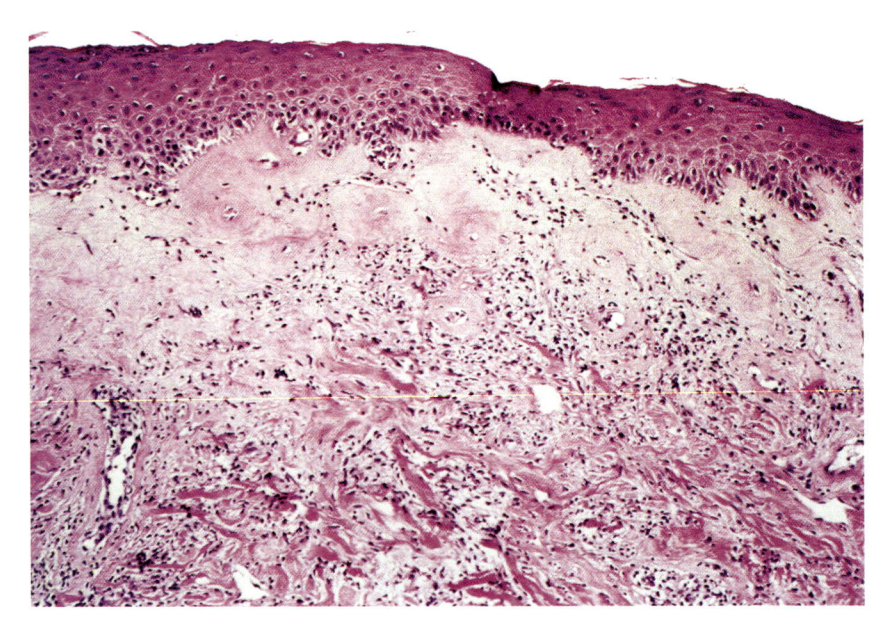

Figure 7-58
LICHEN SCLEROSUS
The whitish plaques bilaterally involve the vulvar skin.

Figure 7-59
LICHEN SCLEROSUS
Early lesions are characterized by a variably dense band of interstitial lymphocytes within the superficial reticular and papillary dermis, focal lichenoid changes along the dermal-epidermal interface, and only focal evidence of papillary dermal sclerosis.

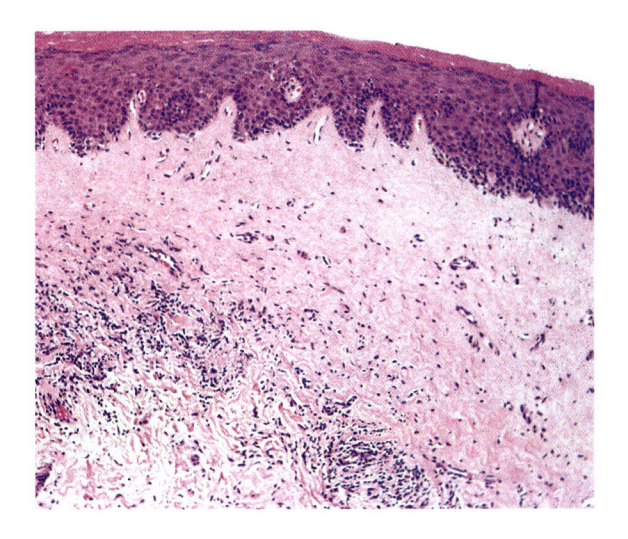

## Figure 7-60
**LICHEN SCLEROSUS: ADVANCED LESIONS**

Above: Over time, the characteristic homogenized and pale sclerosis of the papillary dermis is apparent, with displacement of the interstitial lymphocytic component to the periphery of the sclerotic zone.

Right: At higher magnification, evidence of persistent lymphocyte-mediated interface injury is seen within the basal cell layer and in association with occasional apoptotic keratinocytes.

(94a). In males, circumcision is curative in some cases. Oral retinoids are used for anogenital advanced disease.

### LICHENOID PIGMENTARY PURPURA

**Definition.** *Lichenoid pigmentary purpura* is a subtype of pigmented purpuric dermatosis that clinically is characterized by lichenoid papules, plaques, and sometimes macules. Associated pinpoint hemorrhages give a cayenne pepper–colored appearance to the hemorrhagic areas (95–100). The condition is sometimes referred to as *lichenoid purpura of Gougerot-Blum* (101).

**Clinical Features.** The early tan-brown to red macular lesions occur most commonly on the lower extremities but may occur as well on the trunk or, rarely, the arms (fig. 7-61). They begin insidiously and often without symptoms. The lesions may persist for months to years. If drug induced, the lesions usually resolve after withdrawal of the drug. Drugs that have been associated with this disorder include diuretics, meprobamate, nonsteroidal antiinflammatory drugs, some antibiotics including ampicillin, and acetaminophen and phenacetin. With

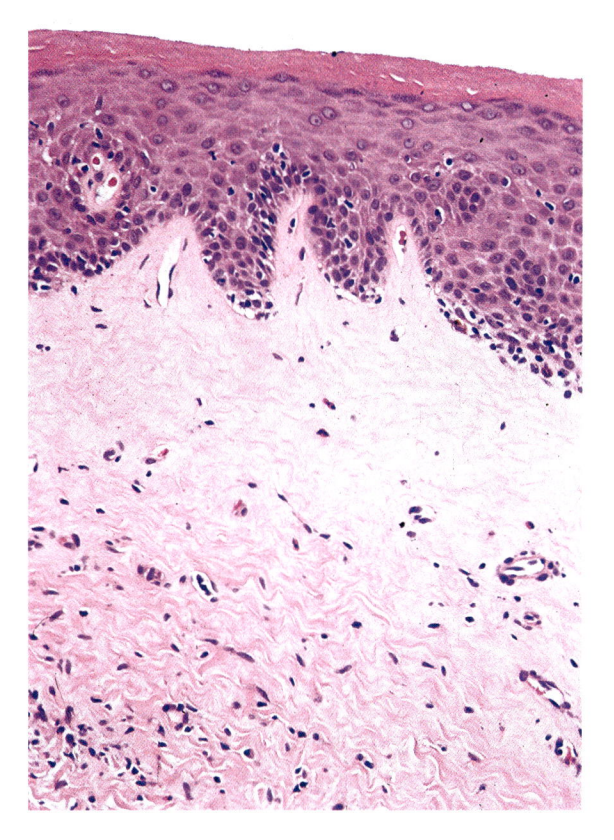

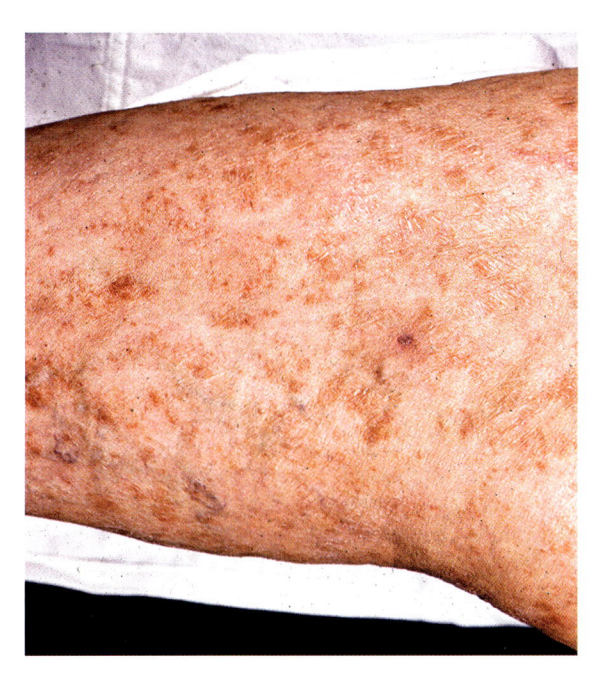

## Figure 7-61
**LICHENOID PIGMENTARY PURPURA**

The maculopapular rash consists of pale pink to tan-brown lesions on extremity skin.

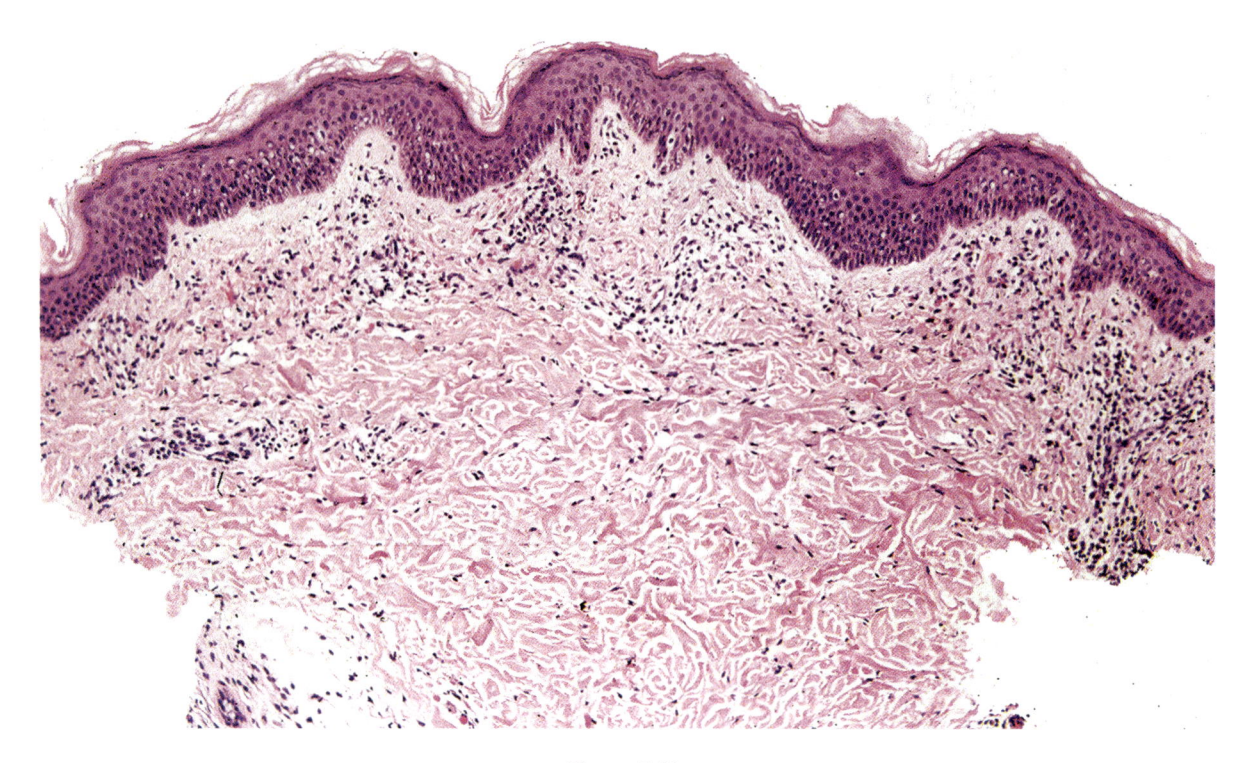

## Inflammatory Disorders of the Skin

**Figure 7-62**
**LICHENOID PIGMENTARY PURPURA: EARLY LESION**
There is a sparse superficial perivascular and focally papillary dermal interstitial lymphocytic infiltrate. At this magnification, the lesion is unimpressive.

progressive development of a lichenoid immune response, early macular lesions may become raised to form papules and plaques.

**Pathologic Findings.** Lichenoid purpuras are related to the progressive pigmentary purpura lesions (e.g., Schamberg disease), and are considered by some to represent variants of these entities. There is a superficial perivascular lymphoid inflammatory infiltrate that rapidly reaches confluence within the papillary dermis, producing a characteristic inflammatory band along the dermal-epidermal interface (figs. 7-62, 7-63). While true cytotoxic alteration to the basal cell layer is generally inconspicuous, acute injury to superficial dermal microvessels is evidenced by foci of papillary dermal erythrocyte extravasation, and chronic injury by the accumulation of siderophages. The latter may only be obvious with iron stains (fig. 7-64). As is the case in other forms of progressive pigmentary purpura, the lymphocytic inflammatory component is intimately associated with capillary loops within dermal papillae, accounting for the belief that this group of disorders represents a form of lymphocytic "capillaritis."

**Differential Diagnosis.** As in all types of pigmentary purpura, any of the causes of non-palpable purpura are possibilities. On the lower extremities, venous insufficiency is probably the most common cause of progressive purpura and pigmentary alterations. Occasionally, pigmentary purpuras are a sign of early cutaneous T-cell lymphoma, scurvy, or senile purpura. The other types of pigmentary purpura, namely, Schamberg disease, the eczematous purpura of Doukas and Kepatanakis, and lichen aureus must be considered (fig. 7-65). Clinicopathologic correlation is often necessary to make the correct diagnosis.

**Treatment and Prognosis.** Withdrawal of the offending drug results in clearing of much of the erythema and pigmentary abnormalities. If the disorder is associated with other diseases, such as stasis dermatitis or cutaneous T-cell lymphoma, then treatment of those entities results in at least partial clearing of the eruption.

*Lichenoid Dermatitis (Subacute to Chronic Cytotoxic Dermatitis)*

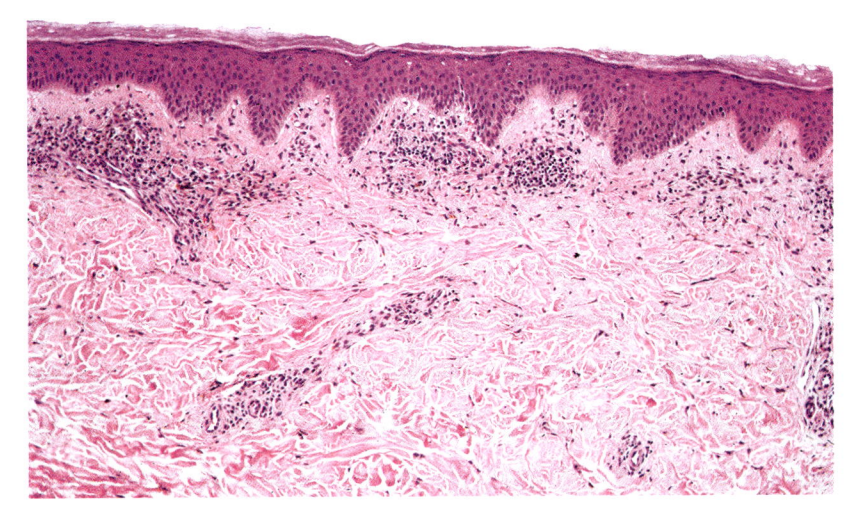

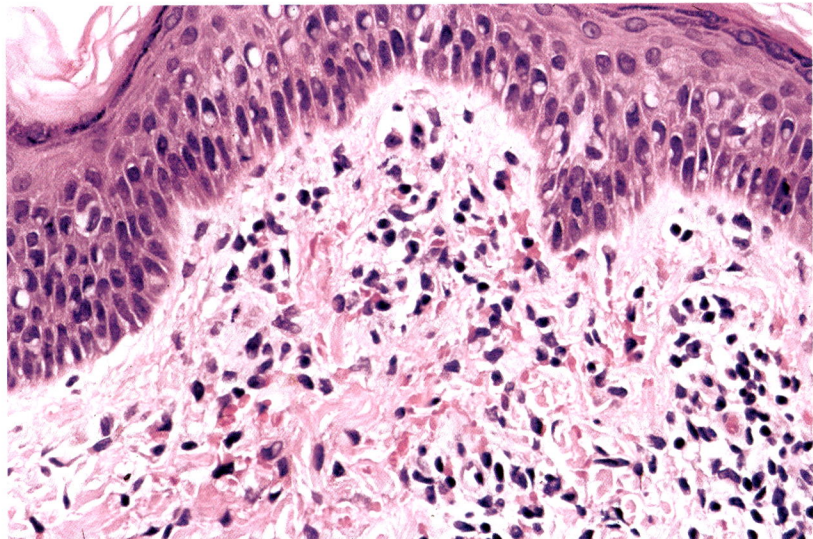

Figure 7-63

**PROGRESSIVE PIGMENTARY PURPURA: LICHENOID VARIANT**

Top: In this advanced lesion, confluent lymphocytes are present within the papillary dermis, focally forming a band-like architecture.

Bottom: At high magnification, an interstitial and focally perivascular infiltrate of lymphocytes extends high within the papillary dermis and focally involves the capillary loops. There is mild vacuolization along the dermal-epidermal junction and evidence of pericapillary hemorrhage. In such lesions, the apparent cytotoxic injury to the basal layer may be the consequence of "capillaritis," rather than true immune-mediated basal layer destruction.

Figure 7-64

**PROGRESSIVE PIGMENTARY PURPURA: LICHENOID VARIANT**

The chronicity of the process is evidenced by the blue iron deposits within the papillary dermis, correlating with the accumulation of hemosiderin (iron stain).

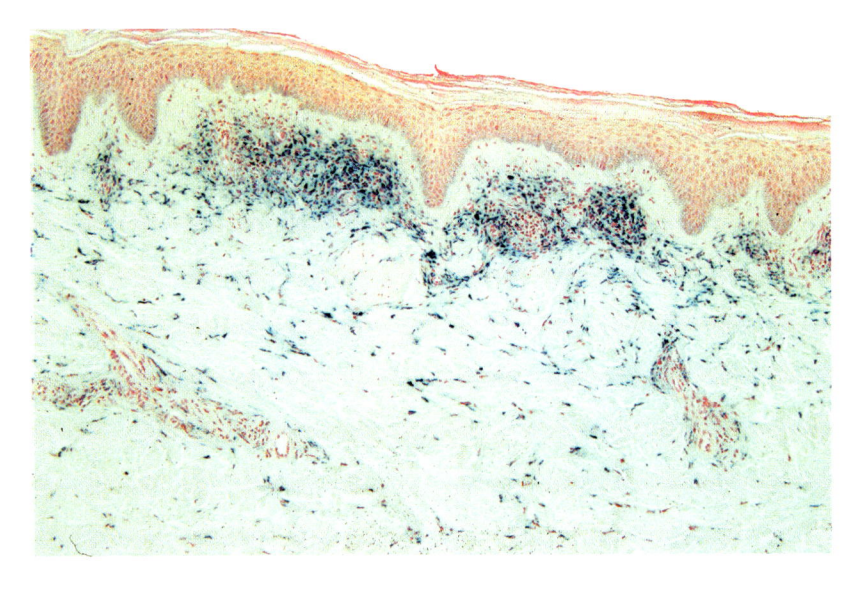

*Inflammatory Disorders of the Skin*

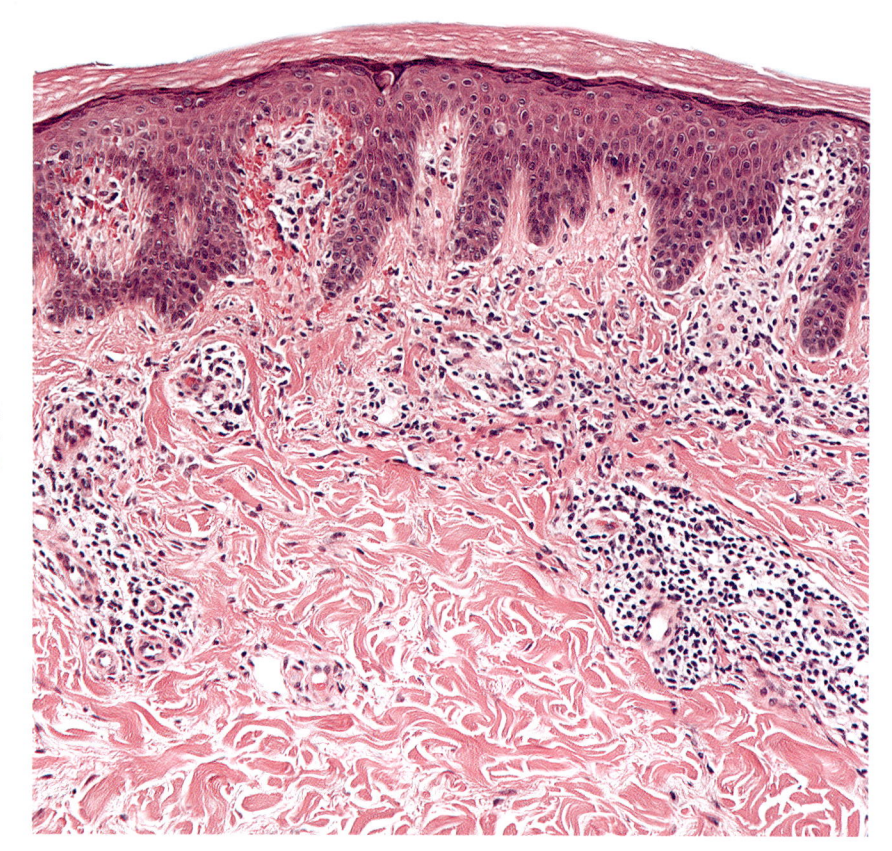

**Figure 7-65**

**LICHEN AUREUS**

A superficial dermal lichenoid lymphocytic infiltrate is associated with papillary dermal fibrosis and hemorrhage.

## REFERENCES

1. Boyd AS. Update on the diagnosis of lichenoid dermatitis. Adv Dermatol 1996;11:287-315.
2. Patterson JW. The spectrum of lichenoid dermatitis. J Cutan Pathol 1991;18:67-74.
3. Boyd AS. New and emerging therapies for lichenoid dermatoses. Dermatol Clin 2000;18:21-9.
4. Christofidou-Solomidou M, Albelda SM, Bennett FC, Murphy GF. Experimental production and modulation of human cytotoxic dermatitis in human-murine chimeras. Am J Pathol 1997;150:631-9.
5. Goldblum OM. Lichen planus. Skinmed 2002;1:52-3.
6. Katta R. Lichen planus. Am Fam Physician 2000;61:3319-24, 3327-8. Erratum in: Am Fam Physician 2000;62:1786.
7. de Moura Castro Jacques C, Cardozo Pereira AL, Cabral MG, Cardoso AS, Ramos-e-Silva M. Oral lichen planus part I: epidemiology, clinics, etiology, immunopathogeny, and diagnosis. Skinmed 2003;2:342-7.
8. DeRossi SS, Ciarrocca KN. Lichen planus, lichenoid drug reactions, and lichenoid mucositis. Dent Clin North Am 2005;49:77-89.
9. Dissemond J. Oral lichen planus: an overview. J Dermatolog Treat 2004;15:136-40.
10. Moyal-Barracco M, Edwards L. Diagnosis and therapy of anogenital lichen planus. Dermatol Ther 2004;17:38-46.
11. Sugerman PB, Savage NW. Oral lichen planus: causes, diagnosis and management. Aust Dent J 2002;47:290-7.
12. Buechner SA. Common skin disorders of the penis. BJU Int 2002;90:498-506.
13. Eisen D. The clinical features, malignant potential, and systemic associations of oral lichen planus: a study of 723 patients. J Am Acad Dermatol 2002;46:207-14.
14. Fleckman P, Omura EF. Histopathology of the nail. Adv Dermatol 2001;17:385-406.

15. Ramrakha-Jones VS, Paul M, McHenry P, Burden AD. Nail dystrophy due to lichen sclerosus? Clin Exp Dermatol 2001;26:507-9.
16. Scardamaglia L, Howard A, Sinclair R. Twenty-nail dystrophy in a girl with incontinentia pigmenti. Australas J Dermatol 2003;44:71-3.
16a. Powell FC, Rogers RS, Dickson ER, Moore SB. An association between HLA DRI and lichen planus. Br J Dermatol 1986;114:473-8.
17. Lodi G, Giuliani M, Majorana A, et al. Lichen planus and hepatitis C virus: a multicentre study of patients with oral lesions and a systematic review. Br J Dermatol 2004;151:1172-81.
18. Nagao Y, Sata M. Hepatitis C virus and lichen planus. J Gastroenterol Hepatol 2004;19:1101-13.
19. Chainani-Wu N, Lozada-Nur F, Terrault N. Hepatitis C virus and lichen planus: a review. Oral Surg Oral Med Oral Pathol Oral Radiol Endod 2004; 98:171-83.
20. Cardozo Pereira AL, Castro Jacques Cde M, Cabral MG, Cardoso AS, Ramos-e-Silva M. Oral lichen planus part II: therapy and malignant transformation. Skinmed 2004;3:19-22.
21. Larsson A, Warfvinge G. Malignant transformation of oral lichen planus. Oral Oncol 2003;39:630-1.
22. Cribier B, Frances C, Chosidow O. Treatment of lichen planus. An evidence-based medicine analysis of efficacy. Arch Dermatol 1998;134:1521-30.
23. Setterfield JF, Black MM, Challacombe SJ. The management of oral lichen planus. Clin Exp Dermatol 2000;25:176-82.
24. Chan ES, Thornhill M, Zakrzewska J. Interventions for treating oral lichen planus. Cochrane Database Syst Rev 2000:CD001168.
25. Carbone M, Goss E, Carrozzo M, et al. Systemic and topical corticosteroid treatment of oral lichen planus: a comparative study with long-term follow-up. J Oral Pathol Med 2003;32:323-9.
26. Hegarty AM, Hodgson TA, Lewsey JD, Porter SR. Fluticasone propionate spray and betamethasone sodium phosphate mouthrinse: a randomized crossover study for the treatment of symptomatic oral lichen planus. J Am Acad Dermatol 2002;47:271-9.
27. Feliciani C, Tulli A. Topical cyclosporin in the treatment of dermatologic diseases. Int J Immunopathol Pharmacol 2002;15:89-93.
28. Demitsu T, Sato T, Inoue T, Okada O, Kubota T. Corticosteroid-resistant erosive oral lichen planus successfully treated with topical cyclosporine therapy. Int J Dermatol 2000;39:79-80.
29. Akyol M, Ozcelik S. Non-acne dermatologic indications for systemic isotretinoin. Am J Clin Dermatol 2005;6:175-84.
30. Henderson RL Jr, Williford PM, Molnar JA. Cutaneous ulcerative lichen planus exhibiting pathergy, response to acitretin. J Drugs Dermatol 2004;3:191-2.
31. Lazarous MC, Kerdel FA. Topical tacrolimus Protopic. Drugs Today (Barc) 2002;38:7-15.
32. Ling MR. Topical tacrolimus and pimecrolimus: future directions. Semin Cutan Med Surg 2001;20:268-74.
33. Bergman J, Rico MJ. Tacrolimus clinical studies for atopic dermatitis and other conditions. Semin Cutan Med Surg 2001;20:250-9.
34. Ruzicka T, Assmann T, Lebwohl M. Potential future dermatological indications for tacrolimus ointment. Eur J Dermatol 2003;13:331-42.
35. MacDonald AJ, Drummond A, Chui D, Holmes S. Lichen nitidus and lichen spinulosus or spinous follicular lichen nitidus? Clin Exp Dermatol 2005;30:452-3.
36. Scheinfeld NS, Lehman D. Condyloma with lichen nitidus. Skinmed 2005;4:177-8.
37. Dobbs CR, Murphy SJ. Lichen nitidus treated with topical tacrolimus. J Drugs Dermatol 2004;3:683-4.
38. Shepherd V, Lun K, Strutton G. Lichen striatus in an adult following trauma. Australas J Dermatol 2005;46:25-8.
39. Hofer T. Lichen striatus in adults or 'adult blaschkitis'? There is no need for a new naming. Dermatology 2003;207:89-92.
40. Hauber K, Rose C, Brocker EB, Hamm H. Lichen striatus: clinical features and follow-up in 12 patients. Eur J Dermatol 2000;10:536-9.
41. Patrizi A, Neri I, Fiorentini C, Bonci A, Ricci G. Lichen striatus: clinical and laboratory features of 115 children. Pediatr Dermatol 2004;21:197-204.
42. Vargas-Diez E, Garcia-Diez A, Marin A, Fernandez-Herrera J. Life-threatening graft-vs-host disease. Clin Dermatol 2005;23:285-300.
43. Penas PF, Fernandez-Herrera J, Garcia-Diez A. Dermatologic treatment of cutaneous graft versus host disease. Am J Clin Dermatol 2004;5:403-16.
44. Sanders JE. Chronic graft-versus-host disease and late effects after hematopoietic stem cell transplantation. Int J Hematol 2002;76(Suppl 2):15-28.
45. Ratanatharathorn V, Ayash L, Lazarus HM, Fu J, Uberti JP. Chronic graft-versus-host disease: clinical manifestation and therapy. Bone Marrow Transplant 2001;28:121-9.
46. Akpek G. Clinical grading in chronic graft-versus-host disease: is it time for change? Leuk Lymphoma 2002;43:1211-20.

47. Callen JP. Collagen vascular diseases. J Am Acad Dermatol 2004;51:427-39.
48. Pramatarov KD. Chronic cutaneous lupus erythematosus—clinical spectrum. Clin Dermatol 2004;22:113-20.
49. Sanders CJ, Van Weelden H, Kazzaz GA, Sigurdsson V, Toonstra J, Bruijnzeel-Koomen CA. Photosensitivity in patients with lupus erythematosus: a clinical and photobiological study of 100 patients using a prolonged phototest protocol. Br J Dermatol 2003;149:131-7.
50. Fabbri P, Cardinali C, Giomi B, Caproni M. Cutaneous lupus erythematosus: diagnosis and management. Am J Clin Dermatol 2003;4:449-65.
51. Patel P, Werth V. Cutaneous lupus erythematosus: a review. Dermatol Clin 2002;20:373-85.
52. Yung A, Oakley A. Bullous systemic lupus erythematosus. Australas J Dermatol 2000;41:234-7.
53. Callen JP. Update on the management of cutaneous lupus erythematosus. Br J Dermatol 2004;151:731-6.
54. Lee L, Gaither KK, Coulter SN, Norris DA, Harley JB. Pattern of cutaneous immunoglobulin G deposition in subacute cutaneous lupus erythematosus is reproduced by infusing purified anti-Ro (SSA) autoantibodies into human skin-grafted mice. J Clin Invest 1989;83:1556-62.
55. Callen JP. Collagen vascular diseases. J Am Acad Dermatol 2004;51:427-39.
56. Greenberg SA, Amato AA. Uncertainties in the pathogenesis of adult dermatomyositis. Curr Opin Neurol 2004;17:359-64.
57. Santmyire-Rosenberger B, Dugan EM. Skin involvement in dermatomyositis. Curr Opin Rheumatol 2003;15:714-22.
58. Dalakas MC, Hohlfeld R. Polymyositis and dermatomyositis. Lancet 2003;362:971-82.
59. Elston DM. What is your diagnosis? Dermatomyositis. Cutis 2003;71:21,39-40.
60. Dourmishev LA, Dourmishev AL, Schwartz RA. Dermatomyositis: cutaneous manifestations of its variants. Int J Dermatol 2002;41:625-30.
61. Pachman LM. Juvenile dermatomyositis: immunogenetics, pathophysiology, and disease expression. Rheum Dis Clin North Am 2002;28:579-602.
62. Sontheimer RD. Dermatomyositis: an overview of recent progress with emphasis on dermatologic aspects. Dermatol Clin 2002;20:387-408.
63. Callen JP. Dermatomyositis: diagnosis, evaluation and management. Minerva Med 2002;93:157-67.
64. Caro I. Dermatomyositis. Semin Cutan Med Surg 2001;20:38-45.
65. Callen JP. Dermatomyositis. Lancet 2000;355:53-7.
66. Ramanan AV, Feldman BM. Clinical outcomes in juvenile dermatomyositis. Curr Opin Rheumatol 2002;14:658-62.
67. Sontheimer RD. The management of dermatomyositis: current treatment options. Expert Opin Pharmacother 2004;5:1083-99.
68. Choy EH, Isenberg DA. Treatment of dermatomyositis and polymyositis. Rheumatology (Oxford) 2002;41:7-13.
69. Ghate J, Katsambas A, Augerinou G, Jorizzo JL. Review article: a therapeutic update on dermatomyositis/polymyositis. Int J Dermatol 2000;39:81-7.
69a. Quain RD, Werth VP. Management of cutaneous dermatomyositis: current therapeutic options. Am J Clin Dermatol 2006;7:341-51.
70. Patel DG, Kihiczak G, Schwartz RA, Janniger CK, Lambert WC. Pityriasis lichenoides. Cutis 2000;65:17-20, 23.
71. Paquet P, Fraiture AL, Pierard-Franchimont C, Pierard GE. [How I explore ... a lichenoid drug reaction.] Rev Med Liege 2001;56:855-8. [French]
72. Singh AE, Romanowski B. Syphilis: review with emphasis on clinical, epidemiologic, and some biologic features. Clin Microbiol Rev 1999;12:187-209.
73. Hollier LM, Cox SM. Syphilis. Semin Perinatol 1998;22:323-31.
74. Golden MR, Marra CM, Holmes KK. Update on syphilis: resurgence of an old problem. JAMA 2003;290:1510-4.
75. Goldmeier D, Guallar C. Syphilis: an update. Clin Med 2003;3:209-11.
76. Baughn RE, Musher DM. Secondary syphilitic lesions. Clin Microbiol Rev 2005;18:205-16.
77. Emmert DH, Kirchner JT. Sexually transmitted diseases in women. Gonorrhea and syphilis. Postgrad Med 2000;107:181-4, 189-90, 193-7.
78. Rosen T, Hwong H. Pedal interdigital condylomata lata: a rare sign of secondary syphilis. Sex Transm Dis 2001;28:184-6.
79. Bruce AJ, Rogers RS 3rd. Oral manifestations of sexually transmitted diseases. Clin Dermatol 2004;22:520-7.
80. Pao D, Goh BT, Bingham JS. Management issues in syphilis. Drugs 2002;62:1447-61.
81. Walker GJ. Antibiotics for syphilis diagnosed during pregnancy. Cochrane Database Syst Rev 2001:CD001143.
82. Rompalo AM. Can syphilis be eradicated from the world? Curr Opin Infect Dis 2001;14:41-4.
83. Fowler VG Jr, Maxwell GL, Myers SA, et al. Failure of benzathine penicillin in a case of seronegative secondary syphilis in a patient with acquired immunodeficiency syndrome: case report and review of the literature. Arch Dermatol 2001;137:1374-6.

84. Birnbaum NR, Goldschmidt RH, Buffett WO. Resolving the common clinical dilemmas of syphilis. Am Fam Physician 1999;59:2233-40, 2245-6.
85. Kingston M, Carlin E. Treatment of sexually transmitted infections with single-dose therapy: a double-edged sword. Drugs 2002;62:871-8.
86. Marra CM. Neurosyphilis. Curr Neurol Neurosci Rep 2004;4:435-40.
87. Augenbraun M. Treatment of latent and tertiary syphilis. Hosp Pract (Minneap) 2000;35:89-95.
88. Yesudian PD, Sugunendran H, Bates CM, O'Mahony C. Lichen sclerosus. Int J STD AIDS 2005;16:465-73.
89. Funaro D. Lichen sclerosus: a review and practical approach. Dermatol Ther 2004;17:28-37.
90. Thami GP, Kaur S. Genital lichen sclerosus, squamous cell carcinoma and circumcision. Br J Dermatol 2003;148:1083-4.
91. Tasker GL, Wojnarowska F. Lichen sclerosus. Clin Exp Dermatol 2003;28:128-33.
92. Regauer S, Liegl B, Reich O, Pickel H, Beham-Schmid C. [Vulvar lichen sclerosus. The importance of early clinical and histological diagnosis.] Hautarzt 2004;55:158-64. [German]
93. Smith YR, Haefner HK. Vulvar lichen sclerosus: pathophysiology and treatment. Am J Clin Dermatol 2004;5:105-25.
94. Neill SM, Tatnall FM, Cox NH; British Association of Dermatologists. Guidelines for the management of lichen sclerosus. Br J Dermatol 2002;147:640-9.
94a. Katsambas AD, Lotti TM, eds. European handbook of dermatologic treatments, 2nd ed. New York: Springer; 2003.
95. Newton RC, Raimer SS. Pigmented purpuric eruptions. Dermatol Clin 1985;3:165-9.
96. Inui S, Itami S, Yoshikawa K. A case of lichenoid purpura possibly caused by diltiazem hydrochloride. J Dermatol 2001;28:100-2.
97. Lor P, Krueger U, Kempf W, Burg G, Nestle FO. Monoclonal rearrangement of the T cell receptor gamma-chain in lichenoid pigmented purpuric dermatitis of gougerot-blum responding to topical corticosteroid therapy. Dermatology 2002;205:191-3.
98. Zaballos P, Puig S, Malvehy J. Dermoscopy of pigmented purpuric dermatoses (lichen aureus): a useful tool for clinical diagnosis. Arch Dermatol 2004;140:1290-1.
99. Aoki M, Kawana S. Lichen aureus. Cutis 2002;69:145-8.
100. Ling TC, Goulden V, Goodfield MJ. PUVA therapy in lichen aureus. J Am Acad Dermatol 2001;45:145-6.
101. Fishman HC. Pigmented purpuric lichenoid dermatitis of Gougerot-Blum. Cutis 1982;29:260-1,264.

# 8  PERFORATING DERMATITIS

## GENERAL CONSIDERATIONS

Perforating disorders are a small group of pathogenetically unrelated conditions that share the common feature of abnormal communication between epidermal and dermal elements that normally do not come into contact (1). The resultant lesions generally are predominated by reactive epidermal and dermal inflammatory changes. Although any condition that can result in transepidermal elimination or perforation (e.g., perforating dermatofibroma) could broadly be included in this category, the present discussion focuses on non-neoplastic conditions that primarily show perforation and associated inflammatory alterations. While it could be argued that the perforating disorders are not primarily dermatitic, their virtually invariable association with a brisk inflammatory response warrants their inclusion in this Fascicle. Certain disorders already described, such as granuloma annulare, also perforate. In this particular instance, the necrobiotic collagen is actually extruded with keratotic debris through the epidermis. A clue to this type of disorder is the superficial location of the focal necrobiotic zones of granuloma annulare in relationship to the epidermis. Likewise, accumulations of urates, as in the tophus of gout, or calcium in calcinosis cutis, are partially eliminated from the skin through the epidermis and may, in the broad sense, be considered under the rubric of perforating disorders.

The pathogenesis of perforating disorders of the skin is varied, and in some instances, is the result of either inherited or acquired abnormalities in extracellular matrix elements (e.g., collagen and elastin) (2). In other instances (e.g., Kyrle disease), epidermal maturation and keratinization are abnormal, resulting in an epithelial layer that is imbalanced with regard to consistently producing a barrier that separates dermal elements from the skin surface. Certain forms of dermatitis, metabolic conditions and neoplasia associated with altered connective tissue elements, occasionally show a tendency for perforation and transepidermal elimination, as in the perforating variants of granuloma annulare and dermatofibroma. The precise molecular signals at the level of epithelial-mesenchymal interaction that mediate this process remain to be defined.

Special diagnostic studies are limited to histochemical stains for extracellular matrix elements, such as elastin. These approaches facilitate localization of these components at sites of perforation, and enhance sensitivity of detection of underlying structural abnormalities that relate to the genesis of the perforation and its associated reactive and inflammatory alterations (e.g., as in elastosis perforans serpiginosa).

## KYRLE DISEASE

**Definition.** *Kyrle disease* is a perforating disorder involving primary alterations in elastic tissue; the cause is unknown (3–6). The fact that it sometimes occurs in siblings raises the possibility of some type of autosomal recessive inheritance. It is a chronic dermatosis that usually occurs in mid life, although there are rare childhood cases, with women more commonly affected than men.

**Clinical Features.** The lesions occur on the extensor surfaces, scapula, and buttocks. Only in later stages of the disease are the head and neck involved. The initial lesion is small and skin colored, and forms a papule that is slightly hyperkeratotic. The lesion becomes gradually larger and elevated, and is seen as a verrucous gray-brown mass. Lesions are a few millimeters to a centimeter in size. The lesions occur in crops, but are asynchronous in their development in different locations.

After the hyperkeratotic component is removed or there is spontaneous healing, the sites develop areas of hyperpigmentation or hypopigmentation, and usually a centrally depressed atrophic scar. The lesion has been traditionally

*Inflammatory Disorders of the Skin*

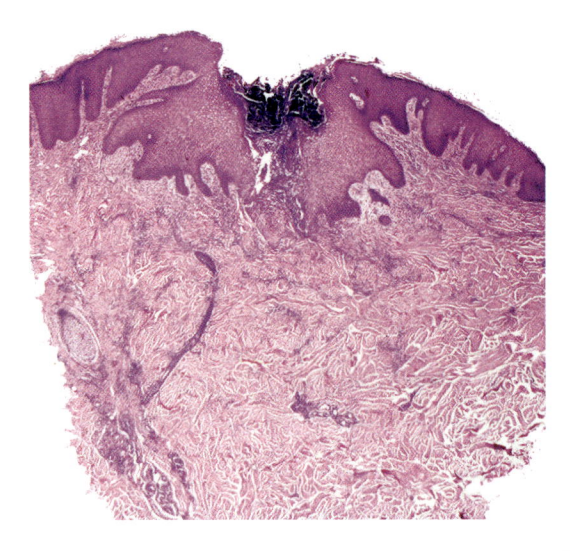

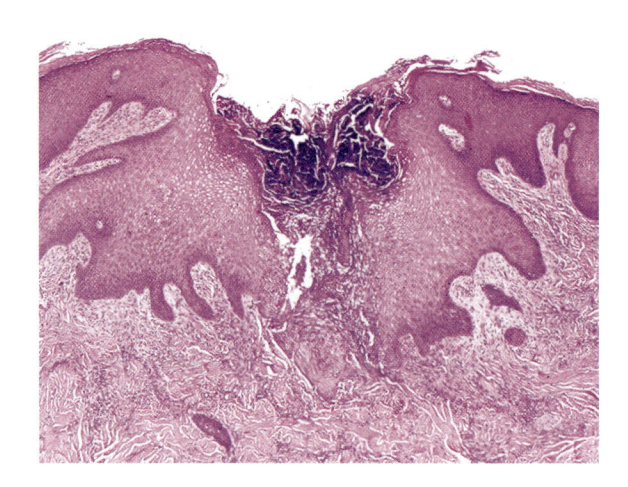

**Figure 8-1**
**KYRLE DISEASE**
Left: A broad zone of epidermal invagination is bordered by endophytic hyperplastic epidermal changes.
Right: At higher magnification, the basophilic material within the invagination and the broad bordering zone of epithelial proliferation are seen.

thought to be associated with diabetes, but this association is not statistically corroborated.

**Pathologic Findings.** A broad, shallow, epidermal invagination forms and generally does not show evidence of follicular association (fig. 8-1). The scale within the invagination is parakeratotic, and the underlying viable epidermis is thinned to the point that scale approximates the underlying dermis. The basal cell layer is unable to keep pace with the rate of overlying epidermal maturation and desquamation. As a result, zones of communication between the keratotic contents of the invagination and the underlying dermis develop, leading to the formation of granulomatous inflammation and basophilic debris that is subsequently transepidermally eliminated into the invagination (fig. 8-2).

**Differential Diagnosis.** The clinical differential diagnosis includes Darier disease, keratosis pilaris, guttate psoriasis, and guttate parapsoriasis depending on the stage of lesional development. The distribution of the lesion is helpful, as well as the histopathologic features. Histopathologically, Kyrle disease must be distinguished from other perforating disorders (the diagnostic criteria for which are provided below).

**Treatment and Prognosis.** The disease is chronic and persistent. When effective treatment of associated systemic disorders results in marked improvement in the cutaneous lesions (7,8), acquired perforating disorder of diabetes or renal failure should be considered.

## ELASTOSIS PERFORANS SERPIGINOSA

**Definition.** *Elastosis perforans serpiginosa* (EPS) is a striking disorder composed of hyperkeratotic papules in an easily discernable, often arcuate array. It is associated with a variety of disorders, including congenital diseases and Down syndrome (9,10).

**Clinical Features.** While the etiology of this disorder is uncertain, it appears to be a type of transepithelial elimination disorder in which long, coarse branching fibers of elastin are located in tracts in the epidermis and intermingled with collagen fibers (11). This characteristic change leads to hyperkeratotic papules (fig. 8-3). Immunopathologic studies have demonstrated a delayed hypersensitivity type reaction at the periphery of the lesion.

Males are affected at least four times more than females, and the lesion occurs during the second decade of life in most affected persons; it can also be found in childhood and congenitally. The lesions occur mainly on the nape and sides of the neck, and on the upper extremities.

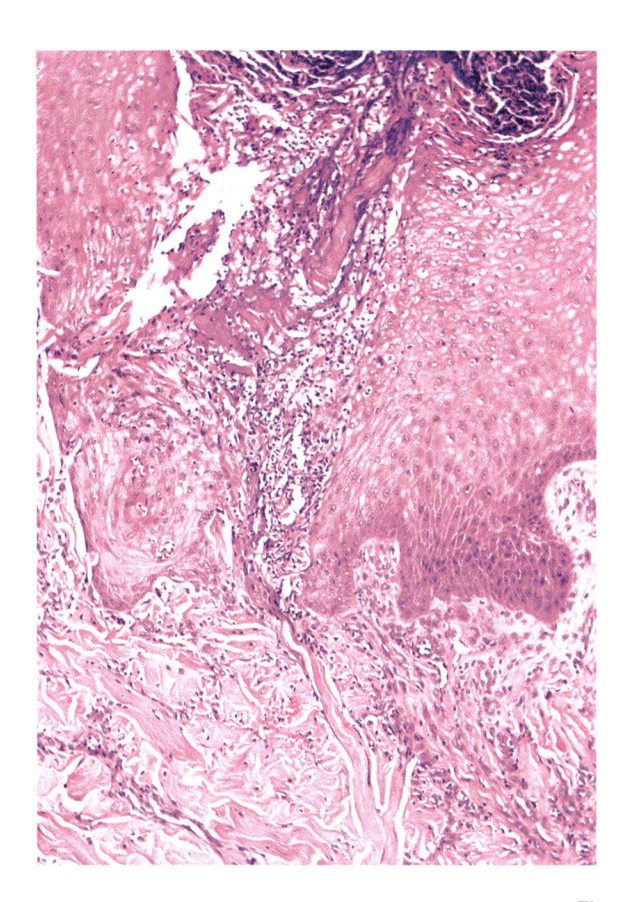

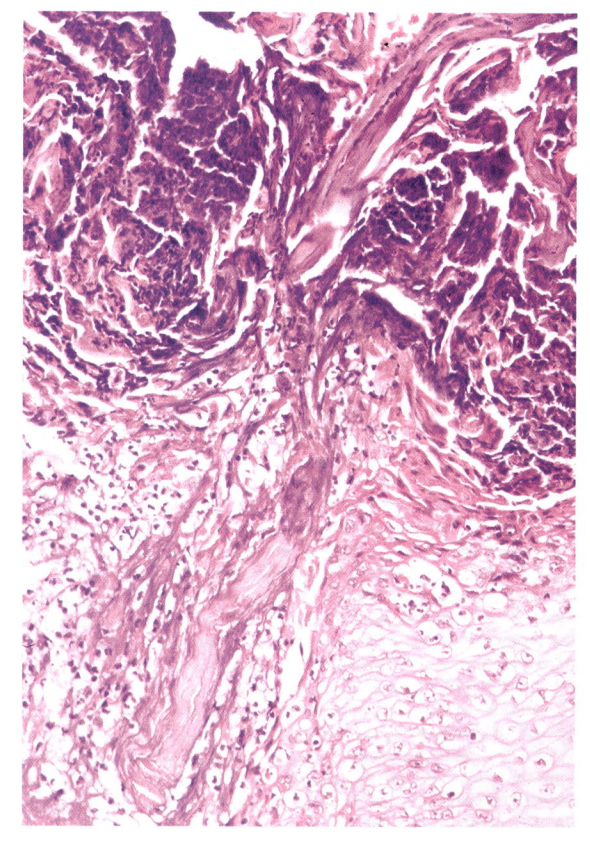

*Perforating Dermatitis*

Figure 8-2
**KYRLE DISEASE: ZONE OF DERMAL-EPIDERMAL COMMUNICATION**

Left: The epidermis is no longer capable of covering the dermal elements at the base, resulting in focal communication of degenerating dermal elements with the overlying invagination and secondary inflammatory changes within the underlying dermis.

Right: At higher magnification, the transepidermally eliminated material consists of strands of degenerating collagen that provoke an inflammatory response within the invagination, contributing to the basophilic hue typical of the extruded material.

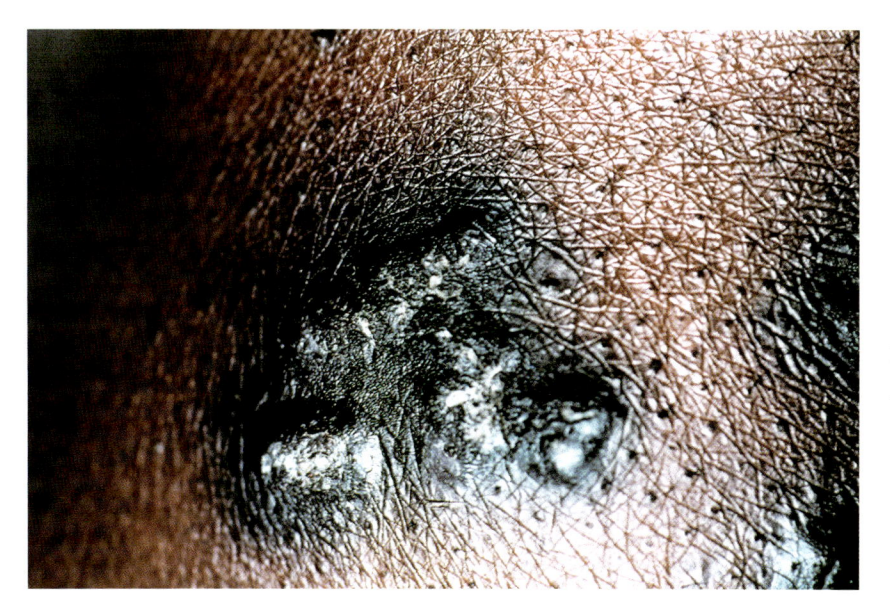

Figure 8-3
**ELASTOSIS PERFORANS SERPIGINOSA**

Annular hyperkeratotic papules have associated postinflammatory hyperpigmentation.

*Inflammatory Disorders of the Skin*

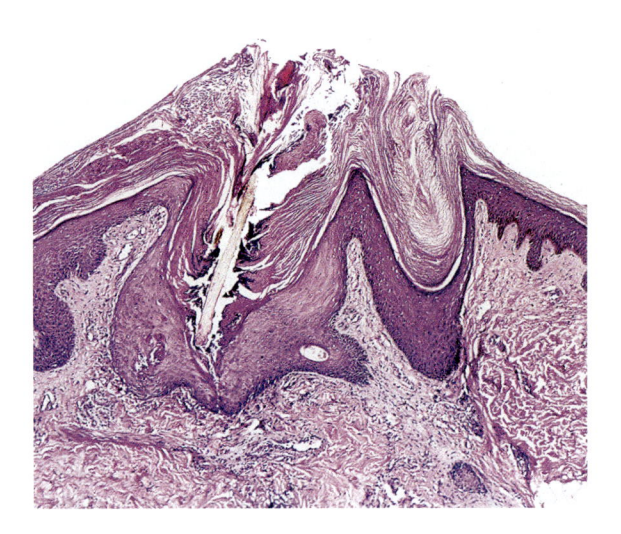

**Figure 8-4**

**ELASTOSIS PERFORANS SERPIGINOSA**

Above: There is a broad, follicle-like invagination associated with hyperkeratosis. At the base of the lesion are foci of perforation.

Right: At high magnification, the transepidermal perforation is associated with extrusion of altered elastic fibers within the underlying dermis. Although a hair shaft is secondarily entrapped here, many lesions are discontinuous with the follicular epithelium.

The lesions are often symmetrically distributed. In some cases they are widespread, especially when associated with Down syndrome or penicillamine therapy. The lesions occur in an arcuate or semicircular array on the affected areas. They gradually evolve, with new lesions forming at the periphery, and with regression of central papules. The regression results in a central wrinkled atrophic area that is often hyperpigmented. The lesions occur over months to years and there is gradual progression.

Most cases are idiopathic, but EPS can be induced by penicillamine therapy. Penicillamine is used to treat Wilson disease and cystinuria. EPS is also associated with Rothmund-Thomson syndrome, Marfan syndrome, osteogenesis imperfecta, Ehlers-Danlos syndrome IV, and occasionally, acrogeria, scleroderma, and Down syndrome. It is unclear whether EPS is associated with pseudoxanthoma elasticum. When associated with these disorders, the lesions are often congenital and are present in an arcuate array, most commonly on the nape of the neck.

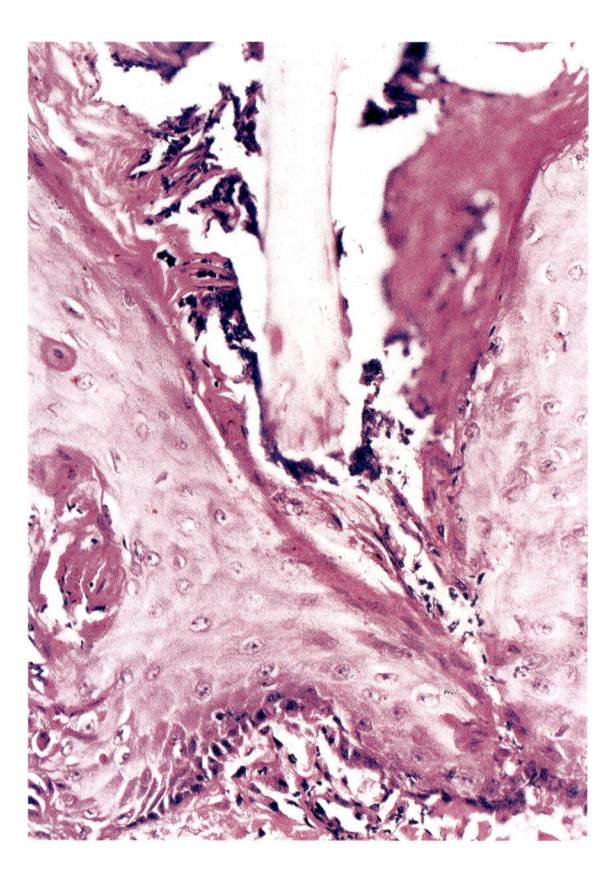

**Pathologic Findings.** Histologically, there is nodular, often endophytic epidermal hyperplasia and hyperkeratosis at sites where altered elastic fibers are extruded upward through perforations, forming either straight or narrow winding channels (fig. 8-4). The material within the channels consists of basophilic degenerated elastic fibers, cellular debris, and keratin, and focally stains with the Verhoeff reagent (fig. 8-5). The epidermal base of the lesion has a broad hyperplastic area, sometimes referred to as a "claw-like structure." The dermis at the base of the perforating channel may contain a reactive chronic inflammatory infiltrate, occasionally with a giant cell response. Increased quantities of altered elastic fibers are detected within adjacent dermal papillae and along the epidermal tract, especially in those lesions associated with heritable disorders. This suggests that the basic defect in this condition is the production of increased amounts of superficial dermal elastin, which undergoes reactive transepidermal elimination. In the acquired lesions, such as those due to penicillamine therapy, this pattern of increased elastic tissue is less evident.

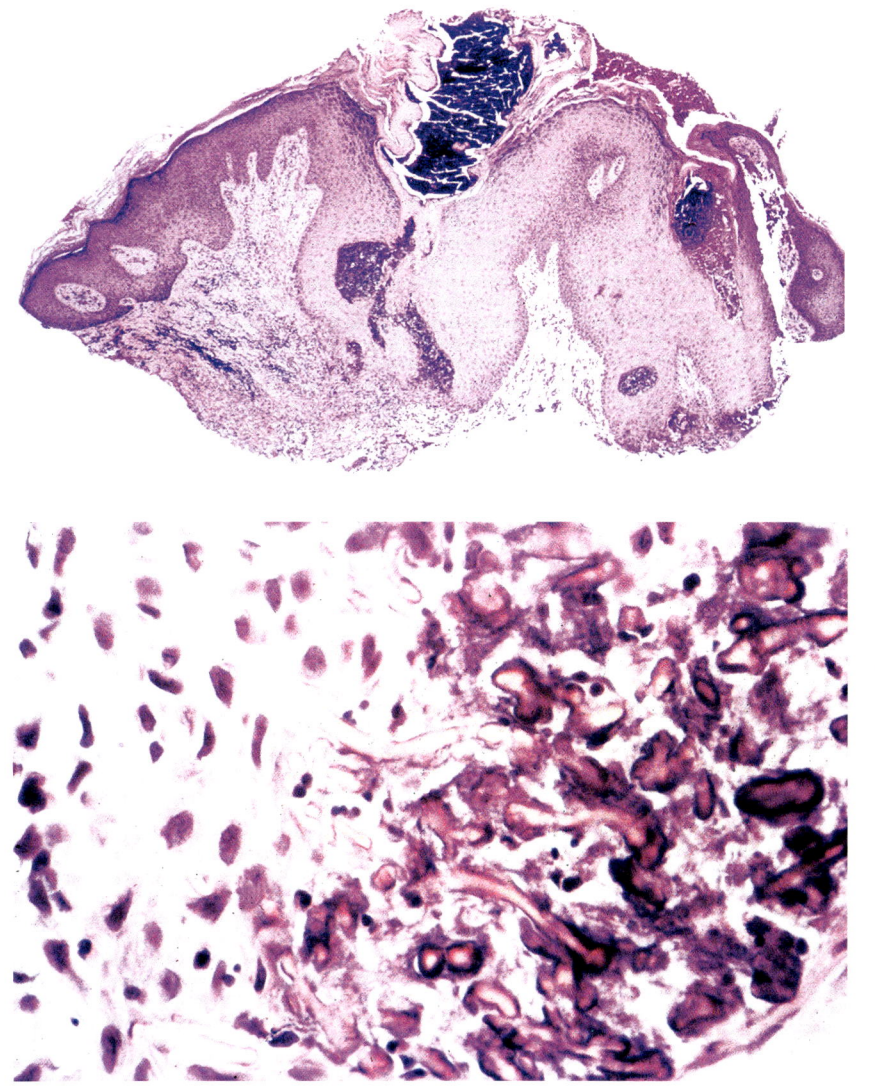

Figure 8-5
ELASTOSIS PERFORANS SERPIGINOSA

Top: The elastic tissue stain shows positive material being extruded from the central cornified plug.

Bottom: At high magnification, altered elastic fibers are present directly beneath the hyperplastic epithelium where they are focally penetrating during the process of transepidermal elimination.

**Differential Diagnosis.** The differential diagnosis includes other perforating disorders, but because of the unusual arcuate or semilunar lesional configurations, porokeratosis and some annular eruptions, such as annular lichen planus, annular lues, and annular sarcoidosis, are considered. Dermatophyte infections are also considered in some cases.

**Treatment and Prognosis.** Cryotherapy is the most useful treatment. Other types of therapy, including superficial destructive measures such as dermabrasion, should be avoided because of the incidence of keloid formation that is associated with this disorder.

## REACTIVE PERFORATING COLLAGENOSIS

**Definition.** *Reactive perforating collagenosis* belongs with the disorders of transepidermal elimination since it is associated with the elimination of collagen fibers through channels in the epidermis (12–16).

**Clinical Features.** Reactive perforating collagenosis is a disorder of unknown etiology. Some cases are familial, and it is possibly inherited as an autosomal recessive trait, but autosomal dominant inheritance cannot be completely excluded. Minor or superficial trauma results in the formation of small, strikingly keratotic papules, a few millimeters in diameter. These

## Inflammatory Disorders of the Skin

**Figure 8-6**

**REACTIVE PERFORATING COLLAGENOSIS**

Hyperkeratotic papules, some with central umbilication, are at sites of trauma (here affecting the skin of the dorsum of the hand).

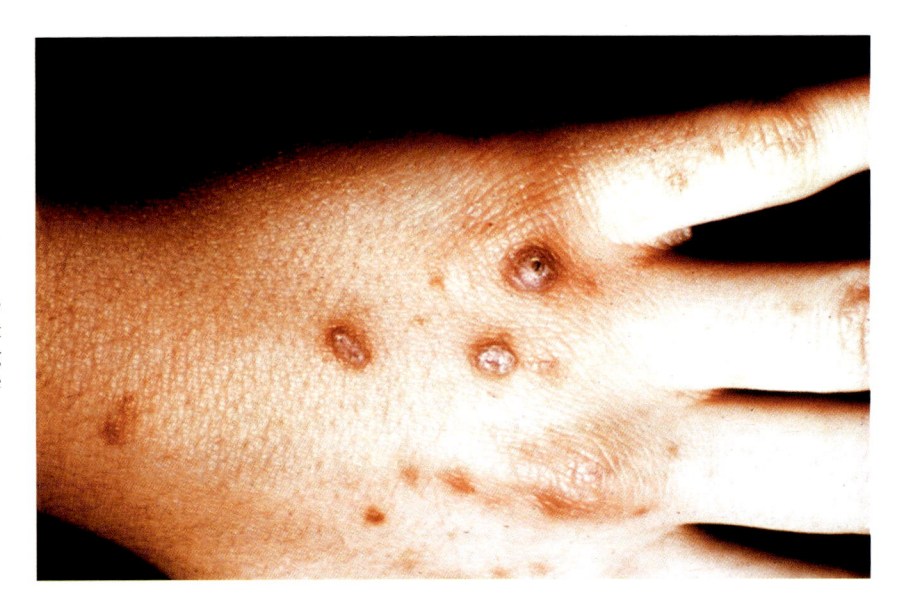

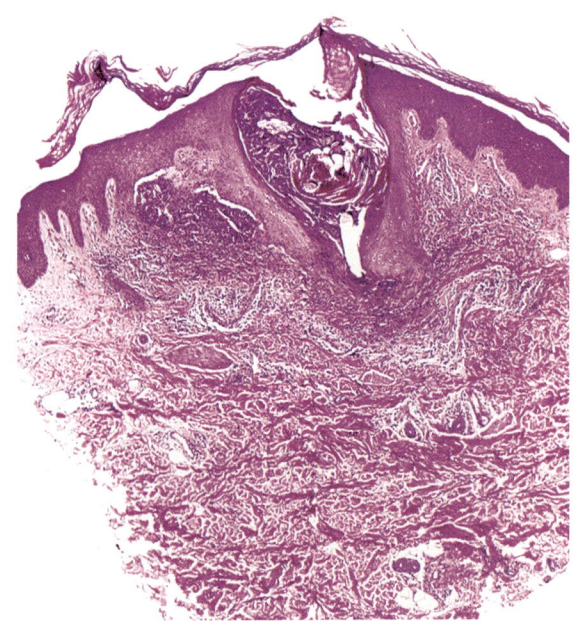

**Figure 8-7**

**REACTIVE PERFORATING COLLAGENOSIS**

The cup-shaped depression is filled with parakeratotic and hyperorthokeratotic scale and inflammatory debris.

develop over the course of a few weeks. At maturation, there is a dense, hyperkeratotic, umbilicated core that can be removed and results in a bleeding ulcer or erosion (fig. 8-6). If the hyperkeratotic area is not removed, the lesions eventually resolve spontaneously, leaving a hypopigmented area or a small, depressed scar.

Onset in childhood is characteristic, and is often associated with an arthropod bite or some other type of trauma. The lesions are asymptomatic, but become troublesome from a cosmetic viewpoint. Lesions are usually located on the hands and forearms, as well as on the trunk or areas of the thighs and face that are subject to trauma.

**Pathologic Findings.** There is either a cup-shaped epidermal depression filled with orthokeratotic scale or a sharply demarcated ulcer filled with basophilic material that includes inflammatory cell debris and collagen fibers (fig. 8-7). In lesions with an intact epidermal depression, the base of the depression communicates with basophilic, degenerating collagen bundles associated with inflammatory debris (fig. 8-8). The basophilic material, which represents degenerating collagen, may also be detected within the cup-shaped invagination as it is eliminated to the epidermal surface. On both sides of the depression or apparent ulceration, collagen fibers penetrate the epidermis. Special stains, such as the trichrome stain, reveal fibers both in the epidermis and the debris-filled area. The findings of reactive perforating collagenosis are similar to those of elastosis perforans serpiginosa; however, in the former condition, altered collagen is eliminated, whereas in the latter, the eliminated material consists of altered elastic fibers.

**Differential Diagnosis.** The differential diagnosis includes elastosis perforans serpiginosa, perforating folliculitis, and the acquired perforating dermatosis of renal failure/diabetes.

**Treatment and Prognosis.** Therapy is difficult and there are no consistently effective therapeutic modalities. Psoralen and ultraviolet A (PUVA) can lead to partial remission in some patients, and topical retinoids result in a diminution in the hyperkeratotic aspects of the disorder (17–19).

## ACQUIRED PERFORATING DISORDER OF DIABETES OR RENAL FAILURE

**Definition.** *Acquired perforating disorder (APD) of diabetes or renal failure* occurs in patients with diabetes mellitus or those with renal failure on hemodialysis (21–22). Previously, these disorders were thought to be Kyrle disease but are now considered distinct from the other disorders of transepidermal elimination.

**Clinical Findings.** APD is a pruritic disorder, although it is unclear as to whether the itching is primarily related to underlying disease (e.g., renal failure) or predominantly related to the effect of transepithelial perforation. The lesions present as hyperkeratotic papules, usually with an umbilicated surface, most commonly over the extensor surfaces of the extremities. APD can also be observed on the trunk and occasionally on the neck, scalp, and face. The lesions are chronic and slowly progressive, but spontaneously heal after several weeks to months, without any striking scarring.

**Pathologic Findings.** The dome-shaped lesion has a central crater filled with variably parakeratotic scale and inflammatory debris. Basophilic acellular material is generally admixed, and fragments of hair shafts are occasionally observed. Individual collagen bundles perforate the base of the crater, a characteristic finding that may require multiple biopsy levels to detect. In addition to the neutrophils within the crater, the adjacent dermis contains a mixed inflammatory infiltrate consisting of lymphocytes, histiocytes, and neutrophils. Lichen simplex chronicus is often present in the adjacent epidermis.

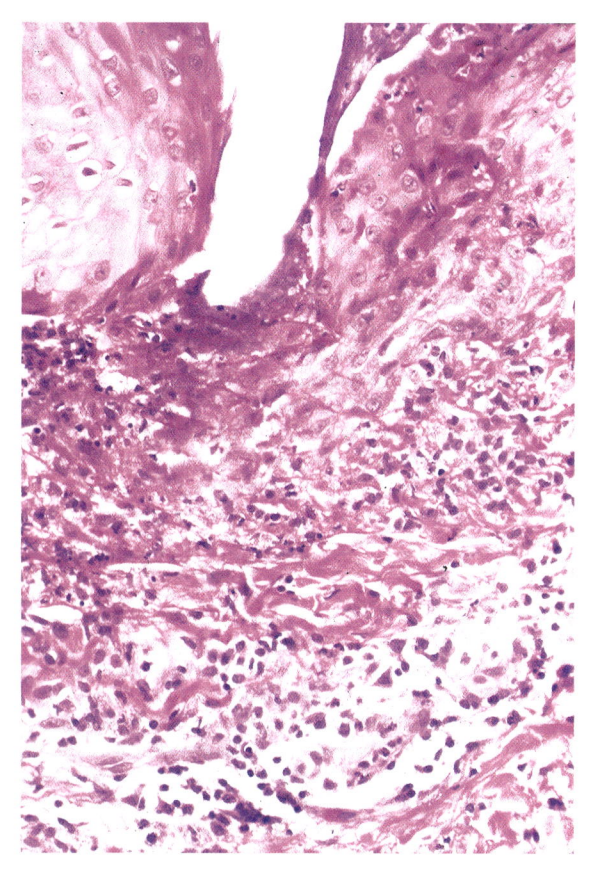

Figure 8-8

**REACTIVE PERFORATING COLLAGENOSIS**

At high magnification, the base of the central depression shows a site of transepithelial perforation involving degenerating basophilic collagen bundles associated with mixed inflammatory infiltrate.

**Differential Diagnosis.** The other perforating disorders must be considered in the differential diagnosis, but the clinical history usually allows for the correct interpretation.

**Treatment and Prognosis.** Topical keratolytics and retinoids, and even narrowband ultraviolet (UV)B and PUVA therapy are helpful for the treatment of this disorder (23). Effective control of the underlying systemic disorder also may result in improvement in cutaneous lesions.

## REFERENCES

1. Sehgal VN, Jain S, Thappa DM, Bhattacharya SN, Logani K. Perforating dermatoses: a review and report of four cases. J Dermatol 1993;20:329-40.
2. Morgan MB, Truitt CA, Taira J, Somach S, Pitha JV, Everett MA. Fibronectin and the extracellular matrix in the perforating disorders of the skin. Am J Dermatopathol 1998;20:147-54.
3. Harman M, Aytekin S, Akdeniz S, Derici M. Kyrle's disease in diabetes mellitus and chronic renal failure. J Eur Acad Dermatol Venereol 1998;11:87-8.
4. Dyall-Smith D. Signs, syndromes and diagnoses in dermatology. Kyrle's disease. Australas J Dermatol 1994;35:101-4.
5. De Mare S, Koopman RJ, Steijlen PM. Acquired perforating dermatosis (Kyrle's disease). Br J Dermatol 1993;129:211.
6. Cunningham SR, Walsh M, Matthews R, Fulton R, Burrows D. Kyrle's disease. J Am Acad Dermatol 1987;16:117-23.
7. Kasiakou SK, Peppas G, Kapaskelis AM, Falagas ME. Regression of skin lesions of Kyrle's disease with clindamycin: implications for an infectious component in the etiology of the disease. J Infect 2005;50:412-6.
8. Saleh HA, Lloyd KM, Fatteh S. Kyrle's disease. Effectively treated with isotretinoin. J Fla Med Assoc 1993;80:395-7. Erratum in: J Fla Med Assoc 1993;80:467.
9. Mehta RK, Burrows NP, Payne CM, Mendelsohn SS, Pope FM, Rytina E. Elastosis perforans serpiginosa and associated disorders. Clin Exp Dermatol 2001;26:521-4.
10. Scherbenske JM, Benson PM, Rotchford JP, James WD. Cutaneous and ocular manifestations of Down syndrome. J Am Acad Dermatol 1990;22:933-8.
11. Lewis KG, Bercovitch L, Dill SW, Robinson-Bostom L. Acquired disorders of elastic tissue: part I. Increased elastic tissue and solar elastotic syndromes. J Am Acad Dermatol 2004;51:1-21.
12. Mahanupab P, Chiewchanvit S. Acquired reactive perforating collagenosis: report of a case and review of the literature. J Med Assoc Thai 2002;85:1019-23.
13. Faver IR, Daoud MS, Su WP. Acquired reactive perforating collagenosis. Report of six cases and review of the literature. J Am Acad Dermatol 1994;30:575-80.
14. Tsuboi H, Mukuno A, Sato N, Katsuoka K, Yanase N. Acquired reactive perforating collagenosis in a patient with lung fibrosis. J Dermatol 2004;31:916-9.
15. Schmults CA. Acquired reactive perforating collagenosis. Dermatol Online J 2002;8:8.
16. Satchell AC, Crotty K, Lee S. Reactive perforating collagenosis: a condition that may be underdiagnosed. Australas J Dermatol 2001;42:284-7.
17. Serrano G, Aliaga A, Lorente M. Reactive perforating collagenosis responsive to PUVA. Int J Dermatol 1988;27:118-9.
18. Berger RS. Reactive perforating collagenosis of renal failure/diabetes responsive to topical retinoic acid. Cutis 1989;43:540-2.
19. Cullen SI. Successful treatment of reactive perforating collagenosis with tretinoin. Cutis 1979;23:187-91,193.
20. Keough GC, Hivnor CM, Elston DM, McCollough ML. Acquired perforating dermatosis in a patient with chronic renal failure and diabetes mellitus. Cutis 1998;62:94-6.
21. Hong SB, Park JH, Ihm CG, Kim NI. Acquired perforating dermatosis in patients with chronic renal failure and diabetes mellitus. J Korean Med Sci 2004;19:283-8.
22. Farrell AM. Acquired perforating dermatosis in renal and diabetic patients. Lancet 1997;349:895-6.
23. Ohe S, Danno K, Sasaki H, Isei T, Okamoto H, Horio T. Treatment of acquired perforating dermatosis with narrowband ultraviolet B. J Am Acad Dermatol 2004;50:892-4.

# 9 ULCERATIVE DERMATITIS

## GENERAL CONSIDERATIONS

In addition to the epidermal alterations that have been outlined in the previous chapters, certain forms of dermatitis present primarily as zones of ulceration. These conditions are usually idiopathic or infectious, and because of the latter consideration, the use of special diagnostic tests is often required to exclude potentially treatable disorders. Because ulceration creates a portal for systemic infection and sepsis, accurate diagnosis and treatment have critical implications for patient care.

The pathogenesis of primary ulcerating forms of dermatitis is highly variable, and often involves multiple factors. The products of inflammatory cells (e.g., neutrophils) result in enzymatic tissue destruction, and alterations in nutrient vessels within the dermis result in ischemia that promotes necrosis. Toxins produced directly by infectious agents cause lysis and necrosis of skin cells. In many instances, the precise causes of ulceration are not well characterized. The ability (or lack thereof) of ulcers to heal is a primary determinant of whether ulcerative dermatitis is persistent or resolvable. Accordingly, models to understand the wound healing response are as germane to the pathophysiology of ulcerative dermatitis as are those that seek to provoke it.

Special studies are used to exclude a primary infectious cause. They include special histochemical and immunofluorescence stains for organisms, polymerase chain reaction (PCR) analysis for specific DNA of infectious agents, and tissue culture for microbes.

Human skin xenografts on immunodeficient mice induce pyoderma gangrenosum–like dermatitis by overexpression of the gene for interleukin 8 (1). The same xenograft model has been used to better understand the molecular determinants and correlates of sequential healing of skin ulcers.

## APHTHOUS STOMATITIS/MUCOSITIS

**Definition.** *Recurrent aphthous stomatitis* is a condition that is frequently brought to the attention of the dermatopathologist for diagnostic evaluation (2–10). Unlike traumatic stomatitis, it produces recurrent, nonvesicular, discrete, painful ulcers of the oral mucosa. The etiology is unknown, although herpes simplex virus (HSV) and autoimmune reactions directed against squamous mucosal epithelium are leading possibilities. Precipitating factors include stress, trauma, and immunologic and nutritional imbalances.

**Clinical Features.** Typically, lesions are round to elliptical ulcers occurring singly or in small numbers. The base is generally covered by gray-white slough surrounded by an edematous and erythematous rim that gradually contracts centripetally with healing (fig. 9-1).

Lesions are characterized into four types: 1) *minor aphthous ulceration*: these lesions are smaller than 1 cm and heal within several weeks without scarring; 2) *major aphthous ulceration*: these lesions are smaller than 1 cm and heal within several weeks, but with scarring; 3) *herpetiform aphthous ulceration*: these clustered small (1 to 3 mm) lesions heal in several weeks and are sensitive to topical tetracycline; and 4) *Behçet syndrome*: these oral and genital ulcerations are associated with ocular and skin lesions, arthritis, and other systemic findings attributable to immune complex formation and deposition (11–13).

**Pathologic Findings.** There is an initial influx of T lymphocytes into the subepithelial zone, followed by epithelial destruction first involving the basal cell layer (fig. 9-2). With resultant erosion of the epithelial surface, a fibrinopurulent membrane forms along the ulcer surface. The edge of the biopsy is well-demarcated in the fully evolved lesion and there is minimal residual inflammation. Submucosal vessels show variable injury, and although some

*Inflammatory Disorders of the Skin*

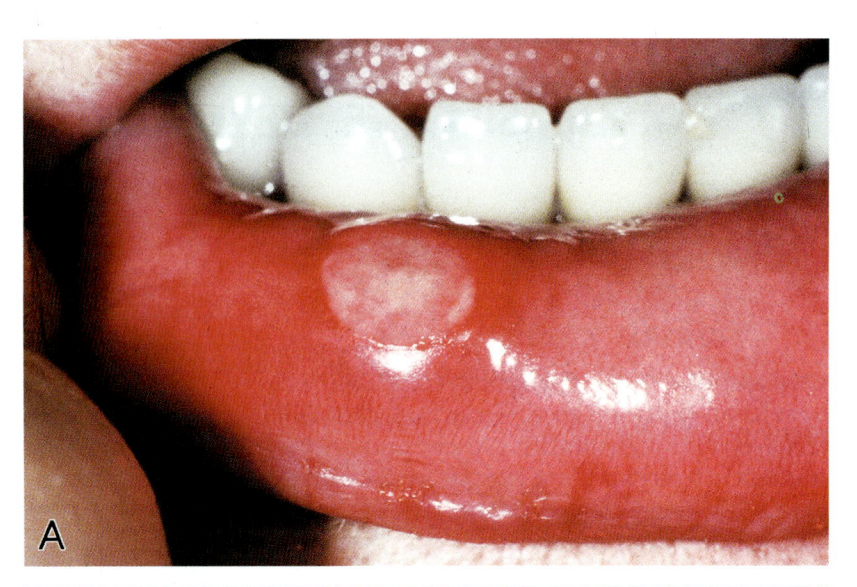

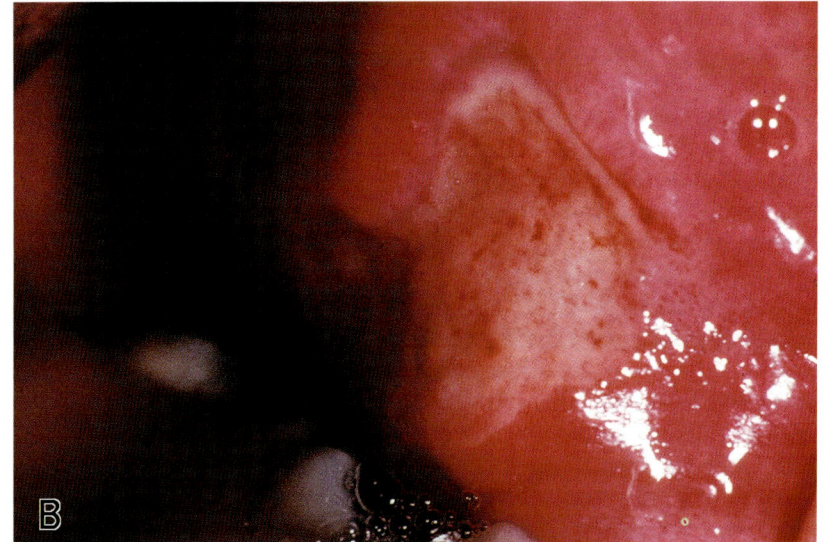

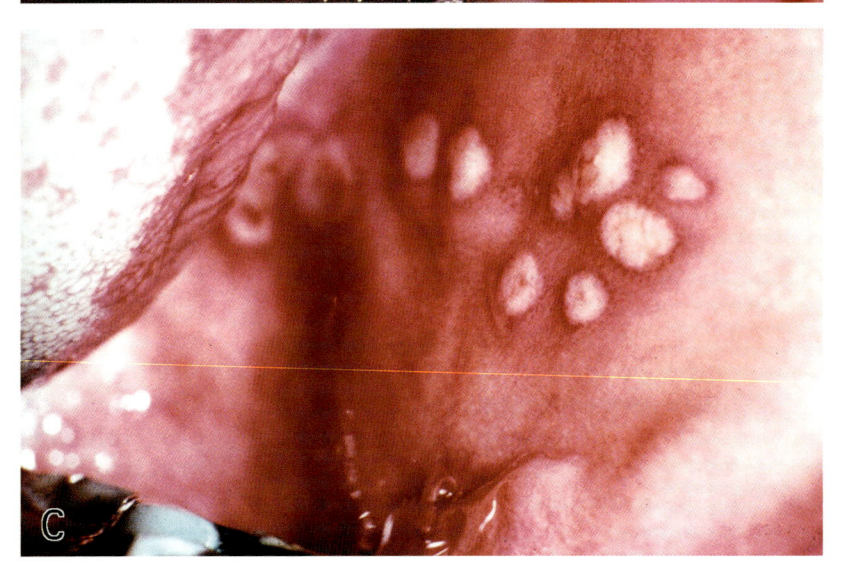

**Figure 9-1**
**APHTHOUS MUCOSITIS**

A: There is a solitary, shallow, round ulcer involving lip epithelium characterized by a gray-white base surrounded by a rim of erythema. Such lesions often heal without scarring and are designated as minor aphthous ulcers.

B: Coalescent lesions involving buccal mucosa show partial resolution, leaving behind zones of superficial fibrosis (major aphthous ulcers).

C: A herpetiform pattern shows multiple discrete ulcers with tan-white bases, surrounded by a rim of erythema in a herpes-like clustering pattern.

262

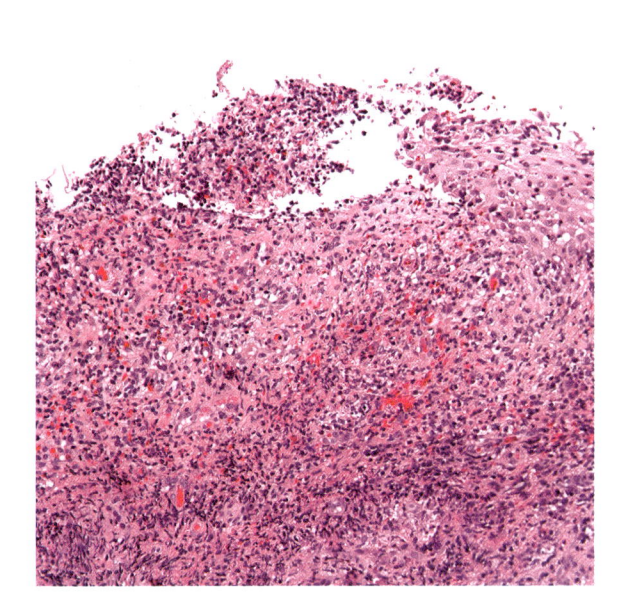

**Figure 9-2**
**APHTHOUS MUCOSITIS**

There is a discrete zone of shallow ulceration and exudation with fibrin, debris, and hemorrhage. On the right is part of the remaining epithelium of the mucosa.

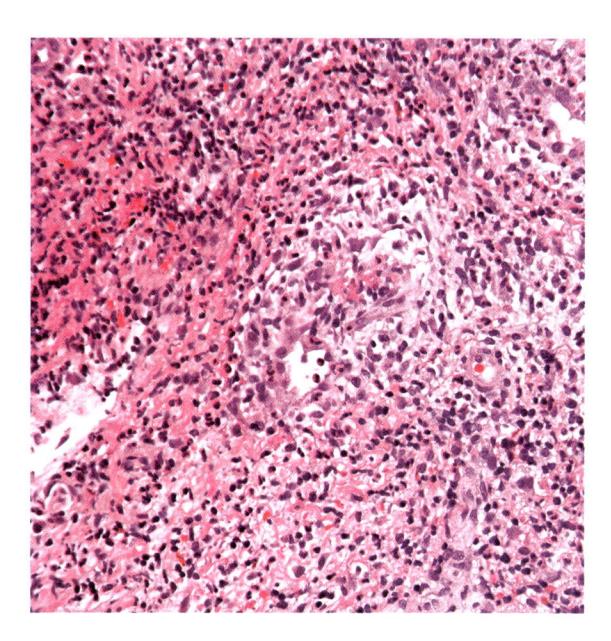

**Figure 9-3**
**APHTHOUS MUCOSITIS**

At high magnification, the ulcer is characterized by a variably dense, subepithelial infiltrate of lymphocytes with extravasation of red blood cells and vasculopathic alterations.

studies suggest a vasculitic component (fig. 9-3), definitive evidence of primary vascular injury in aphthosis is lacking.

**Differential Diagnosis.** The differential diagnosis includes erosive lichen planus and herpetic infection. In the former, there is generally evidence of the subacute to chronic nature of the alterations in the adjacent epithelial layer, which may show stratum corneum formation, focal abortive stratum granulosum formation, or colloid body-like necrotic cells along the mucosal-submucosal interface. Occasionally, direct immunofluorescence is required for the detection of colloid body–like necrotic cells which are immunoglobulin (Ig)M-positive globular bodies within the superficial submucosa.

**Treatment and Prognosis.** Therapy is generally supportive, and lesions resolve spontaneously over time. For extremely painful lesions, a viscous granular paste, benzocaine 20 percent, usually containing a potent steroid, is used topically. Amlexanox is also helpful. A dilute solution of a broad spectrum antibiotic such as tetracycline as an oral retention vehicle alleviates pain and leads to healing in many cases. After a few minutes of retention in the mouth, the liquid is expectorated. Intralesional corticosteroids are also used. Exclusion of infectious causes or chronic or systemic disorders is an important component of patient management. Systemic immunosuppression may be needed for recalcitrant cases, but rigorous trials have not been conducted with these agents; these include thalidomide, cyclosporine, colchicine and azathioprine.

## PYODERMA GANGRENOSUM

**Definition.** *Pyoderma gangrenosum* describes a rapidly evolving cutaneous eruption that begins as a hemorrhagic pustule and rapidly develops into an ulceration (14–18). The disorder is commonly associated with systemic diseases, especially chronic inflammatory bowel diseases such as ulcerative colitis (19–21).

**Clinical Features.** The acute onset of the hemorrhagic pustule or painful nodule is often associated with a history of trauma to the site. The superficial pustule is usually follicular, and rapidly becomes a striking nodule that breaks down with ulcer formation. The borders of the ulcer typically appear undermined and are dusky purple (fig. 9-4). The base of the ulcer is associated

**Figure 9-4**

**PYODERMA GANGRENOSUM**

The ulcers have a sharp, undermined border surrounded by skin of dusky purple coloration. Foci of purulent exudate cover the ulcer bases.

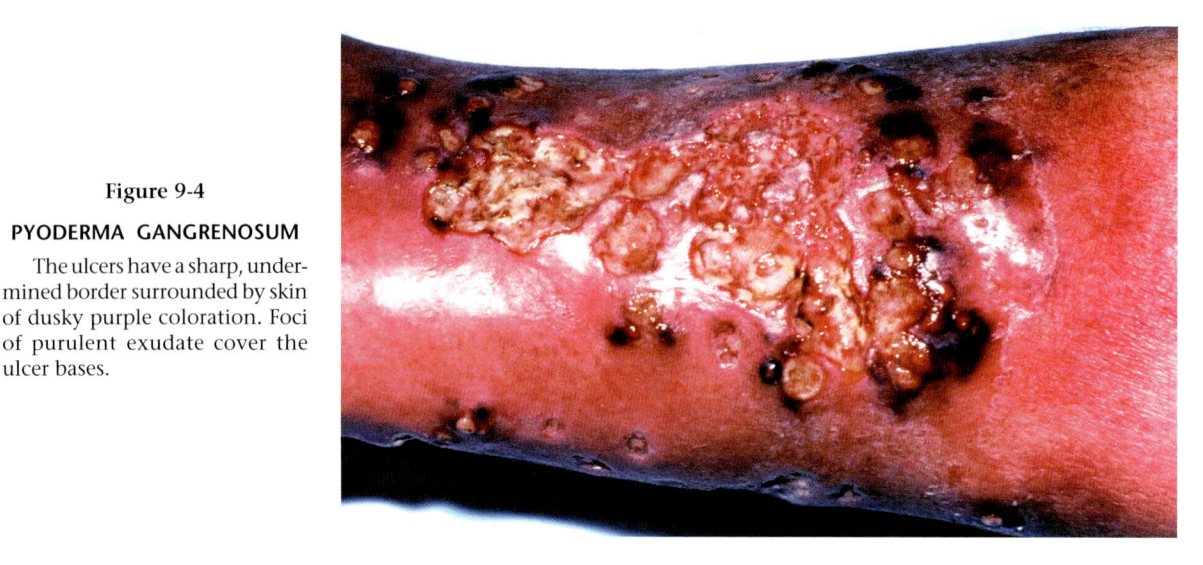

with a purulent exudate and may be partially covered with an eschar. Follicular pustules are observed in the advancing border of the lesion. The lesions are initially solitary, but additional lesions may develop. Most commonly, they affect the lower extremities, but they occur at any site including the face. Lesions heal with the formation of a characteristic cribriform scar.

The patients usually appear systemically ill, with malaise and sometimes fever, in the initial stages of the disease. The most common associations with the disorder are large and small bowel inflammatory diseases, especially Crohn disease and ulcerative colitis. The disorder is also associated with diverticulitis, leukemia, myeloma, chronic active hepatitis, especially with hepatitis B infection, and Behçet syndrome, among others. If untreated, the course may last for months to years and tends to be recurrent. As older lesions are resolving, new lesions appear. Sometimes the lesions are present for months or, rarely, years before the inflammatory bowel disease appears. When ulcerative colitis is preceded for a protracted period by pyoderma gangrenosum, on rare occasion toxic megacolon will herald the onset of the colitis.

**Pathologic Findings.** Biopsy of the earliest lesion reveals a perivascular lymphoid infiltrate around the involved follicle. As the lesion progresses, the ulcer edge shows a mixed inflammatory infiltrate, often with a pronounced perivascular cuff of lymphocytes (fig. 9-5). There is generally overlying epidermal hyperplasia, which grows downward into the well-defined edge of the ulcer base to produce the punched-out, undermined appearance appreciated clinically (fig. 9-5, top). The ulcer base consists of a sea of neutrophils, which replaces the dermal matrix (fig. 9-6) but is not associated with primary neutrophilic vasculitis. Certain clinical variants (e.g., atypical pyoderma gangrenosum; see below) may show neutrophilic involvement of the deep dermis and subcutis. Special stains for bacteria and fungi, as well as cultures, are consistently negative if deep lesional tissue is examined to exclude superficial contamination.

The diagnosis of pyoderma gangrenosum is based on astute clinicopathologic correlation and exclusion of conditions that could mimic florid tissue infiltration by neutrophils, particularly infection. Lesions generally respond favorably to therapy with corticosteroids, making exclusion of infection mandatory before implementation of treatment.

**Differential Diagnosis.** The main entity in the differential diagnosis is usually an infectious process, most commonly ecthyma gangrenosum or even progressive gangrene. Infectious disorders such as deep fungal infections and amebiasis also give rise to similar lesions. Stasis ulceration is commonly misdiagnosed for these lesions, because of the predilection of the lesions on the lower leg. Occasionally, systemic vasculitic disorders, such as Wegener granulomatosis, result in ulceration. The palisading of giant cells around the inflamed area and the presence of granulomatous vasculitis aid in diagnosis of Wegener granulomatosis.

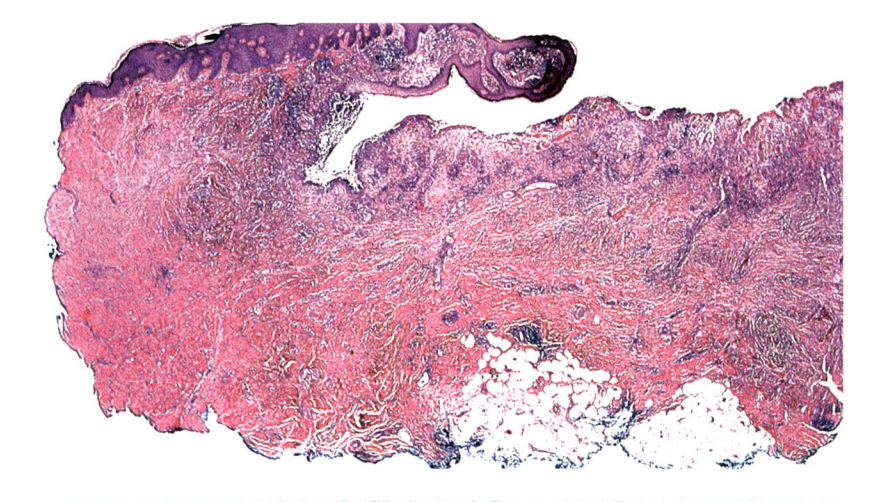

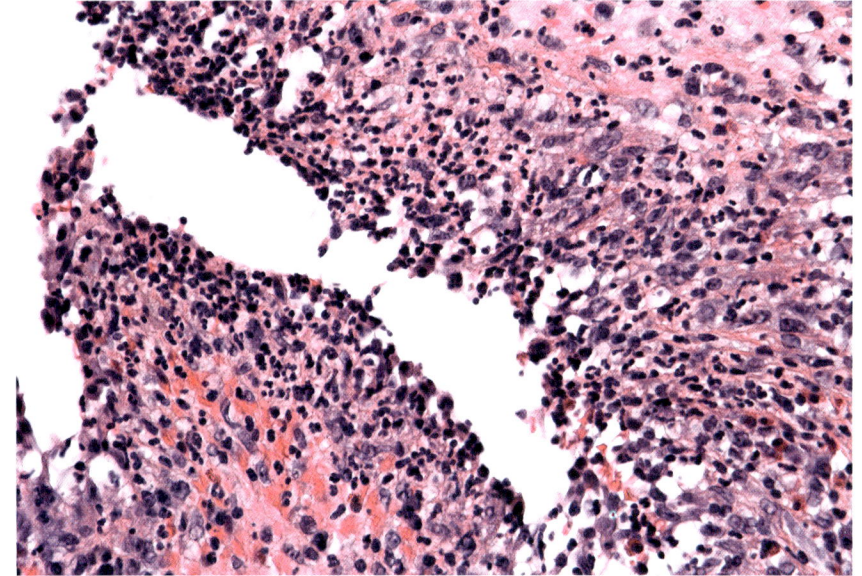

**Figure 9-5**

**PYODERMA GANGRENOSUM**

Top: At scanning magnification, the characteristic overhanging edge is undermined by inflamed and ulcerated dermis.

Bottom: The advancing edge of the lesion is characterized by numerous neutrophils.

*Atypical pyoderma gangrenosum* is an ulcerative lesion with unique features that is associated with systemic disease. For example, acute myelocytic leukemia, myelofibrosis, and Behçet disease can present with pyoderma gangrenosum–like ulcers. The atypical features include unusual locations, such as the trunk, and often a deep nodular component. Histologically, the lesions show extensive infiltration of not only the dermis but even the subcutaneous fat. They are not well-defined lesions but are extensive and diffuse. The possibility of an associated disorder is suspected when such atypical features are noted. We alert the clinician to this situation by an extensive comment that outlines the reasons for concern. We also look carefully for asscociated histologic findings, as in the case of leukemic ulcers, where there are atypical neutrophils with associated nuclear abnormalities within the reactive neutrophilic infiltrate.

**Treatment and Prognosis.** For pyoderma gangrenosum associated with an underlying disorder, such as acute inflammatory bowel disease, the treatment of the disorder often results in clearing of the lesions. For lesions of unknown etiology and even for those associated with other systemic diseases, it is sometimes necessary to treat with oral prednisone (22,23). Dapsone and intralesional triamcinolone injections are used (24,25), as well as sulfasalazine and cyclosporine (26,27). Therapy with antitumor necrosis factor agents, such as infliximab, or with intravenous gammaglobulins, is used for recalcitrant cases. Proper and aggressive wound care and careful debridement are part of the therapeutic regime.

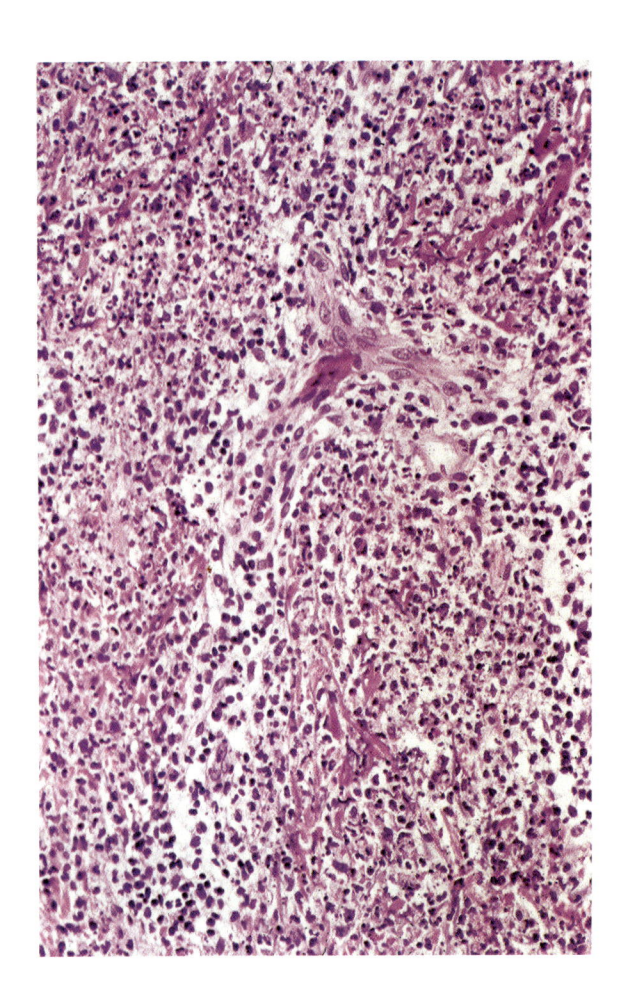

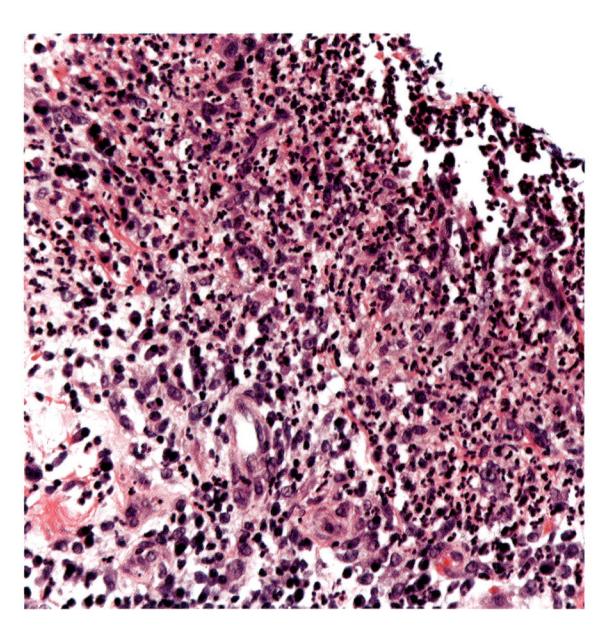

**Figure 9-6**

**PYODERMA GANGRENOSUM: DERMAL INFILTRATE BENEATH ULCER**

Left: There is marked replacement of the dermal matrix by mature neutrophils, without evidence of associated vasculitis. Special stains are always required for such lesions to exclude the possibility of an infectious cause.

Above: At high magnification, the granulation tissue is associated with numerous superficial neutrophils. Primary bacterial elements are not demonstrable.

## ULCERATING INFECTIOUS DISORDERS

Ulcerating infectious disorders share the common clinical and histologic feature of cutaneous ulceration caused by infection with various agents. While comprehensive discussion of all infections that may produce cutaneous ulceration is beyond the scope of this section, the following diseases represent conditions that generally are discussed in differential diagnoses of ulcers that do not fit easily into the categories that have been outlined in the sections above. This review also emphasizes some of the special diagnostic approaches that are useful adjuncts when evaluating dermatitic cutaneous ulcers with potentially infectious causes.

### Ecthyma Gangrenosum

*Ecthyma gangrenosum* is a cutaneous manifestation indicating systemic infection, usually by *Pseudomonas aeruginosa* (28–30). Immunocompromised individuals are preferentially affected (31,32). The lesions begin as erythematous papules and pustules, and then evolve to discrete ulcers with a peripheral rim of erythema and a covering black adherent eschar, also known as a sphacelus.

Histologically, there is extensive necrosis and an associated neutrophil-rich mixed inflammatory infiltrate extending from the epidermal layer often into the subcutaneous fat (figs. 9-7–9-10). Gram-negative bacilli are detected by Gram stain (fig. 9-11), particularly within the walls of reticular dermal blood vessels. Because ecthyma may occur in the setting of profound immunosuppression, it should always be excluded in situations where there is extensive dermal necrosis, even in association with a paucity of inflammatory cells. We recommend stains for organisms in such cases to make certain that infection is not missed because of the minimal amount of inflammation. Intravenous antipseudomonal antibiotics are required, often necessitating double coverage.

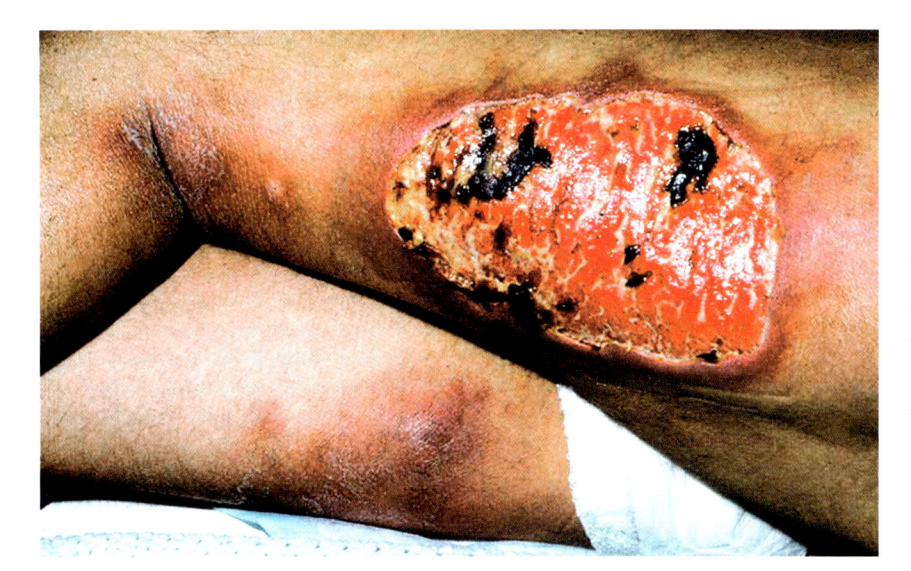

## Figure 9-7
### ECTHYMA GANGRENOSUM
New lesions consist of erythematous nodules with incipient central necrosis and ulceration. The extensive region of ulceration bordered by an erythematous hue is consistent with the persistent evolution of coalescent lesions.

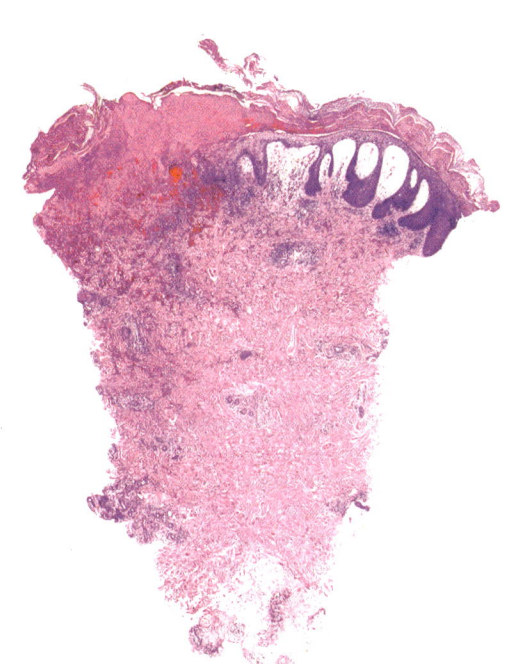

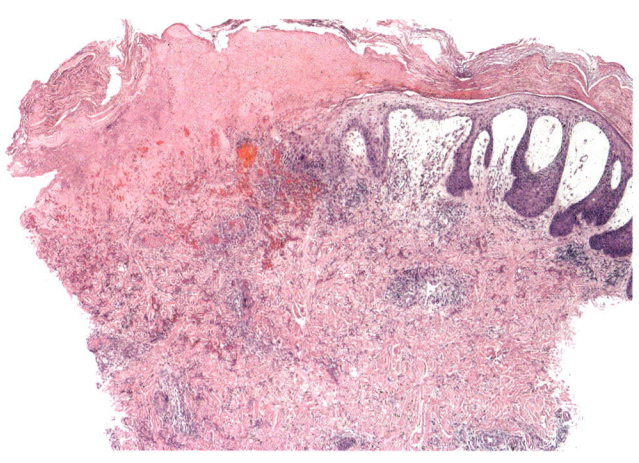

## Figure 9-8
### ECTHYMA GANGRENOSUM
Left: At scanning magnification, extensive necrosis and incipient ulceration with foci of dermal-epidermal separation are seen.

Above: At higher magnification, a zone of epidermal and superficial dermal necrosis (left) and incipient epidermal sloughing (right) are noted.

## Streptococcal Ecthyma

*Streptococcal ecthyma* is a bacterial disease that begins as an impetigo-like pustule and eventuates in ulceration, deep dermal necrosis, and pyoderma. Lesions tend to develop in warm climates and in the setting of poor hygiene and malnutrition. Group A streptococci are the causative organisms. The clinical lesion is a sharply defined ulcer, often on the lower extremity, and generally covered by pus or gray-yellow crust. Secondary lymphangitis and lymphadenopathy are frequent. The histopathology is nonspecific, revealing ulceration with reactive alterations, dermal necrosis, and neutrophil-rich mixed inflammation containing intracellular gram-positive cocci in chains upon special staining. Therapy includes local care, systemic antibiotics, and correction of the underlying systemic and nutritional imbalances. Healing occurs spontaneously with scarring and hyperpigmentation.

*Inflammatory Disorders of the Skin*

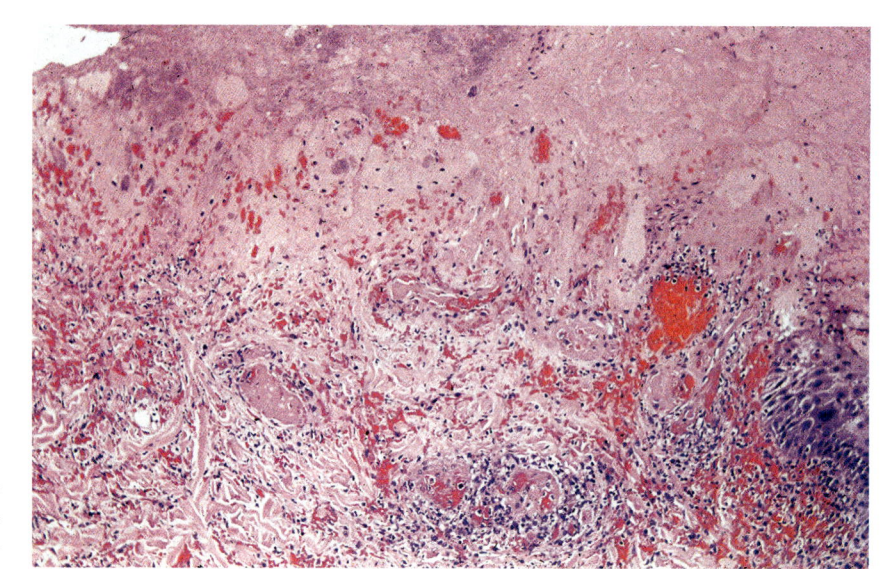

**Figure 9-9**

**ECTHYMA GANGRENOSUM: DERMAL ALTERATIONS**

Top: There is a variably dense, neutrophil-rich inflammatory infiltrate associated with extensive necrosis.

Bottom: At higher magnification, foci of hemorrhage are the result of involvement of dermal vessels in the extensive field of necrosis. Involved microvessels often show causative *Pseudomonas* organisms within the walls.

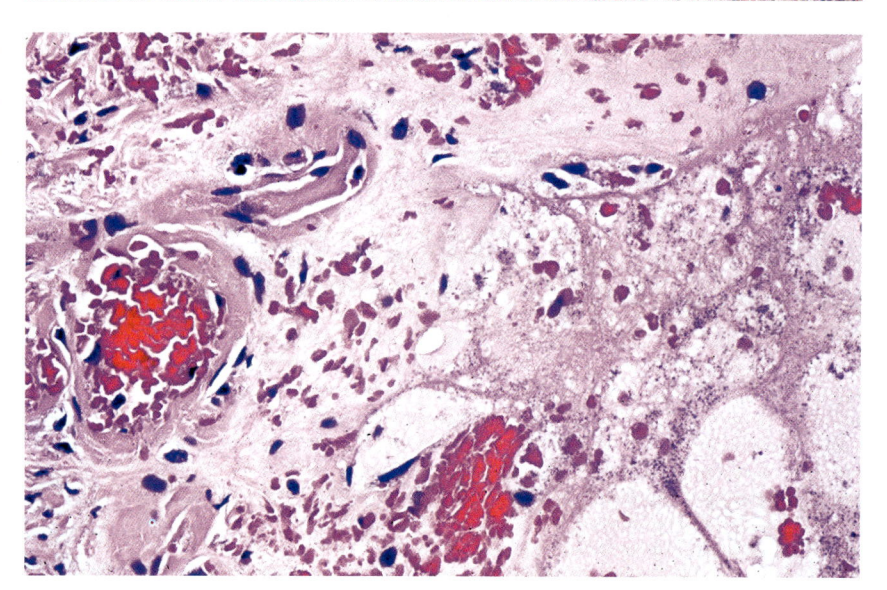

### Anthrax

There has been renewed interest in the histopathologic presentation of *cutaneous anthrax infection* with more recent and immediate threats of bioterrorism. Transmitted by contact with *Bacillus anthracis*, lesions are erythematous papules, hemorrhagic papulovesicles, or ulcerated nodules covered by an adherent eschar or sphacelus (33–36). All stages may be present as lesions evolve.

The histopathology consists of superficial epidermal ulceration with an associated fibrinopurulent exudate, marked dermal edema, hemorrhage, interstitial neutrophilic infiltration, and occasionally, extension into the subcutaneous fat. Organisms are small (3 to 5 μm in length), gram-positive rods that are dispersed within the ulcer base and among collagen fibers, but generally not within inflammatory cells. In the absence of positive cultures or Gram stains, PCR analysis is useful. Conventional disease is treated with penicillin. Bioterrorist regimens include ciprofloxacin and/or doxycycline.

### Tularemia

*Tularemia* is caused by *Francisella tularensis*, which is transmitted from the handling of infected animals (e.g., rodents and rabbits),

*Ulcerative Dermatitis*

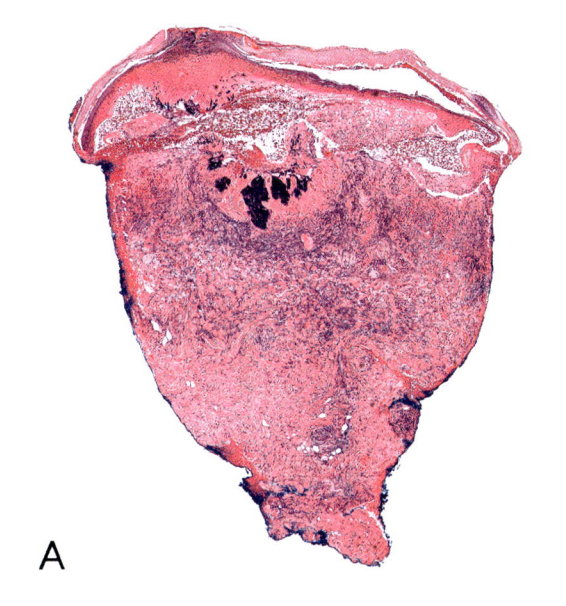

**Figure 9-10**

**ECTHYMA GANGRENOSUM**

A: At scanning magnification, there is extensive epidermal and dermal necrosis with a mixed inflammatory infiltrate.

B: Higher magnification shows that the largely necrotic epidermis and superficial dermis are heavily colonized by bacterial forms.

C: Viable cells are not apparent due to the extensive necrosis.

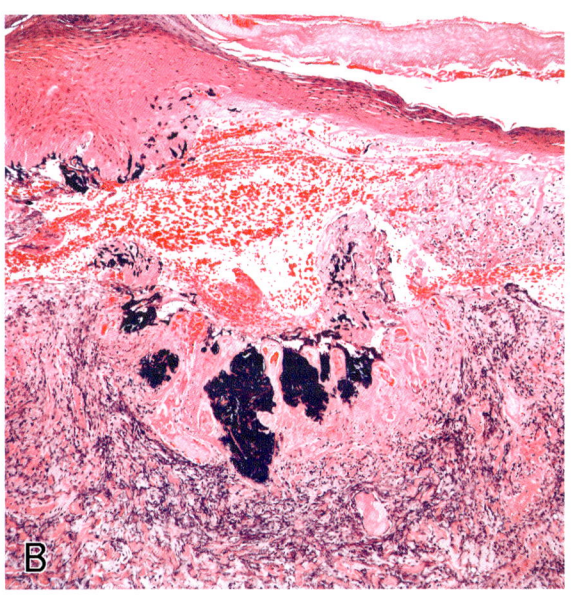

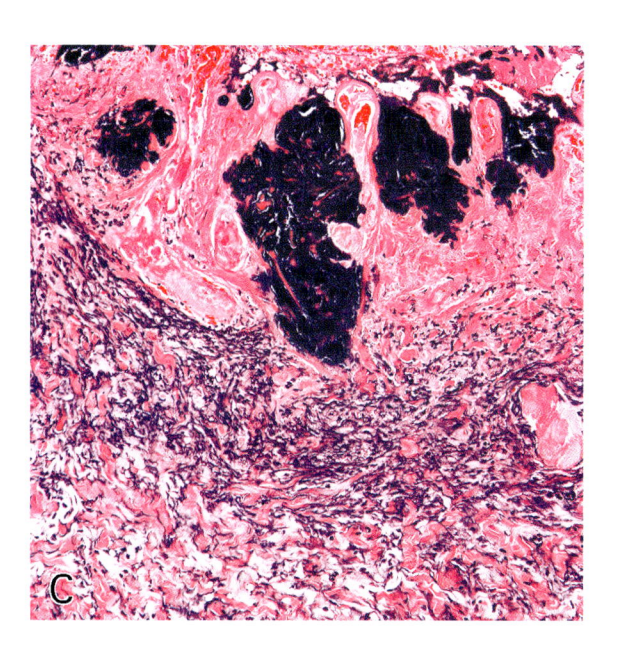

contaminated food or water, or via arthropod bite. Cutaneous tularemia generally presents as a papulonodule with ulceration at the contact site (37–41). Suppurative lymphadenitis may supervene, with the constitutional signs of fever, respiratory symptoms, and muscle aches.

Biopsy of the ulcer discloses adjacent epidermal hyperplasia and underlying alterations consisting characteristically of three distinct zones. Centrally, there is granular necrosis with neutrophil debris and hemorrhage bordered by an epithelioid histiocytic infiltrate, with a more heterogeneous outer mantle of lymphocytes, histiocytes, plasma cells, and extravasated erythrocytes. The latter is a typical finding that is important in the differential diagnosis with other infections potentially resulting in zonal dermal necrobiosis (cat scratch disease and lymphogranuloma venereum). In older lesions, granulomatous inflammation resembling sarcoidosis may dominate the histologic picture. Organisms are difficult to impossible to detect in histologic sections. Treatment is with streptomycin.

*Inflammatory Disorders of the Skin*

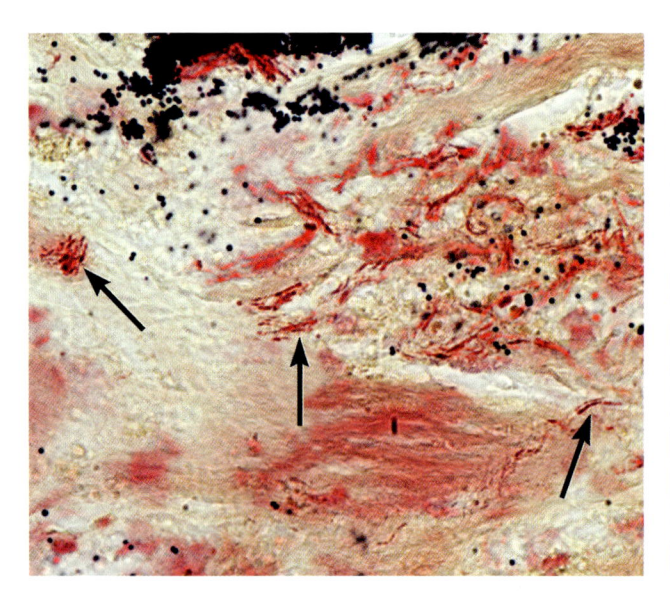

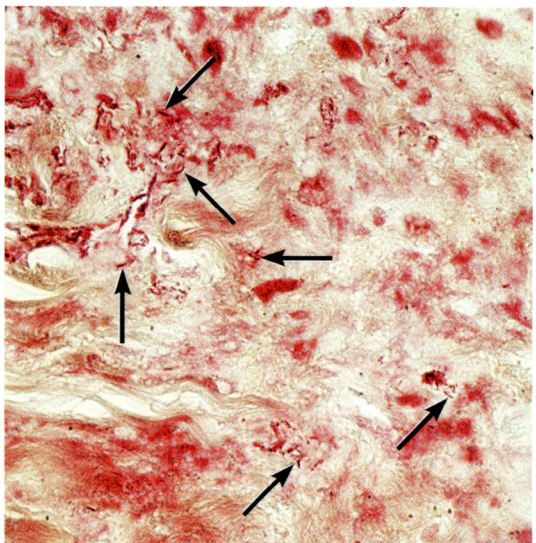

Figure 9-11

**ECTHYMA GANGRENOSUM: GRAM STAIN**

Left: Although the more superficial organisms represent secondary involvement by gram-positive cocci, the pathogenic gram-negative rods are also apparent (arrows).

Right: Gram-negative rods representing *Pseudomonas* are present within the deep dermal tissue.

### Lymphogranuloma Venereum

*Lymphogranuloma venereum* is a venereal chlamydial infection that occurs most commonly in tropical and semitropical climates (42,43). At the site of inoculation (genital skin), there are one to many asymptomatic herpetiform papules that ulcerate. This is followed by the development of inguinal or anorectal lymphadenitis, suppuration, and draining sinuses. In time, lymphatic fibrosis and obstruction may develop, resulting in genital elephantiasis and chronic ischemic ulceration and fistulae.

The histopathology of the ulcerated lesions is not specific, showing fibrin and cellular debris along the ulcer base, and mixed inflammation with epithelioid granuloma formation within the underlying dermis. Although the Giemsa stain may reveal intracellular chlamydia, more specific immunofluorescence assays are generally preferred for the definitive detection of organisms. Culture, however, remains the most sensitive and specific method of diagnosis. Doxycycline is the treatment of choice.

### Cat Scratch Disease

Exposure to cats with *Bartonella henselae* is the primary mode of transmission of *cat scratch disease*. The disease is characterized by the development of solitary or multiple erythematous papules at the scratch inoculation site (44–48). Pustule formation and ulceration may develop in some but not all lesions. Systemic signs include fever and regional lymphadenopathy.

Skin biopsy reveals reactive epidermal alterations sometimes with associated ulceration, granular dermal necrobiosis surrounded by histiocytes occasionally in palisaded array, and multinucleated giant cells, all surrounded by a mantle of lymphocytes with admixed eosinophils and nuclear debris. The zoning of alterations within the dermis is similar to the histologic alterations typical of tularemia, but there is no extravasation of red blood cells, a characteristic feature of that infection. The Warthin-Starry stain is required for the detection of organisms, which appear as rods that are sometimes compared to a safety pin. Immunofluorescence assays are also available for more sensitive and specific detection.

Treatment is not necessary in immunocompetent hosts. For those who are immunosuppressed, erythromycin and doxycycline are used.

### Chancroid

*Chancroid* is a venereal disease seen predominantly in tropical and subtropical climates. It is caused by infection by *Haemophilus ducreyi*, which produces a painful suppurating and ulcerated papule at the genital site of inoculation (49–52). Suppurative lymphadenitis of draining nodes may supervene. Histologically, there are three horizontally aligned zones of alteration: 1) the fibrinopurulent ulcer surface; 2) an underlying stratum of activated granulation tissue; and 3) a deepest layer of diagnostically characteristic dense lymphoplasmacytic inflammation. Gram-negative bacilli in parallel chains are generally demonstrable within the surface layer of the ulcer. Azithromycin, ceftriaxone, ciprofloxacin, and erythromycin have activity against *H. ducreyi*.

### Granuloma Inguinale

Caused by *Calymmatobacterium granulomatis*, *granuloma inguinale* is a venereal disease that is prevalent in tropical and semitropical climates (53,54). At the contact site, an ulcerated papulonodule develops. Biopsy reveals adjacent epidermal hyperplasia and a neutrophil-rich ulcer surface. Beneath the hyperplastic epidermis, there is a prominent mixed, interstitial dermal band-like infiltrate composed of lymphocytes, histiocytes, and plasma cells. A characteristic feature is the presence of multiple small collections of neutrophils in the midst of the band-like inflammatory response. The infiltrate can at times be so dense as to extend even into subcutaneous fat. The histiocytes, typically more within the upper dermis, contain cytoplasmic vacuoles with inclusions, termed Donovan bodies. With the Giemsa or Warthin-Starry stain, these inclusions prove to be formed by aggregated bacilli. Trimethoprim-sulfamethoxazole, doxycycline, erythromycin, or ciprofloxacin are used to irradicate the organism.

### Primary Syphilis

The chancre is the first stage in the evolution of *syphilitic spirochete* (*Treponema pallidum*) *infection*, and represents a direct response to the primary site of inoculation (as opposed to secondary and tertiary manifestations, which are more generalized systemic immune responses to the organism) (55–57). Clinically, there is an indurated painless ulcer with sharply defined margins. The genital skin is most commonly affected, but other mucosal and cutaneous sites are sometimes involved.

Histologically, there is superficial ulceration covered by a fibrinopurulent exudate and overlying a brisk interstitial and perivascular infiltrate composed of lymphocytes, numerous plasma cells, neutrophils, and histiocytes, which may extend into the deep reticular dermis. The infiltrate is often so extensive as to be tumefactive. In addition, there is extensive endothelial cell hypertrophy with luminal obliteration. The vessels affected are of various calibers and their walls are markedly infiltrated by plasma cells, resulting in a plasma cell vasculopathy. Marked dermal edema is generally present. The Warthin-Starry stain is generally positive (unlike lesions of secondary syphilis), revealing spirochetes both within the dermis, especially in a perivascular array, but also interstitially and within the epidermal layer bordering the ulcer. Therapy is with penicillin.

## REFERENCES

1. Oka M, Berking C, Nesbit M, et al. Interleukin-8 overexpression is present in pyoderma gangrenosum ulcers and leads to ulcer formation in human skin xenografts. Lab Invest 2000;80:595-604.
2. Zunt SL. Recurrent aphthous stomatitis. Dermatol Clin 2003;21:33-9.
3. Bruce AJ, Rogers RS 3rd. Acute oral ulcers. Dermatol Clin 2003;21:1-15.
4. Porter SR, Hegarty A, Kaliakatsou F, Hodgson TA, Scully C. Recurrent aphthous stomatitis. Clin Dermatol 2000;18:569-78.
5. Herbert AA, Berg JH. Oral mucous membrane diseases of childhood: I. Mucositis and xerostomia. II. Recurrent aphthous stomatitis. III. Herpetic stomatitis. Semin Dermatol 1992;11:80-7.
6. Sciubba JJ. Herpes simplex and aphthous ulcerations: presentation, diagnosis and management—an update. Gen Dent 2003;51:510-6.
7. Baughman RA. Recurrent aphthous stomatitis vs. recurrent herpes: do you know the difference? J Ala Dent Assoc 1996;80:26-32.
8. Tilliss TS, McDowell JD. Differential diagnosis: is it herpes or aphthous? J Contemp Dent Pract 2002;3:1-15.
9. Stoopler ET, Sollectio TP. Recurrent aphthous stomatitis. Update for the general practitioner. N Y State Dent J 2003;69:27-9.
10. Natah SS, Konttinen YT, Enattah NS, Ashammakhi N, Sharkey KA, Hayrinen-Immonen R. Recurrent aphthous ulcers today: a review of the growing knowledge. Int J Oral Maxillofac Surg 2004;33:221-34.
11. Lee LA. Behcet disease. Semin Cutan Med Surg 2001;20:53-7.
12. Al-Otaibi LM, Porter SR, Poate TW. Behcet's disease: a review. J Dent Res 2005; 84:209-22.
13. Suzuki Kurokawa M, Suzuki N. Behcet's disease. Clin Exp Med 2004;4:10-20.
14. Bennett ML, Jackson JM, Jorizzo JL, Fleischer AB Jr, White WL, Callen JP. Pyoderma gangrenosum. A comparison of typical and atypical forms with an emphasis on time to remission. Case review of 86 patients from 2 institutions. Medicine (Baltimore) 2000;79:37-46.
15. Bhat RM, Shetty SS, Kamath GH. Pyoderma gangrenosum in childhood. Int J Dermatol 2004;43:205-7.
16. Iijima S, Ogawa T, Nanno Y, Tsunoda T, Kudoh K. Pyoderma gangrenosum first presenting as a recalcitrant ulcer of the ear lobe. Eur J Dermatol 2003;13:606-9.
17. Blitz NM, Rudikoff D. Pyoderma gangrenosum. Mt Sinai J Med 2001;68:287-97.
18. Powell FC, Collins S. Pyoderma gangrenosum. Clin Dermatol 2000;18:283-93.
19. Tavarela Veloso F. Review article: skin complications associated with inflammatory bowel disease. Aliment Pharmacol Ther 2004;20 Suppl 4:50-3.
20. Boh EE, al-Smadi RM. Cutaneous manifestations of gastrointestinal diseases. Dermatol Clin 2002;20:533-46.
21. Ujiie H, Sawamura D, Yokota K, Nishie W, Shichinohe R, Shimizu H. Pyoderma gangrenosum associated with Takayasu's arteritis. Clin Exp Dermatol 2004;29:357-9.
22. Gettler S, Rothe M, Grin C, Grant-Kels J. Optimal treatment of pyoderma gangrenosum. Am J Clin Dermatol 2003;4:597-608.
23. Powell FC, O'Kane M. Management of pyoderma gangrenosum. Dermatol Clin 2002;20:347-55.
24. Wenzel J, Gerdsen R, Phillipp-Dormston W, Bieber T, Uerlich M. Topical treatment of pyoderma gangraenosum. Dermatology 2002;205:221-3.
25. Jennings JL. Pyoderma gangrenosum: successful treatment with intralesional steroids. J Am Acad Dermatol 1983;9:575-80.
26. Schofer H, Baur S. Successful treatment of postoperative pyoderma gangrenosum with cyclosporin. J Eur Acad Dermatol Venereol 2002;16:148-51.
27. Shenefelt PD. Pyoderma gangrenosum associated with cystic acne and hidradenitis suppurativa controlled by adding minocycline and sulfasalazine to the treatment regimen. Cutis 1996;57:315-9.
28. Solowski NL, Yao FB, Agarwal A, Nagorsky M. Ecthyma gangrenosum: a rare cutaneous manifestation of a potentially fatal disease. Ann Otol Rhinol Laryngol 2004;113:462-4.
29. Zomorrodi A, Wald ER. Ecthyma gangrenosum: considerations in a previously healthy child. Pediatr Infect Dis J 2002;21:1161-4.
30. Jones SG, Olver WJ, Boswell TC, Russell NH. Ecthyma gangrenosum. Eur J Haematol 2002;69:324.
31. Khan MO, Montecalvo MA, Davis I, Wormser GP. Ecthyma gangrenosum in patients with acquired immunodeficiency syndrome. Cutis 2000;66:121-3.
32. Baro M, Marin MA, Ruiz-Contreras J, de Miguel SF, Sanchez-Diaz I. Pseudomonas aeruginosa sepsis and ecthyma gangrenosum as initial manifestations of primary immunodeficiency. Eur J Pediatr 2004;163:173-4.

33. Godyn JJ, Reyes L, Siderits R, Hazra A. Cutaneous anthrax: conservative or surgical treatment? Adv Skin Wound Care 2005;18:146-50.
34. Wenner KA, Kenner JR. Anthrax. Dermatol Clin 2004;22:247-56.
35. Spencer RC. Bacillus anthracis. J Clin Pathol 2003;56:182-7.
36. Tutrone WD, Scheinfeld NS, Weinberg JM. Cutaneous anthrax: a concise review. Cutis 2002;69:27-33.
37. McGinley-Smith DE, Tsao SS. Dermatoses from ticks. J Am Acad Dermatol 2003;49:363-92.
38. Cronquist SD. Tularemia: the disease and the weapon. Dermatol Clin 2004;22:313-20.
39. Feldman KA. Tularemia. J Am Vet Med Assoc 2003;222:725-30.
40. Ellis J, Oyston PC, Green M, Titball RW. Tularemia. Clin Microbiol Rev 2002;15:631-46.
41. Choi E. Tularemia and Q fever. Med Clin North Am 2002;86:393-416.
42. Mabey D, Peeling RW. Lymphogranuloma venereum. Sex Transm Infect 2002;78:90-2.
43. Brown TJ, Yen-Moore A, Tyring SK. An overview of sexually transmitted diseases. Part I. J Am Acad Dermatol 1999;41:511-32.
44. Chian CA, Arrese JE, Pierard GE. Skin manifestations of Bartonella infections. Int J Dermatol 2002;41:461-6.
45. Lamps LW, Scott MA. Cat-scratch disease: historic, clinical, and pathologic perspectives. Am J Clin Pathol 2004;121:S71-80.
46. Chomel BB, Boulouis HJ, Breitschwerdt EB. Cat scratch disease and other zoonotic Bartonella infections. J Am Vet Med Assoc 2004;224:1270-9.
47. Conrad DA. Treatment of cat-scratch disease. Curr Opin Pediatr 2001;13:56-9.
48. Schutze GE. Diagnosis and treatment of Bartonella henselae infections. Pediatr Infect Dis J 2000;19:1185-7.
49. Sehgal VN, Srivastava G. Chancroid: contemporary appraisal. Int J Dermatol 2003;42:182-90.
50. Lewis DA. Chancroid: clinical manifestations, diagnosis, and management. Sex Transm Infect 2003;79:68-71.
51. Bong CT, Bauer ME, Spinola SM. Haemophilus ducreyi: clinical features, epidemiology, and prospects for disease control. Microbes Infect 2002;4:1141-8.
52. Lewis DA. Chancroid: from clinical practice to basic science. AIDS Patient Care STDS 2000;14:19-36.
53. O'Farrell N. Donovanosis. Sex Transm Infect 2002;78:452-7.
54. O'Farrell N. Donovanosis: an update. Int J STD AIDS 2001;12:423-7.
55. Zeltser R, Kurban AK. Syphilis. Clin Dermatol 2004;22:461-8.
56. Golden MR, Marra CM, Holmes KK. Update on syphilis: resurgence of an old problem. JAMA 2003;290:1510-4.
57. Goldmeier D, Guallar C. Syphilis: an update. Clin Med 2003;3:209-11.

# 10 NONVASCULITIC ANGIOCENTRIC DERMATITIS

## GENERAL CONSIDERATIONS

The term *angiocentric dermatitis* defines those disorders characterized primarily by perivascular inflammatory infiltrates, with or without vasculitis. The term angiocentric emphasizes the trophic tendency for inflammatory cells to concentrate about vessels and has a firm basis in the molecular mechanisms of cellular adhesion. Although all forms of dermatitis, per force, are angiocentric in their earliest evolutionary stages, some are distinguished by subsequent localization of immune cells in nonangiocentric tissue compartments (e.g., the epidermis in the case of spongiotic and cytotoxic dermatitis; the subcutaneous fat in the case of panniculitis). Because the epidermis is basically unaltered in angiocentric dermatitis, these conditions are often diagnosed at scanning magnification after the normal overlying epidermal layer is appreciated. *Vasculitis*, a term that literally implies inflammation of the vessel, describes vessel injury manifested by varying degrees of endothelial degeneration and necrosis. Accordingly, vasculitis is technically present when endothelial cells exhibit little more than degenerative cytoplasmic vacuolization and hypereosinophilia (urticarial vasculitis). Classic *fibrinoid necrosis* defines a condition in which injury has progressed so far that the vessel wall permits more leakage of blood cells and serum components, including fibrin (see chapter 11, Vasculitic Angiocentric Dermatitis).

The term *lymphocytic vasculitis* implies damage to the vessel wall provoked primarily by lymphocytes. It is generally characterized by a perivascular angiocentric pattern with associated hemorrhage but often without the classic fibrinoid necrosis of the vessel wall. Lymphocytic vasculitis is a reaction pattern that is seen in a diverse array of conditions, including erythema multiforme, pityriasis lichenoides et varioliformis acuta, and pigmentary purpura, and in dysplastic/lymphoproliferative angiocentric cutaneous infiltrates (e.g., lymphomatoid papulosis). In the setting of pure angiocentric dermatitis without evidence of epidermal alterations or chronicity, lymphocytic vasculitis may suggest the exanthem of systemic viral infection.

As is expected in a primarily dermal inflammatory process, scaling, crust formation, irregular epidermal topography, and variability in epidermal-derived pigmentation are not primary features because the epidermal layer is not appreciably affected. Rather, the character of the clinical lesion relates primarily to the nature of the dermal inflammatory component. When perivascular and interstitial edema predominate, lesions are generally edematous plaques (i.e., hives or urticaria) that have blanchable erythema and are evanescent. Persistence of such lesions beyond 24 hours often indicates a component of vascular injury (i.e., urticarial vasculitis). Angiocentric infiltrates in which inflammatory cells remain intimately associated with vessel walls may enlarge to become well-circumscribed, erythematous plaques with slightly elevated borders, producing gyrate or polycyclic formations on the skin surface. Erythematous papules and plaques caused by angiocentric lymphocytic infiltrates occasionally appear vesicular and polymorphous when associated with marked superficial dermal edema. Although all of these examples involve blanchable erythema (i.e., redness that disappears on compression), the presence of perivascular hemorrhage caused by injury to vessel walls may result in deep red-purple erythema (i.e., purpura), which does not blanch. Moreover, when perivascular hemorrhage is appreciable, lesions are not only observed, but may be palpated (i.e., palpable purpura). Repeated hemorrhage to skin may result in both transient (i.e., acute) purpura, as well as persistent pigmentation caused by hemosiderin deposition (e.g., pigmentary purpura). In contrast, necrotizing angiocentric injury to superficial dermal vessels produces acute and chronic clinical manifestations of perivascular hemorrhage, whereas similar damage to larger subcutaneous vessels results in gross pathology dominated by secondary ischemia and necrosis of the subcutis, dermis, and epidermis. Because such infarctive lesions often occur at multiple foci along the course of deep vessels, the clinical nodules they produce may be linear or result in indurated, painful plaques that mimic panniculitis.

The earliest phase of angiocentric dermatitis shows both intraluminal and perivascular accumulation of inflammatory cells. An example of this phenomenon is urticaria, which is often only several hours old at the time of biopsy. In urticaria, there characteristically are intraluminal neutrophils as well as scant perivascular collections of lymphocytes, neutrophils, and sometimes eosinophils. Established lesions of angiocentric dermatitis generally show a predominance of perivascular inflammatory cells, as in erythema annulare centrifugum, in which lymphocytes within the perivascular adventitia are tightly apposed to vessel walls. In some but not all forms of angiocentric dermatitis, late lesions demonstrate both perivascular and interstitial infiltrates of inflammatory cells. Established or chronic, dermal delayed-hypersensitivity responses to injected antigens, such as in arthropod bites and stings, commonly result in this interstitial pattern. Although this concept provides a theoretical schema for the evolution of certain conditions in this category, not all types of angiocentric dermatitis evolve through all three phases, and many are characterized by only one or two of the phases throughout their natural progression.

Because the general histology of angiocentric dermatitis is subtle, especially in the absence of overt vasculitis, care must be taken not to confuse the general histology of this group of disorders with "nonspecific chronic inflammation" or even with normal skin. Each of the conditions discussed in the following sections has characteristic findings that facilitate its recognition. Coupled with an understanding of the gross pathology and clinical characteristics of individual lesions, precise clinicopathologic diagnoses are possible. For this reason, throughout this Fascicle, we emphasize the importance of clinical correlation. For example, whereas individual lesions of ordinary urticaria generally occur and regress within 24 hours, urticarial vasculitic lesions commonly persists for several days. Association of polymorphous light eruption with exposure to ultraviolet light, erythema chronicum migrans with tick-bite exposure, and urticarial papular eruptions with pregnancy are among other examples of how knowledge of clinical parameters facilitate diagnosis of this group of often histologically subtle disorders.

## PATHOGENESIS

All forms of angiocentric (perivascular) dermatitis involve inflammatory cell aggregation about postcapillary venules from the outset. While some progress via leukocyte migration from the perivascular space to specific target sites and result in spongiotic, psoriasiform, cytotoxic, bullous, and interstitial forms of dermatitis or panniculitis, pure angiocentric dermatitis begins and ends in the vicinity of the perivascular space. It is now understood that the mast cells that are concentrated about postcapillary venules are major gatekeepers responsible for regulating the influx into skin of macromolecules and leukocytes. Mast cell cytoplasmic granules liberated upon secretory stimulation contain histamine, heparin, serine proteases, and cytokines that collaborate to modify constitutive microvascular permeability to proteinaceous transudates and to circulating inflammatory cells. Mast cell cytokines, such as tumor necrosis factor-alpha (TNFα) influence microvascular endothelium via induction of endothelial proteins that regulate progressive and often selective leukocyte adhesion and diapedesis (1). This precisely orchestrated and complex cascade is likely to differ as a result of numerous factors, including provocative stimuli, systemic immune status, and anatomic site. In addition to mast cells, trophic factors are elaborated by other dermal cells (e.g., macrophages and nerve fibers) and epidermal cells (keratinocytes). Chemotactic and chemokinetic molecules related to provocative antigens also contribute to the microenvironmental cues that give each type of angiocentric dermatitis its distinctive clinical and pathologic characteristics.

## SPECIAL DIAGNOSTIC STUDIES

The mainstay of special testing in angiocentric dermatitis is direct immunofluorescence to document the presence of immune complex deposition in the setting of necrotizing cutaneous vasculitis. Characteristically, granular deposition of complement and/or one or more immunoglobulins is seen within the walls of small, superficial vessels (i.e., postcapillary venules). It is important to ascertain that the immunoglobulin deposition is within vessel walls and not in vascular lumens or in the perivascular space. Fibrin frequently is detected in the perivascular region; although this finding is not diagnostic for vasculitis, it suggests increased vascular permeability and possible vascular damage. Leukocytoclastic vasculitis secondary to various causes (e.g., systemic lupus erythematosus, rheumatoid arthritis, drugs, cryoglobulinemia, livedo vasculitis, hepatitis-associated vasculitis) may show similar results on direct immunofluorescence.

The timing of a skin biopsy to detect vasculitis is critical, because the immune deposits are transitory. The highest yield of detected deposits is in skin lesions that have been present for 18 to 24 hours. Lesions that have been present for more than 48 hours usually show only fibrin deposition and may be negative for evidence of immune complexes. Vascular deposition of immunoreactants is not always diagnostic of leukocytoclastic vasculitis; it has been noted in other inflammatory dermatoses such as erythema multiforme. Immunofluorescence findings should always be correlated with the clinical history and changes on routine histology.

*Henoch-Schönlein purpura* (HSP) is a specific subset of leukocytoclastic vasculitis in which immunoglobulin (Ig)A is the most prominent of the immunoglobulins (1a). Although IgM, IgG, and complement may also be present, IgA usually has the strongest staining intensity. A diagnosis of HSP should be suspected if granular vascular staining with IgA is detected in the absence of all other immunoreactants. In early lesions, the deposition may be punctuate and focal, and the entire specimen must be carefully examined, sometimes with levels, to detect the subtle immunofluorescent changes. Patients with HSP have increased levels of circulating IgA immune complexes and may also have deposition of IgA in renal glomeruli and blood vessels of the gastrointestinal mucosa. These changes correlate with the clinical manifestations of hematuria and abdominal pain frequently seen in these patients.

Patients with *urticarial vasculitis* have persistent urticarial skin lesions that individually last for longer than 24 hours and resolve with purpura or hyperpigmentation. These patients may have associated connective tissue diseases or hypocomplementemia, but drugs and hepatitis C infection are also associated with this disorder. Direct immunofluorescence shows skin lesions indistinguishable from those of leukocytoclastic vasculitis from other causes. Roughly two thirds of patients with urticarial vasculitis have vascular staining with either immunoglobulins or complement.

*Polyarteritis nodosa* is a form of vasculitis involving medium-sized arteries of the skin associated with palpable purpura as well as punched-out cutaneous ulcers, referred to as *macroscopic polyarteritis nodosa* (2). These patients may have associated systemic involvement including the kidneys, liver, heart, and gastrointestinal tract. Histology reveals panarteritis in the deep dermis and subcutaneous tissue. Immunopathologic studies show IgM, C3, and fibrin deposition within the vessel walls; deposition of immunoreactants in small superficial vessels; and the complete absence of immune deposits. There is also a form of polyarteritis associated with vasculitis of the entire spectrum of cutaneous vessels, which presents as large hemorrhagic areas and bullous lesions, designated as *microscopic polyarteritis nodosa*. This form is associated with pANCA (perinuclear antineutrophil cytoplasmic antibody) positivity and has renal and pulmonary involvement. Finally, there is a form of polyarteritis known as the benign cutaneous form associated with recurrent nodules on the lower extremities. No systemic involvement ensues, but there may be underlying inflammatory bowel disease or adult Still disease associated with a prior streptococcal infection.

## ANIMAL MODELS

Angiocentric inflammation may be provoked in the skin of experimental animals using a variety of inflammatory stimuli, including direct cytokine injection. This is because proinflammatory mediators activate endothelial cells, particularly those lining postcapillary venules, to become receptive to adhesive interactions with often specific subsets of circulating leukocytes. Persistence of inflammatory cells within the perivascular space is also likely to involve adhesive pathways and possibly implicates antigen recognition and presentation events by resident dendritic cells in the perivascular space. One animal model for angiocentric inflammation employs human skin that has been xenografted to genetically immune-deficient mice. Injection of provocative cytokines into the grafts, or elicitation of endogenous cytokine release, results in angiocentric inflammation that may then be studied to better define the cellular mechanisms and molecular cascades responsible for this phenomenon critical to the earliest phases of all forms of dermatitis (2a,2b).

## SUPERFICIAL VARIANTS

### Urticaria

**Definition.** *Urticaria*, or *hives*, is a common disorder of the skin resulting in pruritic, pink-white wheals (3–13). These wheals are localized zones of dermal edema that produce isolated, polycyclic, and often coalescent plaques surmounted by a smooth, normal-appearing epidermal surface. About 20 percent of the general population experience at least one episode of urticaria during their lifetime. Clinically, most forms of urticaria are divided into acute and chronic forms. *Acute urticaria* consists of a single, self-limiting episode involving lesions that last for less than 24 hours. *Chronic urticaria* involves repeated episodes of evanescent wheals. Lesions that last more than 24 hours tend to correlate with urticarial vasculitis (see below).

Urticaria and angioedema describe the clinical phenomena associated with a variety of mechanisms, including those of immunologic, inflammatory, or idiopathic etiology. The basic underlying events include an immediate-type hypersensitivity reaction involving IgE, degranulation of mast cells, mechanisms related to complement or arachidonic acid metabolism, or idiopathic mechanisms.

**Clinical Features.** The lesions of urticaria are papules or wheals that are well circumscribed, pruritic, and erythematous. They usually measure a few millimeters in diameter, although coalescence to form plaques, often with arcuate configurations, commonly occurs (fig. 10-1). They are formed by the accumulation of edema fluid in the superficial dermis and are transient, usually not lasting longer than 18 to 24 hours. *Angioedema,* on the other hand, affects the entire skin, including the subcutaneous fat, and therefore presents as large nodular erythematous and pruritic lesions that deform affected areas with marked indurated swelling, usually affecting the head and neck region or large areas of the arms or legs. These lesions, individually, also tend to resolve in a limited period of time. Both urticaria and angioedema tend to recur for varying periods of time, although individual lesions have a limited time frame in evolution. Either occurs as the principal manifestation of the eruption, or they occur together. When angioedema is present, other manifestations of extracutaneous involvement are frequently present, including shortness of breath, wheezing, arthralgias, abdominal pain, vomiting, and diarrhea. Episodes last for a few hours, for weeks to months, or rarely, even years. Acute urticaria describes episodes less than 8 weeks in duration; chronic urticaria refers to those of longer duration. Persons with an acute flare of the disease may show dermographism, the appearance of a wheal after stroking the skin briskly.

A consideration of the different causes of urticaria is helpful in understanding the clinical background of presentations. IgE-dependent urticaria occurs often in the setting of an atopic diathesis and may accompany flares of asthma, hay fever, or eczema. Food allergy is a common example of IgE-dependent urticaria, with shellfish as a frequent inciting agent. Urticaria occurs as a result of physical stimuli, induced by light, cold, pressure, vibration, or direct blunt trauma as in dermographism. In some of these situations, IgE has been shown to be involved; in others, the mechanism is unclear.

Complement-mediated urticarias include hereditary angioedema, which involves the first component of complement. There is a functional deficiency in the inhibitor of this component, when activated. This deficiency is acquired in association with connective tissue disorders and certain malignant disorders.

Urticaria occurs in 70 percent of patients with serum sickness as a part of the complex presentation of this disorder, which presents with pruritus, erythema, and wheals. The symptoms usually last for a few days and occur 1 to 3 weeks

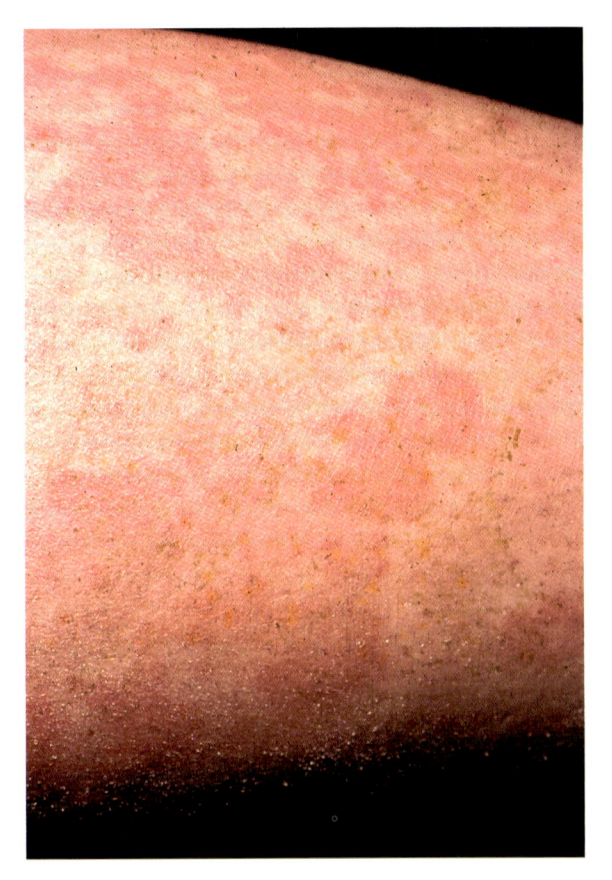

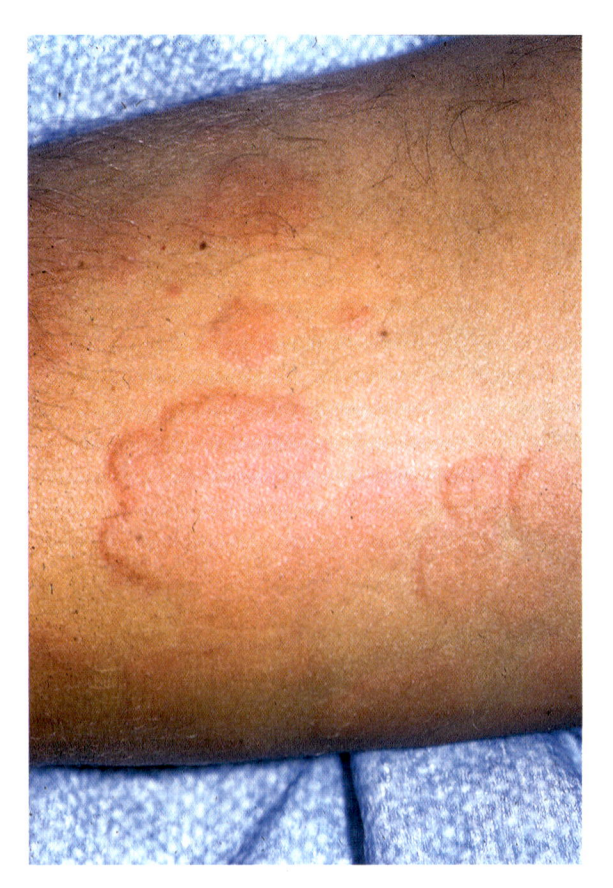

**Figure 10-1**

**URTICARIA**

Left: There are numerous, well-circumscribed, raised erythematous lesions varying from small papules to irregular plaques.

Right: Newer lesions consist of small erythematous papules and plaques. Over time, other lesions exhibit central clearing, producing an arcuate clinical appearance as a result of erythema at the lesion perimeter.

after the administration of the sensitizing agent. Blood product administration, in addition to being a cause of serum sickness, can result in episodic urticaria resulting from the binding of antibodies to these products, culminating in the formation of immune complexes.

Urticaria can result from nonimmunologic and idiopathic causes. Certain agents, such as opiates, radiocontrast material, and some antibiotics, directly cause mast cell and basophil mediator release and result in urticaria. Chronic and recurrent urticaria are of idiopathic cause in about of 70 percent of persons. The diagnosis of idiopathic urticaria should only be made after a careful search for an underlying cause. Occasionally, urticaria can be a paraneoplastic phenomenon.

**Pathologic Findings.** The link between the clinical presentation of urticaria (i.e., localized or diffuse cutaneous swelling) and the histopathology is mast cell degranulation (14). Mast cells are normally situated about small cutaneous venules. When these cells are triggered to degranulate, histamine is liberated, resulting in interendothelial gaps and increased microvascular permeability. This results in progressive accumulation of edema fluid within the intervascular interstitium. Because mast cells also contain other proinflammatory mediators, such as certain cytokines, affected endothelial cells attract circulating leukocytes, resulting in an angiocentric inflammatory pattern (fig. 10-2).

Histologically, the findings may be extraordinarily subtle, leading to confusion with normal

## Inflammatory Disorders of the Skin

**Figure 10-2**

**URTICARIA**

Top: Beneath a normal-appearing epidermis, the dermis is pale because of extravasated edema fluid. Accompanying lymphatic ectasia and a scant perivascular inflammatory infiltrate are also present.

Bottom: At higher magnification of the perivascular inflammatory component, the infiltrate is mixed, consisting of scattered lymphocytes, neutrophils, and rare eosinophils. Neutrophils are often detected within lumens of postcapillary venules surrounded by edema fluid (arrow).

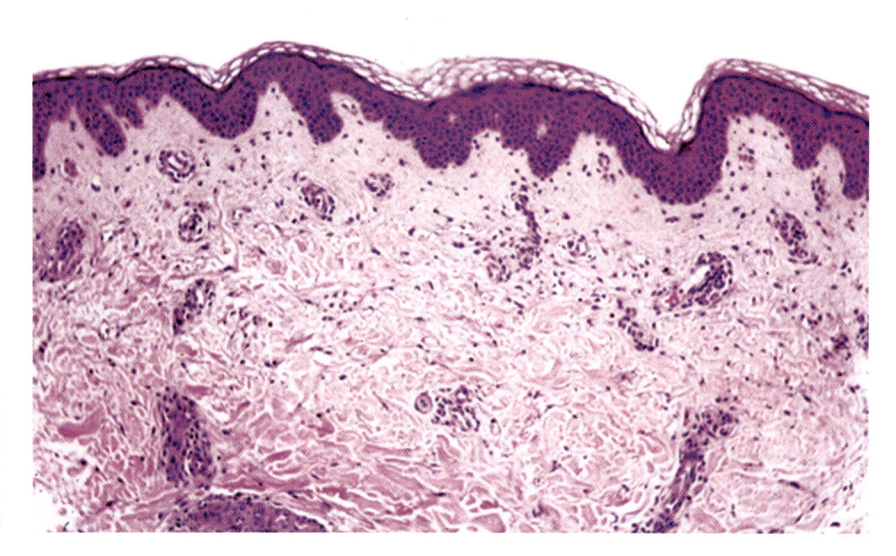

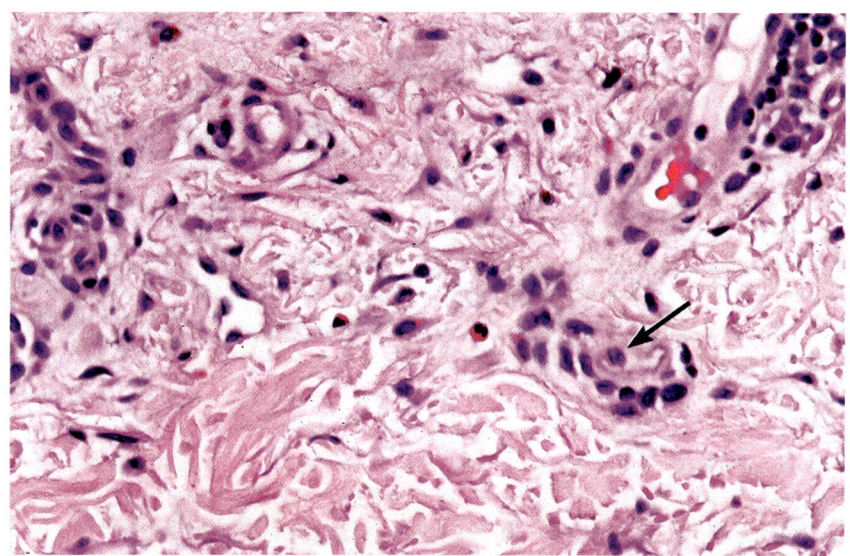

skin. There is, however, always at least superficial dermal edema, manifested by increased spacing between adjacent bundles of collagen (fig. 10-2, top). This edema may be readily appreciated as a diffuse zone of superficial dermal pallor at scanning magnification. A frequently overlooked finding that invariably occurs coincidentally with even subtle dermal edema is dilation of lymphatic channels. At higher magnification, the subtle pattern of angiocentric inflammation consists of a sparse cuff of lymphocytes and sometimes eosinophils about affected venules; a helpful feature is the presence of intraluminal neutrophils adherent to luminal endothelial cells (fig. 10-2, bottom). Certain forms of urticaria are described as neutrophil rich. These lesions usually show diffuse dermal edema with associated interstitial permeation of intervenular collagen by neutrophils, a superficial and often deep, sparse angiocentric infiltrate of lymphocytes and occasional neutrophils, and intraluminal adherent neutrophils.

So-called urticarial vasculitis produces such subtle vascular injury that it is usually difficult to document in routine tissue sections. Occasionally, 1-μm sections permit more sensitive assessment of the subtle vascular injury inherent in urticarial vasculitis. Direct immunofluorescence may also show a pattern of antibody and complement deposition restricted to the walls of superficial postcapillary venules.

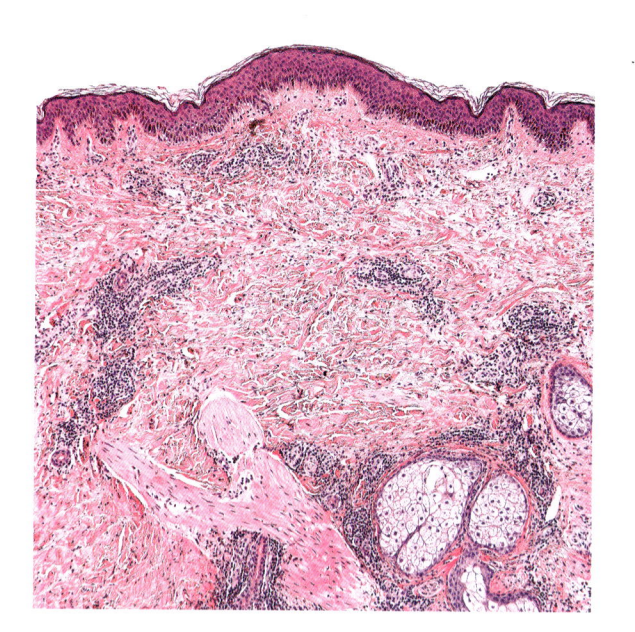

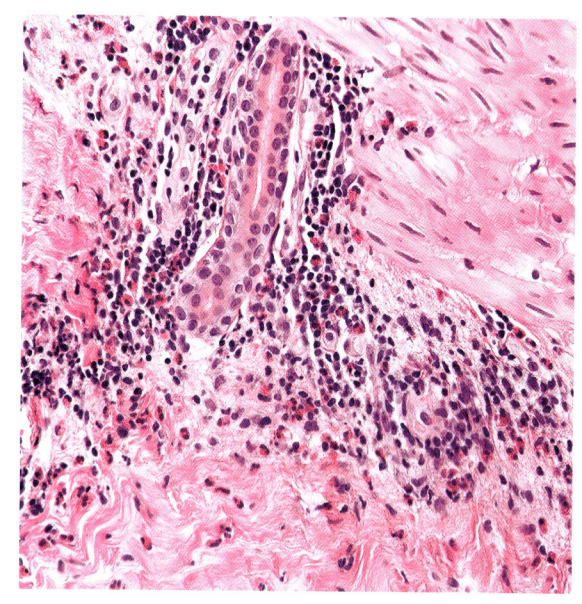

Figure 10-3

**PREDOMINANTLY DERMAL DRUG ERUPTION**

Left: The lesion is characterized by a superficial and deep perivascular inflammatory infiltrate beneath a normal epidermis and dermal edema imparting an urticarial clinical appearance. Histologically, however, the abundance of lymphocytes is more consistent with a delayed, not immediate, hypersensitivity response.

Right: At high magnification, vessels within the perieccrine adventitia are surrounded by a mixture of lymphocytes and numerous eosinophils.

**Clinicopathologic Variants.** Because the urticarial reaction is a clinical and pathologic pattern induced by a wide variety of stimuli, there are potentially as many variants as there are causes. A *neutrophil-rich variant* of urticaria has been described in which interstitial infiltration by neutrophils dominates the histologic picture. Hereditary forms of urticaria include *familial cold urticaria* and *Muckle-Wells syndrome*, consisting of urticaria combined with neural deafness and amyloidosis. *Hereditary angioedema* is a dominantly inherited condition where urticaria not only involves the skin but also oropharyngeal, laryngeal, and gastrointestinal mucosae. *Dermatographism* refers to the induction of cutaneous urticaria at sites of stroking with a pointed object. This common variant may correlate with an atopic diathesis. As mentioned earlier, urticarial lesions that persist for more than 24 hours may indicate *urticarial vasculitis*. Histologically, such lesions superficially resemble ordinary urticaria, although foci of perivascular erythrocyte extravasation, fibrin deposition, and endothelial swelling and degeneration are observed. Urticarial vasculitis does not present with the histologic findings of necrotizing, leukocytoclastic vasculitis. Patients with urticarial vasculitis may have underlying systemic disorders, such as collagen-vascular diseases and certain malignancies, and the diagnosis of urticarial vasculitis may precipitate further evaluation along these lines.

**Differential Diagnosis.** Many disorders have an urticaria-like presentation as part of their clinical picture. Papular bullous pemphigoid can appear urticarial. Polymorphous light eruption can have an urticarial appearance. Many drug reactions can appear urticarial but also persist (fig. 10-3). Insect bite reactions, also known as papular urticaria, reveal a tell-tale punctum and are persistent. They often exhibit a linear pattern. The figurate erythema can have an urticarial appearance. The pruritic papules and plaques of pregnancy can be differentiated by their distribution, the timing of the disorder in pregnancy, and the severe pruritus. Early herpes gestationis can appear urticarial but its relationship to pregnancy and its progression to bulla formation help differentiate it from urticaria. Early mastocytoma in infancy can appear urticarial.

Rarely, cutaneous leukemic infiltrates appear urticarial. Erythema multiforme may exhibit urticaria-like lesions as part of its spectrum, but the presence of target lesions, the lesional distribution, and mucosal involvement allow for correct diagnosis.

Some disorders at first glance appear angioedematous. For example, superficial thrombophlebitis may resemble angioedema of the lower extremity. Myxedema, scleredema adultorum, and especially the superior vena cava syndrome may initially resemble angioedema, but the persistence, the fixed nature of the lesions, and the absence of pruritus and other associated symptoms usually allow for successful discrimination.

**Treatment and Prognosis.** If a causative allergen is responsible for the urticaria, its elimination from the diet or the environment must be effected. Any suspect drug must be discontinued. Antihistamines, especially H1 blockers such as cetirizine or hydroxyzine, may be used (15–19). If they are ineffective, H2 blockers such as cimetidine can be added (20,21). Mast cell stabilizing agents are also employed. For severe cases of angioedema and sometimes severe urticaria, a short course of prednisone is effective (22). Danazol is useful for hereditary angioedema, as is whole fresh plasma (23–26).

## Pruritic Urticarial Papules and Plaques of Pregnancy

**Definition.** *Pruritic urticarial papules and plaques of pregnancy* (PUPPP) describes one of the more common eruptions of pregnancy, which occurs often in the third trimester, is extremely pruritic, and affects primigravida patients most commonly (27–30).

**Clinical Features.** PUPPP occurs in mostly prima gravida women, in the third trimester of pregnancy (often in the 36th week), but occasionally in the immediate postpartum period. It begins as 1- to 2-mm papules, usually in the striae distensae and umbilicus. The papules coalesce to form plaques in the periumbilical area, and then spread to the buttocks and thighs. Some papules exhibit vesiculation. Although the pruritus is severe, erosive excoriations are rarely evident, an unusual finding with pruritus and a helpful clue to the diagnosis. Extension to the arms and legs occurs, but breast involvement is rare. Facial involvement has not been noted.

Predisposing factors related to maternal weight gain, twin pregnancies, and paternal-derived influences expressed in placental cells have been suggested, although a definitive cause has not been elucidated.

**Pathologic Findings.** The histologic findings resemble those of urticaria, as described above. Specifically, there is superficial dermal edema associated with a superficial to mid-dermal, sparse perivascular lymphoid inflammatory infiltrate containing rare neutrophils and often confined to vessel lumens (fig. 10-4). Eosinophils are generally present within the inflammatory infiltrate. Epidermal alterations (mild spongiosis, acanthosis) are not consistently seen and may be a secondary phenomenon due to scratching (fig. 10-4C). There is no interface dermatitis.

**Differential Diagnosis.** Herpes gestationis is the principal eruption of pregnancy to be differentiated from PUPPP. The presence of bullous and vesicular lesions in herpes gestationis aids in diagnosis, as does the history of recurrence in subsequent pregnancy and an onset in the postpartum period. An additional helpful clue in early herpes gestationis is the presence of lymphocytes at the dermal-epidermal junction.

Other eruptions to be considered are urticarial drug eruptions, which are more diffuse (fig. 10-3); urticarial insect bite reactions (figs. 10-5–10-8), which show a characteristic distribution that is usually focal and in linear array; and scabies, which affects the areola and the interdigital spaces. Urticaria and contact dermatitis are also considered in the differential diagnosis. As noted earlier, pemphigoid occasionally occurs in a form that is exclusively urticarial and intensely pruritic (figs. 10-9, 10-10). In such cases, direct immunofluorescence may be required to establish the correct diagnosis.

Impetigo herpetiformis is a variant of pustular psoriasis that also occurs in the third trimester. It commonly affects the groin, the axillae, and the neck. The pustular nature of this eruption allows for differentiation.

**Treatment and Prognosis.** Application of topical steroids, several times daily, leads to resolution. Occasionally, a brief course of oral steroids, rapidly tapered, is necessary for control. Antihistamines are not helpful in most cases. PUPPP generally is self-limiting, often resolving at delivery, and therefore treatment is often not

*Nonvasculitic Angiocentric Dermatitis*

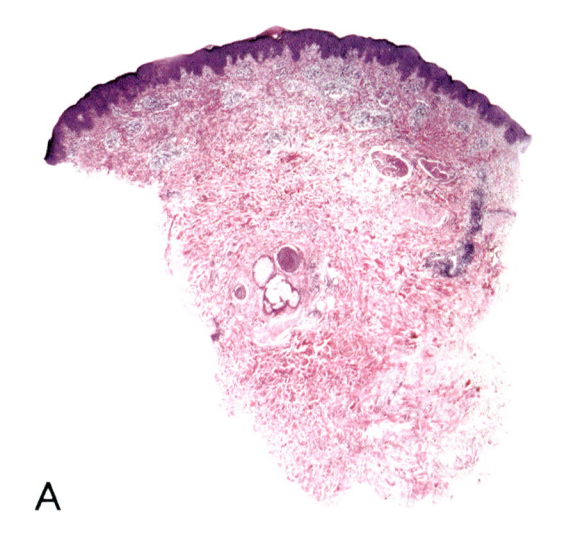

Figure 10-4

PRURITIC URTICARIAL PAPULES
AND PLAQUES OF PREGNANCY

A: At scanning magnification, only mild edema is present within the superficial and mid-dermis, as evidenced by subtle pallor.

B: At higher magnification, a sparse angiocentric inflammatory infiltrate is apparent.

C: The sparse perivascular mixed inflammatory infiltrate typically contains neutrophils and eosinophils. Note the mild epidermal acanthosis and spongiosis, mild secondary alterations due to scratching that are not observed in early lesions.

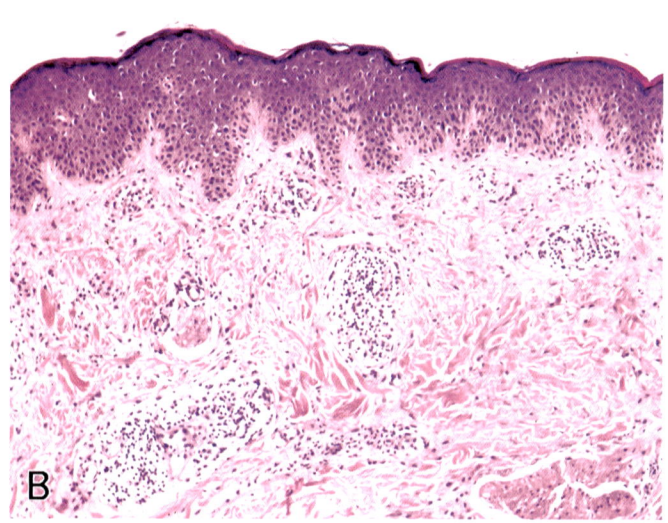

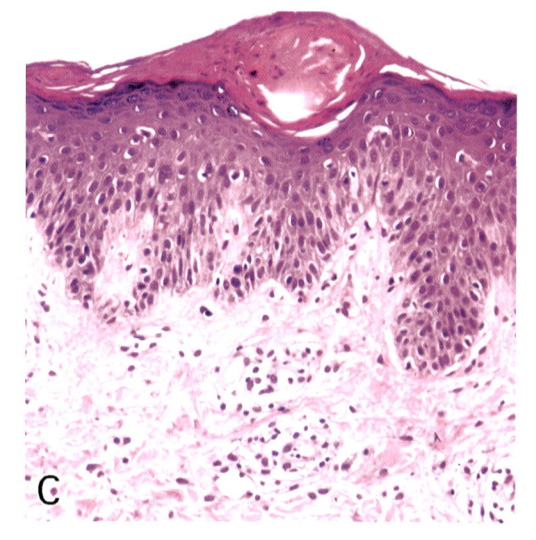

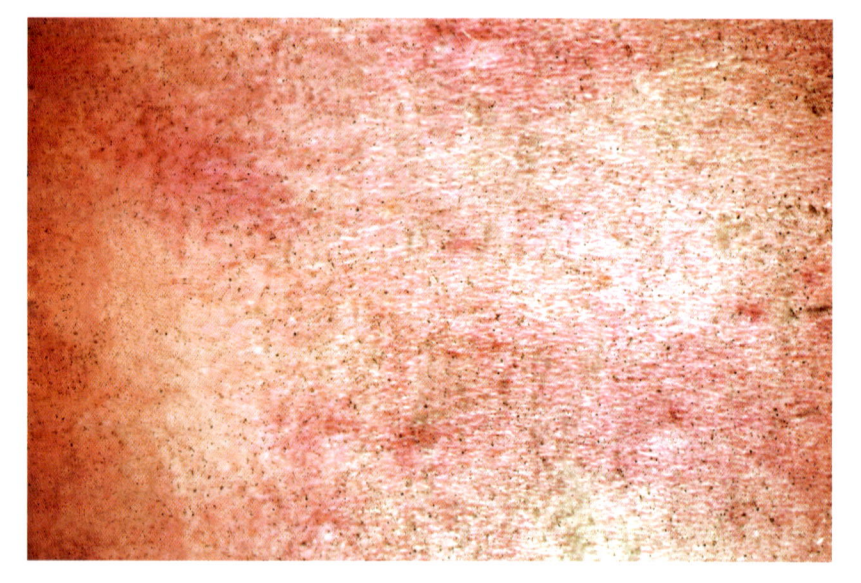

Figure 10-5

URTICARIAL INSECT
BITE REACTION

There are multiple, flesh-colored to slightly erythematous papules and small plaques. These developed after exposure to a stinging insect.

*Inflammatory Disorders of the Skin*

**Figure 10-6**

**PREDOMINANTLY DERMAL INSECT BITE REACTION**

There are clustered and linear aggregates of indurated erythematous papules, including one with a central ecchymotic zone, possibly representing a punctum.

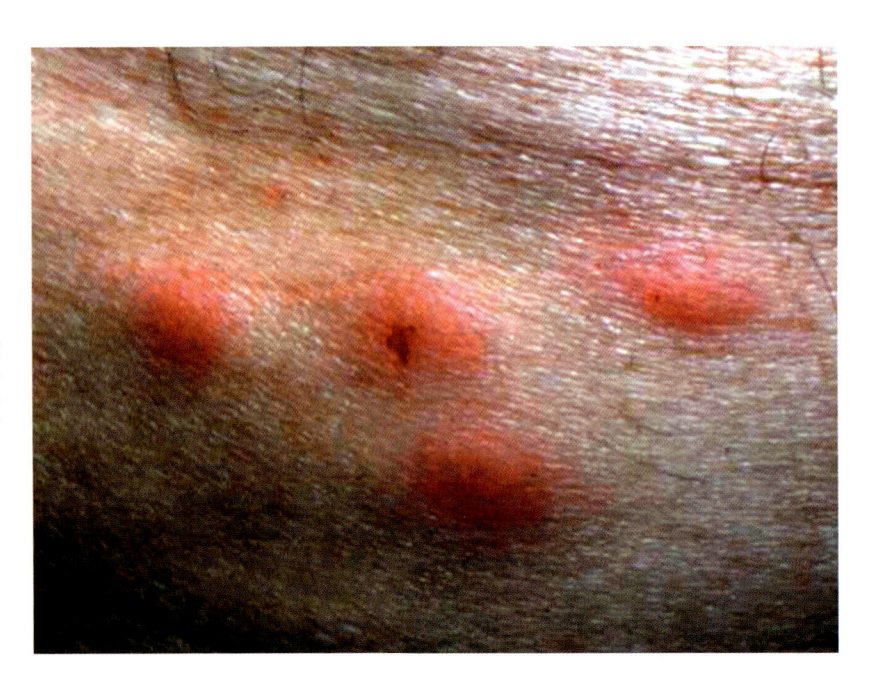

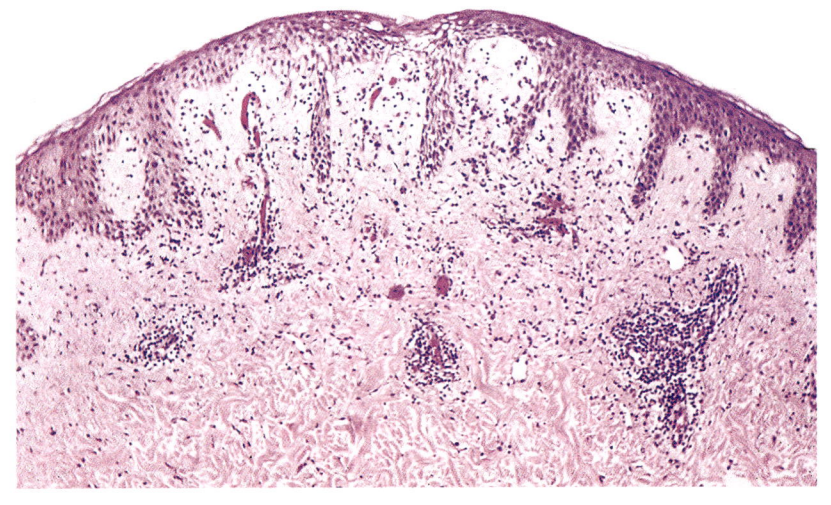

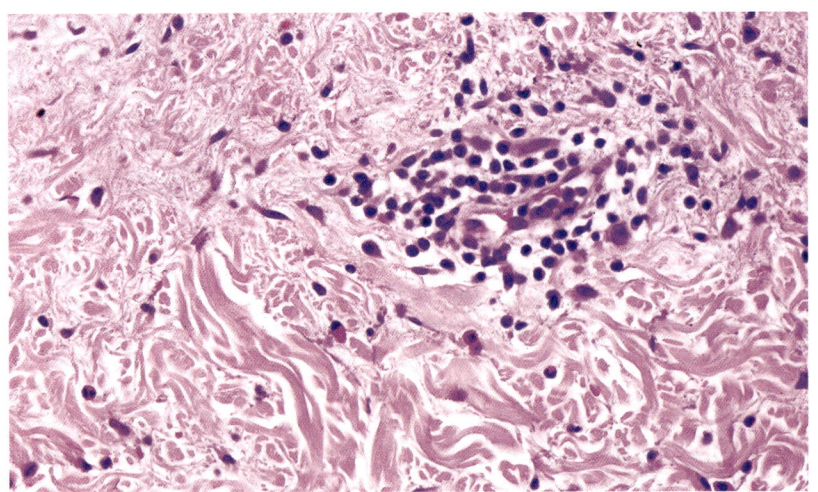

**Figure 10-7**

**URTICARIAL INSECT BITE REACTION**

Top: The epidermis is unremarkable; the underlying dermis shows edema and an angiocentric inflammatory infiltrate.

Bottom: At higher power, the angiocentric inflammatory component shows interstitial eosinophils, rare neutrophils, and perivascular lymphocytes, indicating a delayed-type hypersensitivity reaction.

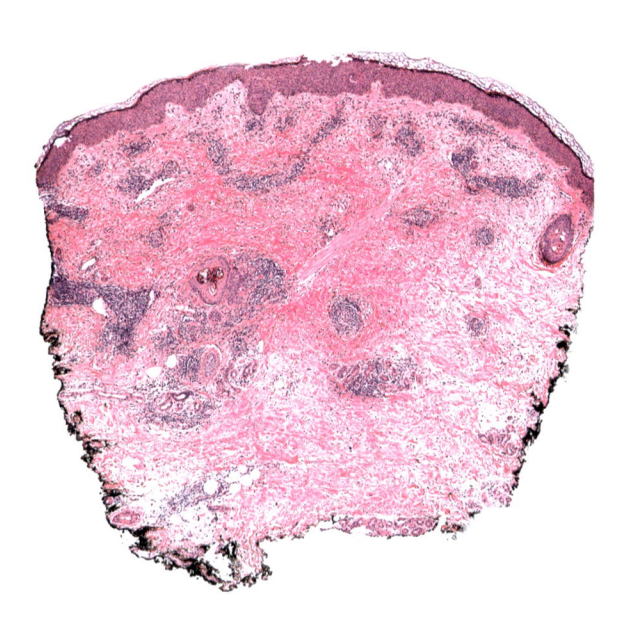

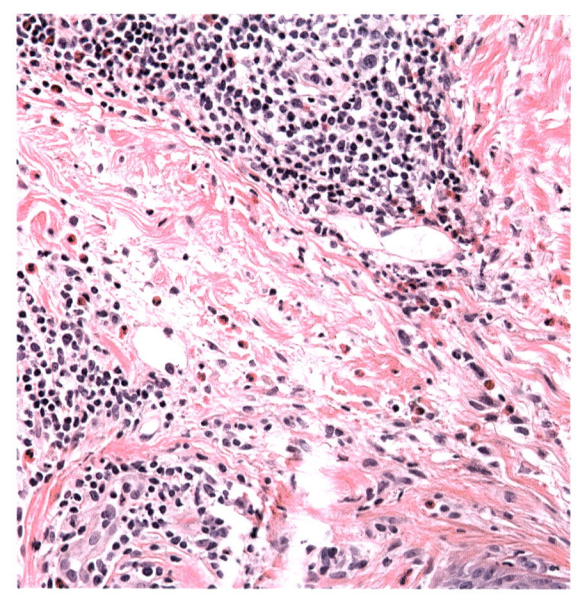

## Figure 10-8

**PREDOMINANTLY DERMAL INSECT BITE REACTION**

Left: At scanning magnification, beneath a normal epidermis there is a wedge-shaped superficial and deep perivascular and periadnexal inflammatory infiltrate with evidence of associated interstitial involvement.

Right: High magnification shows perivascular and interstitial inflammatory cells, the latter dominated by eosinophils.

required. Interestingly, the eruption tends not to recur with subsequent pregnancies. There is no associated fetal mortality or morbidity.

### Dermal Contact Dermatitis

**Definition.** *Dermal contact dermatitis* (DCN) is a type of delayed hypersensitivity reaction caused by a variety of allergens that results in prominent indurated plaques without prominent epidermal involvement (31).

**Clinical Features.** The contact allergens that cause these reactions include nickel, neomycin, sulfur, and some metal haptens including chromates. The lesions occur in the characteristic contact distribution of the offending agent, but they do not progress through the phases of vesiculation and "weeping" associated with the usual type of cutaneous response to contact allergens. Rather, edematous plaques appear and become progressively indurated. In part because of the higher solubility of the antigens, and, therefore, presumed penetration of antigen through the follicle rather than the superficial epidermis, remarkable dermal reactions are seen. Sometimes these reactions are so intense that they present as a nodule that is considered

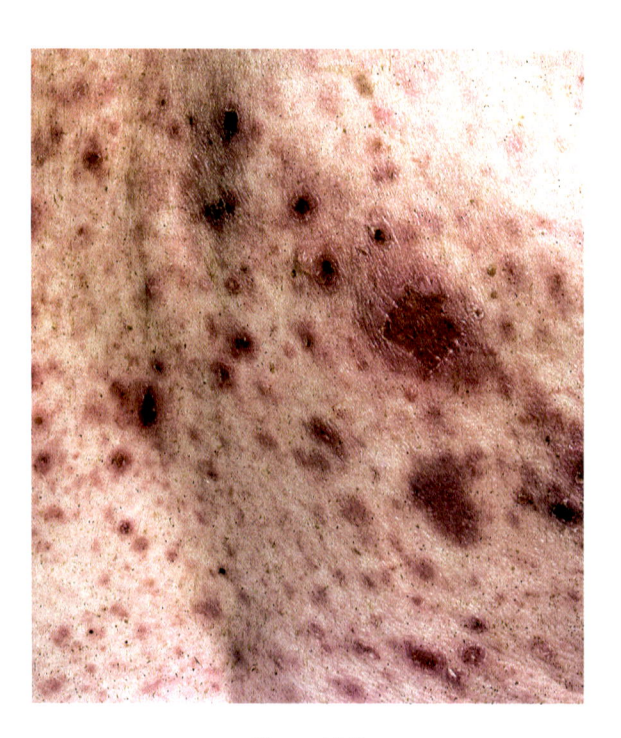

## Figure 10-9

**URTICARIAL PEMPHIGOID**

There are multiple, deeply erythematous, variably sized plaques as well as zones of erosion due to excoriation.

*Inflammatory Disorders of the Skin*

**Figure 10-10**

**URTICARIAL PEMPHIGOID**

Top: There is marked edema within the superficial dermis associated with a cell-poor perivascular and papillary dermal mixed inflammatory infiltrate containing numerous eosinophils.

Bottom: A clue to the diagnosis is the tendency of eosinophils to accumulate directly beneath the basal lamina. A microscopic zone of dermal-epidermal vacuolization is observed overlying a markedly edematous papillary dermis.

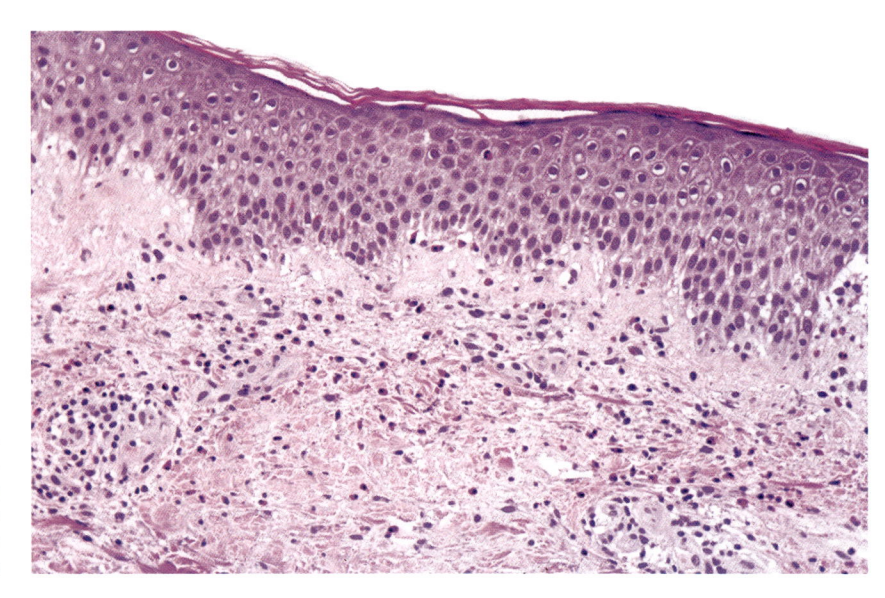

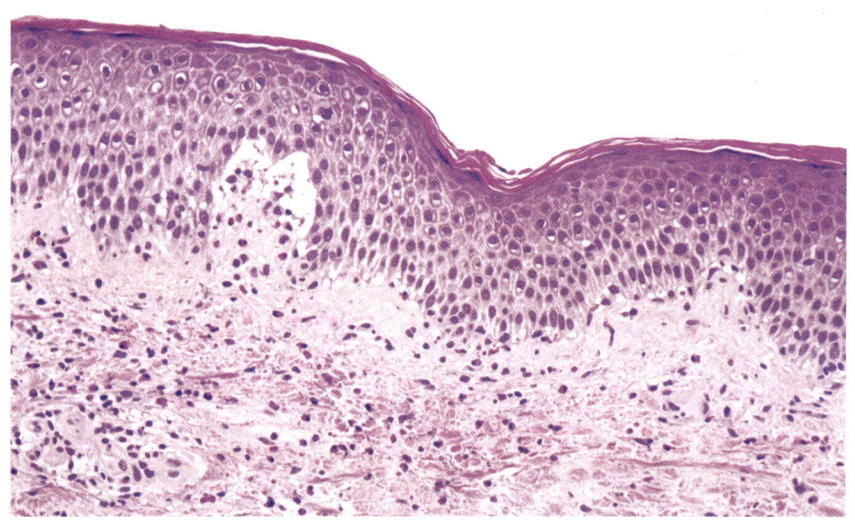

"lymphomatoid." The lesions respond to the usual treatment for contact dermatitis.

**Pathologic Findings.** Delayed hypersensitivity reactions, also discussed in the context of spongiotic dermatitis, all begin as angiocentric infiltrates. As lesions evolve, acute, subacute, and chronic epidermal alterations develop, ranging from spongiotic to hyperplastic. These alterations are generally associated with epidermotropic lymphocyte migration from the dermis into both the follicles and the epidermal layer. Depending on the nature and route of delivery (topical versus systemic) of the antigenic stimulus, certain delayed hypersensitivity reactions show little or no epidermal alteration during their clinical course. These reactions are usually follicle based and have a prominent follicular eczematous response.

Dermal delayed hypersensitivity reactions consist of a superficial and sometimes deep angiocentric infiltrate of lymphocytes and occasional eosinophils beneath a normal epidermal layer. Dermal edema may be observed, as well as intraluminal neutrophils adherent to adjacent endothelial cells, a finding also encountered in urticaria. Because of the nature of some of the antigens and their solubility, the follicle may show the most profound reaction, with prominent spongiosis and infiltration of the epithelium by lymphocytes and often eosinophils. When the reaction is elicited by injected antigen, such as in certain arthropod bites and

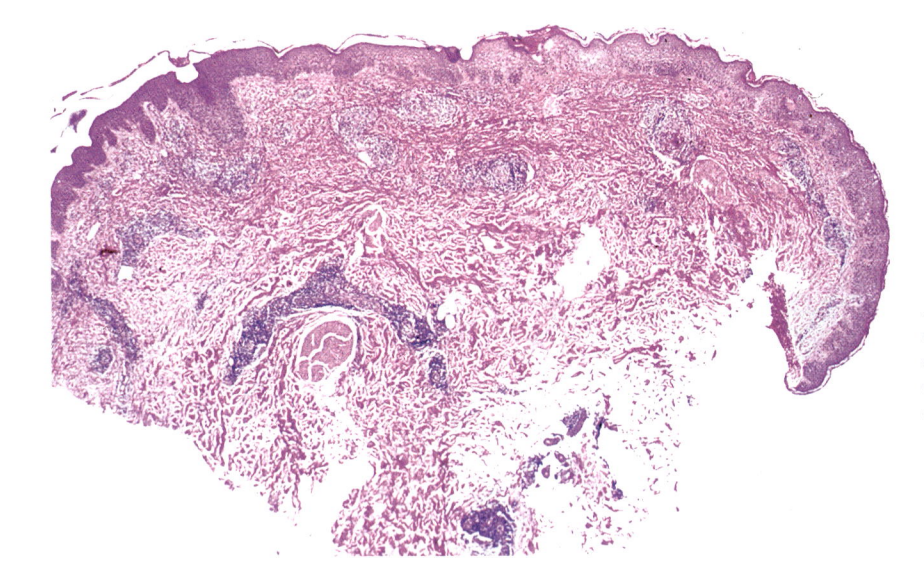

**Figure 10-11**

**ANGIOCENTRIC DERMAL DELAYED HYPERSENSITIVITY REACTION**

This lesion, the result of an arthropod sting, shows a characteristic superficial and deep angiocentric infiltrate composed of lymphocytes and eosinophils.

stings, an interstitial pattern of inflammatory cell migration involving intervenular connective tissue may be observed (fig. 10-11).

**Differential Diagnosis.** Dermal hypersensitivity reactions, especially of the nodular type, raise the differential diagnosis of cutaneous B- or T-cell lymphoma; lymphocytic infiltrates of other causes, such as Jessner lymphocytic infiltrate; or even cutaneous lupus erythematosus. The correct diagnosis depends upon the characteristic clinical features of contact dermatitis, a careful history, and a suspect contact allergen. Appropriate therapeutic response sometimes helps in the correct diagnosis. A biopsy is often necessary to differentiate hypersensitivity from lymphomatoid reactions.

**Treatment and Prognosis.** Treatment includes topical corticosteroid applications and cool soaks. Oral antihistamines are used for the pruritus. Occasionally, systemic steroids are necessary to suppress the reaction.

### Progressive Pigmentary Purpura

**Definition.** *Pigmentary purpura*, also known as *progressive pigmentary purpuric dermatosis*, *Schamberg disease*, the *lichenoid pigmentary purpura of Gougerot-Blum* (see chapter 7), and *lichen aureus*, is a group of disorders associated with patches of yellow-brown pigmentation, usually on the lower extremities, and with a specific type of lichenoid and perivascular lymphoid infiltrate with microscopic hemorrhage (32–38).

**Clinical Features.** The lesions begin as small petechiae that gradually assume the yellow-brown discoloration associated with hemosiderin deposition (fig. 10-12). The lesions are more common in men than women and occur at any age. They are distributed mainly on the lower extremities, but occur occasionally on the arms and even on the trunk. The early petechial eruption, which often has a follicular appearance, gradually resolves, leaving a brown-red to yellow cayenne pepper-like coloration of the affected areas. Although certain drugs can result in pigmentary purpura, most lesions are idiopathic. Sometimes these lesions are the first manifestation of mycosis fungoides.

There are several subgroups of this disorder. Schamberg disease, or progressive pigmentary purpura, is an extensive eruption with multiple areas of discoloration on the legs, arms, and even trunk. The lichenoid purpuras exhibit an eczematous hemorrhagic picture. Lichen aureus presents as a yellow-brown patch that is several centimeters in size and occurs on the thighs, buttocks, or trunk. There have been reports of pigmentary purpura associated with lymphoid atypia or eventuating in mycosis fungoides: in a study of 34 patients with pigmentary purpura, 7 had mycosis fungoides (39). Seventeen cases were related to immune dysregulatory drug ingestion such as calcium channel blockers, angiotensin-converting enzyme (ACE) inhibitors, antidepressants, and other drugs. The conclusion

**Figure 10-12**

**PROGRESSIVE PIGMENTARY PURPURA**

Multiple red-brown petechial lesions and small pigmented macules are observed on extremity skin.

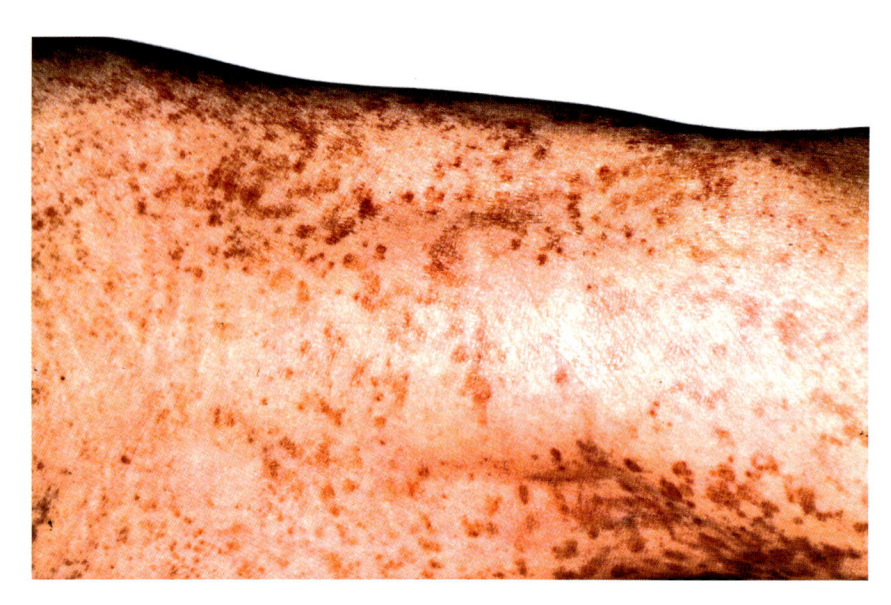

of the study was that a lymphoid infiltrate with atypia and features of pigmentary purpura does not necessarily correlate with progression to mycosis fungoides and that patients must be evaluated carefully and followed if there is any suspicion of possible mycosis fungoides (39).

**Pathologic Findings.** The angiocentric lymphocytic inflammation is sparse and characteristically centered about small capillary loops within dermal papillae (fig. 10-13). Overt vascular injury or fibrinoid necrosis is not encountered; it is presumed that the mechanism that permits chronic erythrocyte extravasation is too subtle to be appreciated by conventional microscopy. Erythrocytes within the perivascular space indicate recent hemorrhage and siderophages (i.e., macrophages containing hemosiderin) indicate chronic hemorrhage. These latter cells are best appreciated with an iron stain. Lichenoid variants of pigmentary purpura show coalescence of the angiocentric pattern to form a band of lymphocytes within the superficial papillary dermis. There may be mild associated spongiosis, but true interface change (i.e., basal cell layer vacuolization, colloid body formation) is not observed.

**Differential Diagnosis.** Clinically, the parafollicular involvement of venules in early Schamberg disease may suggest the possibility of scurvy. The early changes of petechiae suggest cutaneous necrotizing vasculitis or idiopathic thrombocytopenia purpura (ITP). More localized eczematous lesions suggest a dermatophyte or a drug eruption. Lichen aureus may resemble a fixed drug reaction or targetoid hemosiderotic hemangioma. Histologically, because findings are often subtle, care must be taken to note the pericapillary distribution of lymphocytes within dermal papillae, lest findings be regarded as entirely nonspecific.

**Treatment and Prognosis.** If a causative drug is found, withdrawal of this drug can lead to resolution. If an underlying T-cell lymphomatous process is the cause, the lymphomatoid disorder is treated. Topical corticosteroids may partially clear the inflammatory component. Many cases fail to respond to treatment.

### Reticular Erythematous Mucinosis

**Definition.** *Reticular erythematous mucinosis* is a disorder of unknown etiology that affects predominantly women, and may be related to ultraviolet light exposure (39a,40).

**Clinical Features.** This disorder, which presents as plaques and macules in the central chest and upper back, affects adult females most commonly. The erythema has a reticulated appearance; hence, the name reticular erythematous mucinosis. Occasionally, the upper arms and face are involved. More infiltrative plaque-like lesions are termed *plaque-like mucinosis*. The course is persistent, but with waxing and waning, and sometimes spontaneous resolution.

**Pathologic Findings.** There is a sparse, superficial perivascular lymphoid inflammatory infiltrate with associated mucin deposition

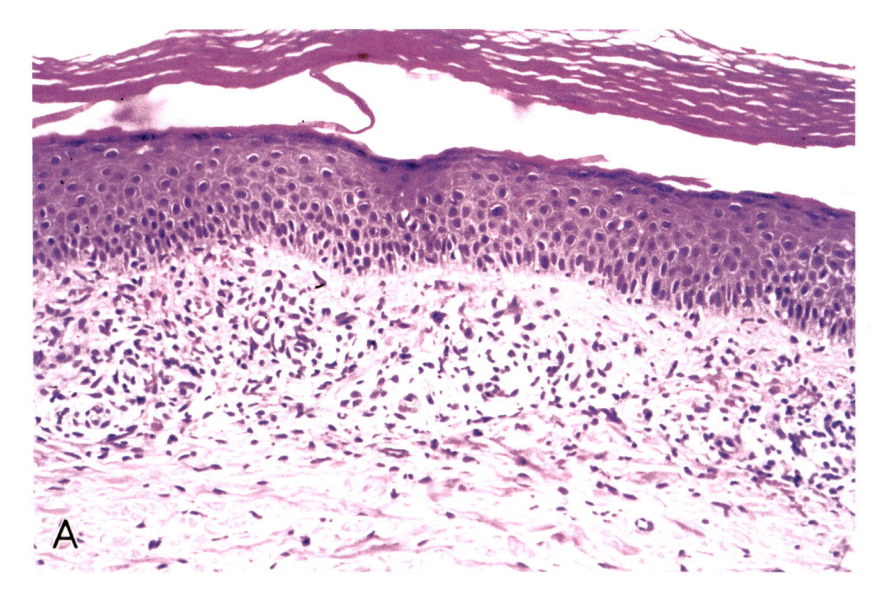

### Figure 10-13
### PROGRESSIVE PIGMENTARY PURPURA

A: The perivascular lymphocytic infiltrate extends into the most superficial layers of the papillary dermis as a consequence of involvement of small capillary loops.

B: The lymphocytic infiltrate extends upward to involve the capillary loops, where recent hemorrhage and remote hemosiderin deposition is observed.

C: Higher magnification of capillary loop involvement shows characteristically extravasated erythrocytes and associated hemosiderin deposition.

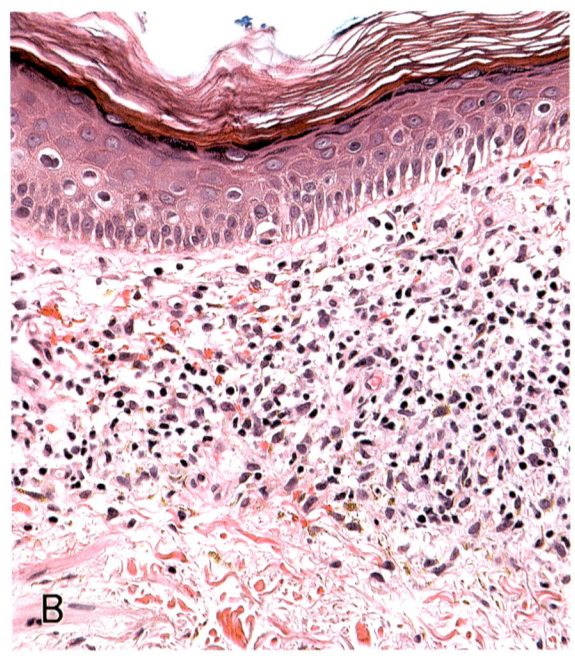

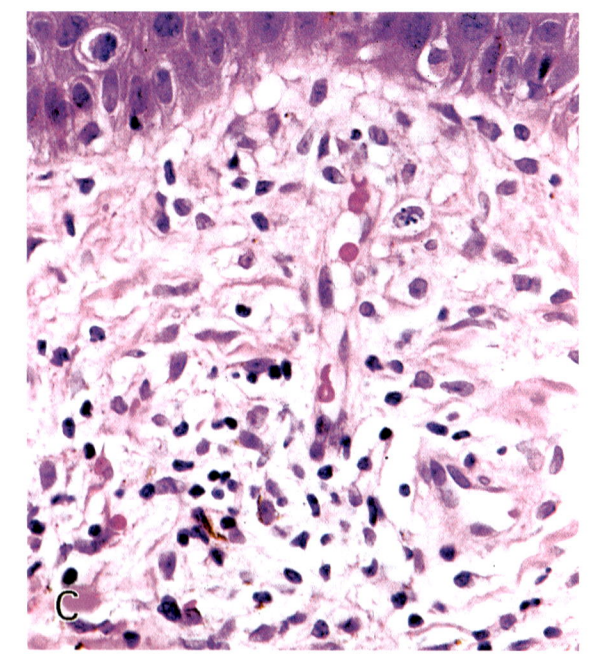

within the superficial reticular and papillary dermis (figs. 10-14, 10–15).

**Differential Diagnosis.** The differential diagnosis includes lupus tumidus, and localized myxedema or mucinosis. Reticular erythematous mucinosis shows neither epidermal atrophy nor absence of the appendages. The perivascular lymphocytic infiltrate is exclusively superficial, in distinction from lupus tumidus (figs. 10-16, 10-17). Clinical parameters differentiate this condition from forms of localized mucinosis.

**Treatment and Prognosis.** Therapy is protection from ultraviolet light, topical steroid application, and steroid injection. Only rarely is further therapy needed (41–44).

### Morbilliform Viral Exanthem

**Definition.** *Morbilliform viral exanthem* is caused by a number of etiologic agents producing systemic viremia, including parvovirus B19, Epstein-Barr virus, hepatitis B, human immunodeficiency virus (HIV), and enteroviruses. The eruption is believed to represent a cutaneous delayed

*Inflammatory Disorders of the Skin*

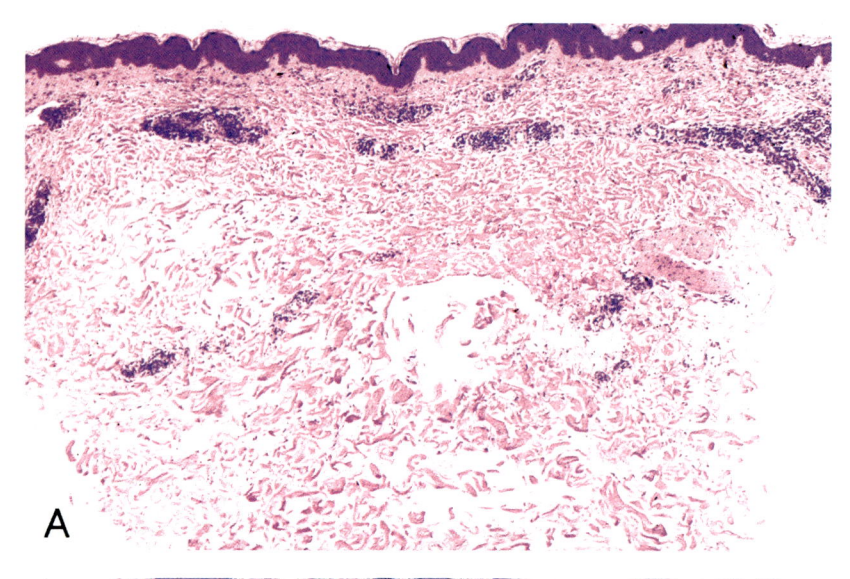

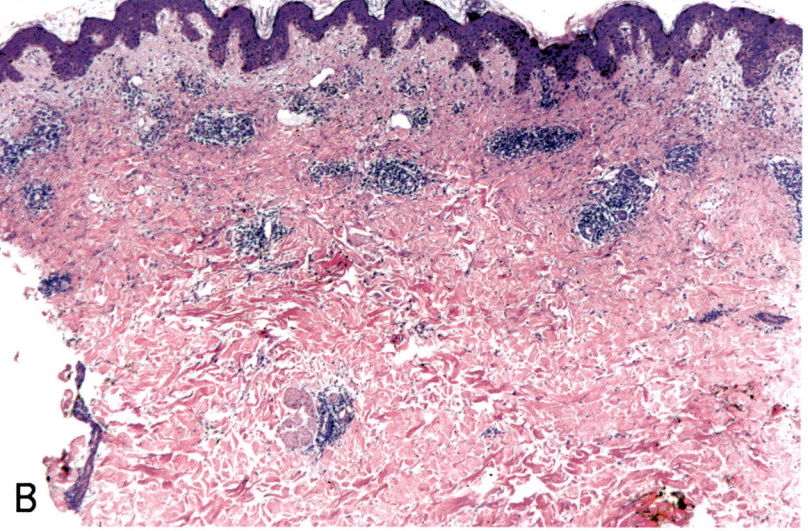

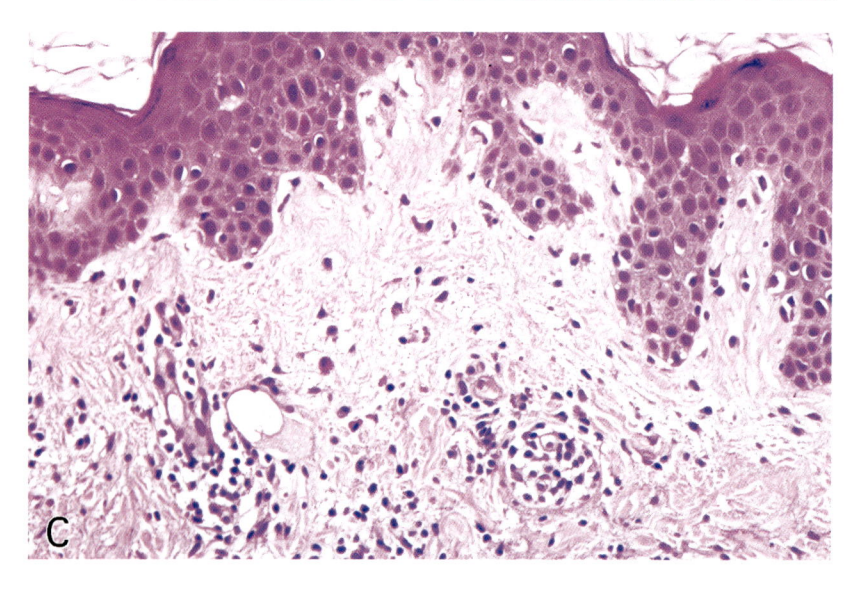

**Figure 10-14**

**RETICULAR ERYTHEMATOUS MUCINOSIS**

A: The sparse, superficial, tightly angiocentric lymphoid inflammatory infiltrate is reminiscent of erythema annulare centrifugum.

B: A deeper angiocentric infiltrate grades off in the reticular dermis, as may be seen in some photoeruptions.

C: At higher magnification, the epidermis appears normal, whereas the papillary dermis is pale as a result of diffuse mucin deposition.

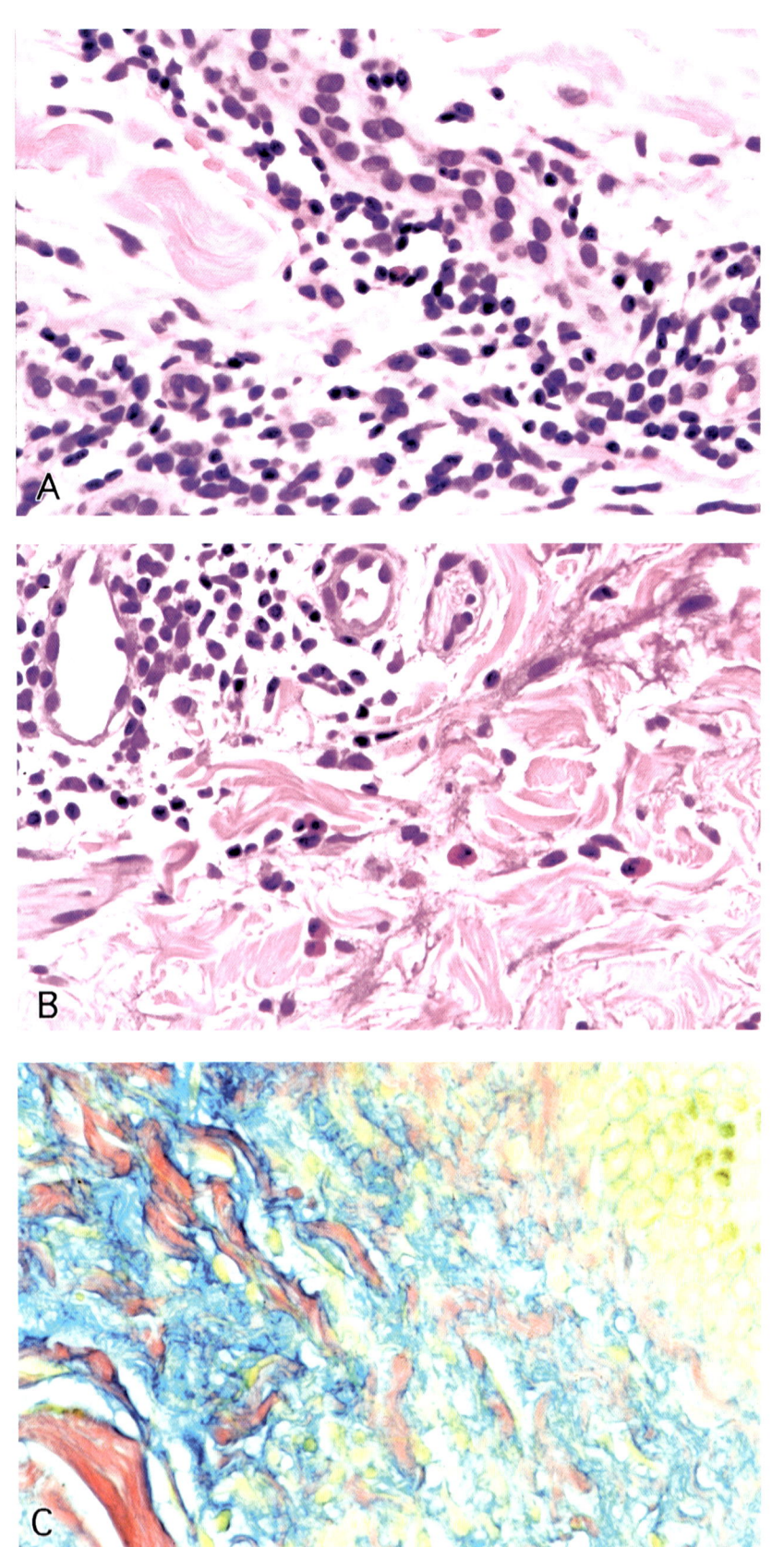

**Figure 10-15**

**RETICULAR ERYTHEMATOUS MUCINOSIS**

A: High magnification of the perivascular lymphoid component.

B: High magnification of the interstitial pathology shows subtle stringy and finely particulate mucin strands splaying apart reticular dermal collagen bundles.

C: The mucin stain is confirmatory (Alcian blue, ph 2.5).

*Inflammatory Disorders of the Skin*

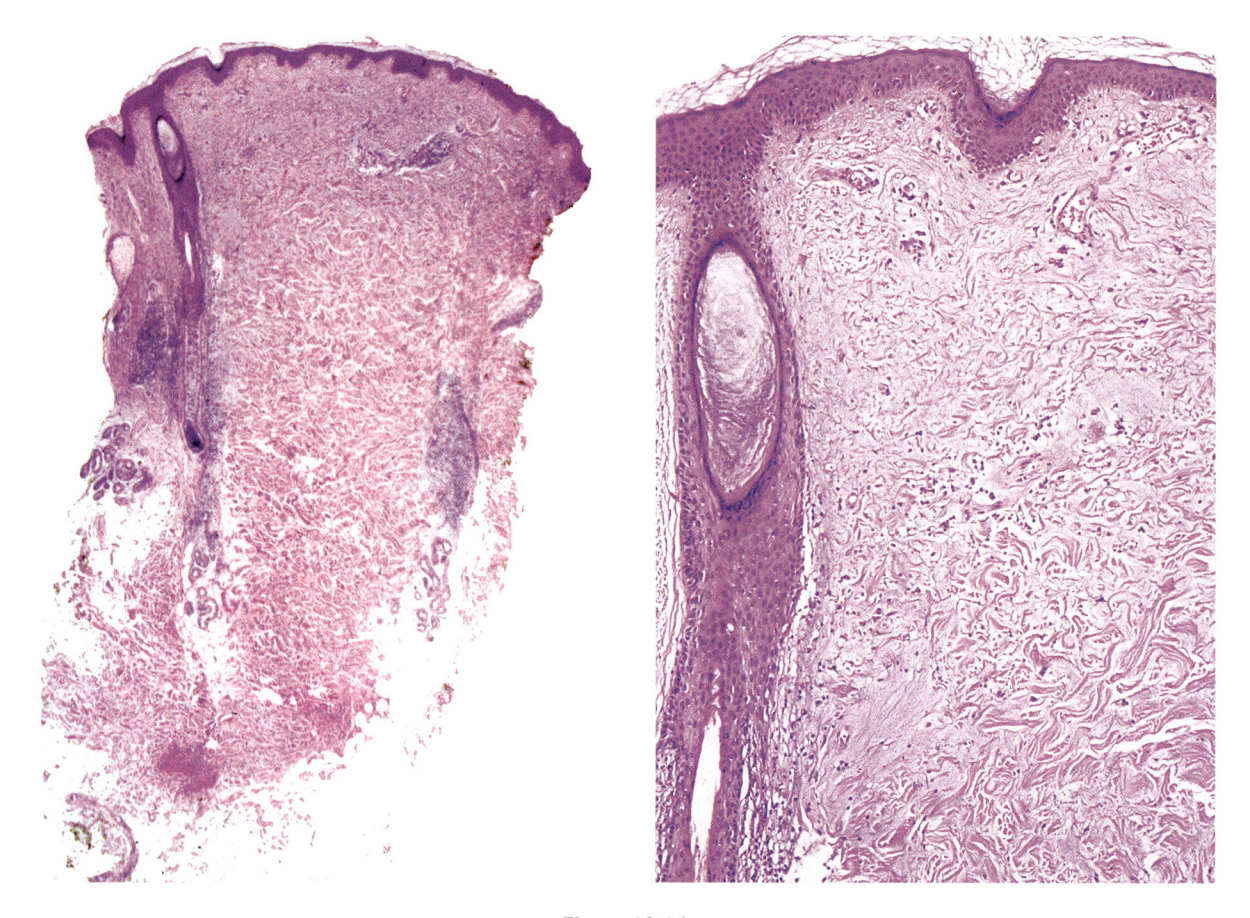

**Figure 10-16**

**PREDOMINANTLY DERMAL (TUMID) LUPUS ERYTHEMATOSUS**

Left: At scanning power, significant abnormalities, aside from a sparse, patchy angiocentric inflammatory infiltrate, are not prominent.

Right: There is a hint of cell-poor interface injury to the basal layer of the hair follicle to the left, providing a clue to the diagnosis. Histochemical staining reveals abundant mucin deposition within the reticular dermis.

hypersensitivity response to viral infection (45). Both children and adults are affected.

**Clinical Features.** There is a usually asymptomatic, erythematous macular to maculopapular eruption that is frequently generalized in distribution. Constitutional symptoms of fever, malaise, muscle aches, and respiratory or gastrointestinal complaints often accompany the exanthem. The clinical differential diagnosis includes drug eruption, and in the period following bone marrow transplantation, acute graft-versus-host disease.

**Pathologic Findings.** The histologic manifestations are characteristic yet nonspecific. There is a superficial perivascular lymphocytic infiltrate with associated endothelial prominence indicative of immune activation (fig. 10-18). There may be focal nuclear alterations with clumped chromatin and at times, ghost-like nuclei in endothelial cells. Often there is scant, focal erythrocyte extravasation about the involved superficial postcapillary venules. Papillary edema is variable, as are epidermal changes. When present, these changes are associated with a focal infiltrate of lymphocytes extending upward from affected venules. The changes include focal basal layer vacuolization, focal apoptosis (dyskeratosis), and slight spongiosis. These subtle changes are often the best clue to the viral exanthema. The absence of eosinophils also helps differentiate morbilliform viral exanthem from drug reaction. In many cases, however, the epidermis appears to be normal.

*Nonvasculitic Angiocentric Dermatitis*

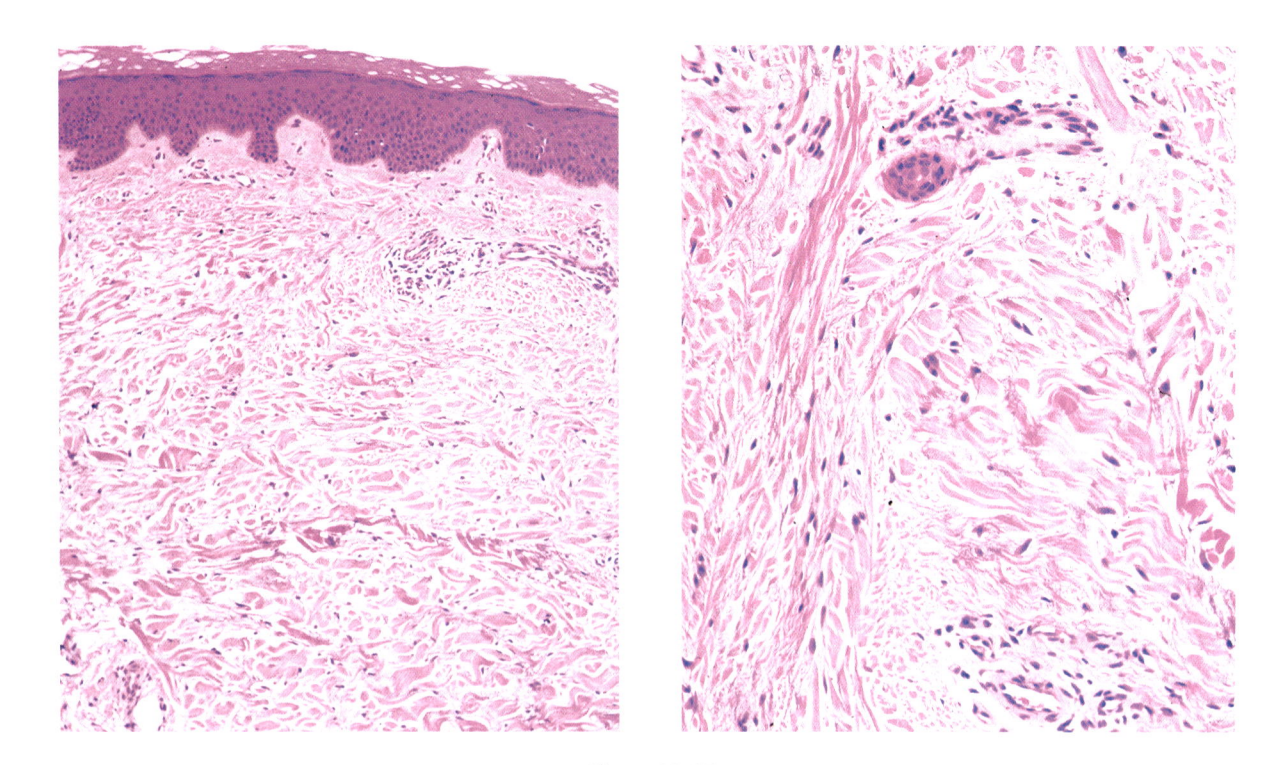

Figure 10-17

**DERMAL (TUMID) LUPUS ERYTHEMATOSUS**

Left: The epidermis appears normal, and the dermis shows the impression of diffuse edema manifested by subtle widening of the spaces between adjacent collagen bundles.

Right: Pale blue-gray mucin is appreciated at high magnification and upon histochemical staining.

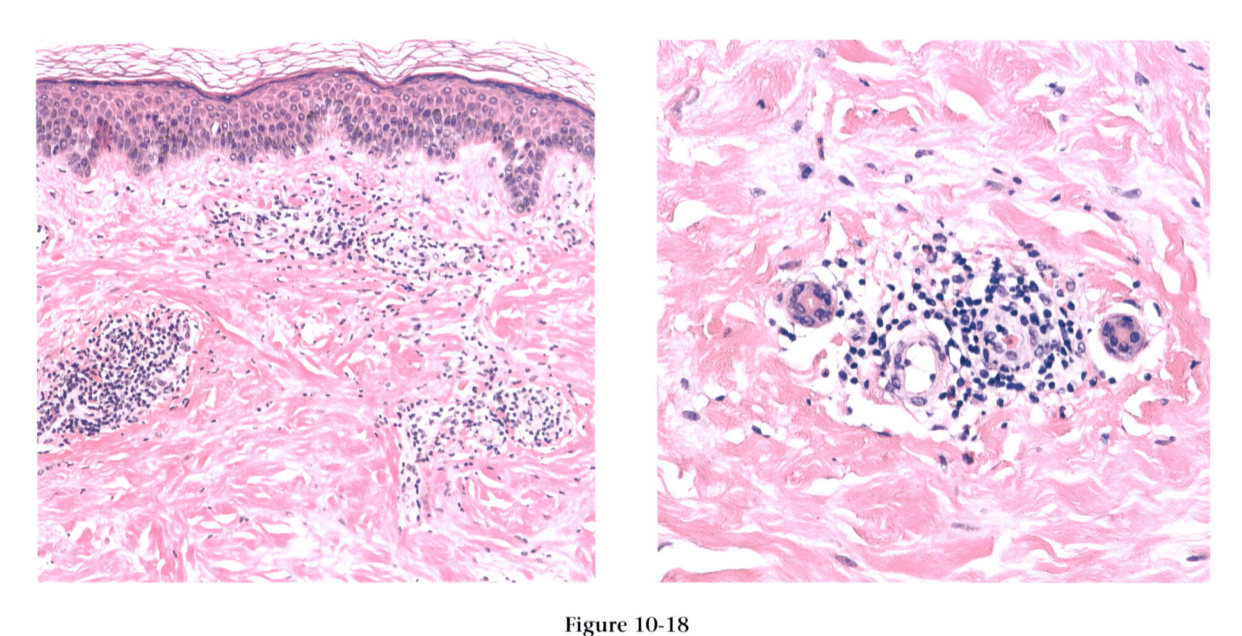

Figure 10-18

**MORBILLIFORM VIRAL EXANTHEM (HUMAN IMMUNODIFICIENCY VIRUS)**

Left: The lesions consist predominantly of a superficial perivascular lymphocytic infiltrate without epidermal changes, and thus resemble a predominantly dermal delayed hypersensitivity reaction.

Right: At high magnification, there is a perivascular lymphocytic infiltrate with rare extravasated erythrocytes.

*Inflammatory Disorders of the Skin*

**Figure 10-19**

**POLYMORPHOUS LIGHT ERUPTION**

There is an admixture of urticarial and erythematous papules, some with incipient vesiculation, as well as several small plaques.

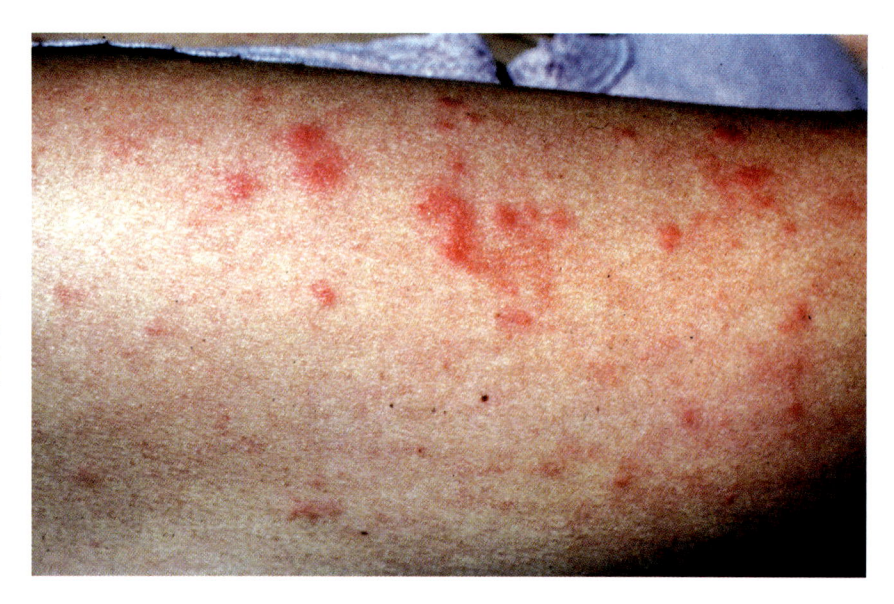

**Differential Diagnosis.** The lesions must be differentiated from superficial drug eruptions, mild predominantly dermal contact allergy, and in the appropriate clinical setting, early evolutionary stages of interface dermatitis (e.g., acute graft-versus-host disease). The absence of eosinophils in most viral exanthems excludes drug eruptions or contact allergy, and the requisite evidence of epidermal apoptosis required for firm histologic suspicion of acute graft-versus-host disease is generally lacking. Efforts to detect viral particles or antigens in lesional tissue have been disappointing, perhaps as a consequence of biopsy timing with respect to the most active stages of viremia/tissue infection.

**Treatment and Prognosis.** Most lesions are self-limiting, and resolve spontaneously with the resolution of the viremia. Treatment is therefore supportive.

## SUPERFICIAL AND DEEP VARIANTS

### Polymorphous Light Eruption

**Definition.** *Polymorphous light eruption* (PMLE) is the most common of the skin diseases induced by exposure to light. It presents initially with inflammatory papules and plaques in light-exposed areas (46–51). Over time, with recurrences, the lesions may exhibit different clinical appearances, and may extend to areas that are not exposed to light.

**Clinical Features.** PMLE appears at any age. Patients experience symptoms of pruritus or burning, associated with redness, after as little as 30 minutes exposure to incident light. Usually, however, symptoms occur in the first 2 hours. The eruption often lasts for a few days but may persist throughout the summer months. Women are more often affected than men. The sites of involvement are the exposed areas, especially the backs of the hands, forearms, face, and back of the neck, as well as the back of the legs of women. The effective light wavelength varies in different patients, and may be ultraviolet (UV)A, UVB, or both. Patients note decreasing sensitivity over the summer, a phenomenon known as "hardening."

Lesions vary from papules, the most common manifestation, to plaques that appear urticarial or eczematous, to a papulovesicular type eruption (fig. 10-19). Less common are lesions that resemble erythema multiforme or lesions that are hemorrhagic.

**Pathologic Findings.** The histology of PMLE, when correlated closely with the clinical appearance and setting in which lesions occur, is characteristic. The eruption, as the name implies, includes multiple erythematous papules and plaques that develop in sun-exposed skin. Because photosensitivity is a cause of lupus erythematosus, lupus is commonly cited in the clinical differential diagnosis. In addition, photoeczematous eruptions and phototoxic eruptions (i.e., exaggerated sunburn reaction) are also frequent diagnostic considerations.

Histologically, PMLE initially mimics lupus erythematosus, and we have seen the former

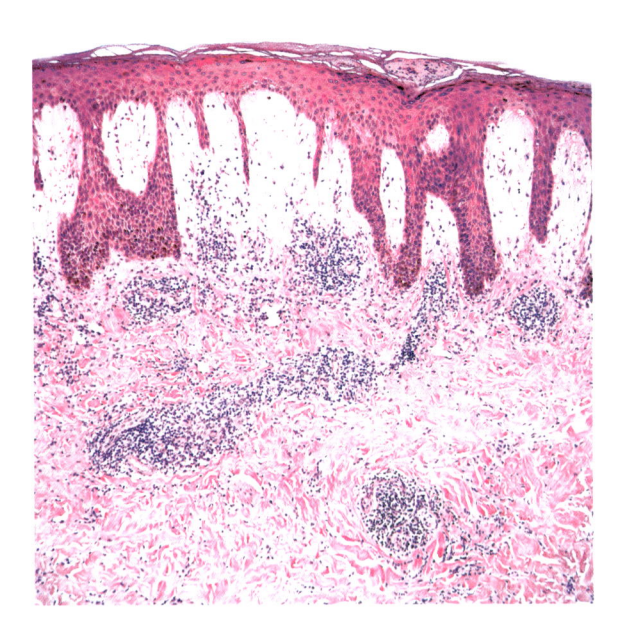

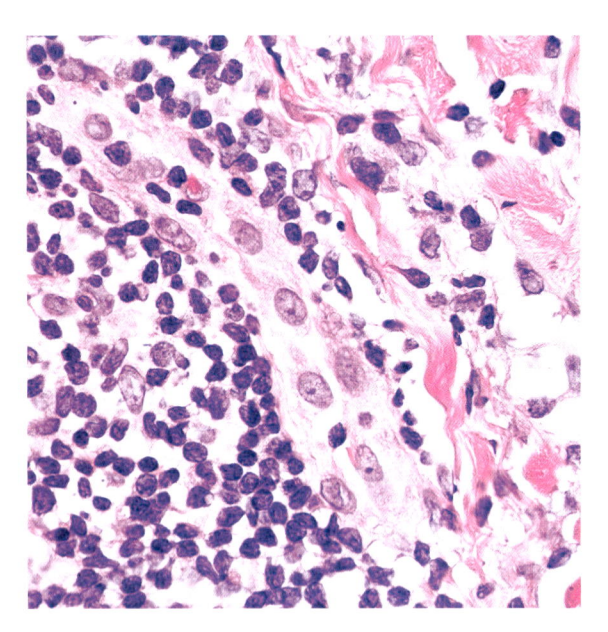

**Figure 10-20**

**POLYMORPHOUS LIGHT ERUPTION**

Left: Marked papillary dermal edema and an underlying superficial and deep perivascular lymphoid inflammatory infiltrate are characteristic. In lesions with less edema, the angiocentric lymphoid component may predominate, resulting in confusion with predominantly dermal forms of lupus erythematosus.

Right: At higher magnification, there is characteristically vacuolated, "bubbly" cytoplasm, a clue to a light-induced immune reaction.

erroneously diagnosed as the latter. At scanning magnification, there is a superficial and deep, dermal angiocentric infiltrate of lymphocytes that gradually fades in intensity from the superficial to deep dermis. In addition, there is often marked papillary dermal edema (fig. 10-20). In contrast to lupus erythematosus, there is absent or minimal basement membrane thickening, dermal mucinosis, or cytotoxic alteration of the basal cell layer of the epidermis or follicular epithelium. The affected venules of the endothelial basement membrane region show a characteristic vasculopathy. There is prominent perivascular edema, with rare extravasation of red blood cells and perivascular neutrophilic debris. Table 7-3 summarizes the salient diagnostic differences between polymorphous light eruption and photoexacerbated lupus erythematosus.

**Differential Diagnosis.** Atopic dermatitis can produce similar papular lesions, but their distribution is different and the pruritic symptomatology more severe. The plaque-like lesion of PMLE most resembles lupus erythematosus, and must be differentiated by biopsy and appropriate immunofluorescence or serologic studies. Clinically, PMLE does not show the follicular plugging or atrophy of lupus. Jessner lymphocytic infiltrate is clinically similar, but persists, and does not show evidence of the tapering of the infiltrate in the deep dermis, endothelial cell vacuolization, red blood cell extravasation, or neutrophilic debris. Also there is no clinical evidence of hardening.

**Treatment and Prognosis.** The most basic treatment is protection from sunlight exposure, especially during times of most solar radiation, from before noon to mid-afternoon. Broad-spectrum sunscreen should be used. For individual lesions, topical steroid application is often useful and results in at least partial resolution.

Phototherapy can be given as a mode of hardening. The skin is treated with progressive controlled exposure to UVB. If unsuccessful, psoralen with UVA (PUVA) can be administered with subsequent controlled progression to exposure to sunlight. Antimalarial drugs given during the summer months are helpful for patients who are resistant to other types of therapy. Ophthalmologic examination is necessary with follow up for patients on antimalarials.

### Erythema Annulare Centrifugum (Deep Variant)

**Definition.** *Erythema annulare centrifugum* is a characteristic dermatosis that occurs at any age and is usually idiopathic (52–57). Along with erythema chronicum migrans and erythema gyratum repens, it is often referred to as a form of deep figurate or gyrate erythema.

Although an association or cause cannot be determined for most occurrences of erythema annulare centrifugum, occasional cases have been related to infection (e.g., dermatophytosis elsewhere) or rarely to internal malignancy. The histologic findings suggest that the process is a predominantly dermal delayed hypersensitivity reaction.

**Clinical Features.** This common but poorly understood disorder typically begins as an erythematous papule that rapidly enlarges to form an erythematous plaque with prominent central clearing. The advancing edge of the lesion is slightly elevated and often retains an adherent zone of scale along the inner aspect of the border (i.e., trailing scale). Lesions are generally asymptomatic or slightly pruritic. The clinical differential diagnosis includes dermatophyte infection, eczematous dermatitis, and other forms of gyrate erythema.

**Pathologic Findings.** Scanning magnification reveals a well-defined, perivascular inflammatory infiltrate composed of lymphocytes and occasionally rare eosinophils tightly clustered about superficial and mid-dermal vessels (fig. 10-21). Often, the apposition of inflammatory cells to affected vessels is so discrete that vascular channels so outlined resemble Chinese figure writing, a finding of assistance in remembering the pattern of "figurate erythema." At higher magnification, the tight perivascular cuff of lymphocytes, often referred to as a "coat-sleeve infiltrate," is better appreciated. The overlying epidermis is often unaffected, although if the area showing the trailing scale is biopsied, focal parakeratosis and mild epidermal hyperplasia and spongiosis may be observed.

**Differential Diagnosis.** The histologic findings of erythema annulare centrifugum must be differentiated from other causes of type IV hypersensitivity reactions, including those directly the result of overlying dermatophytosis, contact dermatitis, and drugs. Periodic acid–Schiff (PAS) stains are often performed, particularly because tinea corporis is also a possibility. The characteristic coat-sleeve nature of the inflammatory infiltrate, although not entirely specific, is the most helpful histologic sign for determining the correct diagnosis. In some cases, there is a focal interstitial component, resulting in a picture that may be identical to the chronic manifestations of the rare condition, erythema gyratum repens (see below), highlighting the importance of accurate correlative clinical information. Erythema gyratum repens, in contrast to erythema annulare centrifugum, is characterized by annular plaques distributed widely and forming concentric rings with a "wood-grain" pattern. This disorder affects middle-aged to elderly individuals, and is highly associated with internal malignancy.

**Treatment and Prognosis.** Treatment is generally for symptoms; lesions eventually regress over time, although new ones may form. Primary therapy is focused on the identification and treatment of the underlying or associated condition. Dapsone is helpful in recalcitrant cases, and although systemic steroids are not used often, topical preparations are effective.

### Erythema Gyratum Repens

**Definition.** *Erythema gyratum repens* is commonly considered a paraneoplastic phenomenon that presents as figurative erythema (58–63).

**Clinical Features.** This figurate type of eruption characteristically has parallel bands of erythema that may occur in an annular, linear, or even gyrate array. The pattern is described as timber bark-like or resembling the skin of a zebra. Lesions begin on the extremities, but most commonly affect the trunk. They spare the hands, feet, and face. Men are twice as commonly involved as women, generally in the sixth to seventh decade of life. The underlying carcinoma is usually of the lung, although carcinomas of the uterus, cervix, breast, esophagus, and stomach have been noted.

**Pathologic Findings.** There is a superficial and deep angiocentric infiltrate of lymphocytes, usually without significant epidermal or interstitial dermal involvement. The lymphocytes are characteristically tightly applied to the vessel walls, producing the coat-sleeve pattern typical of other forms of gyrate erythema. Rarely, in some of the more chronic lesions, there is an interstitial infiltrate that is so marked as to resemble lymphocytoma cutis.

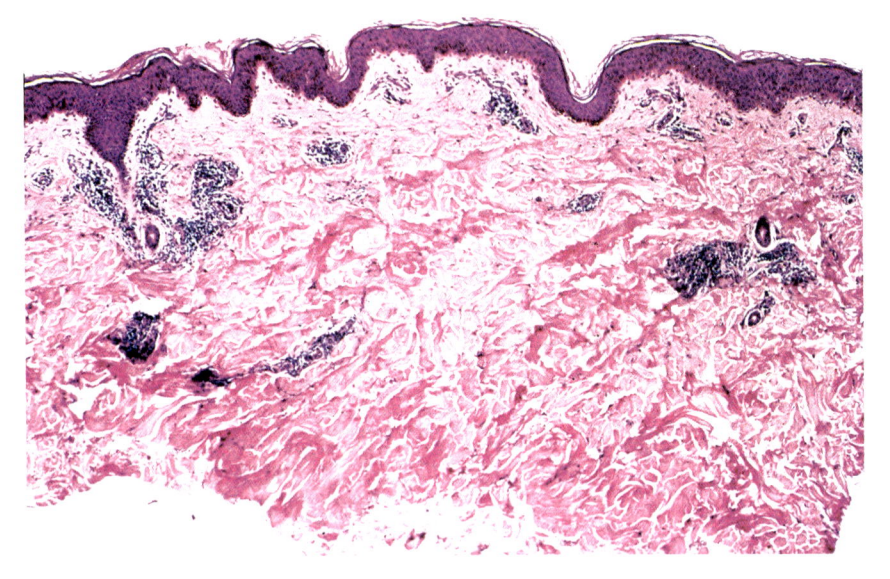

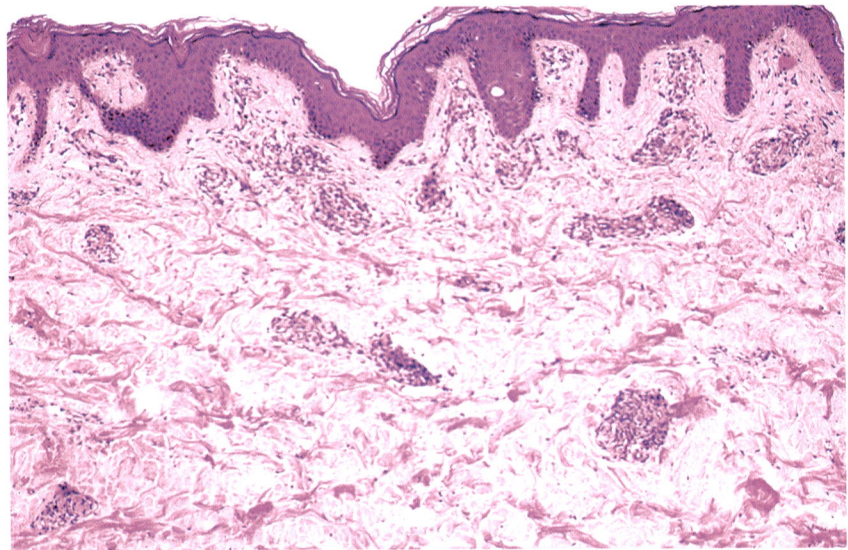

**Figure 10-21**

**ERYTHEMA ANNULARE CENTRIFUGUM**

Top: Unlike polymorphous light eruption, dermal edema is not prominent. Rather, a "coat-sleeve" lymphoid infiltrate accentuates the course of the involved dermal venules.

Bottom: In addition to the lymphocytes that are tightly aggregated about dermal venules, this lesion shows mild epidermal acanthosis and spongiosis.

**Differential Diagnosis.** The differential diagnosis includes other types of gyrate erythema, such as erythema chronicum migrans and the figurate erythemas.

**Treatment and Prognosis.** The lesions resolve with the extirpation of the carcinoma. With recurrence of the carcinoma, the lesions often recur.

### Erythema Chronicum Migrans

**Definition.** A variant of gyrate erythema, along with erythema annulare centrifugum and erythema gyratum repens, *erythema chronicum migrans* represents a local cutaneous immune reaction at the site of a tick bite (64–67).

Erythema chronicum migrans is a delayed hypersensitivity reaction to the local injection of the spirochete *Borrelia burgdorferi* by Ixodes tick inoculation. As such, this condition represents an important potential marker for the development of Lyme disease (68,69). Indeed, erythema chronicum migrans may coexist with the symptom complex of Lyme disease, which includes myalgias, malaise, and arthralgias, and which may eventuate in overt cardiac, neurological, and arthritic lesions.

**Clinical Features.** The clinical appearance of erythema chronicum migrans is a papule that enlarges to form an erythematous plaque with a smooth indurated border and a variable

## Inflammatory Disorders of the Skin

**Figure 10-22**

**ERYTHEMA CHRONICUM MIGRANS**

A papule has enlarged to form a large plaque with indurated erythematous borders and a prominent zone of central clearing.

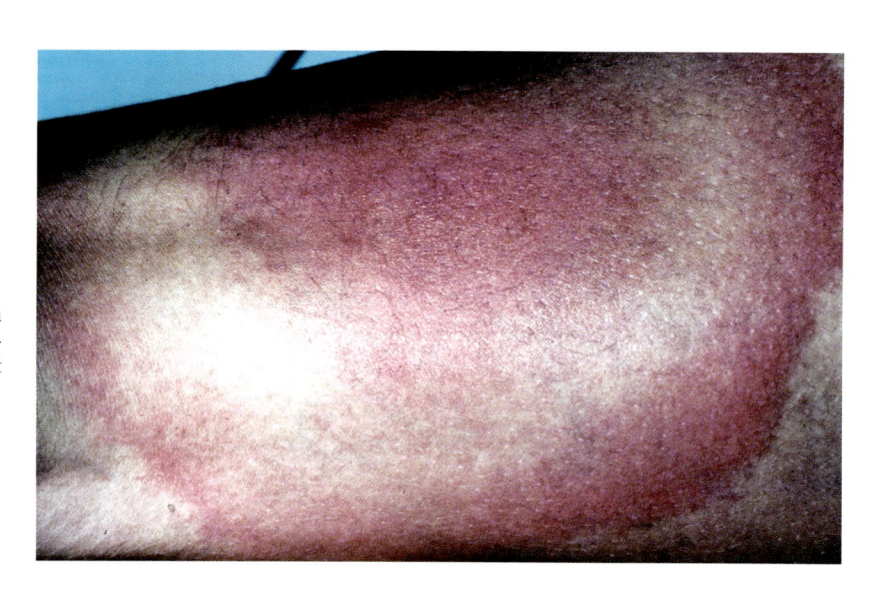

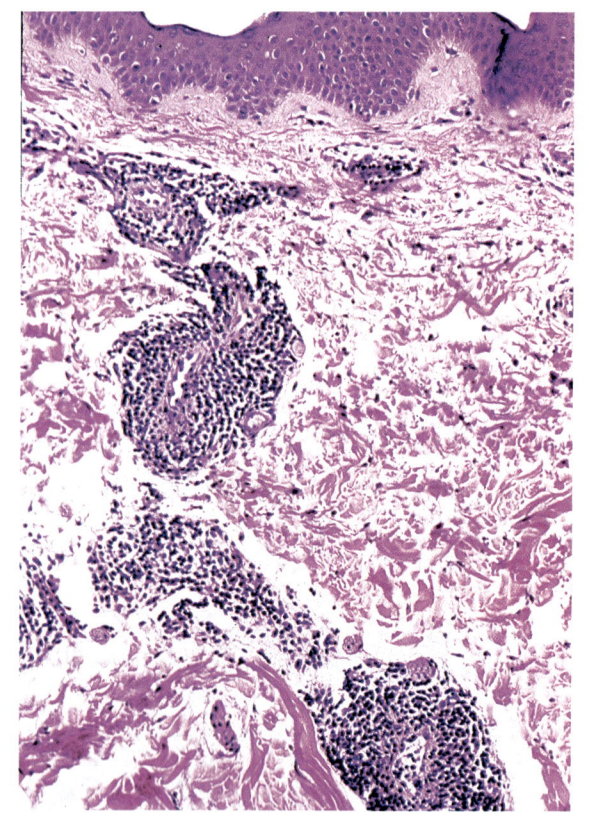

**Figure 10-23**

**ERYTHEMA CHRONICUM MIGRANS**

There is a characteristic coat-sleeve lymphoid infiltrate that tightly cuffs venules within the superficial and deep dermis. Depending on where in the plaque the biopsy is obtained, eosinophils and epidermal alternations may also be encountered. A Lyme titer is often appropriate even when the histopathology is less characteristic of a more classic purely angiocentric presentation of gyrate erythema.

degree of central clearing (fig. 10-22). A trailing scale at the border, as seen in erythema annulare centrifugum, is generally not present. A persistent zone of central erythema or hemorrhage, indicative of the bite punctum, is apparent in some lesions. The lesion develops from days to several months after inoculation.

**Pathologic Findings.** Erythema chronicum migrans, unlike more superficial variants of erythema annulare centrifugum, demonstrates a superficial and deep, intensely angiocentric inflammatory infiltrate composed predominantly of lymphocytes with occasional admixed eosinophils and plasma cells (70). The depth of angiocentric extension into the reticular dermis is an important diagnostic feature of this disorder (figs. 10-23, 10-24). The overlying epidermis is generally unaffected, although biopsy specimens from the central punctum may show epidermal hyperplasia and granulomatous inflammation in sites of retained mouth parts of the offending tick. A helpful sign at or near the bite site is the presence of vasculopathy, especially deeper in the dermis, in which plasma cells, plasmacytoid lymphocytes, and lymphocytes infiltrate the vessel wall and collect within the subendothelial region, with formation of intravascular thrombi. Apposition of the lymphocytes and plasma cells to nerves is a common finding that helps in the diagnosis.

Spirochetes are sometimes, but not invariably, demonstrable in biopsied tissue using silver stains (e.g., Warthin-Starry) or by dark-field microscopy. Polarization microscopy sometimes

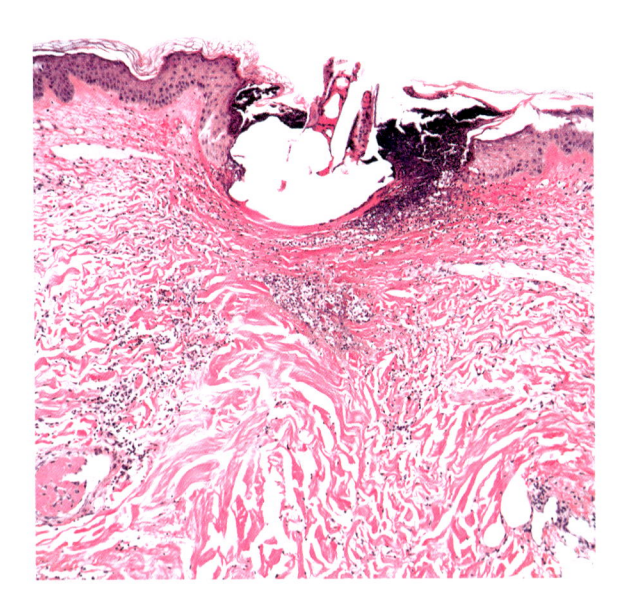

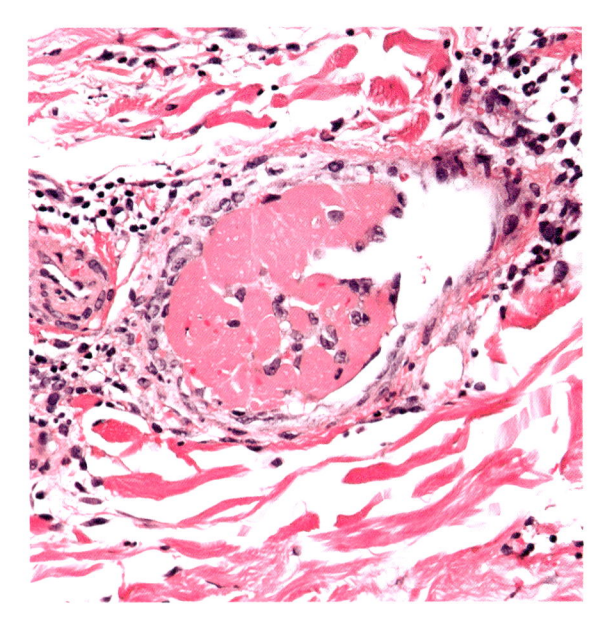

**Figure 10-24**

**TICK BITE REACTION SITE WITHIN ERYTHEMA CHRONICUM MIGRANS LESION**

Left: This predominantly dermal delayed hypersensitivity reaction is causally associated with the partial remnants of a tick retained within a centrally located punctum.
Right: This dermal vessel contains an organizing thrombus, a frequent finding associated with tick bite sites.

identifies birefringent mouthparts at the punctum site. Serologic titers for *Borrelia* are indicated in all suspected cases.

**Differential Diagnosis.** Careful and correlative clinical history and histologic study, as well as ancillary special diagnostic tests, may be required to differentiate erythema chronicum migrans from other forms of localized delayed type hypersensitivity. As with erythema annulare centrifugum, the tight, coat-sleeve pattern of the angiocentric infiltrate, the vasculopathy, and the neural changes are helpful histologic signs.

**Treatment and Prognosis.** Treatment and prognosis are those of the underlying condition (Lyme disease). Adequate antibiotic therapy must be employed. Lesions are generally self-limiting, and slowly regress even if therapy is not instituted.

### Jessner Lymphocytic Infiltrate

**Definition.** The *lymphocytic infiltrate of Jessner* (LIJ) occurs most commonly as clusters of multiple papules or plaques on the face or neck, or occasionally on the trunk.

**Clinical Features.** An asymptomatic group of papules or a plaque appears usually in one affected area of the face, neck, or, rarely, trunk (fig. 10-25). The lesions are pink to red. They usually resolve spontaneously and do not scar, although topical steroid application may hasten their resolution (71–73).

**Pathologic Findings.** There is a superficial and deep perivascular mononuclear cell infiltrate containing an admixture of small lymphocytes and large, pale histiocytes. In more advanced lesions, there is also a prominent interstitial infiltrate (fig. 10-26). Although perifollicular adventitia appear to be involved at scanning magnification, inspection at higher power reveals extension only about periadnexal vessels and the absence of true interface changes. Epidermotropism into the overlying epidermis is not present, and dermal mucin deposition is usually minimal, but may be significant in chronic lesions. While the infiltrate is usually associated with T cells, as determined by immunohistochemical staining, some variants show perivascular T and B cells admixed with monocytoid cells. In chronic lesions, germinal follicles have been described.

**Differential Diagnosis.** PMLE can be distinguished by its recurrent nature and relationship

*Inflammatory Disorders of the Skin*

**Figure 10-25**

**LYMPHOCYTIC INFILTRATE OF JESSNER**

The characteristic lesion is a pink-red plaque involving facial skin without evidence of epidermal changes.

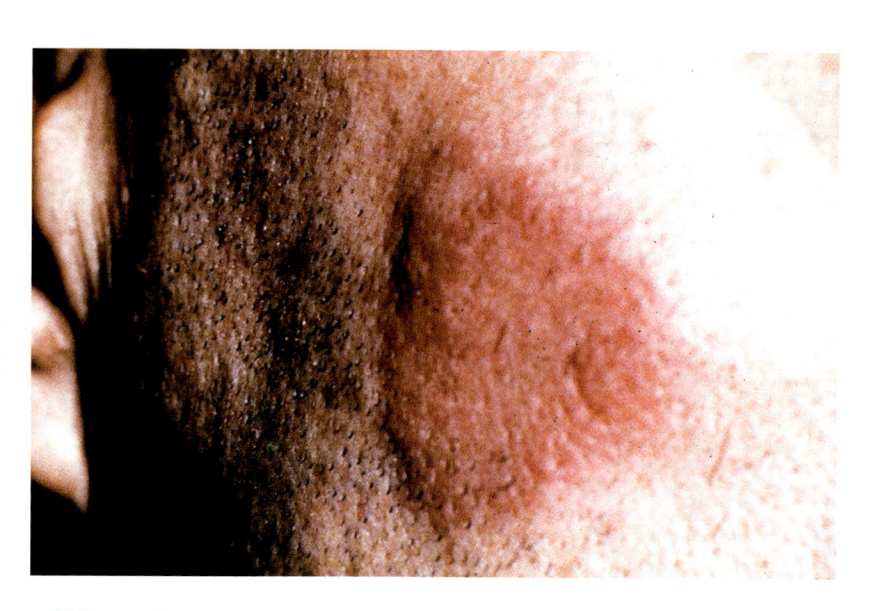

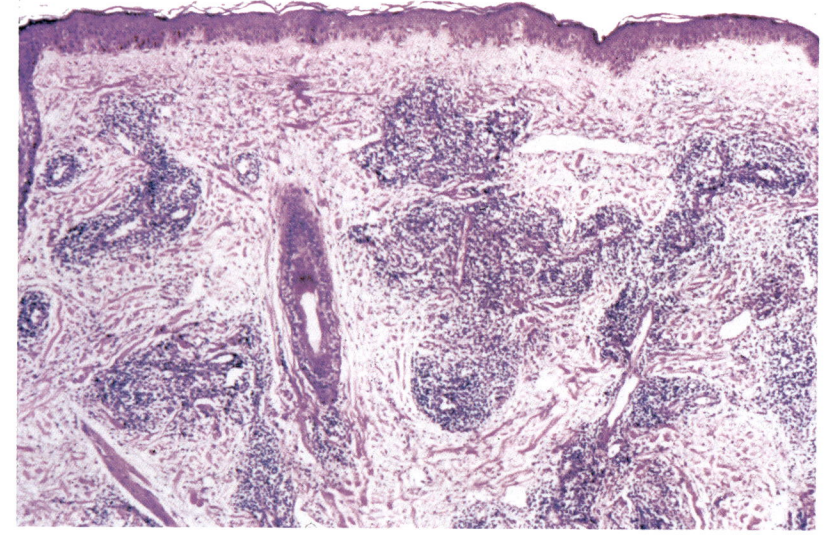

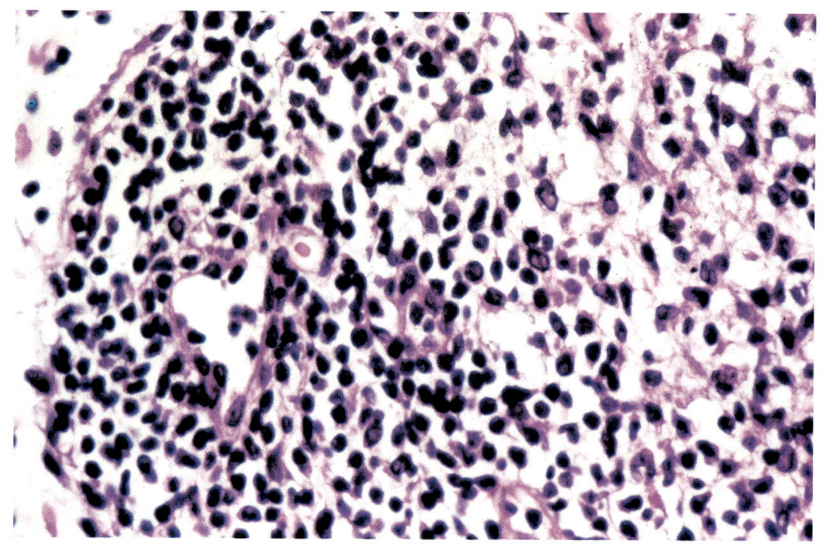

**Figure 10-26**

**LYMPHOCYTIC INFILTRATE OF JESSNER**

Top: There is a superficial and deep perivascular mononuclear cell infiltrate and no evidence of true interface changes in the epidermis of adnexal epithelium.

Bottom: At higher magnification, the inflammatory component is characteristically composed of variably sized lymphocytes with larger, pale admixed histiocytes.

to light exposure, with hardening or desensitization to light with progressive exposure. LIJ does not show the prominent papillary dermal edema, vasculopathy, or debris and extravasation of red blood cells often seen in PMLE.

Cutaneous discoid lupus erythematosus lesions commonly exhibit epidermal atrophy and follicular plugging, unlike LIJ. Histologically, LIJ lacks interface change of the epidermis or follicular epithelium, basement membrane zone thickening, and epidermal thinning.

**Treatment and Prognosis.** Topical corticosteroid therapy often results in at least partial clearing of the lesion (74,75). Corticosteroid lesional injection is helpful in persistent lesions. Some healing with antimalarial drugs has been noted (76).

## Still Disease

**Definition.** *Still disease* is a rash that appears in association with juvenile rheumatoid arthritis early in the course of the disease, but may occur intermittently throughout the course of the disease or precede the other manifestations of the disease for years (77–85).

**Clinical Features.** The characteristic lesions are papules, a few millimeters in diameter and rarely up to several centimeters. When large, there may be central clearing or paleness. The lesions are nonpruritic and are bright pink or salmon-pink. They are often evanescent, in some cases lasting only a few hours. They are characteristically present on the trunk and limbs, but also on the face. Usually they appear in the afternoon and disappear in the evening. Rarely, nodules also occur. Although the rash may occur without other arthritic symptoms and even precede the other symptoms, it most commonly occurs in the first weeks of the disease in patients with lymphadenopathy, splenomegaly, and an elevated sedimentation rate. In some patients, the lesions recur intermittently for years.

**Pathologic Findings.** There is a lymphoid infiltrate tightly disposed about superficial and deep venules with admixed neutrophils (fig. 10-27) (86,87). Neutrophils are likewise distributed, with focal debris, between vessels in the reticular dermis. The presence of the lymphocytes allows for differentiation from erythema marginatum, in which only dermal neutrophils are present. The occasional subcutaneous nodules resemble rheumatoid nodules histologically.

**Differential Diagnosis.** Clinically, the differential diagnosis includes erythema marginatum; the latter never involves the face. Also, the lesions of erythema marginatum are semilunar or arcuate in shape and last for less than an hour.

**Treatment and Prognosis.** The lesions wax and wane with the disease; there is no specific treatment for them. Systemic disease is treated with immunosuppression with prednisone and with steroid-sparing agents such as methotrexate, cyclosporine, hydroxychloroquine, azathioprine, or inhibitors of tumor necrosis factor (TNF).

*Inflammatory Disorders of the Skin*

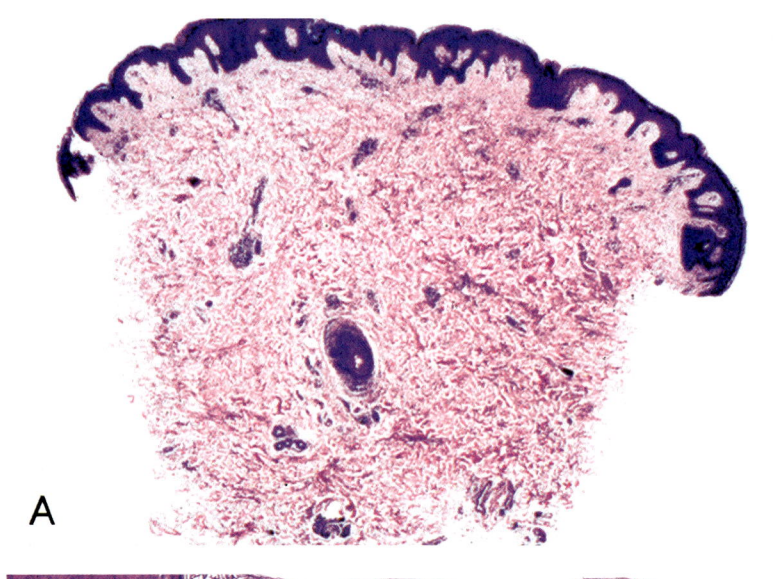

**Figure 10-27**

**STILL DISEASE**

A: At scanning power, the biopsy could qualify as normal skin.

B: At higher magnification, a scant perivascular lymphoid infiltrate is observed.

C: A clue to the correct diagnosis is the presence of rare neutrophils and nuclear fragments in the intervenular connective tissue that separates the microvessels that are surrounded by lymphocytes.

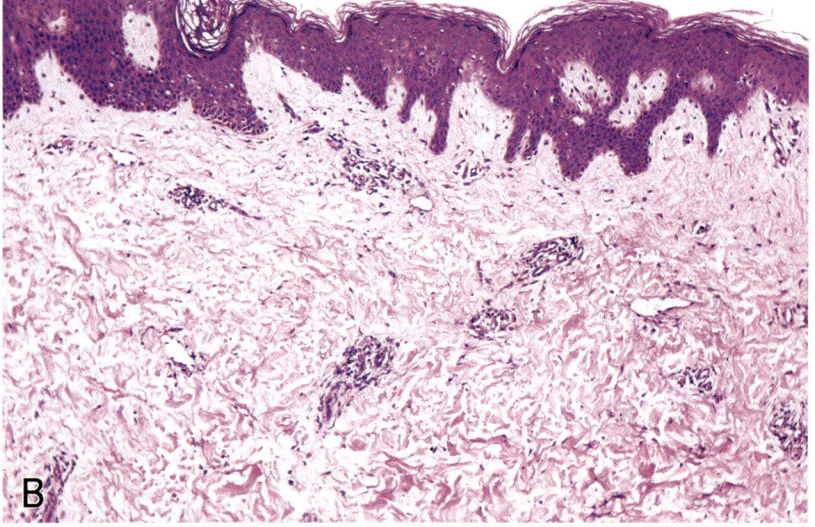

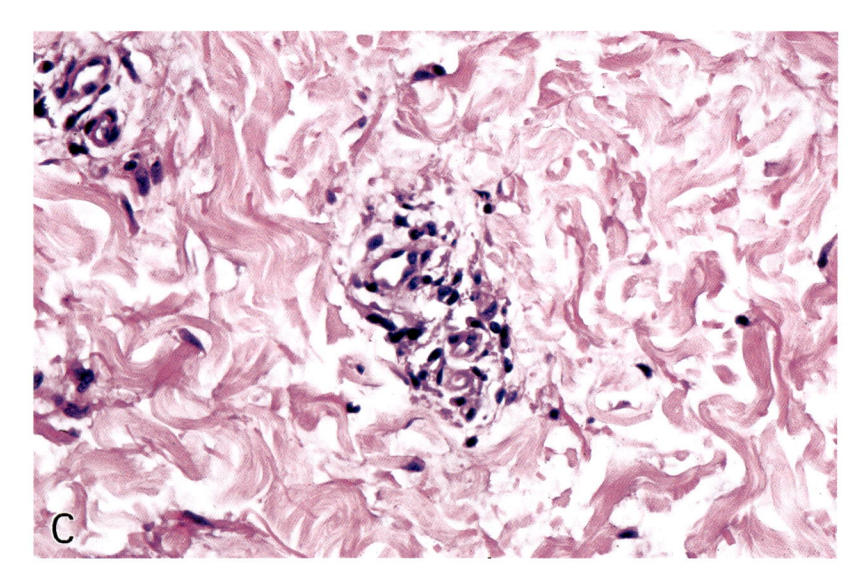

## REFERENCES

1. Walsh LJ, Trinchieri G, Waldorf HA, Whitaker D, Murphy GF. Human dermal mast cells contain and release tumor necrosis factor-alpha which induces endothelial leukocyte adhesion molecule-1. Proc Natl Acad Sci USA 1991;88:4220-4.
1a. Cummins DL, Mimouni D, Rencic A, Kouba DJ, Nousari CH. Henoch-Schönlein purpura in pregnancy. Br J Dermatol 2003;149:1282-5.
2. Chen KR, Toyohara A, Suzuki A, Miyakawa S. Clinical and histopathological spectrum of cutaneous vasculitis in rheumatoid arthritis. Br J Dermatol 2002;147:905-13.
2a. Yan HC, Juhasz I, Pilewski J, Murphy GF, Herlyn M, Albelda SM. Human/severe combined immunodeficient mouse chimeras. An experimenal in vivo model system to study the regulation of human endothelial cell-leukocyte adhesion molecules. J Clin Invest 1993;91:986-96.
2b. Christofidou-Solomidou M, Murphy GF, Albelda SM. Induction of E-selectin-dependent leukocyte recruitment by mast cell degranulation in human skin grafts transplanted on SCID mice. Am J Pathol 1996;148:177-88.
3. Baxi S, Dinakar C. Urticaria and angioedema. Immunol Allergy Clin North Am 2005;25:353-67.
4. Kapp A, Wedi B. Chronic urticaria: clinical aspects and focus on a new antihistamine, levocetirizine. J Drugs Dermatol 2004;3:632-9.
5. Klemens JC, Tripathi A. Urticaria and angioedema. Allergy Asthma Proc 2004;25(Suppl 1):S44-6.
6. Kaplan AP. Chronic urticaria: pathogenesis and treatment. J Allergy Clin Immunol 2004;114:465-74.
7. Beltrani VS. Urticaria: reassessed. Allergy Asthma Proc 2004;25:143-9.
8. Kozel MM, Bossuyt PM, Mekkes JR, Bos JD. Laboratory tests and identified diagnoses in patients with physical and chronic urticaria and angioedema: A systematic review. J Am Acad Dermatol 2003;48:409-16.
9. Grattan CE, Sabroe RA, Greaves MW. Chronic urticaria. J Am Acad Dermatol 2002;46:645-57.
10. Charlesworth EN. Chronic urticaria: background, evaluation, and treatment. Curr Allergy Asthma Rep 2001;1:342-7.
11. Kaplan AP. Clinical practice. Chronic urticaria and angioedema. N Engl J Med 2002;346:175-9.
12. Zuberbier T, Greaves MW, Juhlin L, et al. Definition, classification, and routine diagnosis of urticaria: a consensus report. J Investig Dermatol Symp Proc 2001;6:123-7.
13. Green JJ, Heymann WR. Urticaria and angioedema. Adv Dermatol 2001;17:141-82.
14. Stewart GE 2nd. Histopathology of chronic urticaria. Clin Rev Allergy Immunol 2002;23:195-200.
15. Stanaland BE. Treatment of patients with chronic idiopathic urticaria. Clin Rev Allergy Immunol 2002;23:233-41.
16. Black AK, Greaves MW. Antihistamines in urticaria and angioedema. Clin Allergy Immunol 2002;17:249-86.
17. Juhlin L. Alternative treatments for severely affected patients with urticaria. J Investig Dermatol Symp Proc 2001;6:157-9.
18. Zuberbier T, Greaves MW, Juhlin L, Merk H, Stingl G, Henz BM. Management of urticaria: a consensus report. J Investig Dermatol Symp Proc 2001;6:128-31.
19. Grattan C, Powell S, Humphreys F; British Association of Dermatologists. Management and diagnostic guidelines for urticaria and angio-oedema. Br J Dermatol 2001;144:708-14.
20. Simons FE, Sussman GL, Simons KJ. Effect of the H2-antagonist cimetidine on the pharmacokinetics and pharmacodynamics of the H1-antagonists hydroxyzine and cetirizine in patients with chronic urticaria. J Allergy Clin Immunol 1995;95:685-93.
21. Choy M, Middleton RK. Cimetidine in idiopathic urticaria. DICP 1991;25:609-12.
22. Pollack CV Jr, Romano TJ. Outpatient management of acute urticaria: the role of prednisone. Ann Emerg Med 1995;26:547-51.
23. Brestel EP. Danazol in chronic urticaria. J Allergy Clin Immunol 1990;85:1112.
24. Berth-Jones J, Graham-Brown RA. Cholinergic pruritus, erythema and urticaria: a disease spectrum responding to danazol. Br J Dermatol 1989;121:235-7.
25. Wong E, Eftekhari N, Greaves MW, Ward AM. Beneficial effects of danazol on symptoms and laboratory changes in cholinergic urticaria. Br J Dermatol 1987;116:553-6.
26. Collins P, Ahamat R, Green C, Ferguson J. Plasma exchange therapy for solar urticaria. Br J Dermatol 1996;134:1093-7.
27. Ahmadi S, Powell FC. Pruritic urticarial papules and plaques of pregnancy: current status. Australas J Dermatol 2005;46:53-8.
28. Buccolo LS, Viera AJ. Pruritic urticarial papules and plaques of pregnancy presenting in the postpartum period: a case report. J Reprod Med 2005;50:61-3.
29. Powell FC. Pruritic urticarial papules and plaques of pregnancy and multiple pregnancies. J Am Acad Dermatol 2000;43:730-1.

30. Aronson IK, Bond S, Fiedler VC, Vomvouras S, Gruber D, Ruiz C. Pruritic urticarial papules and plaques of pregnancy: clinical and immunopathologic observations in 57 patients. J Am Acad Dermatol 1998;39:933-9.
31. Katoh N, Hirano S, Kishimoto S, Yasuno H. Dermal contact dermatitis caused by allergy to palladium. Contact Dermatitis 1999;40:226-7.
32. Erbagci Z, Tuncel A, Erkilic S, Ozkur M. Progressive pigmentary purpura related to raloxifene. Saudi Med J 2005;26:314-6.
33. Torrelo A, Requena C, Mediero IG, Zambrano A. Schamberg's purpura in children: a review of 13 cases. J Am Acad Dermatol 2003;48:31-3.
34. Abeck D, Gross GE, Kuwert C, Steinkraus V, Mensing H, Ring J. Acetaminophen-induced progressive pigmentary purpura (Schamberg's disease). J Am Acad Dermatol 1992;27:123-4.
35. Aoki M, Kawana S. Lichen aureus. Cutis 2002;69:145-8.
36. Zaballos P, Puig S, Malvehy J. Dermoscopy of pigmented purpuric dermatoses (lichen aureus): a useful tool for clinical diagnosis. Arch Dermatol 2004;140:1290-1.
37. Price ML, Jones EW, Calnan CD, MacDonald DM. Lichen aureus: a localized persistent form of pigmented purpuric dermatitis. Br J Dermatol 1985;112:307-14.
38. Fishman HC. Pigmented purpuric lichenoid dermatitis of Gougerot-Blum. Cutis 1982; 29:260-1,264.
39. Crowson A, Magro C, Zahorchak R. Atypical pigmentary purpura: a clinical, histopathologic, and genotypic study. Hum Pathol 1999:30:1004-12.
39a. Braddock SW, Davis CS, Davis RB. Reticular erythematous mucinosis and thrombocytopenic purpura. Report of a case and review of the world literature, including plaquelike cutaneous mucinosis. J Am Acad Dermatol 1988;19:859-68.
40. Braddock SW, Kay HD, Maennle D, et al. Clinical and immunologic studies in reticular erythematous mucinosis and Jessner's lymphocytic infiltrate of skin. J Am Acad Dermatol 1993;28(Pt 1):691-5.
41. Meewes C, Henrich A, Krieg T, Hunzelmann N. Treatment of reticular erythematous mucinosis with UV-A1 radiation. Arch Dermatol 2004;140:660-2.
42. Rubegni P, Sbano P, Risulo M, Poggiali S, Fimiani M. A case of reticular erythematous mucinosis treated with topical tacrolimus. Br J Dermatol 2004;150:173-4.
43. Greve B, Raulin C. Treating REM syndrome with the pulsed dye laser. Lasers Surg Med 2001;29:248-51.
44. Yamazaki S, Katayama I, Kurumaji Y, Yokozeki H, Nishioka K. Treatment of reticular erythematous mucinosis with a large dose of ultraviolet B radiation and steroid impregnated tape. J Dermatol 1999;26:115-8.
45. Scott LA, Stone MS. Viral exanthems. Dermatol Online J 2003;9:4.
46. Fesq H, Ring J, Abeck D. Management of polymorphous light eruption: clinical course, pathogenesis, diagnosis and intervention. Am J Clin Dermatol 2003;4:399-406.
47. Stratigos AJ, Antoniou C, Katsambas AD. Polymorphous light eruption. J Eur Acad Dermatol Venereol 2002;16:193-206.
48. Naleway AL. Polymorphous light eruption. Int J Dermatol 2002;41:377-83.
49. Lecha M. Idiopathic photodermatoses: clinical, diagnostic and therapeutic aspects. J Eur Acad Dermatol Venereol 2001;15:499-504.
50. Gonzalez E, Gonzalez S. Drug photosensitivity, idiopathic photodermatoses, and sunscreens. J Am Acad Dermatol 1996;35:871-85.
51. Van Praag MC, Boom BW, Vermeer BJ. Diagnosis and treatment of polymorphous light eruption. Int J Dermatol 1994;33:233-9.
52. Weyers W, Diaz-Cascajo C, Weyers I. Erythema annulare centrifugum: results of a clinicopathologic study of 73 patients. Am J Dermatopathol 2003;25:451-62.
53. Bottoni U, Innocenzi D, Bonaccorsi P, et al. Erythema annulare centrifugum: report of a case with neonatal onset. J Eur Acad Dermatol Venereol 2002;16:500-3.
54. Rosina P, D'Onghia FS, Barba A. Erythema annulare centrifugum and pregnancy. Int J Dermatol 2002;41:516-7.
55. Halevy S, Cohen AD, Lunenfeld E, Grossman N. Autoimmune progesterone dermatitis manifested as erythema annulare centrifugum: Confirmation of progesterone sensitivity by in vitro interferon-gamma release. J Am Acad Dermatol 2002;47:311-3.
56. Thami GP, Sachdeva A, Kaur S, Mohan H, Kanwar AJ. Erythema annulare centrifugum following pancreatico-biliary surgery. J Dermatol 2002;29:347-9.
57. Kim KJ, Chang SE, Choi JH, Sung KJ, Moon KC, Koh JK. Clinicopathologic analysis of 66 cases of erythema annulare centrifugum. J Dermatol 2002;29:61-7.
58. Stone SP, Buescher LS. Life-threatening paraneoplastic cutaneous syndromes. Clin Dermatol 2005;23:301-6.
59. Eubanks LE, McBurney E, Reed R. Erythema gyratum repens. Am J Med Sci 2001;321:302-5.
60. Sabir S, James WD, Schuchter LM. Cutaneous manifestations of cancer. Curr Opin Oncol 1999;11:139-44.

61. Boyd AS, Neldner KH, Menter A. Erythema gyratum repens: a paraneoplastic eruption. J Am Acad Dermatol 1992;26(Pt 1):757-62.
62. Miyagawa F, Danno K, Uehara M. Erythema gyratum repens responding to cetirizine hydrochloride. J Dermatol 2002;29:731-4.
63. Ameen M, Chopra S, Darvay A, Acland K, Chu AC. Erythema gyratum repens and acquired ichthyosis associated with transitional cell carcinoma of the kidney. Clin Exp Dermatol 2001;26:510-2.
64. Lipsker D, Lieber-Mbomeyo A, Hedelin G. How accurate is a clinical diagnosis of erythema chronicum migrans? Prospective study comparing the diagnostic accuracy of general practitioners and dermatologists in an area where Lyme borreliosis is endemic. Arch Dermatol 2004;140:620-1.
65. Ledbetter LS, Hsu S, Lee JB. Large, patchy skin eruptions after a hiking trip. Erythema chronicum migrans hallmarks Lyme disease. Postgrad Med 2000;107:51-3.
66. Sanfilippo AM, Barrio V, Kulp-Shorten C, Callen JP. Common pediatric and adolescent skin conditions. J Pediatr Adolesc Gynecol 2003;16:269-83.
67. Edlow JA. Erythema migrans. Med Clin North Am 2002;86:239-60.
68. Coyle PK. Lyme disease. Curr Neurol Neurosci Rep 2002;2:479-87.
69. Steere AC. Lyme disease. N Engl J Med 2001; 345:115-25.
70. de Koning J. Histopathologic patterns of erythema migrans and borrelial lymphocytoma. Clin Dermatol 1993;11:377-83.
71. Higgins CR, Wakeel RA, Cerio R. Childhood Jessner's lymphocytic infiltrate of the skin. Br J Dermatol 1994;131:99-101.
72. Dippel E, Poenitz N, Klemke CD, Orfanos CE, Goerdt S. Familial lymphocytic infiltration of the skin: histochemical and molecular analysis in three brothers. Dermatology 2002;204:12-6.
73. O'Toole EA, Powell F, Barnes L. Jessner's lymphocytic infiltrate and probable discoid lupus erythematosus occurring separately in two sisters. Clin Exp Dermatol 1999;24:90-3.
74. Hafejee A, Winhoven S, Coulson IH. Jessner's lymphocytic infiltrate responding to oral auranofin. J Dermatolog Treat 2004;15:331-2.
75. Farrell AM, McGregor JM, Staughton RC, Bunker CB. Jessner's lymphocytic infiltrate treated with auranofin. Clin Exp Dermatol 1999;24:500.
76. Trehan M. The use of antimalarials in dermatology. J Dermatol Treat 2000;11:185-94.
77. Hashkes PJ, Laxer RM. Medical treatment of juvenile idiopathic arthritis. JAMA 2005;294:1671-84.
78. Kadar J, Petrovicz E. Adult-onset Still's disease. Best Pract Res Clin Rheumatol 2004;18:663-76.
79. Andres E, Kurtz JE, Perrin AE, et al. Retrospective monocentric study of 17 patients with adult Still's disease, with special focus on liver abnormalities. Hepatogastroenterology 2003;50:192-5.
80. Suzuki K, Kimura Y, Aoki M, et al. Persistent plaques and linear pigmentation in adult-onset Still's disease. Dermatology 2001;202:333-5.
81. Efthimiou P, Paik P, Bielory L. Diagnosis and management of adult onset Still's disease. Ann Rheum Dis 2006;65:564-72.
82. Affleck AG, Littlewood SM. Adult-onset Still's disease with atypical cutaneous features. J Eur Acad Dermatol Venereol 2005;19:360-3.
83. Luthi F, Zufferey P, Hofer MF, So AK. "Adolescent-onset Still's disease": characteristics and outcome in comparison with adult-onset Still's disease. Clin Exp Rheumatol 2002;20:427-30.
84. Perez C, Montes M, Gallego M, Loza E. Atypical presentation of adult Still's disease with generalized rash and hyperferritinaemia. Br J Dermatol 2001;145:187-8.
85. Noyon G, Blanc D, Kienzler JL, Laurent R, Estavoyer JM, Dupont JL. [Skin manifestations of Still's disease in adults. Apropos of 4 cases.] Ann Dermatol Venereol 1983;110:107-11. [French]
86. Lee JY, Yang CC, Hsu MM. Histopathology of persistent papules and plaques in adult-onset Still's disease. J Am Acad Dermatol 2005;52:1003-8.
87. Jeon YK, Paik JH, Park SS, et al. Spectrum of lymph node pathology in adult onset Still's disease; analysis of 12 patients with one follow up biopsy. J Clin Pathol 2004;57:1052-6.

# 11 VASCULITIC ANGIOCENTRIC DERMATITIS

## GENERAL CONSIDERATIONS

This section focuses on angiocentric inflammatory conditions characterized by overt histologic evidence of vessel wall destruction. Such forms of cutaneous necrotizing vasculitis are generally mediated by autoimmune mechanisms and frequently involve inflammatory responses to immune complexes deposited in vessel walls, or other events that culminate in endothelial injury and necrosis.

## SUPERFICIAL VASCULITIC VARIANTS

### Cutaneous Necrotizing Vasculitis (Leukocytoclastic Vasculitis)

**Definition.** *Cutaneous necrotizing vasculitis,* also known as *leukoclastic vasculitis,* describes a group of disorders that are associated with inflammation and necrosis of blood vessels. The presence of palpable purpura, usually on the extremities, is the most characteristic presentation (1–5). Different causes can result in this clinical disorder, from idiopathic, to drug induced, to systemic disease induced.

**Clinical Features.** Cutaneous necrotizing vasculitis affects both sexes and occurs at any age. In children, it is a frequent manifestation of Henoch-Schönlein purpura. The lesions are variable in type, and include papules, pustules, hemorrhagic vesicles, ulcers, and livedo reticularis. The most characteristic lesions are reddened papules with petechiae or frank hemorrhage that do not blanch, and are described as palpable purpura (figs. 11-1, 11-2). These lesions, sometimes asymptomatic, may be associated with burning or itching, or dysesthesia at the sites of involvement.

Cutaneous necrotizing vasculitis most commonly occurs on the lower extremities (fig. 11-1), but may affect the buttocks or back, and extend onto the arms and trunk. Sometimes, there is a generalized distribution that usually spares the palms, soles, face, and mucosa. This type of vasculitis is usually caused by immune complexes. The most common exogenous triggers are drugs and infection, which characteristically result in a superficial vasculitis. The most common endogenous causes are rheumatoid factor, cryoglobulins, and tumor antigens.

**Pathologic Findings.** Necrotizing vasculitis is characterized histologically by the destruction of small dermal venules associated with leukocytoclasia, fibrinoid degeneration of the endothelial wall, and extravasation of erythrocytes (fig. 11-3) (6). Early lesions (which are often best for the detection of immune complex deposits by immunofluorescence) are often subtle by conventional histology, showing only foci of perivascular hemorrhage and a sparse superficial perivascular infiltrate of admixed lymphocytes, neutrophils, and occasionally, eosinophils (fig. 11-4). Multiple levels through the specimen block may be required for the detection of karyorrhexis and karyolysis of neutrophil nuclei (nuclear dust) and early fibrin deposition within the walls of superficial postcapillary venules. Established lesions, by contrast, typically show frank fibrinoid necrosis of vessel walls, sometimes accompanied by fibrin thrombus formation; associated nuclear dust formation; and perivascular hemorrhage. Because the superficial vascular plexus extends within the perivascular adventitia that invests adnexal epithelium, occasional vessels appear to be situated within the deep dermis. In late/advanced lesions, postcapillary venules are almost undetectable due to the extent of their necrosis (fig. 11-5). At this juncture, epidermal necrosis or frank vesiculation may be present as a consequence of ischemia. Involvement of deeper and larger vessels (fig. 11-6) or the finding of intradermal or epidermal micropustule formation (fig. 11-7) should raise the possibility of systemic involvement or infection, respectively.

Cryoglobulinemia types II and III (fig. 11-8) are characterized by multiple, pale, pink,

307

*Inflammatory Disorders of the Skin*

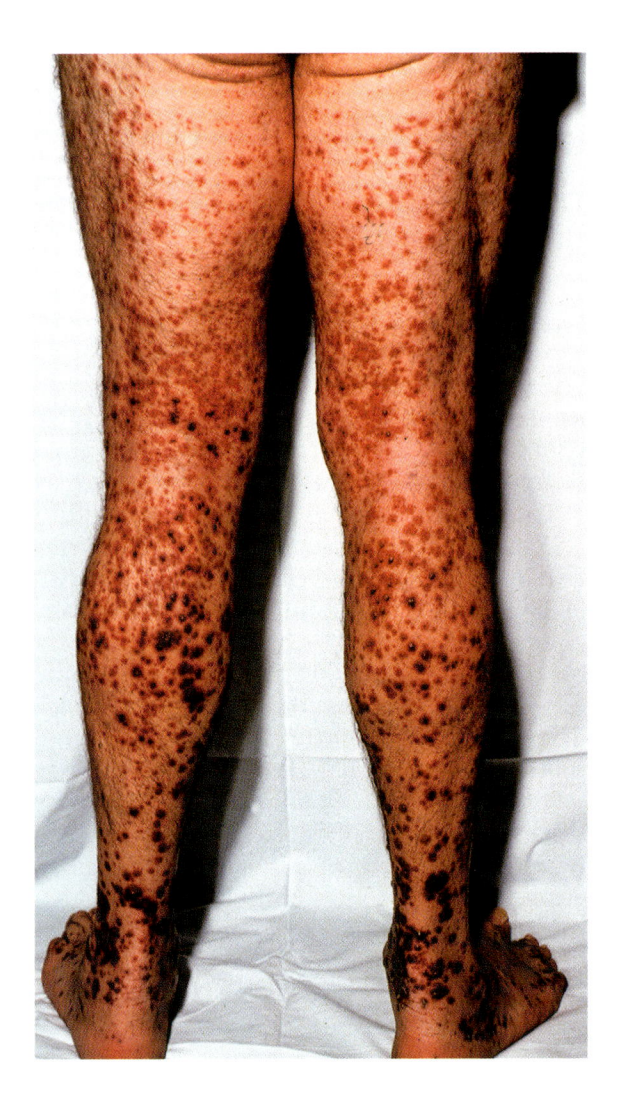

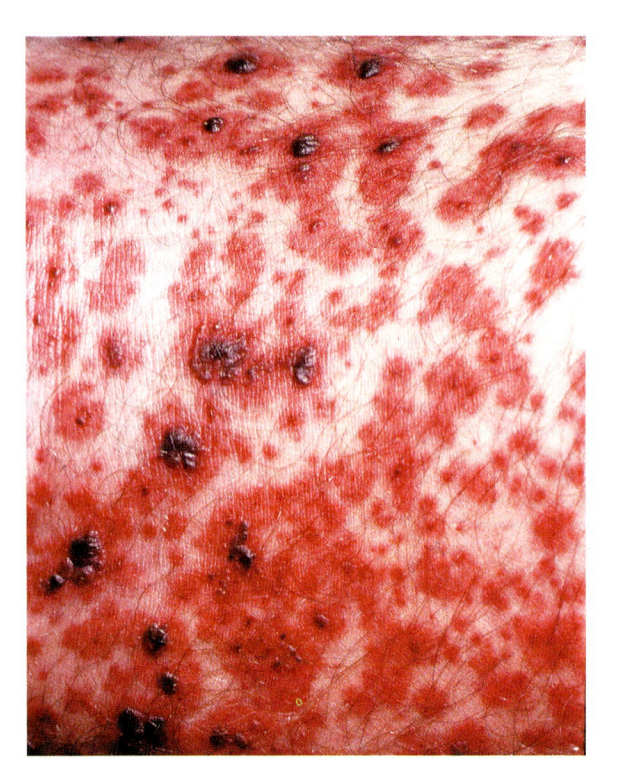

Figure 11-1

CUTANEOUS NECROTIZING VASCULITIS
(LEUKOCYTOCLASTIC VASCULITIS)

Left: The lower extremities are preferentially involved by palpable purpura.

Above: The purpuric lesions are focally coalescing and are palpable as a result of the extravasated fibrin and erythrocytes.

Figure 11-2

DIASCOPY OF PALPABLE PURPURA

Compression of lesions fails to produce blanching, as would occur in inflammatory condition characterized by increased blood flow and inflammation but not by erythrocyte extravasation.

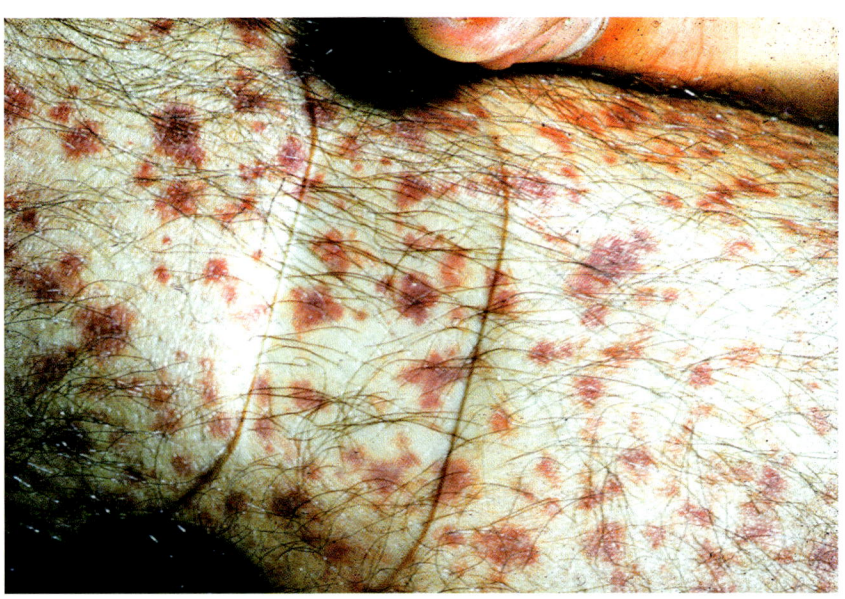

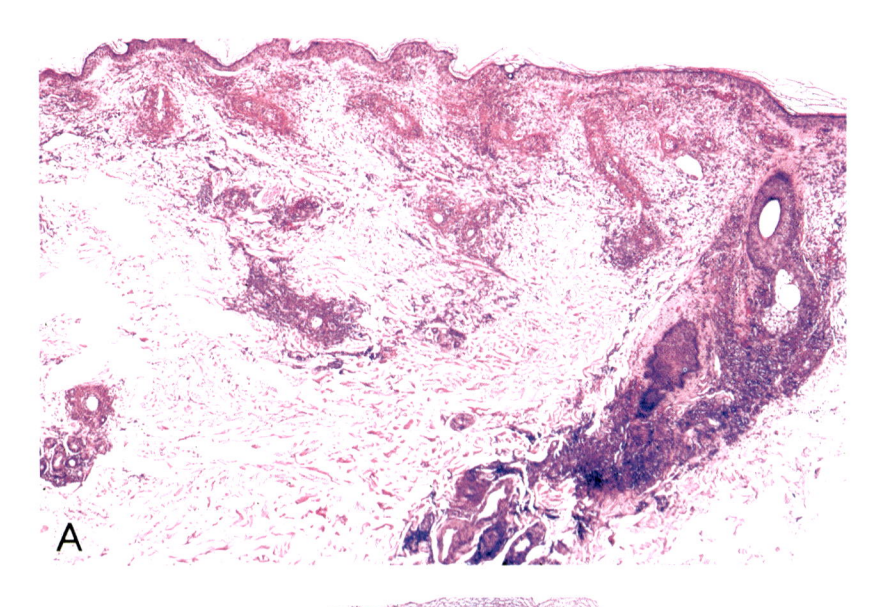

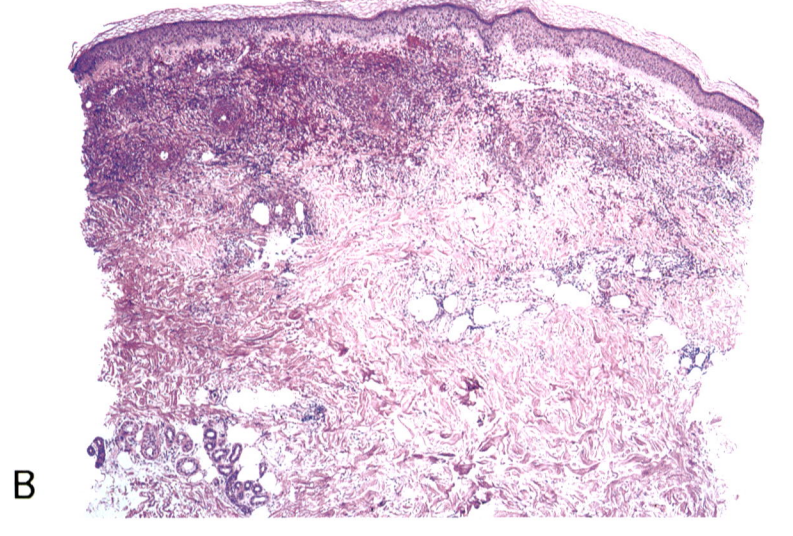

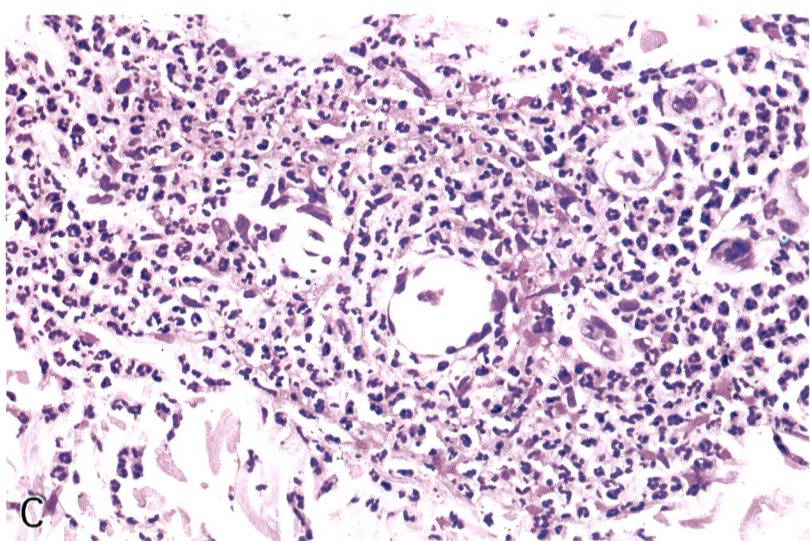

### Figure 11-3
### CUTANEOUS NECROTIZING VASCULITIS

A: Scanning magnification shows preferential involvement of the superficial vascular plexus with foci of periadnexal extension as a consequence of the continuity of the adnexal vessels with those of the superficial plexus.

B: This more advanced lesion, in addition to showing the superficial perivascular localization of the inflammatory infiltrate, discloses patchy erythrocyte extravasation visible even at this magnification.

C: Higher magnification shows intense angiocentric inflammation composed predominantly of neutrophils undergoing early karyorrhexis.

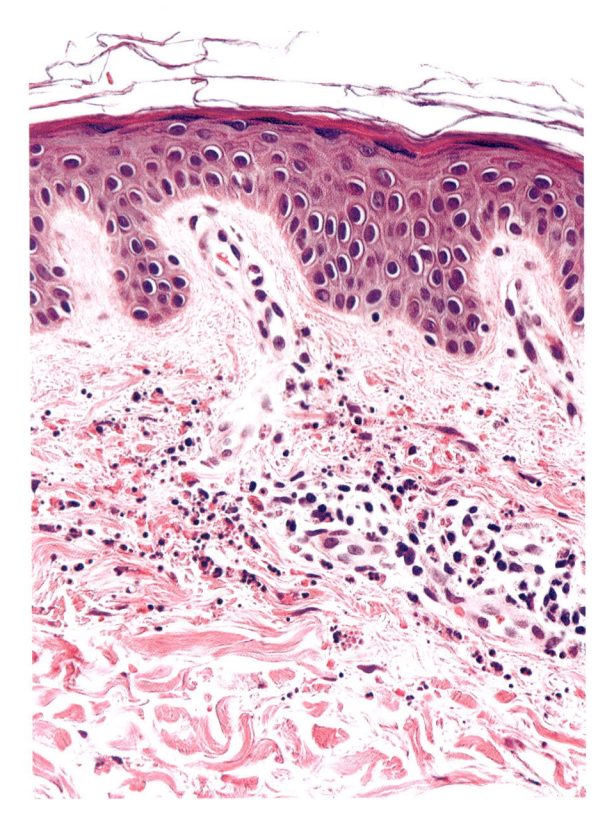

*Inflammatory Disorders of the Skin*

Figure 11-4

**EARLY CUTANEOUS NECROTIZING VASCULITIS**

A mixed inflammatory infiltrate associated with nuclear fragmentation (dust) is present around superficial postcapillary venules that at this stage show little to no necrotizing change.

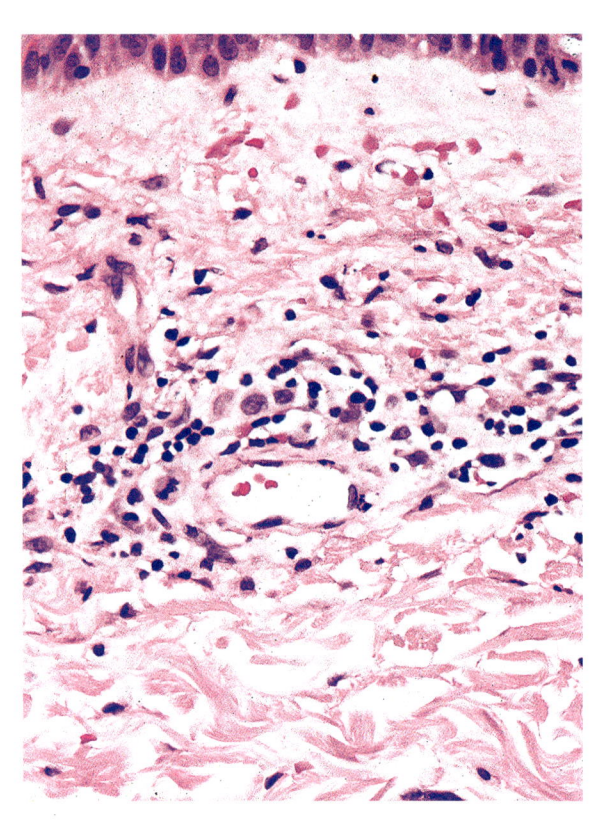

Figure 11-5

**CUTANEOUS NECROTIZING VASCULITIS: ADVANCED-RESOLVING LESION**

The neutrophilic infiltrate has begun to be replaced by lymphocytes and macrophages; residual extravasated erythrocytes are apparent directly beneath the epidermis.

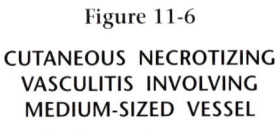

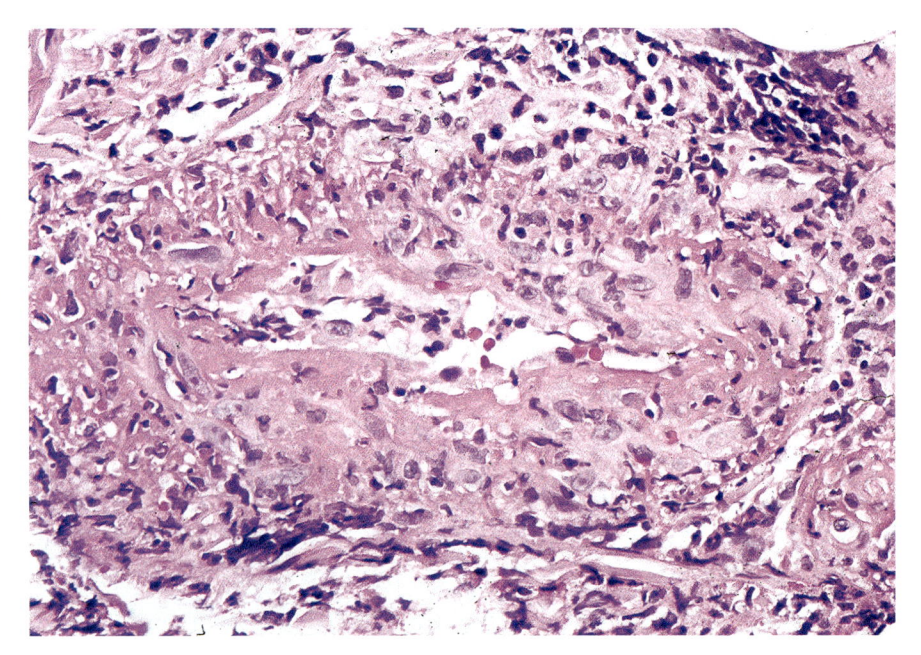

Figure 11-6

**CUTANEOUS NECROTIZING VASCULITIS INVOLVING MEDIUM-SIZED VESSEL**

This larger, deeper, dermal vessel shows characteristic fibrinoid necrosis and deposition of nuclear dust. Involvement of deeper and larger vessels may correlate with the presence of extracutaneous lesions in some instances.

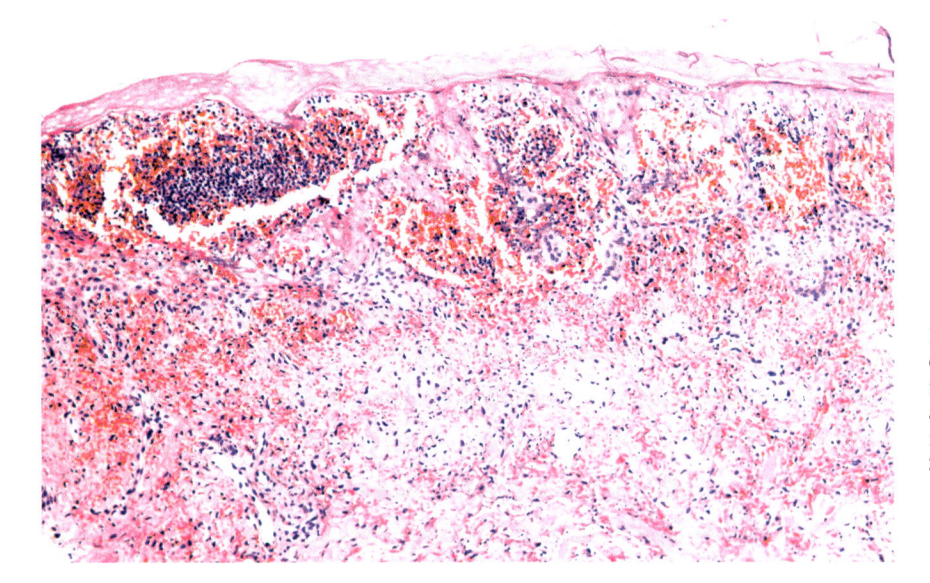

**Figure 11-7**

**CUTANEOUS NECROTIZING VASCULITIS WITH SUBEPIDERMAL AND INTRAEPIDERMAL PUSTULE FORMATION**

In addition to the vasculitic changes and erythrocyte extravasation in the superficial dermis, the presence of accumulating pustules could indicate an infectious etiology. Special stains are indicated.

homogeneous, waxy, intraluminal thrombi associated with perivascular hemorrhage that is often out of proportion to the mild degree of inflammatory vasculitic injury (fig. 11-9). In contrast to fibrin thrombi, which stain with phosphotungstic acid-hematoxylin (PTAH) but not the PAS reagent, the intraluminal thrombi of cryoglobulinemia are PTAH-negative and PAS-positive.

Urticarial vasculitis (see separate section for more detail) should not be confused with cutaneous necrotizing vasculitis and it may be indistinguishable from ordinary urticaria by light microscopy because overt fibrinoid vessel necrosis does not occur. Direct immunofluorescence, examination of plastic-embedded 1-µm–thick sections, and most importantly, clinical correlation are critical for the accurate diagnosis of urticarial vasculitis.

By direct immunofluorescence, granular deposition of complement and/or one or more immunoglobulins is seen within the walls of small, superficial vessels (i.e., postcapillary venules) in early lesions of necrotizing cutaneous vasculitis. It is important to ascertain that the immunoglobulin deposition is within the vessel walls and not in vascular lumens or the perivascular space. Fibrin frequently is detected in the perivascular region. Although this finding is not diagnostic for vasculitis, it suggests increased vascular permeability and possible vascular damage. Cutaneous necrotizing vasculitis secondary to various causes (e.g., systemic lupus erythematosus, rheumatoid arthritis, drug-induced, cryoglobulinemia, livedo vasculitis, hepatitis-associated) may also show similar results on direct immunofluorescence.

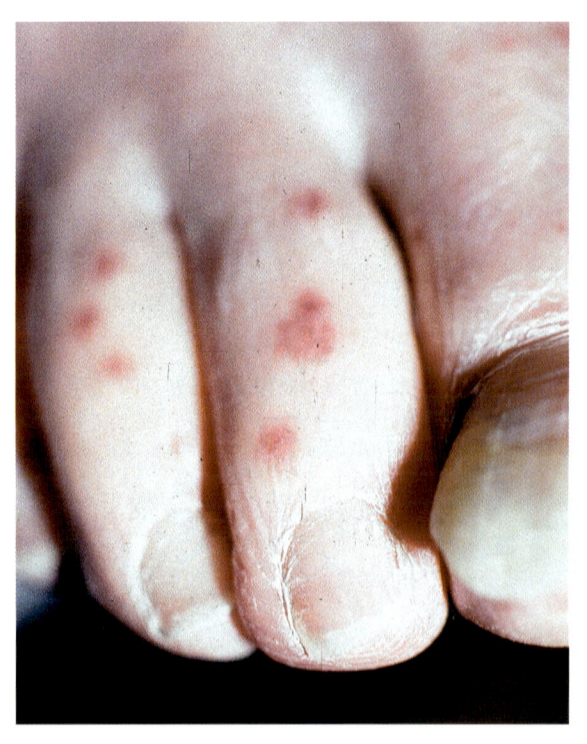

**Figure 11-8**

**CUTANEOUS NECROTIZING VASCULITIS: CRYOGLOBULINEMIA**

Purpuric lesions on the skin of extremities and digits (as seen here) are characteristic.

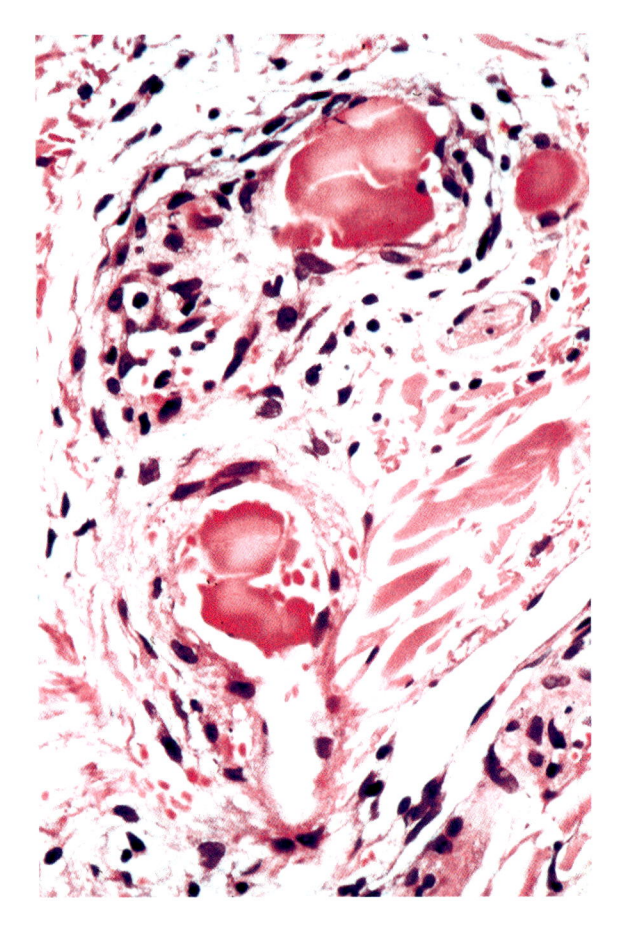

**Figure 11-9**

**CRYOGLOBULINEMIC VASCULITIS**

Waxy, homogeneous thrombi are within the lumens of superficial vessels. The vessels are surrounded by inflammatory cells and extravasated erythrocytes. The significant fibrinoid necrosis of vessel walls may be inconspicuous in such lesions.

The timing of the skin biopsy to detect vasculitis is critical because the immune deposits are transitory. The highest yield of detected deposits is in skin lesions that have been present for 18 to 24 hours. Lesions that have been present for more than 48 hours may be negative. Vascular deposition of immunoreactants is not always diagnostic of cutaneous necrotizing vasculitis; it has been noted in other inflammatory dermatoses such as erythema multiforme. Immunofluorescence findings should always be correlated with the clinical history and changes on routine histology.

*Henoch-Schönlein purpura* (HSP) is a specific subset of necrotizing vasculitis in which immunoglobulin (Ig)A is the most prominent of the immunoglobulins (7,8). Although IgM, IgG, and complement may also be present, IgA usually has the strongest staining intensity. A diagnosis of HSP should be suspected if granular vascular staining with IgA is detected in the absence of other immunoreactants. Patients with HSP have increased levels of circulating IgA immune complexes and may also have deposition of IgA in renal glomeruli and blood vessels of the gastrointestinal mucosa. These changes correlate with the clinical manifestations of hematuria and abdominal pain frequently seen in this patient population.

Patients with *urticarial vasculitis* have persistent urticarial skin lesions that last for longer than 24 hours and resolve with purpura or hyperpigmentation. These patients may have associated connective tissue diseases or hypocomplementemia. Direct immunofluorescence of these skin lesions is indistinguishable from that of necrotizing vasculitis from other causes, and accordingly, correlation with clinical parameters and conventional histology is always required when interpreting direct immunofluorescence as representing necrotizing cutaneous vasculitis. Roughly two thirds of patients with urticarial vasculitis have vascular staining for either immunoglobulins or complement.

**Differential Diagnosis.** Because the lesions are often acutely purpuric clinically, the histologic differential diagnosis is limited, especially when neutrophils with nuclear dust are observed. Extensive thrombus formation, epidermal necrosis, and epidermal pustulation suggest a septic cause, and special stains for bacteria are advisable. Thrombi should be examined for fibrin, since the pale waxy thrombi of cryoglobulinemia/cryofibrinogenemia may mimic the histologic alterations associated with conventional hypersensitivity vasculitis.

**Treatment and Prognosis.** Bouts of cutaneous necrotizing vasculitis may be episodic and last 1 to 4 weeks. They can recur over a period of months to years. Regardless of the etiology, the lesions may be associated with systemic symptoms, including fever, malaise, myalgia, and arthralgias. Systemic steroid therapy is generally employed and is effective (9). The treatment of an associated disorder, such as cryoglobulinemia or systemic vasculitis, improves cutaneous symptoms. Advanced immunosuppression may be needed with azathioprine, cyclosporine, or plasmapheresis. For idiopathic cases that do not respond to conservative therapy, hydroxychloroquine, dapsone, and colchicine are used. If no symptoms are present, clinical observation and follow-up after a thorough review of systems is also a possibility.

## Septic (Bacterial) Vasculitis and Pustular Vasculitis

**Definition.** *Septic vasculitis* is clinically associated with multiple palpable purpuric lesions and often hemorrhagic areas with bullae (10–12). *Pustular vasculitis* is a process that involves pustulation on a purpuric base.

**Clinical Features.** The palpable purpura of septic vasculitis is confined to the lower extremities or the trunk and upper extremities. Areas of extensive hemorrhagic bullae affect the skin in a similar distribution. Pustular vasculitis is the classic presenting form of gonococcemia in which the pustular lesions are usually limited in number. It also occurs as an id reaction to infection, for example, streptococcal pharyngitis. Pustular vasculitis, however, can occur in large numbers of lesions, as with inflammatory bowel disease, the bowel arthritis dermatosis syndrome, or drug reactions.

**Pathologic Findings.** In addition to the features of necrotizing vasculitis, septic vasculitis is characterized by a marked tendency for fibrin thrombus formation within affected postcapillary venules. Pustule formation within the epidermis, epidermal necrosis, and formation of prominent dermal microabscesses associated with fibrin thrombi in inflamed vessels suggest a possible infectious cause (see fig. 11-7). In pustular vasculitis, a subcorneal, intraepidermal, or subepidermal abscess, or an intraadnexal abscess, is associated with diffuse necrotizing vasculitis in the dermis.

**Differential Diagnosis.** A variety of organisms are associated with acute septic vasculitis, including *Pneumococcus*, *Meningococcus*, *Gonococcus*, group A *Streptococcus*, *Staphylococcus*, and *Rickettsia*, among others. A chronic form of septic vasculitis occurs in association with meningococcal and gonococcal infections.

**Treatment and Prognosis.** Appropriate antibiotic therapy guided by microbiologic data and species sensitivities is the usual treatment. If the lesions are severe, oral corticosteroids are added to the antibiotic therapy. For ulcerated areas, local care is often needed to speed the healing.

## Urticarial Vasculitis

**Definition.** *Urticarial vasculitis* is urticaria often surmounted by petechial hemorrhage that lasts longer than 24 hours (13–17).

**Clinical Features.** The unique constellation of findings include urticarial lesions that may show a petechial component, arthralgias, arthritis, at times abdominal pain, and sometimes intracranial hypertension. The erythrocyte sedimentation rate is often elevated. There may be complement abnormalities in some patients.

**Pathologic Findings.** In our experience, the conventional histology of urticarial vasculitis can be extraordinarily subtle and difficult to differentiate from forms of true urticaria. Occasionally, there is focal perivascular hemorrhage and nuclear dust, although frank fibrinoid necrosis is seldom observed (fig. 11-10). Endothelial cells may be prominent and show degenerative alterations, although 1-µm–thick, plastic-embedded sections or ultrastructural analysis is generally required for the detection of such alterations. Specimens are often submitted for direct immunofluorescence in an effort to detect immune complex deposits, although this approach is of limited use due to the incidence of both false-positive and false-negative results.

**Differential Diagnosis.** The primary entity in the differential diagnosis is ordinary urticaria. A presumption of urticarial vasculitis is made when the histopathology of urticaria is present in clinically purpuric lesions that have persisted for greater than 24 hours' duration. Intense infiltration of small vessel walls by neutrophils (fig. 11-10) favors a diagnosis of urticarial vasculitis over ordinary urticaria, where neutrophils are more often within vessel lumens or within perivascular/intervascular connective tissue.

**Treatment and Prognosis.** The treatment is directed primarily at underlying associated conditions, which include connective tissue disorders and hepatitis B infection. A diagnosis of urticarial vasculitis obligates the clinician to a diligent search for an underlying cause. H1 blockers, indomethacin, colchicine, and even systemic steroids may be needed in severe cases.

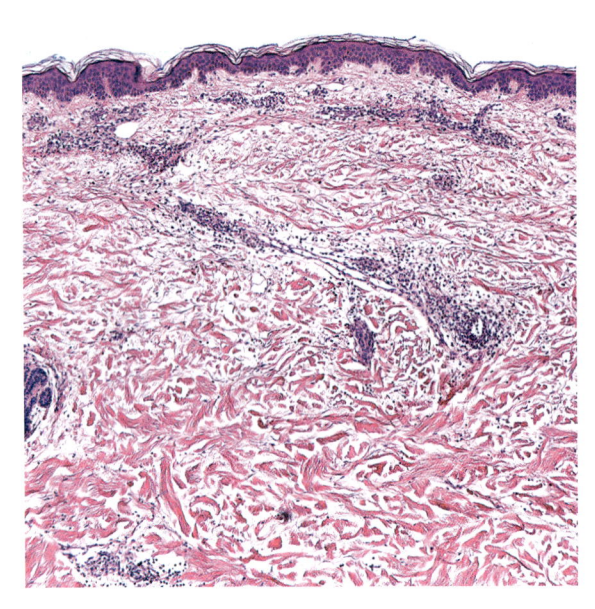

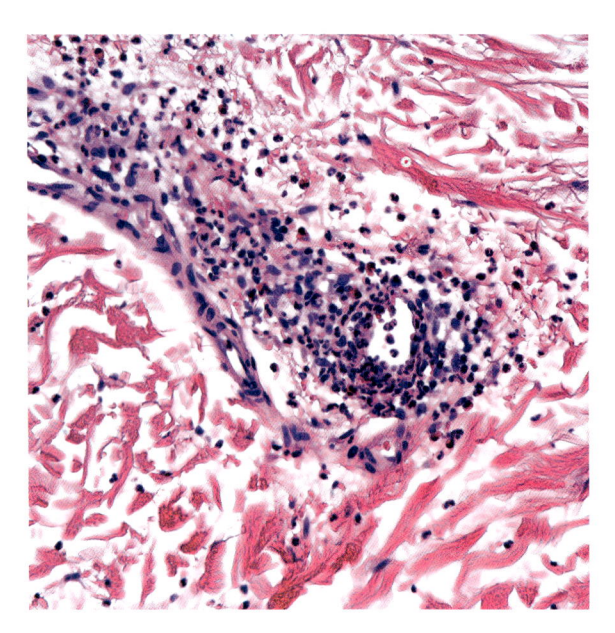

**Figure 11-10**

**URTICARIAL VASCULITIS**

Left: Low magnification shows a superficial and mid-dermal perivascular inflammatory infiltrate and marked superficial dermal edema.

Right: There is striking permeation of involved vessel walls by neutrophils with early nuclear fragmentation; lymphocytes and eosinophils are also noted. Frank vessel wall necrosis, even in this florid example, is lacking.

## Rocky Mountain Spotted Fever

**Definition.** *Rocky Mountain spotted fever* is a tick-borne vasculotropic rickettsiosis occurring primarily in children and producing a systemic disease with a characteristic cutaneous rash (18–25).

**Clinical Features.** The constitutional symptoms include fever, headache, and muscle aches. Within 4 to 5 days, a blanchable erythematous maculopapular rash develops on the distal extremities, including the palms and soles. Central progression of the rash then ensues, with characteristic sparing of facial skin. Lesions become petechial and slowly resolve over several weeks or they progress to coalescent hemorrhagic and necrotic plaques, sometimes with gangrene of skin of the distal extremities, genitalia, and nose. The lesions are clinically variable, however, and in some patients no rash develops. The lesions may be pruritic.

**Pathologic Findings.** There is a superficial perivascular lymphocytic infiltrate with endothelial prominence and focal necrosis. Perivascular hemorrhage is present in late lesions. In severe forms of the disease, extensive intraluminal fibrin thrombus formation with associated epithelial necrosis is present. *Rickettsia* are present in the walls of affected blood vessels and, because they are gram-negative coccobacilli, they may be extremely difficult to visualize, requiring electron microscopy, immunofluorescent staining with specific antibodies, or polymerase chain reaction (PCR) analysis for their definitive identification.

**Differential Diagnosis.** The differential diagnosis includes morbilliform viral exanthems, coagulopathy, and anticardiolipin antibody syndrome.

**Treatment and Prognosis.** Antibiotics may be effective, particularly in the early stages of disease progression. Avoidance of tick vectors and available vaccines are the primary strategies for prophylaxis (26).

## SUPERFICIAL AND DEEP VASCULITIC VARIANTS

### Thrombogenic Vasculopathy

**Definition.** *Thrombogenic vasculopathy* describes a group of disorders in which there are cutaneous thrombosis and clinical hemorrhagic manifestations. It results from a variety of causes including abnormalities in coagulation, increased blood viscosity, and endothelial cell injury, the latter a manifestation of true type II immune reaction in the skin. Superficial, deep, or both vascular strata may be involved.

**Clinical Features.** The lesions most commonly associated with this entity are large areas of hemorrhagic infarction, as seen in coumadin necrosis; ulcers or digital infarcts, as occur sometimes with the antiphospholipid antibody syndrome (APLA); or calciphylaxis. Atrophie blanche and livedo reticularis associated with chronic thrombogenic processes, cryoglobulinemia, and cholesterol emboli may also be responsible. Another cause is hereditary or acquired proteins C and S deficiency, which may be due to a functional defect, as found in factor V Leiden deficiency or as a true quantitative reduction, as in chronic liver disease.

**Pathologic Findings.** The main histologic feature is vascular thrombosis that exhibits little inflammation but may be associated with ischemic changes, such as digital infarcts. There is associated vascular ectasia that often occurs when livedo reticularis is present. Monoclonal cryoglobulinemia type I has these typical features. The thrombi in this disorder are periodic acid–Schiff (PAS) positive, since they are monoclonal proteins and do not stain for fibrin.

In the chronic forms, reactive angioendotheliomatosis is seen. This change, often associated with ulcers of stasis dermatitis, differs by the presence of thrombi in the small vessel lumens, a finding strongly suggestive of a chronic coagulopathy. In calciphylaxis, the size of the involved average vessel is 100 µm. Small venules in subcutaneous fat may show fibrin thrombi speckled with calcium, as well as intimal fibrosis and mural calcification (fig. 11-11).

### Cutaneous Polyarteritis Nodosa

**Definition.** While polyarteritis nodosa usually refers to a systemic disease of blood vessels, which includes a necrotizing vasculitic component affecting arteries of medium size in the skin, viscera, and kidneys, a localized cutaneous form also occurs, so-called *benign cutaneous polyarteritis nodosa* (27–29). Cutaneous polyarteritis nodosa may present as areas of nodularity, often with ulceration secondary to large vessel vasculitis, known as *macroscopic polyarteritis nodosa*. Cutaneous polyarteritis nodosa may also present as large hemorrhagic areas associated with palpable purpura and petechiae, referred to as *microscopic polyarteritis nodosa*. These patients are usually pANCA (perinuclear antineutrophil cytoplasmic antibody) positive; they have antibodies directed against neutrophil primary granules, which demonstrate perinuclear staining with immunofluorescence.

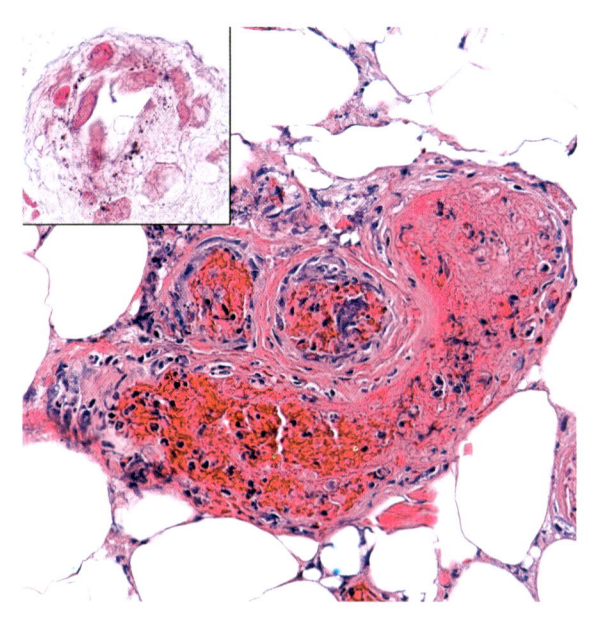

**Figure 11-11**

**CALCIPHYLAXIS**

The involved subcutaneous vessels show intraluminal thrombi, and their walls are stippled by purple-staining material, indicative of calcium salts. Subtle deposits are more sensitively detected with a von Kossa stain (inset).

**Clinical Features.** The localized form of benign cutaneous polyarteritis nodosa affects women more commonly than men. It presents as ulcers and nodules on the lower legs associated with myalgias and arthralgias, and at times paresthesias. The lesions begin as subcutaneous red to blue nodules that go on to ulcerate (fig. 11-12). They are present usually bilaterally and may be associated with livedo reticularis. The lesions may be identical to those of systemic polyarteritis nodosa affecting the skin; however, in the case of the latter, a prominent livedo pattern is observed with livedo vasculitis, or there is palpable purpura with extensive areas of necrotizing hemorrhage on the extremities.

*Inflammatory Disorders of the Skin*

### Figure 11-12
**CUTANEOUS POLYARTERITIS NODOSA**

The lesions are painful and nodular, occurring along the lines of arteries underlying the skin of the dorsum of the foot. A livedo pattern of erythema accompanies the vascular insult.

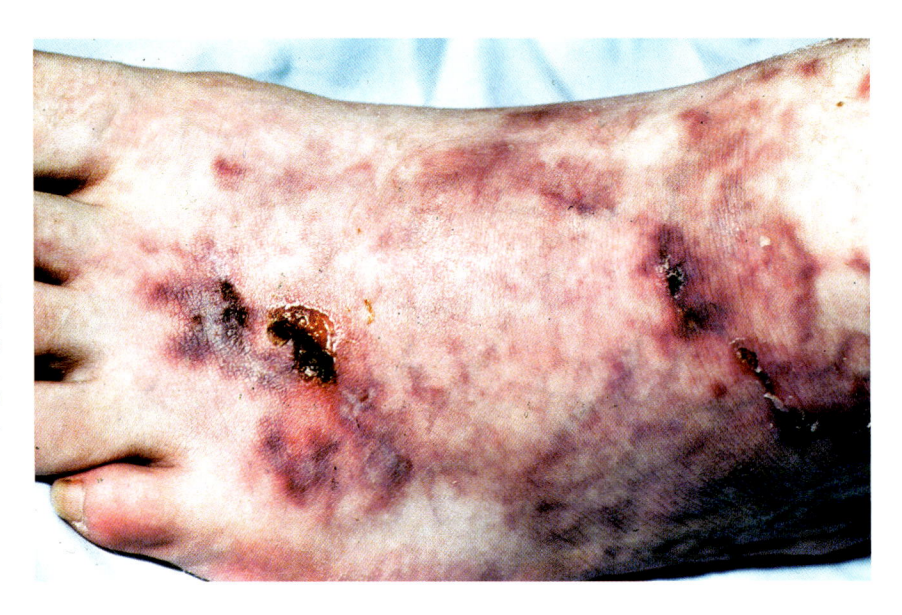

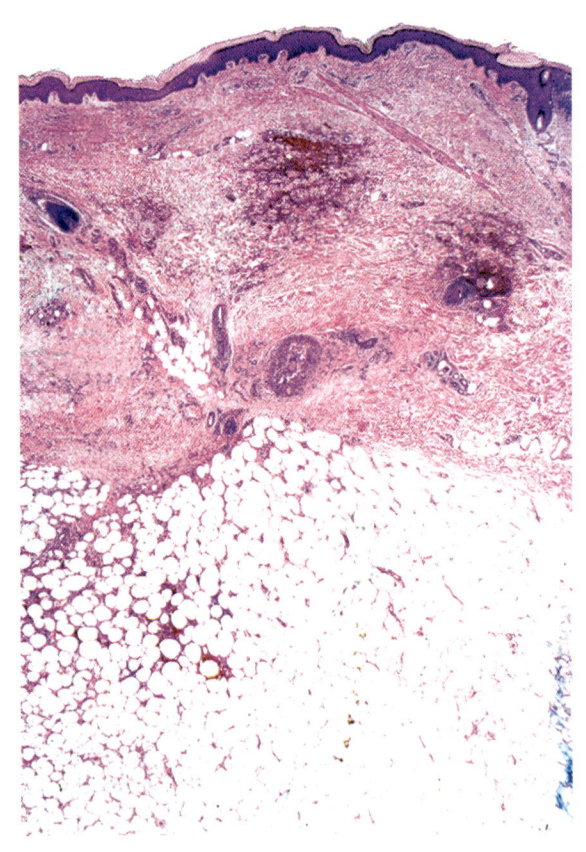

### Figure 11-13
**CUTANEOUS POLYARTERITIS NODOSA**

At scanning magnification, this deep biopsy specimen includes medium-size cutaneous arteries within the deep reticular dermis. These vessels are infiltrated by inflammatory cells, and their presence is critical to an accurate diagnosis.

Systemic disease is also associated with symptoms in other organs, including the central nervous system (stroke), kidney, and peripheral neuropathies, myalgias, and arthralgias. The vasculitis may occur in the eyes and testes.

**Pathologic Findings.** Histologically, a deep biopsy specimen from a well-selected site of involvement is required for the evaluation of polyarteritis nodosa. At scanning magnification, there is an angiocentric inflammatory infiltrate involving small to medium-sized arteries within the deep dermis and subcutis (fig. 11-13). At higher magnification, the walls of the involved arteries are infiltrated primarily by mononuclear cells and neutrophils with foci of nuclear dust. Eosinophils are rarely observed (fig. 11-14). The infiltration may be segmental, with regions of sparing in vessels sectioned longitudinally; it may focally involve only part of the wall of the vessels sectioned transversely. Occlusive intraluminal fibrin thrombi may be present in acute lesions, and with chronicity, these thrombi organize and are associated with obliterative intimal proliferation. The affected vessels are differentiated from inflamed veins with thickened walls by the detection of an internal elastic lamina in routinely stained sections. When the elastic lamina has been fragmented or partially destroyed, elastic tissue histochemistry may be necessary to identify residua of this structure. Secondary inflammatory changes are seen in the adjacent dermis as well as in the subcutaneous fat (fig. 11-15). The secondary panniculitis of

*Vasculitic Angiocentric Dermatitis*

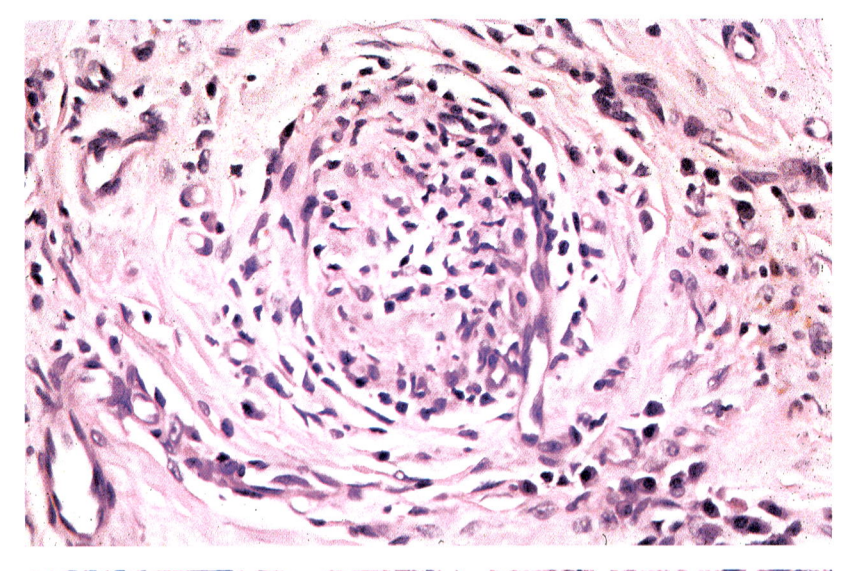

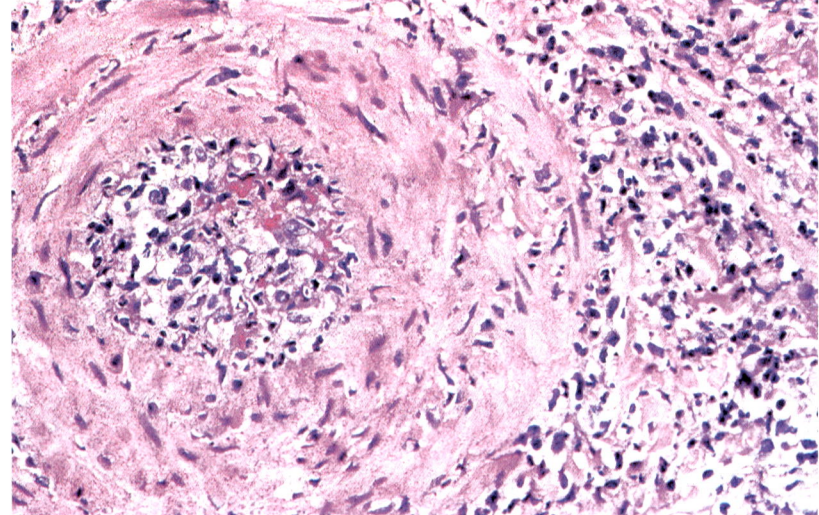

Figure 11-14

VASCULAR INJURY IN CUTANEOUS POLYARTERITIS NODOSA

Top: High magnification shows the infiltration of this deep dermal artery by mixed inflammatory cells.
Bottom: Necrotizing and obliterative changes are present. The involved artery within the subcutaneous fat is heavily infiltrated by inflammatory cells and shows obliterative intimal proliferation.

Figure 11-15

POLYARTERITIS NODOSA WITH SECONDARY PANNICULITIS

This vessel shows typical obliterative and inflammatory changes of polyarteritis nodosa. Inflammatory changes within the adjacent fat were also observed (see fig. 11-16).

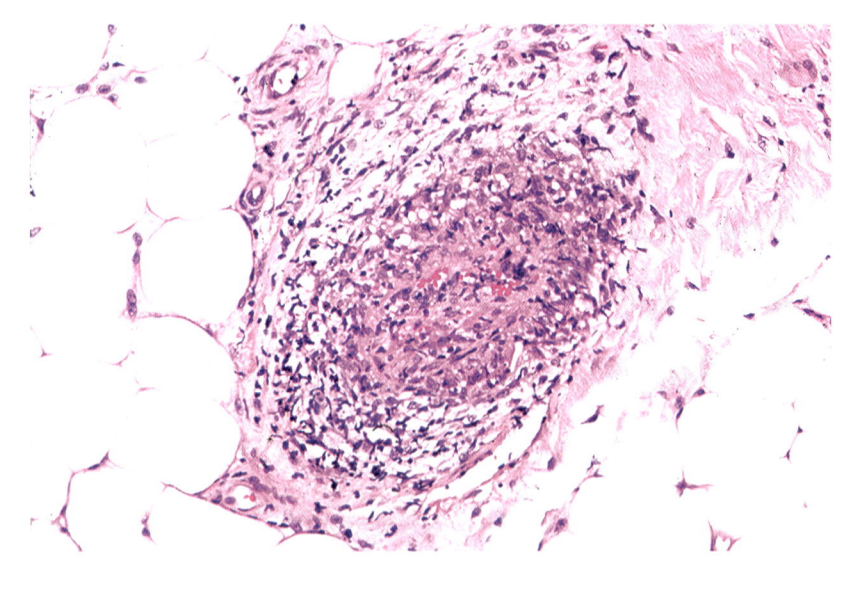

**Figure 11-16**

**PANNICULITIS ASSOCIATED WITH POLYARTERITIS NODOSA**

The adipose tissue adjacent to the vessel depicted in figure 11-15, shows the secondary lobular panniculitis characterized by both neutrophils and mononuclear cells.

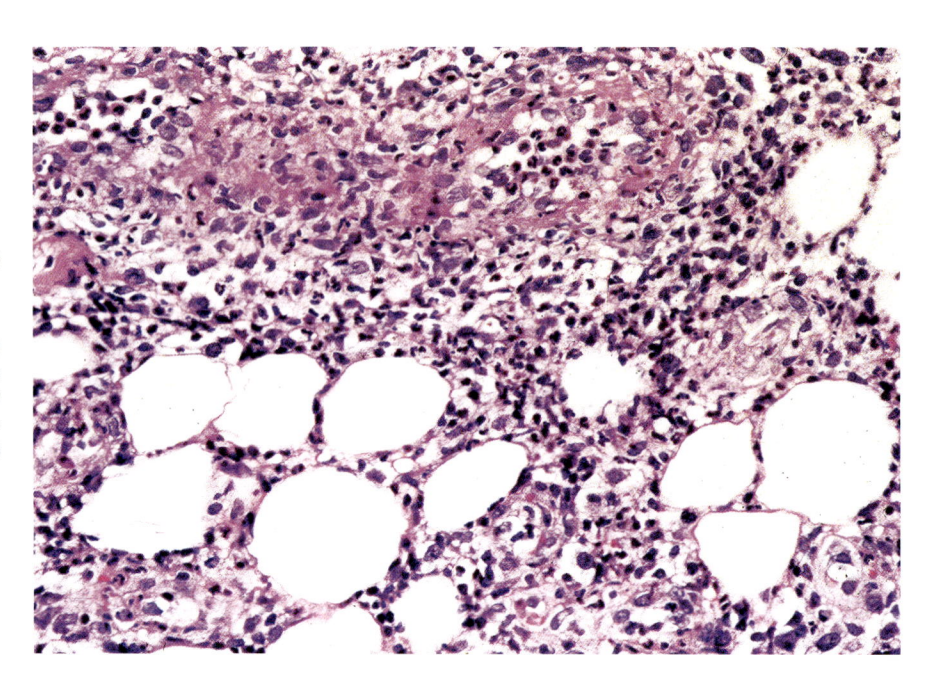

polyarteritis nodosa may assume a lobular pattern and thus be confused with early lesions of nodular vasculitis or erythema induratum, which produce panniculitic changes similar to polyarteritis nodosa (fig. 11-16). Microscopic polyarteritis nodosa presents as vasculitis not only of larger vessels but also of small arterioles and venules throughout the dermis and even extending into subcutaneous fat.

**Differential Diagnosis.** Other forms of vasculitis, including drug-induced, infectious, and postinfectious, must be considered. Disorders such as Wegener granulomatosis or Churg-Strauss disease must be ruled out as well.

**Treatment and Prognosis.** Benign cutaneous polyarteritis nodosa is managed mainly with antiinflammatory drugs, usually of the nonsteroidal type; however, in patients with multiple painful severe lesions, prednisone is necessary. In systemic polyarteritis nodosa, prednisone and cyclophosphamide are used, as are intravenous immunoglobulins. Plasma exchange is reserved for very severe cases or for those in which organ dysfunction is marked.

## Superficial Migratory Thrombophlebitis

**Definition.** *Superficial migratory thrombophlebitis*, also known as *Mondor disease*, consists of multiple coalescent tender nodules and indurated plaques occurring often, but not invariably, on the lower extremities (30–33). In addition to panniculitis, the differential diagnosis often includes cutaneous polyarteritis nodosa.

**Clinical Features.** Often, a cord-like structure can be felt at the site of the thrombophlebitis, and linear tenderness and erythema of the skin overlying a vein may be the first clues to the diagnosis (fig. 11-17). While the lesions most commonly occur on the lower legs, they are often associated with an underlying carcinoma when present on the trunk. Lesions spontaneously resolve in a few weeks.

**Pathologic Findings.** Edema fluid and inflammatory cell infiltration expands the walls of medium-sized subcutaneous veins. The lumens of involved vessels are characteristically occluded by recent or organizing thrombi (fig. 11-18, top). Inflammation may spill over into the surrounding fat, producing a localized mantle of secondary panniculitis. At higher magnification, the inflammatory component within the vessel wall of established lesions consists of lymphocytes and histiocytes, with occasional multinucleated macrophages (fig. 11-18, bottom). Neutrophils may be detected in early phases of this disorder. In healing lesions, in which organization of the luminal thrombus has occurred, multinucleated cells persist, a finding of diagnostic value in reconstructing the earlier inflammatory phase.

**Differential Diagnosis.** Detection of remnants of an internal elastic lamina assists in differentiating some lesions of polyarteritis nodosa from superficial migratory thrombophlebitis. The co-existence of lobular panniculitis favors the nodular vasculitic stage of erythema induratum (fig. 11-19; see also chapter 13). Of course, clinical parameters are also of key differential diagnostic importance.

**Treatment.** The treatment is symptomatic in most cases, with bed rest when possible and antiinflammatory agents.

### Livedo Reticularis, Livedo Vasculitis, and Atrophie Blanche

**Definition.** *Livedo reticularis* is a reaction pattern of the skin that occurs in association with a variety of disorders, and ranges from simple ectasia of vessels to vasculitis (34–40). *Livedo vasculitis* is idiopathic livedo reticularis associated with necrotizing vascular injury and ulceration. *Atrophie blanche* is a combination of livedo reticularis with ulcerations and scarring around the ankles. This variant of livedo vasculitis results in striking purpuric areas that become ulcerated and then develop stellate atrophic scars over the ankle area. Some of these patients have conditions associated with hypercoagulability.

**Clinical Features.** Livedo reticularis usually appears clinically as a network-like array of reddish blue to purple discolorations of the skin, particularly on the lower extremities, but also on the trunk and even the upper extremities. Although livedo reticularis occurs as an idiopathic reaction, it is also a cutaneous reaction pattern incited by various causes. Livedo reticularis is associated with connective tissue diseases and hypercoagulable states that affect the vessels. Antiphospholipid antibody syndrome gives rise to livedo reticularis; patients have elevated anticardiolipin antibodies or the lupus anticoagulant antibody (a misnomer since it predisposes to coagulation). Idiopathic livedo reticularis may have no sequelae or may occur in association with cerebrovascular lesions, a condition called *Sneddon syndrome*, which is probably a manifestation of systemic connective tissue disease. Livedo vasculitis has many of the causes listed above.

The vasculitic disorders and those characterized by vessel wall abnormalities that are associated with livedo include arteriosclerosis,

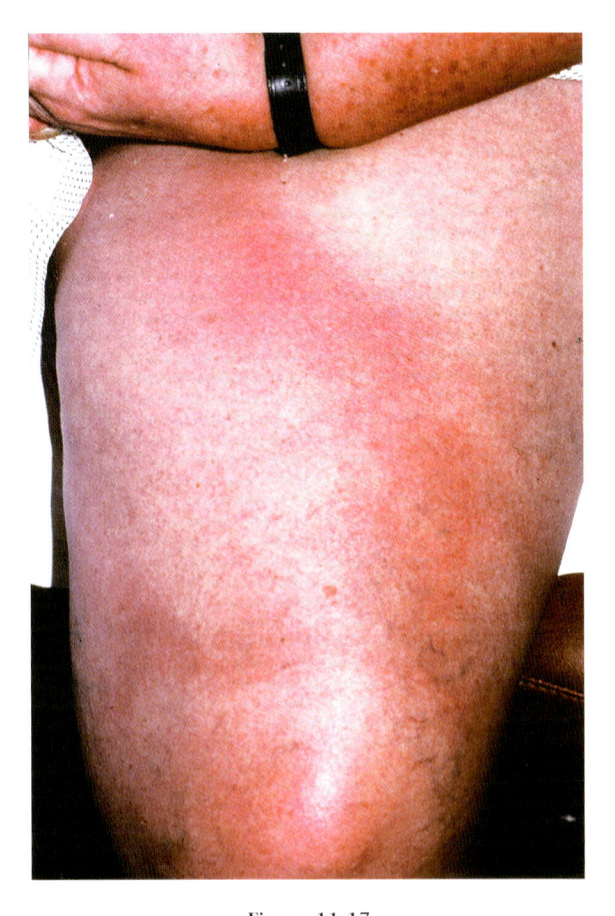

Figure 11-17

**SUPERFICIAL MIGRATORY THROMBOPHLEBITIS**
Coalescent nodules form linear plaques. These lesions tend to be very tender.

a variety of connective tissue diseases with vasculitis, lymphoma, and some infections including syphilis and tuberculosis. Cholesterol emboli are associated with livedo reticularis, especially on the soles of the feet, as are certain drugs, including quinine and quinidine.

**Pathologic Findings.** The morphologic changes of livedo reticularis vary with the underlying disorder. The hypercoagulable syndromes are associated with thrombogenic changes. With cholesterol emboli, the characteristic clefting is due to the loss of the cholesterol content of the embolus during processing. The characteristic features of livedoid vasculitis include hyalinized thickening of vessels in the mid to deep dermis, endothelial prominence and degeneration, and intraluminal thrombosis. Generally, overt cutaneous necrotizing vasculitis

*Inflammatory Disorders of the Skin*

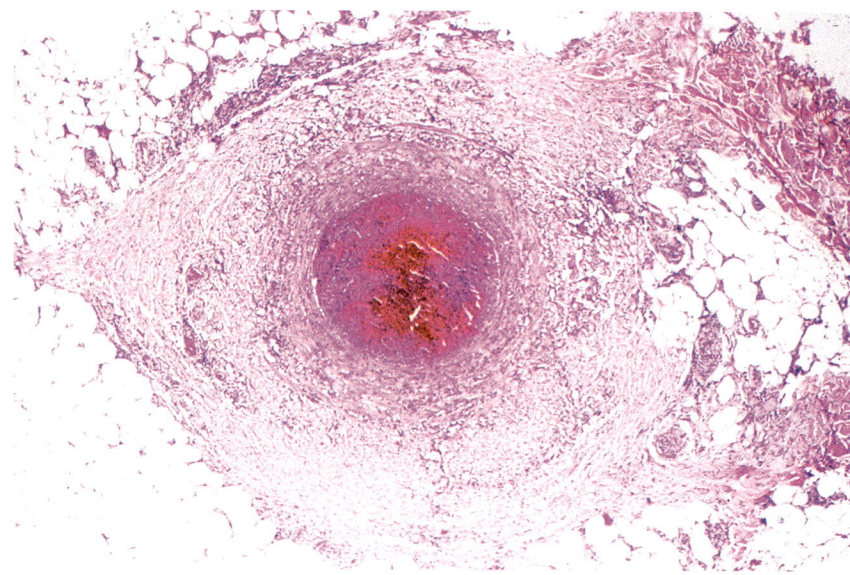

**Figure 11-18**

**SUPERFICIAL MIGRATORY THROMBOPHLEBITIS**

Top: The subcutaneous vein is occluded by a thrombus. Its wall is thickened by associated edema and inflammatory infiltration.

Bottom: Higher magnification shows the wall of the vein infiltrated by mononuclear cells and occasional multinucleated giant cells.

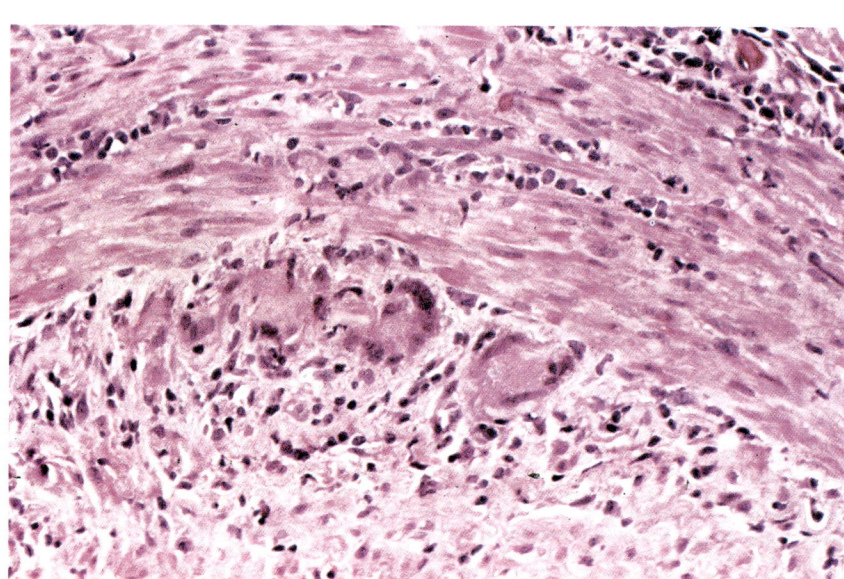

is not observed, except in the earliest phases. With chronicity, there may be considerable fibrosis, correlating with the clinical presentation of atrophie blanche.

**Differential Diagnosis.** The principle differential diagnostic consideration of livedo reticularis is cutis marmorata. Cutis marmorata is a disorder that affects patients exposed to cold. It is a transient reaction that occurs in many normal children, and unlike livedo reticularis, subsides with warming of the skin.

**Treatment and Prognosis.** The underlying disorders, whether arteriosclerotic, cholesterol emboli, hypercoagulable syndromes, or connective tissue disease, must be treated in order to combat livedo reticularis.

### Nodular Vasculitis (Early Erythema Induratum)

This early vasculitic component of the lobular panniculitis, *erythema induratum*, is discussed in chapter 13. Representative images are presented here in figure 11-19.

### Granulomatous Vasculitis

**Definition.** *Granulomatous vasculitis* describes several disorders that may produce purpura, plaques, ulcers, and profound organ

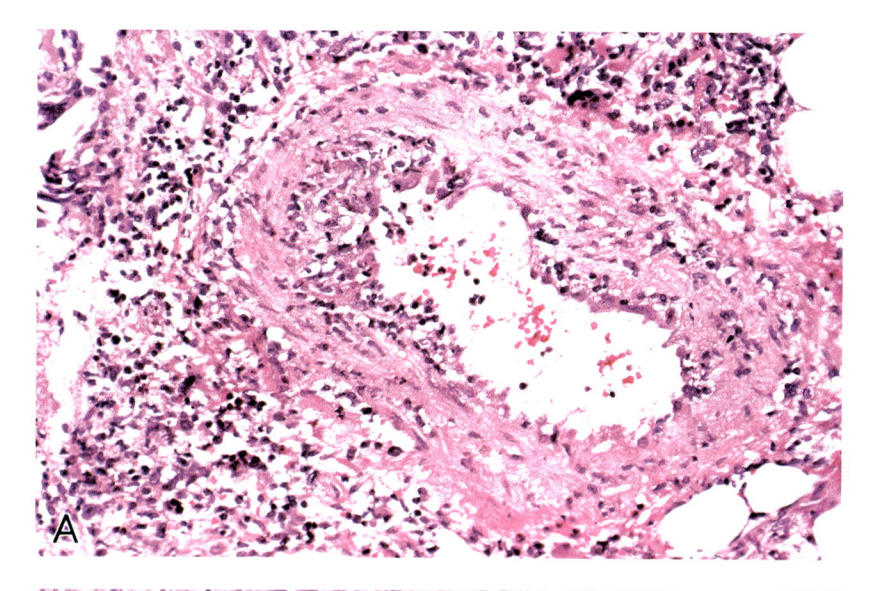

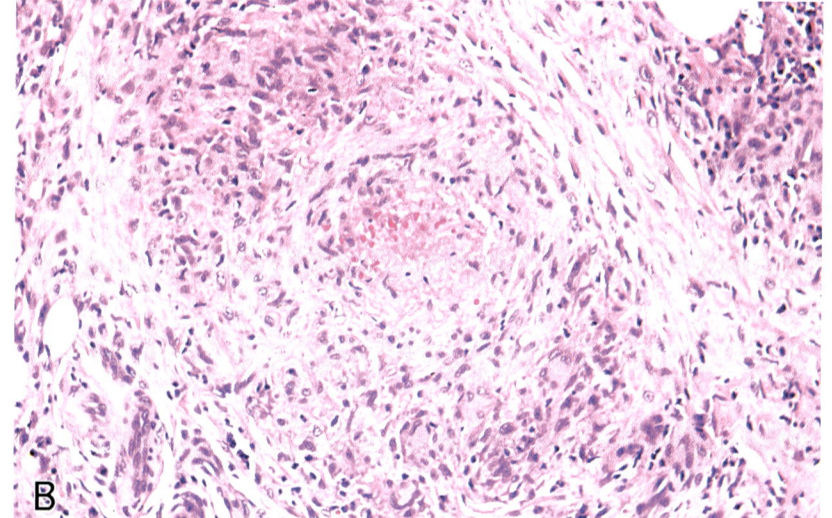

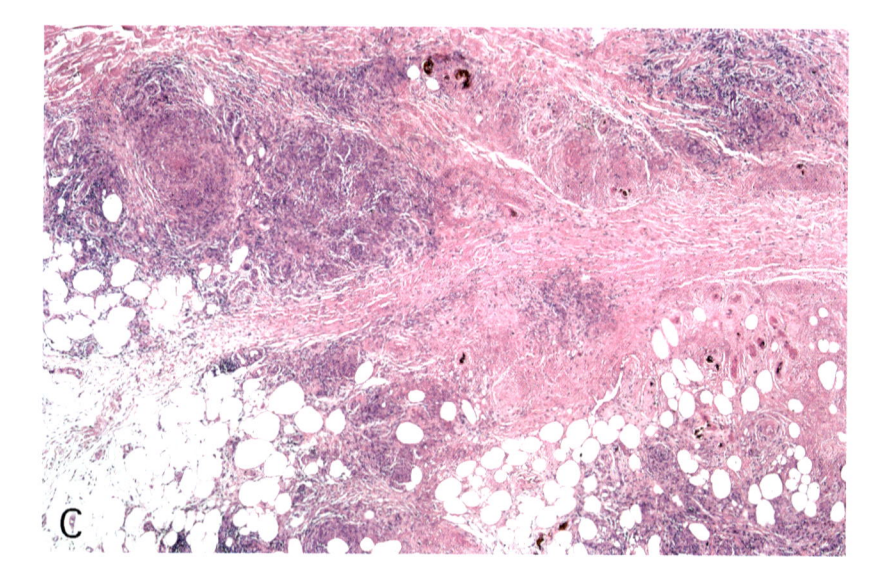

### Figure 11-19

### NODULAR VASCULITIS PHASE OF ERYTHEMA INDURATUM

A: The vasculitis is typically associated with small to medium-sized arteries and veins. Here the vessel wall is infiltrated by lymphocytes and neutrophils, and zones of fibrinoid necrosis and early fibrosis may be observed.

B: This vessel is completely occluded by a fibrin thrombus. Associated inflammatory and fibrosing alterations are seen within the vessel walls.

C: The predominant finding is a lobular inflammatory infiltrate within the subcutis.

dysfunction due to granulomatous infiltration of vessel walls (41–46).

**Clinical Features.** When a large vessel is involved, as in *temporal arteritis*, the changes include a prominent palpable artery that is pulseless in the temporal artery distribution, prominent pain, and in some cases, ulceration of the scalp. Blindness occurs in about 20 percent of the patients.

*Giant cell arteritis* is another type of large vessel granulomatous vasculitis that is associated with rheumatic disease and occasionally with Reiter disease.

*Buerger disease,* also known as *thromboangiitis obliterans,* affects small and medium-sized arteries, especially of the lower extremities, and occurs usually in males who are smokers. Buerger disease is associated with Raynaud syndrome and ischemic pain upon walking.

The small vessel involvement of granulomatous vasculitis is divided into those vessels associated with an extravascular inflammatory component and those without. Conditions without extravascular inflammation present principally as nodules and sometimes ulcerations on the extremities. Typical causes are sarcoidosis, reactions to infections like herpes zoster, and acquired hypogammaglobulinemia. When there is associated granulomatous inflammation that is extravascular, the lesions appear to be granuloma annulare-like or necrobiosis-like. Lesions that are granuloma annulare-like microscopically present as plaques or nodules. Lesions may be few in number and present, for example, on the dorsum of the hands or on the elbows. These lesions are associated with diabetes, thyroiditis, and the arthropathy associated infections from *Streptococcus* or *Mycobacterium* organisms. Parvovirus B-19 and hepatitis C are associated with extravascular reactions, but usually there is also an interface dermatitis. These reactions are id-like to the infectious process and the extravascular inflammation is usually mononuclear. When the extravascular areas are associated with neutrophils, inflammatory bowel disease or sclerosing cholangitis enter into the differential diagnosis. When there is a true suppurative intervascular response with extensive neutrophilic infiltration and necrosis, the etiology is infectious or a systemic disease such as Wegener granulomatosis. Clinically, these lesions are usually ulcerative nodules.

**Differential Diagnosis.** The differential diagnosis of granulomatous vasculitis is broad and includes disorders that resemble the granulomatous vasculitis of the large vessel type, such as polyarteritis nodosa. In granulomatous vasculitis associated with extravascular inflammation, the leading diagnostic entity is a granuloma annulare-like reaction or necrobiosis. Infection is the principal disorder to be distinguished from granulomatous vasculitis with extravascular neutrophilic inflammation.

**Treatment and Prognosis.** The treatment depends upon managing the underlying disorder.

### Wegener Granulomatosis

**Definition.** *Wegener granulomatosis* (WG) is a systemic vasculitic syndrome involving both arteries and veins, and causing necrotizing granulomatous inflammation of the upper respiratory tract, lungs, kidneys, and skin. Cutaneous WG is associated with ulcerating nodules (47–51).

**Clinical Features.** The onset of WG is approximately in the fifth decade of life, and there is a slight male predominance. The disease rarely occurs in African Americans. This disorder is immunologically mediated, but its exact etiology is unknown. Patients present with systemic symptoms including fever, malaise, pain in the region of the sinuses, and purulent or bloody rhinorrhea. There may be cough associated with hemoptysis, shortness of breath, chest pains, and even symptoms of pleurisy. Half of the patients eventually have cutaneous involvement, but less than 20 percent have skin involvement at the time of their initial symptoms. The most characteristic changes are a palpable purpura manifesting as necrotizing vasculitis, ulcerating nodular lesions on the extremities, and nonspecific changes such as a papulovesicular eruption. Subcutaneous nodules occur on the lower extremities; however, involvement of the upper limbs, face, and trunk is also seen. Oral ulcerations are characteristic and are sometimes the initial presenting symptom. Eye involvement includes proptosis due to inflammatory nodules in the orbit, conjunctivitis, and episcleritis. In the nervous system, there may be signs of cerebral vasculitis as well as neuritis. Most patients exhibit signs of glomerulitis. The course of this disease is fatal if untreated.

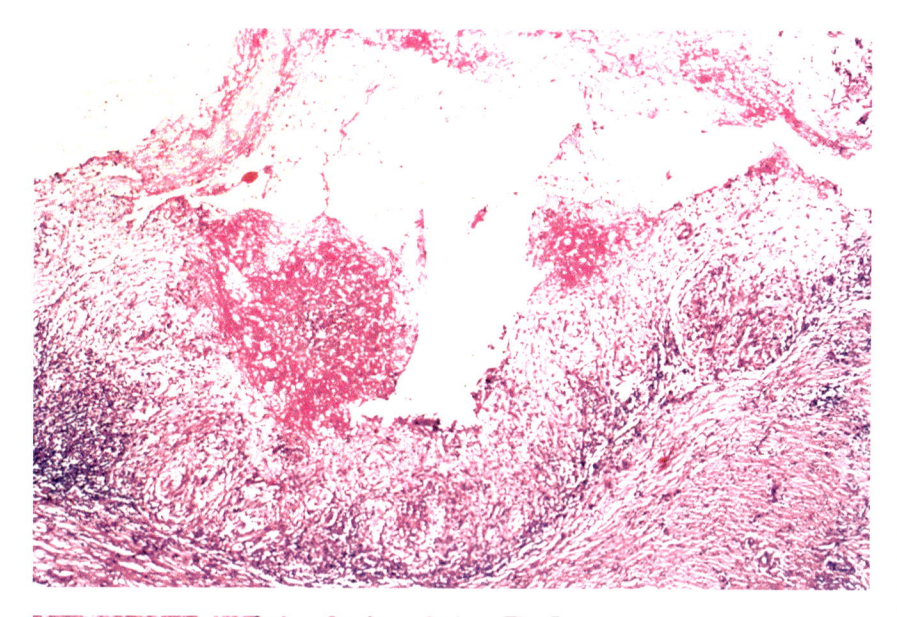

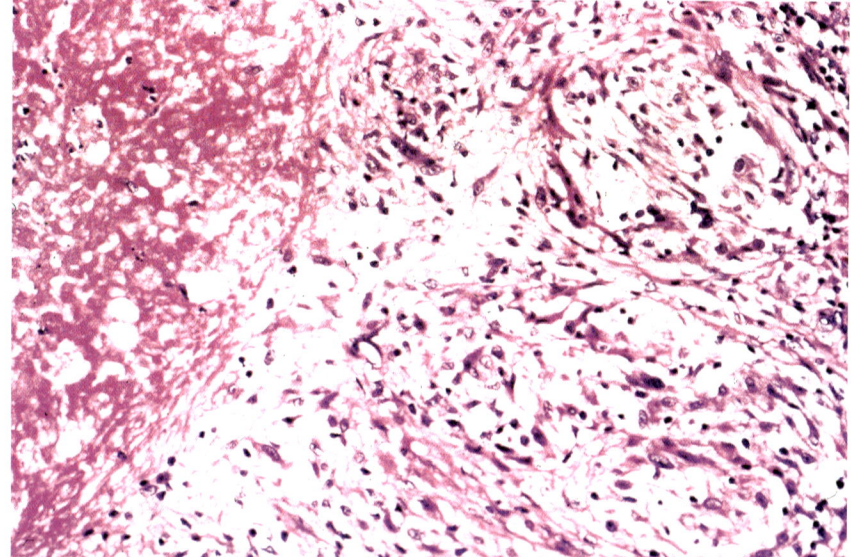

**Figure 11-20**

**WEGENER GRANULOMATOSIS**

Top: At scanning magnification, there is epidermal and dermal ulceration associated with a brisk underlying inflammatory infiltrate.

Bottom: At higher magnification, there are geographic zones of fibrinoid necrosis bordered by an elusive aggregated granulomatous response. Vasculitic changes are also commonly encountered.

**Pathologic Findings.** The dermis is infiltrated by palisaded granulomas and giant cells juxtaposed with zones of fibrinoid necrosis (fig. 11-20). Regions of granular necrosis occasionally form serpentine architectural configurations. Necrotizing vasculitis is also present, with luminal thrombosis. Thus, the findings consist of extravascular interstitial granulomatous inflammation with geographic zones of granular fibrinoid necrosis, and necrotizing vasculitis mediated by neutrophils but also associated with mixed inflammatory elements.

**Differential Diagnosis.** The differential diagnosis includes infectious granulomatous diseases such as blastomycosis, angiocentric lymphoma, mid-line granuloma, and Goodpasture syndrome. An important consideration is Churg-Strauss vasculitis, a form of pulmonary and systemic vasculitis with the potential for cutaneous involvement, which shows granulomatous infiltration of vessel walls with numerous eosinophils and extravascular granulomas, usually without significant necrosis.

**Treatment and Prognosis.** Systemic cyclophosphamide and prednisone are the two most effective agents (52,53). Cutaneous disease can be treated with topical or intralesional corticosteroids and aggressive wound care.

*Inflammatory Disorders of the Skin*

**Figure 11-21**

GRANULOMA FACIALE

This lesion is a typical erythematous, brown-purple facial plaque with patulous follicular openings.

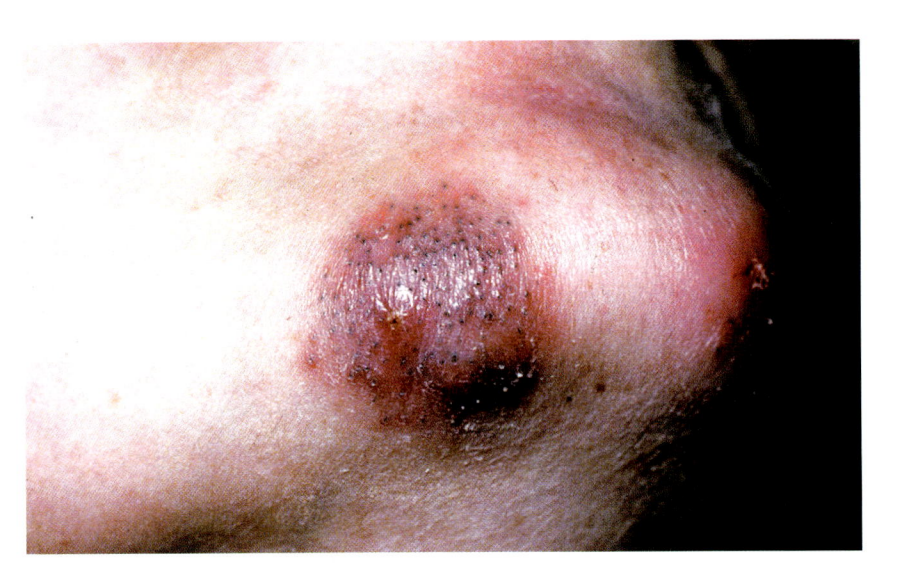

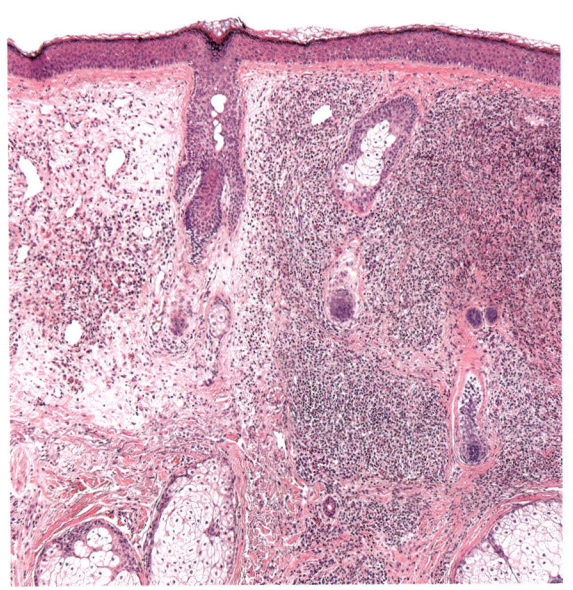

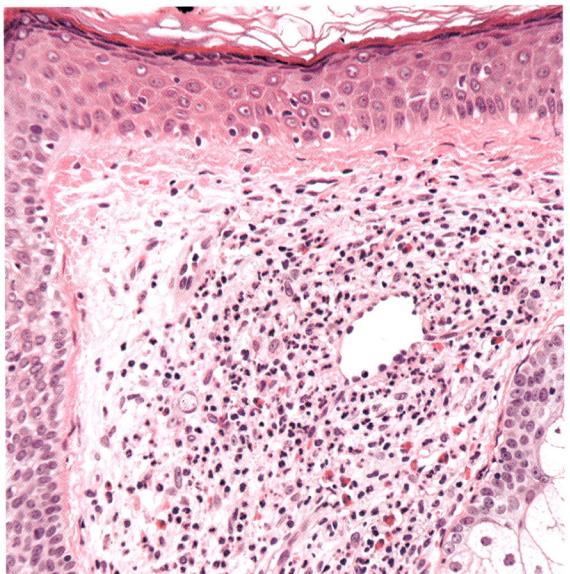

**Figure 11-22**

GRANULOMA FACIALE

Left: At scanning magnification, there are coalescent aggregates of inflammatory cells within the superficial and deep dermis. These aggregates begin as angiocentric foci with associated vasculitis. The characteristic zone of sparing of the dermis is directly beneath the epidermal layer.

Right: Higher magnification shows a mixed inflammatory infiltrate, replete with eosinophils, associated with the formation of nuclear dust and fibrinoid necrosis of involved vessels.

## Granuloma Faciale

**Definition.** *Granuloma faciale* is an idiopathic facial dermatitis consisting of solitary tan-brown to pink-purple plaques and that generally affects middle-aged men (54–57).

**Clinical Features.** Granuloma faciale presents as asymptomatic, soft, brown-red plaques involving the facial skin. Rarely, the upper extremities are involved (fig. 11-21). The lesions characteristically contain dilated follicular ostia.

**Pathologic Findings.** Scanning magnification reveals coalescent, angiocentric infiltration by inflammatory cells within the superficial and deep dermis (fig. 11-22, left). The inflammatory component characteristically spares a thin mantle of dermis directly beneath the epidermal and adnexal basement membrane zones (i.e., Grenz zone, or zone of sparing). Vessels may be nearly totally obliterated by fragmented neutrophils that demarcate their preexisting loci (fig. 11-22, right).

**Differential Diagnosis.** Granuloma faciale must be differentiated from other forms of necrotizing vasculitis, including erythema elevatum diutinum. The presence of a Grenz zone of subepidermal sparing and the clinical site of occurrence and appearance, favor granuloma faciale.

**Treatment and Prognosis.** Lesions may persist for decades, and generally are poorly responsive to therapy. Occasionally, systemic dapsone and chloroquine, injected corticosteroids, or destructive modalities, including surgical excision, radiation therapy, cryotherapy, and argon or pulse-dye lasers are effective (58,59).

### Erythema Nodosum Leprosum

**Definition.** *Erythema nodosum leprosum* is a specific type of vasculitic reaction associated with lepromatous and borderline leprosy (60).

**Clinical Features.** Erythema nodosum leprosum occurs in both men and women with lepromatous and borderline leprosy, usually during treatment. It is also associated with other types of infection, pregnancy, or marked physical or mental stress. Patients present with tender reddish or deep purple nodules that are associated with fever. The nodules are usually present over the extremities but may occur over the entire surface of the skin. There also may be associated arthralgias and arthritis, myalgias, and myositis as well as iritis and orchitis in some severely affected patients. Pain is usually present, especially in the arms and legs.

**Pathologic Findings.** There is an angiocentric inflammatory infiltrate involving the deep dermal vessels. The infiltration of vessel walls by a mixture of inflammatory cells with nuclear dust formation and zones of fibrinoid necrosis is striking. The adjacent dermis often contains foamy histiocytes and admixed lymphocytes; the histiocytes contain numerous *Lepra* bacilli within their cytoplasm.

**Differential Diagnosis.** The entities in the differential diagnosis are drug eruptions, other types of lepromatous reactions such as reversal reactions, and erythema nodosum of other causes.

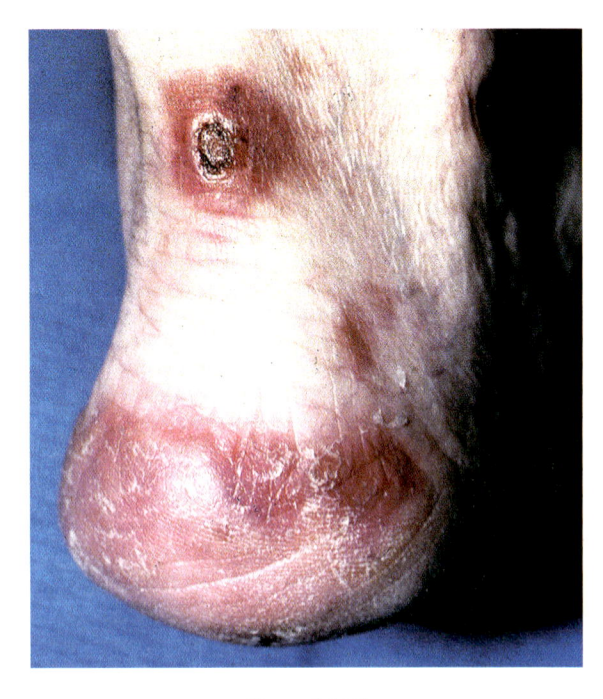

Figure 11-23
ERYTHEMA ELEVATUM DIUTINUM
Chronic necrotizing vasculitis in this lesion is manifested by a longstanding hemorrhagic nodule with ulceration. These lesions typically occur on the distal extremities, as seen here.

**Treatment and Prognosis.** The treatment of erythema nodosum leprosum usually includes steroid therapy to quiet the severely acute episode, but nonsteroidal antiinflammatory drugs are helpful (61). Thalidomide and clofazimine are used in appropriate patients (62–66).

### Erythema Elevatum Diutinum

**Definition.** *Erythema elevatum diutinum* is a chronic skin disease with lesions that are reddish to purple but become firm yellowish nodules or plaques that are acrally distributed, usually symmetrically (67–73). This disease is associated with exacerbations of streptococcal infections.

**Clinical Features.** Erythema elevatum diutinum occurs at any age but is most common in middle to later life. The lesions are reddish to violaceous at first and are multiple and often symmetrical (fig. 11-23). They are present on the extensor surfaces of the extremities and have a predilection for the skin over the metacarpal joints as well as other sites around the hands and knees; lesions also affect the buttocks and

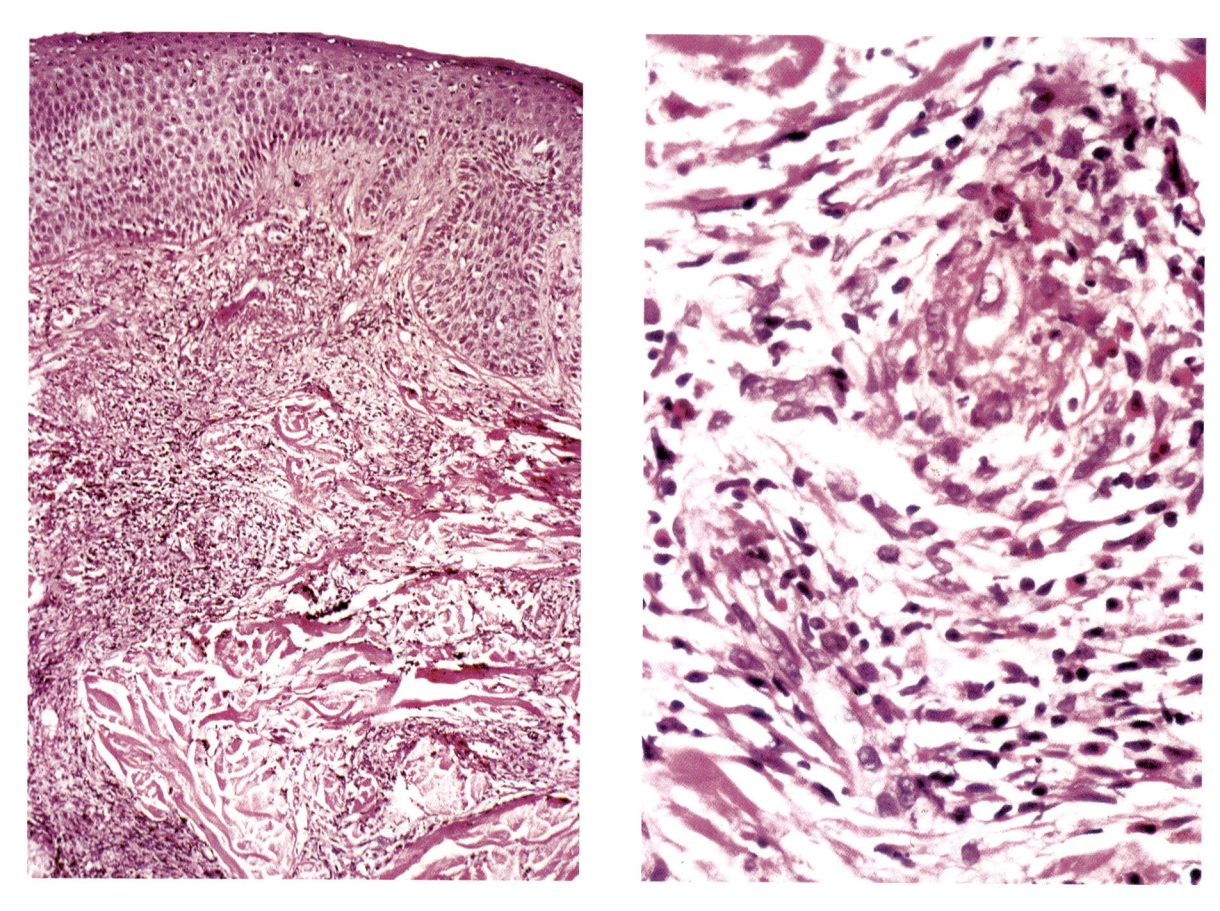

**Figure 11-24**

**ERYTHEMA ELEVATUM DIUTINUM**

Left: Histologically, there is a brisk superficial and mid-dermal inflammatory infiltrate composed of lymphocytes and neutrophils, with associated necrotizing vascular injury.

Right: At higher magnification, the necrotizing vasculitis is associated with characteristic superficial dermal and perivascular fibrosis, indicative of chronicity.

the Achilles tendon, and occasionally the face, ears, and mucous membranes. Petechiae or purpura are sometimes noted on the surface of the lesions. As the lesions become chronic, they become firm and fibrous and turn yellow.

There are few symptoms except for occasional itching or burning. Patients usually have arthralgias. Inflammatory bowel disease and occasionally myeloma are associated with the disorder. Streptococcal infections can exacerbate the disease and there is some evidence that there is an immune basis because of the presence of cutaneous vasculitis.

**Pathologic Findings.** A brisk superficial and mid-dermal mixed inflammatory perivascular infiltrate, composed of lymphocytes and variably fragmented neutrophils, is associated with necrotizing vascular injury (fig. 11-24). The neutrophils infiltrate the collagen fibers, resulting in degenerative changes. In late lesions, hemosiderin deposition and extensive dermal fibrosis that may give an almost plywood-like appearance with scattered neutrophils in the fibrous tissue are seen (figs. 11-25, 11-26). A vaguely concentric perivascular fibrosis, imparting an onion skin-like change, is diagnostically helpful and provides testimony of the chronicity of the vascular injury (fig. 11-25, bottom). Such fibrotic sequelae commonly form tumoral nodules clinically. Lipid-engorged histiocytes may give older lesions a xanthomatous appearance.

**Differential Diagnosis.** Originally these lesions were thought to be variants of granuloma annulare because of their predilection for the

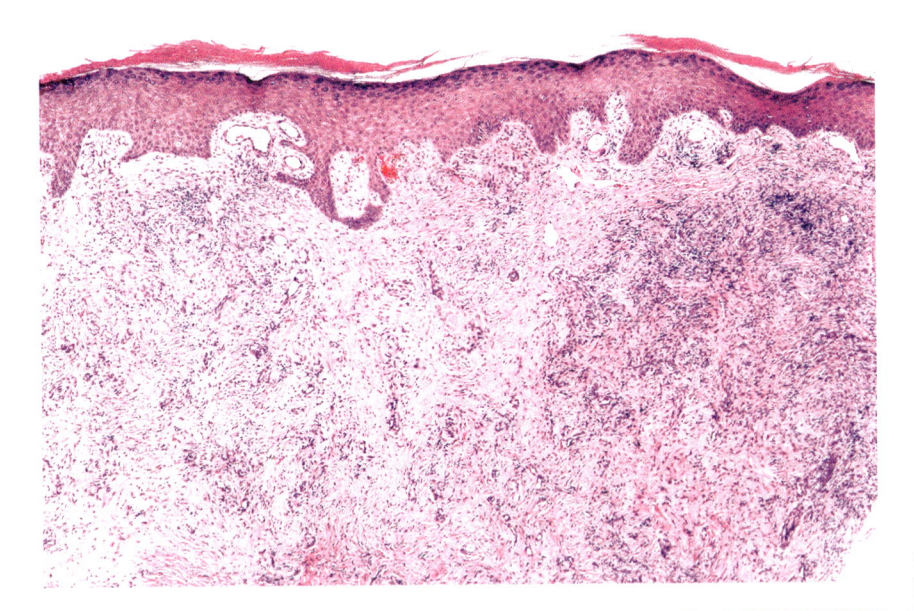

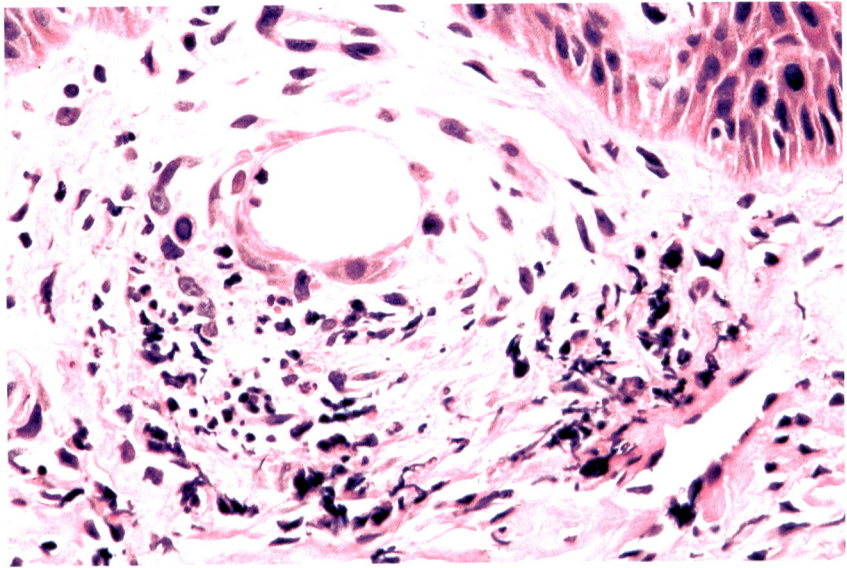

**Figure 11-25**

**ERYTHEMA ELEVATUM DIUTINUM: ADVANCED LESION**

Top: Secondary fibrosing alterations within the dermis are present along with residual foci of necrotizing vascular injury. The fibrosing response may at times produce tumoral nodules.

Bottom: At higher magnification, the chronic vascular injury is associated with marked fibroplasia within the perivascular connective tissue.

extensor surfaces and dorsum of the hands. Sweet syndrome is in the differential diagnosis of edematous lesions. Tuberous xanthoma or multicentric histiocytosis can be confused with the yellow nodular form of erythema elevatum diutinum.

**Treatment and Prognosis.** Patients respond to dapsone and sulfapyridine (74). As soon as the medications are withdrawn, the lesions exacerbate. Oral glucocorticoids are not helpful, but topical and intralesional formulations decrease the size of lesions. Niacinamide sometimes suppresses the eruption (75).

### Lymphocytic Vasculitis Group

**Definition.** *Lymphocytic vasculitis* are those disorders in which there is definite evidence of lymphocyte-mediated vascular injury, with or without fibrin deposition in the vessel walls, or thrombogenic changes within the vessel lumens (76,77). *Dysplastic lymphocytic vasculitis*, or *lymphomatoid vasculitis*, is a variant form in which the involved lymphoid elements are atypical because of immune activation or true dysplasia (e.g., as in lymphomatoid papulosis and angioimmunoblastic lymphadenopathy involving the skin).

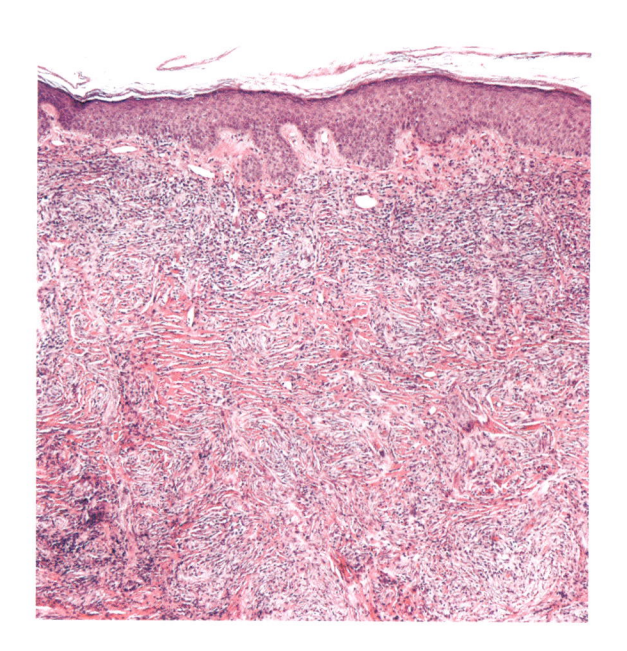

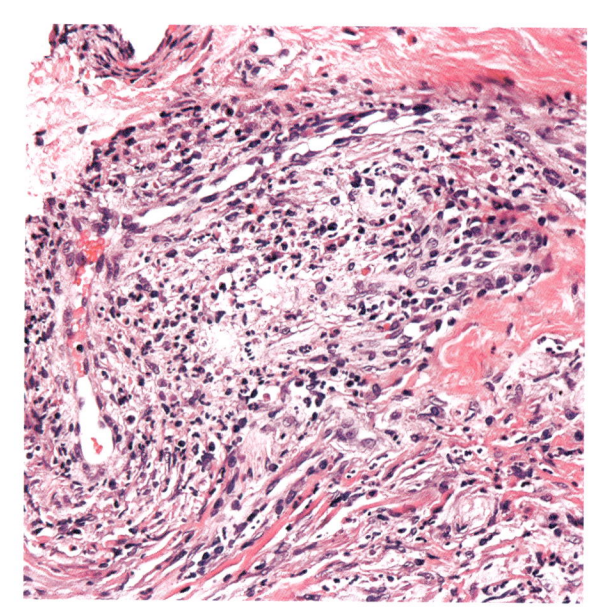

**Figure 11-26**

**ERYTHEMA ELEVATUM DIUTINUM: OLDER LESION**

Left: Chronic necrotizing vasculitis is associated with progressive and laminated fibrosis that extends from the involved superficial and deep blood vessels.

Right: Higher magnification shows blood vessels within the fibrotic dermis that demonstrate necrotizing vasculitis of both acute and chronic duration.

**Clinical Features.** The lesions of lymphocytic vasculitis characteristically are palpable purpura occurring on the lower extremities; the trunk may also be involved. Some lesions present as discrete ulcer nodules, others as hemorrhagic plaques. Several disorders cause lymphocytic vasculitis, with or without thrombosis. Many connective tissue diseases (lupus erythematosus, Sjögren syndrome, rheumatoid arthritis, Behçet disease, and at times relapsing polychondritis) are associated with lymphocytic vasculitis. When there is a thrombogenic vasculopathic process, it usually signals the presence of an associated lupus anticoagulant or cryofibrinogenemia. In such instances, the vasculitis results from an antibody-dependent cell-mediated response. While lupus anticoagulant and cryofibrinogenemia occur in systemic lupus erythematosus, they are also associated with lymphoproliferative processes that may be clinically covert, in which case they are designated as essential cryofibrogenemia or the primary antiphospholipid antibody syndrome.

*Perniosis* connotes often cold-associated, painful or pruritic, erythematous or violaceous papules or nodules occurring in acral sites that can present pathologically as lymphocytic vasculitis. Perniosis is idiopathic or associated with systemic disease. Many persons who have "idiopathic" perniosis may have atopy.

**Pathologic Findings.** Lymphocytic vasculitis defines several disorders in which perivascular cuffs of lymphocytes are associated with vascular damage, to a degree that perivascular hemorrhage may ensue. Insect bite reactions showing lymphocytic vasculitis are excellent examples of the prototypical alterations of this group of lesions. Histologically, superficial, deep, or superficial and deep dermal vessels are cuffed by lymphocytes. There may be perivascular hemorrhage and edema. A hallmark is the permeation of vessel walls by lymphocytes with associated signs of endothelial injury and sloughing (fig. 11-27). In severe cases, overt fibrinoid necrosis and fibrin thrombus formation may be noted.

**Differential Diagnosis.** The differential diagnosis includes palpable purpura of other causes including those associated with cutaneous necrotizing vasculitis, with its variety of etiologic agents. Also, disseminated intravascular

## Vasculitic Angiocentric Dermatitis

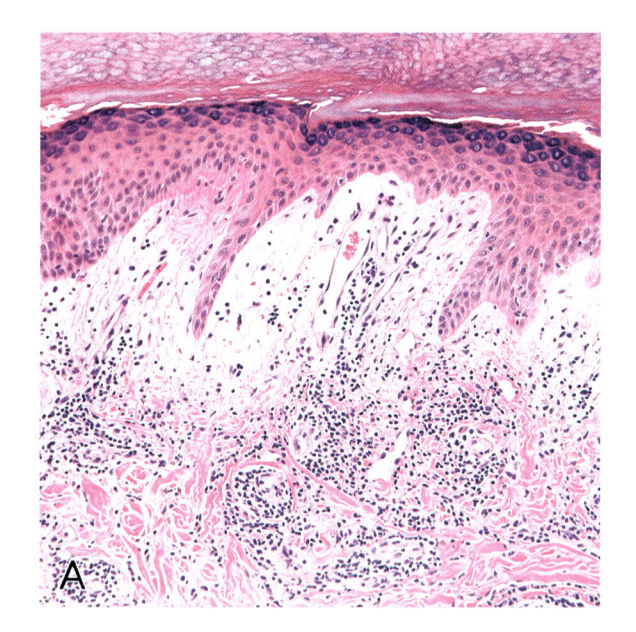

**Figure 11-27**

**LYMPHOCYTIC VASCULITIS (PERNIO)**

A: This biopsy of acral skin shows characteristic lymphocytic vasculitis and superficial dermal edema.

B: The lymphocytic vasculitis (lower left) and perieccrine involvement of the inflammatory component are typical of the deep dermal alterations of perniosis.

C: These small deep dermal vessels are permeated by lymphocytes and show variable endothelial degenerative changes with focal sloughing.

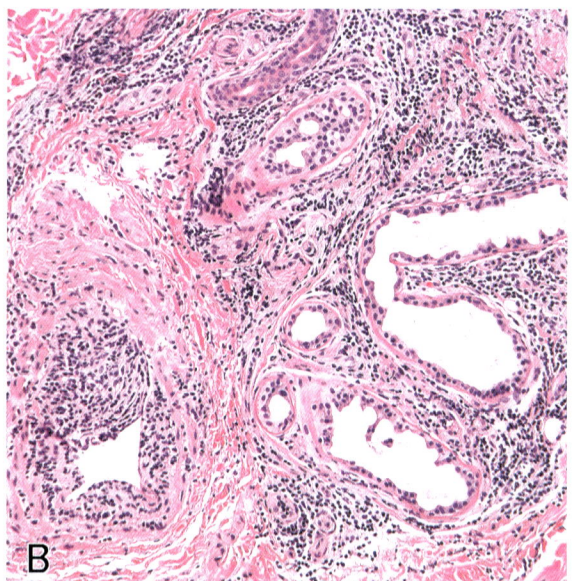

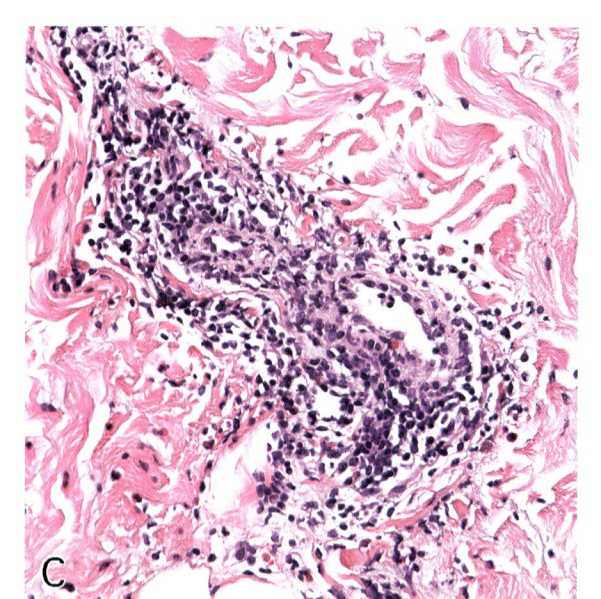

coagulation can present a clinical picture of palpable purpura and must be differentiated. Septic vasculitis may mimic lymphocytic vasculitis. Ulcerated lesions must be differentiated from vasculopathies or other causes of hemorrhagic ulcerative nodules including lymphomatoid vasculitis.

**Treatment and Prognosis.** The treatment is directed toward the underlying cause. Most frequently, prednisone is an appropriate immunosuppressive drug that may be used alone or in combination with other drugs for control of underlying disorders of connective tissue origin. Perniosis is treated with appropriate warm clothing to protect the extremities. Idiopathic lymphocytic vasculitis may only respond to prednisone therapy.

### Lymphomatoid Papulosis

**Definition.** *Lymphomatoid papulosis* is an asymptomatic disorder in which recurrent crops of papulonodular lesions occur and heal spontaneously (78–83). The chronic lesion is associated with cutaneous lymphoma.

**Clinical Features.** Lymphomatoid papulosis occurs any time in life, from childhood to old age, but most cases occur in mid-life. Both sexes

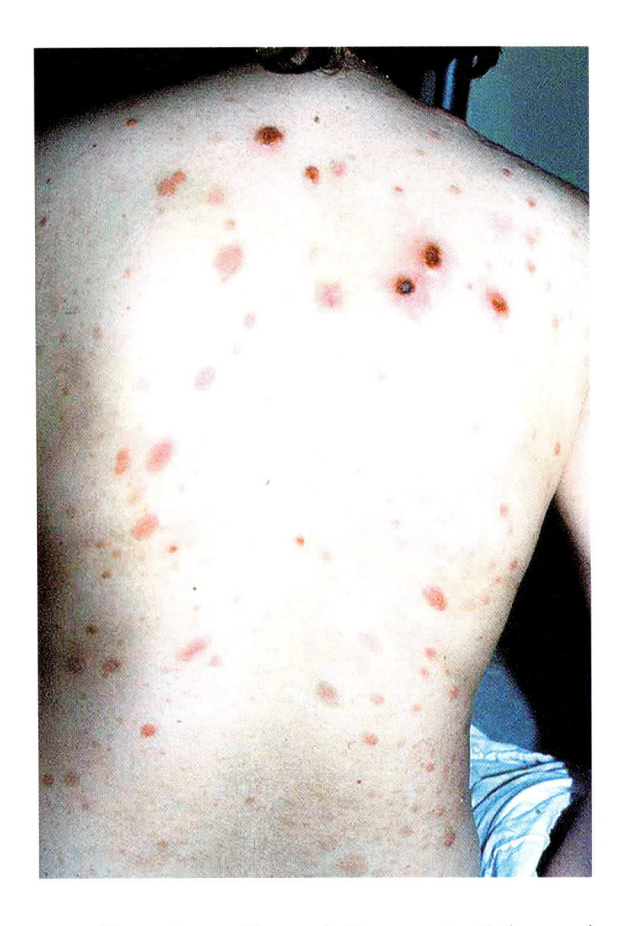

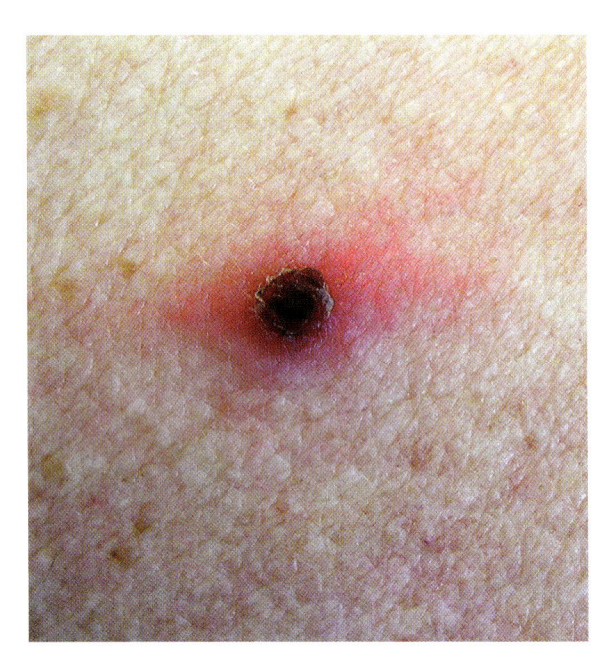

*Inflammatory Disorders of the Skin*

**Figure 11-28**

**LYMPHOMATOID PAPULOSIS**

Left: There are multiple plaques and "juicy" nodules, some with hemorrhagic centers.

Above: The erythematous papulonodule shows a central hemorrhagic crust.

are affected equally and the exact etiology of the disorder is not completely understood. The lesions are papulonodules of approximately 5 mm in diameter but may reach 1 cm or more. They begin as red erythematous and edematous papules and nodules that ulcerate and form a central, necrotic, black crust. There is usually a very polymorphous appearance to the lesions, because as early lesions occur other lesions mature and some spontaneously resolve (fig. 11-28): hence, the lesions of lymphomatoid papulosis are at different stages of development. Scarring sometimes accompanies healing. Most lesions last only a few weeks but the entire eruption may be chronic and recurrent over years, with patients going through lesion-free periods.

Lymphomatoid papulosis is associated with an underlying lymphoma in up to 20 percent of patients, especially mycosis fungoides, cutaneous anaplastic large cell lymphoma, CD30-positive large cell lymphoma and Hodgkin disease, and some consider lymphomatoid papulosis to represent a form of indolent cutaneous T-cell lymphoma.

**Pathologic Findings.** There are three main histologic subtypes of lymphomatoid papulosis: type A, type B, and type C, which represent a spectrum of disease with some overlapping features (84). In *type A lesions*, there is a superficial and deep perivascular and focally interstitial mixed inflammatory infiltrate consisting of variably atypical mononuclear cells, neutrophils, and occasional eosinophils (fig. 11-29). The infiltrate often forms a wedge-shaped pattern when observed at scanning magnification. The dominant atypical cell is an enlarged, 25- to 40-μm Reed-Sternberg (RS)-like cell with prominent nucleoli and occasional binucleation. There is positive staining for CD30. Epidermal infiltration is absent or inconspicuous, although keratinocyte necrosis and secondary inflammatory changes may develop in advanced lesions. The involved dermal vessels show endothelial prominence, focal necrosis, and sometimes perivascular hemorrhage, indicating a level of lymphocytic vasculitis.

The *type B pattern* shows a more monotonous infiltrate of small to medium-sized lymphocytes

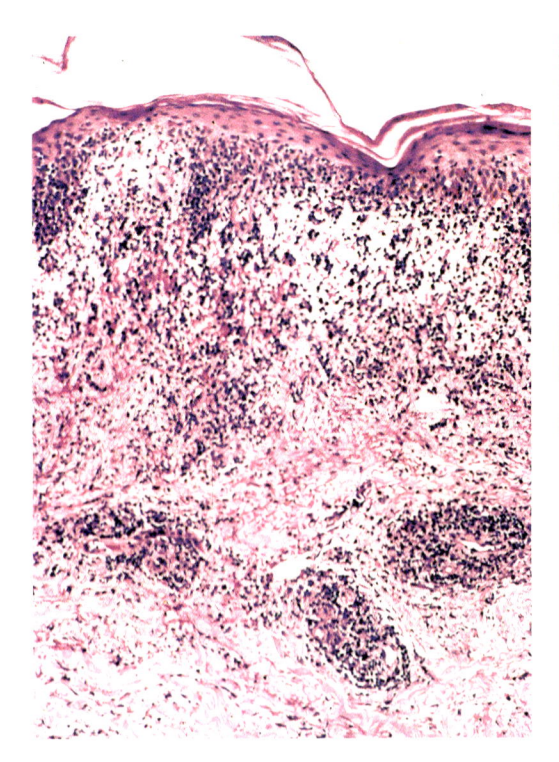

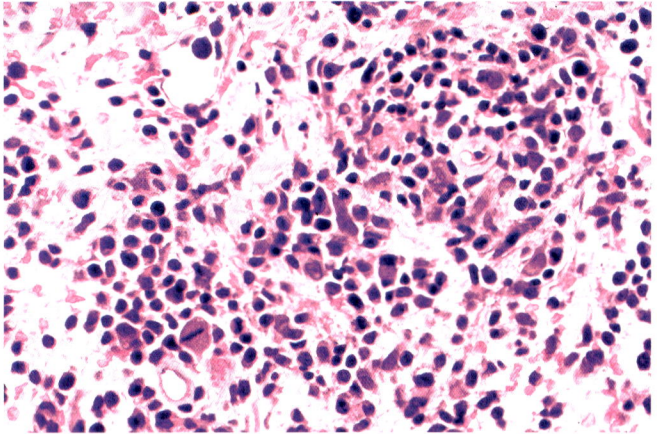

## Figure 11-29
### LYMPHOMATOID PAPULOSIS

Left: The intense angiocentric infiltrate consists of hyperchromatic mononuclear cells. The papillary dermal and epidermotropic involvement is characteristic of some lesions.

Above: Higher magnification shows marked polymorphism of the infiltrating lymphoid cells and associated foci of lymphocytic vasculitis.

about superficial and deep dermal vessels, although occasional neutrophils, histiocytes, eosinophils, and rare RS-like cells are detected. As in type A lesions, the angiocentric component is associated with focal lymphocytic vasculitis, but unlike the type A variant, there is interstitial papillary dermal involvement as well as frequent epidermotropism (fig. 11-30), producing a pattern that may closely mimic the epidermotropic variant of cutaneous T-cell lymphoma. The lymphoid cells in question may also show significant cytologic atypia, with nuclear hyperchromasia and complex contours, similar to the features of malignant T cells. Atypical cells may not express CD30 but are predominantly CD3+, CD4+, and CD8- in their staining pattern.

The *type C pattern* shows a monotonous cytologic population, often of large cells, with scant admixed inflammation. The staining phenotype, as with type A, is similar to cutaneous anaplastic large cell lymphoma.

Although T-cell marker analysis and PCR for T-cell receptor gene rearrangements help exclude overt malignancy when they fail to indicate clonality, positive results (abnormal CD4/CD8 ratios, loss of pan-T-cell maturation markers, and T-cell receptor gamma gene rearrangements) are not helpful, since numerous studies have indicated that such abnormalities are routinely seen in the setting of lymphomatoid papulosis.

**Differential Diagnosis.** Pityriasis lichenoides et varioliformis acuta (PLEVA) may exhibit a similar clinical picture but usually the lesions are small and differ histologically, although they may be difficult to distinguish from type B lymphomatoid papulosis. Other CD30+ lymphoproliferative disorders, particularly in chilren, must also be considered. Lymphoma cutis can present as ulceronodules and early lesions can resemble insect bite reactions.

Histologically, types A and C lymphomatoid papulosis must be differentiated from large cell anaplastic lymphoma. In lymphomatoid papulosis, less than 50 percent of the inflammatory component is represented by CD30+ RS-like cells. Anaplastic large cell kinase (ALK-1), if present, is highly suggestive of systemic disease or the propensity to develop anaplastic large cell lymphoma. Type B lesions must be differentiated from true cutaneous T-cell lymphoma. Since the papulonodular lesions of T-cell lymphoma are generally nonepidermotropic, whereas patch-plaque stages show epidermal involvement, the clinical features help separate the type

## Inflammatory Disorders of the Skin

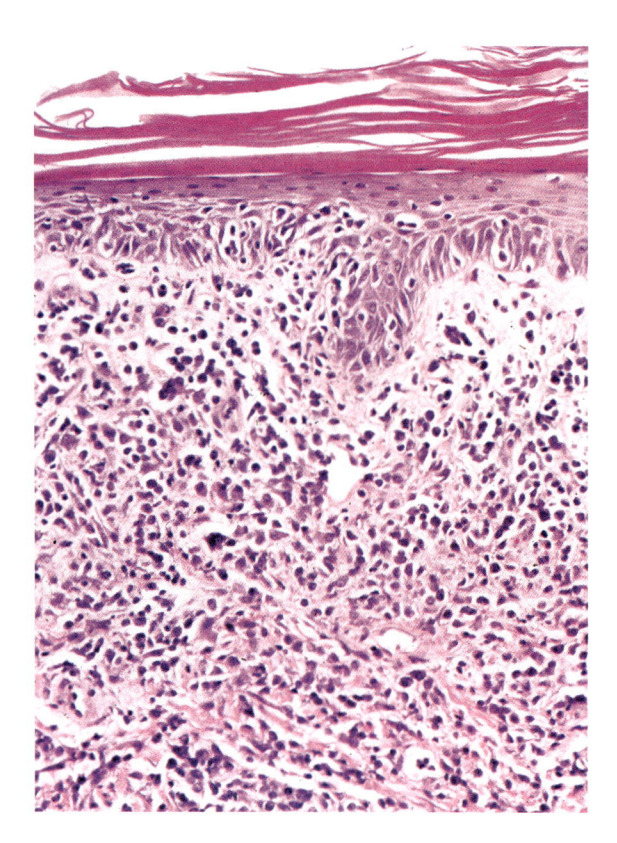

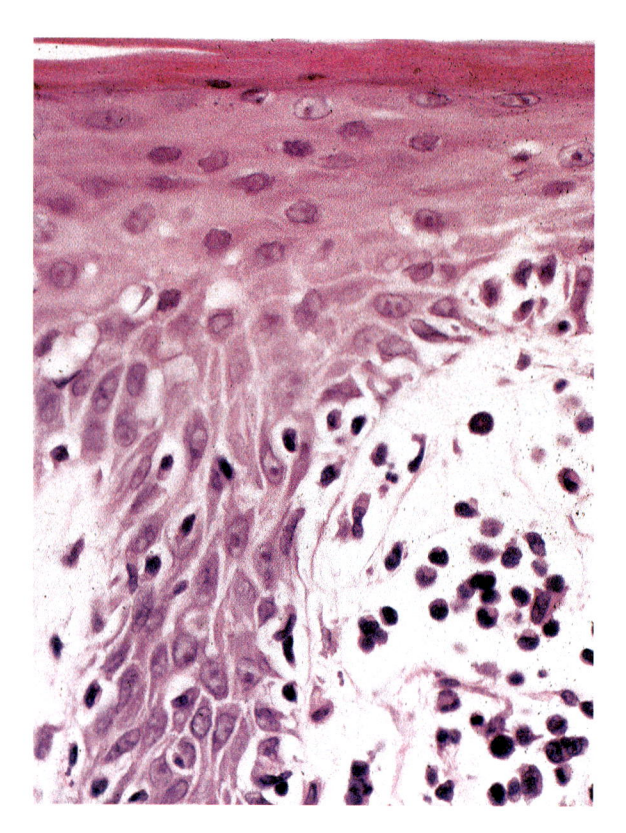

**Figure 11-30**

**LYMPHOMATOID PAPULOSIS**

Left: A markedly polymorphic mononuclear cell infiltrate is observed, with rare associated Reed-Sternberg-like forms. There is associated epidermotropism of atypical cells (type B).

Right: Higher magnification shows early epidermotropism of lymphocytes into the epidermis.

B variant from patch-plaque T-cell lymphoma, particularly in situations where cell marker analyses and PCR studies do not discriminate between these two entities.

**Treatment and Prognosis.** There is no standard successful treatment for this disorder. Electron beam therapy has been useful in some patients; PUVA (psoralen and ultraviolet A) can control local disease (85). Some patients respond to antibiotics, but of the many different types of treatments, including chemotherapeutic agents, none is universally successful in altering the recurrent course of the disease. Even treatment of the underlying lymphoma, when present, does not always result in resolution of the lesions of lymphomatoid papulosis. Low dose methotrexate, topical steroids, nitrogen mustard, and cyclophosphamide have been used in therapy. Excimer laser may be a useful adjunct to systemic therapy (85a).

### Angioimmunoblastic Lymphadenopathy Involving the Skin

**Definition.** *Angioimmunoblastic lymphadenopathy* is a lymphoproliferative disorder of T cells that affects the skin with a generalized eruption (86–92). It is a disease of older individuals and is characterized by generalized lymphadenopathy and hepatomegaly.

**Clinical Features.** This lesion occurs mainly in the sixth or seventh decade of life, and affects both men and women equally. About 40 percent of patients with this disorder develop skin lesions. The clinical symptoms include a rash that is usually maculopapular but sometimes has plaques and nodules. When maculopapular, the lesions often are itchy and may be scaly. There is an association with Epstein-Barr virus (EBV) infection, and with eventual T- and B-cell clonal evolution, with the development of peripheral

T-cell lymphoma and immunoblastic B-cell lymphoma in some patients.

**Pathologic Findings.** Like lymphomatoid papulosis, angioimmunoblastic lymphadenopathy involving the skin is a form of lymphocytic vasculitis with associated T-cell atypia. There is a superficial and deep, perivascular activated lymphocytic infiltrate, with admixed immunoblasts and plasma cells. The affected vessels may show endothelial prominence and necrosis, and perivascular hemorrhage may ensue. EBV is detectable immunohistochemically, and clonal T-cell receptor gene rearrangements are documented by PCR analysis.

**Differential Diagnosis.** The principal clinical differential diagnosis for the plaques and nodules is cutaneous mycosis fungoides or other types of cutaneous lymphoma. The maculopapular rash resembles a drug eruption or a viral exanthem. Histologically, lesions may be confused with lymphomatoid papulosis, although the typical RS cells and epidermotropic T cells of the type A and B variants, respectively, are not seen, and plasma cells are a prominent feature of the lymphocytic vasculitis of angioblastic lymphadenopathy.

**Treatment and Prognosis.** This disorder is a type of T-cell lymphoma and usually responds to appropriate chemotherapeutic agents, including cyclophosphamide, vincristine, daunorubicin, and prednisone. Interferon alpha-2a and radiation therapy have also been used. Some patients with the cutaneous eruption respond to PUVA therapy. With treatment, up to 25 percent of patients enter remission, although most die from disease, with a median survival period of 24 months. As a result, high-dose chemotherapy followed by bone marrow transplantation is gaining a greater role in therapy, particularly early in disease evolution.

## REFERENCES

1. Liao YH, Su YW, Tsay W, Chiu HC. Association of cutaneous necrotizing eosinophilic vasculitis and deep vein thrombosis in hypereosinophilic syndrome. Arch Dermatol 2005;141:1051-3.
2. Lotti TM, Comacchi C, Ghersetich I. Cutaneous necrotizing vasculitis. Relation to systemic disease. Adv Exp Med Biol 1999;455:115-25.
3. Campanile G, Hautmann G, Lotti TM. The etiology of cutaneous necrotizing vasculitis. Clin Dermatol 1999;17:505-8.
4. Curgunlu A, Karter Y, Uyanik O, Tunckale A, Curgunlu S. Leukocytoclastic vasculitis and renal cell carcinoma. Intern Med 2004;43:256-7.
5. Pique E, Palacios S, Santana Z. Leukocytoclastic vasculitis presenting as an erythema gyratum repens–like eruption on a patient with systemic lupus erythematosus. J Am Acad Dermatol 2002;47:S254-6.
6. Bielsa I, Carrascosa JM, Hausmann G, Ferrandiz C. An immunohistopathologic study in cutaneous necrotizing vasculitis. J Cutan Pathol 2000;27:130-5.
7. Gedalia A. Henoch-Schonlein purpura. Curr Rheumatol Rep 2004;6:195-202.
8. Ballinger S. Henoch-Schonlein purpura. Curr Opin Rheumatol 2003;15:591-4.
9. Allen NB, Bressler PB. Diagnosis and treatment of the systemic and cutaneous necrotizing vasculitis syndromes. Med Clin North Am 1997;81:243-59.
10. Mohan N, Kerr G. Infectious etiology of vasculitis: diagnosis and management. Curr Rheumatol Rep 2003;5:136-41.
11. Lie JT. Vasculitis associated with infectious agents. Curr Opin Rheumatol 1996;8:26-9.
12. Millikan LE, Flynn TC. Infectious etiologies of cutaneous vasculitis. Clin Dermatol 1999;17:509-14.
13. Davis MD, Brewer JD. Urticarial vasculitis and hypocomplementemic urticarial vasculitis syndrome. Immunol Allergy Clin North Am 2004;24:183-213, vi
14. Guha B, Youngberg G, Krishnaswamy G. Urticaria and urticarial vasculitis. Compr Ther 2003;29:146-56.
15. Venzor J, Lee WL, Huston DP. Urticarial vasculitis. Clin Rev Allergy Immunol 2002;23:201-16.
16. Black AK. Unusual urticarias. J Dermatol 2001;28:632-4.
17. Wisnieski JJ. Urticarial vasculitis. Curr Opin Rheumatol 2000;12:24-31.
18. Bratton RL, Corey R. Tick-borne disease. Am Fam Physician 2005;71:2323-30.

19. Amsden JR, Warmack S, Gubbins PO. Tick-borne bacterial, rickettsial, spirochetal, and protozoal infectious diseases in the United States: a comprehensive review. Pharmacotherapy 2005;25:191-210.
20. Rizzo M, Mansueto P, Di Lorenzo G, Morselli S, Mansueto S, Rini GB. Rickettsial disease: classical and modern aspects. New Microbiol 2004;27:87-103.
21. Masters EJ, Olson GS, Weiner SJ, Paddock CD. Rocky Mountain spotted fever: a clinician's dilemma. Arch Intern Med 2003;163:769-74.
22. Warner RD, Marsh WW. Rocky Mountain spotted fever. J Am Vet Med Assoc 2002;221:1413-7.
23. Sexton DJ, Kaye KS. Rocky mountain spotted fever. Med Clin North Am 2002;86:351-60.
24. Buckingham SC. Rocky Mountain spotted fever: a review for the pediatrician. Pediatr Ann 2002;31:163-8.
25. Thorner AR, Walker DH, Petri WA Jr. Rocky mountain spotted fever. Clin Infect Dis 1998;27:1353-9.
26. Donovan BJ, Weber DJ, Rublein JC, Raasch RH. Treatment of tick-borne diseases. Ann Pharmacother 2002;36:1590-7.
27. Herbert CR, Russo GG. Polyarteritis nodosa and cutaneous polyarteritis nodosa. Skinmed 2003;2:277-83.
28. Gushi A, Hashiguchi T, Fukumaru K, Usuki K, Kanekura T, Kanzaki T. Three cases of polyarteritis nodosa cutanea and a review of the literature. J Dermatol 2000;27:778-81.
29. Khoo BP, Ng SK. Cutaneous polyarteritis nodosa: a case report and literature review. Ann Acad Med Singapore 1998;27:868-72.
30. Naschitz JE, Kovaleva J, Shaviv N, Rennert G, Yeshurun D. Vascular disorders preceding diagnosis of cancer: distinguishing the causal relationship based on Bradford-Hill guidelines. Angiology 2003;54:11-7.
31. Pena-penabad C, Martinez W, del Pozo J, Garcia-Silva J, Yebra MT, Fonseca E. Guess what! Superficial migratory thrombophlebitis. Thromboangiitis obliterans (Buerger's disease). Eur J Dermatol 2000;10:405-6.
32. Lesher JL Jr. Superficial migratory thrombophlebitis. Cutis 1991;47:177-80.
33. Samlaska CP, James WD, Simel DL. Superficial migratory thrombophlebitis and factor XII deficiency. J Am Acad Dermatol 1990;22:939-43.
34. Gibbs MB, English JC 3rd, Zirwas MJ. Livedo reticularis: an update. J Am Acad Dermatol 2005;52:1009-19.
35. Kraemer M, Linden D, Berlit P. The spectrum of differential diagnosis in neurological patients with livedo reticularis and livedo racemosa A literature review. J Neurol 2005;252:1155-66.
36. Toubi E, Krause I, Fraser A, et al. Livedo reticularis is a marker for predicting multi-system thrombosis in antiphospholipid syndrome. Clin Exp Rheumatol 2005;23:499-504.
37. Sladden MJ, Nicolaou N, Johnston GA, Hutchinson PE. Livedo reticularis induced by amantadine. Br J Dermatol 2003;149:656-8.
38. Calamia KT, Balabanova M, Perniciaro C, Walsh JS. Livedo (livedoid) vasculitis and the factor V Leiden mutation: additional evidence for abnormal coagulation. J Am Acad Dermatol 2002;46:133-7.
39. Maessen-Visch MB. Atrophie blanche. Eur J Obstet Gynecol Reprod Biol 2000;90:1-2.
40. Maessen-Visch MB, Koedam MI, Hamulyak K, Neumann HA. Atrophie blanche. Int J Dermatol 1999;38:161-72.
41. Marquez J, Flores D, Candia L, Espinoza LR. Granulomatous vasculitis. Curr Rheumatol Rep 2003;5:128-35.
42. Callen JP. Cutaneous vasculitis: relationship to systemic disease and therapy. Curr Probl Dermatol 1993;5;50-80.
43. Jennette CJ, Milling DM, Falk RJ. Vasculitis affecting the skin. A review. Arch Dermatol 1994;130:899-906.
44. Sabat M, Leulmo J, Saez A. Cutaneous granulomatous vasculitis in metastatic Crohn's disease. J Eur Acad Dermatol Venereol 2005;19:652-3.
45. Weidner N. Giant-cell vasculitides. Semin Diagn Pathol 2001;18:24-33.
46. Gibson LE. Granulomatous vasculitides and the skin. Dermatol Clin 1990;8:335-45.
47. Kawakami T, Obara W, Soma Y, Mizoguchi M. Palisading neutrophilic granulomatous dermatitis in a Japanese patient with Wegener's granulomatosis. J Dermatol 2005;32:487-92.
48. Kuchel J, Lee S. Cutaneous Wegener's granulomatosis: a variant or atypical localized form? Australas J Dermatol 2003;44:129-35.
49. Crowson AN, Mihm MC Jr, Magro CM. Cutaneous vasculitis: a review. J Cutan Pathol 2003;30:161-73.
50. Stein SL, Miller LC, Konnikov N. Wegener's granulomatosis: case report and literature review. Pediatr Dermatol 1998;15:352-6.
51. Hewins P, Tervaert JW, Savage CO, Kallenberg CG. Is Wegener's granulomatosis an autoimmune disease? Curr Opin Rheumatol 2000;12:3-10.
52. Langford CA. Wegener's granulomatosis: current and upcoming therapies. Arthritis Res Ther 2003;5:180-91.
53. Regan MJ, Hellmann DB, Stone JH. Treatment of Wegener's granulomatosis. Rheum Dis Clin North Am 2001;27:863-86.
54. Narayan J, Douglas-Jones AG. Eosinophilic angiocentric fibrosis and granuloma faciale: analy-

sis of cellular infiltrate and review of literature. Ann Otol Rhinol Laryngol 2005;114:35-42.
55. LeBoit PE. Granuloma faciale: a diagnosis deserving of dignity. Am J Dermatopathol 2002;24:440-3.
56. Inanir I, Alvur Y. Granuloma faciale with extrafacial lesions. Br J Dermatol 2001;145:360-2.
57. Roustan G, Sanchez Yus E, Salas C, Simon A. Granuloma faciale with extrafacial lesions. Dermatology 1999;198:79-82.
58. Dowlati B, Firooz A, Dowlati Y. Granuloma faciale: successful treatment of nine cases with a combination of cryotherapy and intralesional corticosteroid injection. Int J Dermatol 1997;36:548-51.
59. Elston DM. Treatment of granuloma faciale with the pulsed dye laser. Cutis 2000;65:97-8.
60. Meyerson MS. Erythema nodosum leprosum. Int J Dermatol 1996;35:389-92.
61. Girdhar A, Chakma JK, Girdhar BK. Pulsed corticosteroid therapy in patients with chronic recurrent ENL: a pilot study. Indian J Lepr 2002;74:233-6.
62. Sampaio EP, Hernandez MO, Carvalho DS, Sarno EN. Management of erythema nodosum leprosum by thalidomide: thalidomide analogues inhibit M. leprae-induced TNFalpha production in vitro. Biomed Pharmacother 2002;56:13-9.
63. Perri AJ 3rd, Hsu S. A review of thalidomide's history and current dermatological applications. Dermatol Online J 2003;9:5.
64. Nasca MR, Micali G, Cheigh NH, West LE, West DP. Dermatologic and nondermatologic uses of thalidomide. Ann Pharmacother 2003;37:1307-20.
65. Teo SK, Resztak KE, Scheffler MA, et al. Thalidomide in the treatment of leprosy. Microbes Infect 2002;4:1193-202.
66. Okafor MC. Thalidomide for erythema nodosum leprosum and other applications. Pharmacotherapy 2003;23:481-93.
67. Wahl CE, Bouldin MB, Gibson LE. Erythema elevatum diutinum: clinical, histopathologic, and immunohistochemical characteristics of six patients. Am J Dermatopathol 2005;27:397-400.
68. Gibson LE, el-Azhary RA. Erythema elevatum diutinum. Clin Dermatol 2000;18:295-9.
69. Burnett PE, Burgin S. Erythema elevatum diutinum. Dermatol Online J 2003;9:37.
70. Ly H, Black MM. Atypical presentation of erythema elevatum diutinum. Australas J Dermatol 2005;46:44-6.
71. Yamamoto T, Nakamura S, Nishioka K. Erythema elevatum diutinum associated with Hashimoto's thyroiditis and antiphospholipid antibodies. J Am Acad Dermatol 2005;52:165-6.
72. Lisi S, Mussi A, Muscardin L, Carducci M. A case of erythema elevatum diutinum associated with antiphospholipid antibodies. J Am Acad Dermatol 2003;49:963-4.
73. High WA, Hoang MP, Stevens K, Cockerell CJ. Late-stage nodular erythema elevatum diutinum. J Am Acad Dermatol 2003;49:764-7.
74. Grabbe J, Haas N, Moller A, Henz BM. Erythema elevatum diutinum—evidence for disease-dependent leucocyte alterations and response to dapsone. Br J Dermatol 2000;143:415-20.
75. Kohler IK, Lorincz AL. Erythema elevatum diutinum treated with niacinamide and tetracycline. Arch Dermatol 1980;116:693-5.
76. Kossard S. Defining lymphocytic vasculitis. Australas J Dermatol 2000;41:149-55.
77. Oh CW, Lee SH, Heo EP. A case suggesting lymphocytic vasculitis as a presenting sign of early undifferentiated connective tissue disease. Am J Dermatopathol 2003;25:423-7.
78. Aoki E, Aoki M, Kono M, Kawana S. Two cases of lymphomatoid papulosis in children. Pediatr Dermatol 2003;20:146-9.
79. Deroo-Berger MC, Skowron F, Ronger S, et al. Lymphomatoid papulosis: a localized form with acral pustular involvement. Dermatology 2002;205:60-2.
80. Kagaya M, Kondo S, Kamada A, Yamada Y, Matsusaka H, Jimbow K. Localized lymphomatoid papulosis. Dermatology 2002;204:72-4.
81. Bekkenk MW, Kluin PM, Jansen PM, Meijer CJ, Willemze R. Lymphomatoid papulosis with a natural killer-cell phenotype. Br J Dermatol 2001;145:318-22.
82. Van Neer FJ, Toonstra J, Van Voorst Vader PC, Willemze R, Van Vloten WA. Lymphomatoid papulosis in children: a study of 10 children registered by the Dutch Cutaneous Lymphoma Working Group. Br J Dermatol 2001;144:351-4.
83. Drews R, Samel A, Kadin ME. Lymphomatoid papulosis and anaplastic large cell lymphomas of the skin. Semin Cutan Med Surg 2000;19:109-17.
84. Willemze R, Jaffe ES, Burg G, et al. WHO-EORTC classification for cutaneous lymphoma. Blood 2005;105:3768-85.
85. Gambichler T, Maushagen E, Menzel S. Foil bath PUVA in lymphomatoid papulosis. J Eur Acad Dermatol Venereol 1999;13:63-5.
85a. Kontos AP, Kerr HA, Malick F, Fivenson DP, Lim HW, Wong HK. 308-nm excimer laser for the treatment of lymphomatoid papulosis and stage 1A mycosis fungoides. Photodermatol Photoimmunol Photomed 2006;22:168-71.
86. Huang CT, Chuang SS. Angioimmunoblastic T-cell lymphoma with cutaneous involvement: a case report with subtle histologic changes and clonal T-cell proliferation. Arch Pathol Lab Med 2004;128:e122-4.

87. Diabata M, Ido E, Murakami K, et al. Angioimmunoblastic lymphadenopathy with disseminated human herpesvirus 6 infection in a patient with acute myeloblastic leukemia. Leukemia 1997;11:882-5.
88. Yoon GS, Chang SE, Kim HH, Choi JH, Sung KJ, Moon KC. Cutaneous relapse of angioimmunoblastic lymphadenopathy-type peripheral T-cell lymphoma mimicking and exanthematous drug eruption. Int J Dermatol 2003;42:816-8.
89. Brown HA, Macon WR, Kurtin PJ, Gibson LE. Cutaneous involvement by angioimmunoblastic T-cell lymphoma with remarkable heterogeneous Epstein-Barr virus expression. J Cutan Pathol 2001;28:432-8.
90. Mahendran R, Grant JW, Hoggarth CE, Burrows NP. Angioimmunoblastic T-cell lymphoma with cutaenous involvement. J Eur Acad Dermatol Venereol 2001;15:589-90.
91. Murakami T, Ohtsuki M, Nakagawa H. Angioimmunoblastic lymphadenopathy-type peripheral T-cell lypmphoma with cutaneous infiltration: report of a case and its gene expression profile. Br J Dermatol 2001;144:878-84.
92. Suarez-Vilela D, Izquierdo-Garcia FM. Angioimmunoblastic lymphadenopathy-like T-cell lymphoma: cutaneous clinical onset with prominent granulomatous reaction. Am J Surg Pathol 2003;27:699-700.

# 12 NODULAR/INTERSTITIAL DERMATITIS

## GENERAL CONSIDERATIONS

*Nodular/interstitial dermatitis* constitutes a limited number of conditions without *primary* epidermal alterations that present initially with interstitial to nodular dermal inflammatory infiltrates rather than angiocentric patterns. It encompasses most of the neutrophilic and histiocytic/granulomatous forms of dermatitis.

There are relatively few dermatoses that are dominated by granulocytes. The prototypical cause of granulocytic infiltration of the skin is bacterial infection. Neutrophils within a scale-crust associated with superficial forms of bacterial infection (e.g., impetigo) produce a clinical and histologic picture often referred to as impetiginization. Pustules are generally associated with microabscesses, which are small, tumor-like aggregates of granulocytes. Microabscesses occur within or beneath the stratum corneum, within the epidermis or follicular epithelium, or within the dermis. Pyoderma is the diffuse, extensive, and permeative infiltration of the dermis by granulocytes.

The clinical spectrum of granulocytic dermatitis is variable. Small lesions associated with microabscess formation often present as pinpoint pustules, whereas large, deep abscesses may appear as painful erythematous nodules. Considerable edema and fibrin extravasation often accompany less localized granulocytic infiltrates, producing indurated, erythematous plaques. The potent proteolytic enzymes released by activated granulocytes frequently cause secondary injury to surrounding cells and structures, especially in chronic lesions. In these instances, it is not unusual for epidermal breakdown and frank ulceration to ensue. Tumoral aggregates of malignant granulocytes result in a clinical lesion termed *chloroma*, which characteristically appears as a greenish nodule.

The term *granulomatous dermatitis* is used in this chapter to designate diverse cutaneous inflammatory disorders characterized by dermal and sometimes subcutaneous granulomas. A granuloma is a localized collection of activated histiocytes which may be rimmed by lymphocytes and/or show central necrosis. Activated histiocytes are macrophage-derived cells that ingest either foreign particulates or protein antigens, resulting in attempted lysosomal degradation or antigen processing and presentation. Activated histiocytes often become enlarged, sometimes exhibit multinucleation, and generally show conspicuous eosinophilic cytoplasm that resembles that of epithelial cells. Thus, such cells are often referred to as epithelioid histiocytes.

Particulate material ingested by histiocytes may be birefringent and detectable by polarization microscopy within cytoplasmic granules. Stimuli for epithelioid cell transformation may not be detected, although certain features presumably related to provocative agents may be visible, as is seen with lysosomal intracellular arrays (e.g., asteroid bodies in sarcoidosis). The pattern of multinucleation within granulomas may be of diagnostic significance, as is the case in cutaneous tuberculosis, in which these cells often have wreath-like configurations of nuclei about the cell perimeter (i.e., Langhans giant cells). Foreign-body giant cells, on the other hand, tend to have more centrally clustered nuclei without a well-defined wreath-like configuration. A marked arrangement of the nuclei in an arrow-like or bizarre irregularly shaped figure characterizes the multinucleate cells of necrobiotic xanthogranuloma. The presence or absence of central necrosis within granulomas is of limited diagnostic assistance, although the prototypical lesion of sarcoidosis is often described as composed of predominantly noncaseating, naked (i.e., free of surrounding lymphocytes) granulomas. Granulomas with extensive necrosis, conversely, often suggest the presence of causative organisms, as is the case in mycobacterial and deep mycotic infections.

Such granulomas form aggregates about degenerating, or necrobiotic, collagen. Necrobiosis may be associated with mucin deposition, as in granuloma annulare; fibrinoid degeneration of collagen, as seen in a rheumatoid nodule; or sclerosis and homogenization of collagen bundles, as is typical in necrobiosis lipoidica. In all of these disorders, well-formed granulomas are characterized by an array of histiocytes radially arranged about the perimeter of the necrobiotic zone, with the long axes of each cell in parallel (i.e., palisaded granulomas).

The pattern formed by granulomatous inflammation in the skin may be of diagnostic assistance. In sarcoidosis, granulomas are randomly scattered throughout the superficial and deep dermis, whereas in leprosy, they tend to wind around neurovascular bundles in a serpiginous manner. Granulomas in secondary syphilis are poorly formed and tend to be concentrated within the papillary dermis in association with cytotoxic alterations of the basal cell layer. In the granulomatous inflammation that accompanies follicular perforation, the histiocytic aggregates are centered about the offending pilar epithelium.

The gross pathology of granulomatous dermatitis is highly variable. Often, early lesions are covered by a smooth epidermal surface that is unaffected by the underlying dermal inflammation. In advanced disease, ulceration may be present, particularly if there is transepidermal elimination of granulomatous foci or underlying vascular compromise. Although erythema may be present as a result of varying degrees of secondary angiocentric lymphocytic inflammation, the granulomatous foci themselves are not red. Rather, they tend to display a green-yellow hue like apple jelly, especially when background erythema is eliminated by diascopy (i.e., downward compression over the lesion with a flat glass slide).

The clinical appearance of granulomatous dermatitis helps in the differential diagnostic assessment. Chromomycosis, for example, often exhibits numerous black dots on the lesion surface, the result of transepidermal elimination of pigmented spores. Leprosy may present as a plaque with associated anesthesia, indicative of extensive involvement and destruction of underlying cutaneous nerves. Localization of plaques to anatomic sites of environmental and occupational contact provides important clues to the diagnosis, as is the case in zirconium-induced granulomatous dermatitis of axillary skin due to the application of antiperspirants. Finally, certain forms of granulomatous dermatitis have a characteristic gross pathologic presentation, as is the case with the circinate dermal papules of granuloma annulare.

## PATHOGENESIS

The general histologic appearance of granulocytic dermatitis depends on the predominant cell type (e.g., neutrophil or eosinophil) and the architectural pattern produced by the cutaneous infiltration (e.g., aggregated versus diffuse, association with preexisting structures such as hair follicles). Although acute lesions generally show only infiltrating granulocytes and edema, both of which are often extensive, chronic lesions often demonstrate secondary tissue injury and fibrosis. The presence of secondary injury is important because certain differential diagnoses hinge on reconstruction of the chronology of events within a biopsy specimen. For example, similar patterns of neutrophilic infiltration may be produced in septic vasculitis and acute febrile neutrophilic dermatitis. The former, however, is characterized by primary vascular injury, which is present at very early stages of lesion formation and is often detected at the edge of a given lesion. The latter, conversely, shows foci of secondary vessel injury in established regions, but zones of early neutrophil infiltration, at the margin of a lesion, are devoid of vessel degeneration or necrosis.

Early phases of granulomatous dermatitis may exhibit a remarkably nonspecific histologic picture, often dominated by an angiocentric lymphocytic inflammatory infiltrate, with few aggregated epithelioid histiocytes. Histiocytic infiltration may be insidious in the early stages, as is the case in palisaded granulomatous dermatitis, in which histiocytes are present in small numbers among collagen bundles. As histiocytes begin to aggregate to form discrete granulomas, epithelioid cell transformation, accompanied by cytoplasmic eosinophilia and multinucleation, becomes increasingly apparent. With chronicity, granulomas become associated with zones of fibrosis and collagen deposition, as is the case in the longstanding lesions of silicosis.

Cytokine networks are believed to play a major role in the pathogenesis of both granulocytic and granulomatous dermal infiltrates, although the provocative antigens are highly variable and most remain to be elucidated. Recently, overexpression of interleukin 8 has been shown to produce cutaneous lesions similar to the pyodermal gangrenosum form of neutrophilic dermatosis in a murine-human skin xenograft model (1).

## SPECIAL DIAGNOSTIC STUDIES

Tissue Gram stain is helpful in assessing the presence of bacteria in granulocytic dermatitis, and periodic acid–Schiff (PAS), silver, and acid fast bacillus (AFB) stains, as well as polarization microscopy, are useful for excluding fungi, mycobacteria, and birefringent particulates. Culture of fresh tissue is often more sensitive than histochemical staining for detecting organisms, and culture is requisite for establishing sensitivities to appropriate antibiotic agents.

## PRIMARILY GRANULOCYTIC NODULAR/INTERSTITIAL INFILTRATES

### Acute Febrile Neutrophilic Dermatitis (Sweet Syndrome)

**Definition.** *Acute febrile neutrophilic dermatitis*, or *Sweet syndrome*, is a recurrent skin disorder that is associated with inflammatory, often edematous bright red plaques that are associated with the systemic symptoms of fever and arthralgia. Peripheral neutrophilia is striking and the syndrome is associated with many other diseases (1a–8).

**Clinical Features.** This uncommon disorder usually occurs in the fourth to the seventh decade, but may occur at any time. Women are more commonly affected than men. Although the exact etiology is unknown, it is associated with a variety of other disorders including connective tissue disease, *Yersinia* infection, hematologic malignancies, both leukemia and lymphoma, and underlying visceral carcinomas (9–12).

Characteristically, the lesion begins with an upper respiratory tract infection, gastrointestinal symptoms such as diarrhea, or a flu-like illness that occurs a few weeks before the skin lesion. Fever may be present. The bright red smooth-topped lesions coalesce to form markedly erythematous and edematous plaques (fig. 12-1). There is so much edema that many of the lesions appear vesicular. At the height of the eruption, the lesions are tender. They appear rapidly and resolve with central clearing and a resultant irregular pattern with an arcuate contour. Pustules may occur. There is a bullous form of this disorder that more commonly occurs in association with acute leukemia.

The areas of most striking involvement are the face, neck, and upper extremities, which are affected asymmetrically. Lower extremity involvement is noted but often appears as a panniculitis. The lesions usually resolve spontaneously in a few days to a few weeks but recur unless the underlying cause is found and treated.

**Pathologic Findings.** Acute febrile neutrophilic dermatitis is characterized by coalescent interstitial aggregates of neutrophils, some arranged in a perivascular array, within the superficial and deep dermis (figs. 12-2–12-4) (12). Closer inspection reveals nuclear fragmentation (i.e., "nuclear dust") and occasional fibrin deposits but no evidence of true primary necrotizing vasculitis. Malone et al. (13) have reported that in up to 30 percent of biopsies of neutrophilic dermatosis, a secondary vasculitis is observed as the result of the neutrophilic activity. Although the presence of secondary vasculitis-like changes does not rule out the diagnosis of neutrophilic dermatosis, evidence of primary vasculitis should suggest an alternative diagnosis (14). Although the epidermis is generally spared, some lesions show spongiosis and upward percolation of individual neutrophils between adjacent keratinocytes. The papillary dermis may be markedly edematous, accounting for the superficial dermal vesicles that occur in blistering variants (fig. 12-5).

**Differential Diagnosis.** Lesions most commonly on the extremities, face, and neck resemble erythema multiforme. Some lesions resemble the acute phase of pyodermic gangrenosum. Lesions on the lower extremities must be differentiated from erythema nodosum. Drug eruptions have similar features. Histologically, early neutrophilic dermatosis should be distinguished from Still disease (fig. 12-6). Bacterial infection resulting in cellulitis, and primary vasculitis (as discussed above) also must be considered.

**Treatment and Prognosis.** These lesions usually respond to oral prednisone in a moderate

*Inflammatory Disorders of the Skin*

**Figure 12-1**

**ACUTE FEBRILE NEUTROPHILIC DERMATITIS (SWEET SYNDROME)**

There are multiple, focally coalescent, tender, raised erythematous plaques.

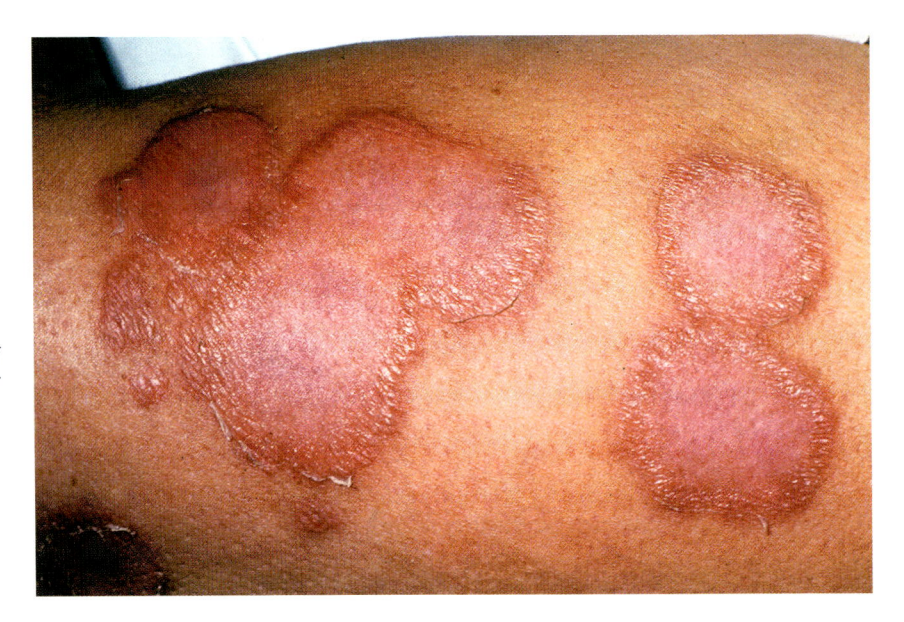

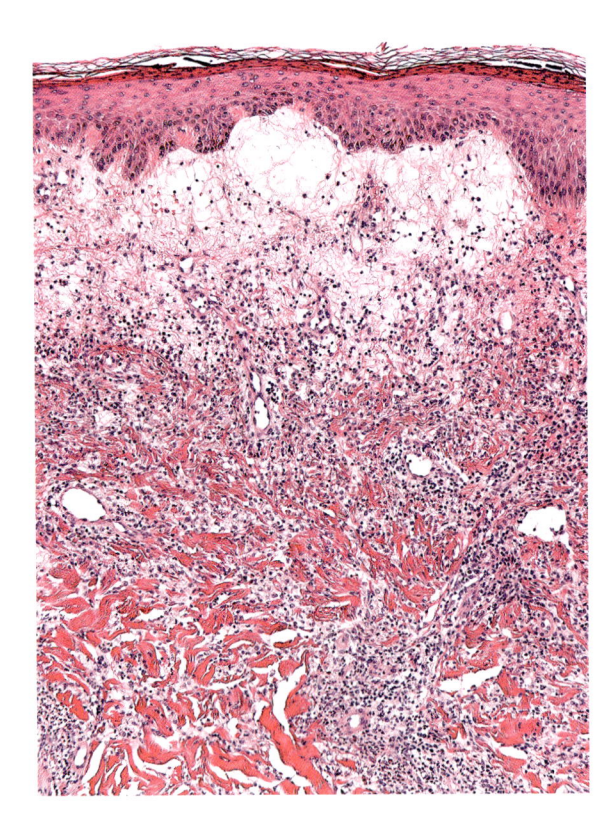

**Figure 12-2**

**ACUTE FEBRILE NEUTROPHILIC DERMATITIS**

There is a nodular interstitial infiltrate composed of neutrophils within the superficial and deep dermis. Advanced lesions, as seen here, may resemble the early evolutionary stages of pyoderma gangrenosum.

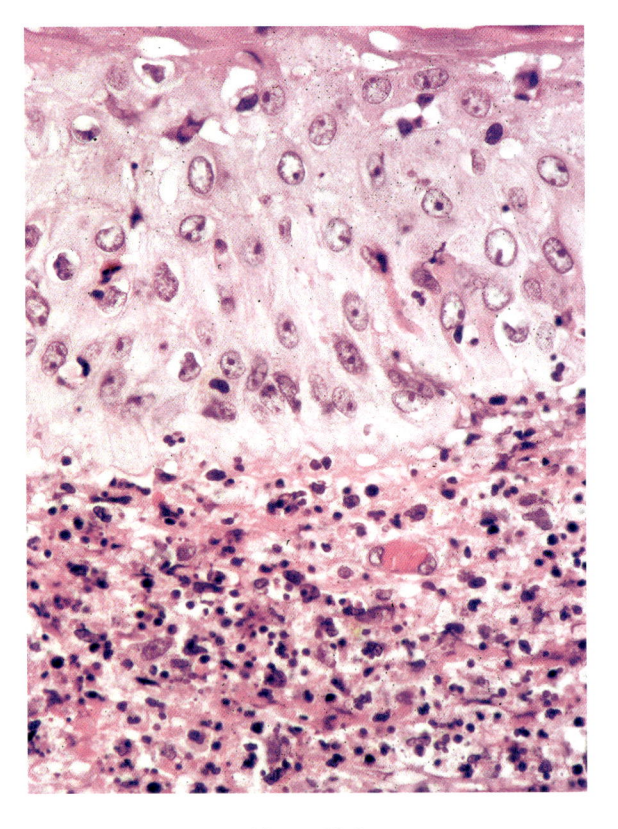

**Figure 12-3**

**ACUTE FEBRILE NEUTROPHILIC DERMATITIS**

At the dermal-epidermal junction, the neutrophilic infiltrate occupies the papillary dermis, although primary epidermal alterations are lacking. Infiltration of the epidermis and ulceration are generally absent.

treatment dose (13). Occasionally, potassium iodide has been used. Eruptions associated with infections respond to antibiotic therapy while dapsone, doxycycline, and clofazimine are used in idiopathic cases. The use of colchicine and cyclosporine has been reported in the literature.

### Eosinophilic Cellulitis (Wells Syndrome)

**Definition.** The uncommon *eosinophilic cellulitis*, or *Wells syndrome*, is associated with recurrent cutaneous plaque-like lesions and swelling that resolve after days to weeks and may, rarely, occur in a familial setting (14–20).

**Clinical Features.** There is often a prodrome of burning or itching, which is then followed rapidly by prominent erythema and swelling. It occurs anywhere on the skin but most commonly on the trunk. The lesions may be single or multiple, and evolve into large areas of edema with violaceous borders resembling morphea. The lesions last for days to weeks, and as they evolve, progress from bright red to rusty colored to finally blue-gray. The etiology of this disorder is unknown but it is occasionally associated with atopic dermatitis, some parasitic diseases, and drug reactions. In most cases an underlying cause is not discovered.

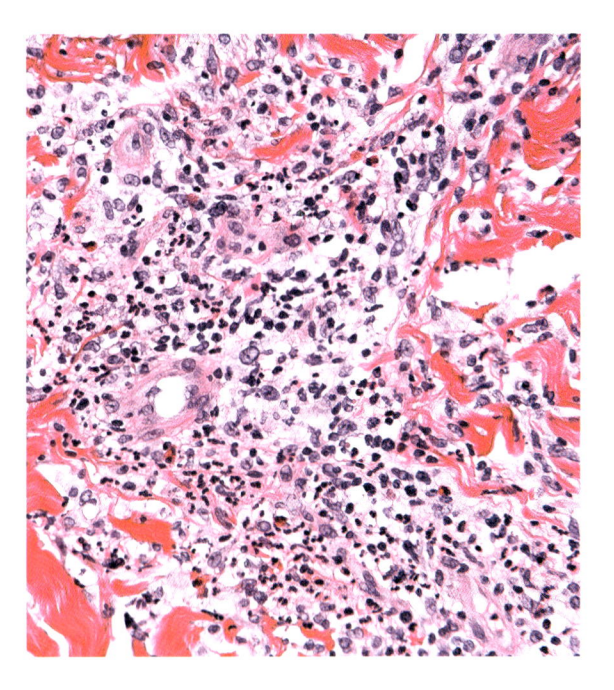

Figure 12-4
ACUTE FEBRILE NEUTROPHILIC DERMATITIS
Although the neutrophilic infiltrate is marked and secondary vascular injury may occur, evidence of primary vasculitis is lacking at high magnification.

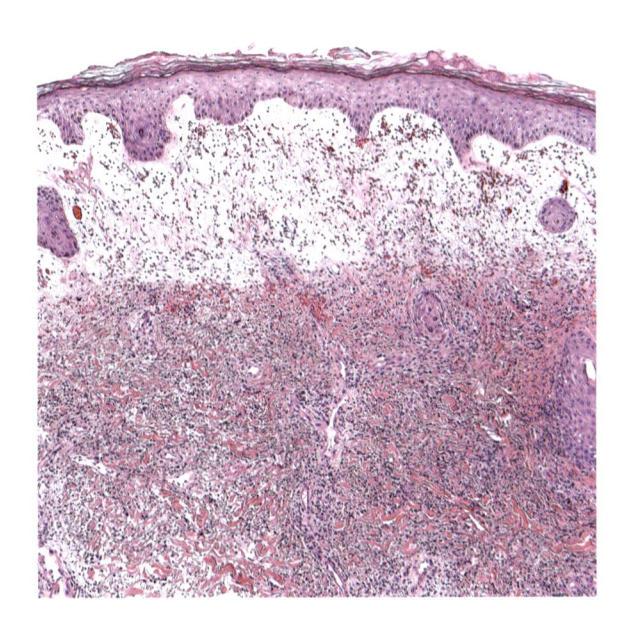

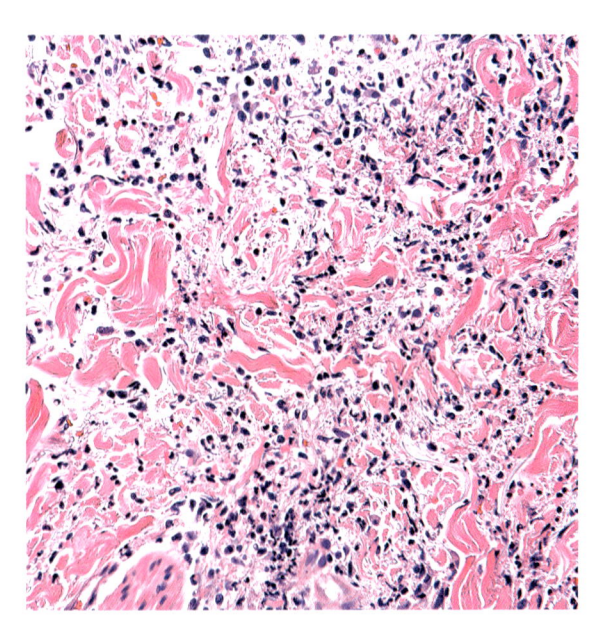

Figure 12-5
ACUTE FEBRILE NEUTROPHILIC DERMATITIS
Left: Scanning magnification shows marked dermal inflammation and striking papillary dermal edema.
Right: At high magnification, the interstitial inflammatory component is dominated by neutrophils.

*Inflammatory Disorders of the Skin*

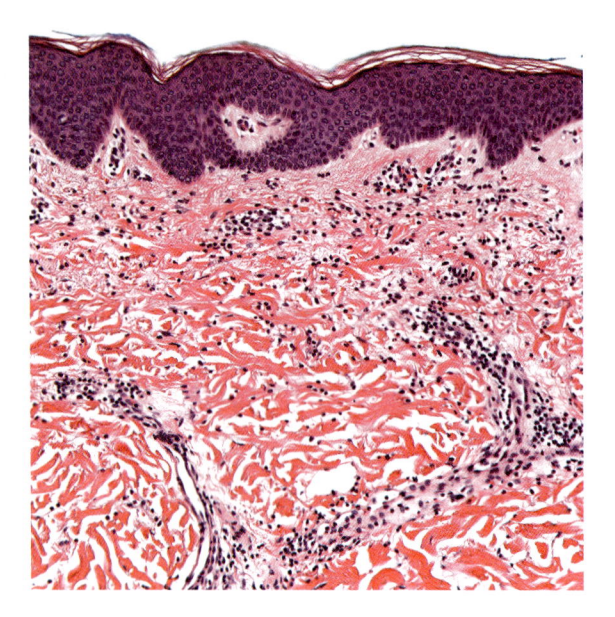

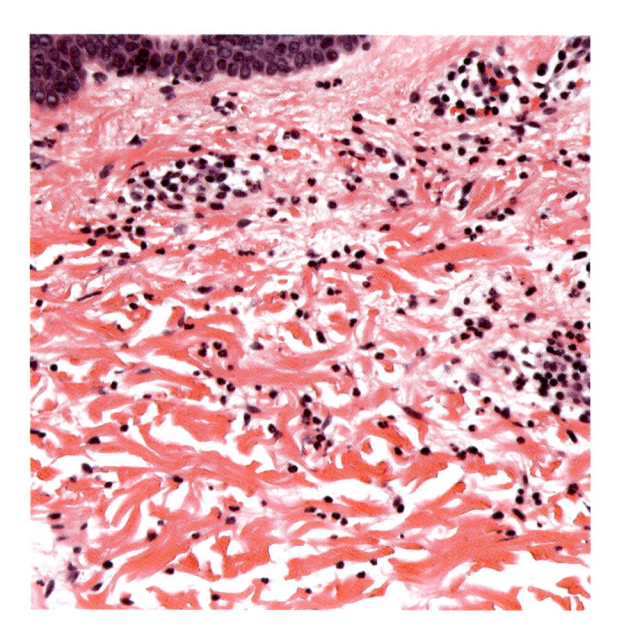

**Figure 12-6**
**STILL DISEASE**

Left: The characteristic cutaneous lesions show a sparse interstitial and perivascular infiltrate containing numerous neutrophils.

Right: At higher magnification, the interstitial neutrophilic component is focally admixed with lymphocytes. Dermal edema is present.

**Pathologic Findings.** The superficial and deep dermis are infiltrated by diffuse to vaguely nodular collections of degranulating eosinophils (figs. 12-7, 12-8). These cells are not associated with primary vasculitis, although marked superficial dermal edema and even dermal bulla formation may be observed (fig. 12-7). Degranulation is characterized by recognizable hypereosinophilic cytoplasmic granules within the extracellular matrix immediately adjacent to the plasma membrane of eosinophils. As these cells persist within the dermis, characteristic flame figures become prominent (fig. 12-8). Flame figures are jagged clusters of degenerating, hypereosinophilic collagen rimmed by degranulating eosinophils and imparting the impression of a burst of fire within the otherwise normal tinctorial quality of the background matrix. With chronicity, flame figures eventually become surrounded by a palisade of giant cells. Flame figures are characteristic of eosinophilic cellulitis, although florid eosinophil-rich arthropod bite reactions occasionally show similar alterations.

**Differential Diagnosis.** Urticarial plaques can resemble eosinophilic cellulitis but are transient. Dermal contact dermatitis and early eczematous patches in atopics resemble eosinophilic cellulitis. The presence of altered collagen resembling flame figures but surrounded by epithelioid cells suggests the possibility of Churg-Strauss syndrome.

**Treatment and Prognosis.** For severe cases, oral prednisone is usually effective. For less severe cases, topical steroid application is used with success. Griseofulvin, cyclosporine, and dapsone are second line agents.

### Pyoderma Gangrenosum

**Definition.** *Pyoderma gangrenosum* is a rapidly evolving cutaneous eruption that begins as a hemorrhagic pustule and rapidly develops into an ulceration (21–27). The disorder is commonly associated with other diseases, especially chronic bowel diseases such as ulcerative colitis (28–30). Clinical and histologic images of pyoderma gangrenosum are presented in chapter 9 (Ulcerative Dermatitis); the discussion here considers lesions that present in a biopsy specimen as primarily nodular/interstitial inflammatory infiltrates.

## Nodular/Interstitial Dermatitis

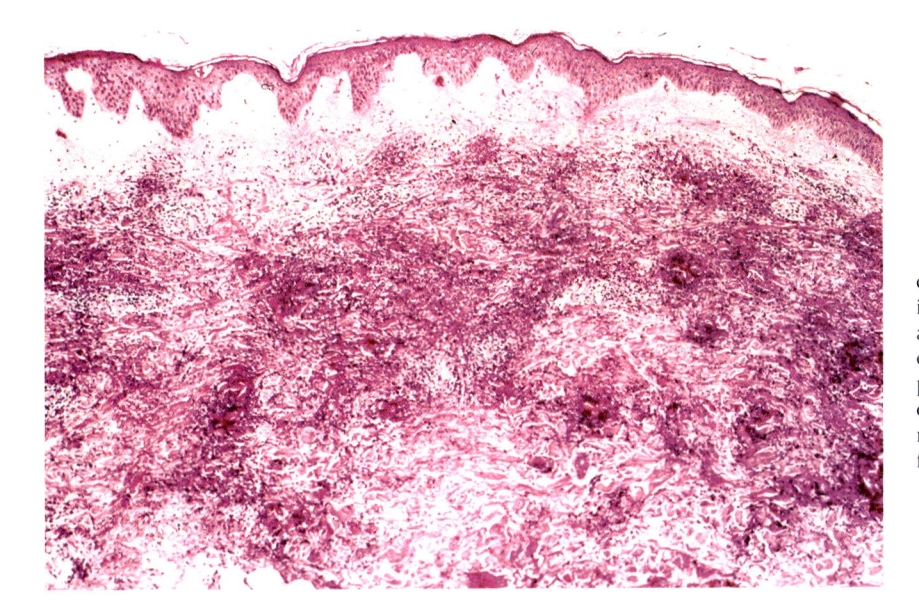

Figure 12-7

**EOSINOPHILIC CELLULITIS (WELLS SYNDROME)**

In this advanced lesion, the dermis is heavily infiltrated by inflammatory cells, with an abundance of degranulating eosinophils. The infiltrate is punctuated by discrete zones of hypereosinophilic collagen representing well-formed flame figures.

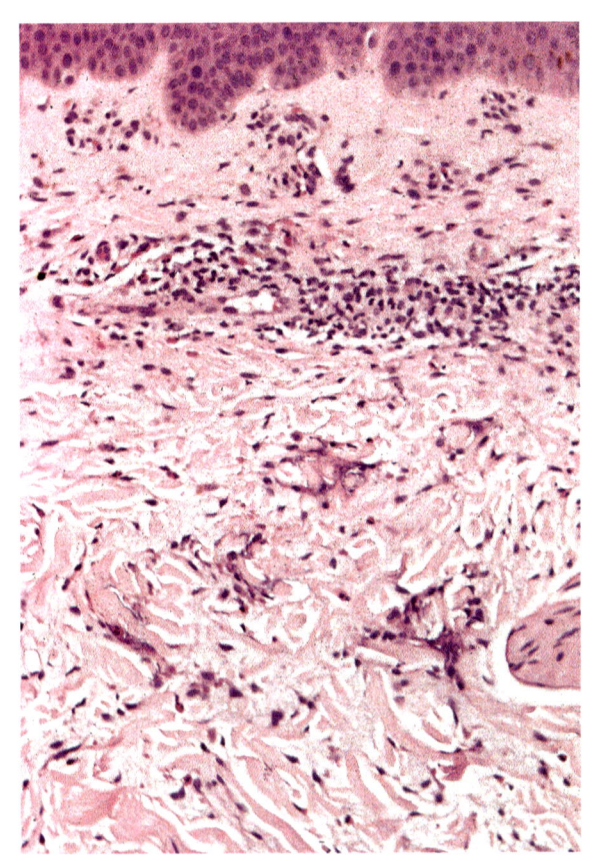

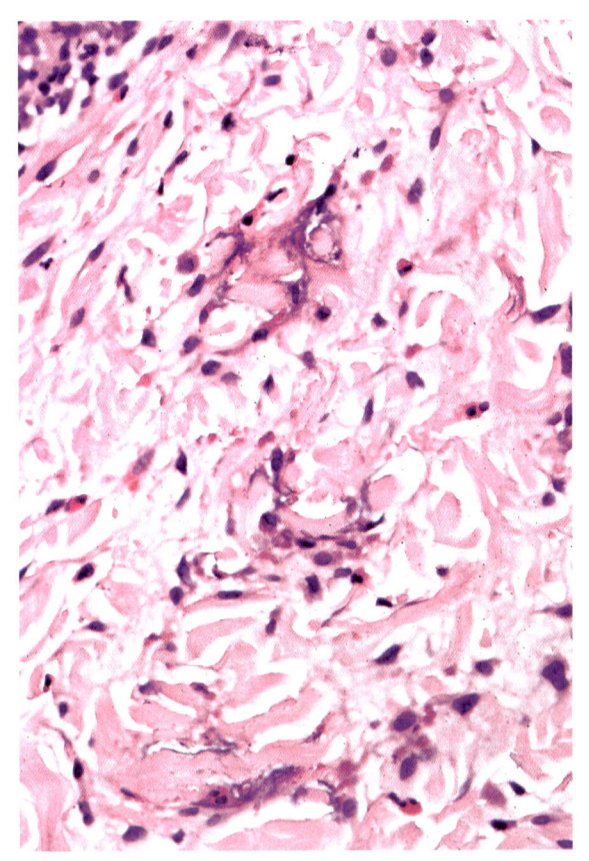

Figure 12-8

**EOSINOPHILIC CELLULITIS**

Left: This early lesion shows perivascular infiltration by inflammatory cells, including eosinophils, as well as the formation of early flame figures.

Right: Higher magnification of early flame figures. Central zones of hypereosinophilic collagen are surrounded by compressed and degranulating eosinophils.

**Clinical Features.** The acute onset of a hemorrhagic pustule or painful nodule is often associated with a history of trauma to the site. The superficial pustule is usually follicle-associated and rapidly goes on to become a striking nodule that breaks down with ulcer formation. The borders of the ulcer typically appear undermined and have a dusky purple coloration. The base of the ulcer is associated with a purulent exudate and may be partially covered with an eschar. In the advancing border of the lesion, follicular pustules may be observed. The lesions are solitary and most commonly affect the lower extremities, but may occur at any site including the face. Lesions heal with the formation of a characteristic cribriform scar.

The patients usually appear systemically ill with malaise and sometimes fever in the initial stages of the disease. The most common associations are with large and small bowel inflammatory diseases, especially Crohn disease and ulcerative colitis. The disorder also is associated with diverticulitis, leukemia, myeloma, chronic active hepatitis, especially with hepatitis B infection, and Behçet syndrome. If untreated, the lesion will last for months to years and tends to be recurrent; as older lesions are resolving, new lesions appear.

**Pathologic Findings.** Early lesions and alterations at the edge of an ulcer show a mixed inflammatory infiltrate, often with a pronounced perivascular cuff of lymphocytes. In the earliest phases, lymphocytes alone are present. Their distribution is about vessels in a parafollicular array. Then neutrophils enter the dermis. There is generally secondary overlying epidermal hyperplasia, which in more advanced disease, grows downward into the well-defined edge of the ulcer base to produce the punched-out, undermined appearance appreciated clinically. The ulcer base consists of many neutrophils, which replace the dermal matrix but are not associated with primary neutrophilic vasculitis. Special stains for bacteria and fungi, as well as cultures, are negative if deep lesional tissue is examined to exclude superficial contamination.

**Differential Diagnosis.** The diagnosis of pyoderma gangrenosum is based on tight clinicopathologic correlation and the exclusion of conditions that mimic florid tissue infiltration by neutrophils, particularly infection. The differential diagnosis usually includes an infectious process, most commonly ecthyma gangrenosum or even progressive gangrene. Deep fungal infections and amebiasis are also similar lesions. Stasis ulceration, because of the predilection of the lesions on the lower leg, is a condition commonly misdiagnosed clinically as pyoderma gangrenosum. Occasionally, systemic vasculitic disorders result in ulceration, such as Wegener granulomatosis.

**Treatment and Prognosis.** For pyoderma gangrenosum associated with an underlying disorder, treatment of the disorder, such as acute inflammatory bowel disease, often clears the lesions. Pyoderma gangrenosum can precede the onset of the bowel disease by several years. For lesions of unknown etiology and even for those associated with other systemic diseases, it is sometimes necessary to treat with oral prednisone (31–35). Dapsone is successful in some cases, as is intralesional triamcinolone injections (36). Sulfa sulfasalazine and cyclosporine have had some success (37–39). Intravenous immunoglobulin and antitumor necrosis factor (TNF) agents such as infliximab are used in recalcitrant cases.

### Infectious Causes of Nodular/Interstitial Granulocytic Infiltrates: Pyoderma

**Definition.** *Bacterial pyoderma* is discussed here because it is common and often misdiagnosed as disorders ranging from vasculitis to squamous cell carcinoma. In classic cases, there is a predisposing condition that favors bacterial invasion and growth within the dermis. There usually is associated diabetes mellitus or ischemic changes due to peripheral vascular disease.

**Clinical Features.** Zones of cellulitis become painful, warm, and indurated due to cellular infiltration and edema (fig. 12-9). *Erysipelas* is an excellent example of a diffuse edematous cellulitis that forms a large plaque-like lesion with a firm advancing edge. Epidermal bullae and sloughing may be seen in advanced lesions. A variant form, *blastomycosis-like pyoderma*, is associated with the development of vegetating, verrucous plaques and pustules superficially resembling cutaneous blastomycosis. Although most forms of pyoderma are associated with ordinary pathogenic bacteria, such as *Staphylococcus aureus*, others result from less common

*Nodular/Interstitial Dermatitis*

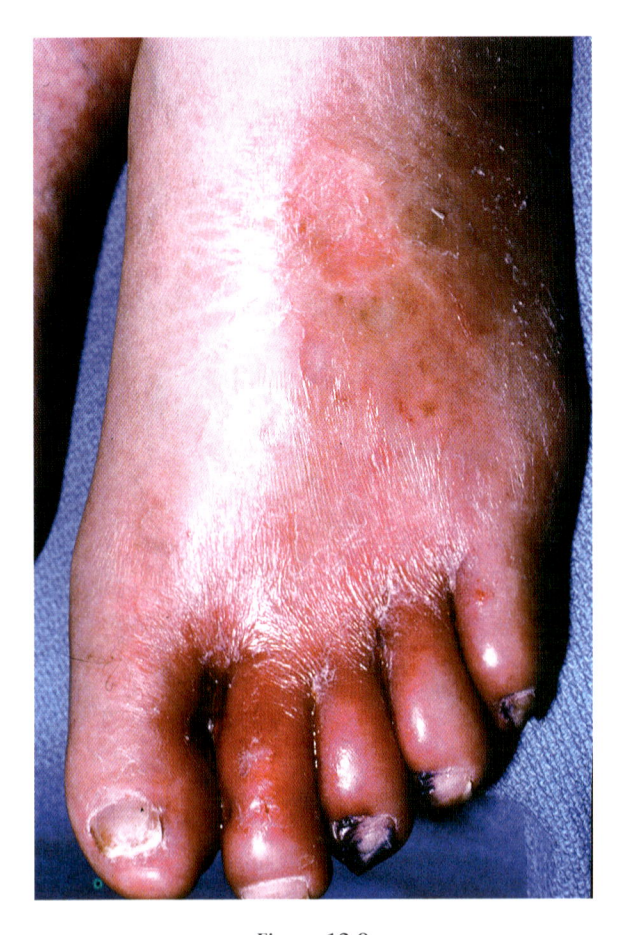

Figure 12-9

**BACTERIAL PYODERMA**

This ischemic foot from a patient with diabetes mellitus has become superinfected by bacteria, resulting in erythema, edema, and localized pain.

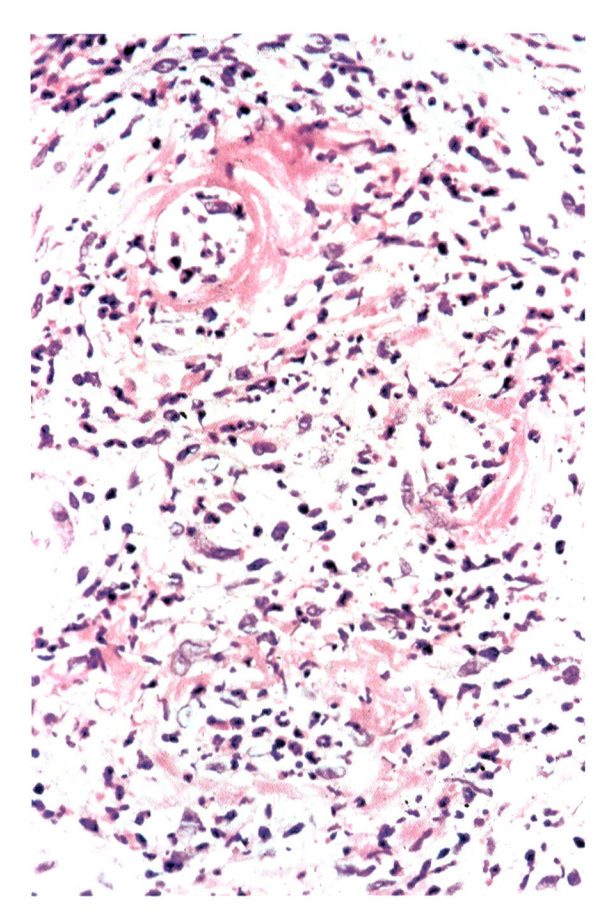

Figure 12-10

**BACTERIAL PYODERMA**

The inflammatory infiltrate is composed predominantly of neutrophils. The tissue Gram stain (not shown) revealed numerous intracellular bacteria.

gram-positive forms, such as *Actinomyces israelii*. *Cervicofacial actinomycosis* results in indurated plaques containing abscesses and draining sinuses from which characteristic sulfur granules occasionally extrude.

**Pathologic Findings.** A biopsy of pyoderma is often nonspecific, with neutrophils and mononuclear cells infiltrating diffusely throughout a markedly edematous dermal layer (fig. 12-10). Secondary injury to small vessels may result in the mistaken diagnosis of necrotizing vasculitis if the clinical features and gross appearance of the lesion are not fully considered. In erysipelas, the edema is severe, with marked dissection of collagen fibers and scattered neutrophils. The lymphatic vessels are easily visible, as are the causative gram-positive streptococcal organisms. The overlying epidermis may show ischemic necrosis, basal cell layer vacuolization with incipient or evolving blister formation, and marked pseudocarcinomatous hyperplasia, as is the case in blastomycosis-like pyoderma, in which dermal and intraepidermal microabscesses are also prominent. Dermal abscesses and sinus tracts should always suggest infection, and the possibility of unusual as well as ordinary infectious causes should be considered in each patient. In cervicofacial actinomycosis, there is an admixture of granulation tissue and chronic inflammatory cells, with discrete dermal abscesses and sinus tracts (figs. 12-11, 12-12, left). Within the aggregated neutrophils that form these structures there are colonies of basophilic filamentous bacteria of around 0.3

*Inflammatory Disorders of the Skin*

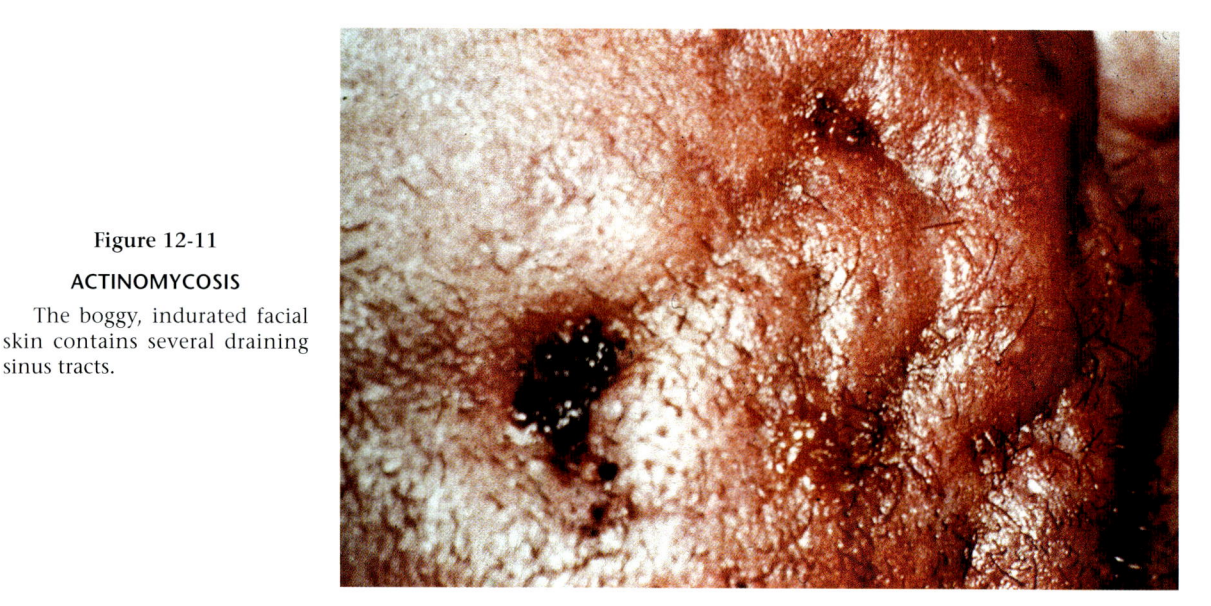

**Figure 12-11**

**ACTINOMYCOSIS**

The boggy, indurated facial skin contains several draining sinus tracts.

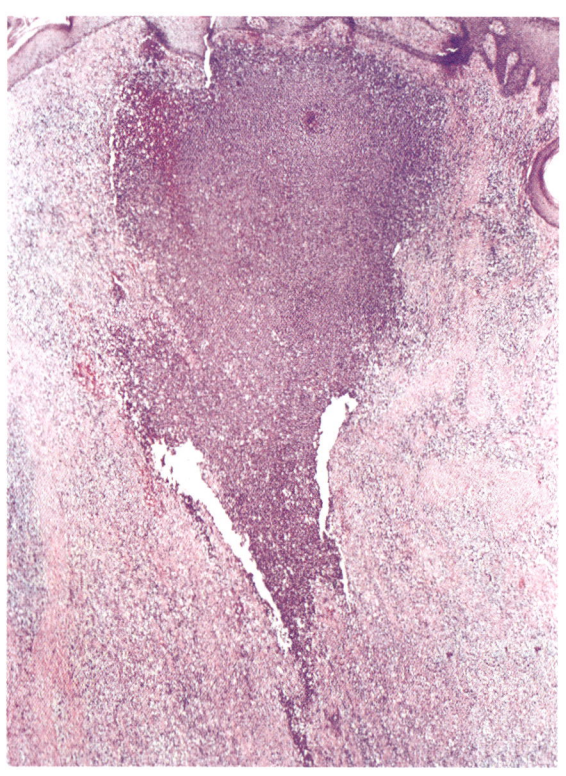

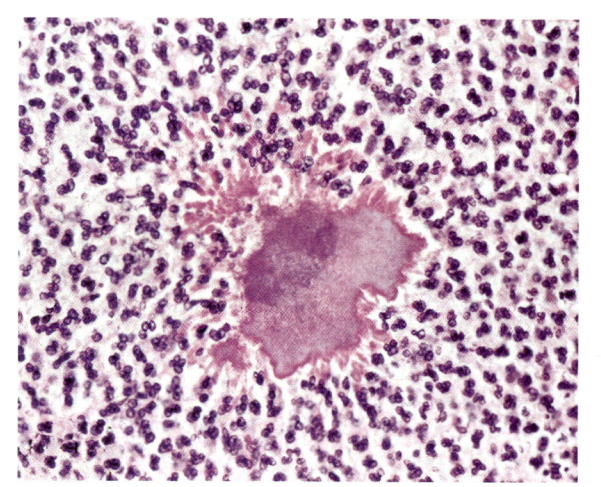

**Figure 12-12**

**ACTINOMYCOSIS**

Left: There is a sinus tract that extends from the epidermal surface into the subcutis. The tract is expanded by abscess-like accumulation of neutrophils bordered by granulation tissue.

Above: At higher magnification, the characteristic sulfur granules of *Actinomyces* are present within the neutrophilic infiltration filling the sinus tract.

to 0.8 µm in diameter (fig. 12-12, right). These colonies have a granular appearance with gray-yellow coloration, and hence are named sulfur granules. These structures are highlighted by use of Gram or silver stains (fig. 12-13).

**Differential Diagnosis.** Bacterial infection in immunologically normal individuals may mimic neutrophilic dermatoses, and if clinical parameters support the possibility of infection, special stains and cultures are mandatory.

**Treatment and Prognosis.** The prognosis is generally favorable with the rapid institution of antibiotics after appropriate microbiological culture and sensitivity testing.

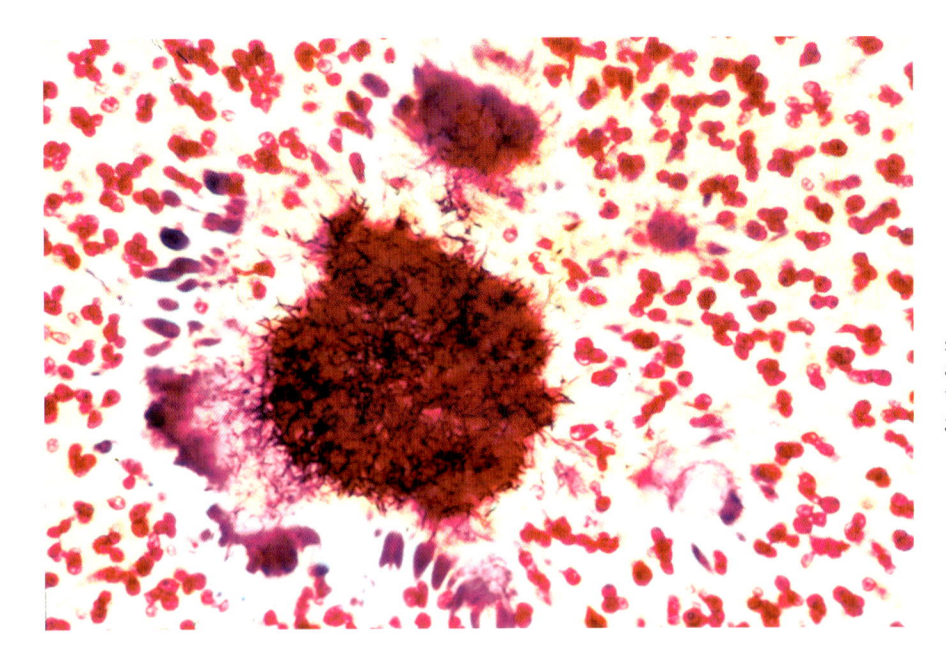

**Figure 12-13**
**ACTINOMYCOSIS**
Gram stain shows the slender filaments that characteristically extend from the perimeter of the sulfur granule.

## PRIMARILY LYMPHOCYTIC NODULAR/INTERSTITIAL INFILTRATES

### Morphea (Early/Inflammatory Stage)

**Definition.** *Morphea* is a localized area of sclerosis of the skin that occurs as a single lesion, as multiple isolated lesions, or as a linear lesion (40–42).

**Clinical Features.** Usually asymptomatic, the lesion begins as an area of thickening of the skin that is ill defined, and may be erythematous and edematous. The initial lesion, when isolated, varies from a few centimeters to 15 to 20 cm in size. As the lesion progresses, the hair follicles and the orifices of the sweat ducts become inapparent and disappear. The lesion may extend deeply into the skin and be associated with bone and muscle changes, including atrophy in adults, as well as flexion contractures and abnormalities in growth in children.

Morphea forms localized single plaques, bands, or a linear type of lesion, as along an extremity. In frontoparietal scalp lesions, striking alopecia results, which, when extending on the forehead, has been given the designation of a "sword's stroke" or "en coup de sabre."

A generalized form of morphea includes multiple lesions on the trunk and extremities. Early lesions are skin colored, but become erythematous and edematous, and as they progress, become paler or ivory colored with a violaceous edge.

The lesions are usually gradually progressive. Late lesions are firm, white, and scar-like. Rarely, spontaneous remissions occur.

**Pathologic Findings.** Early morphea/scleroderma is histologically subtle, since sclerosis is often in its incipient stages and inflammation dominates the histologic picture. There is an interstitial infiltrate of lymphocytes and occasional plasma cells within the deep dermis (fig. 12-14). Lymphocytes typically surround collagen bundles in a pattern reminiscent of the association of infiltrating histiocytes to collagen fibers in early lesions of palisaded granulomatous dermatitis (e.g., granuloma annulare or necrobiosis lipoidica).

At scanning magnification, biopsy specimens of advanced lesions, which must include the full-thickness dermis and a portion of underlying subcutis, are often squared-off rather than trapezoidal as a result of the diffuse replacement of the normally elastic dermis by abnormal connective tissue. The dermal thickness appears markedly increased as a result of downward replacement of subcutaneous tissue by altered collagen. A helpful indicator of this feature in advanced lesions is the location of entrapped eccrine coils, which normally demarcate the junction between the reticular dermis and subcutis. Extension of altered collagen down widened subcutaneous septa may also be observed.

*Inflammatory Disorders of the Skin*

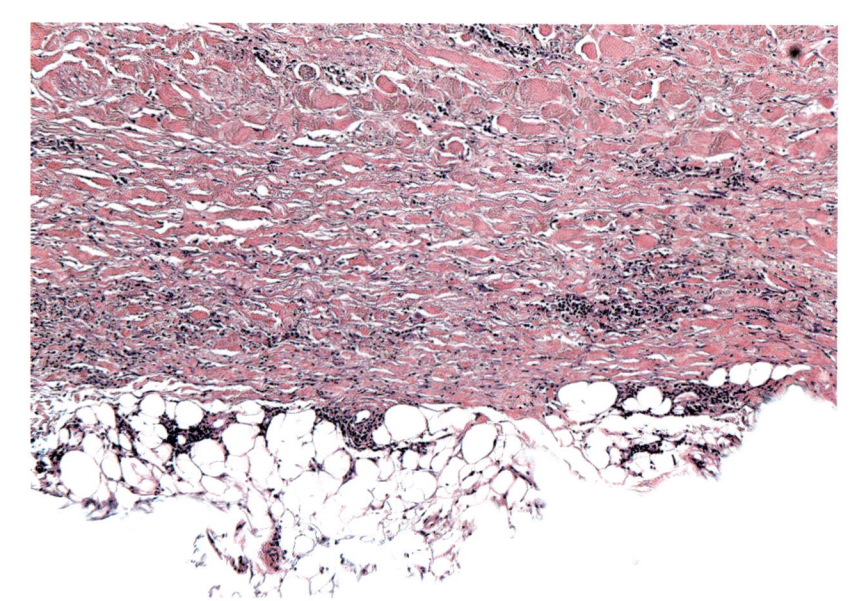

**Figure 12-14**

**MORPHEA, INFLAMMATORY STAGE**

Top: At scanning magnification, there is a patchy perivascular and interstitial inflammatory infiltrate within the deep dermis.

Bottom: At higher magnification, there is interstitial permeation of the dermal collagen by mononuclear cells to form a vaguely micronodular pattern.

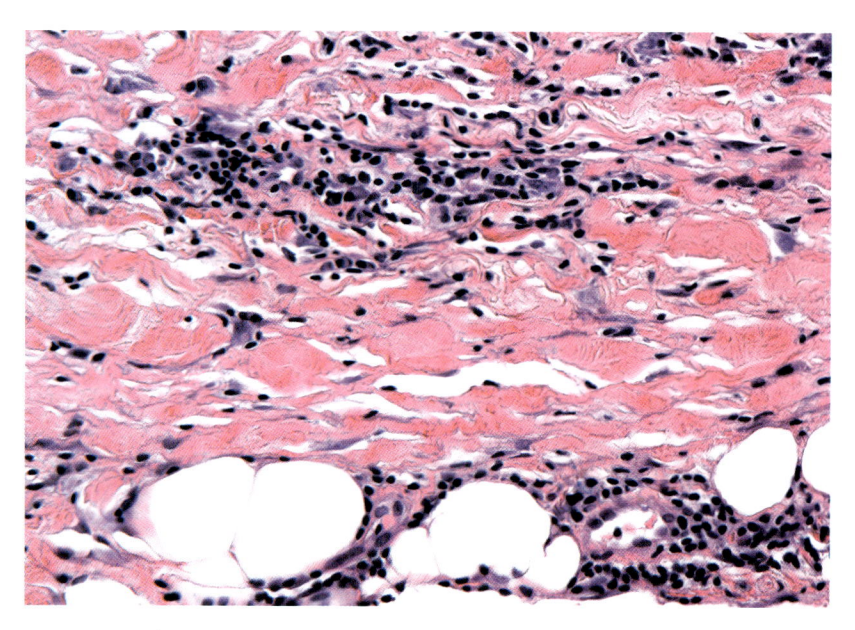

At higher magnification, collagen bundles are thickened and pale, and they display a homogeneous rather than a finely fibrillar quality. Spaces that normally separate adjacent collagen bundles are attenuated. Angiocentric cuffs of lymphocytes and plasma cells, associated with thickening of vessel walls, endothelial cell hypertrophy, and apparent degeneration (i.e., lymphocytic vasculitis), are commonly observed in the deep dermis. Inflammation may also show an interstitial pattern among altered collagen bundles, particularly at the advancing edges of established lesions. In some cases, the predominant infiltrating cell is the plasma cell; morphea then is considered in the differential diagnosis of plasma cell panniculitis. Dermal eccrine coils and neurovascular bundles are no longer surrounded by a cuff of loose adventitial connective tissue as in normal skin; rather, they are entrapped within the altered sclerotic dermal matrix. In the very advanced lesions, all adnexal structures are absent, and the epidermis is diffusely atrophic.

*Eosinophilic fasciitis* is an unusual variant of morphea characterized by the acute onset of painful, firm, swollen regions, usually affecting the skin of one or several extremities.

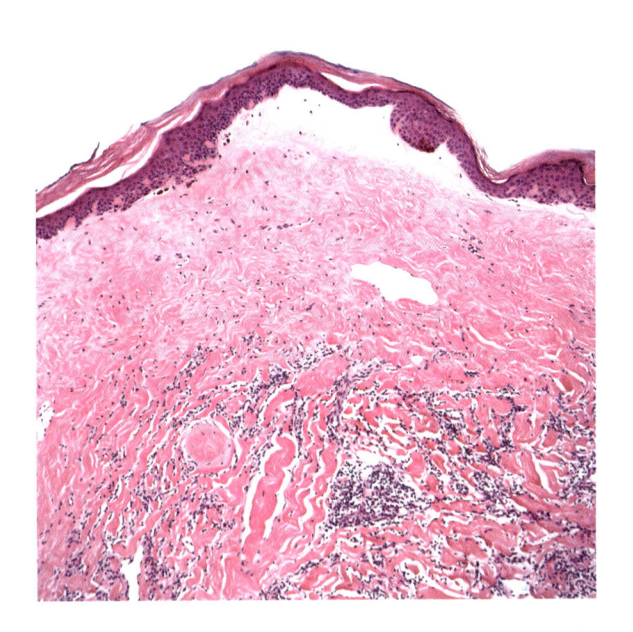

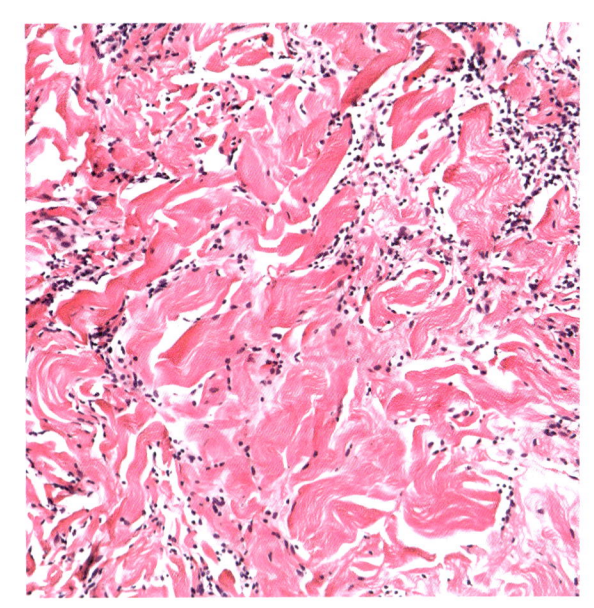

**Figure 12-15**

**LICHEN SCLEROSUS**

Left: This active lesion shows degenerative changes within the superficial dermis consisting of hyalinized sclerosis and associated underlying interstitial lymphoplasmacytic inflammation.

Right: At higher magnification, the active interstitial inflammatory component is similar to granuloma annulare, although it is composed of lymphocytes and plasma cells rather than histiocytes.

Occasionally, there are surface irregularities in these regions, suggesting variable fibrosis and the tethering of skin to underlying fascial planes. Most affected individuals also have peripheral blood eosinophilia and hypergammaglobulinemia. Internal disease involving viscera, however, is unusual. The histologic evaluation, which requires wide, deep surgical excision, reveals abnormal collagen, primarily within the lowermost reticular dermis, within widened septa of the subcutaneous fat, and involving the underlying fascia. Qualitatively, the altered collagen within the subcutaneous septa, replacing the fat lobules, and within the fascia is similar to that observed in ordinary morphea, although most of the reticular dermis is spared. The inflammatory infiltrate in eosinophilic fasciitis may be brisk and is composed of lymphocytes, occasional plasma cells, and occasional eosinophils in a perivascular and interstitial array. Examination of the fascia reveals a mixed lymphocytic and eosinophilic infiltrate around vessels with often prominent mast cells. Skeletal muscle, if present, may also be infiltrated by inflammatory cells and show foci of fibrous replacement. The similarities between morphea and eosinophilic fasciitis have prompted some dermatopathologists to suggest the name *morphea profunda* for the latter condition, although it should be remembered that the two disorders have distinct clinical presentations and well-defined histologic differences.

**Differential Diagnosis.** The differential diagnosis includes systemic scleroderma, which has systemic involvement. Lichen sclerosus et atrophicus may resemble morphea, but is not as firm (fig. 12-15). There is a lichen sclerosus/morphea overlap syndrome, and because of histopathologic similarities, some consider lichen sclerosus et atrophicus to represent a superficial form of morphea. Eosinophilic fasciitis must likewise be considered in the differential diagnosis. This localized lesion is associated with deep inflammation and can result in flexion contractions. Finally, *Borrelia burgdorferi* infection can result in localized sclerotic plaques.

**Treatment and Prognosis.** The treatment for morphea has been consistently unsatisfactory. The process may resolve spontaneously over 3 to 5 years. Topical steroids and calcipotriene have been used with variable success. Some patients respond to antibiotic therapy, such as penicillin and tetracycline, given over a prolonged period of time (several weeks to months) (43). This therapy is more effective when associated with oral corticosteroids (44). Recalcitrant cases have been treated with oral corticosteroids, hydroxychloroquine, mycophenolate, and cyclosporine. Phototherapy with ultraviolet A has been successful in some patients (45,46).

## PRIMARILY HISTIOCYTIC NODULAR/INTERSTITIAL INFILTRATES

### Granulomatous Reactions to Drugs and Foreign Substances

**Definition.** Certain drugs can cause a *granulomatous response* in the skin as a form of delayed hypersensitivity. Some foreign substances elicit a striking granulomatous infiltrate in the skin, known as *foreign body granulomas*.

**Clinical Features.** Drug-induced lesions vary from a lichen planus-like eruption to granulomatous slack skin. At times, the lesions are diagnosed as cutaneous T-cell lymphoma. Drugs that cause a granulomatous response include antibiotics, lipid lowering agents, antihistamines, angiotensin-converting enzyme inhibitors, nonsteroidal antiinflammatory drugs, and tricyclics. These lesions respond to the withdrawal of the drug. Approximately one third of patients with a granulomatous reaction to drugs have associated medical illnesses with a granulomatous diathesis, including rheumatoid arthritis, Crohn disease, hepatitis C, diabetes mellitus, and thyroiditis. Occasionally, an infectious agent triggers the reaction, such as herpesvirus, Epstein-Barr virus, streptococci, and mycobacteria.

Dermal and subcutaneous nodules at the site of trauma should always suggest a foreign body granuloma. Characteristic agents that cause this reaction are silica, zirconium, and beryllium that enter the skin from an external source and result in striking nodules. Zirconium is present in some deodorants. Beryllium is present in fluorescent lights and a broken fluorescent light that penetrates the skin results in a beryllium foreign body granuloma.

**Pathologic Findings.** Granulomatous reactions to drugs show a number of patterns, including localized and diffuse histiocytic dermal infiltrates, frank granuloma formation, lichen planus-like interface alterations, and granulomatous vasculitis. A combination of granulomatous and lichenoid dermatitis with vascular injury suggests a drug-related reaction pattern.

Granulomatous reactions to foreign substances include the formation of epithelioid granulomas, either within the superficial dermis at sites of topical contact, or in the deep dermis at injection sites (figs. 12-16–12-19). If pigment is present, as in a granulomatous delayed hypersensitivity reaction to a tattoo, the diagnosis is easy. Substances such as mineral particulates or contaminants of injected materials, however, may be difficult to detect. Some are birefringent with polarized light, such as silica, and examination by polariscopy is mandatory for granulomatous dermatitis for which the diagnosis is uncertain. Occasionally, elemental analysis by scanning-transmission electron microscopic X-ray probe technology is useful.

**Differential Diagnosis.** Insect bite reactions can result in a striking granulomatous response, although interstitial eosinophils are generally prominent. Other granulomatous disorders, such as sarcoid or infections, are in the differential diagnosis.

**Treatment and Prognosis.** In granulomatous delayed hypersensitivity reactions to drugs, elimination of the offending agent is of both diagnostic and therapeutic importance. Excision is the only effective therapy for reactions elicited by foreign materials.

### Sarcoidosis

**Definition.** *Sarcoidosis* is a chronic granulomatous disorder that has widespread systemic significance, especially involving the lymph nodes, lungs, liver, spleen, and skin (47–59). The lesions can remain confined to the skin without extracutaneous involvement.

**Clinical Features.** The age range at presentation is from as early as 12 years of age to the eighth decade. Most cases, however, occur before 40 years of age. Males and females are equally affected, and the lesion occurs in all races worldwide. The etiology is not known. There are three specific types of lesions. The first type erupts in days. An erythema nodosum–like presentation occurs concurrent with bilateral hilar adenopathy, especially in young women,

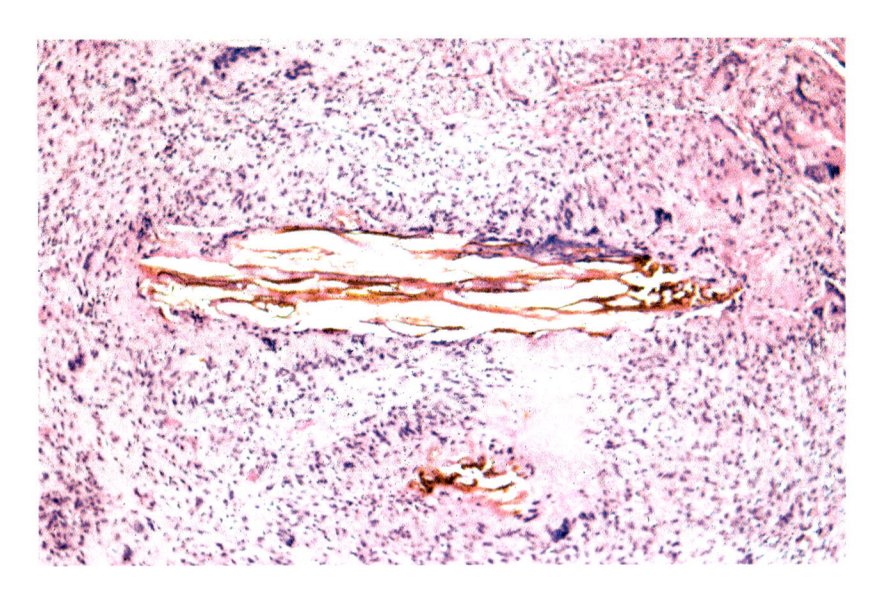

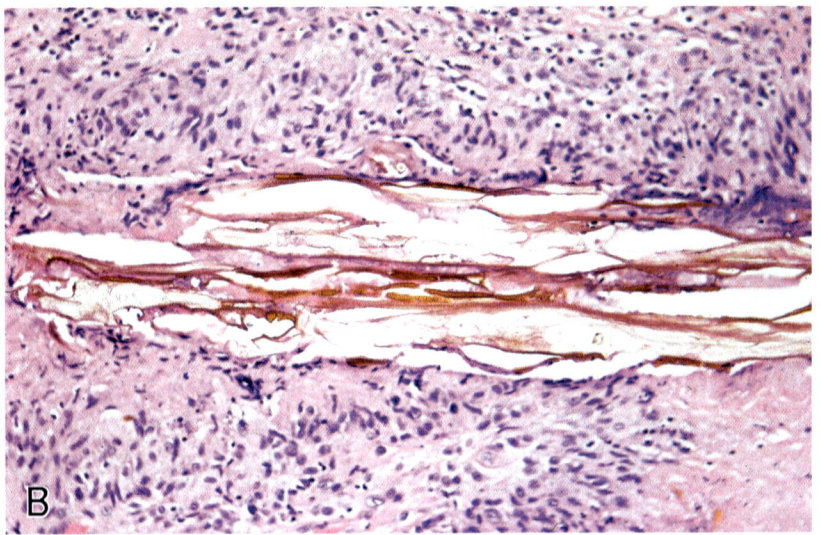

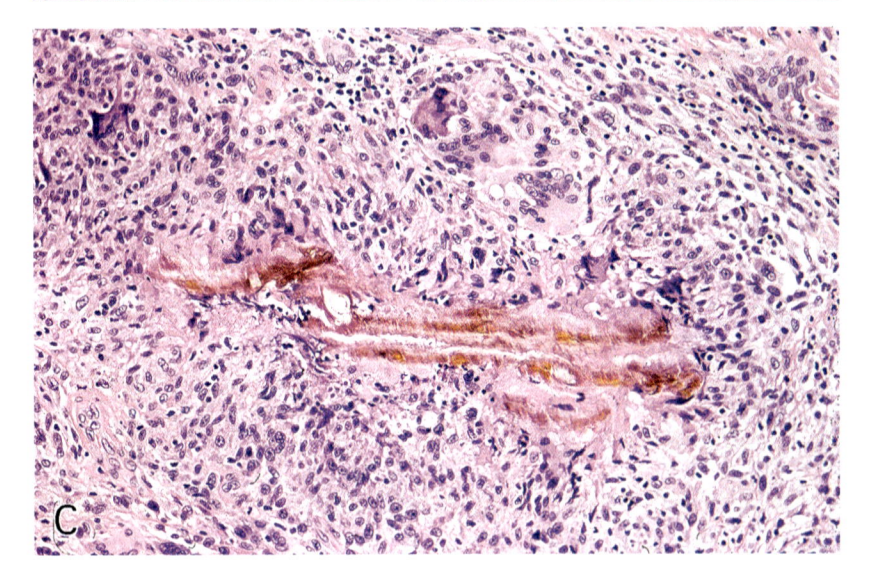

### Figure 12-16

### NODULAR REACTION TO FOREIGN MATERIAL (WOOD SPLINTER)

A: This nodular granulomatous dermal infiltrate is focally centered about elongated particles that exhibit birefringence with polarized light.

B: At higher magnification, the laminated internal structure of the fragmented plant material is readily apparent.

C: The granulomatous infiltrate is tightly applied to this splinter fragment, which is undergoing active enzymatic degradation, ultimately leaving a zone of nodular granulomatous inflammation devoid of the provocative structure.

## Inflammatory Disorders of the Skin

**Figure 12-17**

**NODULAR GRANULOMATOUS INFILTRATE TO SPLINTER**

The traumatically introduced wood particles were contaminated by fungi, here rendered visible with the Grocott methenamine silver (GMS) stain.

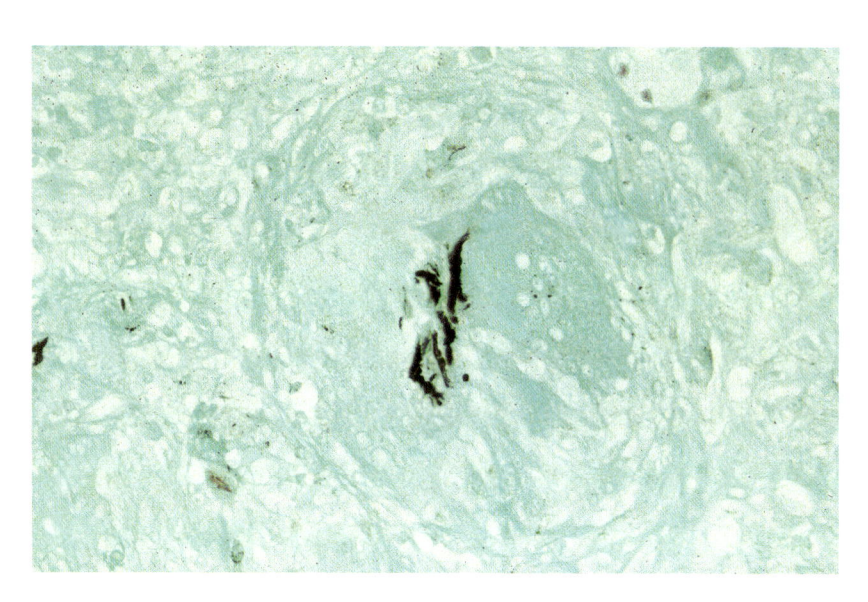

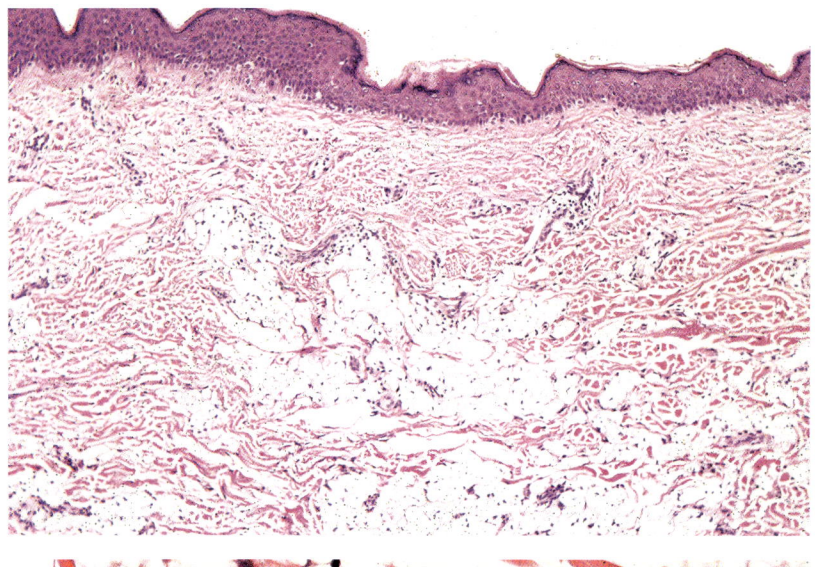

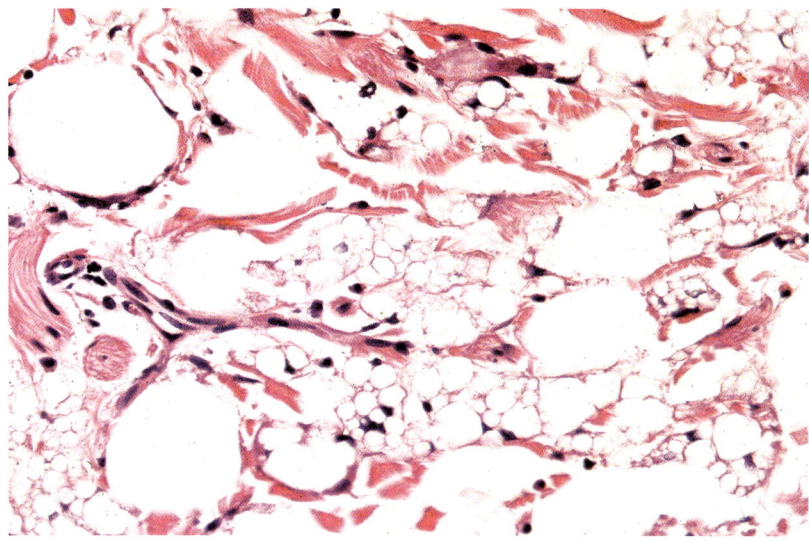

**Figure 12-18**

**SILICONE GRANULOMA**

Top: The nodular dermal pattern is formed by the sparse infiltration of mononuclear cells associated with multiple lucent vacuoles.

Bottom: At higher magnification, the characteristic clear vacuoles of variable size are readily apparent.

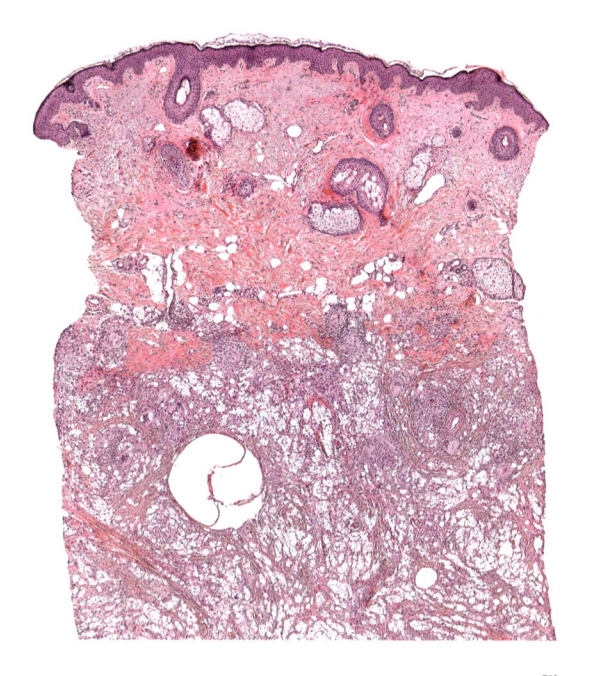

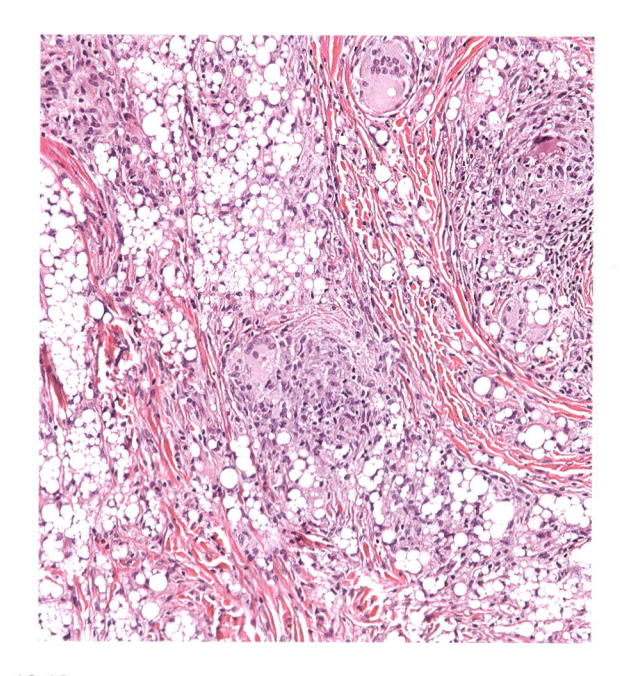

## Figure 12-19
### SILICONE GRANULOMA

Left: At scanning magnification, the granulomatous inflammation is centered in the deep dermis and subcutaneous fat.

Right: Higher magnification shows the characteristic, variably sized rounded vacuoles within the often multinucleated histiocytic component.

with fever, malaise, and painful nodules on the legs. Arthritis and arthralgias are often associated with this type. This syndrome may follow the sarcoidal involvement of the parotid gland. The second type occurs as papules or plaques on the skin that are gradual in appearance and often associated with chronic pulmonary disease and hepatosplenomegaly. Finally, there is a type of sarcoidosis that remains isolated to the skin for years, without evidence of systemic involvement.

The cutaneous lesions are often annular or serpiginous, and occur principally on the extremities but may occur on the buttocks and trunk (fig. 12-20). Central clearing occurs with slight atrophy. There is a disseminated form of sarcoidosis in which there are small papules (a few millimeters) on the face, trunk, and extremities. A variant of nodular sarcoidosis that appears on the face as a violaceous boggy infiltrate, especially on the nose, is known as *lupus pernio*. This lesion also may occur on the cheeks or ears. Rarely, sarcoidosis appears as erythematous patches, sometimes extensively involving the skin. This variant is known as *erythrodermic sarcoid*.

A characteristic indicator of sarcoidosis is the diascopy sign, which is performed by blanching the skin with a clear glass slide. The lesions, which have a reddish brown appearance, show an "apple jelly" coloration on diascopy. Sarcoidosis may be associated with alopecia.

**Pathologic Findings.** Scanning magnification reveals coalescent pale pink granulomas within the superficial and deep dermis (fig. 12-21). At this power, a differential diagnosis of infection, including tuberculoid leprosy, is often entertained. On closer inspection, the granulomas are composed of eosinophilic epithelioid histiocytes, some of which are multinucleated (fig. 12-22). Generally, the rim of lymphocytes that surrounds the granulomatous foci is inconspicuous to absent, although exceptions exist (fig. 12-23). Many of the granulomas are devoid of central necrosis, although small foci of caseation are detected in about 10 percent of cases. Nerves in neurovascular bundles are not infiltrated by inflammatory cells, nor do they exhibit degenerative alterations, as is the case in tuberculoid leprosy. Sarcoidal granulomas, in

*Inflammatory Disorders of the Skin*

**Figure 12-20**

SARCOIDOSIS

These discrete erythematous plaques raise a differential diagnosis that includes, in addition to sarcoidosis, lupus erythematosus and infection, warranting biopsy to reach a final diagnosis.

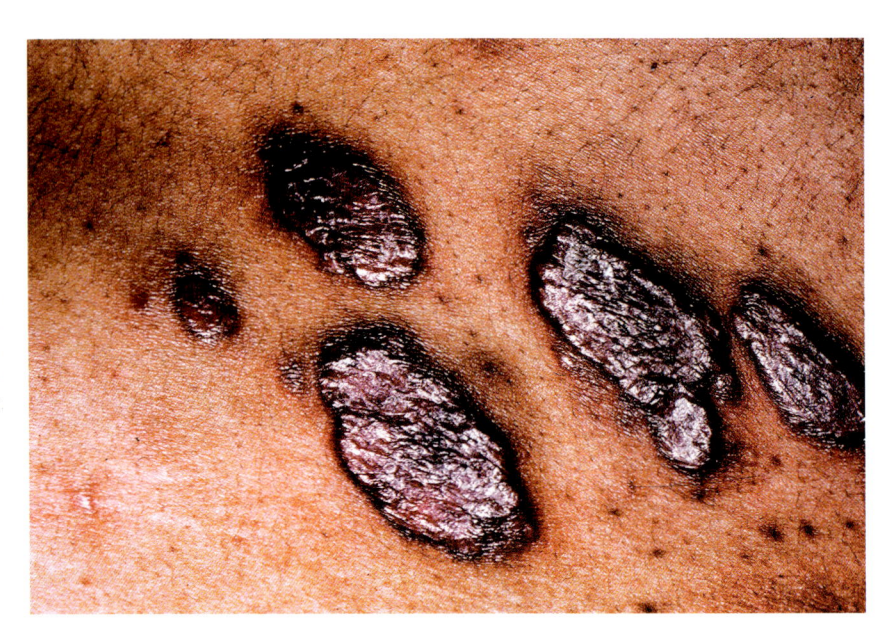

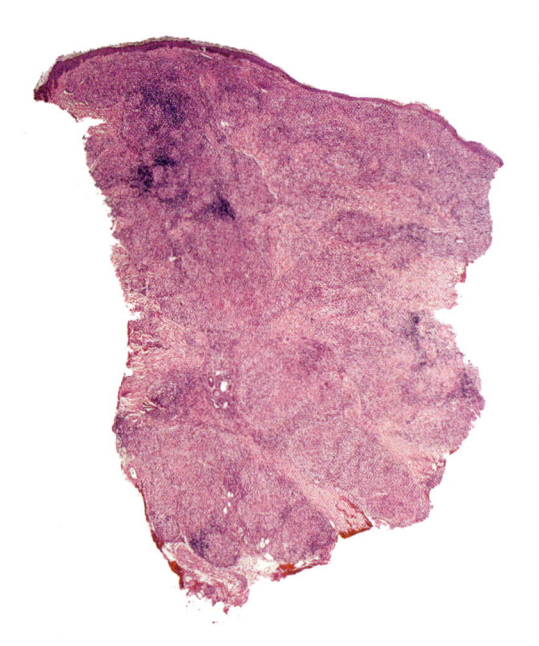

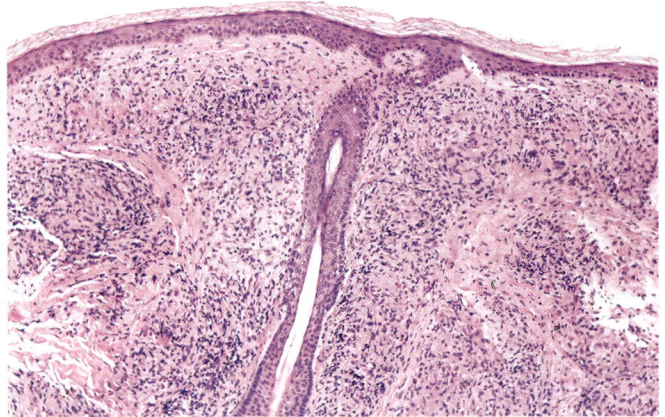

**Figure 12-21**

SARCOIDOSIS

Left: There are numerous confluent granulomas within the superficial and deep dermis, producing a multinodular inflammatory pattern.
Above: The granulomas are noncaseating and in this lesion associated with lymphocytes at their peripheries.

contrast to tuberculoid leprosy and granulomatous vasculitis, abut nerves and vessels without altering them in any way and without associated inflammatory cells. Multinucleated histiocytes may contain eosinophilic stellate inclusions (i.e., asteroid bodies), and rounded, laminated inclusions (i.e., Schaumann bodies).

**Differential Diagnosis.** The differential diagnosis of sarcoidosis is broad and includes, in the localized form, necrobiosis lipoidica and erythema chronicum migrans, granuloma annulare in the papular form, and secondary syphilis in the papular annular form. The disseminated form must be distinguished from granuloma annulare, which at times shows granuloma formation. In such instances, clinicopathologic correlation is paramount. Histologically, sarcoidosis is generally a diagnosis of exclusion, as other infectious and particulate causes of granulomatous dermatitis must always be excluded.

**Treatment and Prognosis.** The treatment of sarcoidosis relates to the degree of involvement

*Nodular/Interstitial Dermatitis*

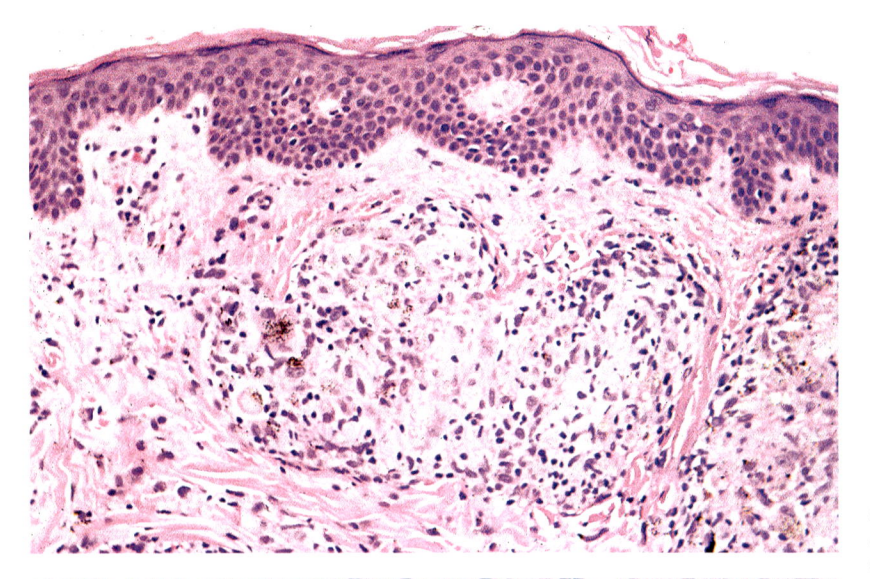

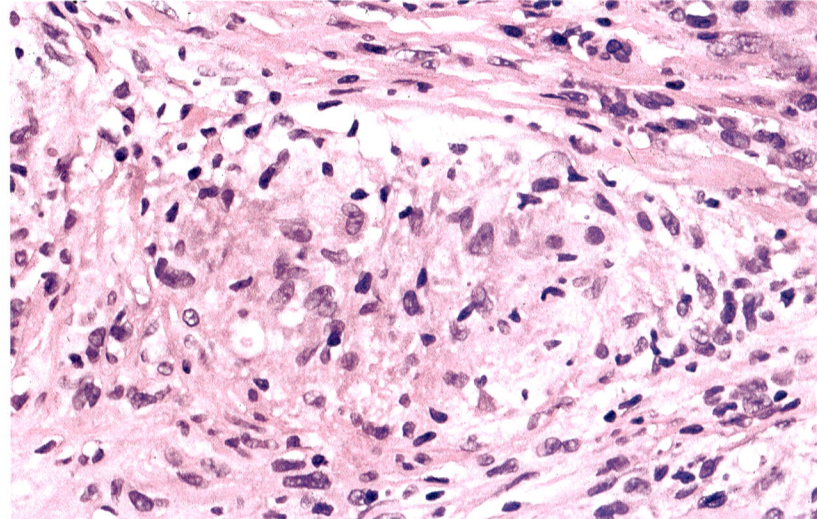

Figure 12-22

SARCOIDOSIS

Top: These granulomas are selectively involving the site of a tattoo in a patient with known sarcoidosis. The differential diagnosis includes a granulomatous immune response to tattoo pigment.
Bottom: At high magnification, the histiocytic cells have abundant, "epithelioid" cytoplasm with an almost syncytial quality.

Figure 12-23

SARCOIDOSIS: NON-NECROTIZING GRANULOMA

Although often described as "naked granulomas," some lesions of sarcoidosis have abundant lymphocytes at the perimeter of the aggregated epithelioid histiocytes, as seen here.

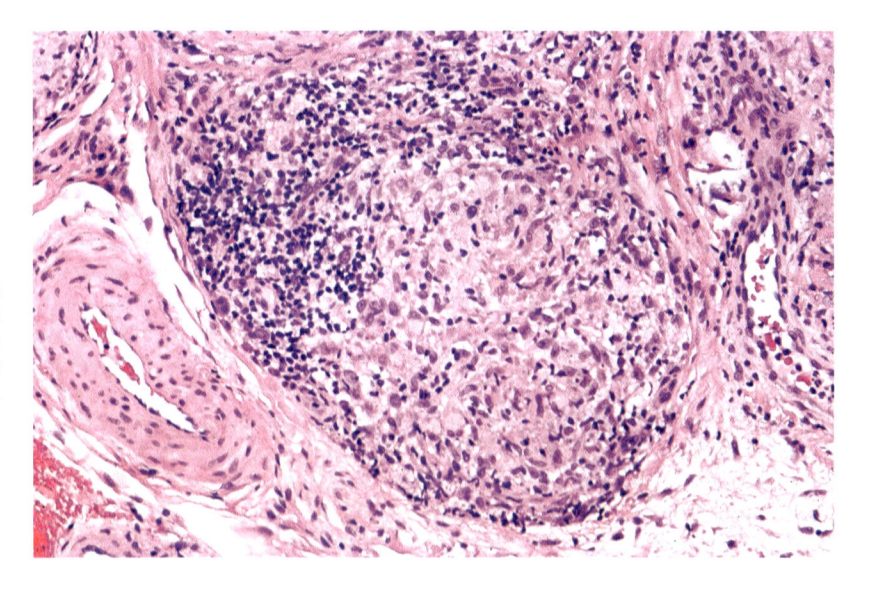

*Inflammatory Disorders of the Skin*

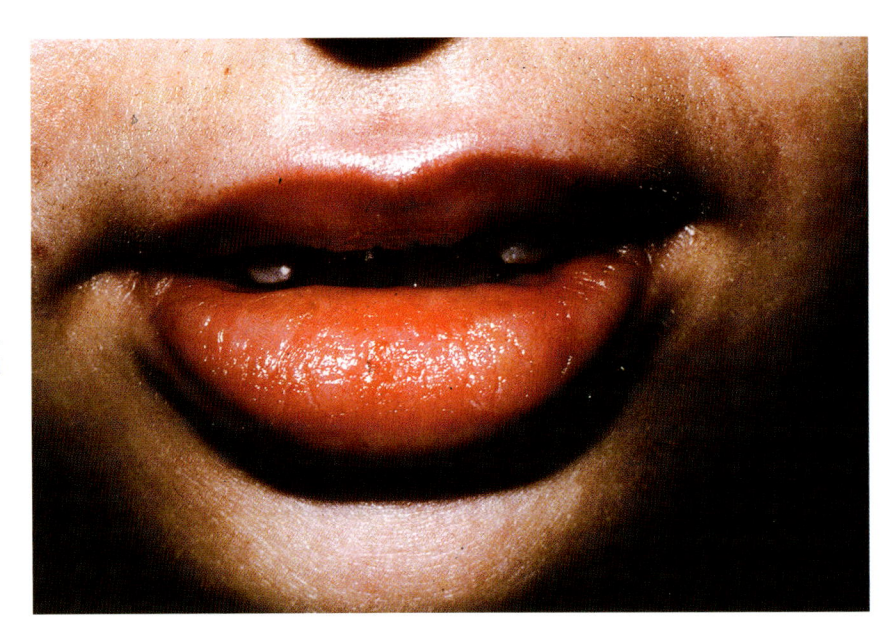

**Figure 12-24**

**CHEILITIS GRANULOMATOSA**

Clinical manifestations include permanent swelling and induration of the lips.

(60). Systemic sarcoidosis is usually treated with oral corticosteroids (61). Lesional steroid injections are sometimes successful in treating cutaneous lesions. Hydroxychloroquine is often effective for cutaneous lesions (62). Methotrexate is used as a systemic agent for both visceral and cutaneous sarcoidosis, but with limited effect (63).

### Cheilitis Granulomatosa

**Definition.** *Cheilitis granulomatosa,* or *Miescher cheilitis*, is an idiopathic disorder that presents as recurrent angioedema and eventually results in permanent swelling of the lips, often with nodularity (64–68).

**Clinical Features.** Cheilitis granulomatosa is an idiopathic disorder. It first begins as angioedema often localized to either the lips or one side of the face (fig. 12-24). The lesions occur mostly in adults, although some late childhood cases have been noted. The recurrent angioedema gives way to persistent swelling of the lips and cheek. Occasionally, the forehead is involved. In chronic disease, there is a nodularity that occurs in the lips. This nodularity is associated with a granulomatous infiltrate in many cases. Bell palsy is associated with this disorder, and it is then designated as the *Melkersson-Rosenthal syndrome* (69,70). The Bell palsy remits, but the swelling persists.

**Pathologic Findings.** There are multiple nonnecrotizing epithelioid granulomas within the submucosal connective tissue, which is often variably edematous (fig. 12-25). Poorly formed granulomas are detected directly beneath the squamous mucosa in early lesions, and may extend into skeletal muscle with advanced disease. Perivascular lymphoid infiltrates are commonly encountered, and sometimes are the only finding. When the clinical lesions appear to be diagnostic, the pathologist can render a diagnosis of "changes consistent with cheilitis granulomatosa."

**Differential Diagnosis.** Hereditary angioedema or angioedema caused by a hypersensitivity reaction must be differentiated. Sarcoidosis does not affect the oral mucosa. Occasionally, leprosy or tuberculosis result in nodular granulomatous lesions of the oral mucosa. Crohn disease may present as lip swelling and must also be considered (see below).

**Treatment and Prognosis.** Topical steroids are used as first-line therapy. Steroid injections reduce lip swelling and clofazimine has shown therapeutic benefit. Long-term use of antibiotics such as penicillin, minocycline, and erythromycin also has shown therapeutic benefit (71–75). Cases that do not respond to medical therapy have been treated with surgical reduction.

### Cutaneous Crohn Disease

**Definition.** *Crohn disease* is a chronic inflammation that can affect any portion of the digestive tract, most frequently involving the small bowel,

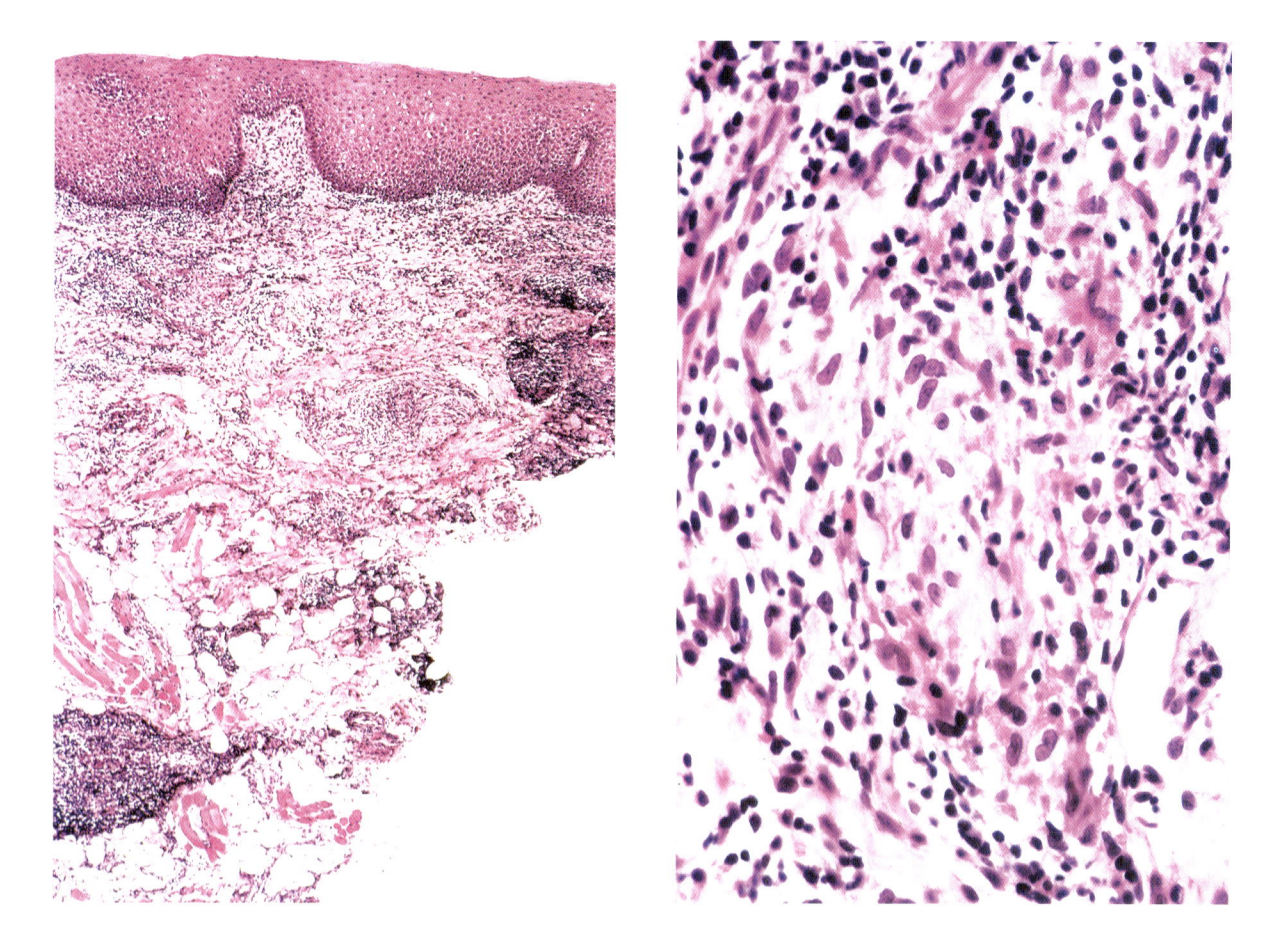

Figure 12-25
**CHEILITIS GRANULOMATOSA**
Left: There are multiple noncaseating granulomas within the submucosal connective tissue. Extension into the fat and underlying muscle also occurs.
Right: At higher magnification, the granulomas consist of aggregated epithelioid histiocytes rimmed by numerous lymphocytes. Plasma cells may also be encountered, owing to the paramucosal location.

that is occasionally associated with cutaneous granulomatous infiltrates (76–78).

**Clinical Features.** The nodules of Crohn disease are most commonly in the mouth or the perioral area. These nodules histologically reveal granulomatous inflammation. Sometimes the nodules are so extensive that they give a cobblestone appearance to the mucosa. In some instances, there is a granulomatous cheilitis in which the lips are swollen by the granulomatous infiltrate. Granulomatous cheilitis may precede by years the involvement of the small bowel. Nodular lesions also occur around the anus and vulva, at sites of colostomy or ileostomy, and in association with the scars, sinus tracts, or fistula tracts that occur as part of Crohn disease. Cutaneous-enteric fistulas are common. There may be nodules in the skin away from oral or perineal sites, in a widespread distribution. This condition is known as *metastatic granulomas of Crohn disease*.

**Pathologic Findings.** There are non-necrotizing epithelioid granulomas surrounded by lymphocytes within the superficial and/or deep dermis and subcutis. As in the intestinal pathology, some of the granulomas are poorly formed and difficult to detect. Associated granulomatous vasculitis has been described. The presence of granulomas in lymphatics is characteristic, when present, but rarely found in these lesions.

**Differential Diagnosis.** The appearance of Bell palsy helps differentiate cheilitis granulomatosis. Clinical-pathologic correlation may be necessary

*Inflammatory Disorders of the Skin*

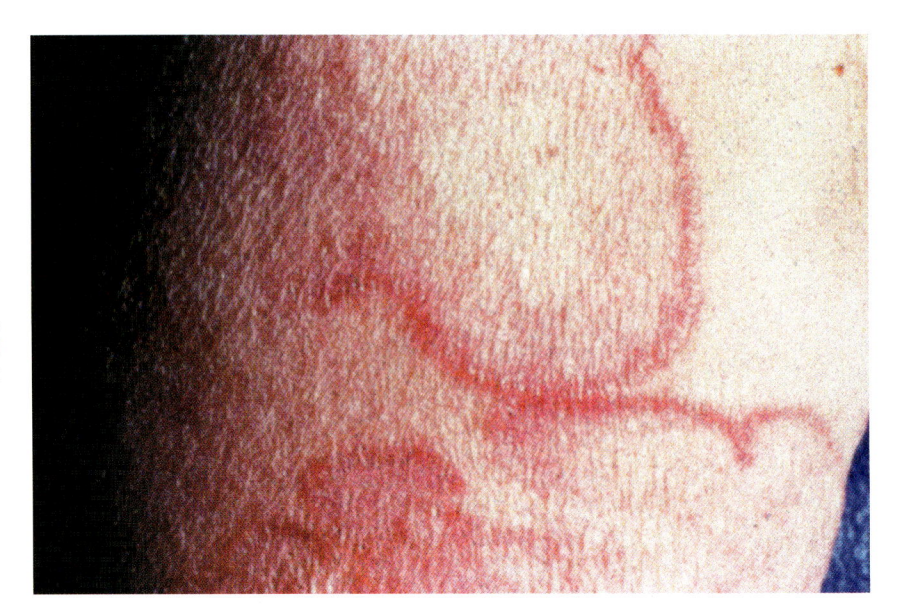

**Figure 12-26**

GRANULOMA ANNULARE

There are multiple elevated, dermal plaques with peripheral erythema, resulting in an annular or polycyclic appearance.

for successful discrimination. Metastatic lesions of Crohn disease must be differentiated from sarcoidosis. Infection, especially tuberculosis or atypical mycobacteria, can cause oral or perineal lesions that must be differentiated as well.

**Treatment and Prognosis.** The treatment of the local lesions is best directed at the underlying disorder. Intralesional steroid injections into the granulomatous nodules may result in partial resolution of the lesions. Systemic treatment with prednisone, cyclosporine, and infliximab is used for cutaneous and metastatic disease.

### Granuloma Annulare

**Definition.** *Granuloma annulare* is a chronic but self-limited and usually asymptomatic disorder that presents as multiple papules in an annular or arciform array. It appears to be related to the delayed-type hypersensitivity reaction in the skin (79–82). The lesion commonly involves the hands and feet, and the elbows and knees.

**Clinical Features.** Granuloma annulare is usually an asymptomatic eruption that occurs principally in children and young adults. Women are almost twice as often affected as men. The lesions first present as small aggregates of dermal papules that, as they progress, form annular papules and plaques between 1 and 5 cm in size, although larger lesions are seen (fig. 12-26). The lesions occur principally on the dorsa of the hands and feet but may develop around the elbows and knees or may be generalized.

There are several variants. *Perforating granuloma annulare* presents as papules in an annular or arciform array with hyperkeratotic excrescences surmounting their surface. A deep *nodular form* of granuloma annulare also occurs. The lesions may be isolated, for example, to the dorsum of the foot or the hand, or may be multiple. In some patients, especially in later life, the lesions are generalized. The nodular form most commonly occurs near the joints, especially around the elbows and knees. Patients who have generalized granuloma annulare often have an associated systemic disorder such as diabetes mellitus. Occasionally, sarcoidosis is associated with granuloma annulare as a granulomatous variant.

**Pathologic Findings.** The lesions of granuloma annulare, along with rheumatoid nodule and necrobiosis lipoidica, are referred to as palisaded granulomas because of the vague suggestion of parallel alignment of histiocytes and lymphoid cells that form at the perimeter of zones of altered collagen in established lesions. Each of these conditions has a distinctive clinical and histologic appearance, and each represents a different cutaneous disorder. Early lesions of granuloma annulare are subtle, consisting of perivascular cuffs of lymphocytes and foci of interstitial infiltration of intervening collagen by lymphocytes and histiocytes (fig. 12-27). Over time, these interstitial foci evolve to zones where degenerating collagen bundles are infiltrated by delicate strands of mucin (figs.

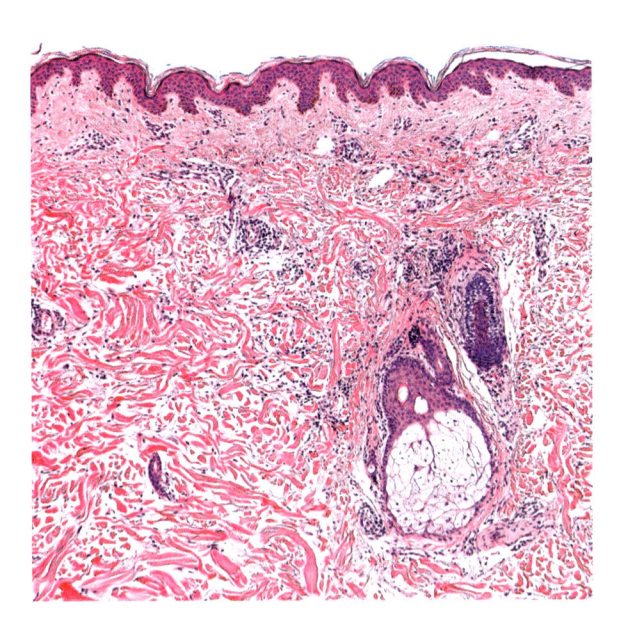

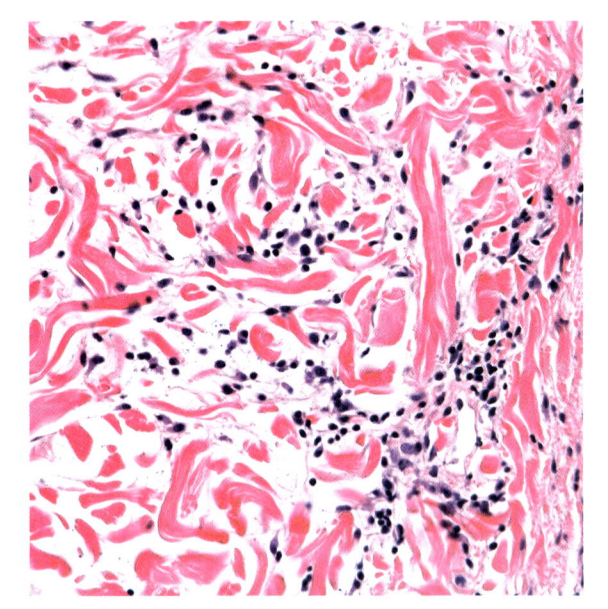

**Figure 12-27**

**GRANULOMA ANNULARE: EARLY LESION**

Left: At scanning magnification, initial sections show a nonspecific perivascular lymphocytic infiltrate with a subtle interstitial component.

Right: At higher magnification, the interstitial component consists of lymphocytes and histiocytes with early mucin deposition.

12-27, 12-28) and become surrounded by histiocytes in a palisaded array (fig. 12-28).

The perforating variant of granuloma annulare is associated with an altered zone of collagen abutting the basement membrane zone and often partially passing into the epidermis and even into the stratum corneum. Below the necrobiotic areas is a mixed infiltrate of lymphocytes and histiocytes. Usually the epidermis on both sides of the altered collagen exhibits reactive hyperplasia and hyperkeratosis. The subcutaneous or nodular variant usually exhibits central fibrinoid necrosis and resembles a small rheumatoid nodule (fig. 12-29). The nodules affect the dermis and subcutaneous fat of children and rarely adults. In the interstitial or generalized variant, a diffuse increase in dermal cellularity is observed. The infiltrate is mainly composed of histiocytes that surround collagen fibers and are accompanied by mucin deposition (fig. 12-30).

**Differential Diagnosis.** The clinical differential diagnosis that accompanies a biopsy specimen of granuloma annulare is diverse, including dyshidrotic eczema, scabies, folliculitis, and insect bites. Superficial annular lesions suggest dermatophytosis, annular lichen planus, or sarcoidosis. Erythema chronicum migrans is in the differential diagnosis of lesions of the trunk or the upper portions of the extremities. The histologic differential diagnosis of the small papules of granuloma annulare includes papular sarcoidosis, a lymphocytic infiltrate, or even early necrobiosis lipoidica. The differential diagnosis of the subcutaneous form includes rheumatoid nodules.

**Treatment and Prognosis.** Spontaneous remission occurs in most persons over the course of months to sometimes 1 or 2 years; however, the lesions tend to recur. Topical therapy with steroid creams, usually of high potency, especially under occlusion, is useful. Cryotherapy is used for localized disease. Topical immunomodulators, such as tacrolimus and pimecrolimus, are often helpful. Successful treatment with imiquimod cream can also be seen. PUVA (psoralen and ultraviolet A) photochemotherapy is successful (83,84). For persistent lesions, injection with triamcinolone may result in resolution. Oral therapy with

*Inflammatory Disorders of the Skin*

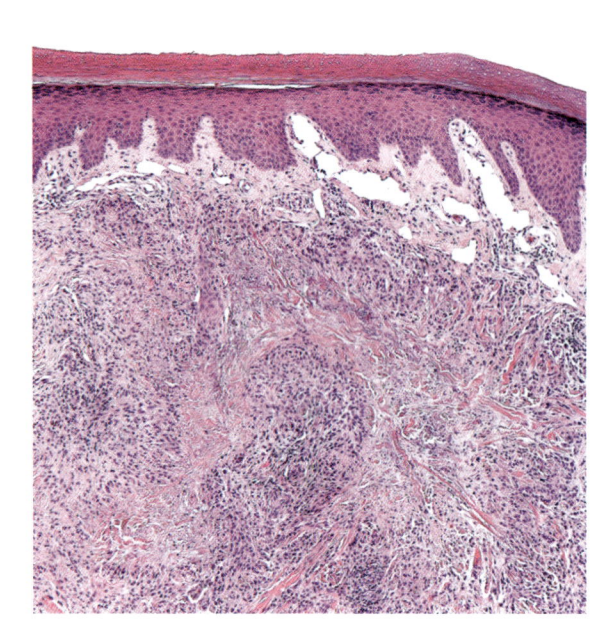

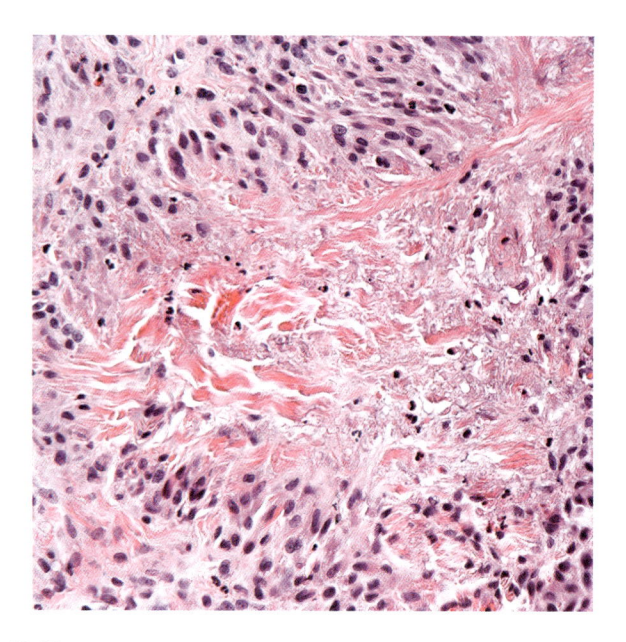

Figure 12-28
**GRANULOMA ANNULARE: LATE LESION**
Left: Multiple palisaded necrobiotic granulomas form a geographic pattern within the dermis of this acral site.
Right: The palisaded granuloma is characteristically formed by a central region of mucinous necrobiosis and surrounded by a "picket-fence" of responding histiocytes.

Figure 12-29
**GRANULOMA ANNULARE: SUBCUTANEOUS VARIANT**
The central zone of necrobiosis lacks the pale pink hue observed in figure 12-28 right, a tinctorial characteristic in part the result of localized mucin deposition. Rather, the region of necrobiosis is intensely eosinophilic, or fibrinoid, resembling the necrobiosis seen in a rheumatoid nodule.

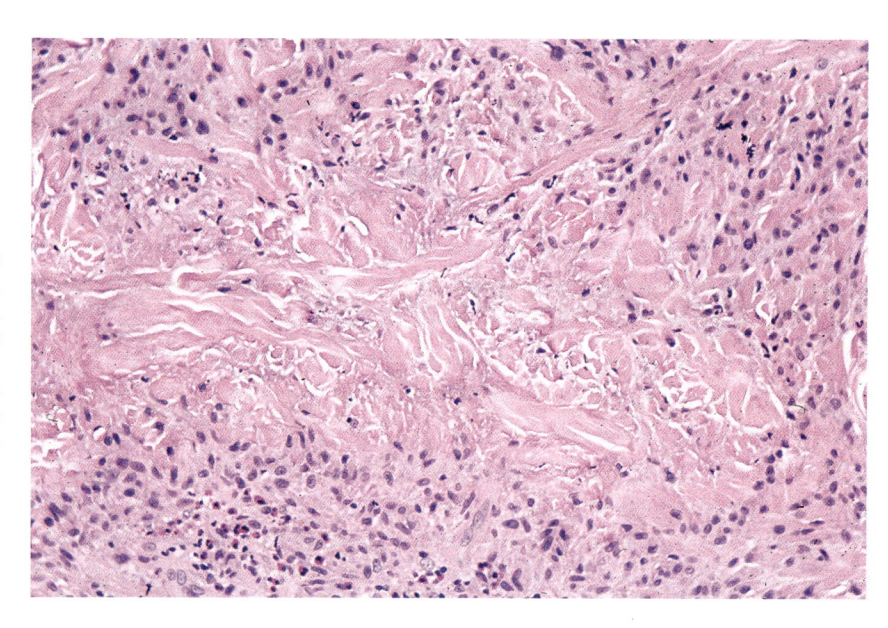

dapsone, hydroxychloroquine, isotretinoin, and TNF blockers is used for disseminated cases.

## Necrobiosis Lipoidica

**Definition.** *Necrobiosis lipoidica* is a striking and unique cutaneous disease that in many cases is associated with diabetes mellitus (85–90). This disease occurs as plaques on the lower surface of the legs. The etiology is unknown.

**Clinical Features.** Necrobiosis lipoidica is a disorder that affects young adults but worsens in early middle life. There is a striking female to male ratio in both the diabetic and the nondiabetic forms. In childhood, an association with diabetes

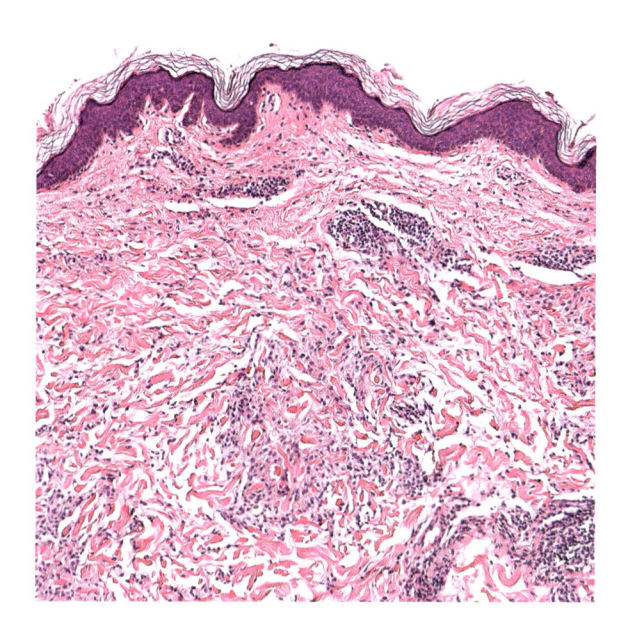

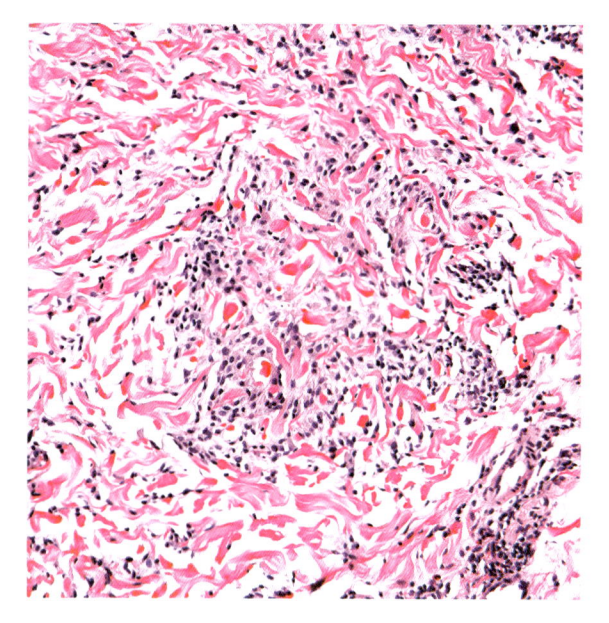

**Figure 12-30**

**INTERSTITIAL GRANULOMA ANNULARE**

Left: There is a variably cellular diffuse infiltrate of histiocytes involving the superficial reticular dermis.
Right: At higher magnification, the infiltrating lymphocytes and histiocytes characteristically surround collagen bundles and are associated with mucin deposition.

is uncommon. The incidence of this disorder is less than 1 percent of diabetic patients. When associated with diabetes, necrobiosis lipoidica usually occurs in a setting of chronic longstanding disease, especially diabetes with onset in the early years of life. The lesions gradually evolve over the course of years and persist. Approximately one third of patients with necrobiosis lipoidica have diabetes mellitus; another third show abnormal glucose tolerance testing; and the remaining third do not have any detectable abnormality of glucose metabolism.

The lesion starts as a small waxy or brown-red papule that slowly and gradually extends into a well-demarcated plaque of variable size (fig. 12-31). Most plaques are a few centimeters in size; however, larger lesions occur. The well-defined lesion has a prominently elevated, brown-red, well-demarcated border. The central area of the lesion is depressed and yellow-brown. There is marked central atrophy imparting a shiny appearance to this portion of the lesion.

The evolution of the lesion results in centrifugal spread with enlargement of the initial plaque or the presence of multiple smaller papules around the initial plaque. In approximately 20 percent of patients, ulcers form, and as they heal, they leave depressed areas (91). Most lesions occur on the shins, but also on the arms, trunk, scalp and face, and rarely, feet.

**Pathologic Findings.** At scanning magnification, the biopsy specimen has a square or rectangular contour, similar to that typically seen in scleroderma, the localized form of which (morphea) necrobiosis lipoidica may clinically resemble (fig. 12-32). An important diagnostic feature at this magnification is the tendency for the inflammatory and sclerotic mesenchymal components of the lesion to be demarcated into horizontal strata, or layers, beneath the atrophic overlying epidermis. At higher magnification, the inflammatory strata are composed of an admixture of histiocytes, lymphocytes, and occasional plasma cells. The altered dermal matrix of the strata consists of sclerotic collagen bundles exhibiting widening and homogenization. Vasculopathic changes may also be present (fig. 12-33).

**Differential Diagnosis.** The clinical differential diagnosis of necrobiosis lipoidica includes granuloma annulare, sarcoidosis, necrobiotic xanthogranuloma, and xanthomatous infiltrates.

*Inflammatory Disorders of the Skin*

**Figure 12-31**

NECROBIOSIS LIPOIDICA

There are several coalescent pink-tan, waxy, indurated plaques involving skin of the lower extremity.

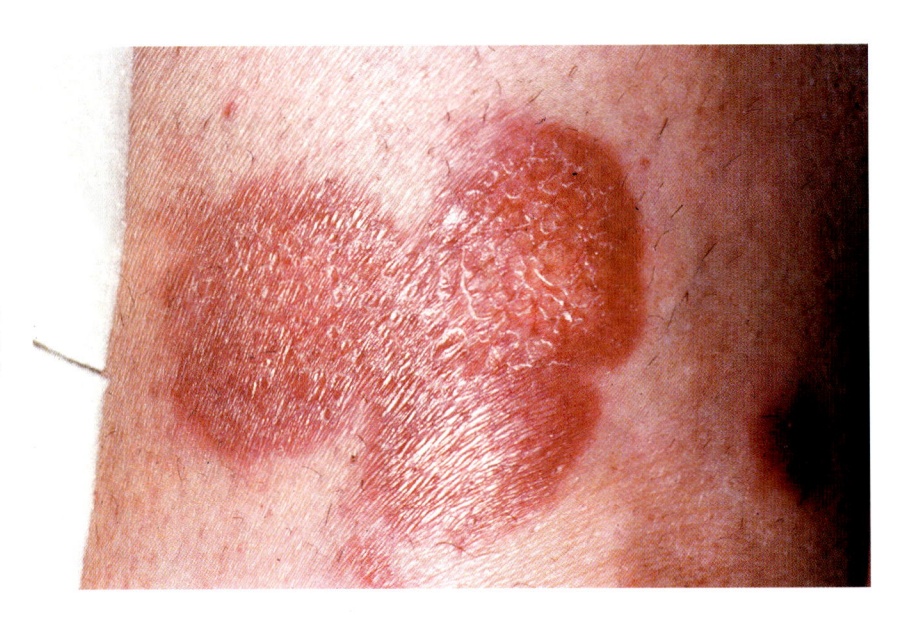

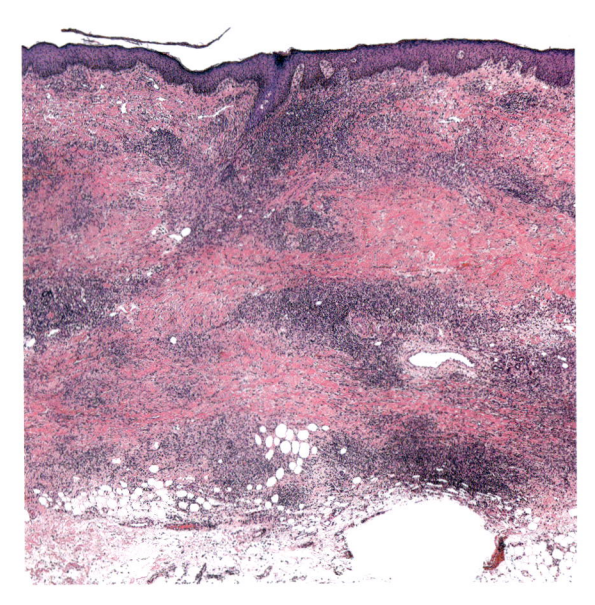

**Figure 12-32**

NECROBIOSIS LIPOIDICA

At scanning magnification, the interstitial pattern of necrobiosis lipoidica is less organized and nodular than seen in granuloma annulare at similar magnification (see fig. 12-27, left). Instead, there is an impression of horizontal stratification involving the superficial and deep dermis, a pattern that has been likened to a layer cake.

Ulcerated lesions on the face may suggest lupus vulgaris. Because necrobiosis lipoidica histologically involves dermal sclerosis and interstitial infiltration by lymphocytes and plasma cells, inflammatory morphea is also in the differential diagnosis for some lesions.

**Treatment and Prognosis.** These lesions do not resolve and the most effective treatment is both topical and intralesional steroid application (92). Ulcerated lesions need appropriate wound care. Persistent ulcerated lesions usually must be excised followed by skin grafting (93).

### Rheumatoid Nodule

**Definition.** *Rheumatoid nodules* are nontender, well-defined subcutaneous lesions that occur in 20 to 25 percent of patients with rheumatoid arthritis or with positive rheumatoid and antinuclear factors, especially around joints or on extensor surfaces (fig. 12-34) (94–98).

**Clinical Features.** Rheumatoid nodules, which are usually subcutaneous and nontender, occur especially at sites of repeated trauma, including the area around the elbows, the ulnar surface of the forearms, around the knees, heels, back of the hands, sacrum, buttocks, and even occasionally on the ears. Blunt trauma may result in ulceration. In some patients, the appearance of nodules presages the appearance of joint changes and symptoms by years.

**Pathologic Findings.** Biopsy specimens of rheumatoid nodules reveal geographic zones of fibrinoid necrobiosis within the dermis (figs. 12-35, 12-36). In these zones, normal reticular dermal collagen is transformed to a granular to amorphous, highly eosinophilic material that resembles fibrin. Mucin deposition, as seen in dermal forms of granuloma annulare, is not present. Some lesions have nuclear debris in the foci

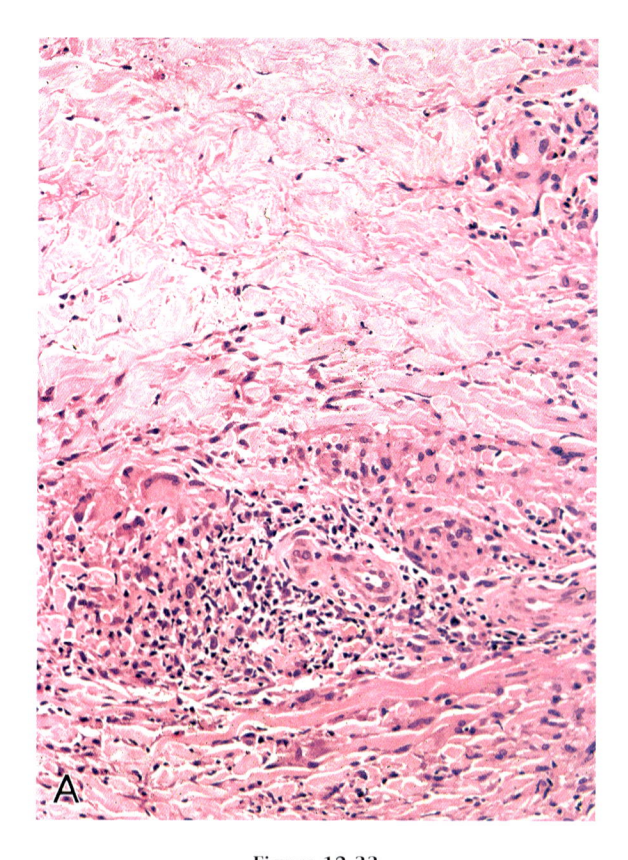

**Figure 12-33**

**NECROBIOSIS LIPOIDICA**

A: At intermediate magnification, as with granuloma annulare, there are vague zones of necrobiotic collagen bordered by more cellular regions of interstitial mononuclear cell infiltration.

B: High magnification shows an active granulomatous and vasculopathic component adjacent to frank necrobiosis of connective tissue.

C: The interstitial inflammatory component is composed of an admixture of lymphocytes and histiocytes. The necrobiotic zone is formed by sclerotic bundles of collagen. The inflammatory and sclerosing changes often extend into the subcutaneous fat (bottom of field).

of degenerating collagen. The granulomatous component consists of a mantle of histiocytes and lymphocytes identical to that described for the fully evolved lesions of granuloma annulare. In lesions that have been chronically traumatized, striking fibrovascular proliferation may accompany some of the inflammatory foci.

**Differential Diagnosis.** The most common lesion to differentiate from rheumatoid nodule is granuloma annulare, the subcutaneous variant. Other nodules that may occur in sites of predilection for rheumatoid nodules as clinical lesions include lymphoma, reticulohistiocytomas, erythema elevatum diutinum, and foreign body reactions.

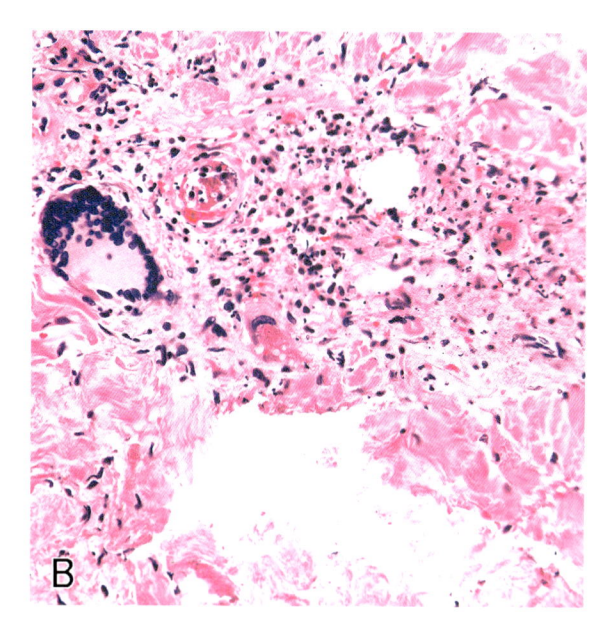

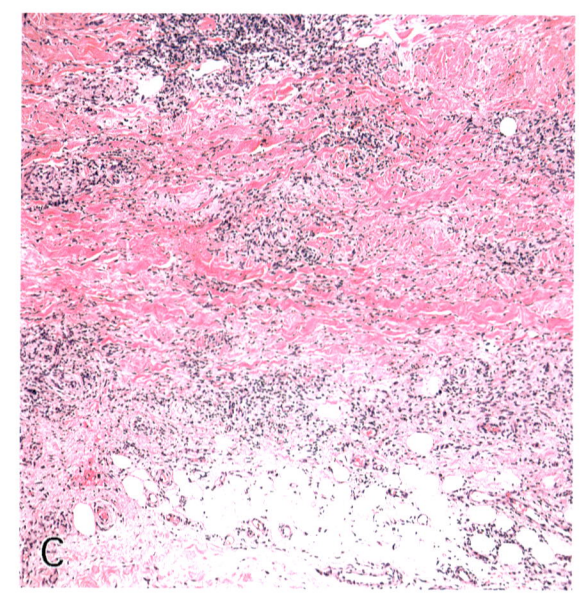

**Treatment and Prognosis.** There is no consistently successful treatment for these lesions. Some occasionally respond to intralesional injection of steroids. Usually, the lesions must be surgically excised (99).

### Annular Elastolytic Giant Cell Granuloma

**Definition.** *Annular elastolytic giant cell granuloma* is an eruption of chronically sun-exposed skin in which there are annular arrays of papules that gradually develop and persist (100–106).

*Inflammatory Disorders of the Skin*

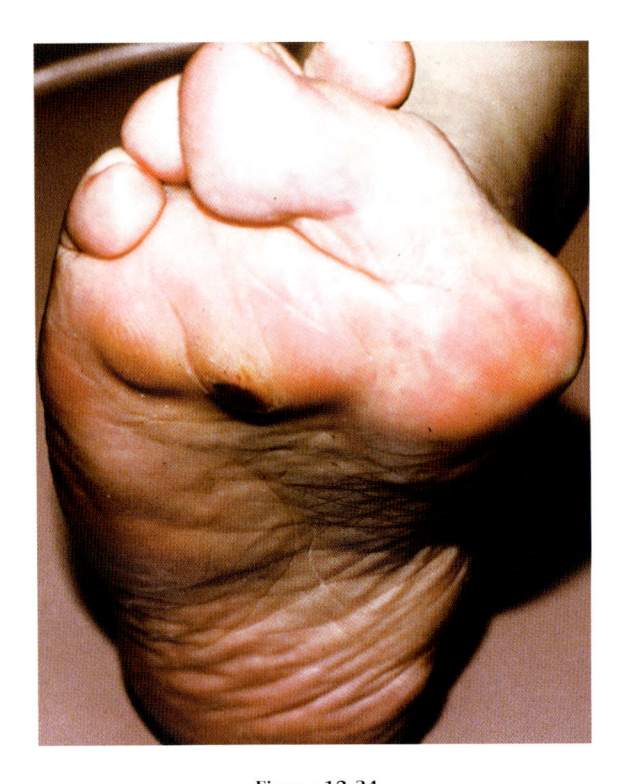

**Figure 12-34**

**RHEUMATOID NODULE**

Firm intradermal and subcutaneous nodules are here associated with the metacarpophalangeal joint.

The original descriptions of elastolytic granuloma used the term actinic granuloma, implying that this unusual inflammatory process was incited by actinically-altered dermal elastic tissue. It is now recognized that this process also rarely affects nonsun-exposed skin, and that severe actinic elastosis is not common to all lesions.

**Clinical Features.** The clinical picture is variable, ranging from solitary to grouped annular patches with elevated borders. The center is often depressed and atrophic. Both genders are affected, although middle-aged Caucasian women are more frequently affected. When lesions develop on sun-damaged skin, there is often a background of dermatoheliosis, with criss-crossed wrinkling, freckling, and "pebbles" of nodular elastosis, as may occur on the posterior neck (so-called cutis rhomboidalis nuchae).

**Pathologic Findings.** Histologically, there is a patchy mononuclear cell infiltrate within the superficial dermis (figs. 12-37–12-39). Multinucleated histiocytes within the infiltrate may contain asteroid bodies, similar to those

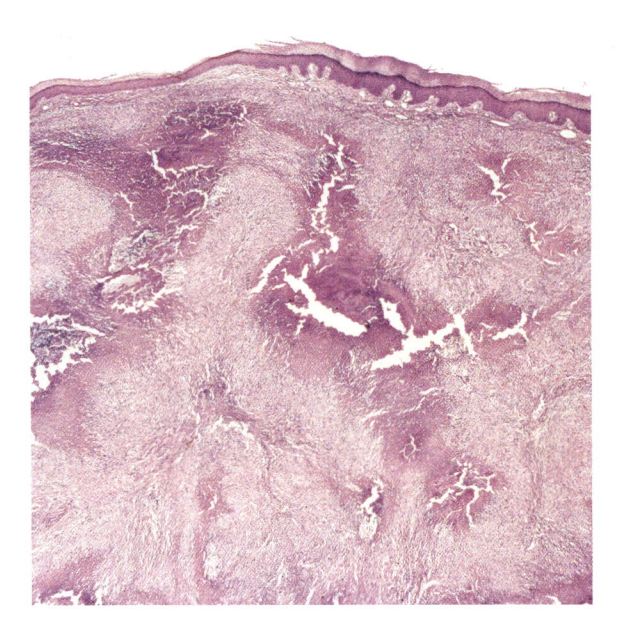

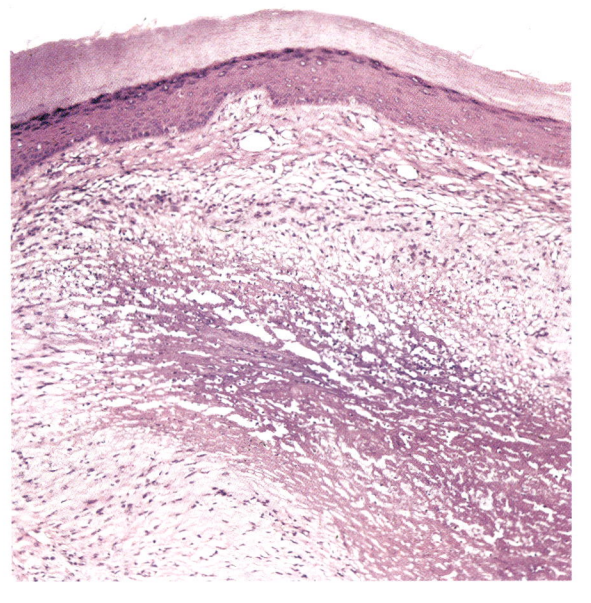

**Figure 12-35**

**RHEUMATOID NODULE**

Top: At scanning magnification, there are discrete geographic zones of fibrinoid necrobiosis within the superficial and mid-dermis.

Bottom: At higher magnification, the zone of necrobiosis is deep red-purple, resembling fibrin; the adjacent dermal stroma shows an interstitial histiocytic infiltrate and fibrosis.

observed in sarcoidosis. The diagnostic hallmark is the incorporation of dermal elastic fibers into the cytoplasm of the histiocytes via phagocytosis. As the lesion expands, it leaves behind an area free of altered elastic fibers.

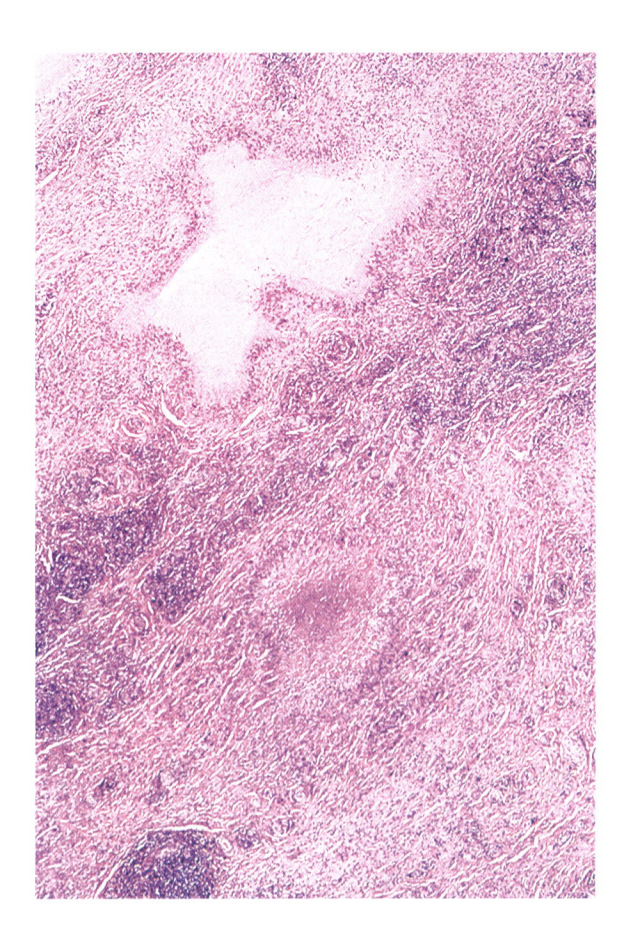

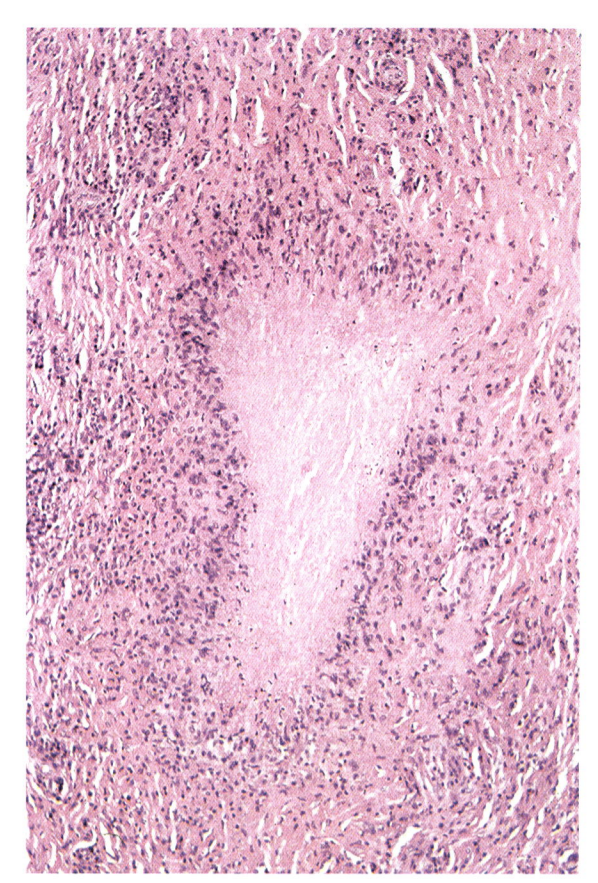

**Figure 12-36**

**WELL-DEVELOPED RHEUMATOID NODULE**

Left: There are multiple foci of geographic necrobiosis here indicated by pallor of the extracellular matrix.

Right: At higher power, the zone of necrobiosis is bordered by a well-formed palisade of elongated histiocytes arranged in a parallel array.

**Differential Diagnosis.** Granuloma annulare is the principal disorder to differentiate; it is distinguished by histopathologic examination. Secondary syphilis and papular sarcoidosis are also distinguished by histology and by the clinical course.

Although localized plaques of elastolytic granulomatous dermatitis are uncommon, the reaction pattern is observed as an incidental finding in a number of disorders, including actinic keratoses, persistent insect bite reactions, and certain variant forms of cutaneous T-cell dyscrasia (i.e., granulomatous slack skin). It is important to recognize the pattern of granulomatous elastolysis, so as not to confuse it with other forms of granulomatous dermatitis. The presence of elastic fiber phagocytosis is a prominent feature of the histiocytic response of elastotic granulomatous dermatitis and important for diagnosis.

**Treatment and Prognosis.** Further evolution of many lesions can be impeded by sun protective creams or lotions. Intralesional injection of corticosteroids results in some diminution of the lesions.

### Necrobiotic Xanthogranuloma

**Definition.** *Necrobiotic xanthogranuloma* is a rare condition in which there are striking papules and plaques that are yellow to yellow-brown. These occur on the extremities especially but may be widespread. Necrobiotic xanthogranuloma is sometimes associated with paraproteinemia, but without paraproteinemia, may be associated with lymphoproliferative disorders (107–109).

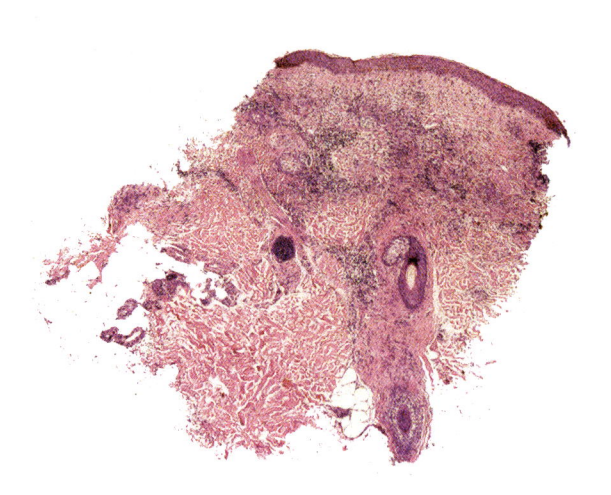

## Inflammatory Disorders of the Skin

### Figure 12-37
**ANNULAR ELASTOLYTIC GIANT CELL GRANULOMA**

Above: At scanning magnification, there is a patchy, ill-defined inflammatory infiltrate within the superficial and mid dermis.

Right: At medium power, the central zone is composed of an interstitial infiltrate of epithelioid histiocytes; the perimeter is formed primarily by infiltrating lymphocytes.

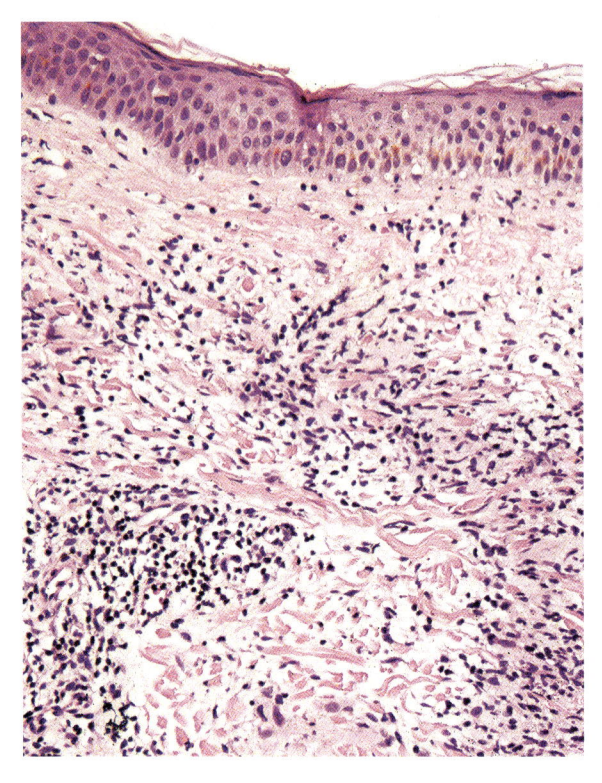

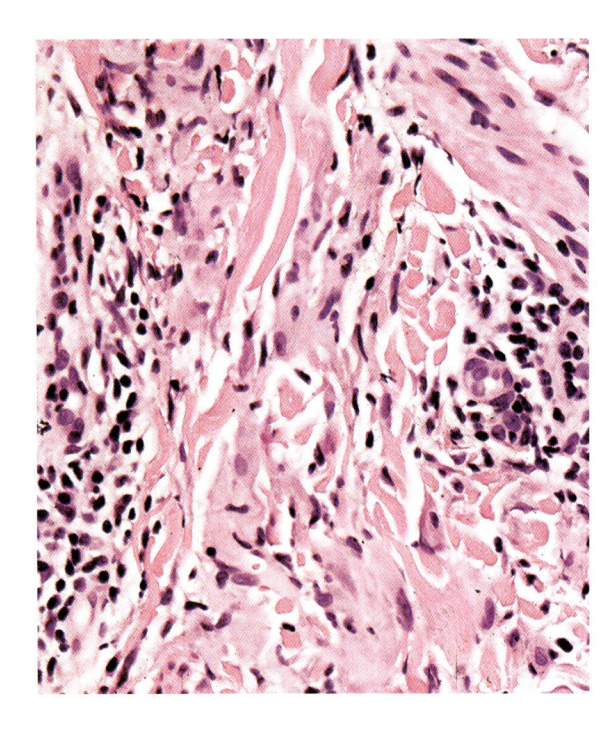

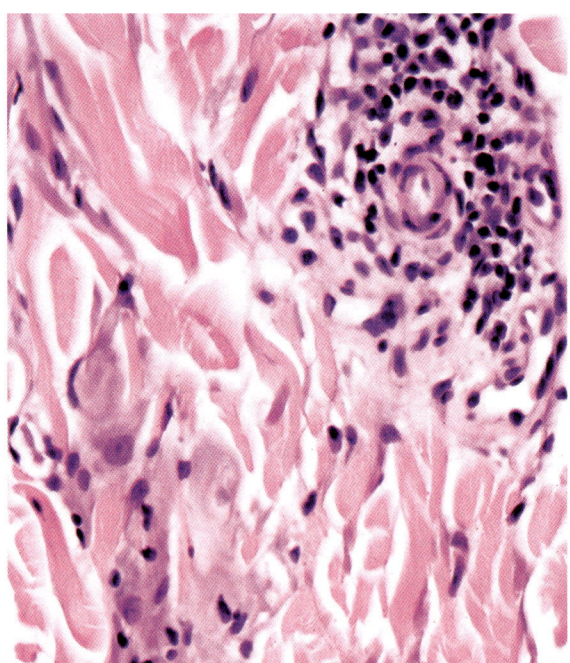

### Figure 12-38
**ELASTOLYTIC GRANULOMA**

Left: At this high power magnification, the interstitial infiltrative pattern of the histiocytes and lymphocytes is better appreciated.

Right: At higher magnification, the histiocytic component focally is associated with degenerating elastic fibers, with zones of fiber phagocytosis that are best demonstrated by elastic tissue stains.

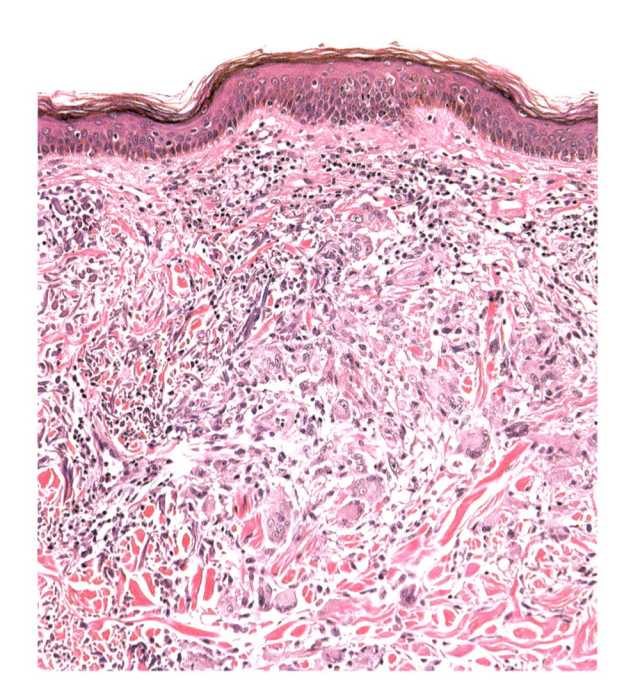

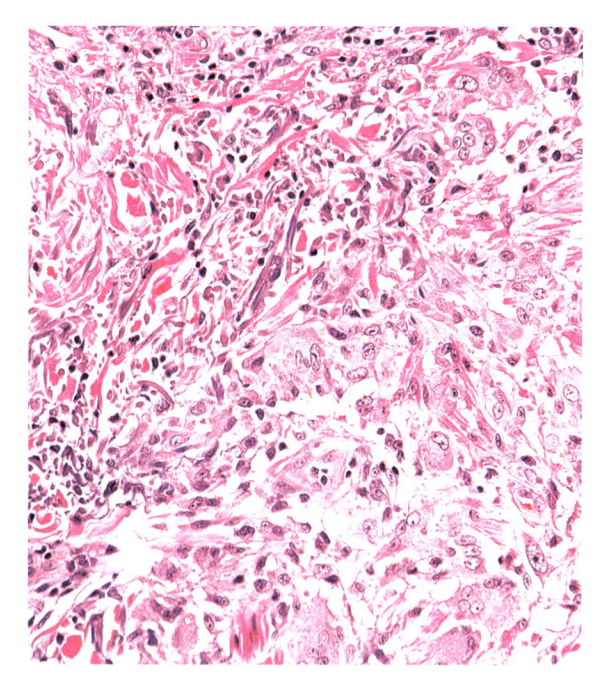

**Figure 12-39**

**ELASTOLYTIC GRANULOMA**

Left: A loosely formed granuloma containing multinucleated histiocytes is present in the superficial dermis.
Right: At high magnification, gray-blue elastin fibers are within the multinucleated histiocytes.

**Clinical Features.** The lesion characteristically shows papules, nodules, and plaques, many of which ulcerate. Lesions occur in the periorbital area most characteristically and may result in eye symptoms and signs such as keratitis, iritis, and uveitis, leading even to blindness. The papules and plaques, when over the extensor surfaces of the arms, result eventually in an infiltrative, deeply destructive disorder extending into tendons and muscles.

**Pathologic Findings.** There is a dermal and subcutaneous nodular and interstitial infiltrate of histiocytes and lymphocytes, with focal granuloma formation. Multinucleated giant cells of the Touton and foreign body types are present, and many histiocytes contain foamy cytoplasm. The intervening stroma consists of broad bands of hyalinized necrobiosis containing cholesterol clefts (fig. 12-40) and nodular accumulations of lymphocytes and plasma cells.

**Differential Diagnosis.** The differential diagnosis includes xanthogranulomas of other causes including hyperlipidemia, reticulohistiocytomas, and erythema elevatum diutinum. Histologically, the lesions must be differentiated from necrobiosis lipoidica, which also may show hyalinized necrobiosis. The presence of cholesterol clefts, lymphoid nodules, and prominent giant cells in necrobiotic xanthogranuloma facilitates the correct diagnosis.

**Treatment and Prognosis.** Patients usually respond when the lymphoproliferative causative disorder or the paraproteinemia is controlled (110). For lesions not responsive to topical or intralesional steroid therapy, excision with grafting may be necessary (111,112).

## Nephrogenic Systemic Fibrosis

**Definition.** *Nephrogenic systemic fibrosis* (NSF) is a recently identified systemic fibrosing disorder that affects patients with renal insufficiency and prior exposure to gadolinium-containing radiographic contrast agents (113). Although the cellular pathogenesis remains unclear, it is discusssed here in reference to other conditions it may mimic.

**Clinical Features.** Clinically, there is frequent symmetrical involvement of the distal extremities and trunk, with associated pain and debilitating joint contractures. Cutaneous

*Inflammatory Disorders of the Skin*

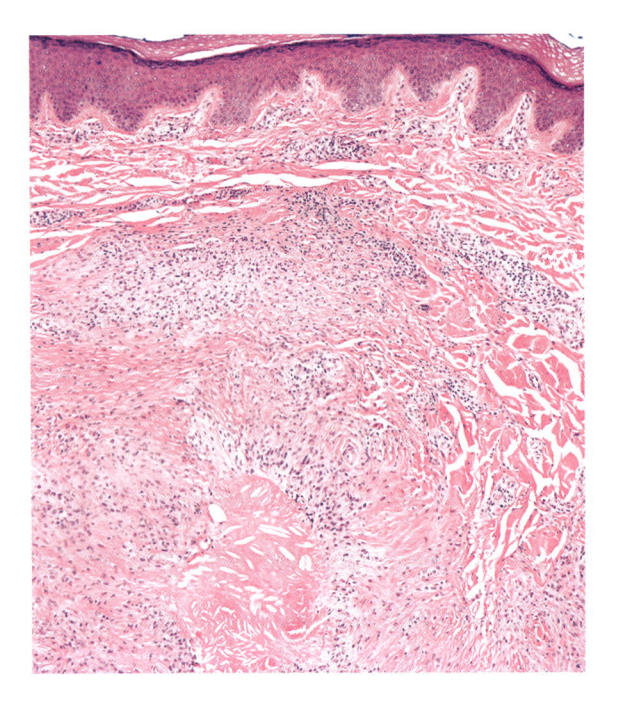

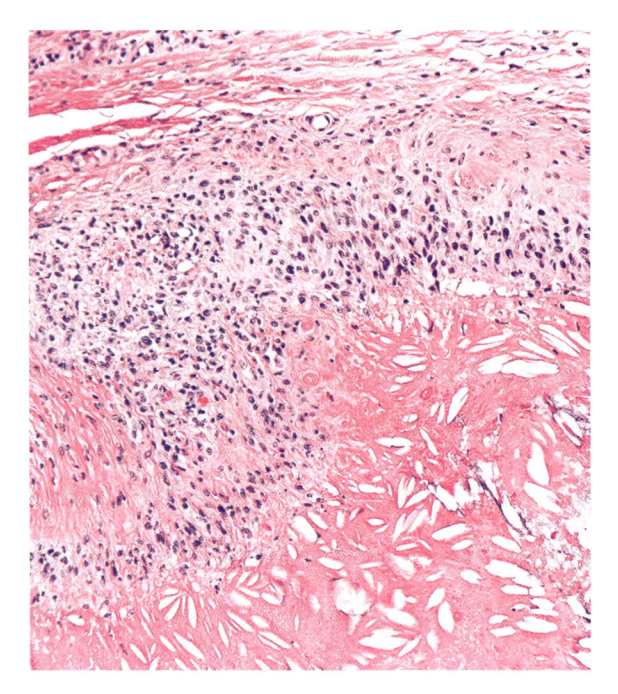

Figure 12-40

**NECROBIOTIC XANTHOGRANULOMATOUS REACTION**

Left: There is a histiocytic infiltrate in the dermis with zones of necrobiosis.
Right: Higher magnification shows a zone of necrobiosis containing cholesterol clefts; giant cells are not prominent in this field.

manifestations include skin hardening, hyperpigmentation, and thickening, and tethering to the underlying fascia (114).

The disorder was first reported as a scleromyxedema-like lesion in the literature in 2000 (115). With increased recognition of the link between the characteristic skin findings and a history of renal disease and lack of an associated paraproteinemia, the disorder was later termed nephrogenic fibrosing dermopathy (116). Several postmortem studies in patients diagnosed with this skin disorder revealed more widespread fibrosis than previously recognized, leading to a change in the nomenclature from nephrogenic fibrosing dermopathy to nephrogenic systemic fibrosis (117). Many extracutaneous sites of involvement by this emerging systemic disorder have been reported, including the dura mater, myocardium, lung, diaphragm, and skeletal muscle (118–120).

**Pathologic Findings.** Definitive diagnosis of NSF requires a deep punch biopsy of the skin in the appropriate clinical context. Histologic sections of affected skin and other anatomic sites reveal increased cellularity in the superficial and deep dermis without associated inflammation (figs. 12-41, 12-42). Other commonly reported histopathologic findings are a slight increase in dermal mucin deposition, thickened eosinophilic dermal collagen bundles with characteristic adjacent clefting, and elongated dermal elastic fibers (highlighted by Verhoeff-van Gieson stain) (114). Immunohistochemical studies reveal dual immunoreactivity of dermal fibrocyte-like cells for CD34 and procollagen-I, and an increased number of CD68/factor XIIIa-positive dendritic cells throughout the dermis (121,122). Calcification, ossification, histiocytes, and osteoclast-like giant cells may be present (123).

**Differential Diagnosis.** NSF shows histologic overlap with other fibrosing dermopathies including scleromyxedema, eosinophilic fasciitis, systemic sclerosis, and sclerodermatous chronic graft-versus-host disease. Differentiating NSF from these potential diagnostic pitfalls involves consideration of the dermal cellularity, quality of dermal collagen alteration, degree of dermal

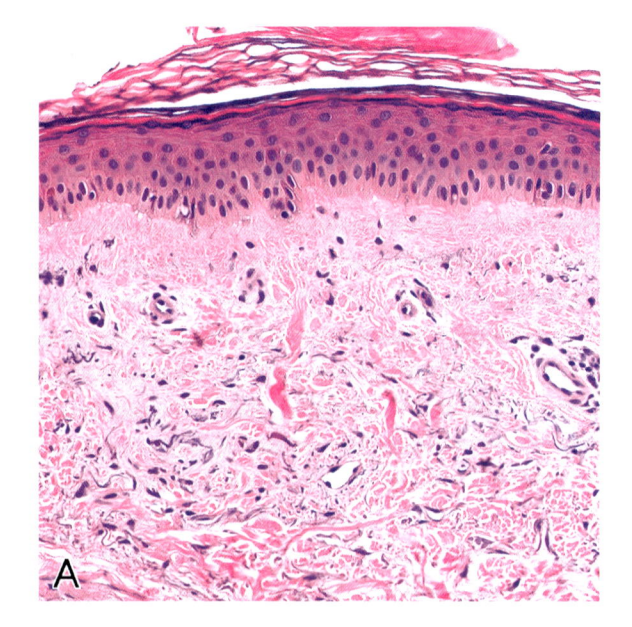

### Figure 12-41
### NEPHROGENIC SYSTEMIC FIBROSIS

A: The epidermis is totally unaffected although some basilar pigmentation, acanthosis, and blunting of rete can occasionally be seen.

B: Increased cellularity is present in the dermis without associated inflammation and no significant mucin deposition.

C: Increased dermal cellularity and thickened eosinophilic collagen bundles with characteristic adjacent clefting are seen.

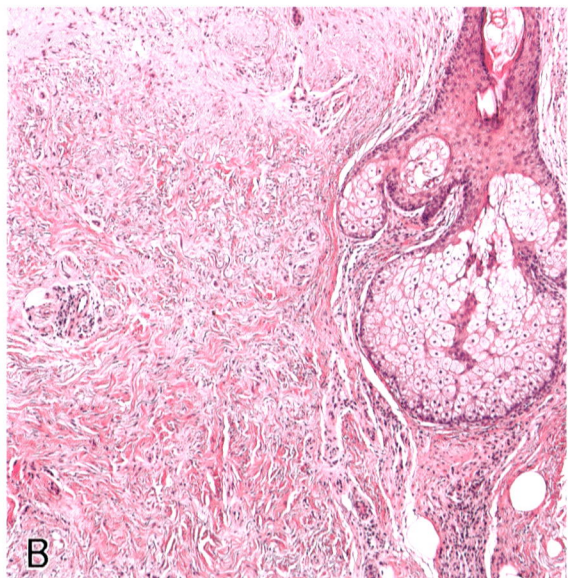

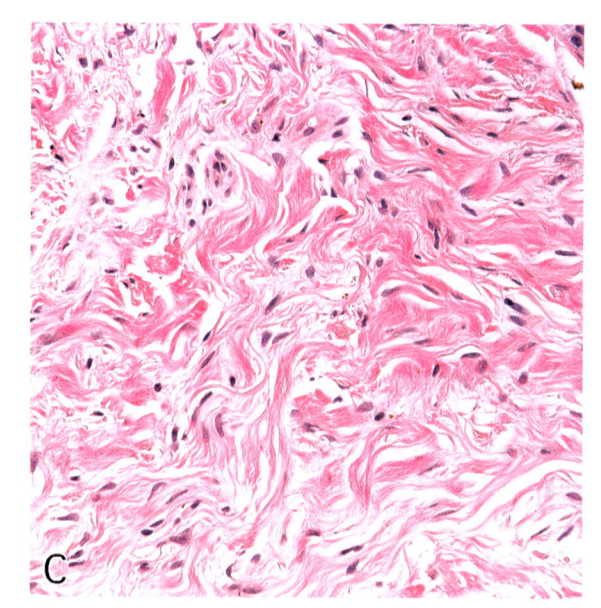

mucin, and presence of inflammatory cells (123). In addition to these histologic features, consideration of the clinical history is paramount in rendering the appropriate diagnosis.

Increased dermal cellularity is observed in NSF, scleromyxedema, and eosinophilic fasciitis. Scleromyxedema can be differentiated from NSF by the presence of dermal mucin "pools" and an associated monoclonal paraproteinemia. Eosinophilic fasciitis is differentiated by the presence of peripheral eosinophilia and polyclonal hypergammaglobulinemia. Systemic sclerosis/morphea and sclerodermatous chronic graft-versus-host disease are histologically characterized by a decrease in dermal cellularity and homogenization of dermal collagen fibers in contrast to NSF. Clinically, the finding of circulating autoantibodies and a history of bone marrow transplantation are useful for differentiating these entities from NSF (123).

**Treatment and Prognosis.** NSF is a rapidly progressive disorder with a high mortality rate that is potentially preventable but with no proven effective therapies. Treatment with topical

*Inflammatory Disorders of the Skin*

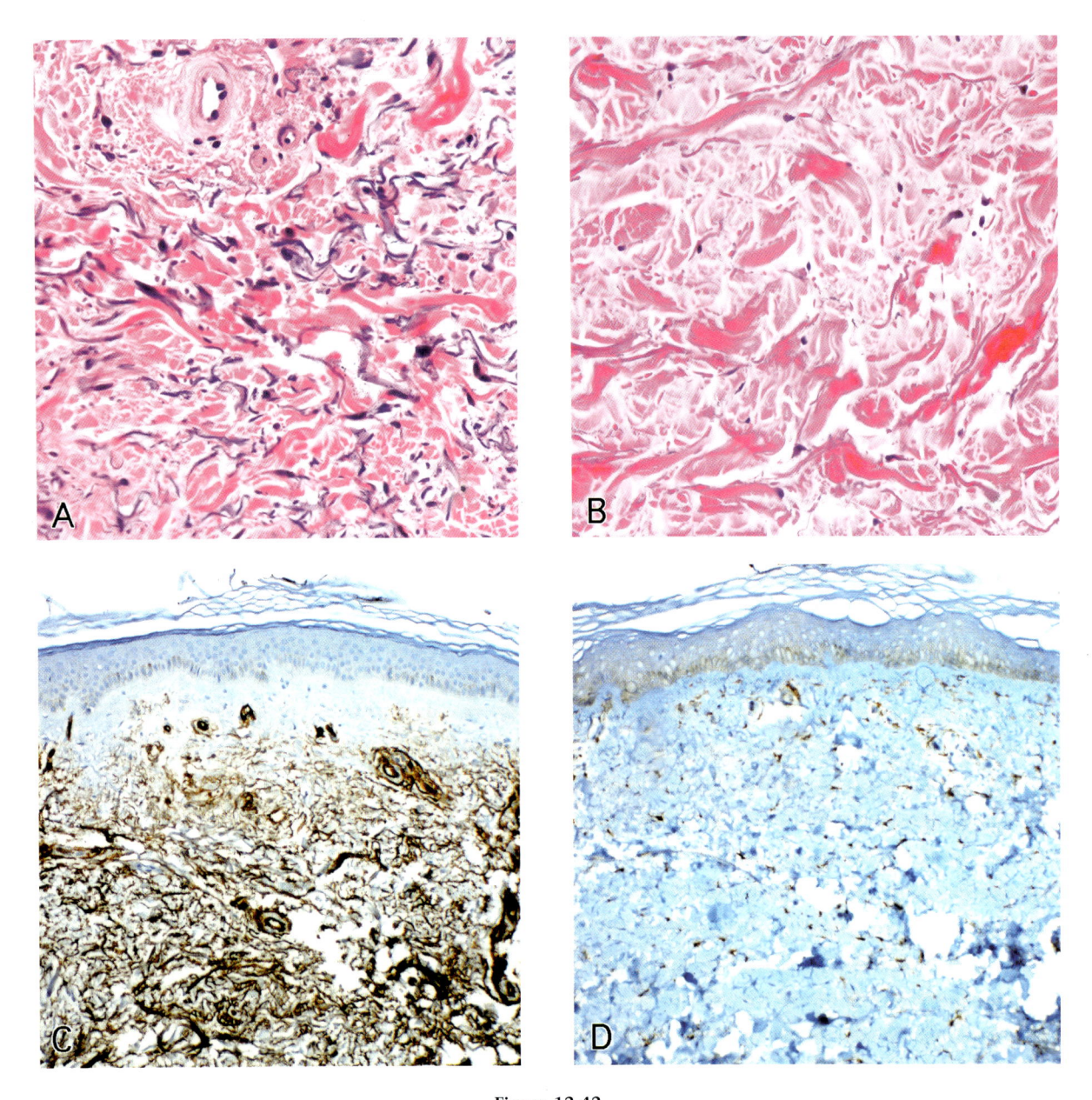

**Figure 12-42**

**NEPHROGENIC SYSTEMIC FIBROSIS**

A,B: Increased dermal cellularity and thickened eosinophilic collagen bundles with characteristic adjacent clefting (A) is compared to normal skin (B) (H&E stain).

C: Immunohistochemical staining for CD34 highlights increased dermal spindle-shaped cells (and normal vascular channels).

D: Immunohistochemical staining for factor XIII shows scattered mononuclear cells in the dermis.

or oral steroids, immunosuppressive agents (methotrexate, cyclosporine, interferon-alpha), thalidomide, oral retinoids, intravenous sodium thiosulfate, intravenous immune globulins, PUVA light, and plasmapheresis have not been shown to be effective (114,124,125). Mild improvement in skin thickening and joint contracture has been reported following treatment with extracorporeal photopheresis and pentoxiphylline, although large trials systematically evaluating the effectiveness of various treatment modalities are lacking (114,124). Recently, lessening of skin tethering and joint contractures with histopathologically decreased cutaneous fibrosis have been shown following treatment with imatinib mesylate, a tyrosine kinase inhibitor of platelet-derived growth factor receptor and transforming growth factor receptor-beta (125,126).

## Granulomatous and Interstitial Inflammatory Reactions to Infectious Agents

Granulomas due to infectious agents result from a variety of organisms. A partial listing of offending agents that must be considered and excluded as causes of granulomatous dermatitis is presented in Table 12-1. Dermal involvement by such infectious agents often produces a nodular and/or interstitial inflammatory reaction (summarized in Table 12-2). Accordingly, one must be cognizant of infection as one cause of such patterns of inflammation, and where appropriate, attempt to identify and classify potentially causative infectious agents (Table 12-3).

As a general rule, granulomatous dermatitis resulting from infection is rare, although it is frequently considered and excluded by special stains in the differential diagnosis of sarcoidosis, panniculitis in immunocompromised hosts, and even in certain atypical granulomatous responses to foreign material or follicular rupture. The clinical appearance of infectious granulomas is highly variable, ranging from erythematous plaques and nodules to frank ulcers with purulent drainage and sinus tract formation. Histologically, suspicion of infection is heightened by zones of necrosis, microabscesses, or the general absence of evidence supporting an obvious cause (e.g., the pattern and composition of a specific granulomatous panniculitis, or clear evidence of material that may elicit granuloma formation, such as keratin). Infectious granulomas may be well formed, as is the case in tuberculoid leprosy, or they may be composed of vague aggregates of vacuolated histiocytes, as in leishmaniasis. Infectious granulomas in immunocompromised hosts may be so poorly formed that only foci of necrosis and admixed acute and chronic inflammatory cells with the vague appearance of loosely aggregated granulomas suggest procuring appropriate special stains that could result in a lifesaving diagnosis.

Table 12-1

**ORGANISMS RESPONSIBLE FOR GRANULOMATOUS DERMATITIS**

| Organisms | Disorders |
| --- | --- |
| Fungi | |
| *Aspergillus* sp | Aspergillosis |
| *Blastomyces dermatitides* | Blastomycosis |
| *Candida albicans* | Candidiasis |
| *Fonsecaea, Phialophora,* and *Cladoporium* sp | Chromomycosis |
| *Coccidioides immitis* | Coccidioidomycosis |
| *Cryptococcus neoformans* | Cryptococcosis |
| *Histoplasma capsulatum* | Histoplasmosis |
| *Rhizopus* and *Mucor* sp | Mucormycosis |
| *Rhinosporidium seeberi* | Rhinosporidiosis |
| *Sporothrix schenckii* | Sporotrichosis |
| Bacteria | |
| *Calymmatobacterium granulomatis* | Granuloma inguinale |
| *Treponema pallidum* | Granulomatous syphilis |
| *Mycobacterium tuberculosis* | Lupus vulgaris |
| *Mycobacterium marinum* | Swimming-pool granuloma |
| *Mycobacterium leprae* | Leprosy |
| Protozoa | |
| *Leishmania* sp | Leishmaniasis and kala-azar |

There are a number of clinical and histologic differential diagnostic features that are helpful in the evaluation of granulomatous dermatitis due to infection. In *cutaneous cryptococcosis*, for example, a biopsy specimen from a cutaneous plaque studded with small papules may reveal diffuse granulomatous inflammation replete with multinucleated giant cells, alternating with zones of gelatinous material that is devoid of significant inflammation but contains numerous spores, each surrounded by mucinous capsules. In *histoplasmosis*, similar granulomatous dermal inflammation containing multinucleated giant cells reveals spores even smaller than cryptococci, devoid of surrounding mucinous alteration. Pigmented organisms that do not require PAS or silver stains for visualization characterize the granulomatous dermal foci of *chromomycosis*. In *mucormycosis*, vague granulomas within inflamed granulation tissue harbor large, ribbon-like hyphae that characteristically branch at right angles. *Aspergillosis*, on the other hand, produces variable degrees of granulomatous dermal inflammation containing hyphae that branch at acute angles. *Coccidioides immitis* (*coccidioidomycosis*) results in giant cells containing large spores which, during multiplication,

## Inflammatory Disorders of the Skin

Table 12-2

### INFECTIOUS AGENTS PRODUCING NODULAR/INTERSTITIAL HISTIOCYTIC INFILTRATES

| | Clinical Features | Histologic Features | Diagnostic Clues |
|---|---|---|---|
| Primary inoculation tuberculosis (e.g., "prosector's paronychia") | Papule, nodule, or painless ulcer with adenopathy of draining nodes | Suppuration leading to dermal infiltration by epithelioid giant cells and histiocytes | Positive AFB[a] stain in early stages |
| Lupus vulgaris | Solitary red-brown papule or nodule on head or neck | Well-formed tuberculoid granulomas in dermis; little or no caseation | AFB rare; PCR for AFB DNA may be positive |
| Scrofuloderma | Cervical lymphadenitis with draining sinus tracts | Tuberculoid granulomas with necrosis and sinus tract formation in dermis | AFB numerous by acid-fast stains |
| Atypical mycobacteria | Papules, nodules, ulcers at inoculation site | Mixed histiocytic infiltrate with lymphocytes and neutrophils; ulceration; no granulomas | Mycobacteria by acid-fast stain; type by culture |
| Leprosy | Anesthetic plaques to diffuse dermal infiltration (leonine facies) | Granulomas in tuberculoid form; diffuse infiltrate of vacuolated histiocytes in lepromatous form | Acid-fast bacilli in lepromatous form; rare or no organisms in tuberculoid form |
| Deep fungus | Erythematous nodules to plaques with reactive epidermal changes/ulceration | Granulomatous infiltrate in dermis; necrosis; occasional microabscess formation | Organisms by PAS or silver stains; culture |
| Chronic leishmaniasis | Tan-brown nodules at periphery of central scar | Tubercles or diffuse dermal infiltrates of parasitized histiocytes | Characteristic organisms within cytoplasm of histiocytes |
| Rhinosporidiosis | Papules, nodules, and polyps involving nasal mucosa | Interstitial histiocytes and giant cells with mixed inflammation | Cysts containing characteristic fungal spores |
| Rhinoscleroma | Papules of nose and respiratory mucosa | Granulomas with many plasma cells | Foamy histiocytes (Mikulicz cells) with intracellular gram-negative *Klebsiella* |
| Cutaneous malakoplakia | Coalescent papules and plaques | Interstitial histiocytes with blue cytoplasmic granules (Michaelis-Gutman bodies) | Intracytoplasmic bacilli by electron microscopy |

[a]AFB = acid-fast bacillus; PCR = polymerase chain reaction; PAS = periodic acid–Schiff.

may contain numerous internal endospores. In ulcerated or draining lesions, diagnostic organisms may be detected near the skin surface as a result of extrusion of dermal inflammatory cells. The organisms of *rhinosporidiosis* are characteristically 6- to 10-μm spores, often within 250- to 350-μm rounded sporangia surrounded by a mixed cellular infiltrate containing granulomatous foci. Unlike the other organisms listed previously, rhinosporidiosis preferentially affects nasal skin and mucosa, producing pruritus and coryza. *Sporothrix schenckii* infection also has a characteristic clinical picture, with ascending lymphatic involvement from the inoculation site often resulting in linear dermal nodules. The organisms of sporotrichosis are 4- to 6-μm, round to ovoid spores, sometimes accompanied by characteristic cigar-shaped or radially arranged buds.

All mycobacterial infections of skin are characterized by small, variably beaded, acid-fast bacilli within histiocytes comprising granulomatous lesions. The organisms may be few in number, and are often best detected in zones that border regions of necrosis or in the setting of immunosuppression. The most common form of *cutaneous tuberculosis*, *lupus vulgaris*, is characterized by well-formed tuberculoid dermal granulomas on head and neck skin. Atypical mycobacterial infections, such as *swimming-pool granuloma* caused by *Mycobacterium marinum*, show mixed inflammatory infiltrates containing neutrophils and little granulomatous inflammation at sites of dermal inoculation. The clinical hallmark of *tuberculoid*

Table 12-3

**DIFFERENTIAL FEATURES IN GRANULOMATOUS DERMATITIS**

| Disorder | Organisms | Inflammation | Clinical Appearance |
|---|---|---|---|
| **Fungi** | | | |
| Aspergillosis | Silver-positive septate mycelia, 45-degree angle branching | May be minimal; vessel emboli and intramural growth | Necrotic eschar |
| Blastomycosis | PAS[a]- and silver-positive 10 μm spores with broad-based buds | Granulomas, microabscesses, epidermal hyperplasia | Verrucous plaques, pustules, ulceration |
| Candidiasis | PAS- and silver-positive pseudoseptate mycelia, 90-degree angle branching, 4-6 μm spores | Granulomas, epidermal hyperplasia, subcorneal pustules | Beefy red scaling plaque, peripheral pustules |
| Chromomycosis | Copper-colored, 6-12 μm spores, division by septation | Mixed inflammation, epidermal hyperplasia; transepidermal elimination of spores | Verrucous plaque covered with black dots (i.e., surface spores) |
| Coccidioidomycosis | PAS- and silver-positive spherule ≤80 μm containing 2-5 μm endospores | Mixed inflammation, variable epidermal hyperplasia | Verrucous papules and plaques |
| Cryptococcosis | PAS- and silver-positive 3-20 μm spores with narrow-based buds, mucin-positive capsule | Granulomatous or noninflammatory, gelatinous | Plaques, ulcers, molluscum-like papules |
| Histoplasmosis | 3-μm H&E- and Giemsa-positive encapsulated spores (capsule is silver-positive) | Mixed inflammation with granulomas, or sheets of histiocytes when immunity impaired | Ulcerated papules and plaques |
| Mucormycosis | PAS- and silver-positive 30 μm nonseptate mycelia, 90-degree angle branching | Mixed inflammation, vessel invasion | Indurated nodules and ulcers |
| Rhinosporidiosis | H&E-positive 250 to 350 μm sporangia containing 6-12 μm spores | Mixed inflammation, epithelial hyperplasia | Papules, nodules, and polyps of nasal epithelium |
| Sporotrichosis | PAS-positive 4-6 μm spores, cigar-like bodies, asteroid-like bodies | Mixed inflammation, microabscesses, organisms difficult to find | Cutaneous nodules with lymphatic distribution, plaques |
| **Bacteria** | | | |
| Granuloma inguinale | Giemsa- or silver-positive intracellular 10-20 μm bacilli (i.e., Donovan bodies) | Mixed inflammation with large histiocytes containing organisms | Ulcerated genital, inguinal, perianal nodules |
| Granuloma syphilis | Silver-positive corkscrew-like spirochetes, mostly within epidermis | Superficial dermal granulomas, cytotoxic pattern, plasma cells | Multiple nodules or plaques |
| Lupus vulgaris (*Mycobacterium tuberculosis*) | Acid-fast beaded bacilli within giant cells or at zones of necrosis | Tuberculoid granulomas, Langhans giant cells | Red-brown nodule or plaque on head or neck |
| Swimming-pool granuloma (*M. marinum*) | Acid-fast beaded bacilli, slightly larger than *Mycobacterium tuberculosis* | Mixed inflammation, tuberculoid granulomas rare, focal necrosis | Nodule or plaque often on arm or hand, may show lymphatic spread |
| Leprosy | Acid-fast intracellular bacilli | Tuberculoid cells or sheets of foam cells (i.e., lepromatous), nerve destruction | Anesthetic plaque or diffuse skin thickening |
| **Protozoa** | | | |
| Chronic leishmaniasis | Giemsa-positive 2-4 μm round intracellular organisms | Microtubercles with epithelioid histiocytes and Langhans cells | Scaling plaques |

[a]PAS = periodic acid–Schiff; H&E = hematoxylin and eosin.

*leprosy*, the anesthetic patch or plaque, may contain coalescent, noncaseating granulomas that course along dermal neurovascular bundles in a serpiginous pattern. Organisms are generally not detected by special histologic stains. The more diffuse infiltrative lesions of *lepromatous leprosy* are characterized by poorly organized dermal infiltrates of finely vacuolated histiocytes, or lepra cells, replete with clusters of *M. leprae* organisms known as globi.

It is beyond the scope of this chapter to provide specific details concerning the many forms of granulomatous dermatitis caused by infectious agents. When faced with granulomatous inflammation that is either suspected clinically of being of infectious origin or has histologic features that do not fit well with noninfectious causes of granulomatous inflammation, special stains for fungi (e.g., PAS and silver) as well as acid-fast reagents for mycobacteria should be used. Table 12-3 is a summary of the salient features of the more common causes of infectious granulomatous inflammation in skin and can be used as an adjunct when evaluating the results of these stains within the context of histologic and clinical parameters.

Infectious causes of granulomatous dermatitis are important to keep in mind, because accurate diagnosis often relies on ordering a special stain, and such a measure may result in lifesaving therapeutic intervention. It is recommended that infectious granulomatous dermatitis be strongly considered when histologic evidence of granuloma formation is encountered in the following settings: clinical suspicion of infection, unusual occupational or travel history, immunocompromised patient, dermal granulomas without obvious cause, granulomatous panniculitis without a clearcut clinicopathologic diagnosis of primary panniculitis, and microabscesses or necrosis.

The definitive exclusion of an infectious cause for granulomatous dermatitis does not depend solely on obtaining negative special stains. The culture of fresh biopsied tissue is generally a much more sensitive means of excluding organisms. Therefore, cultures should be a component of the diagnostic evaluation of potentially infectious forms of granulomatous infiltration of the skin when infection is suspected based on existing clinical or histologic parameters.

The reader is referred to other Fascicles and sources dealing with infectious diseases for a comprehensive review of the correlative clinical and histopathologic aspects of infectious agents that result in granulomatous and nodulointerstitial inflammatory reactions in the dermis and subcutis. In the spirit of a diagnositc atlas, and for purposes of a visual overview, the following examples of infectious agents that may produce nodular/interstitial inflammatory responses are provided in the following figures: leprosy: indeterminate (figs. 12-43, 12-44), tuberculoid (figs. 12-45, 12-46), lepromatous (fig. 12-47); mycetoma (fig. 12-48); necrotizing fasciitis (fig. 12-49); coccidioidomycosis (fig. 12-50); histoplasmosis (fig. 12-51); cryptococcosis (fig. 12-52); aspergillosis (figs. 12-53, 12-54); chromomycosis (fig. 12-55); mucormycosis (fig. 12-56); sporotrichosis (fig. 12-57); fusarium (fig. 12-58); mycobacterial infection (figs. 12-59–12-62); postherpetic granulomatous reaction (fig. 12-63); cutaneous larva migrans (fig. 12-64); cutaneous leishmaniasis (fig. 12-65); and blastomycosis (fig. 12-66).

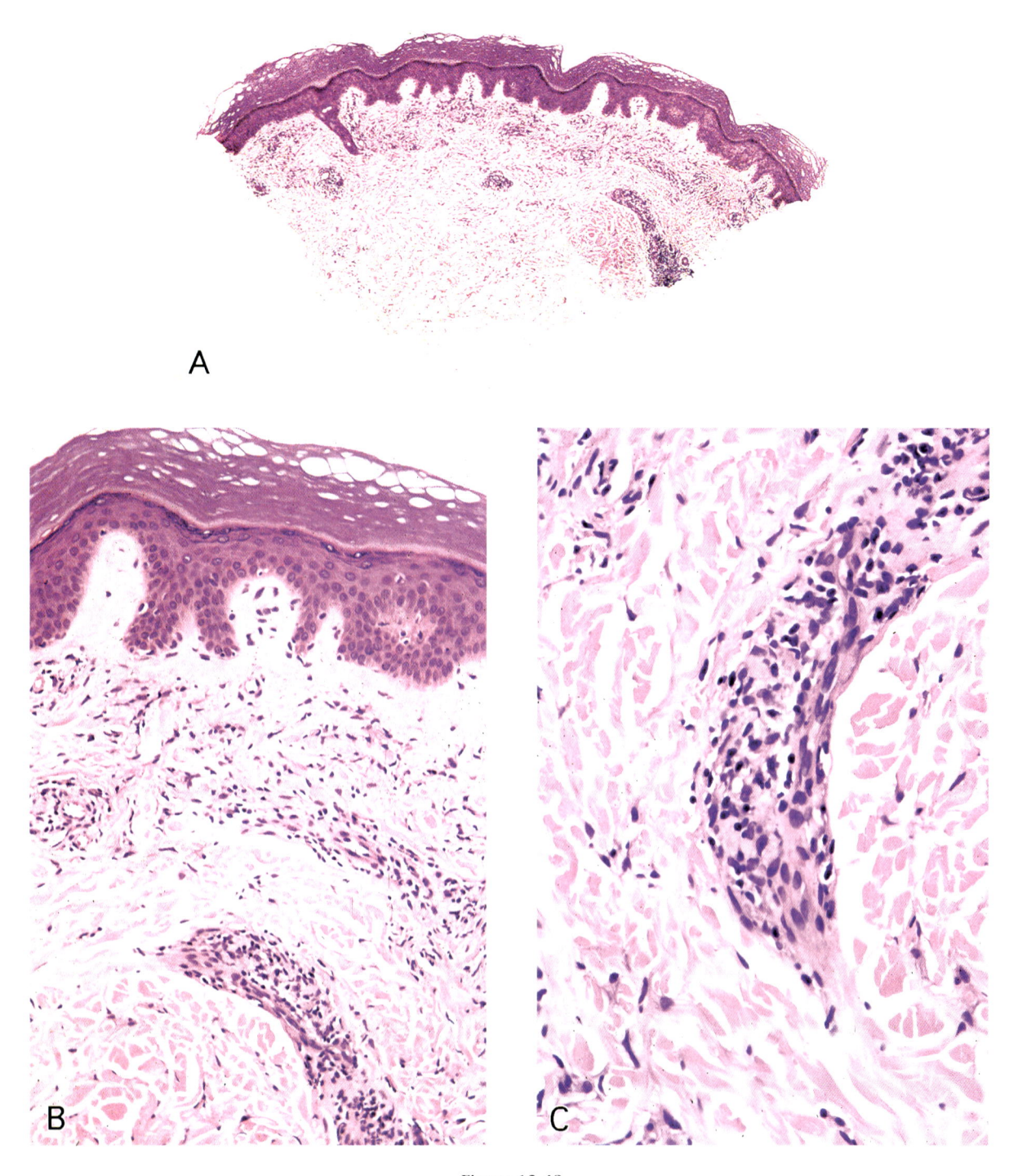

Nodular/Interstitial Dermatitis

Figure 12-43
INDETERMINATE LEPROSY

A: At scanning magnification, the first impression is a superficial dermal delayed hypersensitivity reaction.
B: At higher magnification of the superficial component, the perivascular and papillary dermal interstitial architecture of the lymphohistiocytic infiltrate is appreciated.
C: High magnification of the perivascular infiltrate shows lymphocytes intimately admixed with histiocytes.

*Inflammatory Disorders of the Skin*

**Figure 12-44**

**INDETERMINATE LEPROSY**

Acid-fast bacilli are observed (arrows) in the angiocentric histiocytic component with the Fite stain.

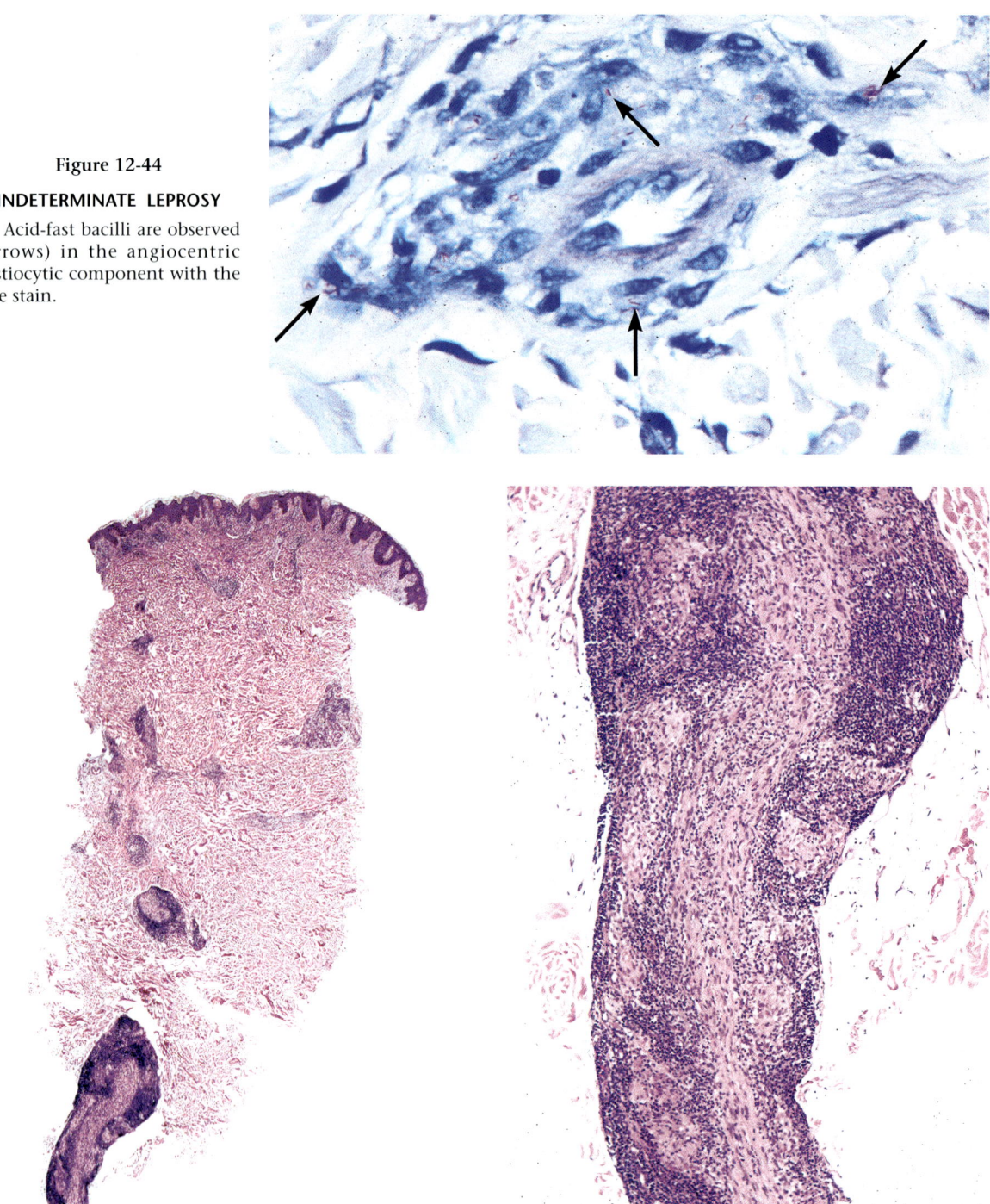

**Figure 12-45**

**TUBERCULOID LEPROSY**

Left: The architecture of the infiltrate is serpiginous as a result of its association with its neurovascular bundles, which extend from the superficial dermis into subcutaneous fat.

Right: Higher magnification of the subcutaneous fat shows the infiltrate centered about partially destroyed nerves. It is formed by coalescent granulomas composed of aggregated epithelioid histiocytes and admixed lymphocytes.

### Nodular/Interstitial Dermatitis

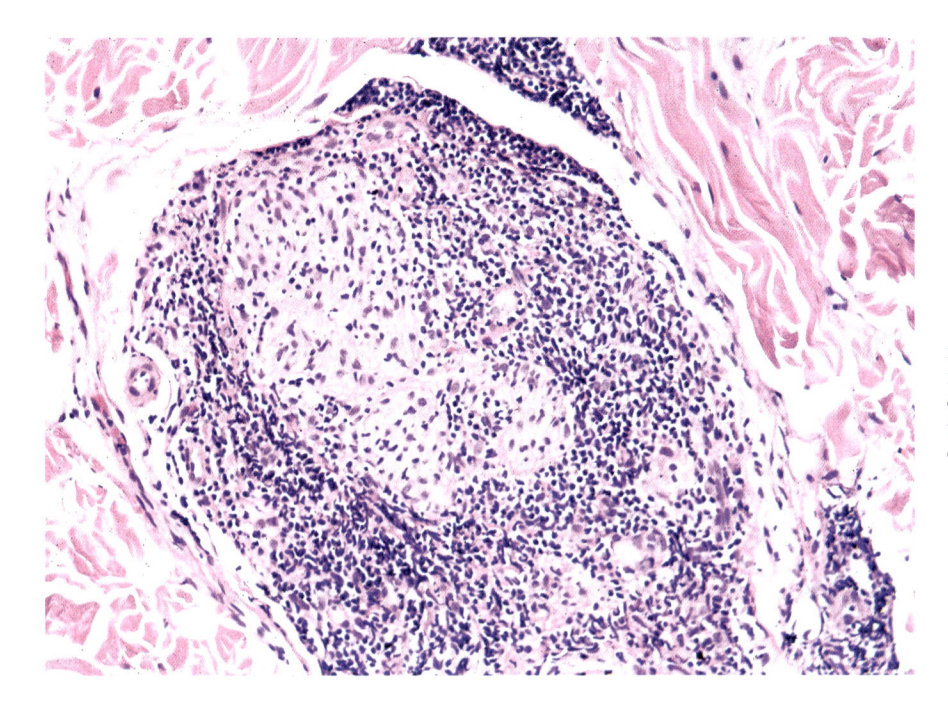

**Figure 12-46**
**TUBERCULOID LEPROSY**
This well-formed micronodule represents a non-necrotizing granuloma composed of epithelioid histiocytes rimmed by numerous lymphocytes.

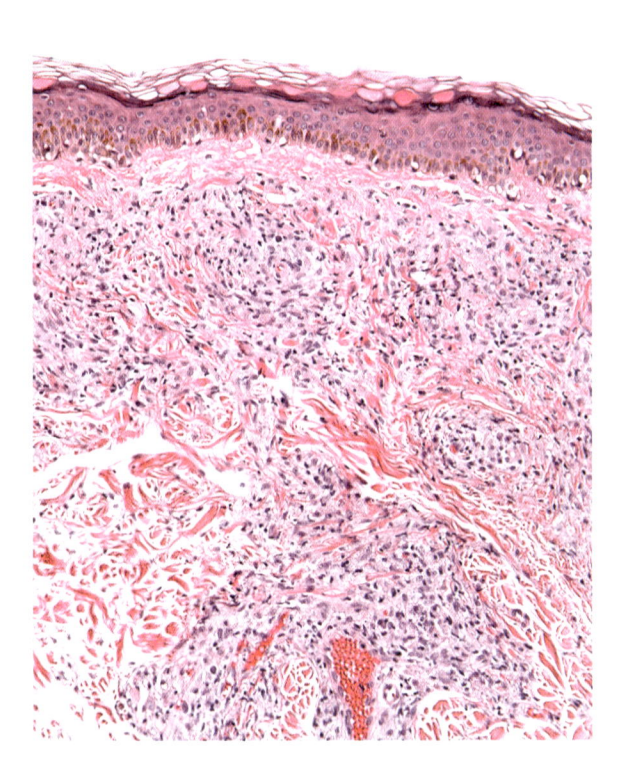

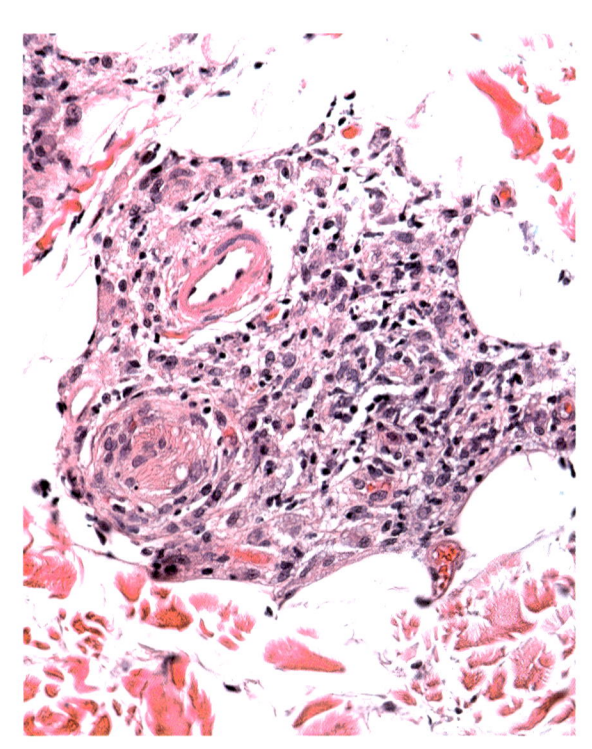

**Figure 12-47**
**LEPROMATOUS LEPROSY**
Left: The superficial and deep perineurovascular infiltrate is composed of lymphocytes and prominent histiocytes.
Right: High magnification of the histiocytic cells shows early infiltration of the perineurium.

*Inflammatory Disorders of the Skin*

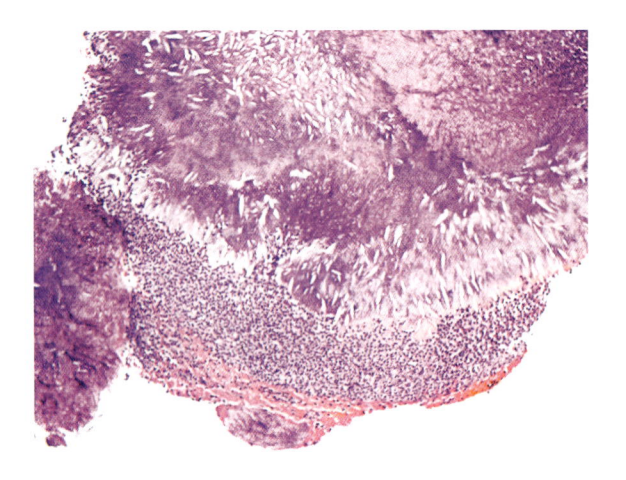

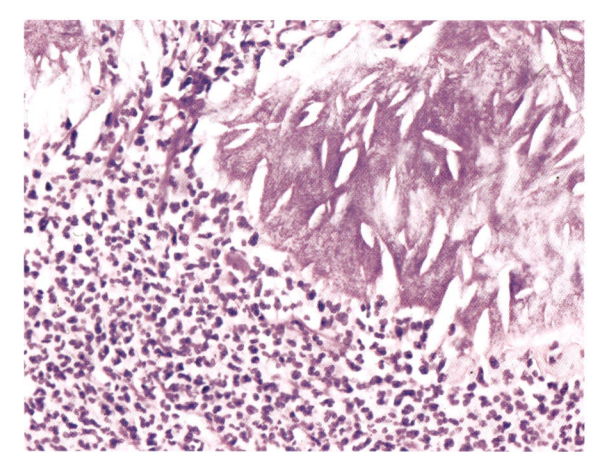

Figure 12-48

MYCETOMA

Left: The tissue reaction is characterized by prominent acute inflammation, necrosis, and reactive mesenchymal alterations (the latter not shown).
Right: Higher magnification of the neutrophilic component.

Figure 12-49

NECROTIZING FASCIITIS

A: At low magnification, there is a seemingly nonspecific admixture of interstitial inflammatory and reactive changes, with associated zones of necrosis.

B: At higher magnification, extensive coagulative necrosis is revealed within connective tissue associated with intravascular thrombosis.

C: Numerous particulate bacterial forms are evident in this necrotizing fasciitis with prominent intravascular thrombosis.

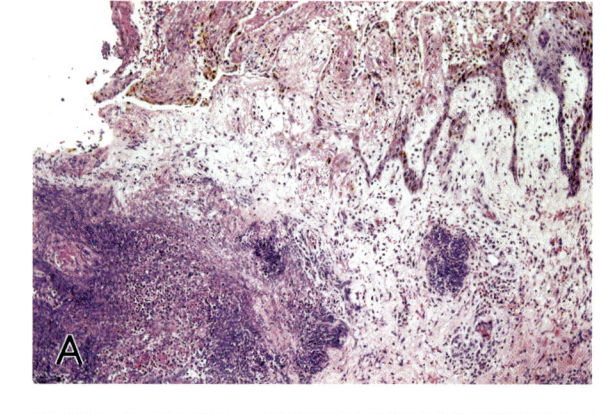

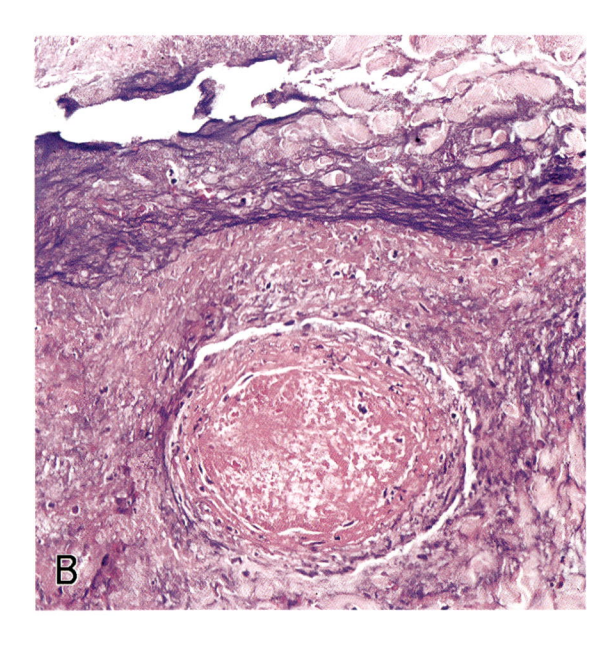

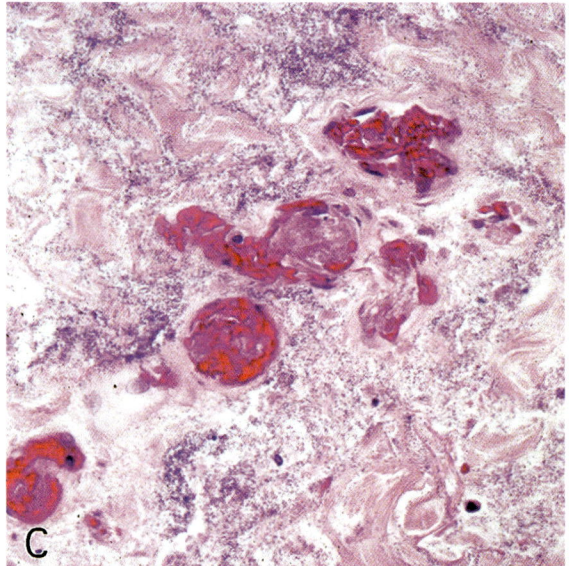

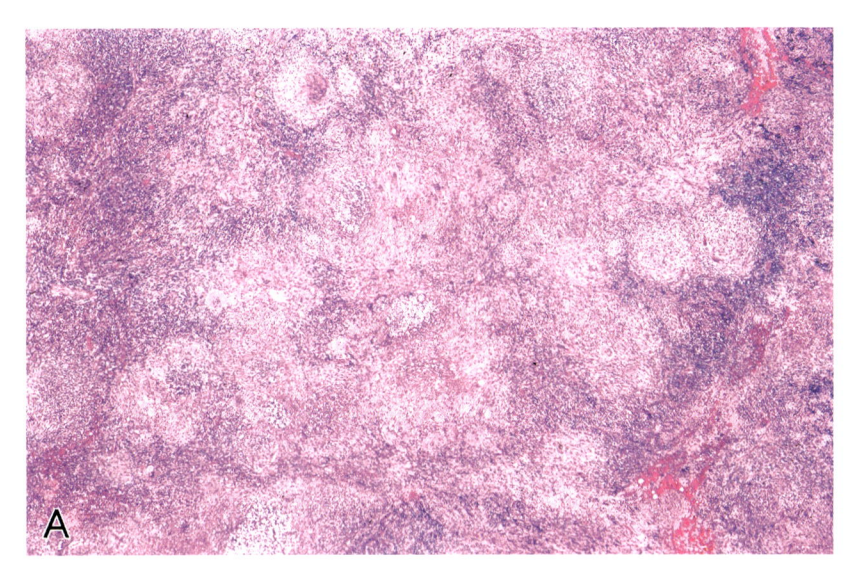

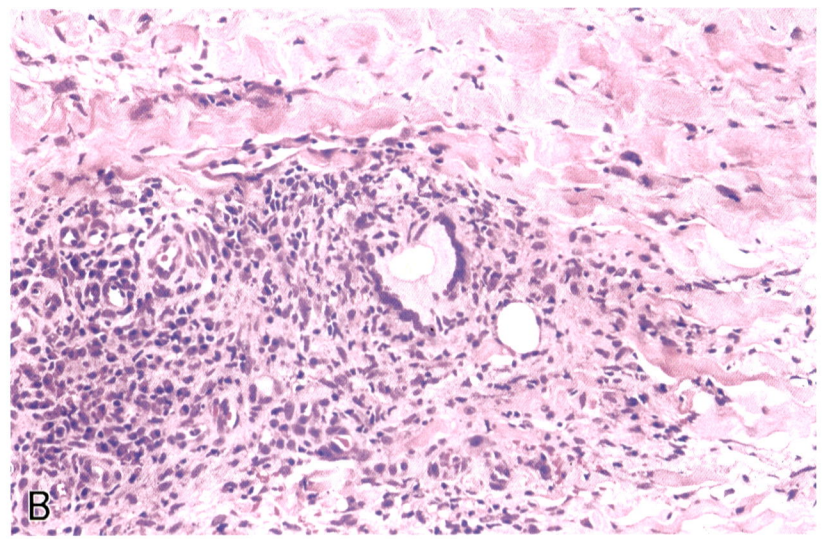

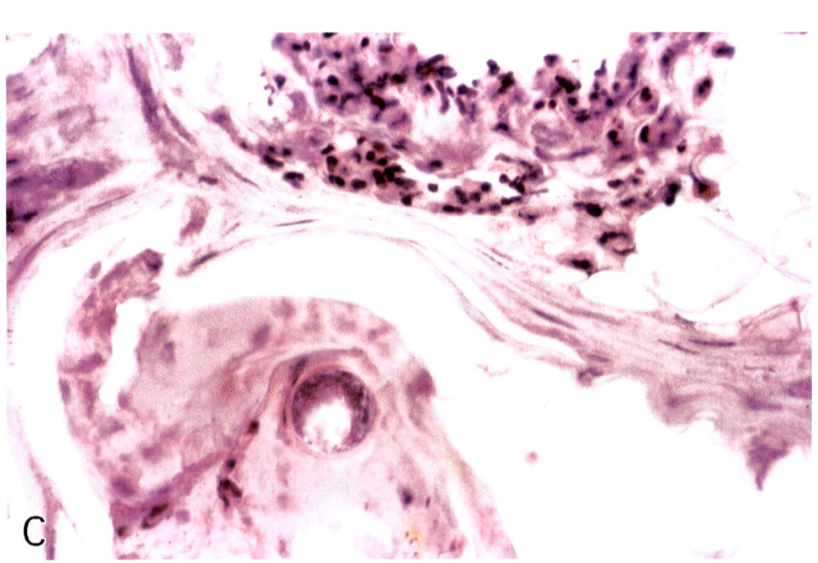

**Figure 12-50**

**COCCIDIOIDOMYCOSIS**

A: The dermis and subcutis are largely replaced by coalescent granulomas.

B: At higher magnification, organisms are detected within vacuoles in the multinucleated histiocytes forming the granulomas.

C: A sporangium containing endospores is observed.

## Inflammatory Disorders of the Skin

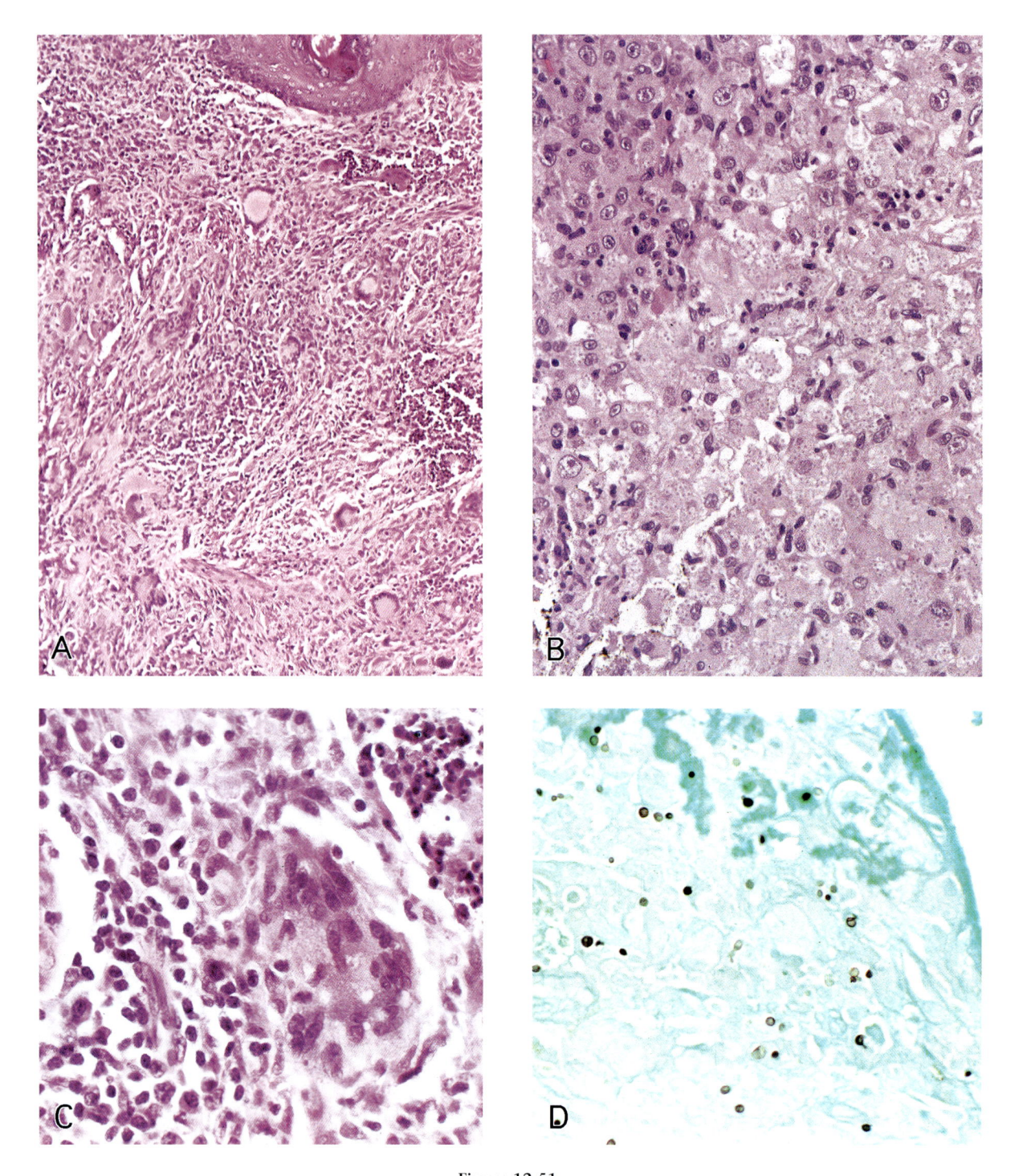

**Figure 12-51**

**HISTOPLASMOSIS**

A: This lesion shows coalescent nodules within the superficial and deep dermis formed by granulomatous inflammation replete with multinucleated histiocytes.

B: Higher magnification of the granulomatous inflammation, dominated by epithelioid histiocytes.

C: High magnification of multinucleated giant cells shows subtle rounded clear zones within cytoplasm that correlate with ingested organisms.

D: With a silver stain, numerous 2- to 4-µm spores are revealed.

Nodular/Interstitial Dermatitis

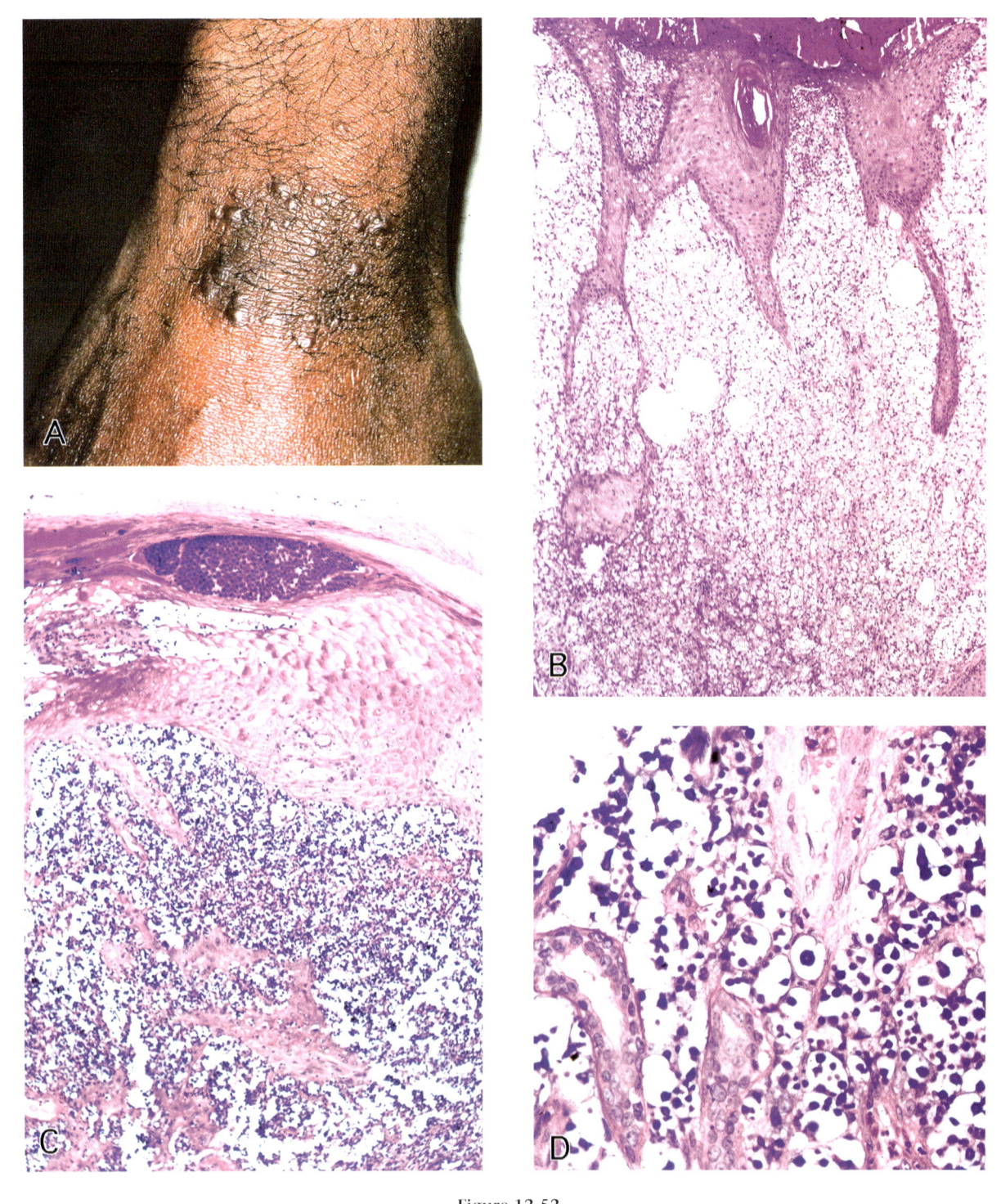

Figure 12-52
**CRYPTOCOCCOSIS**

A: The wrist skin of this immunosuppressed individual shows a hyperpigmented plaque studded by small, firm papules.

B: There is a nodular to focally diffuse granulomatous infiltrate throughout the dermis, with associated overlying epidermal hyperplasia.

C: There are numerous narrow-necked, budding spores surrounded by a mucinous capsule (PAS/Alcian blue stain).

D: The morphology of the budding spores is better appreciated at high power (PAS/Alcian blue stain).

*Inflammatory Disorders of the Skin*

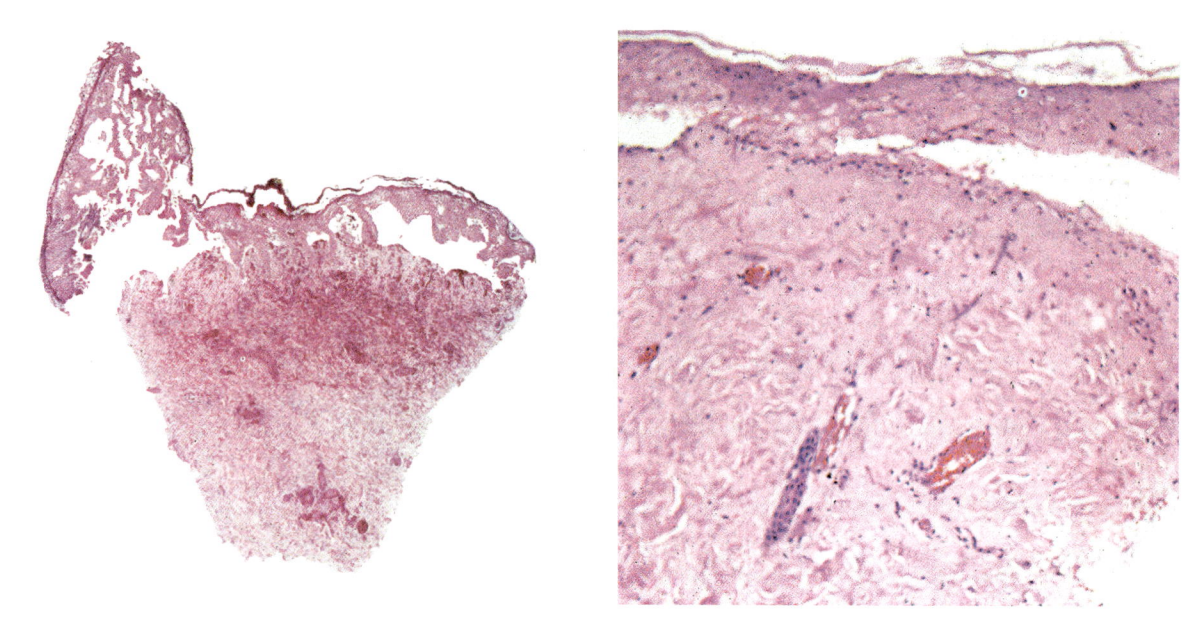

**Figure 12-53**

**ASPERGILLOSIS**

Left: At scanning magnification, there is a patchy inflammatory infiltrate involving the superficial and mid-dermis, with incipient epidermal necrosis.

Right: At higher magnification, coagulative epidermal necrosis and a paucicellular inflammatory component are seen.

**Figure 12-54**

**ASPERGILLOSIS**

A: There is diffuse hemorrhage and infarction associated with what appears to be a remnant of a damaged blood vessel.

B: Hyphae are within the lumen of a blood vessel, indicative of thromboembolic dissemination to the skin.

C: There are numerous septate hyphae that branch at acute angles (silver stain).

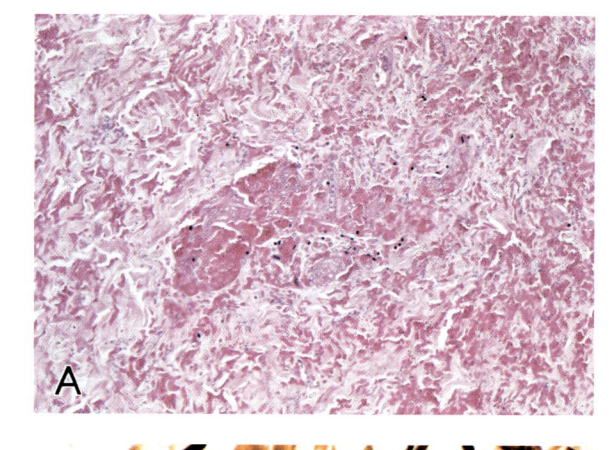

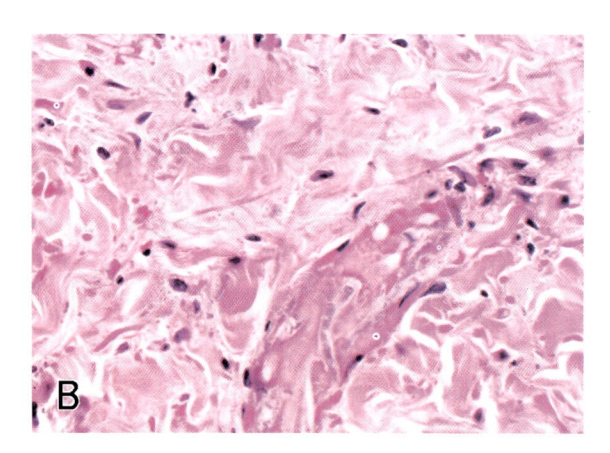

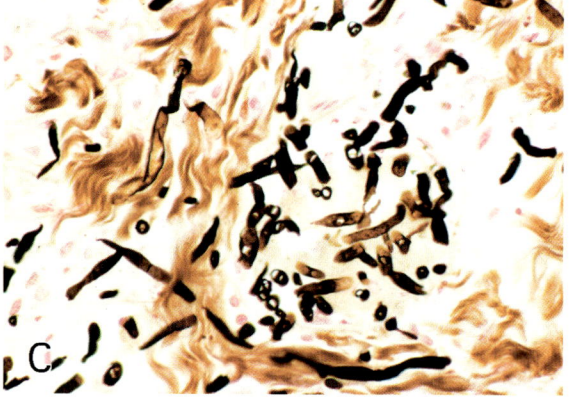

## Nodular/Interstitial Dermatitis

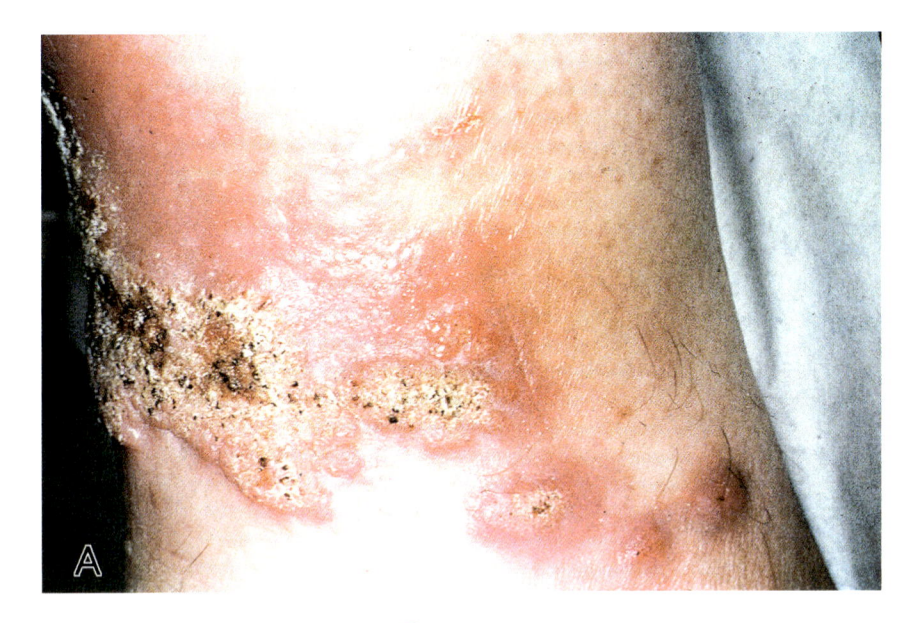

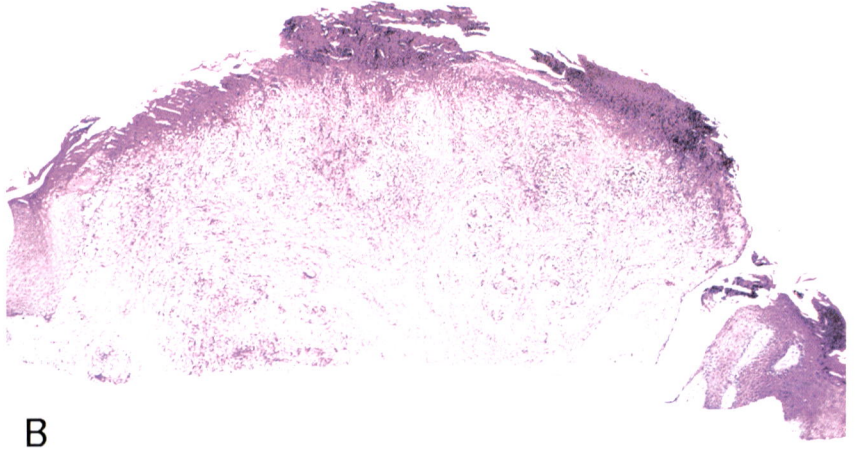

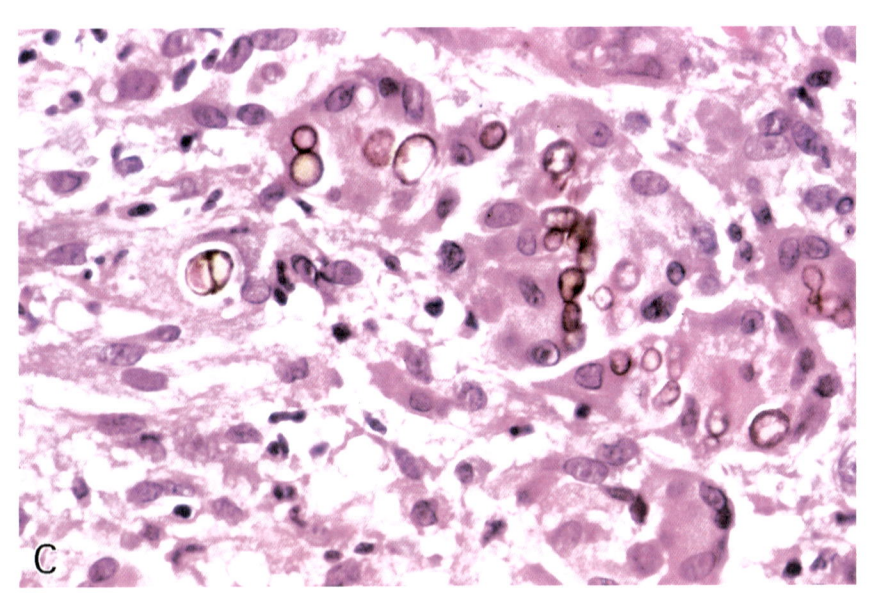

**Figure 12-55**

**CHROMOMYCOSIS**

A: There are multiple, coalescent, verrucous plaques and nodules on the lower extremity.

B: Scanning magnification reveals epidermal alterations bordered by acanthosis, a dense dermal inflammatory infiltrate composed of noncaseating granulomas, and aggregates of neutrophils.

C: At higher magnification, multiple endogenously pigmented spores are present within multinucleated histiocytes. They do not reproduce by budding, but by the formation of septa within individual spores.

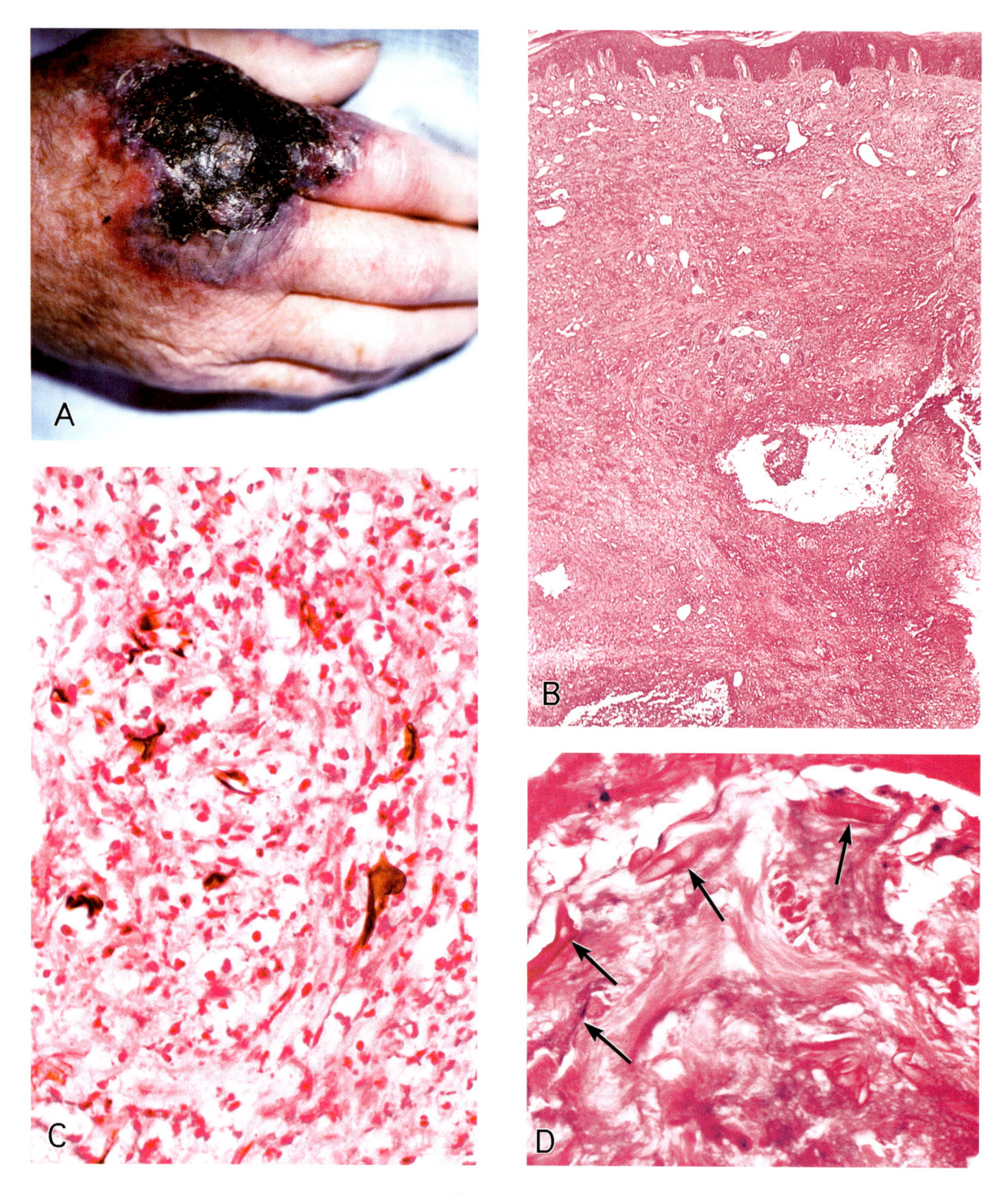

## Inflammatory Disorders of the Skin

**Figure 12-56**
**MUCORMYCOSIS**

A: There is a necrotic and ulcerated plaque on the dorsum of the hand of this immunocompromised patient.

B: At scanning magnification, there is a diffuse, vaguely granulomatous infiltrate within the superficial and deep dermis admixed with granulation tissue and zones of cystic necrosis.

C: The silver stain highlights the twisted, ribbon-like hyphae associated with the dermal granulomatous infiltrate.

D: In this necrotic region, nonseptate organisms are highlighted by PAS (arrows).

Nodular/Interstitial Dermatitis

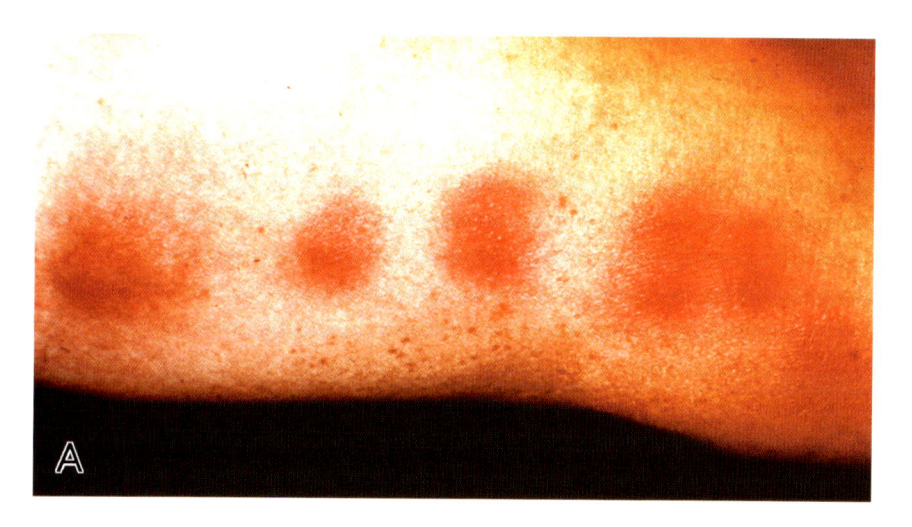

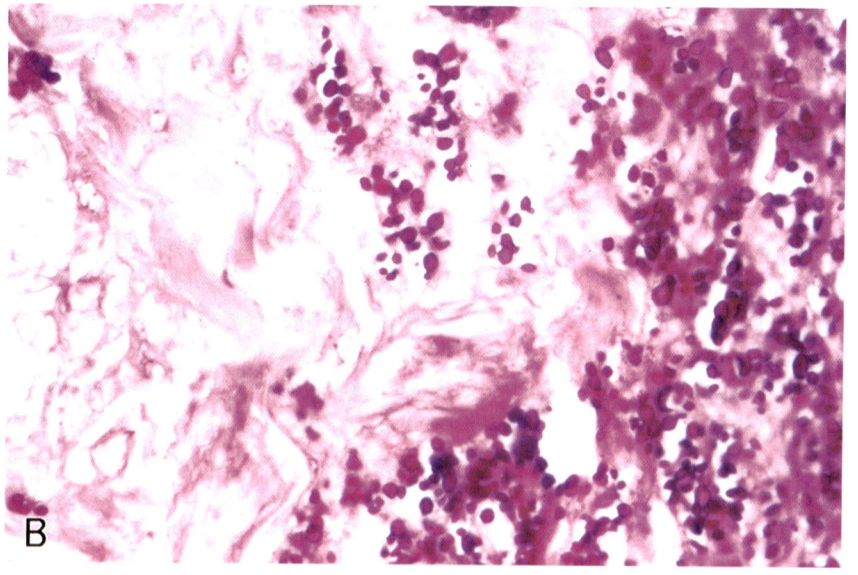

Figure 12-57
SPOROTRICHOSIS

A: There is a linear array of erythematous nodules, correlating with drainage of a primary site of infection in this patient with lymphocutaneous involvement.

B: At high magnification, multiple stained organisms are observed (PAS stain).

C: This granulomatous focus shows an asteroid body, which here represents central spores with homogenous eosinophilic radiations.

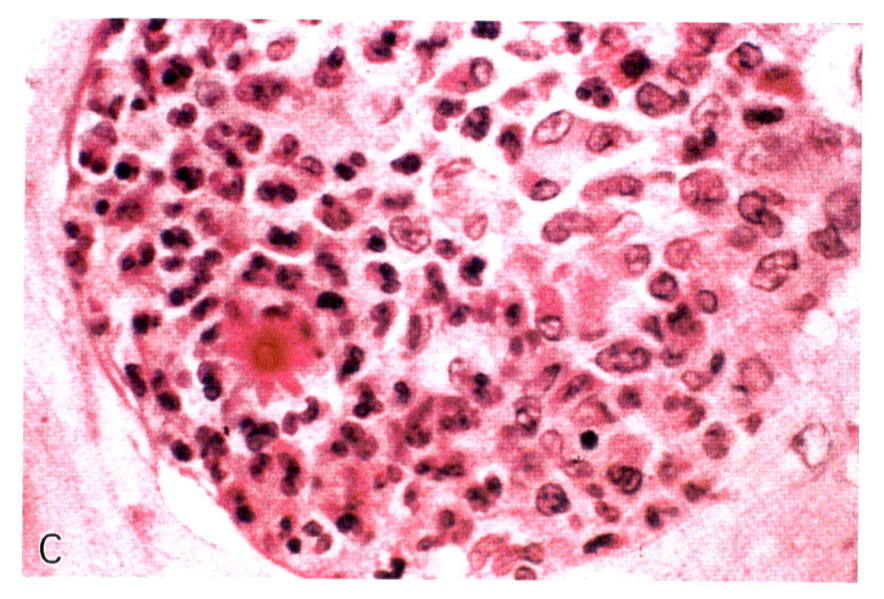

385

*Inflammatory Disorders of the Skin*

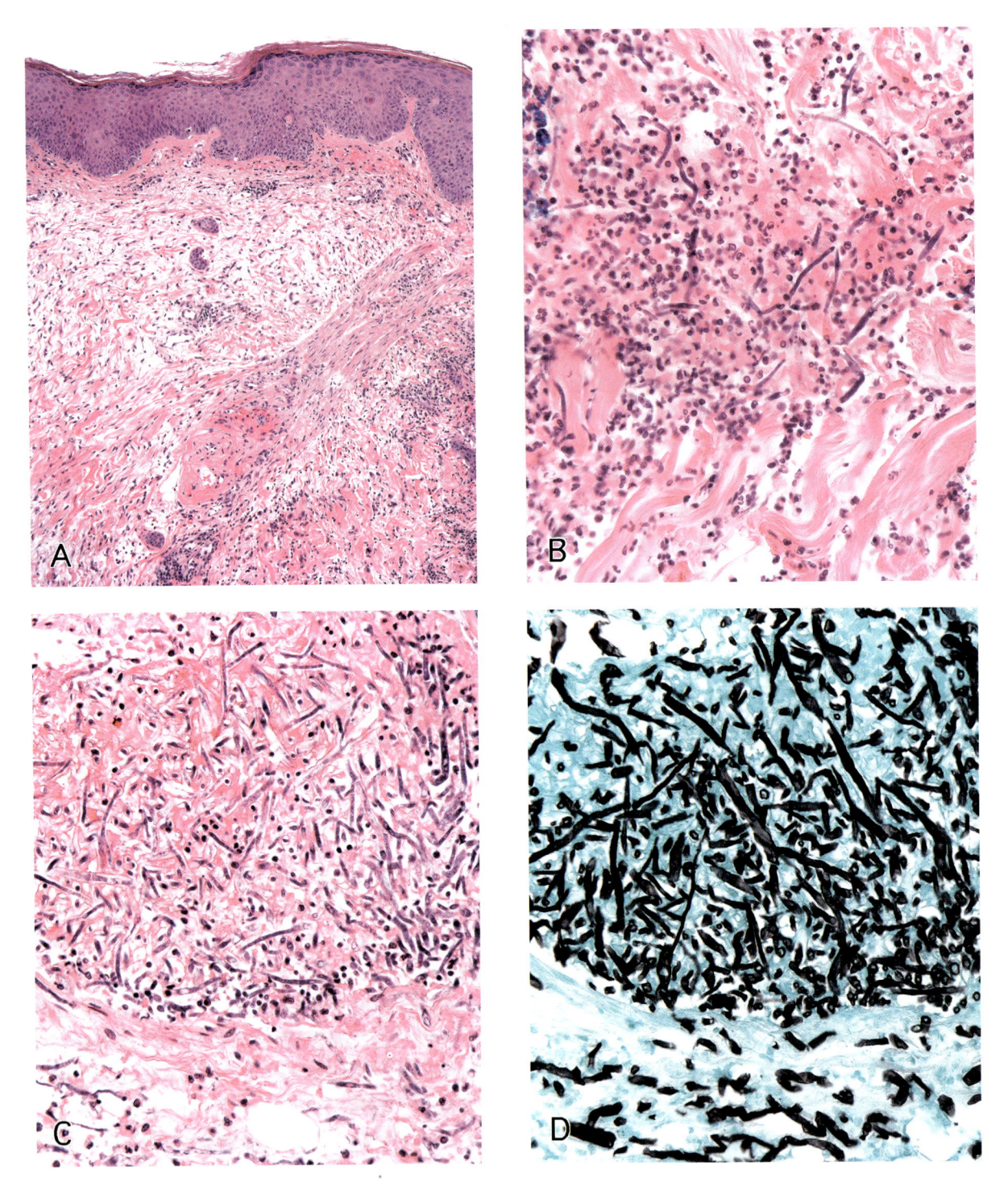

**Figure 12-58**

**FUSARIUM**

A: There is a seemingly nonspecific dermal inflammatory infiltrate with associated edema.

B: Higher magnification shows a mixed interstitial inflammatory component associated with numerous basophilic hyphae.

C: This vessel is almost totally obliterated by a thromboembolus containing numerous hyphae.

D: The hyphal forms are present both within the intravascular thrombus as well as within the vessel wall (silver stain).

*Nodular/Interstitial Dermatitis*

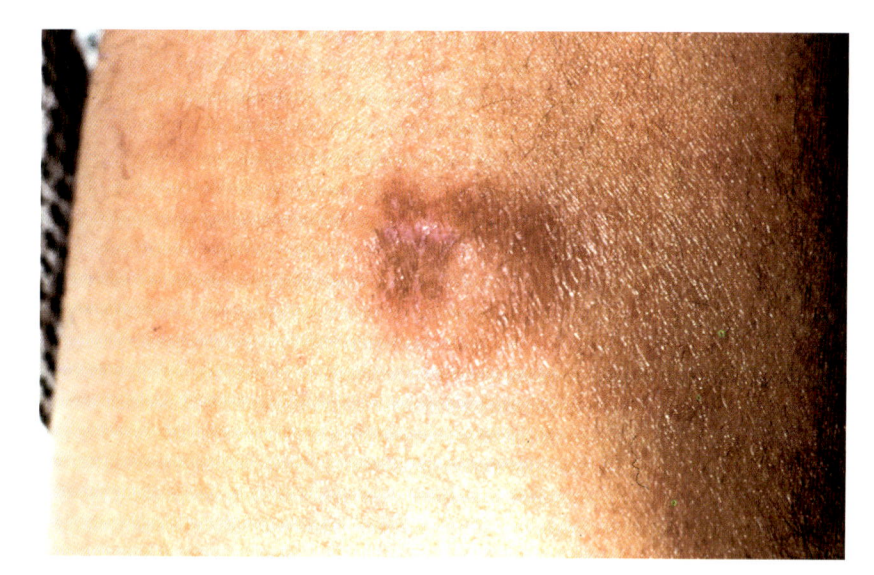

**Figure 12-59**
**CUTANEOUS TUBERCULOSIS**
There is an erythematous nodule without significant epidermal changes.

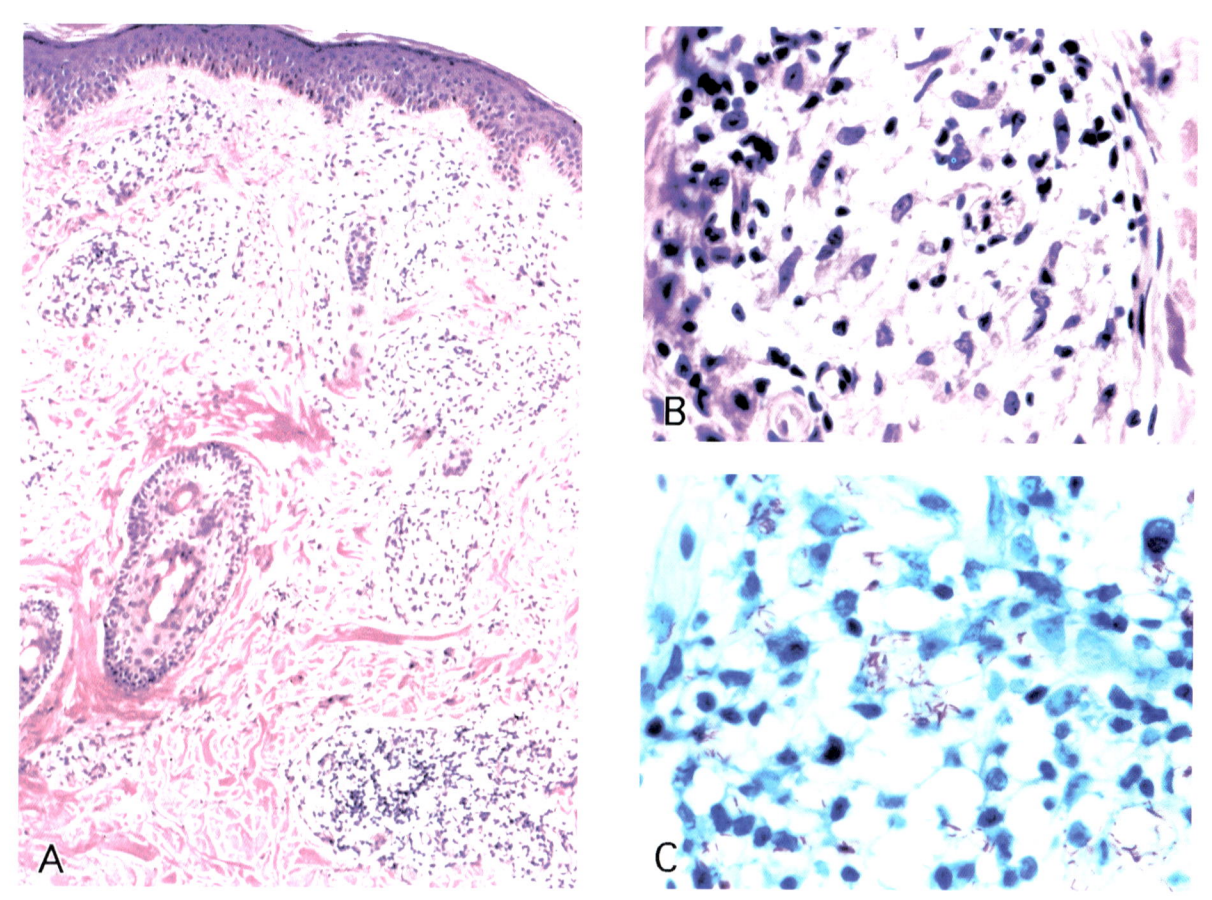

**Figure 12-60**
**CUTANEOUS MYCOBACTERIAL INFECTION**
A: At scanning magnification, numerous superficial and deep dermal inflammatory micronodules are seen.
B: At higher magnification, the micronodules are composed predominantly of epithelioid histiocytes and lymphocytes. In contrast to leprosy, the surrounded dermal nerve branch is unaltered.
C: Characteristically stained beaded bacilli are plentiful within dermal histiocytes (acid-fast stain).

*Inflammatory Disorders of the Skin*

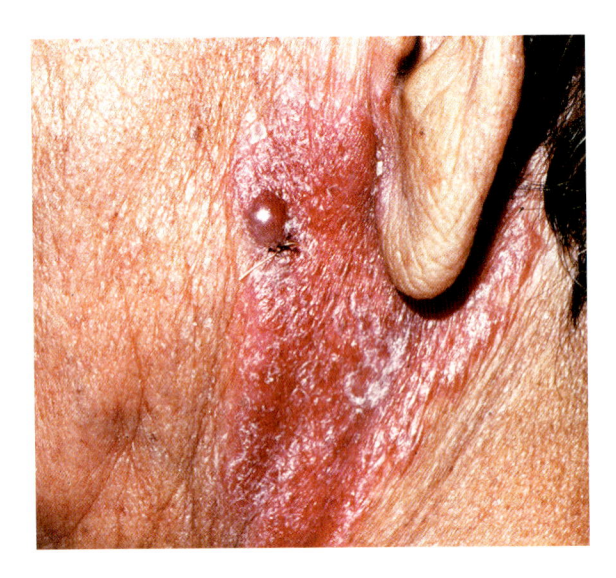

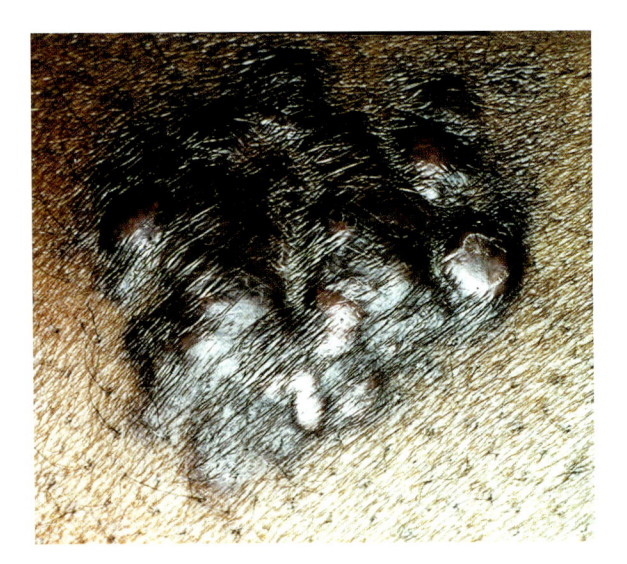

Figure 12-61

**ATYPICAL MYCOBACTERIAL INFECTION**

Left: Primary inoculation sites manifest as solitary nodules or as multiple nodules in linear array, occasionally mimicking sporotrichosis.

Right: Multiple coalescent hyperpigmented nodules are observed on darkly pigmented skin.

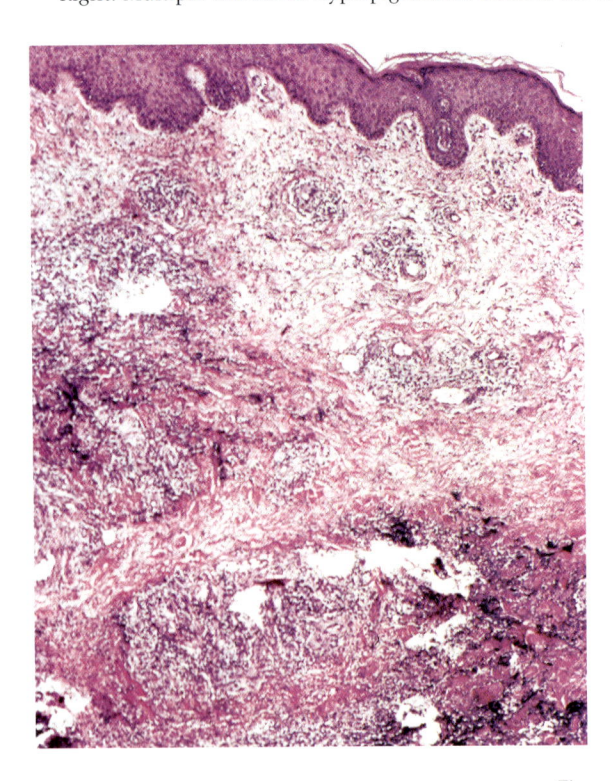

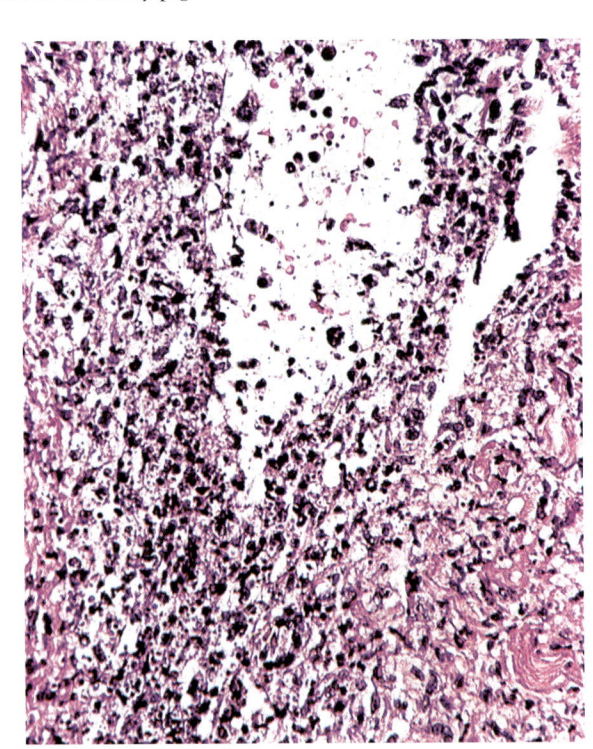

Figure 12-62

**ATYPICAL MYCOBACTERIAL INFECTION**

Left: At scanning magnification, there is a poorly defined, vaguely nodular mixed inflammatory infiltrate within the superficial and deep dermis.

Right: At higher magnification, the vaguely granulomatous foci and necrosis may evolve over time to form more characteristic epithelioid granulomas.

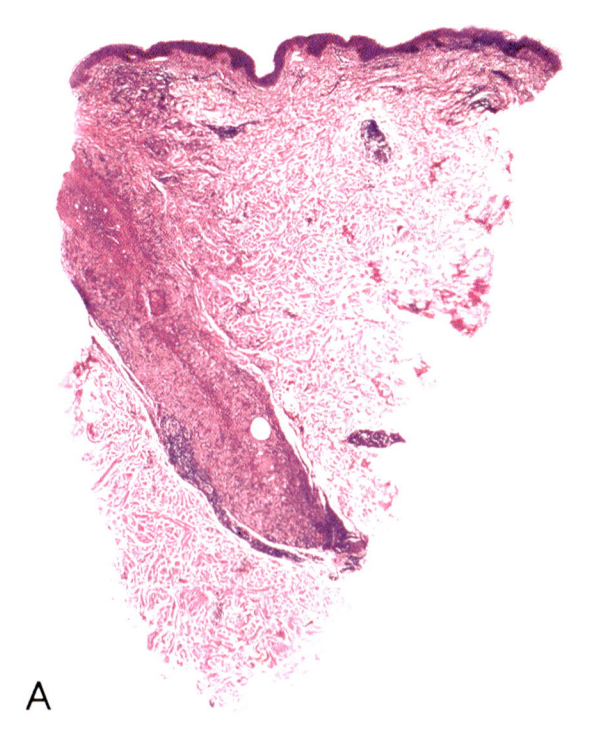

### Figure 12-63
**POSTHERPETIC GRANULOMATOUS DERMATITIS**

A: At scanning magnification, a coalescent zone of granulomatous inflammation spans the superficial and deep dermis.

B: At higher magnification, the granulomatous zones formed by epithelioid histiocytes are associated with adjacent necrosis.

C: Multinucleated epithelioid histiocytes are observed within the granulomatous foci. The clinical history was important in making the diagnosis.

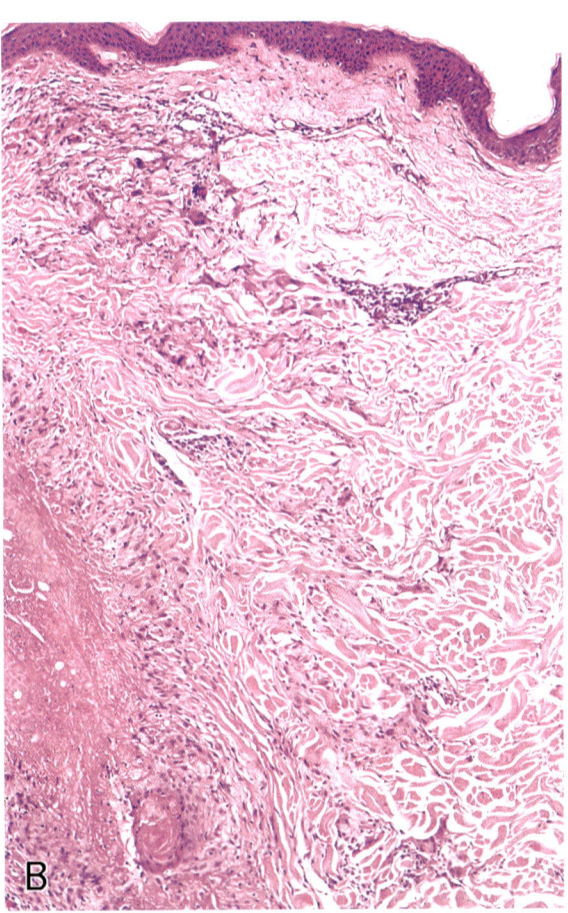

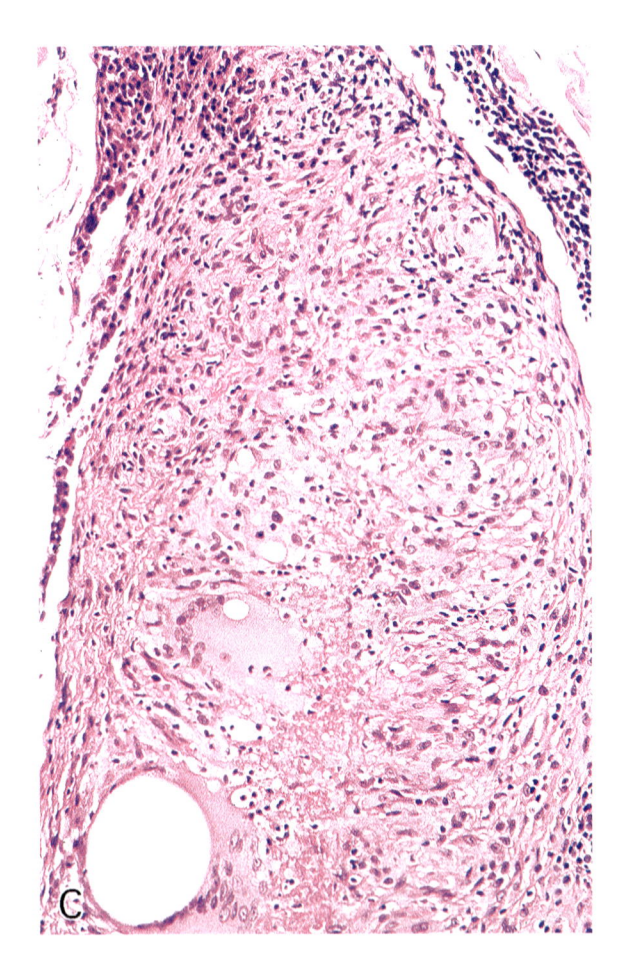

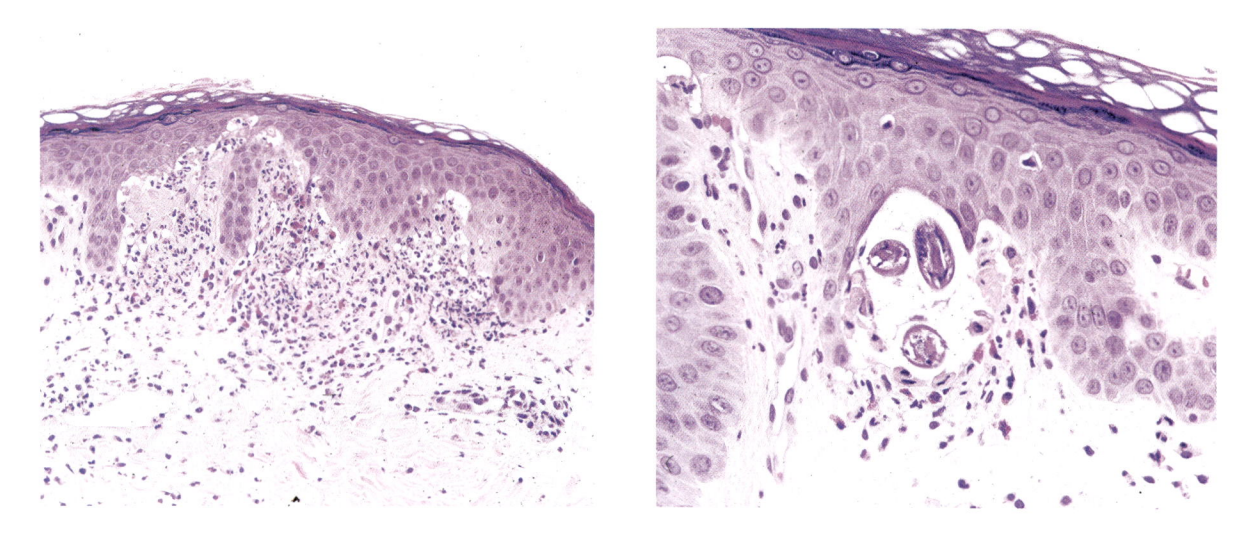

**Figure 12-64**

**CUTANEOUS LARVA MIGRANS**

Left: At scanning magnification, there is a mixed inflammatory infiltrate with a vaguely nodular interstitial pattern composed of lymphocytes, neutrophils, and eosinophils.

Right: At higher magnification, the burrow within the lower epidermis contains the skin-penetrating nematode larvae.

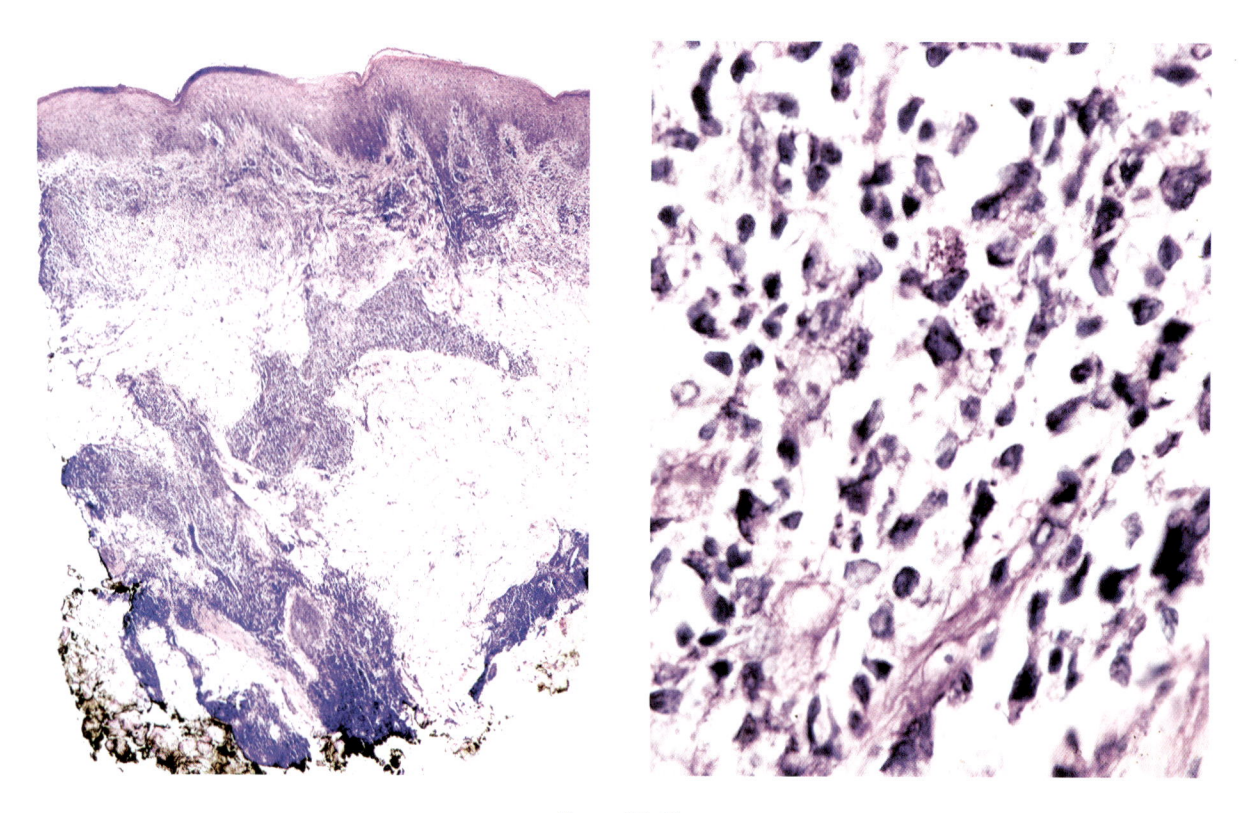

**Figure 12-65**

**CUTANEOUS LEISHMANIASIS**

Left: There is a dense, coalescent, nodular inflammatory infiltrate within the superficial and deep dermis.
Right: At higher magnification, multiple intracellular amastigotes are observed.

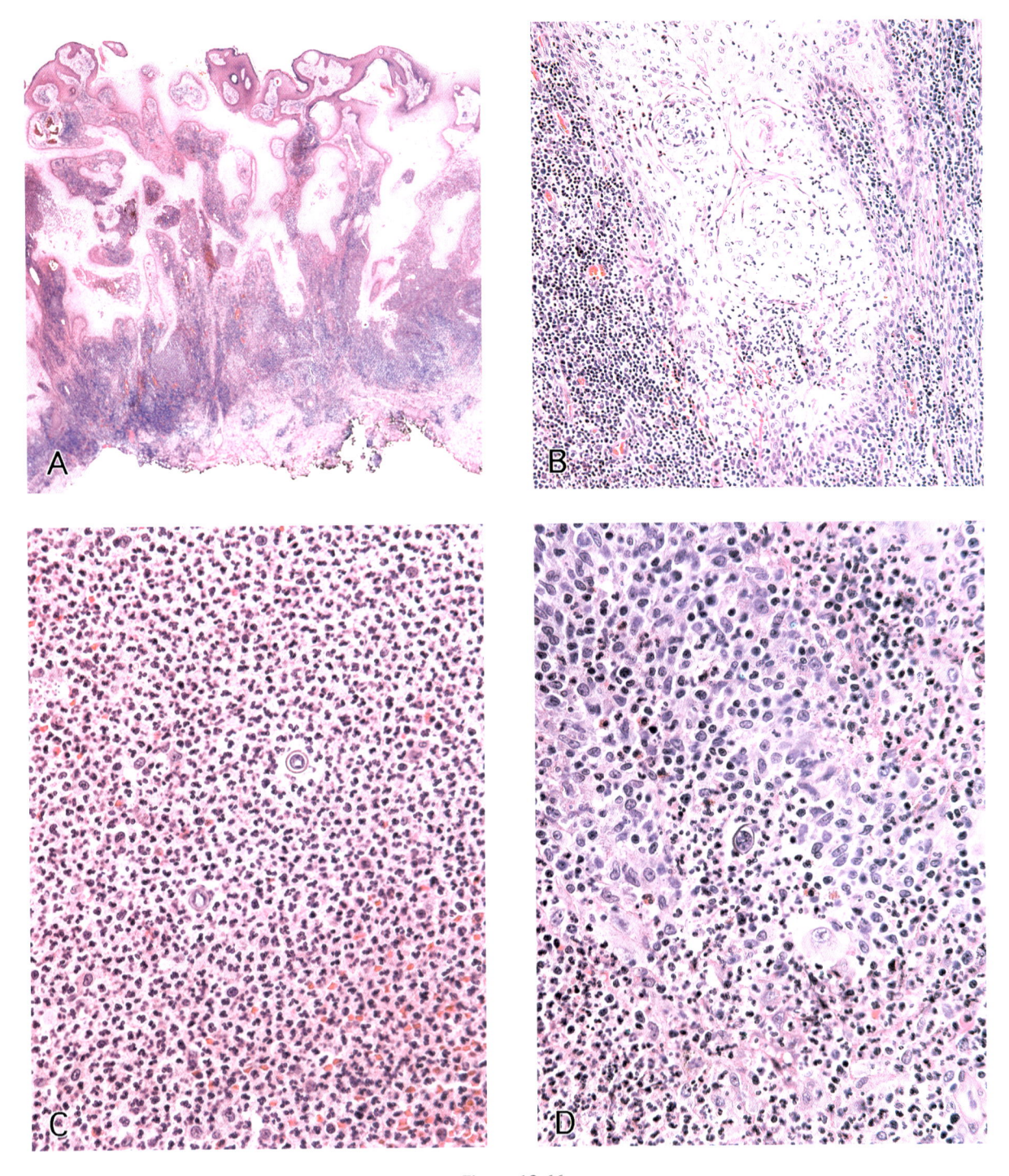

**Figure 12-66**

**BLASTOMYCOSIS**

A: At scanning magnification, the prominent pseudocarcinomatous hyperplasia was mistaken in this sample for invasive squamous cell carcinoma.

B: Pseudocarcinomatous epithelial proliferation with an intraepithelial microabscess.

C: Prominent abscess formation and scattered yeast forms.

D: The prominent neutrophilic component forms confluent microabscesses with admixed histiocytes. A large yeast form is present in the center of the field.

## REFERENCES

1. Oka M, Berking G, Nesbit M, et al. Interleukin-8 overexpression is present in pyodermal gangrenosum ulcers and leads to ulcer formation in human skin xenografts. Lab Invest 2000;80:595-604.
1a. Callen JP. Neutrophilic dermatoses. Dermatol Clin 2002;20:409-19.
2. Jovanovic M, Poljacki M, Vujanovic L, Duran V. Acute febrile neutrophilic dermatosis (Sweet's syndrome) after influenza vaccination. J Am Acad Dermatol 2005;52:367-9.
3. Saez M, Garcia-Bustinduy M, Noda A, et al. Drug-induced Sweet's syndrome. J Eur Acad Dermatol Venereol 2004;18:233.
4. Cohen PR, Kurzrock R. Sweet's syndrome revisited: a review of disease concepts. Int J Dermatol 2003;42:761-78.
5. Nobeyama Y, Kamide R. Sweet's syndrome with neurologic manifestation: case report and literature review. Int J Dermatol 2003;42:438-43.
6. Cohen PR, Kurzrock R. Sweet's syndrome: a neutrophilic dermatosis classically associated with acute onset and fever. Clin Dermatol 2000;18:265-82.
7. Burrall B. Sweet's syndrome (acute febrile neutrophilic dermatosis). Dermatol Online J 1999;5:8.
8. O'Brien MC. Sweet's syndrome. J Emerg Med 2005;29:341-2.
9. Paydas S, Sahin B, Zorludemir S. Sweet's syndrome accompanying leukaemia: seven cases and review of the literature. Leuk Res 2000;24:83-6.
10. Vignon-Pennamen MD, Aractingi S. Sweet's syndrome and leukemia cutis: a common skin homing mechanism? Dermatology 2003;206:81-4.
11. Inomata N, Sasaki T, Nakajima H. Sweet's syndrome with gastric cancer. J Am Acad Dermatol 1999;41:1033-4.
12. Malone JC, Slone SP. Sweet syndrome: a disease in histologic evolution? Arch Dermatol 2005;141:893-5.
13. Malone JC, Slone, SP, Will-Frank LA, et al. Vascular inflammation (vasculitis) in Sweet syndrome: A clinicopathologic study of 28 biopsy specimens from 21 patients. Arch Dermatol 2002;138:345-9.
14. Ferreli C, Pinna AL, Atzori L, Aste N. Eosinophilic cellulitis (Well's syndrome): a new case description. J Eur Acad Dermatol Venereol 1999;13:41-5.
15. Moossavi M, Mehregan DR. Wells' syndrome: a clinical and histopathologic review of seven cases. Int J Dermatol 2003;42:62-7.
16. Holme SA, McHenry P. Nodular presentation of eosinophilic cellulitis (Wells' syndrome). Clin Exp Dermatol 2001;26:677-9.
17. Ghislain PD, Van Eeckhout P. Eosinophilic cellulitis of papulonodular presentation (Wells' syndrome). J Eur Acad Dermatol Venereol 2005;19:226-7.
18. Afsahi V, Kassabian C. Wells syndrome. Cutis 2003;72:209-12
19. Steffen C. The man behind the eponym. George Crichton Wells: eosinophilic cellulitis (Wells syndrome). Am J Dermatopathol 2002;24:164-5.
20. Kuwahara RT, Randall MB, Eisner MG. Eosinophilic cellulitis in a newborn. Pediatr Dermatol 2001;18:89-90.
21. Su WP, Davis MD, Weenig RH, Powell FC, Perry HO. Pyoderma gangrenosum: clinicopathologic correlation and proposed diagnostic criteria. Int J Dermatol 2004;43:790-800.
22. Bhat RM, Shetty SS, Kamath GH. Pyoderma Gangrenosum in childhood. Int J Dermatol 2004;43:205-7.
23. Crowson AN, Mihm MC Jr, Magro C. Pyoderma gangrenosum: a review. J Cutan Pathol 2003;30:97-107.
24. Weenig RH, Davis MD, Dahl PR, Su WP. Skin ulcers misdiagnosed as pyoderma gangrenosum. N Engl J Med 2002;347:1412-8.
25. Mlika RB, Riahi I, Fenniche S, et al. Pyoderma gangrenosum: a report of 21 cases. Int J Dermatol 2002;41:65-8.
26. Wines N, Wines M, Ryman W. Understanding pyoderma gangrenosum: a review. MedGenMed 2001;3:6.
27. Blitz NM, Rudikoff D. Pyoderma gangrenosum. Mt Sinai J Med 2001;68:287-97.
28. Abdelrazeq AS, Lund JN, Leveson SH. Pouchitis-associated pyoderma gangrenosum following restorative proctocolectomy for ulcerative colitis. Eur J Gastroenterol Hepatol 2004;16:1057-8.
29. Menachem Y, Gotsman I. Clinical manifestations of pyoderma gangrenosum associated with inflammatory bowel disease. Isr Med Assoc J 2004; 6:88-90.
30. Ujiie H, Sawamura D, Yokota K, Nishie W, Shichinohe R, Shimizu H. Pyoderma gangrenosum associated with Takayasu's arteritis. Clin Exp Dermatol 2004;29:357-9.
31. Ehling A, Karrer S, Klebl F, Schaffler A, Muller-Ladner U. Therapeutic management of pyoderma gangrenosum. Arthritis Rheum 2004;50:3076-84.

32. Gettler S, Rothe M, Grin C, Grant-Kels J. Optimal treatment of pyoderma gangrenosum. Am J Clin Dermatol 2003;4:597-608.
33. Powell FC, O'Kane M. Management of pyoderma gangrenosum. Dermatol Clin 2002;20:347-55.
34. Wollina U. Clinical management of pyoderma gangrenosum. Am J Clin Dermatol 2002;3:149-58.
35. Rozen SM, Nahabedian MY, Manson PN. Management strategies for pyoderma gangrenosum: case studies and review of literature. Ann Plast Surg 2001;47:310-5.
36. Fukuhara K, Urano Y, Kimura S, Hori K, Arase S. Pyoderma gangrenosum with rheumatoid arthritis and pulmonary aseptic abscess responding to treatment with dapsone. Br J Dermatol 1998;139:556-8.
37. Shenefelt PD. Pyoderma gangrenosum associated with cystic acne and hidradenitis suppurativa controlled by adding minocycline and sulfasalazine to the treatment regimen. Cutis 1996;57:315-9.
38. Park HJ, Han BG, Kim YC, Cinn YW. Recalcitrant oral pyoderma gangrenosum in a child responsive to cyclosporine. J Dermatol 2003;30:612-6.
39. Patrone P, Bragadin G, De Francesco V, Frattasio A, Stinco G. Pyoderma gangrenosum of the scalp treated with cyclosporine A. Int J Dermatol 2002;41:916-8.
40. Sehgal VN, Srivastava G, Aggarwal AK, Behl PN, Choudhary M, Bajaj P. Localized scleroderma/morphea. Int J Dermatol 2002;41:467-75.
41. Krafchik BR. Localized morphea in children. Adv Exp Med Biol 1999;455:49-54.
42. Hawk A, English JC 3rd. Localized and systemic scleroderma. Semin Cutan Med Surg 2001;20:27-37.
43. Möhrenschlager M, Jung C, Ring J, Abeck D. Effect of penicillin G on corium thickness in linear morphea of childhood: An analysis using ultrasound technique. Pediatr Dermatol 1999;16:314-6.
44. Kreuter A, Gambichler T, Breuckmann F, et al. Pulsed high-dose corticosteroids combined with low-dose methotrexate in severe localized scleroderma. Arch Dermatol 2005;141:847-52.
45. Dutz J. Treatment options for localized scleroderma. Skin Therapy Lett 2000;5:3-5.
46. Simon JC, Pfieger D, Schopf E. Recent advances in phototherapy. Eur J Dermatol 2000;10:642-5.
46a. Magro CM, Crowson AN, Shapiro BL. The interstitial granulomatous drug reaction: a distinctive clinical and pathological entity. J Cutan Pathol 1998;25:72-8.
47. Epstein WL. Cutaneous sarcoidosis. Semin Respir Crit Care Med 2002;23:571-7.
48. Huang CL, Mutasim DF. Sarcoidosis mimicking lipodermatosclerosis. Cutis 2005;75:322-4.
49. Antonovich DD, Callen JP. Development of sarcoidosis in cosmetic tattoos. Arch Dermatol 2005;141:869-72.
50. Kim C, Long WT. Sarcoidosis. Dermatol Online J 2004;10:24.
51. Chong WS, Tan HH, Tan SH. Cutaneous sarcoidosis in Asians: a report of 25 patients from Singapore. Clin Exp Dermatol 2005;30:120-4.
52. Singal A, Thami GP. Localization of cutaneous sarcoidosis: from trauma to scars. J Am Acad Dermatol 2004;51:841.
53. Pascual JC, Belinchon I, Albares P, Vergara G, Betlloch I, Banuls J. Cutaneous sarcoidosis and polycythemia vera. J Eur Acad Dermatol Venereol 2004;18:700-1.
54. Yoo SS, Mimouni D, Nikolskaia OV, Kouba DJ, Sauder DN, Nousari CH. Clinicopathologic features of ulcerative-atrophic sarcoidosis. Int J Dermatol 2004;43:108-12.
55. Yanardag H, Pamuk ON, Karayel T. Cutaneous involvement in sarcoidosis: analysis of the features in 170 patients. Respir Med 2003;97:978-82.
56. Giuffrida TJ, Kerdel FA. Sarcoidosis. Dermatol Clin 2002;20:435-47.
57. Katta R. Cutaneous sarcoidosis: a dermatologic masquerader. Am Fam Physician 2002;65:1581-4.
58. Young RJ 3rd, Gilson RT, Yanase D, Elston DM. Cutaneous sarcoidosis. Int J Dermatol 2001;40:249-53.
59. English JC 3rd, Patel PJ, Greer KE. Sarcoidosis. J Am Acad Dermatol 2001;44:725-43.
60. Mosam A, Morar N. Recalcitrant cutaneous sarcoidosis: an evidence-based sequential approach. J Dermatolog Treat 2004;15:353-9.
61. Fazzi P. Pharmacotherapeutic management of pulmonary sarcoidosis. Am J Respir Med 2003;2:311-20.
62. Jones E, Callen JP. Hydroxychloroquine is effective therapy for control of cutaneous sarcoidal granulomas. J Am Acad Dermatol 1990;3(Pt 1):487-9.
63. Webster GF, Razsi LK, Sanchez M, Shupack JL. Weekly low-dose methotrexate therapy for cutaneous sarcoidosis. J Am Acad Dermatol 1991;24:451-4.
64. van der Waal RI, Schulten EA, van de Scheur MR, Wauters IM, Starink TM, van der Waal I. Cheilitis granulomatosa. J Eur Acad Dermatol Venereol 2001;15:519-23.
65. Camacho-Alonso F, Bermejo-Fenoll A, Lopez-Jornet P. Miescher's cheilitis granulomatosa. A presentation of five cases. Med Oral Patol Oral Cir Bucal 2004;9:427-9, 425-7.

66. Kovich OI, Cohen DE. Granulomatous cheilitis. Dermatol Online J 2004;10:10.
67. van der Waal RI, Schulten EA, van der Meij EH, van de Scheur MR, Starink TM, van der Waal I. Cheilitis granulomatosa: overview of 13 patients with long-term follow-up—results of management. Int J Dermatol 2002;41:225-9.
68. Rogers RS 3rd. Granulomatous cheilitis, Melkersson-Rosenthal syndrome, and orofacial granulomatosis. Arch Dermatol 2000;136:1557-8.
69. Shapiro M, Peters S, Spinelli HM. Melkersson-Rosenthal syndrome in the periocular area: a review of the literature and case report. Ann Plast Surg 2003;50:644-8.
70. Ziem PE, Pfrommer C, Goerdt S, Orfanos CE, Blume-Peytavi U. Melkersson-Rosenthal syndrome in childhood: a challenge in differential diagnosis and treatment. Br J Dermatol 2000;143:860-3.
71. Coskun B, Saral Y, Cicek D, Akpolat N. Treatment and follow-up of persistent granulomatous cheilitis with intralesional steroid and metronidazole. J Dermatolog Treat 2004;15:333-5.
72. Perez-Calderon R, Gonzalo-Garijo MA, Chaves A, de Argila D. Cheilitis granulomatosa of Melkersson-Rosenthal syndrome: treatment with intralesional corticosteroid injections. Allergol Immunopathol (Madr) 2004;32:36-8.
73. Ridder GJ, Fradis M, Lohle E. Cheilitis granulomatosa Miescher: treatment with clofazimine and review of the literature. Ann Otol Rhinol Laryngol 2001;110:964-7.
74. Fdez-Freire LR, Serrano Gotarredona A, Bernabeu Wittel J, et al. Clofazimine as elective treatment for granulomatous cheilitis. J Drugs Dermatol 2005;4:374-7.
75. Camacho F, Garcia-Bravo B, Carrizosa A. Treatment of Miescher's cheilitis granulomatosa in Melkersson-Rosenthal syndrome. J Eur Acad Dermatol Venereol 2001;15:546-9.
76. Tavarela Veloso F. Review article: skin complications associated with inflammatory bowel disease. Aliment Pharmacol Ther 2004;20(Suppl 4):50-3.
77. Gilson MR, Elston LC, Pruitt CA. Metastatic Crohn's disease: remission induced by mesalamine and prednisone. J Am Acad Dermatol 1999;41:476-9.
78. Ulnick KM, Perkins J. Extraintestinal Crohn's disease: case report and review of the literature. Ear Nose Throat J 2001;80:97-100.
79. Marty CL, Cheng JF. Granuloma annulare presenting as contact dermatitis. Dermatitis 2005;16:34-7.
80. Hsu S, Le EH, Khoshevis MR. Differential diagnosis of annular lesions. Am Fam Physician 2001;64:289-96.
81. Barron DF, Cootauco MH, Cohen BA. Granuloma annulare. A clinical review. Lippincotts Prim Care Pract 1997;1:33-9.
82. Muhlbauer JE. Granuloma annulare. J Am Acad Dermatol 1980;3:217-30.
83. Schmutz JL. PUVA therapy of granuloma annulare. Clin Exp Dermatol 2000;25:451.
84. Setterfield J, Huilgol SC, Black MM. Generalised granuloma annulare successfully treated with PUVA. Clin Exp Dermatol 1999;24:458-60.
85. Jabbour SA. Cutaneous manifestations of endocrine disorders: a guide for dermatologists. Am J Clin Dermatol 2003;4:315-31.
86. Ferringer T, Miller F 3rd. Cutaneous manifestations of diabetes mellitus. Dermatol Clin 2002;20:483-92.
87. Wee SA, Possick P. Necrobiosis lipoidica. Dermatol Online J 2004;10:18.
88. Marinella MA. Necrobiosis lipoidica diabeticorum. Lancet 2002;360:1143.
89. Szabo RM, Harris GD, Burke WA. Necrobiosis lipoidica in a 9-year-old girl with new-onset type II diabetes mellitus. Pediatr Dermatol 2001;18:316-9.
90. Yigit S, Estrada E. Recurrent necrobiosis lipoidica diabeticorum associated with venous insufficiency in an adolescent with poorly controlled type 2 diabetes mellitus. J Pediatr 2002;141:280-2.
91. Evans AV, Atherton DJ. Recalcitrant ulcers in necrobiosis lipoidica diabeticorum healed by topical granulocyte-macrophage colony-stimulating factor. Br J Dermatol 2002;147:1023-5.
92. Goette DK. Resolution of necrobiosis lipoidica with exclusive clobetasol propionate treatment. J Am Acad Dermatol 1990;22(Pt 2):855-6.
93. Cummins DL, Hiatt KM, Mimouni D, Vander Kolk CA, Cohen BA, Nousari CH. Generalized necrobiosis lipoidica treated with a combination of split-thickness autografting and immunomodulatory therapy. Int J Dermatol 2004;43:852-4.
94. Turesson C, Jacobsson LT. Epidemiology of extraarticular manifestations in rheumatoid arthritis. Scand J Rheumatol 2004;33:65-72.
95. Yamamoto T, Matsunaga T, Nishioka K. Rheumatoid neutrophilic dermatitis, rheumatoid papules, and rheumatoid nodules in a patient with seronegative rheumatoid arthritis. J Am Acad Dermatol 2003;48:634-5.
96. Magro CM, Crowson AN. The spectrum of cutaneous lesions in rheumatoid arthritis: a clinical and pathological study of 43 patients. J Cutan Pathol 2003;30:1-10.
97. Bittenbender S, Telang GH, Benedetto EA. Symmetrical nasal bridge nodules. Rheumatoid nodule. Arch Dermatol 2001;137:1647-52.

98. McGrath MH, Fleischer A. The subcutaneous rheumatoid nodule. Hand Clin 1989;5:127-35.
99. Kai Y, Anzai S, Shibuya H, et al. A case of rheumatoid nodulosis successfully treated with surgery. J Dermatol 2004;31:910-5.
100. Tock CL, Cohen PR. Annular elastolytic giant cell granuloma. Cutis 1998;62:181-7.
101. Pock L, Blazkova J, Caloudova H, Varjassyova I, Konkolova R, Hercogova J. Annular elastolytic giant cell granuloma causes an irreversible disappearance of the elastic fibres. J Eur Acad Dermatol Venereol 2004;18:365-8.
102. Limas C. The spectrum of primary cutaneous elastolytic granulomas and their distinction from granuloma annulare: a clinicopathological analysis. Histopathology 2004;44:277-82.
103. Klemke CD, Siebold D, Dippel E, Hildenbrand R, Bleyl U, Goerdt S. Generalised annular elastolytic giant cell granuloma. Dermatology 2003;207:420-2.
104. Doulaveri G, Tsagroni E, Giannadaki M, et al. Annular elastolytic giant cell granuloma in a 70-year-old woman. Int J Dermatol 2003;42:290-1.
105. Herron MD, Coffin CM, Vanderhooft SL. Annular elastolytic giant cell granuloma. Pediatr Dev Pathol 2002;5:305-9.
106. Meadows KP, O'Reilly MA, Harris RM, Petersen MJ. Erythematous annular plaques in a necklace distribution. Annular elastolytic giant cell granuloma. Arch Dermatol 2001;137:1647-52.
107. Russo GG. Necrobiotic xanthogranuloma with scleroderma. Cutis 2002;70:311-6.
108. Chave TA, Hutchinson PE. Necrobiotic xanthogranuloma with two monoclonal paraproteins and no periorbital involvement at presentation. Clin Exp Dermatol 2001;26:493-6.
109. Mehregan DA, Winkelmann RK. Necrobiotic xanthogranuloma. Arch Dermatol 1992;128:94-100.
110. Meyer S, Szeimies RM, Landthaler M, Hohenleutner S. Cyclophosphamide-dexamethasone pulsed therapy for treatment of recalcitrant necrobiotic xanthogranuloma with paraproteinemia and ocular involvement. Br J Dermatol 2005;153:443-5.
111. Schaudig U, Al-Samir K. Upper and lower eyelid reconstruction for severe disfiguring necrobiotic xanthogranuloma. Orbit 2004;23:65-76.
112. Wells J, Gillespie R, Zardawi I. Case of recalcitrant necrobiotic xanthogranuloma. Australas J Dermatol 2004;45:213-5.
113. Thomsen HS. Nephrogenic systemic fibrosis: a serious late adverse reaction to gadodiamide. Eur Radiol 2006;16:2619-21.
114. Todd DJ, Kagan A, Chibnik LB, Kay J. Cutaneous changes of nephrogenic systemic fibrosis: predictor of early mortality and association with gadolinium exposure. Arthr Rheum 2007;56:3433-41.
115. Cowper SE, Robin HS, Steinberg SM, Su LD, Gupta S, LeBoit PE. Scleromyxedema-like cutaneous disease in renal-dialysis patients. Lancet 2000;356:1000-1.
116. Pryor JG, Poggioli G, Galaria N, et al. Nephrogenic systemic fibrosis: A clinicopathologic study of six cases. J Am Acad Dermatol 2007;57:105-11.
117. Ting WW, Stone MS, Madison KC, Kurtz K. Nephrogenic fibrosing dermopathy with systemic involvement. Arch Dermatol 2003;139:903-6.
118. Saenz A, Mandal R, Kradin R, Hedley-White ET. Nephrogenic fibrosing dermopathy with involvement of the dura mater. Virchows Arch 2006;449:389-91.
119. Kucher C, Steere J, Elenitstsas R, Siegel DL, Xu X. Nephrogenic fibrosing dermopathy/nephrogenic systemic fibrosis with diaphragmatic involvement in a patient with respiratory failure. J Am Acad Dermatol 2006;54(Suppl):S31-4.
120. Koreishi AF, Nazarian RM, Saenz AJ, et al. Nephrogenic systemic fibrosis: a pathologic study of autopsy cases. Arch Pathol Lab Med 2009;133:1943-8.
121. Cowper Se, Su LD, Bhawan J, Robin HS, LeBoit PE. Nephrogenic fibrosing dermopathy. Am J Dermatopathol 2001;23:383-93.
122. Thakral C, Abraham, JL. Gadolinium-induced nephrogenic systemic fibrosis is associated with insoluble Gd deposits in tissue: in vivo transmetallation confirmed by microanalysis. J Cut Pathol 2009;36:1244-54.
123. Kroshinsky D, Kay J, Nazarian RM. Case record of the Massachusetts General Hospital. Case 37-2009. A 46-year-old woman with chronic renal failure, leg swelling, and skin changes. N Engl J Med 2009;361:2166-76.
124. Richmond H, Zwerner J, Kim Y, Fiorentino D. Nephrogenic systemic fibrosis: relationship to gadolinium and response to photopheresis. Arch Dermatol 2007;143:1025-30.
125. Chandran S, Petersen J, Jacobs C, Fiorentino D, Doeden K, Lafayette RA. Imatinib in the treatment of nephrogenic systemic fibrosis. Am J Kid Dis 2009;53:129-32.
126. Kay J, High WA. Imatinib mesylate treatment of nephrogenic systemic fibrosis. Arth Rheum 2008;58:2543-8.

# 13 PANNICULITIS

## GENERAL CONSIDERATIONS

The term *panniculitis* implies a primary inflammatory process involving the subcutaneous fat. Panniculitis may arise as an immunologic disorder in which antigenic targets specifically located in characteristic regions of the subcutis (e.g., septa or lobules) are attacked by host inflammatory cells. Alternatively, it may be the result of ischemia to the subcutis, with secondary invasion by inflammatory cells. In addition, panniculitis may arise when endogenous enzymes (e.g., as in the case of pancreatitis or pancreatic carcinoma) or exogenous toxic substances gain access to subcutaneous tissue. Finally, infectious processes centered predominantly within the fat or infiltrative processes involving the hematopoietic system may result in secondary inflammatory changes in subcutaneous fat that closely mimic primary immunologic insults.

Like the epidermis and dermis, the subcutaneous fat reacts to inflammation and trauma in a limited number of ways. Fat does not become hyperplastic or hypertrophied in response to trauma, and extracellular fluid within the fat is usually localized to the adventitial connective tissue that courses through the thin septa that separate lobules composed of confluent aggregates of adipocytes. Fat undergoing necrosis frequently provokes a histiocytic inflammatory response whereby lipid is engulfed by macrophages to form lipophages, which are foamy cells similar to xanthoma cells. Zones of fat necrosis frequently resolve with fibrosis, although microcysts may form in regions of fat necrosis prior to infiltration by fibroblasts and vessels. Dissolution of the cell membranes of adipocytes produces pooled regions of lipid, frequently referred to as liquefactive fat necrosis. These zones may have a pale blue hue. Accumulation of pale pink material between intact adipocytes often signifies atrophy and a peculiar associated form of fibrosis referred to as hyalinization, which is typically encountered in lupus panniculitis. Degenerating and necrotic adipocytes also undergo saponification whereby calcium salts are deposited in zones of fat necrosis. Occasionally, the lipid within the degenerating adipocytes form needle-shaped clefts, as seen in the rare disorder, subcutaneous fat necrosis of the newborn, and sclerosing lipogranuloma, an iatrogenic disorder representing a response to injected oils or paraffin.

The clinical presentation of most forms of panniculitis is not as characteristic or helpful as the epidermal and dermal alterations that characterize the various forms of superficial dermatitis. Panniculitis is frequently experienced symptomatically before it is a defined clinical lesion. In general, panniculitis is at least tender and, in some cases, exquisitely painful, and may first be appreciated as a tender zone of deep induration. Such zones tend to be nodular in the early stages, although confluence may result in plaque-like zones of cutaneous hardening. Vague erythema often accompanies panniculitis and is testimony to the inflammatory component within the deep tissue. Because most forms of primary panniculitis fail to show significant dermal or epidermal alterations, the cutaneous surface is generally smooth and unremarkable. In disorders such as panniculitis resulting from connective tissue disease (e.g., lupus panniculitis), dermal and epidermal alterations are present, providing diagnostic information that paradoxically occasionally masks the presence of an underlying component within the subcutis.

Early acute lesions of panniculitis are characterized by exquisitely painful zones of nodular induration, with or without accompanying erythema. Chronic lesions are less symptomatic. Because panniculitis frequently resolves with some degree of lobular or septal sclerosis, the induration may persist long after the onset of tenderness and erythema. Although panniculitis occurs anywhere on the body, there is

*Inflammatory Disorders of the Skin*

**Figure 13-1**

**PATTERNS OF SEPTAL AND LOBULAR PANNICULITIS**

The top panels show the temporal progression of septal panniculitis from a paucicellular infiltrate (left) to a fibrosing septal reaction (right). The lower panel depicts fully developed lobular panniculitis.

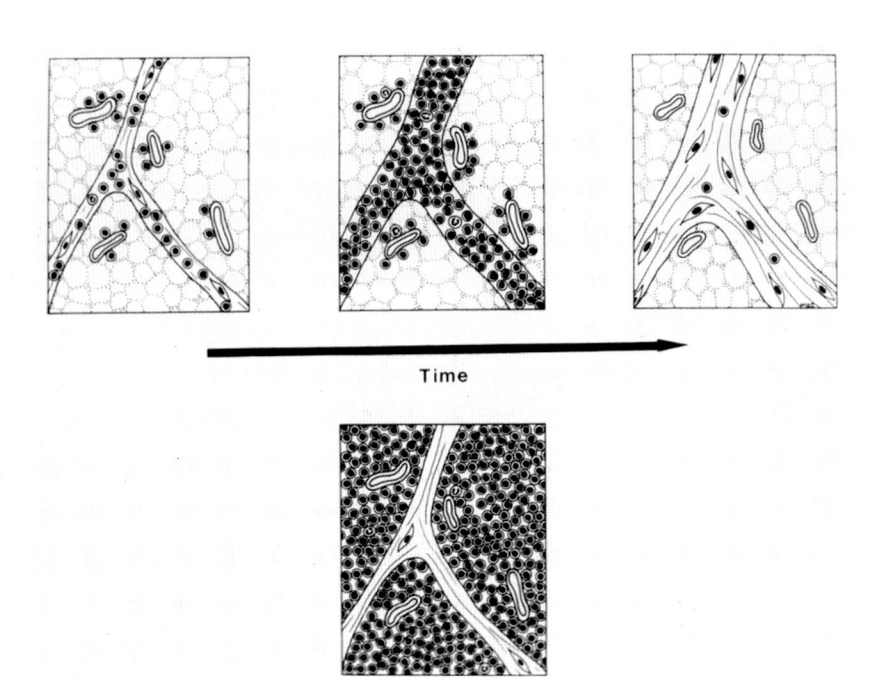

a predisposition for involvement of the lower extremities. Although fundamental differences between the subcutaneous fat and adipose tissue at extracutaneous sites (e.g., pericardium, omentum) have not been identified, the primary panniculitides discussed here have a predisposition for selective involvement of the adipose layer that underlies the dermis. Systemic forms of panniculitis in which fat cells at extracutaneous sites are also targeted by inflammatory mechanisms are extremely rare.

## PATHOGENESIS

Panniculitis is histologically divided into *septal* and *lobular* forms (fig. 13-1). The prototype of septal panniculitis is erythema nodosum, and the prototype of lobular panniculitis is erythema induratum. In septal panniculitis, the earliest inflammatory cells are generally neutrophils admixed with lymphocytes and monocytes. These inflammatory cells infiltrate about small venules, which are present in greatest concentration within the connective tissue septa separating lobules and within the paraseptal regions of the lobule. The early inflammatory infiltrate may diffusely involve the septa and be accompanied by significant edema and fibrin, which expand the septa to many times their normal width. Within these expanded septa, subacute and chronic lesions show a predominance of mononuclear cells, which may produce vaguely granulomatous aggregates. Epithelioid histiocytes and multinucleated cells are observed at this juncture. With chronicity, fibrosis generally follows septal panniculitis, and the deposition of abnormal collagen conforms to the architecture of the zones of the previous inflammatory infiltration. Old septal panniculitis shows septal expansion by fibroblasts, proliferating vessels, and collagen.

Early forms of lobular panniculitis are also composed of neutrophils admixed with mononuclear cells, but these inflammatory components infiltrate more diffusely throughout the central portions of the fat lobule. Although the septa may be involved, most of the inflammatory cells in lobular panniculitis are not present in the peripheral regions of lobules or septal components of the affected subcutis. As time passes, mononuclear cells may predominate, and in certain forms of lobular panniculitis (e.g., erythema induratum), there are frank epithelioid granulomas with caseation necrosis, identical to those occurring in pulmonary tuberculosis. Although vasculitis may be observed in some forms of lobular panniculitis, the affected vessels usually reside within the septa. Inflammatory infiltration of the lobule frequently results in secondary degeneration and necrosis of adipocytes, and in such regions, lipid-laden macrophages (lipophages), microcysts, and fibrosis are commonly identified. Chronic lesions of lobular panniculitis may show diffuse fibrosis of the lobule, and in extreme cases, lobules are almost entirely replaced by collagen and proliferating fibroblasts. In more subtle forms of lobular panniculitis, in which atrophy predominates over necrosis, hyalinized sclerosis between adipocytes is observed, as in lupus panniculitis.

The stimuli for panniculitis are diverse, with provocative factors including hypersensitivity reactions to systemic antigens (e.g., erythema nodosum and erythema induratum), ischemia (e.g., lipodermatosclerosis), vasculitis (e.g., polyarteritis nodosa with secondary panniculitis), enzymatic alterations (e.g., pancreatic panniculitis), connective tissue disease, injected materials, trauma, and direct infection.

We have found that a convenient way to classify panniculitis is based on the structures involved. The lesions are septal, lobular, vascular, and mixed (combining at least two elements in the classification scheme). This scheme is offered for convenience of approach and does not imply that, for example, in a septal panniculitis the lobule is not secondarily, and to a lesser extent, involved. Likewise, in lobular panniculitis, the septa are often secondarily involved or become part of the process as the lesions resolve.

The age of a biopsied lesion may be important in the diagnosis of panniculitis. In erythema nodosum, for example, the earliest changes in the first day or two may not be sufficient to allow for diagnosis. On the other hand, a late lesion, of 3 to 4 weeks' duration, may be very difficult to diagnose because of the extensive fibrosis that obscures the lobular and septal contributions to the lesional characteristics. The chronic changes that occur in almost any type of panniculitis usually include fibrosis that involves septa and lobules. Our approach to chronic lesions is to diagnose the lesion as "panniculitis, see note." After studying the lesion carefully in all aspects, we attempt to determine what the principal features are. For example, in late erythema nodosum giant cells are found in widened septa, a clue to the diagnosis. We then describe the changes in a note and comment that they are most consistent with erythema nodosum.

## SPECIAL DIAGNOSTIC STUDIES

Usually, panniculitis is a diagnosis made by conventional histologic analysis and clinical-pathologic correlation. In cases associated with connective tissue disease or vasculitis, direct immunofluorescence is useful. Panniculitis due to infection may require stains for fungi and mycobacteria, and lesions potentially associated with the introduction of foreign material may be examined by polarized light. Panniculitis associated with lymphoma (e.g., cytophagic panniculitis with subcutaneous T-cell lymphoma) requires examination by antibodies to assess T-cell phenotype and maturation, and potentially by polymerase chain reaction (PCR) to detect possible T-cell receptor gene rearrangements.

## ERYTHEMA NODOSUM, A SEPTAL PANNICULITIS

**Definition.** *Erythema nodosum* is one of the more common and acute types of panniculitis. It usually has a characteristic presentation with strikingly painful nodules on the lower extremities (1–3). The nodules extend to the arms and trunk. The disorder may be associated with numerous underlying conditions or causes (4–8).

**Clinical Features.** Erythema nodosum occurs characteristically in the second to the third decade, but may occur at any time in life. It is more common in females than males. The etiology may be idiopathic or associated with infection, drug ingestion, or a variety of other inflammatory granulomatous diseases, especially with sarcoidosis and some lymphoproliferative disorders.

The lesions usually occur abruptly and evolve over a few days into tender, erythematous, bruise-like areas or nodules on the lower extremities (fig. 13-2). In approximately half the cases there are systemic symptoms including fever, malaise, and arthralgias, especially of the ankle joints. The nodules, which vary from 3 to 30 cm in diameter, are poorly defined, plaque-like, and in the earliest manifestation, appear as a bruise. As they evolve, they become markedly red and exquisitely tender. The lesions are usually round to oval but are sometimes arciform. As they resolve, they become brownish, yellow-green, or even violaceous. They occasionally occur on the upper extremities and trunk, and in some

## Inflammatory Disorders of the Skin

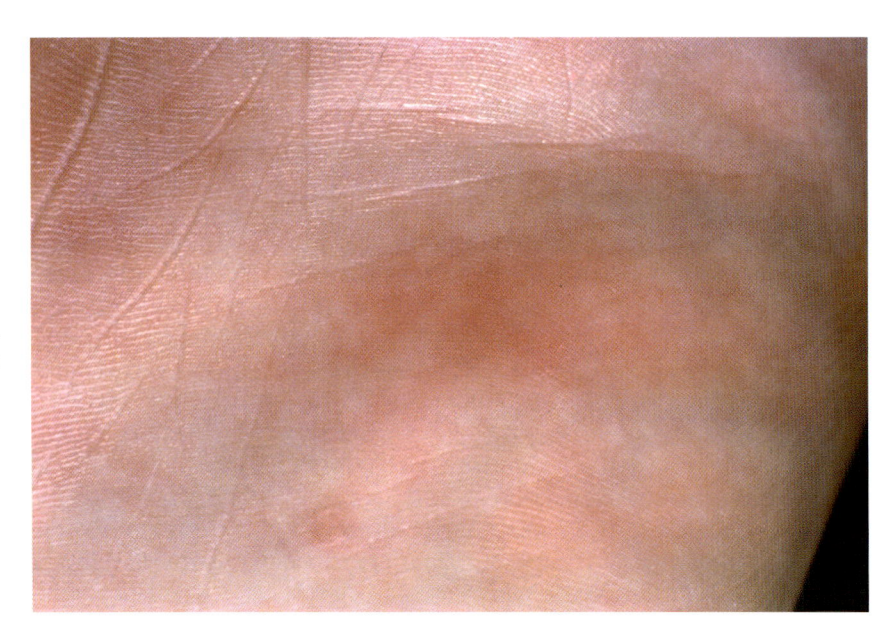

**Figure 13-2**

**ERYTHEMA NODOSUM**

There is a vaguely erythematous zone of painful nodular induration.

unusual instances even on the face. Erythema nodosum usually resolves spontaneously in 4 to 6 weeks. The course, however, depends on the etiology. When there is a chronic underlying disease, erythema nodosum may go on to become a chronic lesion. Ulceration does not occur in these lesions and healing is without clinical scarring. About 20 percent of cases of erythema nodosum have an atypical presentation, usually as a single erythematous, usually painless, nodule. Biopsy reveals the correct diagnosis.

There are multiple etiologies associated with erythema nodosum; the most common are postinfectious and drug-induced types. The most frequent infectious agent is streptococcal, although tuberculosis and other bacterial organisms are associated with this disorder. Deep fungal infections also are associated with erythema nodosum. In coccidiomycosis, the development of erythema nodosum is a sign of the patient's capacity to muster a delayed hypersensitivity reaction. This finding is associated with a better prognosis. Blastomycosis and histoplasmosis are also associated with erythema nodosum. Rarely, inflammatory dermatophyte reactions cause erythema nodosum. Hepatitis B, cat scratch disease, lymphogranuloma venereum, and infectious mononucleosis are among other infectious causes. Chronic bowel disease, often in the early phase in Crohn disease or ulcerative colitis, can give rise to this type of panniculitis. Acute erythema nodosum commonly occurs in the early phases of sarcoidosis, characteristically with the presence of hilar node involvement; chronic sarcoidosis is associated with a chronic type of erythema nodosum. Sweet syndrome, Behçet syndrome, lymphoproliferative disorders, leukemia, and an underlying carcinoma are also associated with erythema nodosum.

**Pathologic Findings.** At scanning magnification, erythema nodosum is the prototypical septal panniculitis (fig. 13-3). There is an inflammatory infiltrate which preferentially tracks down the branching septa that separate the lobules of the subcutaneous layer (fig. 13-4). This inflammatory infiltrate results in prominence and widening of the subcutaneous septa and is best appreciated when the septa are perpendicularly sectioned; tangential sections through widened septa occasionally give the false impression of a more lobular infiltrative process. Because accurate representation of septa within sections is critical to the appreciation of septal panniculitis by scanning magnification, biopsy specimens that include the bulk of the subcutaneous tissue are required. Although inflammatory cells are most typically concentrated within septa, aggregates of inflammatory cells, generally lymphocytes and plasma cells, are also seen about small venules within the paraseptal fat. These perivenular inflammatory aggregates may give the impression, at scanning magnification, that the inflammatory infiltrate has spilled over from the septa into the adjacent

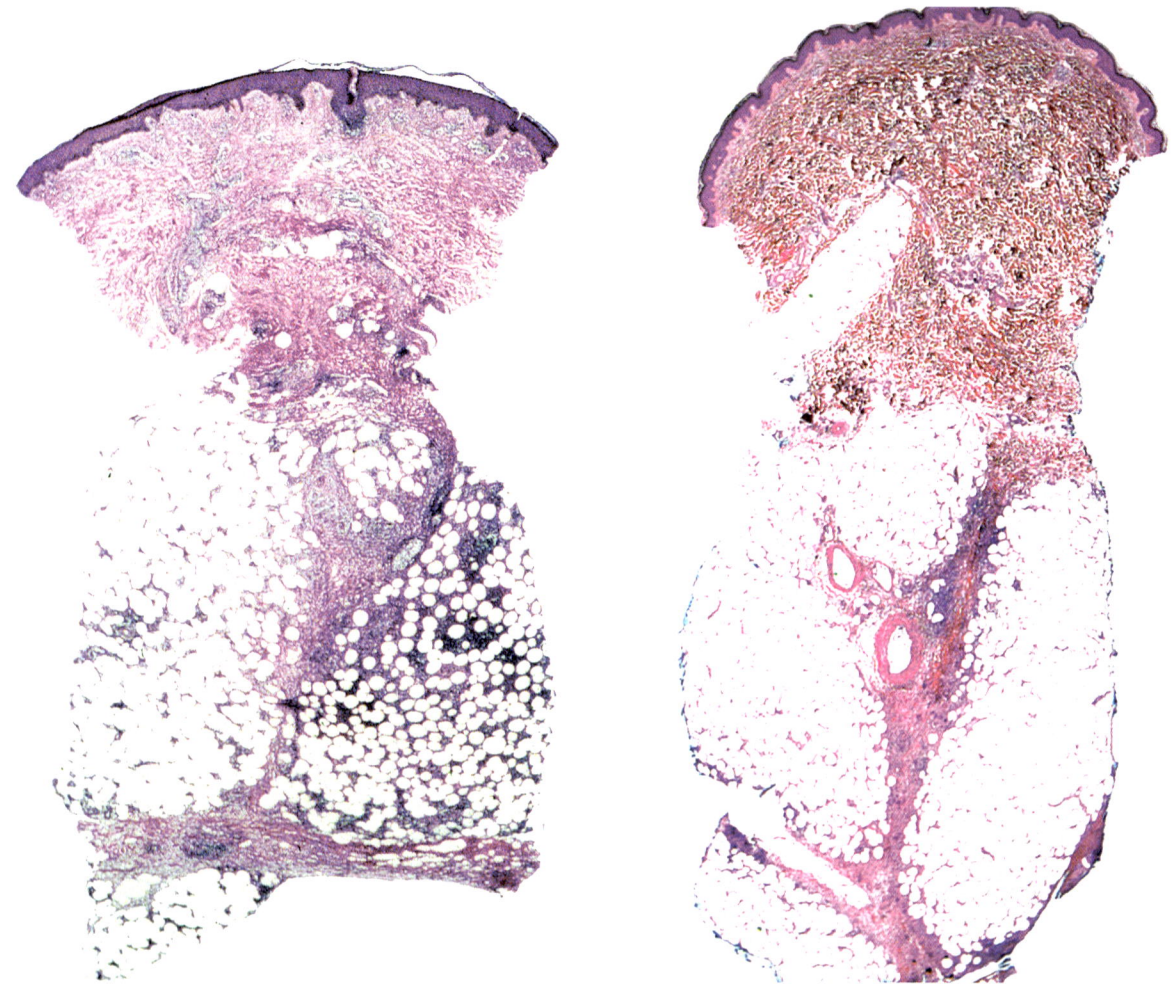

#### Figure 13-3
#### ERYTHEMA NODOSUM

Left: The subcutaneous septa are widened by inflammatory infiltration and some paraseptal involvement is seen. Upon tangential sectioning, this is similar to lobular panniculitis.

Right: The subcutaneous septa are widened by inflammation and early fibrosis.

fat or that the panniculitis is both septal and lobular (fig. 13-3, left).

At higher magnification, the septa are involved by neutrophils, lymphocytes, mononuclear cells, and plasma cells, and vasculitis is usually absent. The initial expansion of septa in acute lesions is the result of the inflammatory infiltration, edema fluid, and fibrin splaying apart adjacent collagen fibers. Over time, mononuclear cells and lymphocytes predominate, and epithelioid cells with multinucleation are seen. Although these zones may suggest tuberculoid granulomas, frank caseation necrosis, as is typical in erythema induratum, is not observed. Latter stages also show the beginning of septal fibrosis. The fibrosis typically involves deposition of collagen bundles centrally within widened septa, with the persistence of inflammatory infiltrates and granulomatous foci at the perimeter of the septa and in the paraseptal fatty tissue. With the exception of focal slight perivenular infiltrates with occasional eosinophils in the lower dermis, the overlying epidermis, the dermis, and the adnexal structures within the dermis are uninvolved by the inflammatory infiltrate. This is an important negative finding

*Inflammatory Disorders of the Skin*

**Figure 13-4**

**ERYTHEMA NODOSUM**

A: At high magnification, the septum is widened by inflammation composed of lymphocytes and histiocytes.

B: At intermediate magnification, the inflammatory component is an admixture of lymphocytes, histiocytes, and occasional eosinophils with focal granuloma formation.

C: At high magnification, significant vasculitis is generally not seen; early active lesions may show minor vasculopathic changes.

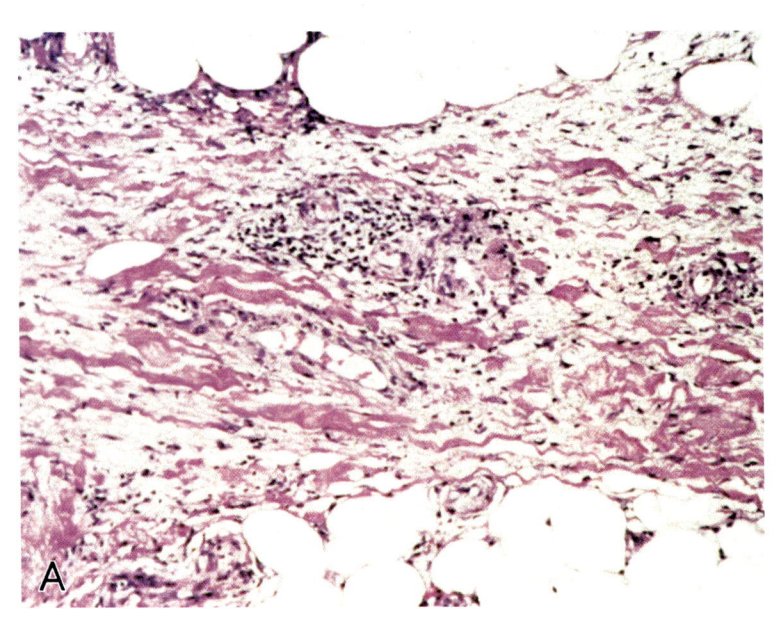

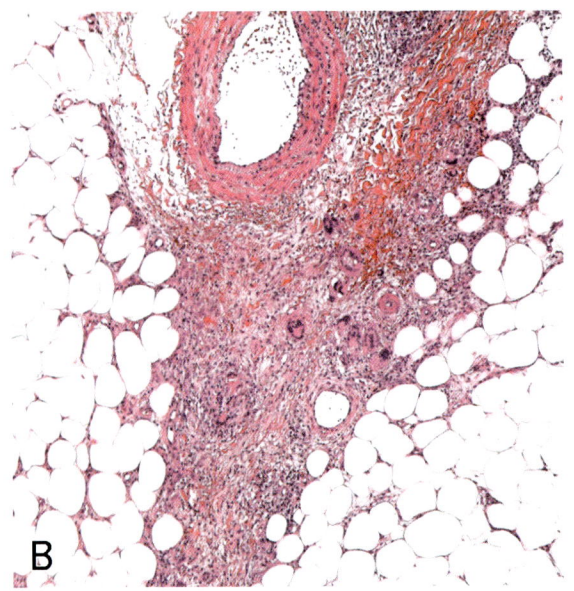

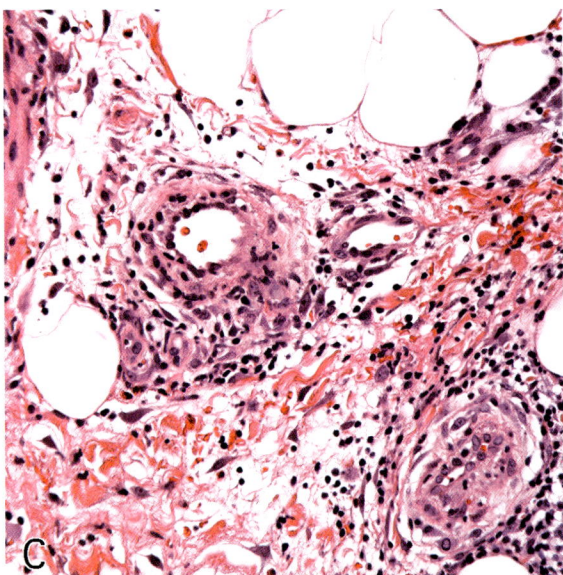

because certain infections and secondary inflammatory processes involving the subcutis closely mimic erythema nodosum with regard to the changes within the subcutaneous layer. These mimics, discussed primarily under infectious panniculitis and factitial panniculitis, generally also show involvement of the dermis and epidermis, providing important and clinically critical diagnostic clues.

**Clinicopathologic Variants.** *Subacute nodular migratory panniculitis* is a variant of erythema nodosum. This condition frequently occurs unilaterally on the lower legs and is observed predominantly in middle-aged women. Grossly, small nodular lesions enlarge to form, by confluence, sharply circumscribed, asymptomatic, indurated plaques with central clearing. The histology is remarkably similar to that of erythema nodosum but there may be prominent paraseptal granulation tissue-like changes. The diagnosis depends on clinical factors (e.g., age, unilateral occurrence) and a more chronic course in subacute nodular migratory panniculitis. This variant responds to oral ingestion of iodides, a therapeutic test to confirm the suspected diagnosis.

*Panniculitis*

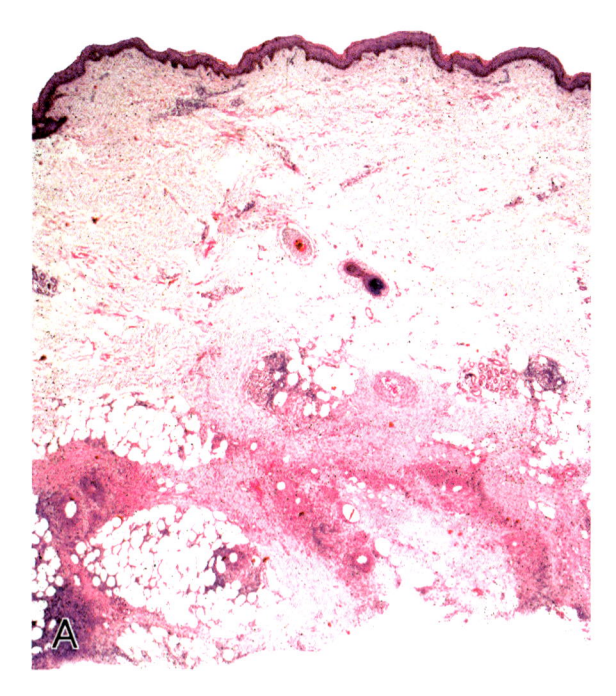

**Figure 13-5**

**BEHÇET DISEASE WITH ERYTHEMA NODOSUM–LIKE LESIONS**

A: The subcutaneous septa are dramatically widened by inflammatory cells and collagen deposition.

B: At higher magnification, the septa show prominent collagen deposition, which is evidence of chronicity.

C: Paraseptal involvement with fibrosis and "spilling" of inflammatory cells into paraseptal adipose tissue.

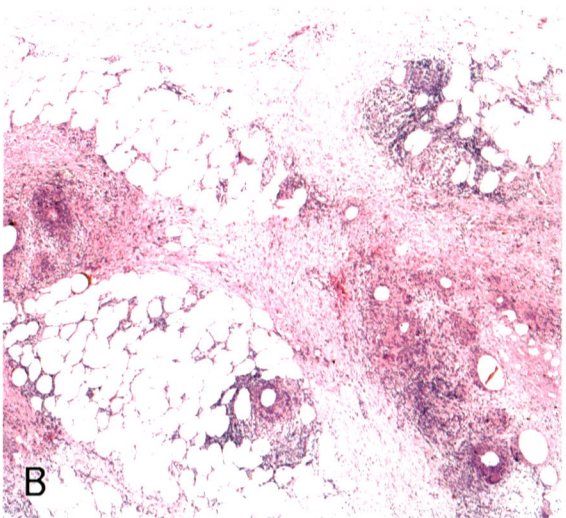

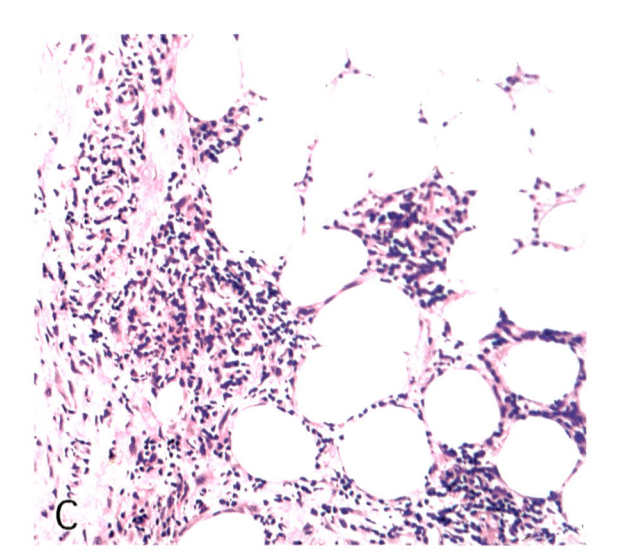

Erythema nodosum-like lesions develop in the setting of Behçet disease (fig. 13-5), and clinical consideration for this possibility is recommended in the routine evaluation of septal panniculitis. On rare occasion, infection of the subcutis (e.g., by fungi in the setting of immunocompromise) may mimic any pattern of panniculitis, and this should be considered and excluded by special stains and culture.

**Differential Diagnosis.** The differential diagnosis includes mainly other types of inflammation of the subcutaneous fat including nodular vasculitis and some forms of systemic vasculitis including Wegener disease and polyarteritis nodosa. Nodular lymphomas, pretibial myxedema, nodular necrobiosis, gummas, and subcutaneous granuloma annulare nodules are considered in the clinical differential diagnosis. The isolated nodular presentation of erythema nodosum is usually clinically considered a cyst, an appendage tumor, or even a metastatic tumor in the correct setting.

There are a group of disorders that variably involve the septa. Among these are scleroderma, necrobiosis lipoidica, eosinophilic fasciitis, and subcutaneous granuloma annulare.

*Inflammatory Disorders of the Skin*

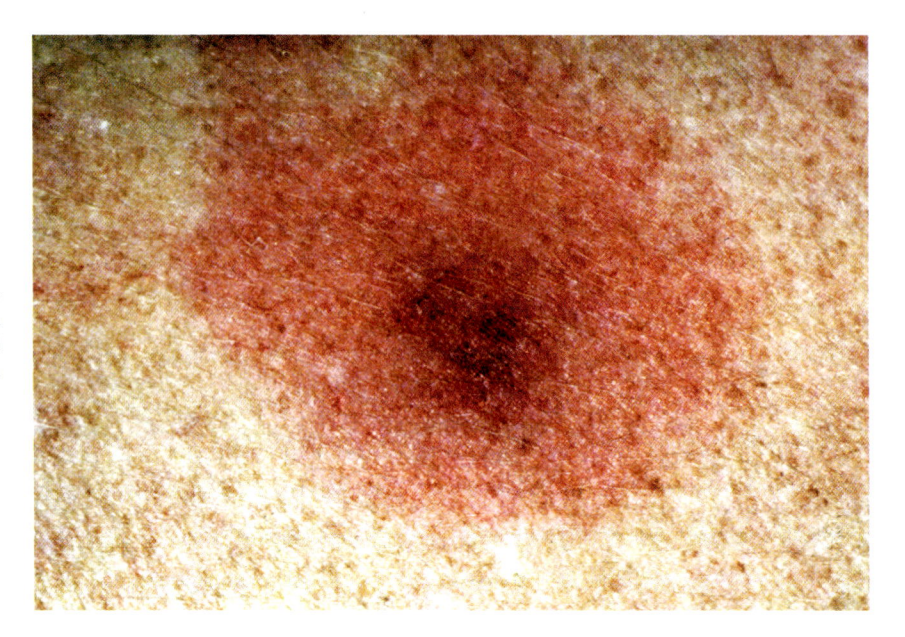

**Figure 13-6**

ERYTHEMA INDURATUM

There is an indurated, erythematous lesion characterized by a dusky purple center surrounded by a pale pink halo. The lesion is painful.

Approximately 20 percent of patients with morphea/scleroderma exhibit fibrosis with widening of the septa. A similar number of patients with necrobiosis show necrobiotic changes of the subcutaneous septa with lipogranuloma formation. Eosinophilic fasciitis often exhibits septal widening and fibrosis similar to morphea/scleroderma. Finally, in some cases of granuloma annulare there is a focal palisading granulomatous reaction in the septa with the changes characteristic of granuloma annulare in the dermis.

**Treatment and Prognosis.** The treatment is basically symptomatic with bed rest and wet dressings along with antiinflammatory agents (9). Erythema nodosum characteristically responds to salicylates, indomethacin, and naproxen. For more severe cases, topical and systemic glucocorticoids are necessary. Potassium iodide is also used.

## ERYTHEMA INDURATUM (NODULAR VASCULITIS), A MIXED PANNICULITIS

**Definition.** *Erythema induratum* (*nodular vasculitis*) is associated with ulceronodular lesions on the legs that are probably due to an immunologically mediated mechanism (10–12). Certain cases are associated with infections with *Mycobacterium tuberculosis* (13–16).

**Clinical Features.** Erythema induratum usually occurs in patients in middle to late life; most are women. It is believed that this condition is immune complex mediated because of the finding of immunoglobulin, complement and evidence of mycobacterial infection by PCR. Cultures for appropriate bacteria are negative. The disorder presents as chronic, recurrent nodules and plaques that ulcerate (fig. 13-6). They may be single or multiple; when multiple, they are often bilateral. Most lesions are asymptomatic but some patients complain of tenderness and discomfort. The erythematous nodular lesions most commonly occur on the calves but also on the shins and upper thighs. As the lesions evolve they become bluish and fluctuant, and ulcerate. These lesions persist for months, sometimes without healing and often with a course marked by recurrences. Patients do not usually have systemic symptoms. Deep scarring often occurs.

**Pathologic Findings.** Histologically, erythema induratum is the prototypical disorder of lobular panniculitis. At scanning magnification, early lesions show a patchy inflammatory infiltrate within the fat lobules, without specific or preferential involvement of septa (fig. 13-7, left). At higher magnification, the inflammatory infiltrate is seen between adipocytes, and as lesions progress, the infiltrate becomes diffusely present throughout the lobule (figs. 13-7–13-11). The inflammatory cells are initially composed of an admixture of neutrophils and lymphocytes. Later, lymphocytes and mononuclear cells with epithelioid forms predominate. Early lesions are typically associated with necrotizing vasculitis involving small- to medium-sized arteries and

404

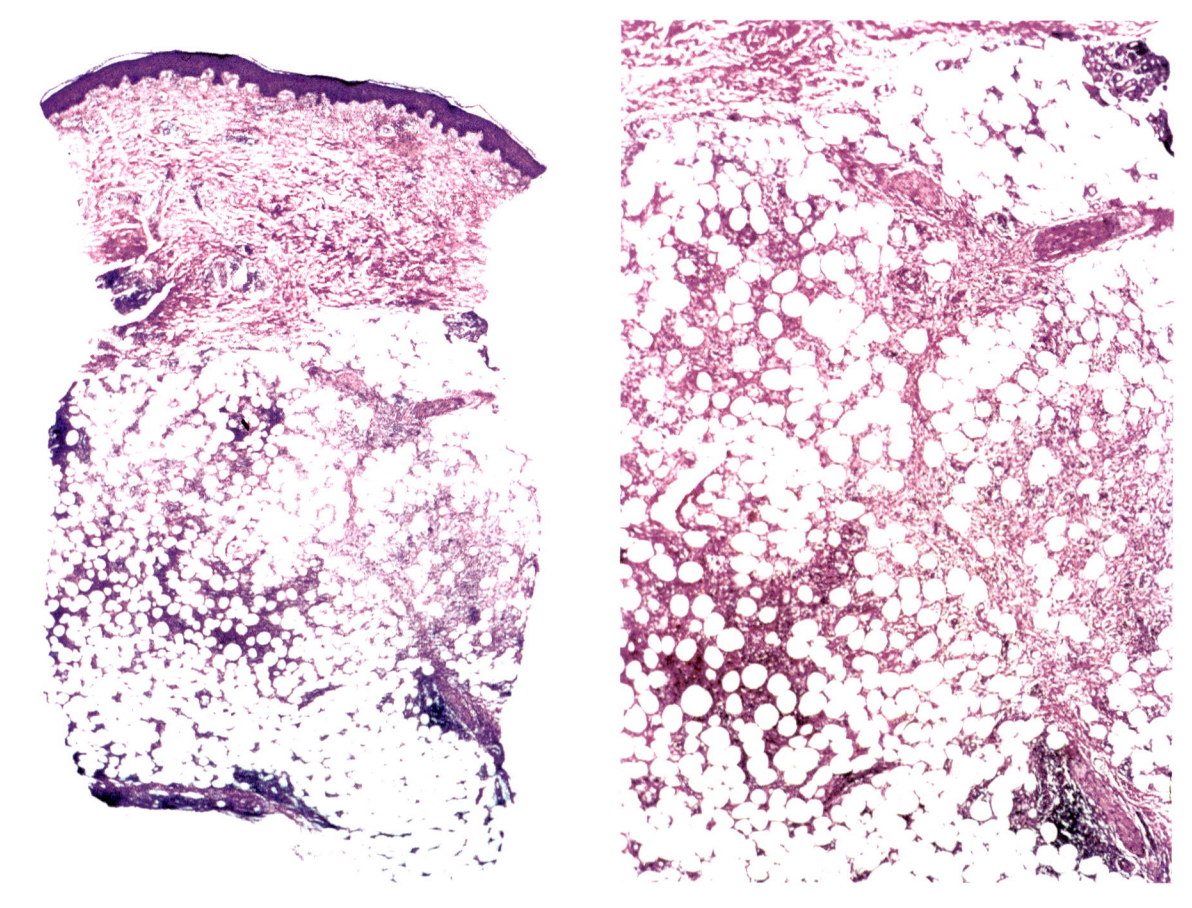

**Figure 13-7**

**ERYTHEMA INDURATUM**

Left: Diffuse inflammation primarily involves the lobule without evidence of septal accentuation.
Right: At higher magnification, vascular lesions may be observed early in the course of the disease in addition to lobular panniculitis.

veins (figs. 13-9, 13-11). The vessel walls are infiltrated by lymphocytes and neutrophils, and zones of fibrinoid necrosis and fibrosis are observed. Vascular thrombosis is focally present.

In older lesions, vasculitic involvement is more difficult to identify. With chronicity, the lobular panniculitis of erythema induratum is predominated by lymphocytes and epithelioid histiocytes with variable degrees of fibrosis (fig. 13-8, top). On close inspection, zones of caseous necrosis may be observed; occasionally, these zones are extensive and geographic. These zones may be rimmed by epithelioid histiocytes with solitary or multiple nuclei. The chronic manifestations are indistinguishable from involvement of fat by tuberculosis infection. For many years, erythema induratum was regarded as a direct manifestation of pulmonary tuberculosis involving subcutaneous fat. Intact organisms, however, are not identified in the caseating granulomas of erythema induratum. On the other hand, it remains unknown whether erythema induratum represents an unusual allergic manifestation stimulated by a number of environmental antigens, including those related to tuberculosis infection.

Although with chronicity, the lobular panniculitis that typifies erythema induratum results in diffuse fibrosis of the subcutaneous fat, residual inflammatory foci may persist, providing a diagnostic clue to the preceding inflammatory insult. In end-stage lesions, however, diffuse fibrosis of the lobule is not considered sufficiently specific to permit a diagnosis of

## Inflammatory Disorders of the Skin

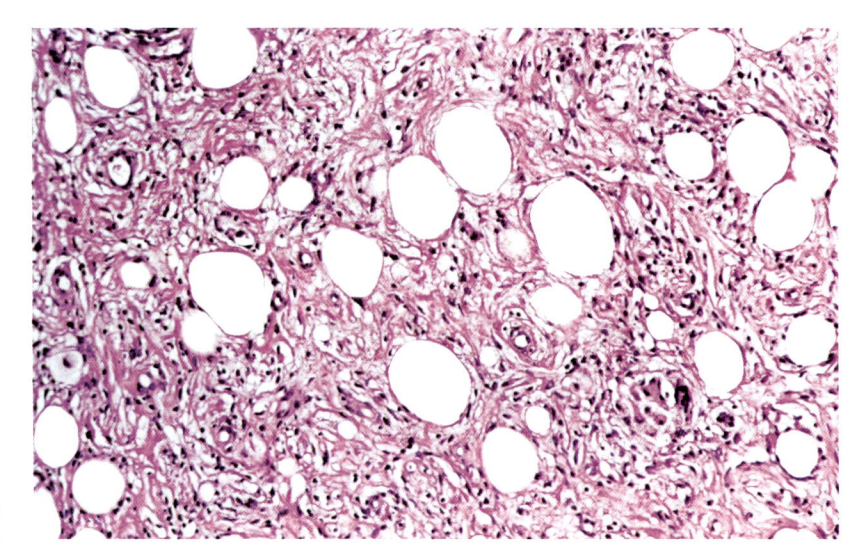

**Figure 13-8**

**ERYTHEMA INDURATUM**

Top: In this older lesion, some of the inflammatory infiltrate has been replaced by collagen fibers.

Bottom: At high magnification, there is both focal necrosis and granulomatous inflammation associated with residual adipocytes.

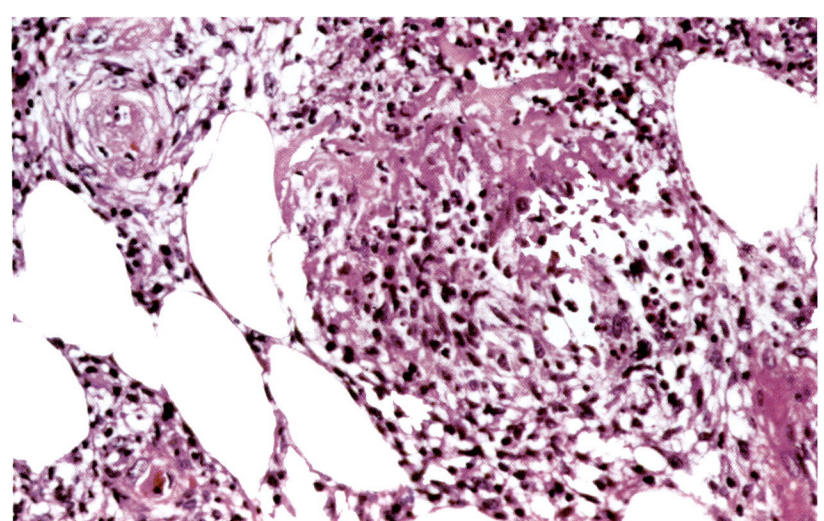

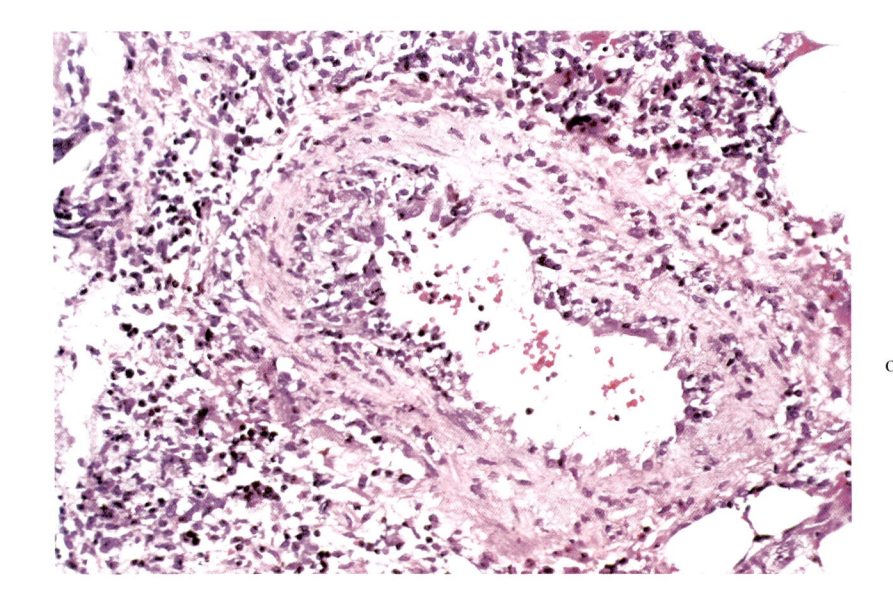

**Figure 13-9**

**ERYTHEMA INDURATUM: VASCULAR INJURY**

This early lesion shows evidence of nodular vasculitis.

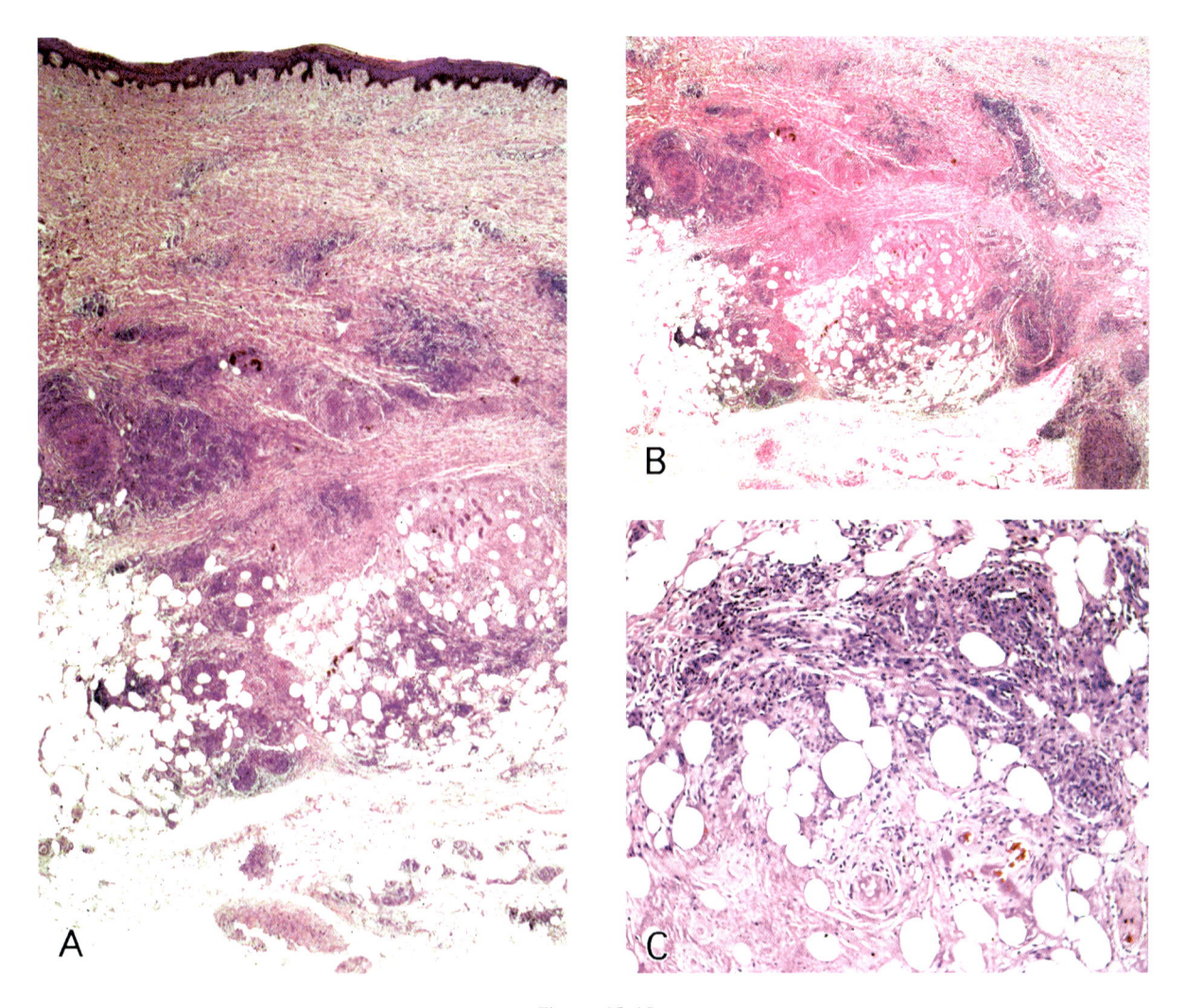

## Figure 13-10
### ERYTHEMA INDURATUM

A: In this early lesion, the inflammatory infiltrate involves primarily the superficial subcutis. Some secondary involvement of the dermis is also evident.

B: At scanning magnification, the inflammatory infiltrate shows a lace-like, or "honeycomb" pattern of infiltration within the fat lobule and scattered vessels (two in lower right) are infiltrated by inflammatory cells.

C: The interstitium of the fat lobule is expanded by numerous lymphocytes and mononuclear cells associated with early collagen deposition.

erythema induratum. In such cases, additional sampling of more recent lesions is recommended for definitive diagnostic evaluation.

As is the case in erythema nodosum, erythema induratum may be mimicked by a number of traumatic or infectious insults to adipose tissue. It is important to note the absence of alterations within the overlying epidermis and at least the upper half of the dermis in erythema induratum, signifying primary panniculitis centered exclusively within the subcutaneous layer.

**Differential Diagnosis.** Multiple lesions must be differentiated from erythema nodosum and the so-called Weber-Christian disease. Ulcerated lesions clinically may resemble pyoderma gangrenosum, deep fungal infection, atrophie blanche, or even neoplasms such as lymphoma. Because lesions histologically show granulomatous lobular inflammation, the differential diagnosis includes infection and factitial panniculitis. The granulomas are seldom so well formed as to suggest subcutaneous sarcoid, however.

*Inflammatory Disorders of the Skin*

**Figure 13-11**

**ERYTHEMA INDURATUM: VASCULITIC AND GRANULOMATOUS FOCI**

A focus showing nodular vasculitis is surrounded by granulomatous inflammation.

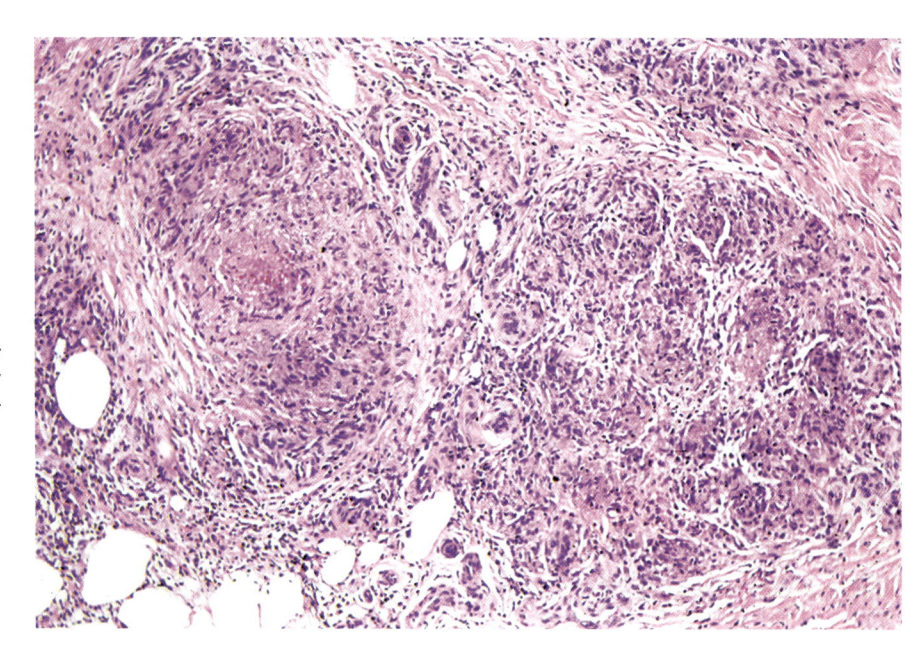

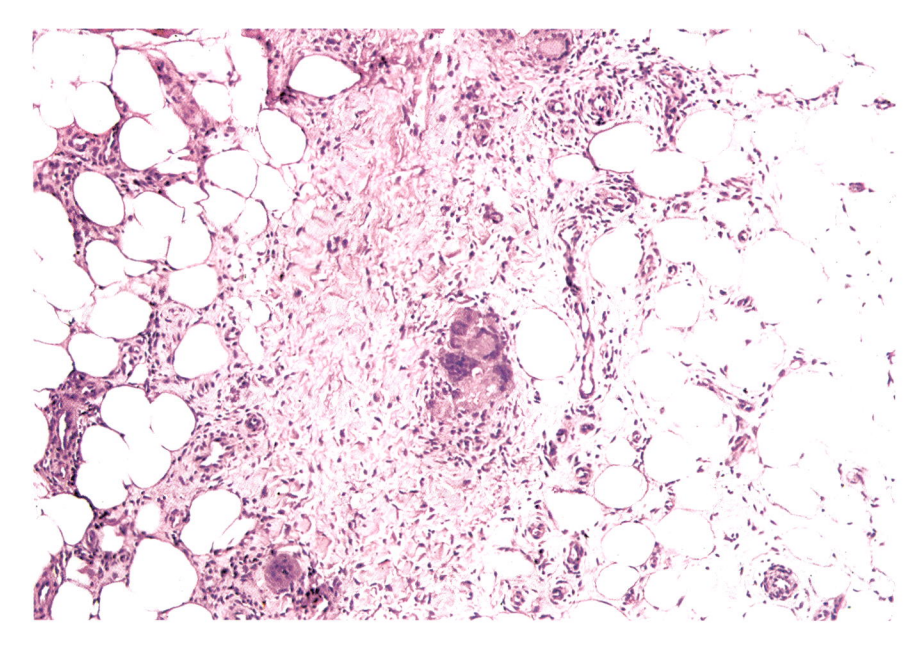

**Figure 13-12**

**ERYTHEMA NODOSUM: LOBULAR INVOLVEMENT**

Although the paraseptal portion of the lobule may be involved, the central region of the lobule is invariably spared.

Erythema nodosum frequently shows paraseptal involvement (fig. 13-12) that, upon tangential sectioning of a small biopsy sample, may appear to represent a lobular pattern. Another diagnostic consideration is polyarteritis nodosa with secondary panniculitis mimicking lobular panniculitis with associated vascular injury (as is seen in erythema induratum) (figs. 13-13, 13-14). In such cases, confirmation of the characteristic restriction of vasculitic involvement of small to medium-sized arteries in polyarteritis nodosa, often facilitated by an elastic tissue stain, is helpful.

**Treatment and Prognosis.** When the lesions are associated with tuberculous infection, they resolve with antituberculous therapy. Symptomatic care with bed rest and wet dressings sometimes resolves the lesions. Antibiotics including tetracyclines and at times even potassium iodide are occasionally associated with remissions. Systemic corticosteroids may be necessary in some patients.

*Panniculitis*

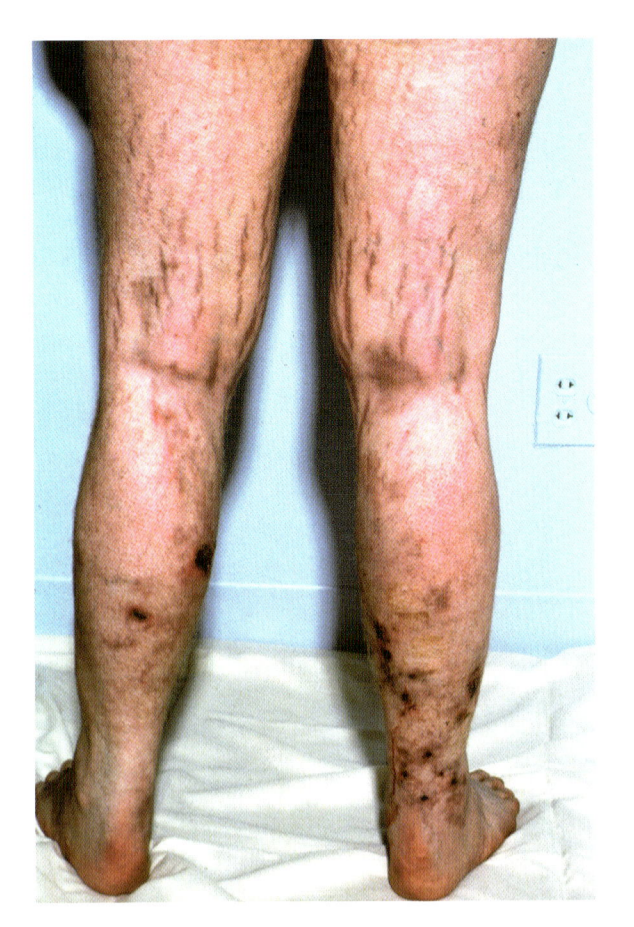

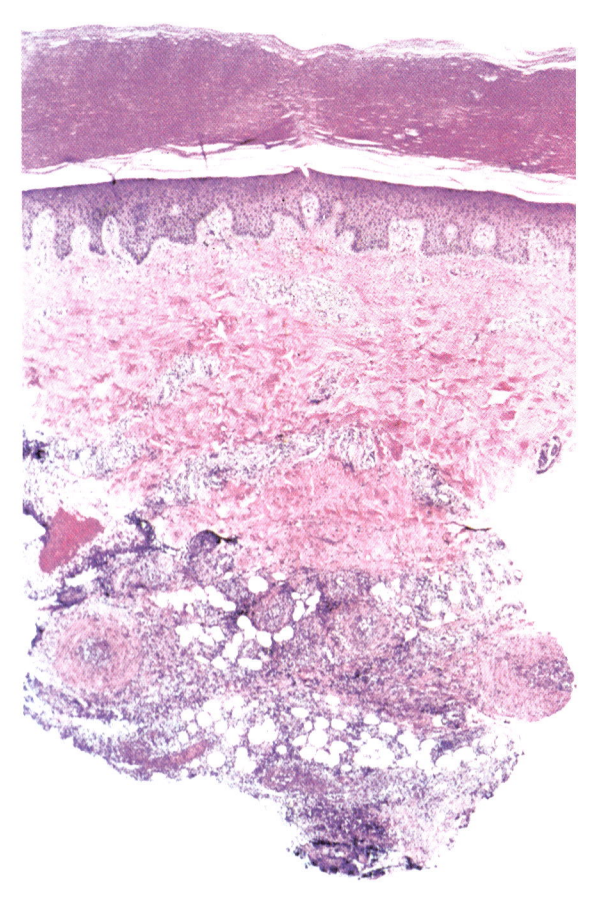

**Figure 13-13**

**POLYARTERITIS NODOSA WITH SECONDARY PANNICULITIS**

Left: The lower extremities of this patient are swollen and indurated due to diffuse panniculitis. The distal legs show zones of nodular ulceration consistent with ischemia. The prominent striae on the posterior side are a complication of chronic steroid administration.

Right: The adipose tissue shows both septal and lobular inflammation by inflammatory cells, mimicking primary panniculitis.

## PANNICULITIS DUE TO CONNECTIVE TISSUE DISEASE

### Lupus Profundus, a Mixed Panniculitis

**Definition.** *Lupus profundus* is a manifestation of lupus erythematosus that occurs in association with systemic disease and as an isolated manifestation of cutaneous disease (17–25).

**Clinical Features.** While the age range is from childhood to late life, the earliest cases are reported in the first 2 to 3 years of life and the median age is in the fourth to fifth decade. Women are more commonly affected than men. The lesions appear principally over the extremities and buttocks, but also occur on the trunk and rarely, the face (fig. 13-15). The lesions are plate-like nodules that are better palpated than visually appreciated if there are no overlying skin changes. While most cases exhibit some changes of discoid lupus erythematosus or poikiloderma, occasionally the skin appears normal over these lesions. Systemic lupus erythematosus is present in about one third of the patients, but the systemic signs are usually mild. Lesions often evolve into depressed atrophic areas.

**Pathologic Findings.** Lupus panniculitis typically produces a characteristic type of hyalinized necrosis of lobular adipocytes, resulting in zones of pale, homogeneous coagulation of the lobule associated with patchy lymphoplasmacytic infiltrates (figs. 13-16–13-18). Variable deposition

409

## Inflammatory Disorders of the Skin

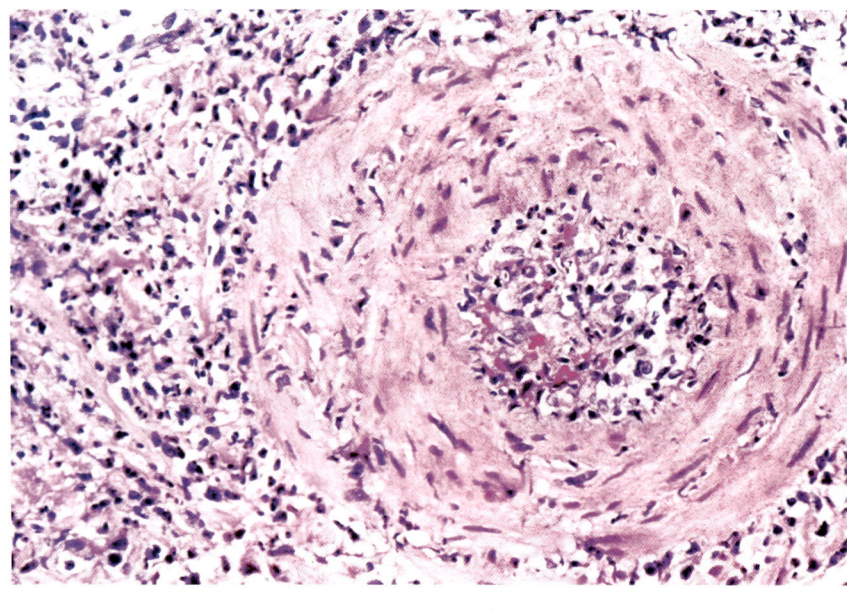

**Figure 13-14**

**POLYARTERITIS NODOSA**

Top: High magnification shows primary vascular involvement. The vessel wall is infiltrated by neutrophils and mononuclear cells. These are medium-sized muscular arteries, a feature that may be confirmed by elastic tissue staining.

Bottom: The remnant of a vessel at the bottom of the field is associated with adjacent secondary lobular panniculitis.

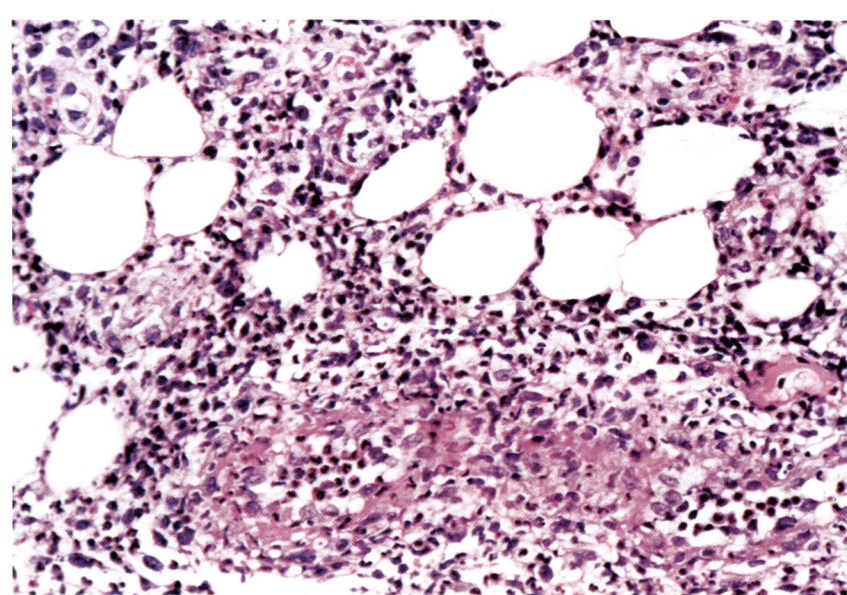

of collagen and mucin is observed, and the inflammatory and sclerosing alterations occasionally extend into the overlying dermis. A lymphocytic hyalinizing vasculitis, often with a redundant annular ring of connective tissue surrounding the vessel, is characteristic. Interface alterations involving the dermal-epidermal junction and other dermal changes of lupus erythematosus are observed in half of the patients. Direct immunofluorescence is often positive, revealing a granular band of immunoglobulin and complement within the basement membrane region.

**Differential Diagnosis.** Clinically, erythema nodosum, subcutaneous inflammatory forms of morphea, and pancreatic fat necrosis are the three prominent lesions in the differential diagnosis, although other panniculitides must also be considered. Prominent septal involvement with giant cell formation and perivenular paraseptal aggregates distinguishes erythema nodosum. The deep inflammatory lesions of morphea may initially mimic lupus profundus; however, the former shows greater hyalinized fibrosis rather than necrosis of the fat lobule, and sclerosing alterations in the overlying dermis and subjacent

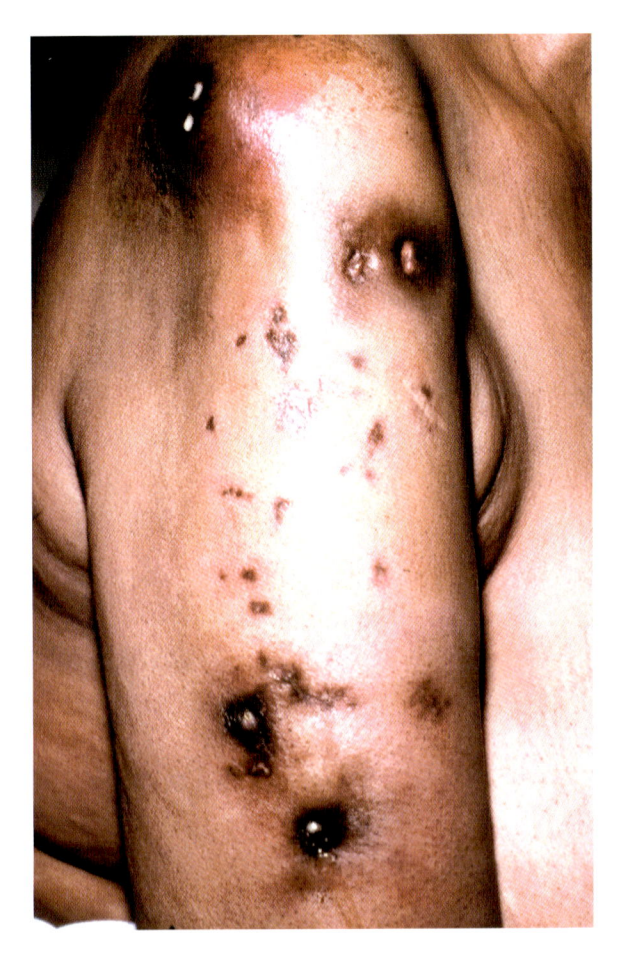

### Figure 13-15
**LUPUS PANNICULITIS**
There are multiple erythematous nodules, some with central zones of ulceration.

fascia typical of morphea are generally observed. Furthermore, the infiltrate of morphea usually has a prominent plasmacellular component and there is no vasculitis. Although pancreatic fat necrosis may produce ghost adipocytes that are pale and focally hyalinized, the degree of inflammation is usually less, and foci of enzymatic fat necrosis with calcification tend to be more localized than is typical of the diffuse lobular involvement of lupus profundus.

## Connective Tissue Panniculitis

*Connective tissue panniculitis* is a lobular lymphocytic panniculitis that presents as a nodule or nodules on limbs and trunk (26). Lesions may be associated in some cases with the development of subcutaneous T-cell lymphoma.

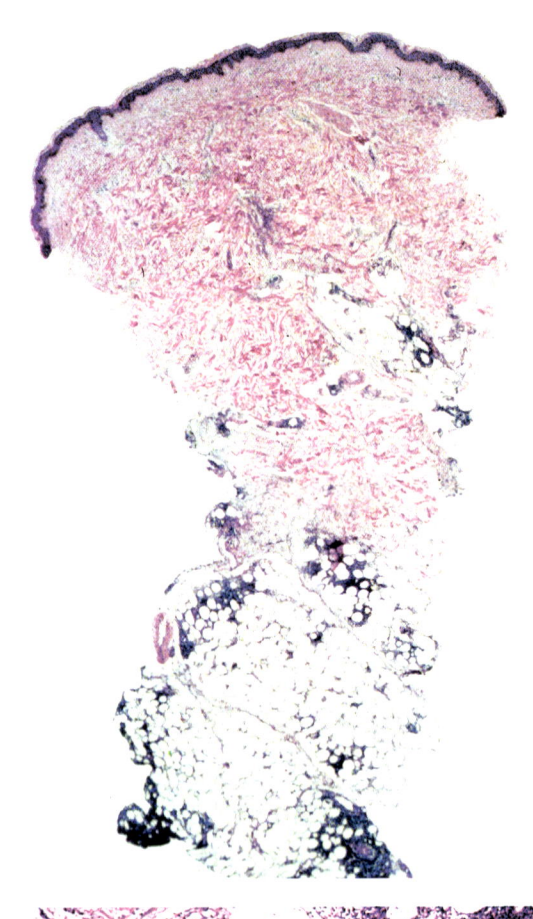

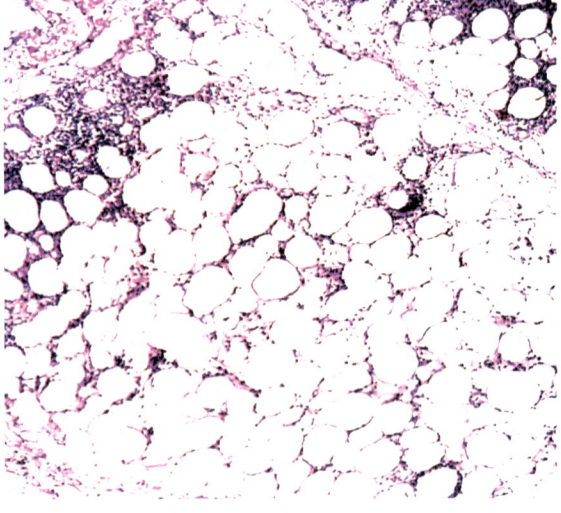

### Figure 13-16
**LUPUS PANNICULITIS**
Top: This early lesion shows deep dermal and subcutaneous aggregates of mononuclear cells.
Bottom: At high magnification, the lymphocytes and plasma cells predominate in this focus. Lobular adipocytes are variably atrophic and separated by a characteristically pale and hyalinized matrix.

# Inflammatory Disorders of the Skin

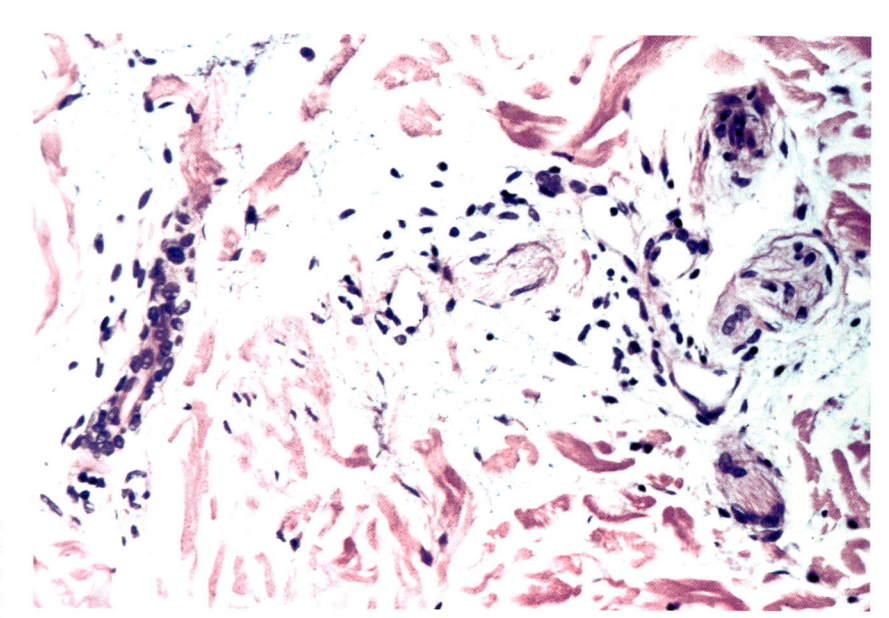

**Figure 13-17**

**LUPUS PANNICULITIS**

Top: High-power view of the dermis shows strands of pale blue mucin expanding spaces that separate collagen bundles from adjacent neurovascular structures, as in other forms of lupus.

Bottom: The infiltrate involves both septa and the lobule; lymphoid follicle formation is seen. Hyalinization of the lobules is prominent.

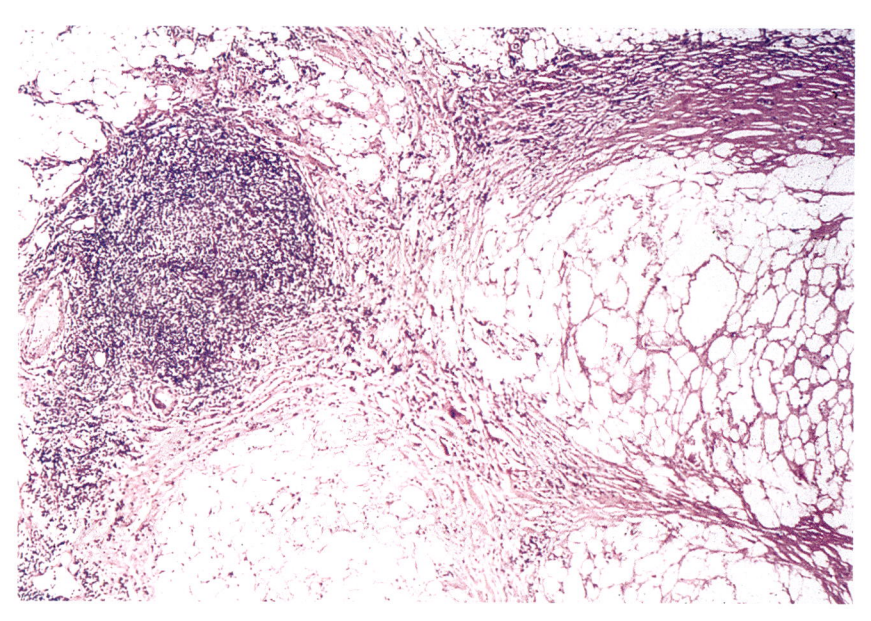

## Panniculitis of Dermatomyositis and Polymyositis, Morphea, and Scleroderma

In *dermatomyositis* and *polymyositis*, there may be prominent focal subcutaneous nodules that are usually asymptomatic (27–29). Sometimes there is evidence of a lymphocytic inflammation of the subcutaneous fat. *Morphea* may present as a striking subcutaneous nodule before evidence of superficial atrophy occurs. This type of panniculitis is usually associated with a dense plasmacellular infiltrate. In *scleroderma*, approximately 25 percent of patients have thickened areas of skin that are associated with hyalinization of the septa, a type of septal panniculitis (30).

Inflammatory morphea with panniculitis shows extension of dermal sclerosis into the subcutaneous fat in association with patchy perivenular and interstitial lymphocytic and plasmacytic infiltrates (fig. 13-19). The sclerosis that affects both the deep reticular dermis and subcutis is characterized by deposition of pale, thickened, homogenous bands of collagen, with marked encroachment upon the intercollagenous spaces and associated mesenchymal hypocellularity.

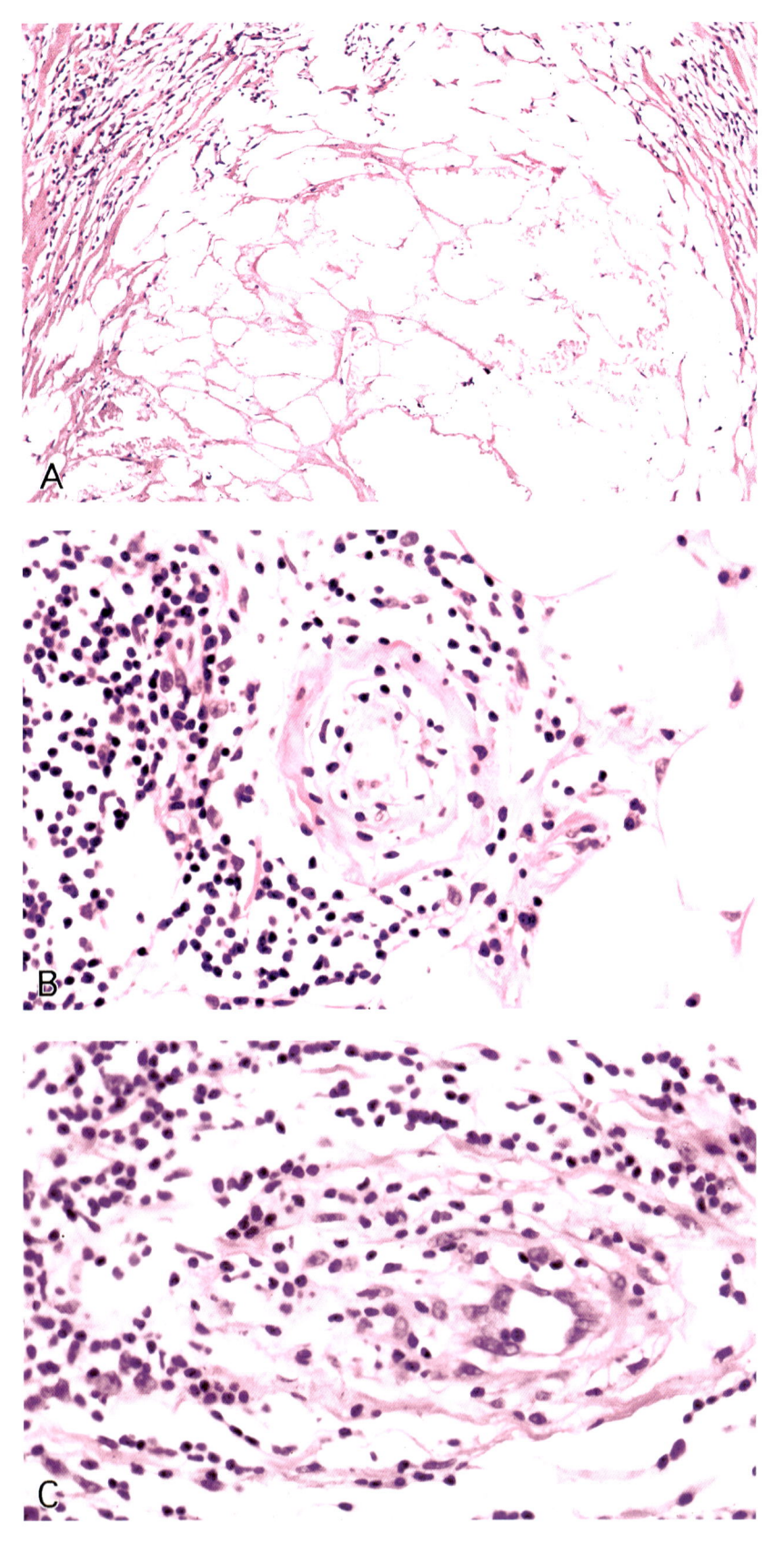

**Figure 13-18**

**LUPUS PROFUNDUS: LOBULAR INVOLVEMENT**

A: The characteristic pale, hyalinized interstitial fibrosis that has begun to separate adjacent adipocytes typifies lupus profundus. Feathery early lipomembranous degenerative changes are also present.

B: High magnification of lymphocytic vasculitis shows a lymphocytic infiltrate that contains occasional plasma cells and focally permeates vessel walls. Granulomatous inflammation, as seen in erythema nodosum and erythema induratum, is absent.

C: This vessel shows endothelial prominence and degenerative alterations in association with a permeative infiltrate that involves the vessel wall. Also note redundant rings of hyalinized matrix surrounding the vessel (also seen in B).

**Figure 13-19**

**SUBCUTANEOUS INFLAMMATORY MORPHEA**

Discrete zones of hyalinized fibrosis that replace adipocytes along septal planes, as well as the patchy lymphoplasmacytic infiltrate, are seen. The hyalinized fibrosis is pale, with swollen and indistinct collagen bundles, as opposed to the coarse fibrosis that may involve septa as a late sequela of erythema nodosum.

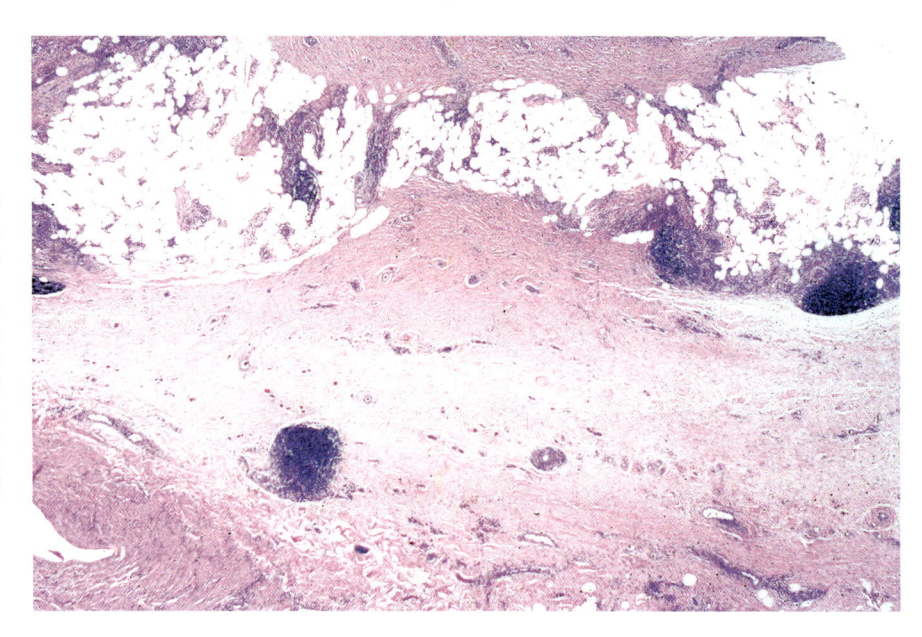

## EOSINOPHILIC FASCIITIS, WITH SEPTAL OR MIXED PANNICULITIS

*Eosinophilic fasciitis* is a distinctive entity of unknown cause (31–37). The extremities are most commonly involved and exhibit marked sleeve-like edematous induration that is extensive. At times, however, there may be a linear band-like area of induration and firmness. This disorder, also called *Shulman syndrome* (fasciitis with eosinophilia), may be associated with normal-appearing skin overlying the area or changes of morphea or scleroderma in the fascia.

There is sclerosis of the deep subcutaneous fat with involvement of the underlying fascia. Often, there is infiltration by lymphocytes and plasma cells, which may form small aggregates, especially at the interface between areas of sclerosis and subcutaneous fat. Eosinophils may be present in the tissue; if tissue eosinophilia is not present, the histologic features may be identical to those of subcutaneous morphea. The patient should have a history of peripheral blood eosinophilia and the above clinical presentation to establish a diagnosis of eosinophilic fasciitis.

## RELAPSING FEBRILE NODULAR NONSUPPURATIVE PANNICULITIS (WEBER-CHRISTIAN DISEASE)

**Definition.** *Relapsing febrile nodular nonsuppurative panniculitis*, also known as *Weber-Christian disease*, is a disorder of unknown etiology that predominantly occurs in women in the fourth to the seventh decade. The characteristic course consists of eruptive crops of nodules that are tender, occasionally break down, and may have systemic involvement (38–43).

Most authors today consider this lesion to represent a variety of different disorders. In our experience, however, there are rare persons in whom this disorder presents and who have no evidence of causation. The uniqueness of the histology of this disorder that allows for a consideration of the evolution of a classic nodular panniculitis leads us to include it here.

**Clinical Features.** Tender inflammatory subcutaneous nodules are on the lower extremities but also on the trunk, arms, and rarely, neck. The lesions become fluctuant, break down, and emit a serous or yellow-brown oily liquid. The disorder is associated with fever, malaise, arthralgias, and occasionally, myalgias. Systemic involvement can lead to involvement of mediastinal or peritoneal, pericardial, or retroperitoneal fat, features uncommon for other causes of primary cutaneous panniculitis. Recorded cases of pericardial involvement have been mistaken for coronary artery thrombosis. Abdominal involvement may lead to a mistaken diagnosis of acute appendicitis or other acute intraabdominal catastrophes. Some persons consider this to be a "waste basket" type of disorder, which is understood when additional causes of panniculitis, such as alpha-1-antitrypsin deficiency, are discovered.

## Figure 13-20

### LOBULAR NEUTROPHILIC PANNICULITIS

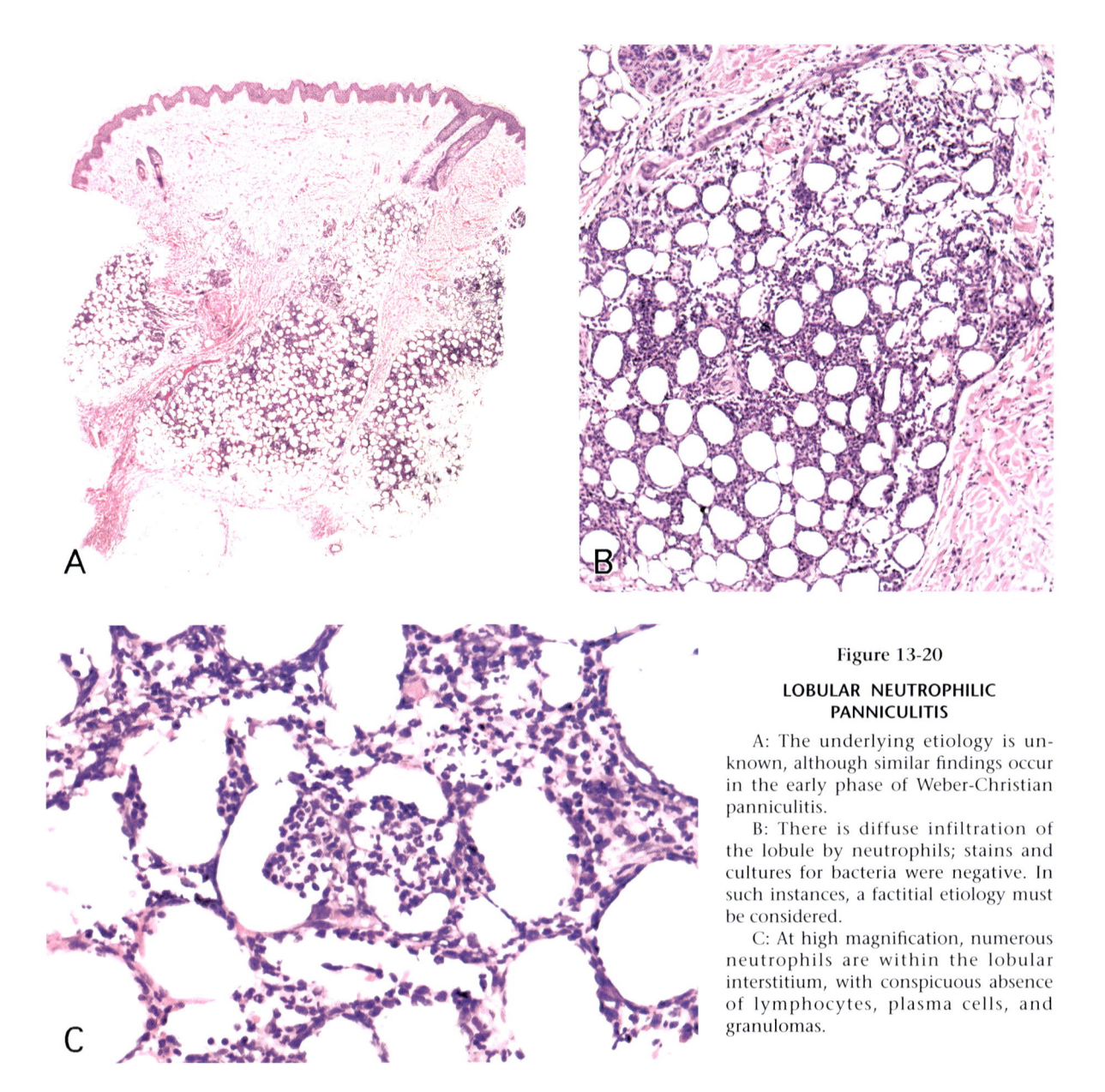

A: The underlying etiology is unknown, although similar findings occur in the early phase of Weber-Christian panniculitis.

B: There is diffuse infiltration of the lobule by neutrophils; stains and cultures for bacteria were negative. In such instances, a factitial etiology must be considered.

C: At high magnification, numerous neutrophils are within the lobular interstitium, with conspicuous absence of lymphocytes, plasma cells, and granulomas.

**Pathologic Findings.** Relapsing nodular panniculitis evolves through three phases, all showing lobular involvement. The first consists of a lobular neutrophilic panniculitis with neutrophil infiltration of lobules with foci of adipocyte degeneration and death (fig. 13-20). The second, arguably the most characteristic, involves infiltration by histiocytes and lipophages almost entirely replacing the lobules. The third stage is resolution of the second, with foci of fibroblastic proliferation and collagen deposition. In this phase, there may be some involvement of the septa, but it is secondary to the prominent changes occurring in the lobule.

**Differential Diagnosis.** Alpha-1-antitrypsin deficiency and pancreatic panniculitis are two considerations. They can be distinguished by clinical-pathologic correlation.

**Treatment and Prognosis.** The treatment has included chloroquine, azathioprine, and even thalidomide (44–46). Cyclophosphamide and cyclosporine have been tried with variable success (47,48).

## PANCREATIC (ENZYMATIC) PANNICULITIS

**Definition.** *Pancreatic panniculitis* is important because it heralds pancreatitis and even adenocarcinoma of the pancreas (49–53).

**Clinical Features.** Painful, red nodules occur at any site on the body but are most common on the lower extremities and abdomen. The lesions are more common in middle age to elderly men than women. There is usually an associated history of abdominal pain, weight loss, the onset of diabetes mellitus, or a history of alcoholism. The tender cutaneous nodules fluctuate and break down, emitting a granular oily type of material. There may be pleural involvement with effusion. The correct diagnosis is made by histologic examination; elevated lipase or amylase levels in the blood confirm the diagnosis. Sometimes these lesions occur after acute episodes of pancreatitis so that the laboratory findings may not be conclusive. All patients must be worked up for pancreatic disease.

**Pathologic Findings.** The panniculitis involves lobules and septa, with predominance of the former, by lymphocytes, histiocytes, eosinophils, and in acute lesions, neutrophils. The inflammatory elements are generally peripheral to focal zones within the lobules showing necrosis and enzymatic degeneration of adipocytes. Affected adipocytes within the lobules show characteristic changes: loss of nuclear detail and pale, homogeneous cytoplasm surrounded by a thickened, eosinophilic cell membrane (ghost cells) (fig. 13-21). Saponification of the necrotic adipocytes causes deposition of finely particulate basophilic calcium salts within the cytoplasm of affected cells. Resolving lesions show accumulation of lipophages, lymphocytes, and histiocytes, producing a granulomatous appearance. Zones of fibrosis may be seen.

**Differential Diagnosis.** The Weber-Christian group of disorders and the alpha-1-antichymotrypsin group of disorders must be considered in the differential diagnosis. Early erythema nodosum must be considered, especially when multiple lesions are present. Rarely, when fat necrosis is extensive, stasis must be excluded.

**Treatment and Prognosis.** The treatment must be directed at elimination of the underlying disease if possible. Local measures to control ulcerated areas and prevent infection are usually instituted. Analgesia may be needed for pain control.

## SCLEREMA NEONATORUM

**Definition.** *Sclerema neonatorum* is associated with abnormalities of the subcutaneous fat that occur because infant fat has a higher saturated to unsaturated fatty acid ratio than adult fat (54). This results in easy solidification of the infant's subcutaneous fat at a higher temperature than adult fat. Prematurity and possibly an associated incompletely formed enzyme system may be involved, leading to altered desaturation of fatty acids. Most affected infants are premature and may be subject to other factors that inhibit the enzyme system including cold exposure, infection, sepsis, and dehydration.

**Clinical Features.** There is rapid, diffuse hardening of the skin and subcutaneous fat. Lesions characteristically begin on the trunk and buttocks in the first few days of life. The extensive involvement of the skin spares only scrotum, palms, and soles. The patients are premature and often debilitated or septic. While cold exposure is not clearly associated with this disorder, there have been sclerema-like findings in children who have been subjected to cold environments. In contrast, *subcutaneous fat necrosis of the newborn* (see below) is a discrete disorder that involves either a plaque or multiple plaques or nodules within the first few days of life, characteristically on the back, buttocks or thighs, and cheeks. In contrast to sclerema neonatorum, subcutaneous fat necrosis of the newborn is benign and self limited, and is rarely associated with hypocalcemia and death.

**Pathologic Findings.** The most striking finding is enlargement of adipocytes due to the development of needle-shaped intracytoplasmic clefts. These are birefringent with polariscopy of frozen tissue sections (fig. 13-22). There is generally some degree of septal fibrosis. Inflammation is scarce, and if present, is mixed and observed within affected lobules. Because of the absence of inflammatory changes, some observers do not classify sclerema neonatorum as a true panniculitis.

**Differential Diagnosis.** The findings are characteristic, and few entities enter into the differential diagnosis. Subcutaneous fat necrosis of the newborn may show similar alterations within lobular adipocytes, although true panniculitis is present and septal fibrosis is not observed.

### Figure 13-21
### PANCREATIC PANNICULITIS

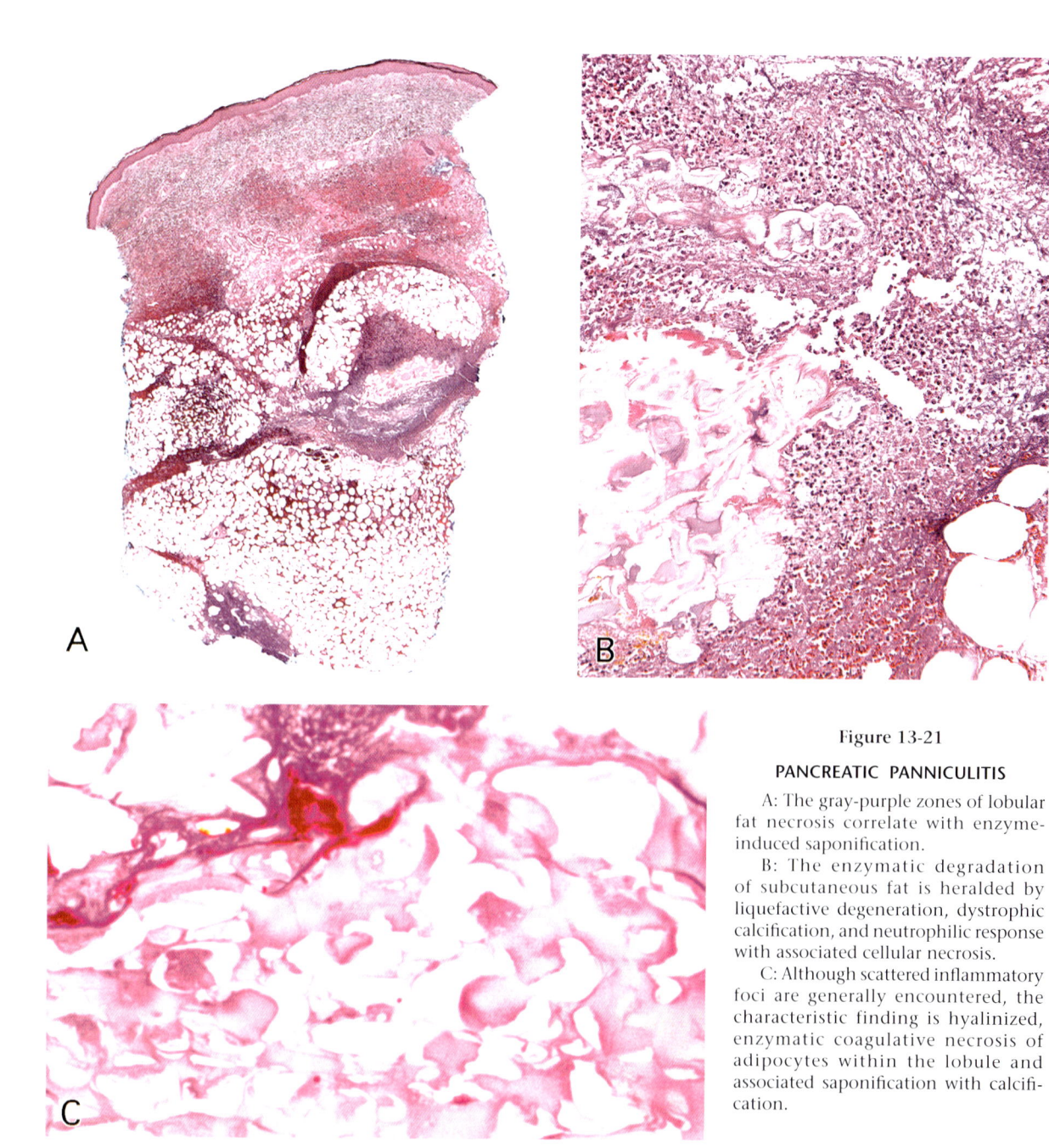

A: The gray-purple zones of lobular fat necrosis correlate with enzyme-induced saponification.

B: The enzymatic degradation of subcutaneous fat is heralded by liquefactive degeneration, dystrophic calcification, and neutrophilic response with associated cellular necrosis.

C: Although scattered inflammatory foci are generally encountered, the characteristic finding is hyalinized, enzymatic coagulative necrosis of adipocytes within the lobule and associated saponification with calcification.

**Treatment and Prognosis.** If patients are not septic at the time of the onset of the disease, sepsis often supervenes and the prognosis is poor. Corticosteroids have been used with variable success.

## SUBCUTANEOUS FAT NECROSIS OF THE NEWBORN

**Definition.** *Subcutaneous fat necrosis of the newborn* consists of abnormalities of the subcutaneous fat similar to those observed in sclerema neonatorum (55–59). Premature infants are more commonly affected.

**Clinical Features.** Subcutaneous fat necrosis of the newborn is characterized by discrete lesions consisting of either a plaque or multiple plaques or nodules, characteristically on the back, buttocks or thighs, and cheeks that occur within the first few days of life. In contrast to sclerema neonatorum, this disorder is benign and self limited. It has rarely been associated

*Inflammatory Disorders of the Skin*

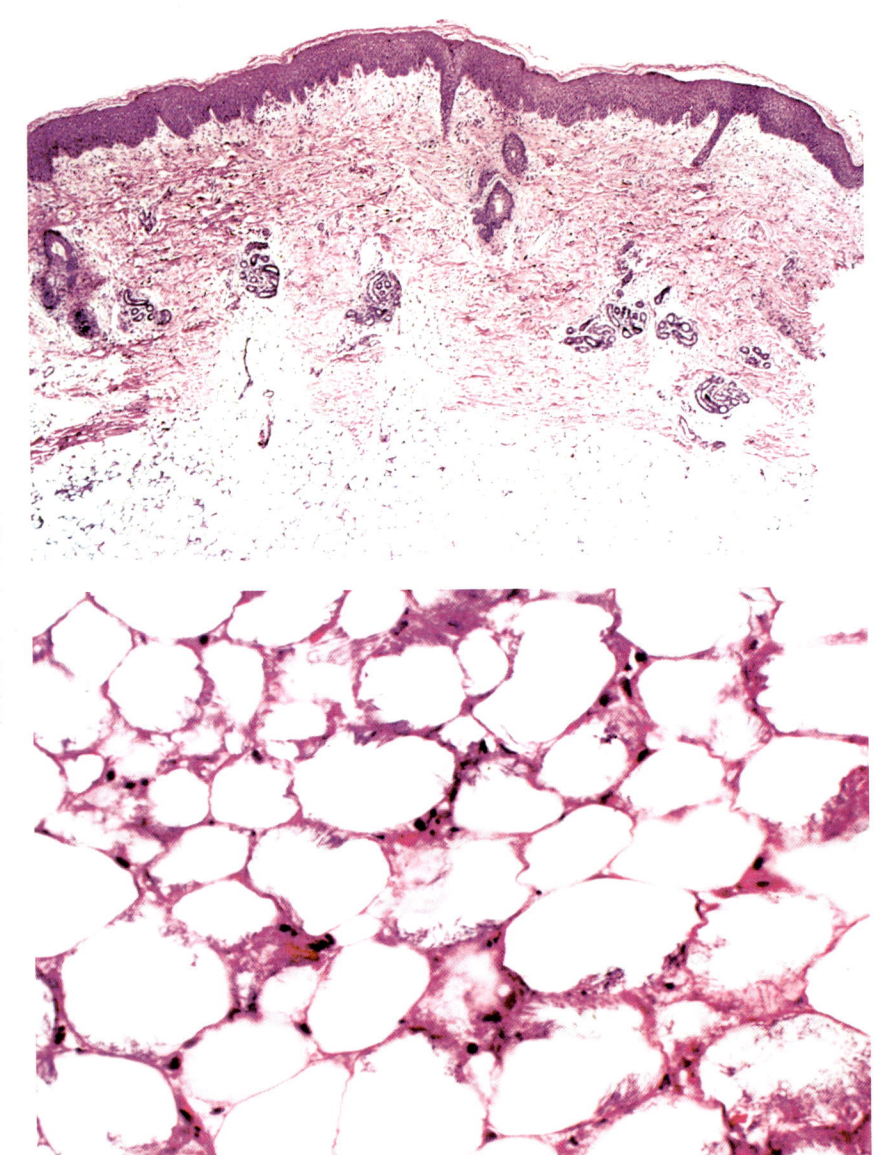

**Figure 13-22**

**SCLEREMA NEONATORUM**

Top: Inflammation is inconspicuous to absent, and unlike subcutaneous fat necrosis of the newborn, this disorder may not represent a true form of panniculitis.

Bottom: At high magnification, individual adipocytes contain fine, needle-shaped clefts concentrated at the cell perimeters.

with hypocalcemia and death. The exact relationship to cold is not clear but certainly physical stress, such as exposure to a cold environment, debilitation due to poor nutrition, and sepsis, result in the increased occurrence of these lesions.

**Pathologic Findings.** There is both lobular and septal panniculitis mediated by lymphocytes, histiocytes, and multinucleated giant cells (fig. 13-23, left). Adipocytes contain characteristic, radially aligned, intracytoplasmic clefts in conventionally fixed and embedded tissue, and phagocytosis of these clefts by multinucleated giant cells is observed (fig. 13-23, right). These clefts are similar to those identified in lesions of sclerema neonatorum. Older lesions may show foci of dystrophic calcification.

**Differential Diagnosis.** The primary differential consideration is sclerema neonatorum, a condition with considerably less inflammation than subcutaneous fat necrosis. Sclerema may be associated with septal fibrosis. The only other panniculitis that exhibits needle-shaped clefts is poststeroid panniculitis, which occurs in children when there is rapid withdrawal of oral steroids. As steroids are now gradually tapered, this phenomenon is no longer seen.

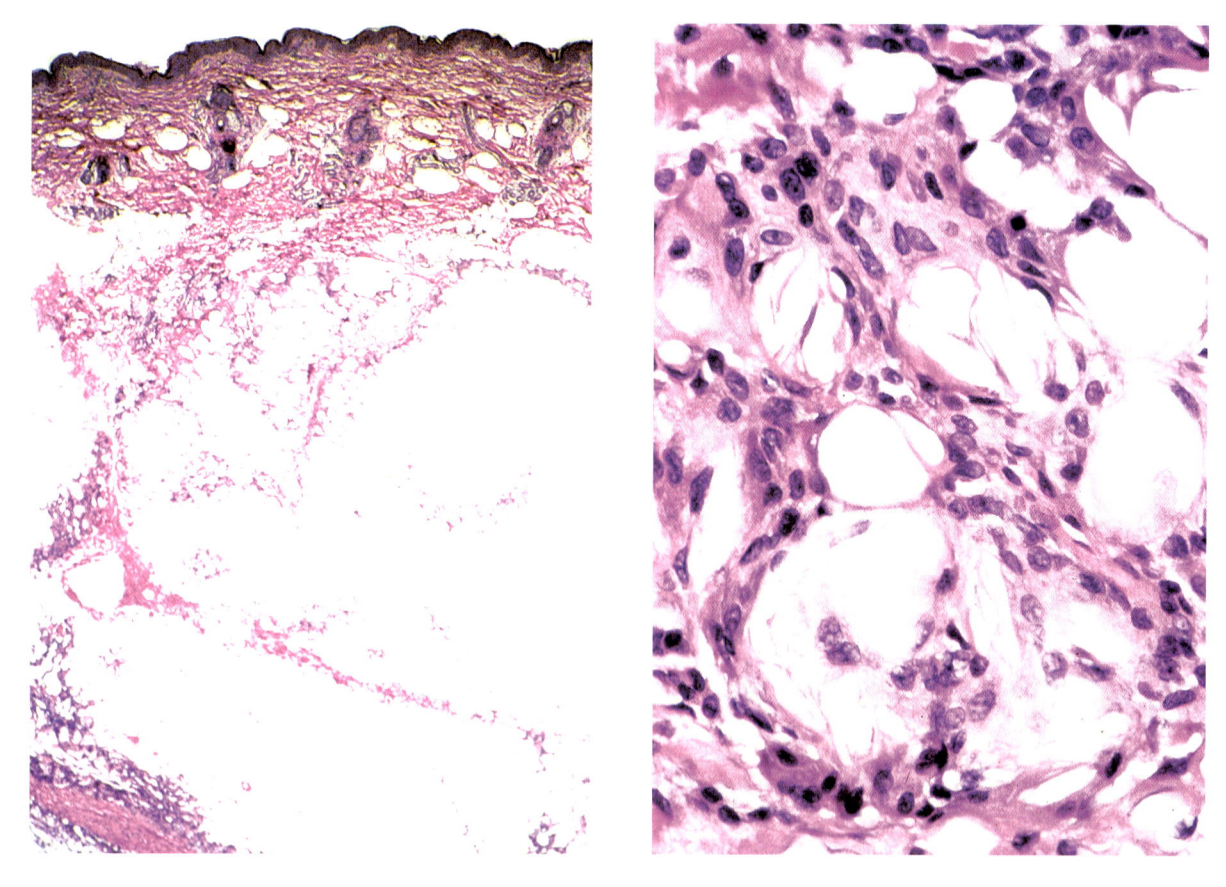

**Figure 13-23**

**SUBCUTANEOUS FAT NECROSIS OF THE NEWBORN**

Left: Mixed inflammatory cells are concentrated at the perimeter of lobules and are associated with degenerating adipocytes (most pronounced in the lower left corner).

Right: High magnification shows individual adipocytes that contain characteristic clefts within their cytoplasm and that are associated with an inflammatory response. On polarization of frozen sections, these clefts are revealed to represent birefringent crystals.

**Treatment and Prognosis.** The course of subcutaneous fat necrosis is spontaneous resolution after a few weeks but there may be temporary hyperpigmentation.

## LIPODERMATOSCLEROSIS, A MIXED PANNICULITIS

**Definition.** *Lipodermatosclerosis* is a disorder associated with venous insufficiency that has a characteristic clinical picture in its chronic fully developed form (60–63).

**Clinical Features.** This lesion is observed in adult women much more frequently than men. Patients have a history of stasis dermatitis of the lower extremities and marked venous insufficiency. The disorder may be a result of superficial and deep thrombosis of varicose veins. The distal third of the lower extremity becomes completely encircled by edematous erythematous plaques that are hyperpigmented, indurated, and depressed. When fully evolved, the lesions have an "inverted bottle-like" or "champagne glass-like" appearance caused by the striking sclerosis of the lower extremity and the ample broad areas of the unaffected proximal portions of the legs above.

**Pathologic Findings.** There is a mixed lymphohistiocytic inflammatory infiltrate involving both subcutaneous septa and lobules. The histiocytic component is frequently lipophagic. The most characteristic feature is the formation of microcysts within the lobules lined by PAS-positive, diastase-resistant cuticle-like membranes, often showing corrugated or

## Inflammatory Disorders of the Skin

**Figure 13-24**

**LIPOMEMBRANOUS PANNICULITIS**

This manifestation of chronic venous stasis shows a mixed pattern of inflammatory panniculitis, with characteristic "feathery" degenerative alterations in the remaining adipocytes.

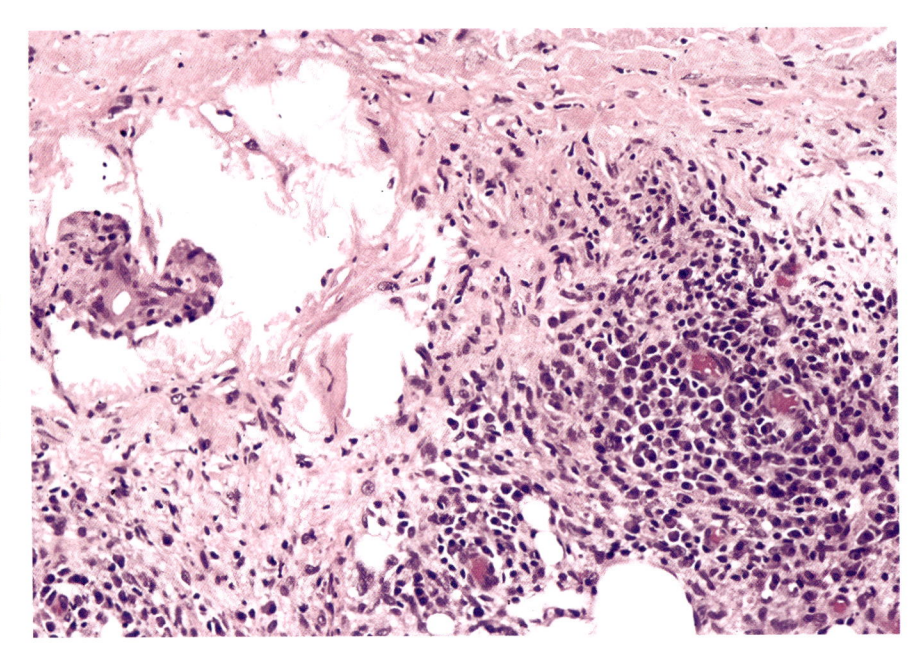

fern-like endophytic projections (fig. 13-24). An alternative name, *lipomembranous panniculitis,* is sometimes applied to this distinctive histologic appearance. When stasis is the primary cause, typical alterations within the overlying dermis are apparent. These include focal hyperplasia of microvessels within the superficial dermis creating glomerulus-like formations, dermal fibrosis, and variable epidermal alterations, including psoriasiform and spongiotic changes.

**Differential Diagnosis.** The presence of nodules on the lower extremities raises the possibility of other panniculitides such as erythema nodosum; however, the marked venous insufficiency and stasis point to lipodermatosclerosis. As the lesions become more expansive, they may resemble cellulitis or chronic fat necrosis induced by an injection.

**Treatment and Prognosis.** There is no effective treatment other than vigorous antistasis measures. Local measures are used to treat dryness, ulcerations, or any cellulitis (64). Acute lipodermatosclerosis may respond to intralesional steroids or stanazol.

## HISTIOCYTIC CYTOPHAGIC PANNICULITIS, A LOBULAR PANNICULITIS

**Definition.** *Histiocytic cytophagic panniculitis* is a lobular type of panniculitis that usually occurs as a reaction to various systemic diseases (65–68). There is often a hemorrhagic diathesis that is related to hemophagocytosis. This lesion must be separated from subcutaneous T-cell lymphoma, a primary T-cell disorder (69).

**Clinical Features.** Multiple large erythema nodosum–like plaques occur on extremities, occasionally on the trunk, and rarely on the face. The patients usually have fever, lymphadenopathy, and enlargement of the spleen and liver. There is frequently associated pancytopenia. This disease is often fatal and is associated with viral infections and some types of connective tissue disease. Similar lesions are observed in subcutaneous T-cell lymphoma but are classified separately because of the histologic and cytogenetic evidence of lymphoma.

**Pathologic Findings.** There is a lobular infiltrate of lymphocytes and histiocytes, with foci of fat necrosis. The lymphocytes are small, uniform, and benign in appearance (as opposed to the atypical lymphocytes of cytophagic panniculitis associated with lymphoma). Also, unlike lymphomas, angiocentric or angiodestructive patterns are not observed. The histiocytes characteristically show phagocytosis of lymphocytes and erythrocytes, called emperipolesis, occasionally producing a "bean-bag" appearance. Cell marker analysis generally fails to disclose abnormalities of the lymphoid component, which is dominated by T cells.

**Differential Diagnosis.** Other types of panniculitis must be considered in the differential diagnosis, since focal cytophagic activity by histiocytes may be observed in any lesion in which histiocytes and lymphocytes are associated with fat necrosis. True cytophagic histiocytic panniculitis shows this feature in a dominant, repeated pattern throughout the affected lobules.

Subcutaneous T-cell lymphoma affects principally the subcutaneous fat and thus mimics a lobular panniculitis. It may have a very aggressive course or may be indolent, and has been previously classified with the histiocytic cytophagic panniculitis group of disorders. With the elaboration of marker and cytogenetic studies, however, subcutaneous T-cell lymphoma is identified as a neoplastic process, which presents findings similar to those of histiocytic cytophagic panniculitis: prominent erythema nodosum–like nodules that are usually dusky to purple and occur on the extremities, sometimes on the trunk, and rarely on the face. These lesions may show scaling and ulceration. When there is disseminated involvement, organomegaly and adenopathy may be present. Patients with subcutaneous T-cell lymphoma characteristically present with a history of fever and malaise, and then the evolution of these nodules. They also report a history of weight loss associated with the systemic symptoms. The diagnosis of true lymphoma is made based on cytology as well as immunophenotypic and genotypic analyses.

**Treatment and Prognosis.** Treatment is of the underlying disorder. Without therapy, the disease can lead to death. Corticosteroids are used, as are chemotherapeutic agents and intravenous gammaglobulin. Infections that have been implicated involve viral, bacterial, and fungal organisms. Bone marrow transplantation is also associated with this syndrome as is connective tissue disease, especially lupus erythematosus and Sjögren syndrome (70–72).

## EOSINOPHILIC PANNICULITIS

**Definition.** *Eosinophilic panniculitis* is a predominantly lobular panniculitis exhibiting inflammation of the subcutaneous fat with eosinophils, which occurs secondary to other disorders of systemic or local nature (73,74). Primary causes of eosinophilic panniculitis include Wells syndrome, polyarteritis nodosa,

Table 13-1

DIFFERENTIAL DIAGNOSTIC CONSIDERATIONS IN EOSINOPHILIC PANNICULITIS

| Diagnostic Finding | Suspected Primary Lesion |
|---|---|
| Necrotizing arteritis | Polyarteritis nodosa |
| Deep necrotizing venulitis | Systemic vasculitis |
| Dermal eosinophils; "flame figures" | Wells syndrome |
| Birefringent material | Contaminants at injection site |
| Dermal interstitial eosinophils and histiocytes resembling granuloma annulare | Deep insect bite reaction |
| Lymphoid atypia | Associated T- or B-cell lymphoma |
| Complex organisms | Parasitosis |

systemic vasculitis, insect bite reactions, drug injection sites containing foreign proteins, and parasitic infestation (e.g., *Toxocara canis* and *Gnathostoma*) (75,76). There is also an association with both T- and B-cell lymphoma, including mycosis fungoides. Atopic patients and those with hypereosinophilic syndrome may also exhibit eosinophilic panniculitis.

**Clinical Features.** The subcutaneous nodules affect predominantly the extremities but also the trunk. There may be evidence of superficial edema. Rarely, there is vesiculation, bullae, or pustulosis overlying the nodules. The nodules are usually asymptomatic.

**Pathologic Findings.** The lobular panniculitis is dominated by eosinophils, but also contains other forms of admixed inflammatory elements. In cases associated with vasculitis, subcutaneous vessel injury may be apparent, or revealed only after obtaining deeper biopsy levels. A clue to the underlying cause may be apparent upon inspection of the overlying dermis, which is significantly involved in some cases (as opposed to primary panniculitis, which generally shows little or no dermal involvement).

**Differential Diagnosis.** The challenge of eosinophilic panniculitis is the determination of its cause. In cases where there is dermal involvement, the features of a primary dermatosis may be apparent. Table 13-1 provides clues to the diagnosis of eosinophilic panniculitis and the differential diagnostic considerations.

## MISCELLANEOUS PANNICULITIDES

### Hypogammaglobulinemia

A nodular panniculitis has been described in association with *hypogammaglobulinemia* of different etiologies. Characteristically, the lesions occur on the lower extremities and are nodular and nontender, and may ulcerate. They appear on the calves and sometimes on the shins. The location is more toward the lower portion of the lower extremities but lesions occur anywhere on the lower and upper extremities, and sometimes on the trunk.

A *postherpetic granulomatous dermatitis* or a granulomatous dermatitis associated with other types of viral, mycobacterial, or even spirochetal infection, may give rise to cutaneous nodules of this sort. The differential diagnosis includes nodular vasculitis/erythema induratum.

These lesions sometimes respond to injection of corticosteroids. Any treatment that is directed toward the cause of the hypogammaglobulinemia or restoration of globulins by infusion usually results in some clearing of the lesion.

### Migratory Panniculitis

*Migratory panniculitis*, also called *subacute nodular migratory panniculitis*, is a variant of erythema nodosum but is discussed separately because it is associated with fewer lesions and often has a specific therapeutic response (also see erythema nodosum, clinicopathologic variants) (77–79).

One or a few lesions occur, usually unilaterally. The lesions appear to migrate, that is to extend gradually peripherally. They are usually less tender than lesions of erythema nodosum and have a boggy sensation to palpation. Often, they appear arciform with an erythematous border and a brownish or violaceous center.

Erythema induratum, nodular vasculitis, and erythema nodosum must be differentiated. The subcutaneous form of necrobiosis lipoidica associated with granulomatous panniculitis is also in the differential diagnosis.

Migratory panniculitis responds to potassium iodide therapy, which is a diagnostic test of this particular type of panniculitis.

### Panniculitis of Rothman-Makai

*Panniculitis of Rothman-Makai* is a spontaneously resolving variant of relapsing febrile nodular nonsuppurative panniculitis (Weber-Christian disease). It has similar clinical features although some authors emphasize the presence of truncal involvement with this disorder. There are usually no systemic signs or symptoms or any visceral manifestations.

Atypical erythema nodosum is probably the most significant differential diagnostic consideration. The work-up and treatment are the same as for Weber-Christian disease.

### Alpha-1-Antitrypsin Deficiency

*Alpha-1-antitrypsin deficiency* is a recurrent chronic disorder in which the patients have a documented decrease in serum alpha-1-antitrypsin (80–85). The lesions are recurrent erythematous subcutaneous nodules that are tender and eventually ulcerate. The lesions are multiple, 1 to 5 cm in size, and occur predominantly on the trunk and proximal extremities. As the nodules break down, they emit either a serous or oily fluid. Healing is associated with the formation of depressed areas at the involved sites.

Histologically, there is lobular panniculitis mediated primarily by neutrophils, although lymphocytes and histiocytes may accumulate at the perimeter of lobular lesions. Within the subcutis, the panniculitis is focal, but interstitial extension of the neutrophilic infiltrate into the overlying dermis is often seen. Necrosis of adipocytes in the regions of lobular neutrophilic infiltration is frequent, a phenomenon possibly potentiated by the absence of enzymatic inhibition of neutrophil proteinases.

The differential diagnosis includes the idiopathic type of relapsing nodular nonsuppurative panniculitis and pancreatic panniculitis. Patients with alpha-1-antitrypsin deficiency often respond to dapsone (86). The direct administration intravenously of human alpha-1-proteinase inhibitor concentrate is also effective treatment.

### Panniculitis Secondary to Covert Fungal or Mycobacterial Infection

Some types of cutaneous deep fungal infections present with a panniculitis that is granulomatous with abscess formation. The presence of abscesses with granulomas should always suggest a panniculitis due to a deep fungal infection or other infectious etiology, such as mycobacterial infection. These panniculitides should always be

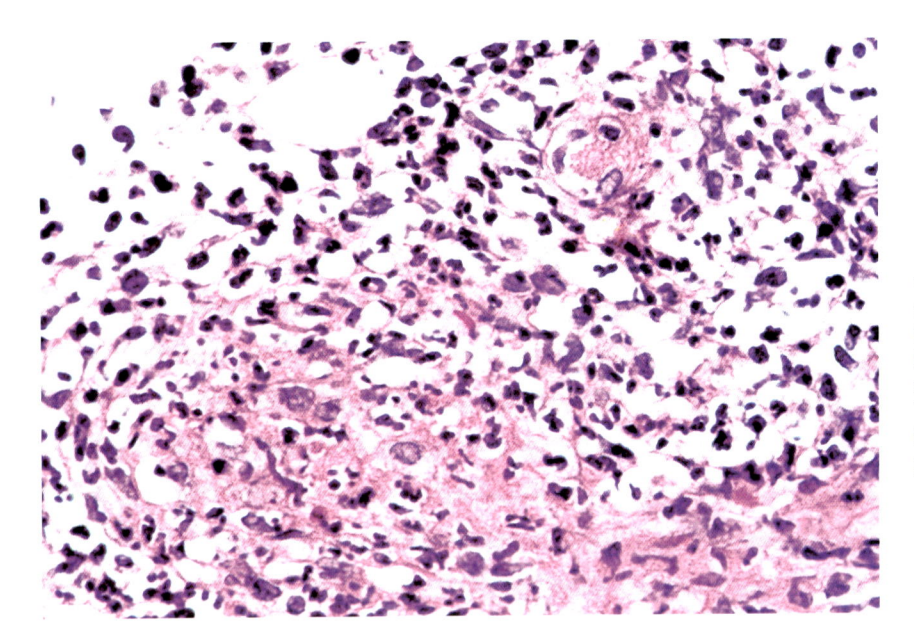

**Figure 13-25**

**INFECTIOUS PANNICULITIS**

Mixed inflammation involving the fat lobule in the absence of alterations characteristic of one of the primary forms of panniculitis prompted stains for fungi and mycobacteria. This approach is recommended in any immunocompromised patient with panniculitis.

evaluated with special stains and cultures. *Infectious panniculitis* should be especially suspected in immunosuppressed individuals, who have a particular diathesis to this complication.

There may be granulomas, microabscesses, and an admixture of septal and lobular inflammation (figs. 13-25, 13-26). We have seen cases that have precisely mimicked erythema nodosum and erythema induratum in the setting of immunocompromise. With profound immunosuppression, the inflammation may be minimal, even with numerous organisms. Conditions that should be excluded in suspected cases of infectious panniculitis include histoplasmosis, sporotrichosis, nocardiosis, atypical mycobacterial infection, and candidiasis. Accordingly, special stains include those for acid-fast organisms (fig. 13-27) and for fungi (PAS and silver).

Granulomatous panniculitis may also develop as a secondary phenomenon in association with a systemic granulomatous disorder, such as sarcoidosis (fig. 13-28), and this diagnostic possibility should be kept in mind in the appropriate clinical settings. Factitial panniculitis (figs. 13-29–13-31) can mimic any form of panniculitis described in this chapter. It is a presumptive diagnosis of exclusion, and cannot be made definitively based on the histopathology alone unless injected materials are identified and defined (87).

*Inflammatory Disorders of the Skin*

**Figure 13-26**

**INFECTIOUS PANNICULITIS**

A: At scanning magnification, there is a densely inflammatory lobular panniculitis, with some secondary involvement of the overlying dermal layer.

B: At higher magnification, the fat lobule is largely replaced by neutrophils with microabscess formation and zonal necrosis (lower right).

C: These microabscesses were positive for bacteria upon Gram staining.

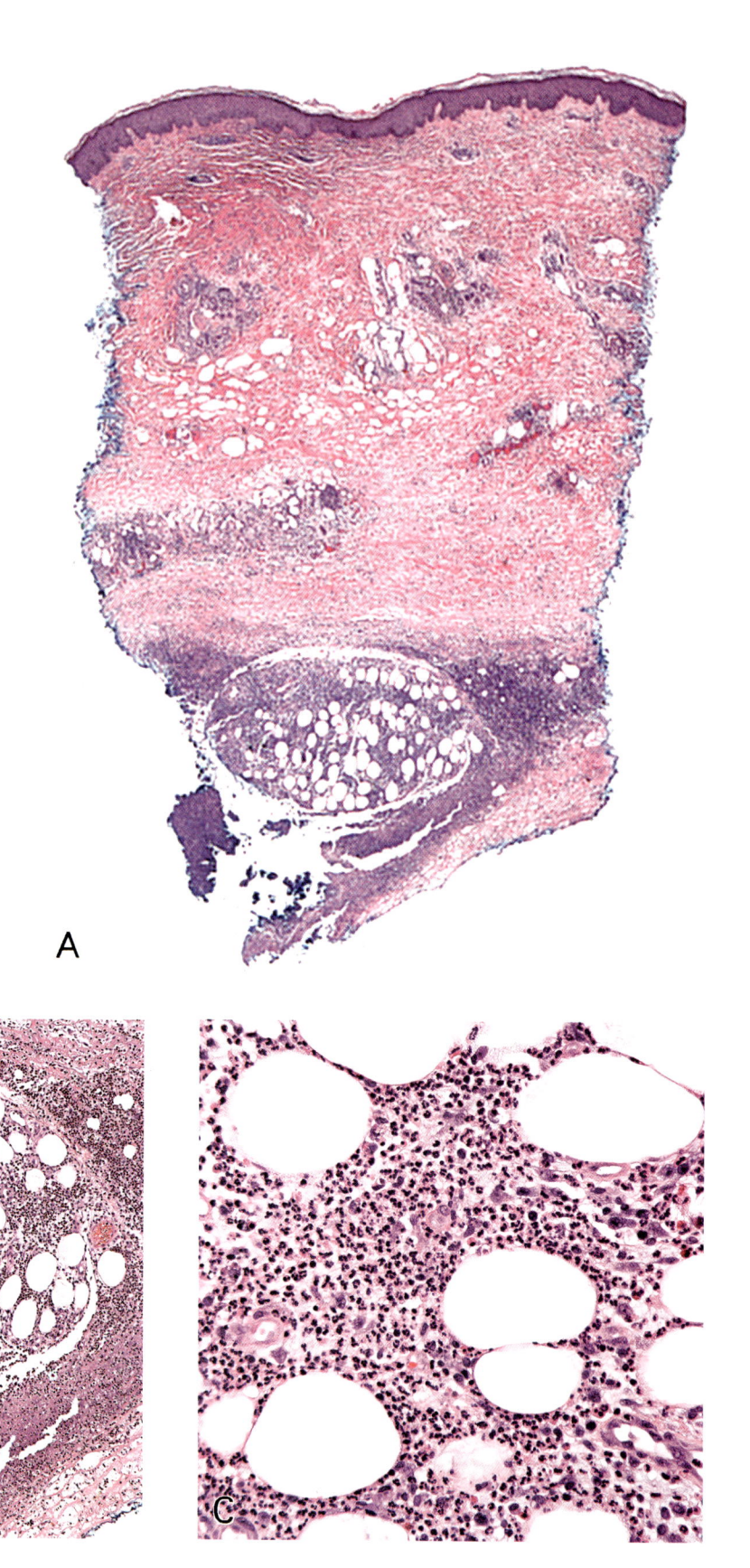

*Panniculitis*

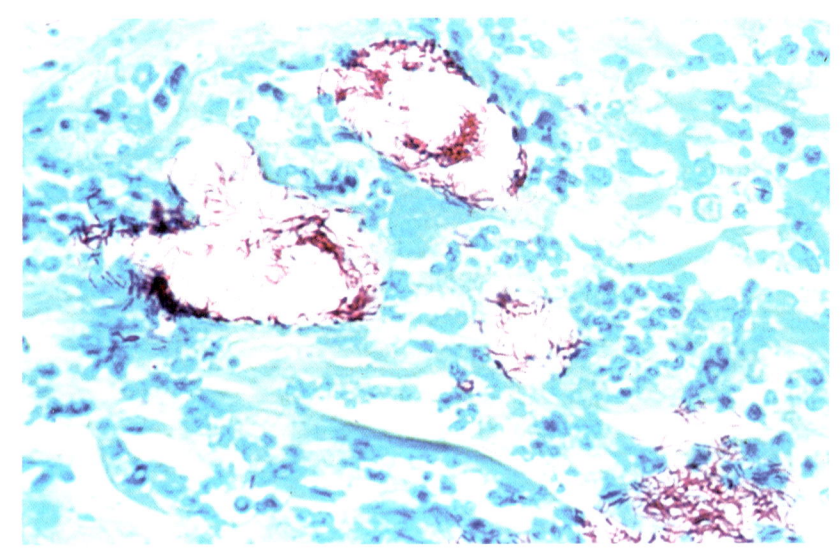

Figure 13-27

INFECTIOUS PANNICULITIS: ACID-FAST STAIN

Numerous atypical mycobacteria are revealed in the subcutaneous lobules (section is adjacent to that depicted in fig. 13-25).

Figure 13-28

SUBCUTANEOUS SARCOIDOSIS

Multiple coalescent, primarily non-necrotizing epithelioid granulomas have replaced the fat lobules. The diagnosis, as with other variants of this condition, is one of exclusion (after other forms of primary and secondary panniculitis have been excluded).

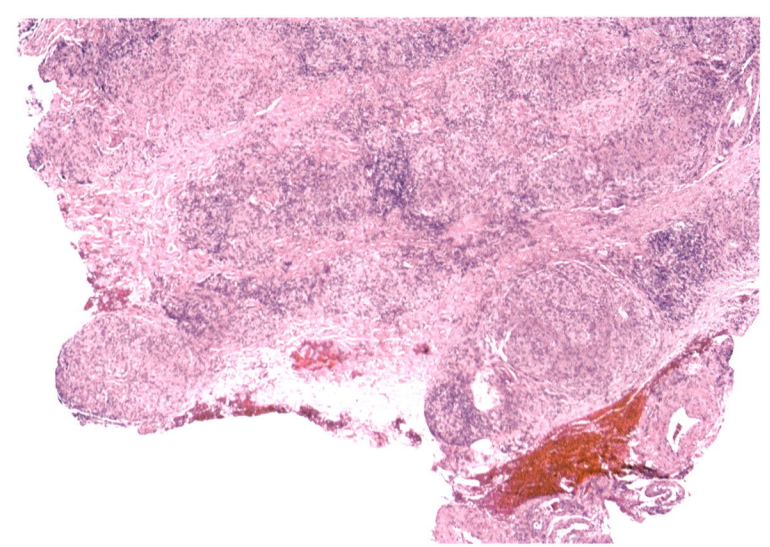

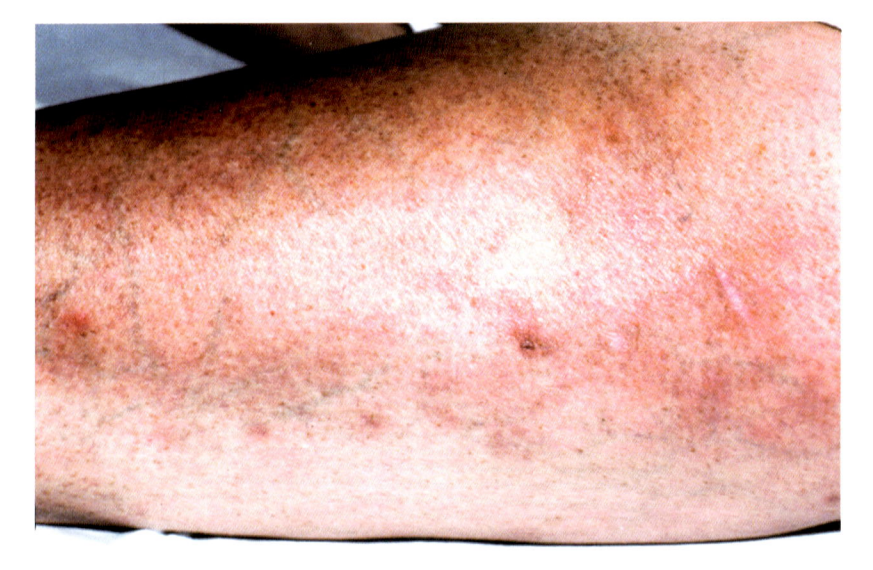

Figure 13-29

FACTITIAL PANNICULITIS

Indurated, erythematous skin with residual small papules. Pinpoint scabs represent injection sites.

## Inflammatory Disorders of the Skin

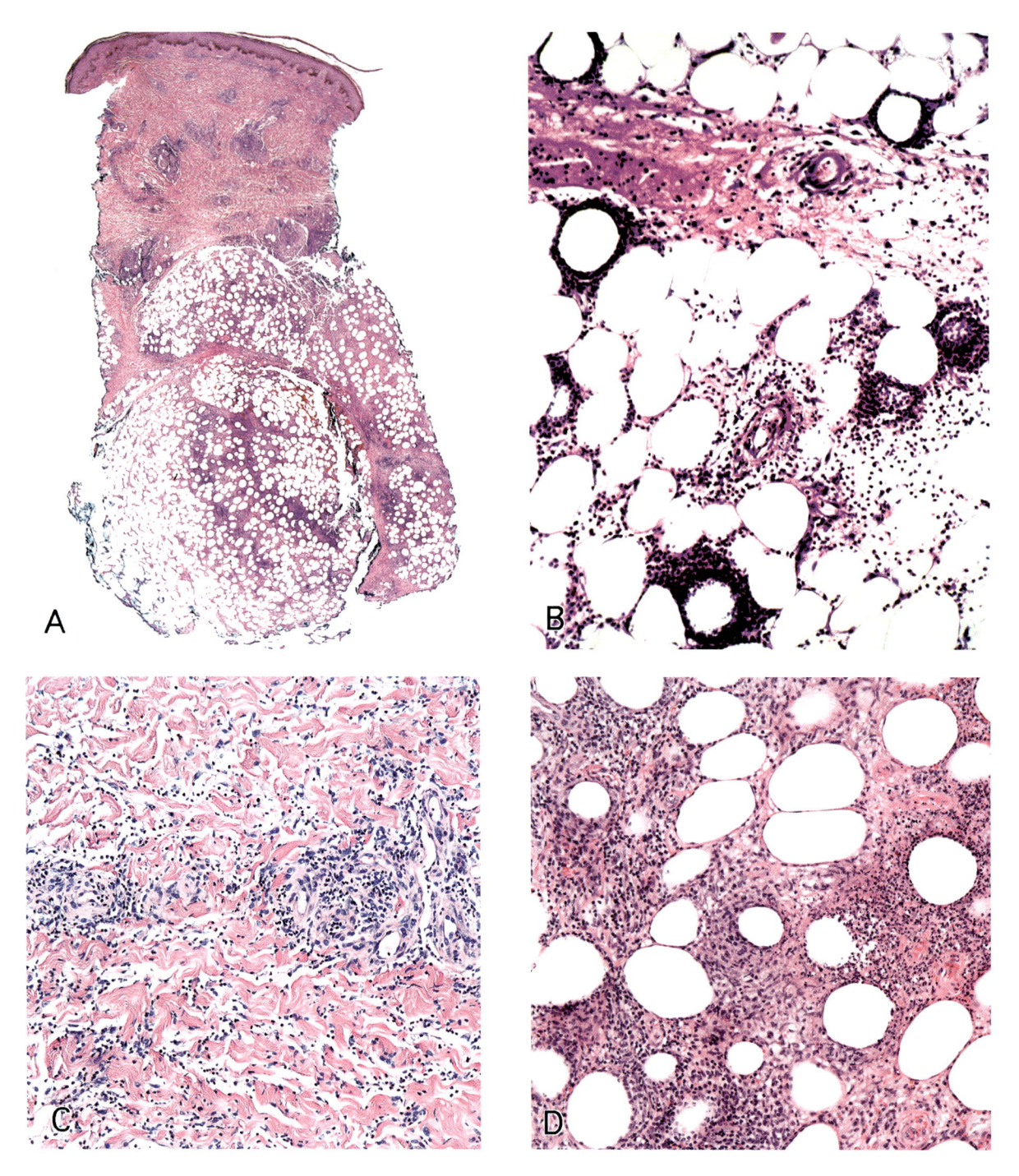

**Figure 13-30**

**FACTITIAL PANNICULITIS**

A: There is a mixed lobular and septal inflammatory component that also involves the overlying dermis.

B: The inflammatory cells are tightly and unevenly clustered about individual adipocytes, suggesting a reaction to variable concentrations of the injected toxin.

C: At higher magnification, a mixed inflammatory component is present both around the vessels and in interstitial loci in the overlying dermis.

D: Within the lobule of adipose tissue, there is a spectrum of acute and chronic granulomatous inflammation with zones of necrosis and microabscess formation.

## REFERENCES

1. Requena L, Requena C. Erythema nodosum. Dermatol Online J 2002;8:4.
2. Gonzalez-Gay MA, Garcia-Porrua C, Pujol RM, Salvarani C. Erythema nodosum: a clinical approach. Clin Exp Rheumatol 2001;19:365-8.
3. Mert A, Ozaras R, Tabak F, Pekmezci S, Demirkesen C, Ozturk R. Erythema nodosum: an experience of 10 years. Scand J Infect Dis 2004;36:424-7.
4. Anan T, Imamura T, Yokoyama S, Fujiwara S. Erythema nodosum and granulomatous lesions preceding acute myelomonocytic leukemia. J Dermatol 2004;31:741-7.
5. Bonci A, Di Lernia V, Merli F, Lo Scocco G. Erythema nodosum and Hodgkin's disease. Clin Exp Dermatol 2001;26:408-11.
6. Brodell RT, Mehrabi D. Underlying causes of erythema nodosum. Lesions may provide clue to systemic disease. Postgrad Med 2000;108:147-9.
7. Sullivan R, Clowers-Webb H, Davis MD. Erythema nodosum: a presenting sign of acute myelogenous leukemia. Cutis 2005;76:114-6.
8. Bartyik K, Varkonyi A, Kirschner A, Endreffy E, Turi S, Karg E. Erythema nodosum in association with celiac disease. Pediatr Dermatol 2004;21:227-30.
9. Friedman ES, LaNatra N, Stiller MJ. NSAIDs in dermatologic therapy: review and preview. J Cutan Med Surg 2002;6:449-59.
10. Requena L, Sanchez Yus E. Panniculitis. Part II. Mostly lobular panniculitis. J Am Acad Dermatol 2001;45:325-61
11. Khachemoune A, Longo MI, Phillips TJ. Nodular vasculitis as a paraneoplastic presentation? Int J Dermatol 2003;42:639-42.
12. Chen YH, Yan JJ, Chao SC, Lee JY. Erythema induratum: a clinicopathologic and polymerase chain reaction study. J Formos Med Assoc 2001;100:244-9.
13. Vieites B, Suarez-Penaranda JM, Perez Del Molino ML, et al. Recovery of Mycobacterium tuberculosis DNA in biopsies of erythema induratum—results in a series of patients using an improved polymerase chain reaction technique. Br J Dermatol 2005;152:1394-6.
14. Bayer-Garner IB, Cox MD, Scott MA, Smoller BR. Mycobacteria other than Mycobacterium tuberculosis are not present in erythema induratum/nodular vasculitis: a case series and literature review of the clinical and histologic findings. J Cutan Pathol 2005;32:220-6.
15. Heinemann C, Kaatz M, Elsner P. Erythema induratum of Bazin and Poncet's disease—successful treatment with antitubercular drugs. J Eur Acad Dermatol Venereol 2003;17:334-6.
16. Lee YS, Lee SW, Lee JR, Lee SC. Erythema induratum with pulmonary tuberculosis: histopathologic features resembling true vasculitis. Int J Dermatol 2001;40:193-6.
17. Massone C, Kodama K, Salmhofer W, et al. Lupus erythematosus panniculitis (lupus profundus): clinical, histopathological, and molecular analysis of nine cases. J Cutan Pathol 2005;32:396-404.
18. Wimmershoff MB, Hohenleutner U, Landthaler M. Discoid lupus erythematosus and lupus profundus in childhood: a report of two cases. Pediatr Dermatol 2003;20:140-5.
19. Pichardo RO, Lu D, Sangueza OP, Selim MA. What is your diagnosis? Lupus profundus. Am J Dermatopathol 2002;24:507-8.
20. Strober BE. Lupus panniculitis (lupus profundus). Dermatol Online J 2001;7:20.
21. Grossberg E, Scherschun L, Fivenson DP. Lupus profundus: not a benign disease. Lupus 2001;10:514-6.
22. Magro CM, Crowson AN, Kovatich AJ, Burns F. Lupus profundus, indeterminate lymphocytic lobular panniculitis and subcutaneous T-cell lymphoma: a spectrum of subcuticular T-cell lymphoid dyscrasia. J Cutan Pathol 2001;28:235-47.
23. Kundig TM, Trueb RM, Krasovec M. Lupus profundus/panniculitis. Dermatology 1997;195:99-101.
24. Cassis TB, Fearneyhough PK, Callen JP. Subcutaneous panniculitis-like T-cell lymphoma with vacuolar interface dermatitis resembling lupus erythematosus panniculitis. J Am Acad Dermatol 2004;50:465-9.
25. Ng PP, Tan SH, Tan T. Lupus erythematosus panniculitis: a clinicopathologic study. Int J Dermatol 2002;41:488-90.
26. Winkelmann RK, Padilha-Goncalves A. Connective tissue panniculitis. Arch Dermatol 1980;116:291-4.
27. Solans R, Cortés J, Selva A, et al. Panniculitis: a cutaneous manifestation of dermatomyositis. J Am Acad Dermatol 2002;46:S148-50.
28. Chao YY, Yang LJ. Dermatomyositis presenting as panniculitis. Int J Dermatol 2000;39:141-4.
29. Ghali FE, Reed AM, Groben PA, McCauliffe DP. Panniculitis in juvenile dermatomyositis. Pediatr Dermatol 1999;16:270-2.
30. Marzano AV, Tanzi C, Caputo R, Alessi E. Sclerodermic linear lupus panniculitis: report of two cases. Dermatology 2005;210:329-32.

31. Schaffer JV, McNiff JM, Seropian S, Cooper DL, Bologna JL. Lichen sclerosus and eosinophilic fasciitis as manifestations of chronic graft-versus-host disease: expanding the sclerodermoid spectrum. J Am Acad Dermatol 2005;53:591-601.
32. Hur JW, Lee HS, Uhm WS, et al. Eosinophilic fasciitis associated with autoimmune thyroiditis. Korean J Intern Med 2005;20:180-2.
33. Agnew KL, Blunt D, Francis ND, Bunker CB. Magnetic resonance imaging in eosinophilic fasciitis. Clin Exp Dermatol 2005;30:435-6.
34. Carneiro S, Brotas A, Lamy F, Lisboa F, Lago E, Azulay D, Cuzzi T, Ramos-e-Silva M. Eosinophilic fasciitis (Shulman syndrome). Cutis 2005;75:228-32.
35. Bukiej A, Dropinski J, Dyduch G, Szczeklik A. Eosinophilic fasciitis successfully treated with cyclosporine. Clin Rheumatol 2005;24:634-6.
36. Agarwal V, Wakhlu A, Aggarwal A, Pal L, Misra R. Eosinophilic fasciitis. J Assoc Physicians India 2004;52:244-5.
37. Cardozo TJ. Eosinophilic fasciitis. Dermatol Online J 2003;9:33.
38. Yoshida T, Ito H, Matsubara Y, et al. Weber-Christian disease presenting with ocular manifestations. Clin Rheumatol 2003;22:339-42.
39. Steffen C. The men behind the eponym: Frederick Parkes Weber and Henry A. Christian: Weber-Christian disease. Am J Dermatopathol 2002;24:514-7.
40. Negalur VG, Negalur BV. Weber Christian disease. J Assoc Physicians India 2003;51:724-5.
41. Ter Poorten MA, Thiers BH. Systemic Weber-Christian disease. J Cutan Med Surg 2000;4:110-2.
42. White JW Jr, Winkelmann RK. Weber-Christian panniculitis: a review of 30 cases with this diagnosis. J Am Acad Dermatol 1998;39:56-62.
43. Khan GA, Lewis FI. Recognizing Weber-Christian disease. Tenn Med 1996;89:447-9.
44. Sorensen RU, Abramowsky C, Stern RC. Corticosteroid-sparing effect of hydroxychloroquine in a patient with early-onset Weber-Christian syndrome. J Am Acad Dermatol 1990;23(Pt 1):1172-4.
45. Hotta T, Wakamatsu Y, Matsumura N, et al. Azathioprine-induced remission in Weber-Christian disease. South Med J 1981;74:234-7.
46. Eravelly J, Waters MF. Thalidomide in Weber-Christian disease. Lancet. 1977;1:251.
47. Iwasaki T, Hamano T, Ogata A, Hashimoto N, Kakishita E. Successful treatment of a patient with febrile, lobular panniculitis (Weber-Christian disease) with oral cyclosporin A: implications for pathogenesis and therapy. Intern Med 1999;38:612-4.
48. Hinata M, Someya T, Yoshizaki H, Seki K, Takeuchi K. Successful treatment of steroid-resistant Weber-Christian disease with biliary ductopenia using cyclosporin A. Rheumatology (Oxford) 2005;44:821-3.
49. Marsh Rde W, Hagler KT, Carag HR, Flowers FP. Pancreatic panniculitis. Eur J Surg Oncol 2005;31:1213-5.
50. Freireich-Astman M, Segal R, Feinmesser M, David M. Pancreatic panniculitis as a sign of adenocarcinoma of unknown origin. Isr Med Assoc J 2005;7:474-5.
51. Shehan JM, Kalaaji AN. Pancreatic panniculitis due to pancreatic carcinoma. Mayo Clin Proc 2005;80:822.
52. Beltraminelli HS, Buechner SA, Hausermann P. Pancreatic panniculitis in a patient with an acinar cell cystadenocarcinoma of the pancreas. Dermatology 2004;208:265-7.
53. Cutlan RT, Wesche WA, Jenkins JJ 3rd, Chesney TM. A fatal case of pancreatic panniculitis presenting in a young patient with systemic lupus. J Cutan Pathol 2000;27:466-71.
54. Fretzin DF, Arias AM. Sclerema neonatorum and subcutaneous fat necrosis of the newborn. Pediatr Dermatol 1987;4:112-22.
55. Dudink J, Walther FJ, Beekman RP. Subcutaneous fat necrosis of the newborn: hypercalcemia with hepatic and atrial myocardial calcification. Arch Dis Child Fetal Neonatal Ed 2003;88:343-5.
56. Tran JT, Sheth AP. Complications of subcutaneous fat necrosis of the newborn: a case report and review of the literature. Pediatr Dermatol 2003;20:257-61.
57. Burden AD, Krafchik BR. Subcutaneous fat necrosis of the newborn: a review of 11 cases. Pediatr Dermatol 1999;16:384-7.
58. Fenniche S, Daoud L, Benmously R, et al. Subcutaneous fat necrosis: report of two cases. Dermatol Online J 2004;10:12.
59. Chuang SD, Chiu HC, Chang CC. Subcutaneous fat necrosis of the newborn complicating hypothermic cardiac surgery. Br J Dermatol 1995;132:805-10.
60. Demitsu T, Okada O, Yoneda K, Manabe M. Lipodermatosclerosis—report of three cases and review of the literature. Dermatology 1999;199:271-3.
61. Herouy Y, Nockowski P, Schopf E, Norgauer J. Lipodermatosclerosis and the significance of proteolytic remodeling in the pathogenesis of venous ulceration. (Review). Int J Mol Med 1999;3:511-5.
62. Kirsner RS, Pardes JB, Eaglstein WH, Falanga V. The clinical spectrum of lipodermatosclerosis. J Am Acad Dermatol 1993;28:623-7.

63. Bruce AJ, Bennett DD, Lohse CM, Rooke TW, Davis MD. Lipodermatosclerosis: review of cases evaluated at Mayo Clinic. J Am Acad Dermatol 2002;46:187-92.
64. Yosipovitch G, Mengesha Y, Facliaru D, David M. Topical capsaicin for the treatment of acute lipodermatosclerosis and lobular panniculitis. J Dermatol Treat 2005;16:178-80.
65. Craig AJ, Cualing H, Thomas G, Lamerson C, Smith R. Cytophagic histiocytic panniculitis--a syndrome associated with benign and malignant panniculitis: case comparison and review of the literature. J Am Acad Dermatol 1998;39(Pt 1):721-36.
66. Secmeer G, Sakalli H, Gok F, et al. Fatal cytophagic histiocytic panniculitis. Pediatr Dermatol 2004;21:246-9.
67. Wick MR, Patterson JW. Cytophagic histiocytic panniculitis—a critical reappraisal. Arch Dermatol 2000;136:922-4.
68. Marzano AV, Berti E, Paulli M, Caputo R. Cytophagic histiocytic panniculitis and subcutaneous panniculitis-like T-cell lymphoma: report of 7 cases. Arch Dermatol 2000;136:889-96.
69. Yung A, Snow J, Jarrett P. Subcutaneous panniculitic T-cell lymphoma and cytophagic histiocytic panniculitis. Australas J Dermatol 2001;42:183-7.
70. Galende J, Vazquez ML, Almeida J, et al. Histiocytic cytophagic panniculitis: a rare late complication of allogeneic bone marrow transplantation. Bone Marrow Transplant 1994;14:637-9.
71. Tsukahara T, Horiuchi Y, Iidaka K. Cytophagic histiocytic panniculitis in systemic lupus erythematosus. Hiroshima J Med Sci 1995;44:13-6.
72. Tsukahara T, Fujioka A, Horiuchi Y, et al. A case of cytophagic histiocytic panniculitis with sicca symptoms and lupus nephritis. J Dermatol 1992;19:563-9.
73. Adame J, Cohen PR. Eosinophilic panniculitis: diagnostic considerations and evaluation. J Am Acad Dermatol 1996;34(Pt 1):229-34.
74. Samlaska CP, de Lorimier AJ, Heldman LS. Eosinophilic panniculitis. Pediatr Dermatol 1995;12:35-8.
75. Perez C, Vives R, Montes M, Ostiz S. Recurrent eosinophilic panniculitis associated with Fasciola hepatica infection. J Am Acad Dermatol 2000;42(Pt 2):900-2.
76. Panizzon R. Well's syndrome (eosinophilic cellulitis): additional cases in the literature. J Am Acad Dermatol 1989;20:1136-7.
77. Lee UH, Yang JH, Chun DK, Choi JC. Erythema nodosum migrans. J Eur Acad Dermatol Venereol 2005;19:519-20.
78. de Almeida Prestes C, Winkelmann RK, Su WP. Septal granulomatous panniculitis: comparison of the pathology of erythema nodosum migrans (migratory panniculitis) and chronic erythema nodosum. J Am Acad Dermatol 1990;22:477-83.
79. Campalani E, Higgins E. Erythema nodosum migrans. Clin Exp Dermatol 2003;28:679-80.
80. Ranes J, Stoller JK. A review of alpha-1 antitrypsin deficiency. Semin Respir Crit Care Med 2005;2:154-66.
81. Ortiz PG, Skov BG, Benfeldt E. Alpha1-antitrypsin deficiency-associated panniculitis: case report and review of treatment options. J Eur Acad Dermatol Venereol 2005;19:487-90.
82. Walling H, Geraminejad P. Determine alpha-1 antitrypsin level and phenotype in patients with neutrophilic panniculitis. J Am Acad Dermatol 2005;52:373-4.
83. Geraminejad P, DeBloom JR 2nd, Walling HW, Sontheimer RD, VanBeek M. Alpha-1-antitrypsin associated panniculitis: the MS variant. J Am Acad Dermatol 2004;51:645-55.
84. Smith KC. Alpha-1-antitrypsin deficiency-associated panniculitis. Int J Dermatol 2004;43:698.
85. McBean J, Sable A, Maude J, Robinson-Bostom L. Alpha1-antitrypsin deficiency panniculitis. Cutis 2003;71:205-9.
86. Yesudian PD, Dobson CM, Wilson NJ. Alpha1-antitrypsin deficiency panniculitis (phenotype PiZZ) precipitated postpartum and successfully treated with dapsone. Br J Dermatol 2004;150:1222-3.
87. Morrison LK, Rapini R, Willison CB, Tyring S. Infection and panniculitis. Dermatol Ther 2010;23:328-40.

# 14 INFLAMMATORY DISORDERS WITH PRIMARY ADNEXAL ALTERATIONS: FOLLICULAR CONDITIONS

## GENERAL CONSIDERATIONS

Based on detailed studies of the normal and pathologic anatomy of the pilar apparatus, it has long been recognized that the hair follicle is amazingly complex. The deepest portion (proximal from the vantage point of trichogenesis), or bulb, is rooted in a mast cell- and axon-rich fibrovascular mesenchyme, embraced by basaloid epithelial cells that form the follicular papilla and hair matrix, respectively. From this emerge several layers of specialized epithelium devoted to genesis and support of the hair shaft. Progressing upward toward the epidermal layer, the insertion of the arrector pili muscle and the origin of the sebaceous duct and gland from the wall of the follicular canal are seen. A functionally critical yet structurally subtle structure, the follicular bulge, is here. It is within this aggregate of undifferentiated basaloid epithelial cells that the ability of the underlying pilar apparatus to regenerate in a cyclic manner appears to reside. This bulge region represents a stem cell–rich repository that is capable of giving rise to mature anagen follicles after dramatic involution termed catagen and telogen (fig. 14-1). In this way, mature anagen follicles periodically regress, involving a process where the entire follicle retracts toward the epidermal layer. As the base of the foreshortened follicle approximates the bulge region, the hair shaft is no longer supported by the nutrient-rich anagen bulb, and the hair shaft falls out of the resting telogen follicle. The persistent bulge gives rise to a new anagen follicle and hair shaft.

The follicular bulge and what lies above it are, therefore, regarded as permanent portions of a normal follicle, whereas the subjacent canal and shaft are expressed in relation to the hair cycle. The infundibulum forms much of what is regarded as the permanent portion of the follicular canal. Incapable of hair shaft formation, the infundibulum is a reservoir for melanocytes and dendritic immune cells which reside in a microenvironmental niche protected from noxious environmental agents that predominate more superficially. It is not surprising that early repigmentation in treated vitiligo often begins about follicular ostia, and that Langerhans cells that resist depletion by chronic exposure to sunlight tend to cluster in the recesses of infundibular epithelium. If a time comes when naked apes are totally alopecic, we suspect that

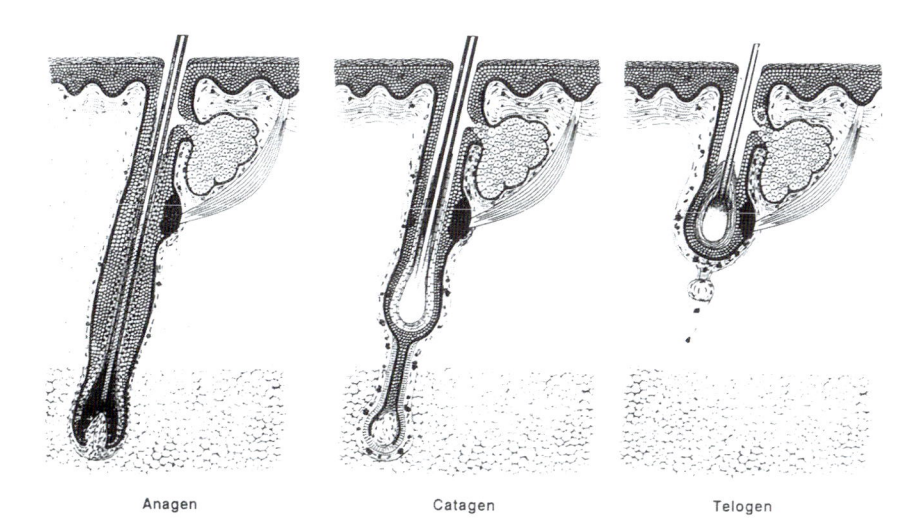

Figure 14-1

MAJOR COMPONENTS OF HAIR AND THE THREE PHASES OF THE HAIR CYCLE (ANAGEN, CATAGEN, AND TELOGEN)

the infundibuli would persist long after the loss of trichogenic capacity of human follicles.

## PATHOGENESIS

The precise pathogenesis of most follicular inflammatory disorders remains unknown. This is perhaps best emphasized by our as yet incomplete understanding of the pathogenesis of acne vulgaris (1) and alopecia areata. Some disorders formerly believed to be wholly noninflammatory are now recognized to have a subtle yet reproducible early inflammatory phase potentially integral to pathogenesis. The target site of inflammation may correlate with the tendency for alopecia to be either reversible or irreversible. For example, when inflammation is centered primarily about the deepest portion of the follicle, the bulb, as in alopecia areata, the potential for reversibility exists. In contrast, when inflammation targets the lowermost portion of the infundibulum where the stem cell–rich bulge resides, as is the case in lupus erythematosus and lichen planopilaris, hair loss tends to be irreversible. These observations further emphasize the key importance of the follicular bulge region in supplying the stem cells necessary for normal follicular cycling.

## SPECIAL DIAGNOSTIC STUDIES

Specific tests for the evaluation of inflammatory follicular pathology are limited to histochemical evaluation to exclude organisms (bacteria or fungi), cell marker analysis to exclude clonal T-cell proliferation as a cause of follicular mucinosis, and hair plucks to evaluation shaft morphology (as with "exclamation point" hairs in alopecia areata). Vertical and horizontal sections are both helpful to the dermatopathologist in rendering a diagnosis. In our opinion, the use of each method is mostly determined by the preference and training of the pathologist.

## ANIMAL MODELS

The cellular and molecular basis for follicular cycling, requisite knowledge for understanding how inflammation may result in temporary or permanent alopecia, has been recently advanced by the development of a number of relevant transgenic and knock-out murine models. Animal models for acne include rodents with a genetic tendency to form follicular cysts and comedones (rhino mice) (1a). Human follicles have recently been maintained in xenografts to immunodeficient mice, an approach of potential future significance for better understanding the effects of inflammation on follicular homeostasis and cycling (1b). Mice receiving bone marrow transplants develop a form of cytotoxic folliculitis that appears to target the bulge region of the follicle (1c,1d), thus providing a model of potential importance for understanding the mechanisms of irreversible inflammatory alopecia.

## ACNE VULGARIS

**Definition.** *Acne vulgaris* is a common disorder that affects especially the face, less often the trunk, and occasionally the buttocks with inflammation of the follicular apparatus (1–5). The clinical features are characteristic. The inflammatory lesions may result in deforming scars.

**Clinical Features.** Acne vulgaris occurs most commonly in puberty, beginning around 10 years of age in females and 14 years in males, but also occurs in adult life, sometimes even in those in the thirties and forties. The lesions are usually more extensive and disfiguring in males than in females and affect Caucasians more commonly than African Americans or Asians. The disease has a hereditary predisposition, especially when cystic, and most affected persons give a history of parents and siblings with severe acne.

There are a variety of factors that are associated with acne. These include principally endocrine factors; drugs of certain types; exposure to environmental substances, such as oils, dioxin, or others associated with certain occupations; and an association with the XYY syndrome.

Pressure and occlusion exacerbate acne and may cause acne in localized areas, for example, in those who have a tendency of "cupping" their chin with their hands or leaning with their chin on their hands. Excessive telephone use on one ear can lead to acne in that area.

Individual lesions usually last for weeks to months, and the condition may last for years. Characteristically, exacerbations occur in the fall and winter, and improve during the summer months. Three types of lesions occur in acne vulgaris. The lesions that are most characteristic are comedones, which are either open (so-called blackheads) or closed (so-called whiteheads).

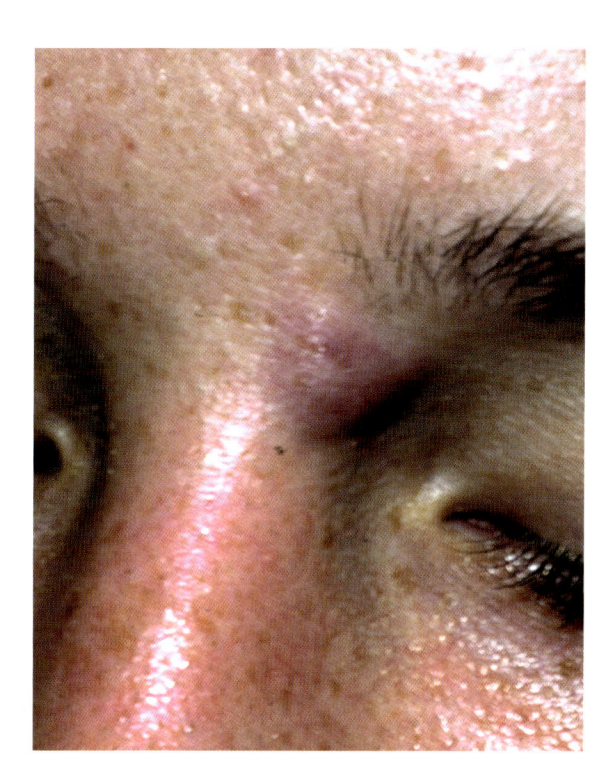

### Figure 14-2

**ACNE VULGARIS**

There are multiple, variably erythematous small papules involving oily skin that shows increased surface lipid secretion.

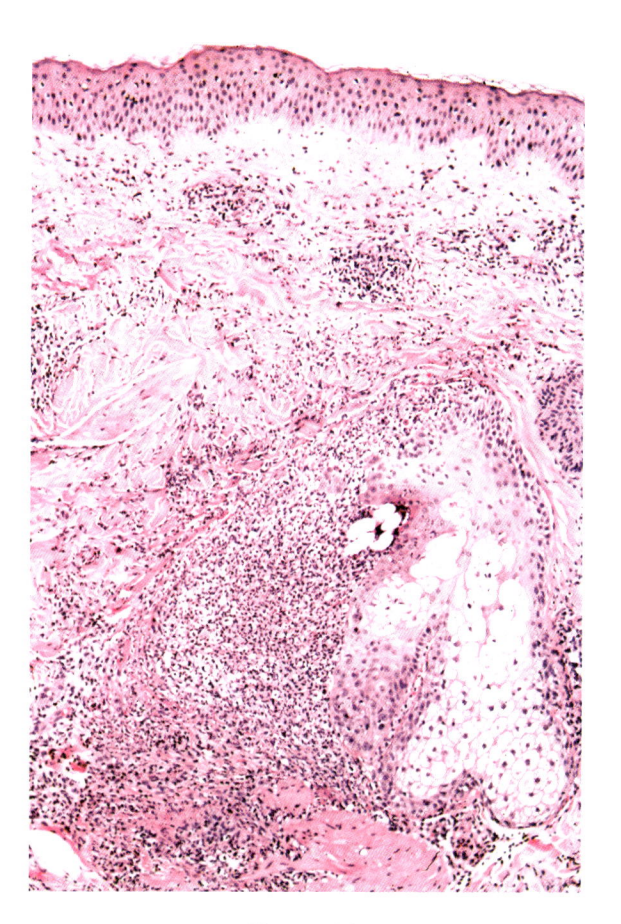

### Figure 14-3

**SUPPURATIVE ACNE: ADVANCED STAGE**

As a consequence of follicular rupture, there is a well-formed dermal abscess.

Papules are the second lesion and occur with or without pustules (fig. 14-2). Nodules, or cysts, are the third type of lesion. These lesions can be very large, even up to several centimeters in size, and may be associated with pain.

Severe acne may be associated with draining sinuses in the involved areas, and leads to scars, which are either depressed or keloidal. One type of acne, in young men especially, is *acne fulminans,* so designated because it is associated with severe cystic acne occurring rapidly and leading to extensive pustulation, and even ulceration of some of the lesions. These patients are ill and have lassitude, malaise, arthralgias, and sometimes fever. *Follicular occlusion syndrome* is a type of severe nodular cystic acne associated with hidradenitis suppurativa, severe nodulocystic acne (acne conglobata), dissecting cellulitis of the scalp (perifolliculitis capitis abscedens et suffodiens), and sometimes pilonidal sinus formation.

**Pathologic Findings.** Common to all forms of acne is the formation of the infundibular cyst, or comedone. This involves dilation of the infundibular canal, which is impacted with keratin and lipid secretions. It is in this environment that bacteria flourish. Melanin pigment tends to accumulate within the more superficial portion of the follicular keratotic plug, producing the characteristic appearance of a blackhead. In time, the periinfundibular adventitia becomes inflamed by lymphocytes and histiocytes, and after rupture and extrusion of follicular contents, with frank microabscesses and granulomas (fig. 14-3). Extension of the follicular keratotic accumulation and associated inflammation into the deeper portion of the follicle results in the appearance of cystic acne (fig. 14-4); rupture into the reticular dermis with abscess formation may result in sinus tracts.

*Inflammatory Disorders of the Skin*

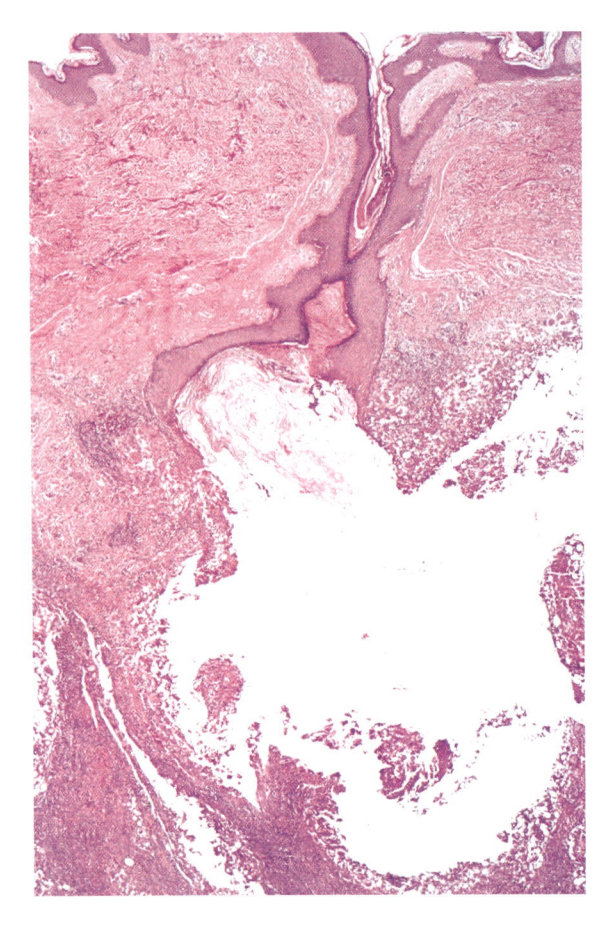

**Figure 14-4**

CYSTIC ACNE/HIDRADENITIS SUPPURATIVA

There is a deep-seated zone of follicular rupture with abscess formation. The granulation tissue response contributes to the sinus tract formation.

**Differential Diagnosis.** The differential diagnosis of acne is quite broad, and includes rosacea, perioral dermatitis, and infectious folliculitis for facial acne. *Pityrosporum* folliculitis and "hot tub" folliculitis due to *Pseudomonas* infection occur on the trunk and resemble acne. Steroid folliculitis, which occurs with either the application of topical steroids or with oral corticosteroids, features papulopustules. A single, painful cyst in acne includes an inclusion cyst, or at times, a dental sinus cyst in the differential diagnosis. One type of truncal acne that is infectious and always considered in the differential diagnosis is cryptococcosis folliculitis. This lesion, however, does not usually exhibit pustules and is associated with immunosuppression.

Many acneiform variants of folliculitis are identified by careful clinicopathologic correlation. These include folliculitis decalvans, a scarring form of scalp acne that leads to alopecia (figs. 14-5, 14-6); acne keloidalis nuchae, a scarring form of folliculitis that involves the posterior scalp of patients of African descent (fig. 14-7); and pseudofolliculitis barbae, follicular papules that develop in the beard region of men after shaving hair shafts too close to the epidermal surface (figs. 14-8, 14-9).

**Treatment and Prognosis.** The treatment of acne is directed at allowing pilar drainage and treating any underlying infection that results in the pustulation and subsequent destructive cystic changes (6–16). Acne treatment varies with the degree of involvement. For more mild cases,

**Figure 14-5**

FOLLICULITIS DECALVANS

Perifollicular pustules and crusting surround intact hair follicles and are present in a background of erythema and localized decreased hair density.

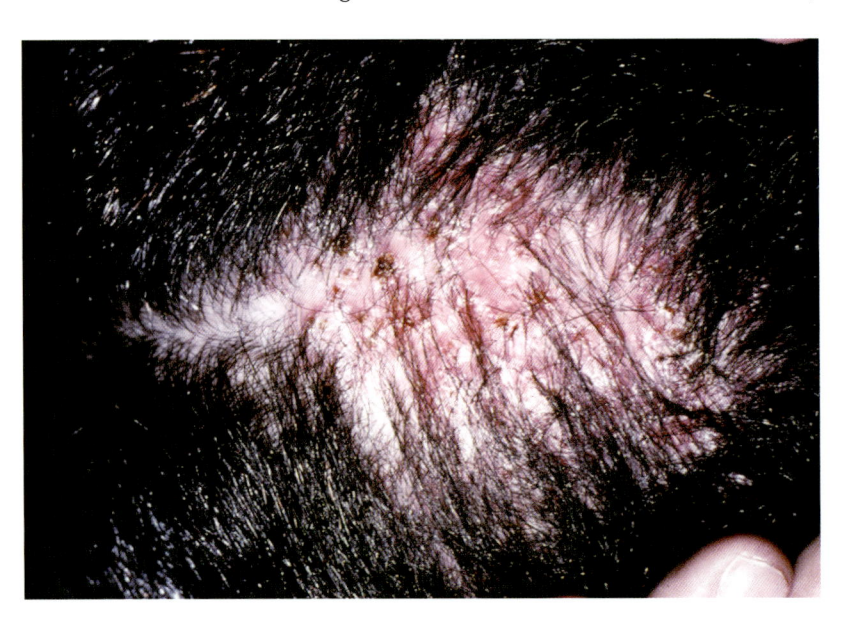

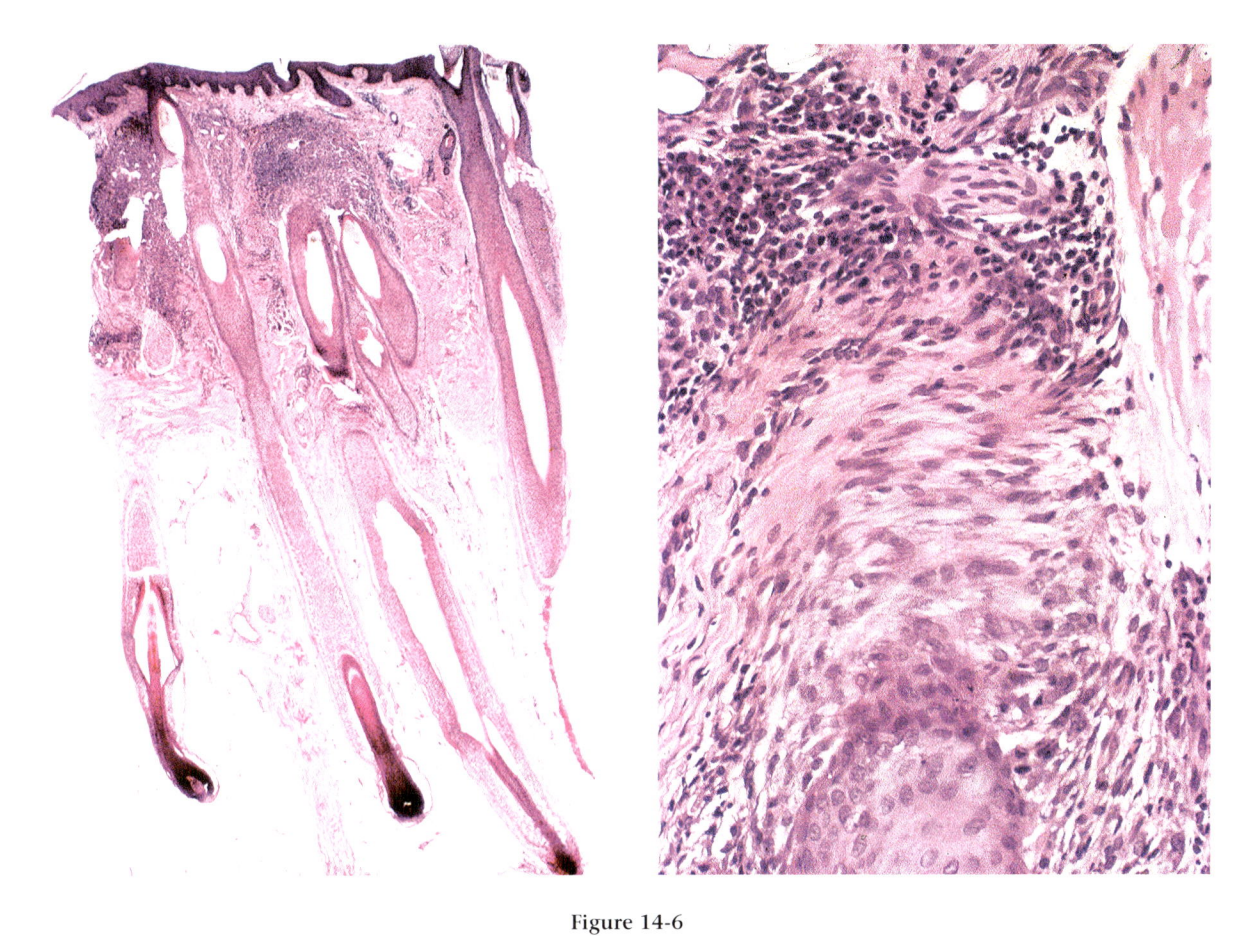

*Inflammatory Disorders with Primary Adnexal Alterations: Follicular Conditions*

Figure 14-6

**FOLLICULITIS DECALVANS**

Left: There is dense inflammation about the superficial portions of multiple hair follicles.
Right: At high magnification, this advanced lesion shows perifollicular fibrosis and an associated lymphoplasmacytic infiltrate.

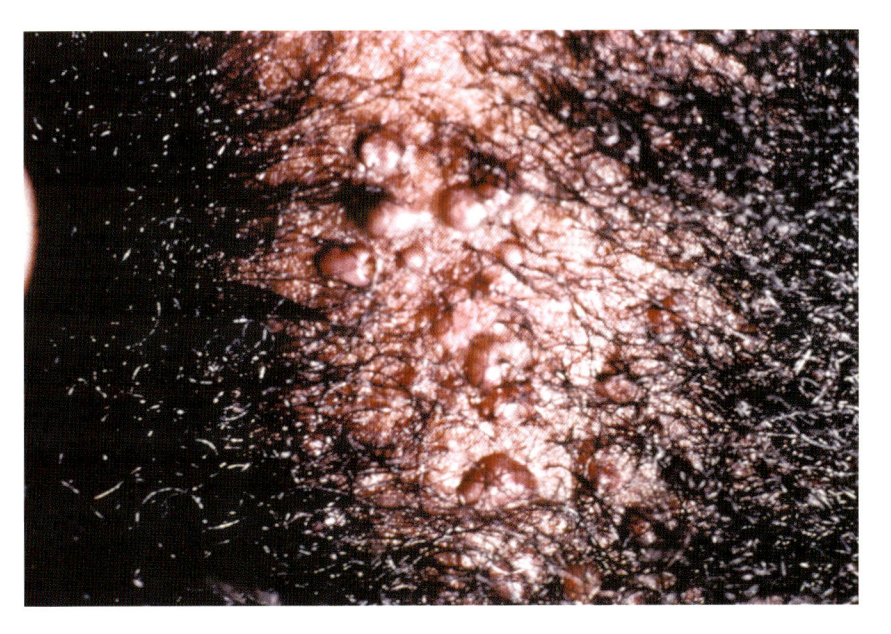

Figure 14-7

**ACNE KELOIDALIS**

There are multiple, firm, flesh-colored perifollicular papules concentrated in regions of hair-bearing skin on the posterior neck.

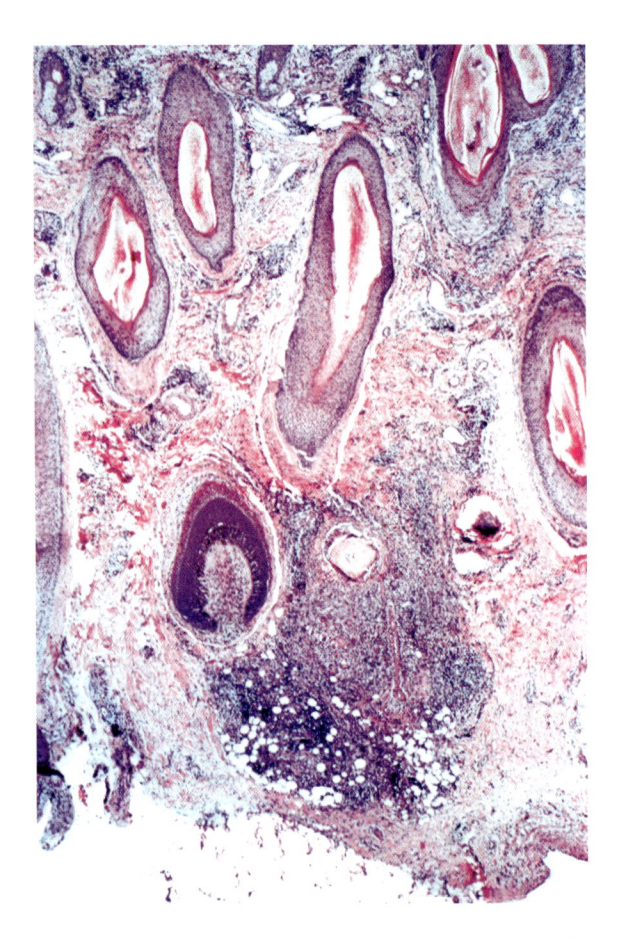

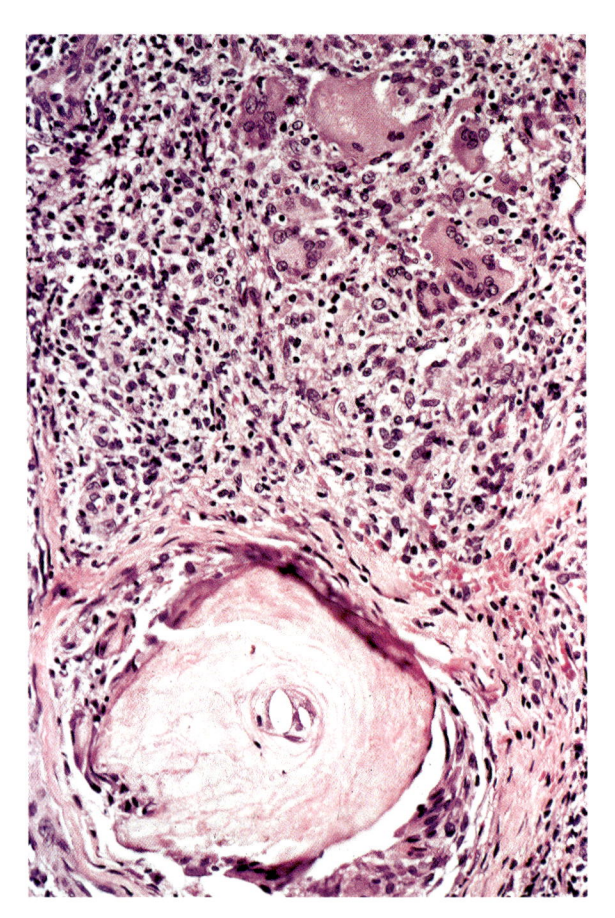

### Figure 14-8
**PSEUDOFOLLICULITIS BARBAE**
Left: This biopsy specimen from the beard area of facial skin shows a focus of dense inflammation in the deep dermis.
Right: At high magnification, a granulomatous infiltrate surrounds the remnants of the follicular contents that have been extruded into the dermis.

topical benzoyl peroxide, retinoids, and antibiotics usually result in improvement. A combination of antibiotic and gel benzoyl peroxide with one of the topical retinoids gives the best result. Azelaic acid is helpful, particularly in patients who hyperpigment. For more advanced lesions, oral antibiotics, such as the tetracyclines and the macrolides, seem to be necessary for control. Isotretinoin both impedes the sebaceous gland function and the keratinization of the pilar orifice and is often quite effective, especially in nodular acne and recalcitrant acne. This drug is teratogenic, and cannot be used in patients who may become pregnant. There are a variety of other complications to isotretinoin therapy including hepatotoxicity and alterations in lipid metabolism. Both tetracycline and isotretinoin are associated with pseudotumor cerebri. Hormonal therapy with spironolactone or its analogues as well as with oral contraceptives is helpful in females with disease of the lower face or with disease associated with endocrinopathies. Laser therapy and photodynamic therapy are new additions to available treatment modalities.

## INFECTIOUS FOLLICULITIS

**Definition.** *Infectious folliculitis* encompasses a number of inflammatory disorders of the hair follicle caused by viruses, bacteria, or fungi (17–21). It occurs in facial areas and in hair-bearing areas, and can, depending upon location, be confused with any other follicular pustular eruption.

**Clinical Features.** *Herpes folliculitis* occurs in the distribution of herpes simplex, usually as

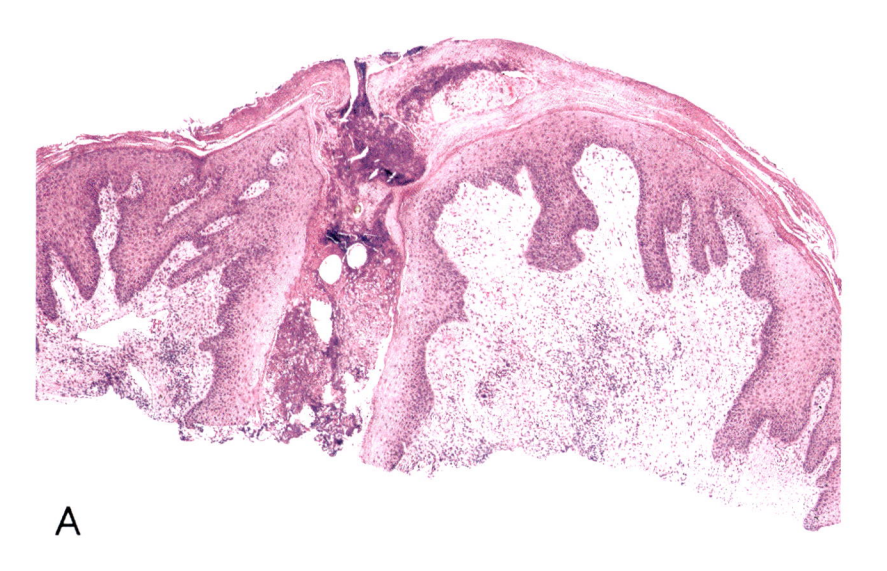

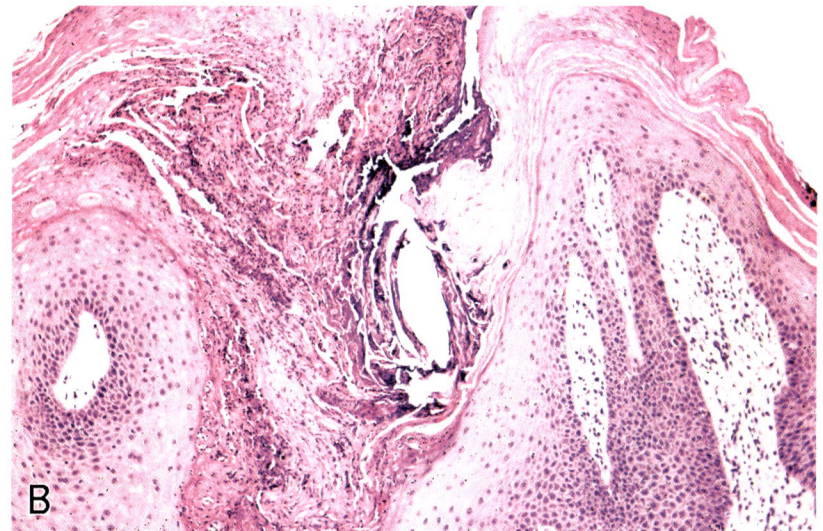

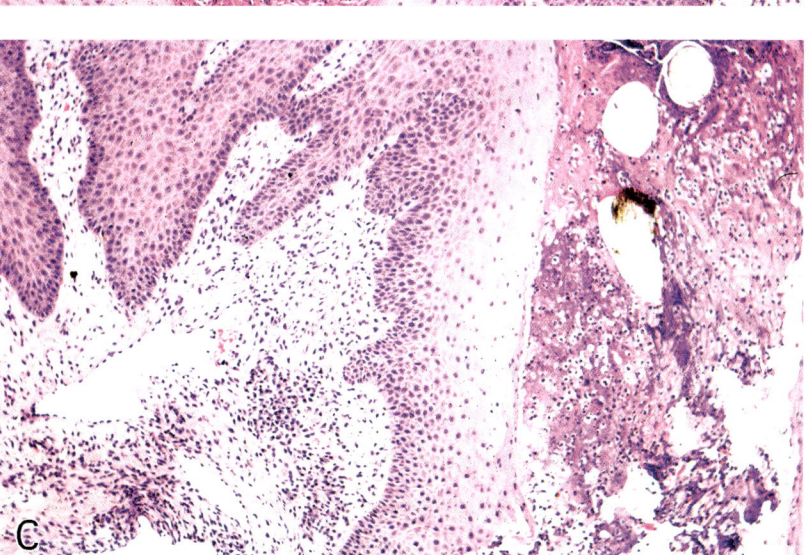

*Inflammatory Disorders with Primary Adnexal Alterations: Follicular Conditions*

Figure 14-9

PSEUDOFOLLICULITIS BARBAE

A: Marked follicular distortion is associated with a pustular inflammatory infiltrate within the follicular canal of a twisted and contorted hair shaft.

B: At higher magnification, the inflammatory infiltrate is seen at the follicular surface and correlates with the formation of a pustule.

C: In a zone of deeper follicular involvement, the follicular wall is markedly hyperplastic and abuts a zone of intrafollicular abscess formation provoked by the twisted hair follicle.

*Inflammatory Disorders of the Skin*

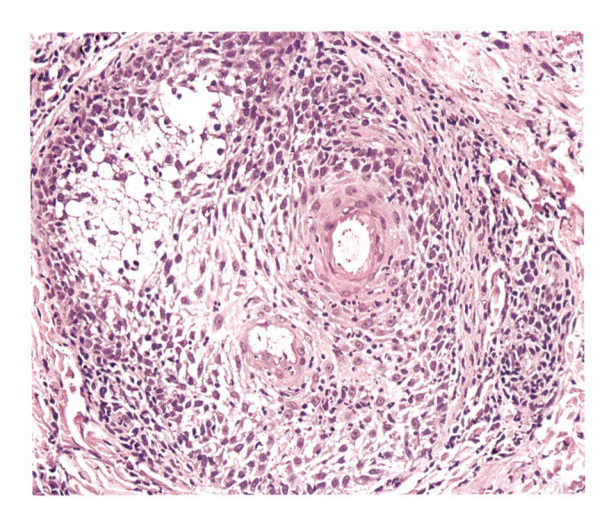

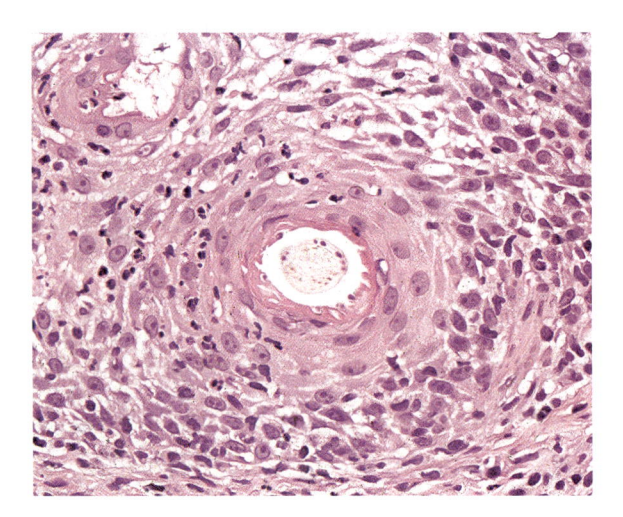

Figure 14-10

DERMATOPHYTIC FOLLICULITIS

Left: There is marked spongiosis and lymphoid infiltration involving the follicular epithelium.
Right: At higher magnification, fungal organisms are apparent within the inner root sheath and at the perimeter of the centrally located hair shaft.

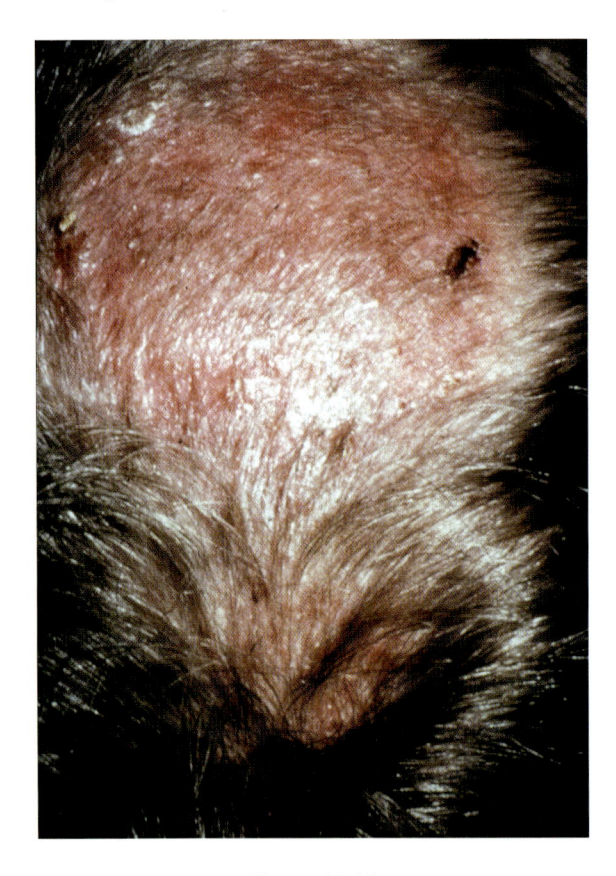

Figure 14-11

TINEA CAPITIS

There is significant fragmentation of hair shafts because of fungal infection. Erythema and scaling are present.

very itchy papules. Fungal and bacterial folliculitis generally present with pustules. Expression of the pustular contents and smearing of the material on an appropriately stained microscope slide allows for identification of the offending agent. Bacterial folliculitides may be associated with secondary lues, and are diagnosed in the appropriate clinical setting with dark field microscopy, by staining for spirochetes, or by serologic studies.

Other organisms that cause folliculitis include dermatophytes, *Pityrosporum ovale*, and other fungi (figs. 14-10–14-15). Some mites, such as *Demodex*, also may cause a folliculitis-like picture.

**Pathologic Findings.** Common to all forms of infectious folliculitis is inflammation. Purely neutrophilic folliculitis generally indicates a bacterial cause, particularly when intrafollicular and perifollicular abscesses involve the infundibulum. When plasma cells and histiocytes are prominently admixed, in association with deeper follicular involvement and destructive alterations, the rare occurrence of *luetic alopecia* should be suspected (fig. 14-15). An admixture of lymphocytes, histiocytes, and neutrophils ("dirty infiltrate") should prompt careful inspection for herpetic cytopathic alterations (acantholysis, multinucleation, intranuclear inclusions) within the follicular or sebaceous epithelium

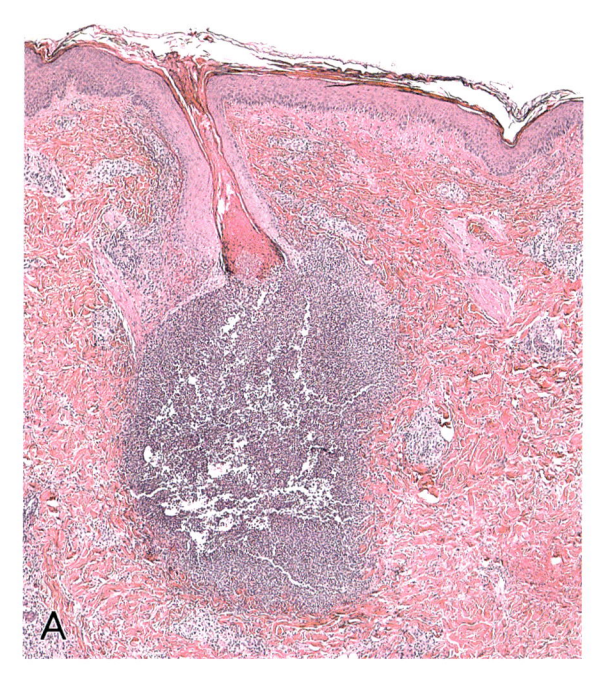

*Inflammatory Disorders with Primary Adnexal Alterations: Follicular Conditions*

Figure 14-12

**FUNGAL FOLLICULITIS**

A: There is inflammatory destruction of the lower two-thirds of this hair follicle.

B: Numerous yeast forms are associated with follicular rupture and incipient microabscess formation.

C: Fungal elements are highlighted within the newly ruptured hair follicle (periodic acid–Schiff [PAS] stain).

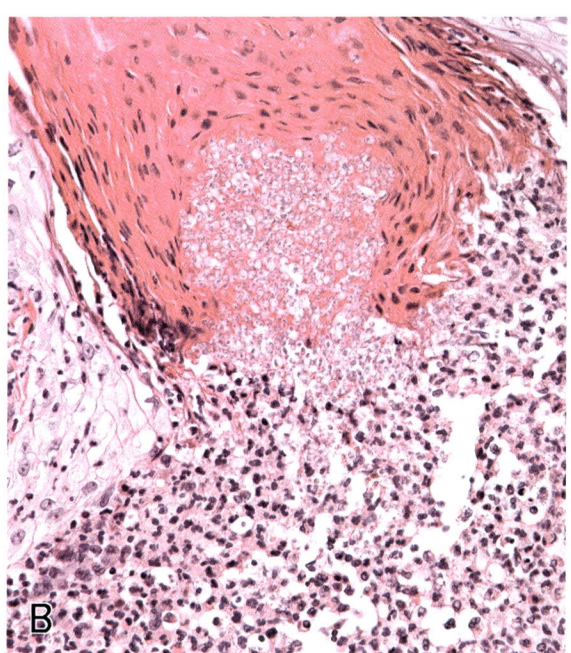

(fig. 14-16). Occasionally, follicular destruction is so profound that the site previously occupied by the pilosebaceous apparatus is replaced by inflammatory cells and cellular debris, with only focal clues of herpetic cytopathology, potentially requiring multiple levels for identification. *Pityrosporon folliculitis* shows nonspecific inflammatory alterations and foci of follicular rupture centered primarily about the infundibulum. Organisms may be detected by the periodic acid–Schiff (PAS) stain either within the affected follicle or free within the perifollicular mixed inflammatory response. Folliculitis induced by opportunistic fungi (e.g., *Cryptococcus*) results in deep-seated granulomas and follicular destruction. This rare form of infectious folliculitis must be kept in mind, especially in immunocompromised patients.

*Inflammatory Disorders of the Skin*

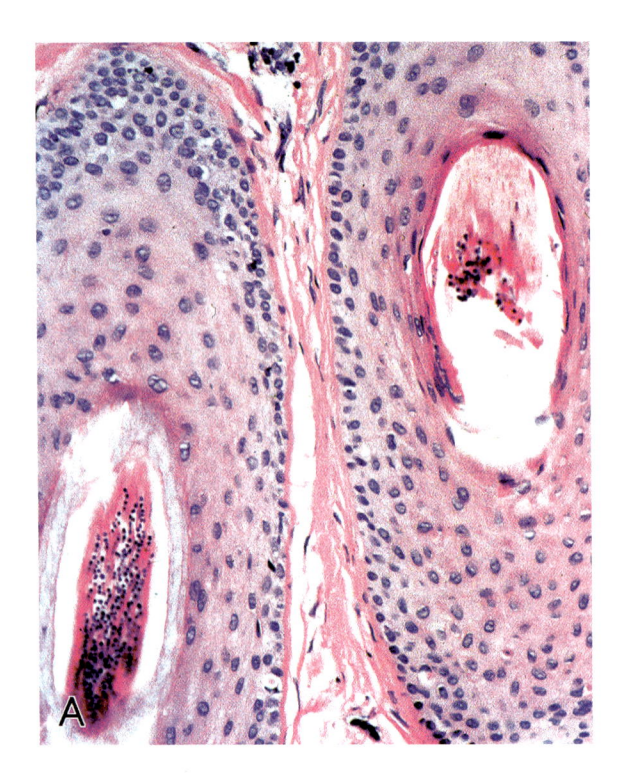

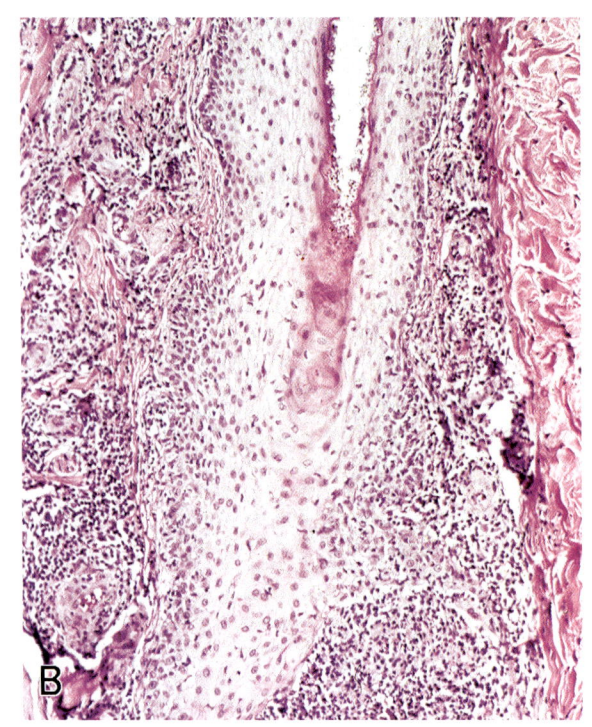

**Figure 14-13**

**TINEA CAPITIS**

A: Numerous basophilic yeast forms are present within the hair shafts, with only sparse associated inflammation of the surrounding dermis.

B: In the inflammatory variant, the intrafollicular and perifollicular abscess is composed of aggregated neutrophils.

C: Higher magnification shows numerous yeast forms lining the follicular canal.

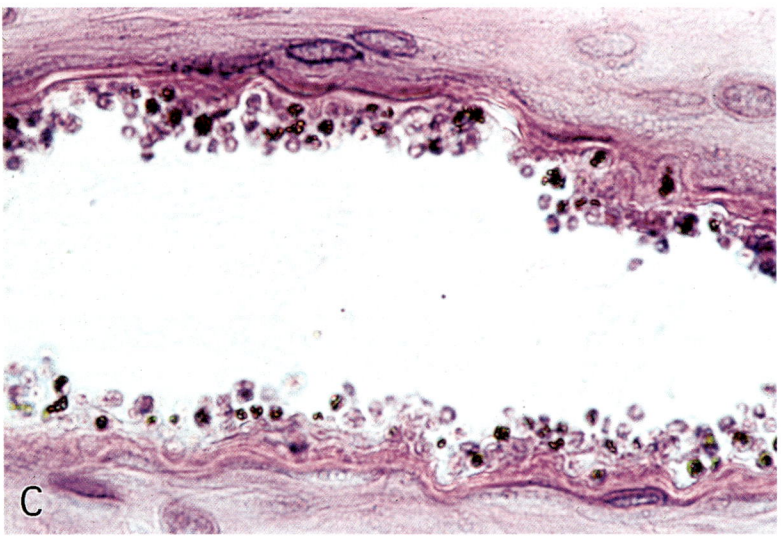

**Differential Diagnosis.** Any type of follicular process with pustules that is not easily explained on the basis of the clinical features must be considered. In such instances, folliculitis should be appropriately examined by special stains to observe bacteria, fungi, or appropriate organisms. Some of the differential diagnostic considerations for pustular folliculitis are provided in Table 14-1.

**Treatment and Prognosis.** The prognosis is generally favorable in immunocompetent individuals, with treatment focused on appropriate antibiotic administration (22). In immunocompromised patients, accurate diagnosis and therapy may be lifesaving, emphasizing the importance of a thorough differential consideration of infectious agents when folliculitis is documented in a skin biopsy.

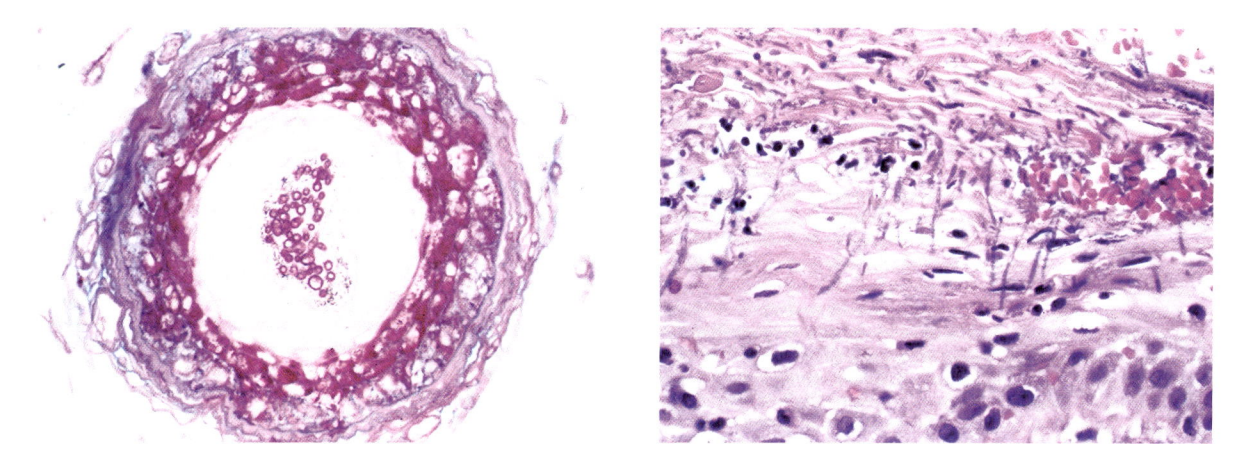

Figure 14-14
**FUNGAL FOLLICULITIS**
Left: In this endothrix type, PAS stain highlights the clustered organisms present within the central portion of the hair shaft.
Right: In this ectothrix type, even in routinely stained sections, large numbers of branching hyphae are apparent as they traverse the follicular epithelium and enter the adjacent dermal stroma.

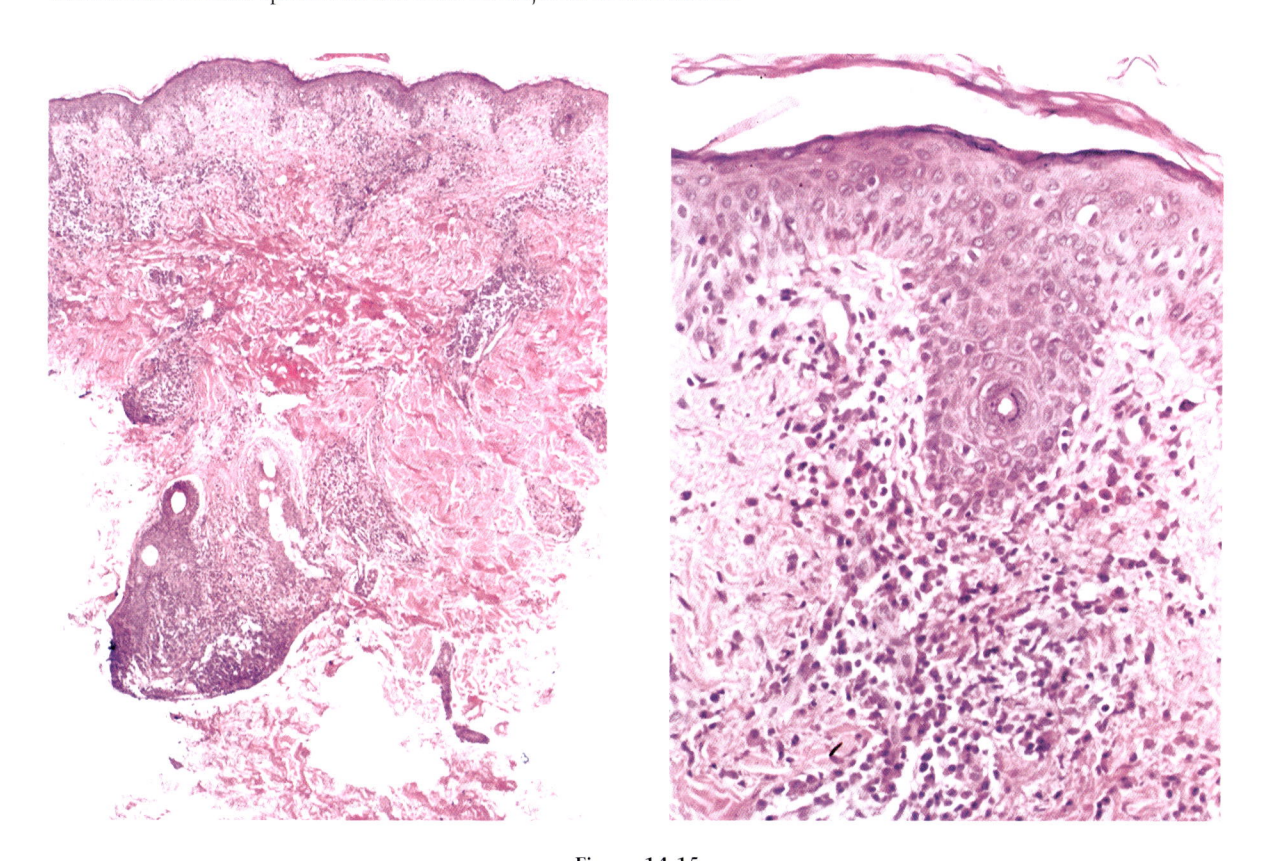

Figure 14-15
**FOLLICULAR INVOLVEMENT IN SECONDARY SYPHILIS**
Left: The mixed inflammatory pattern shows a perivascular, perifollicular, and lichenoid distribution with evidence of deep dermal perifollicular involvement.
Right: At higher magnification, the inflammatory infiltrate forming the lichenoid component is composed of lymphocytes, plasma cells, and histiocytes, with associated vacuolar degeneration of the basal cell layer.

*Inflammatory Disorders of the Skin*

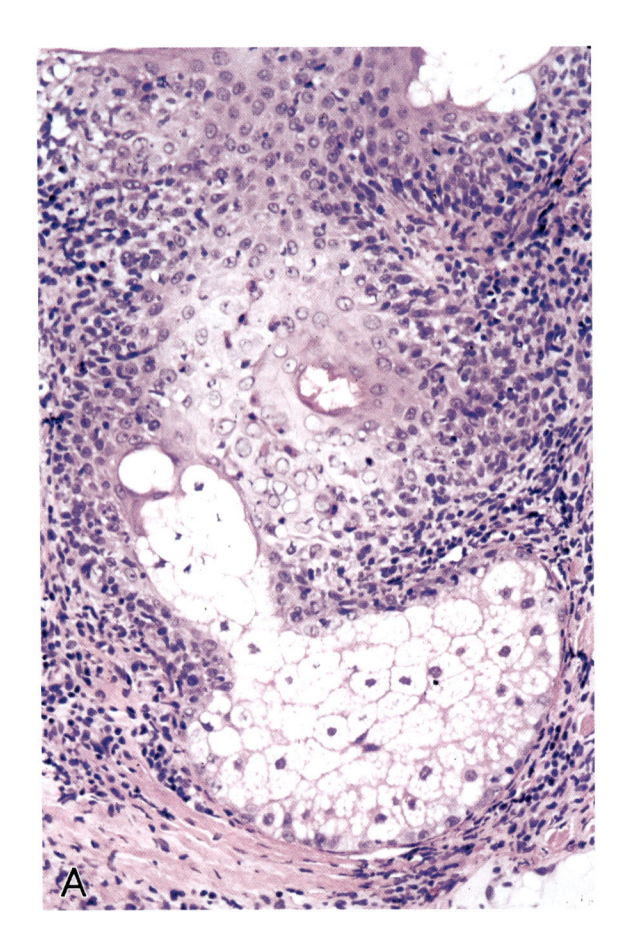

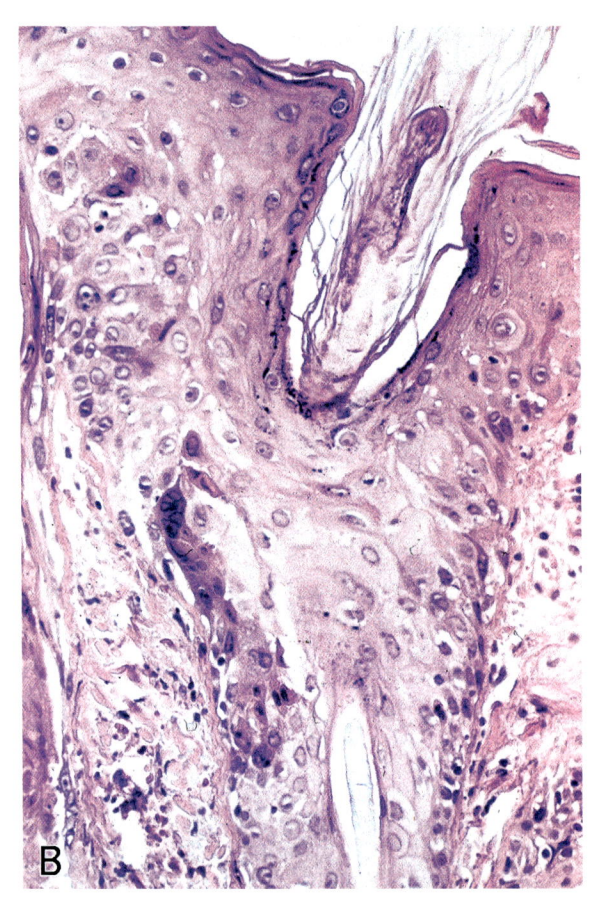

### Figure 14-16
**HERPETIC FOLLICULITIS**

A: In this early lesion, the intact yet inflamed follicular epithelium bordering the sebaceous duct shows the characteristic cytoplasmic alterations of herpesvirus.

B: High magnification of the involved follicular infundibulum shows keratinocytes that have acquired a wind-blown, disarrayed appearance. The formation of multinucleation and associated hypereosinophilia are indicative of early necrosis of the affected cells.

C: In an old lesion, the virally infected follicular epithelial cells show nuclear pyknosis, hypereosinophilic cytoplasm, and residual evidence of multinucleation.

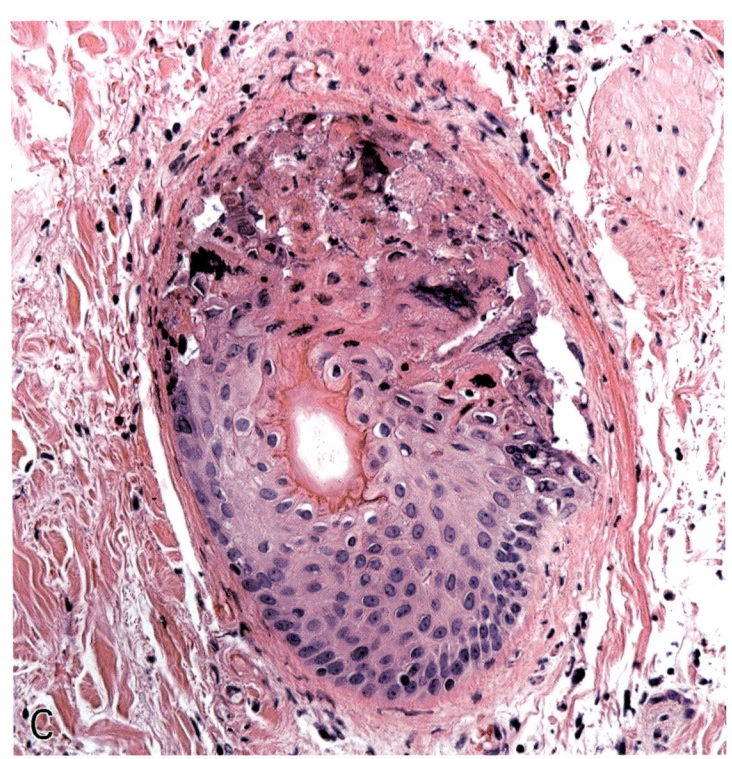

## Table 14-1
### DISTINGUISHING FEATURES OF COMMON FORMS OF PUSTULAR FOLLICULITIS

| Disorder | Clinical Appearance | Histology |
| --- | --- | --- |
| Acute folliculitis | Tender, red pustules or tender nodules | Infundibular microabscess or dermal abscess with perforation |
| Eosinophilic pustular folliculitis | Often annular arrangements of follicular papules and pustules; AIDS[a] or AIDS-related complex (ARC) | Spongiosis about the sebaceous duct; mixed infiltrate with eosinophils; *Demodex* mite may be entrapped |
| Perforating folliculitis | Painful erythematous nodules; some may drain | Thinning and disruption of follicular epithelium; dermal abscess with foreign body response |
| *Pityrosporum* folliculitis | Erythematous small papules and pustules often on trunk; may also have lacrimal obstruction | Acute folliculitis with microperforations containing 2- to 4-μm budding yeast forms |
| *Pseudomonas* folliculitis | Pruritic pustules after exposure to water (e.g., hot tubs) | Pilar canal distended by neutrophils; gram-negative rods on Gram stain |

[a]AIDS = acquired immunodeficiency syndrome.

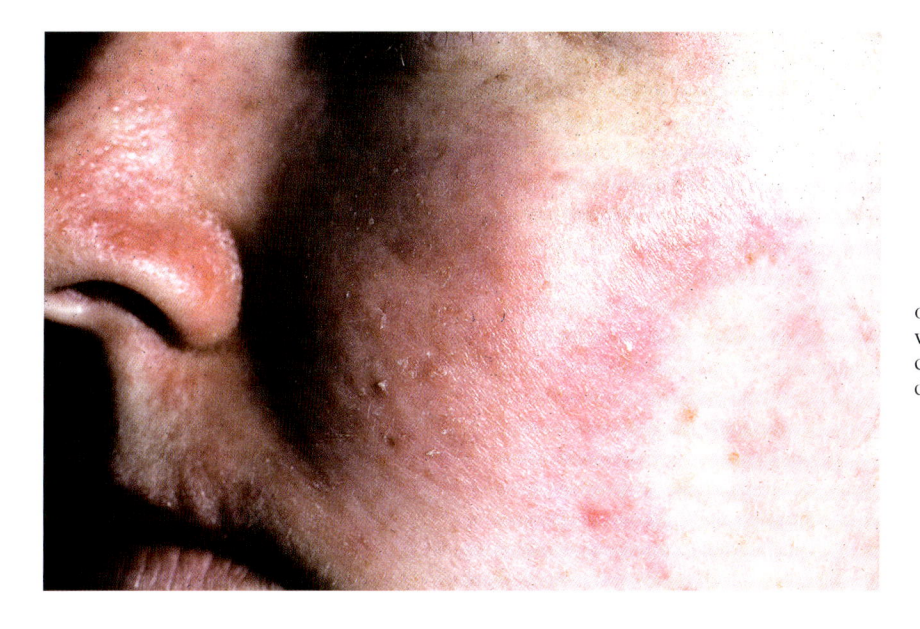

**Figure 14-17**

**ACNE ROSACEA**

There are numerous papules on an erythematous base involving the cheek skin. With chronicity, telangiectasia may develop.

## ACNE ROSACEA

**Definition.** *Acne rosacea* is a chronic disorder of the hair follicles that is associated with increased sensitivity to heat and an increased "blush" reaction (23–28). The lesions may be striking and very problematic to the patient.

**Clinical Features.** This disorder occurs mainly in patients in the fourth to the sixth decade and affects women more commonly than men. One form of rosacea, called *rhinophyma*, typified by enlargement of nasal skin due to sebaceous hyperplasia, is much more common in men (29). Persons with light skin are affected more commonly than those with darker skin. There usually is a history of increased blush reaction, especially upon changes in temperature, such as entering a warm environment, upon ingesting spicy foods, or upon ingesting alcohol. Exposure to sunshine or to the heat emitted from a stove, for example, exacerbates this eruption.

The earliest phases of rosacea are the "flushing and blushing" diathesis; that is, a recurrent erythema that leads with chronicity to telangiectasias. Subsequently, the erythema becomes chronic and the telangiectasias more obvious, with the appearance of tiny papules (fig. 14-17). Eventually, the erythema may become much more prominent, almost disfiguring, and the patients develop central pustules, papules, and nodules. At times, there may be prominent edema of the central face.

*Inflammatory Disorders of the Skin*

**Figure 14-18**

**ACNE ROSACEA**

Well-formed zones of lymphohistiocytic inflammation involve the superficial dermis. Focal aggregation of epithelioid histiocytes form perifollicular granulomas. There is also associated sebaceous hyperplasia.

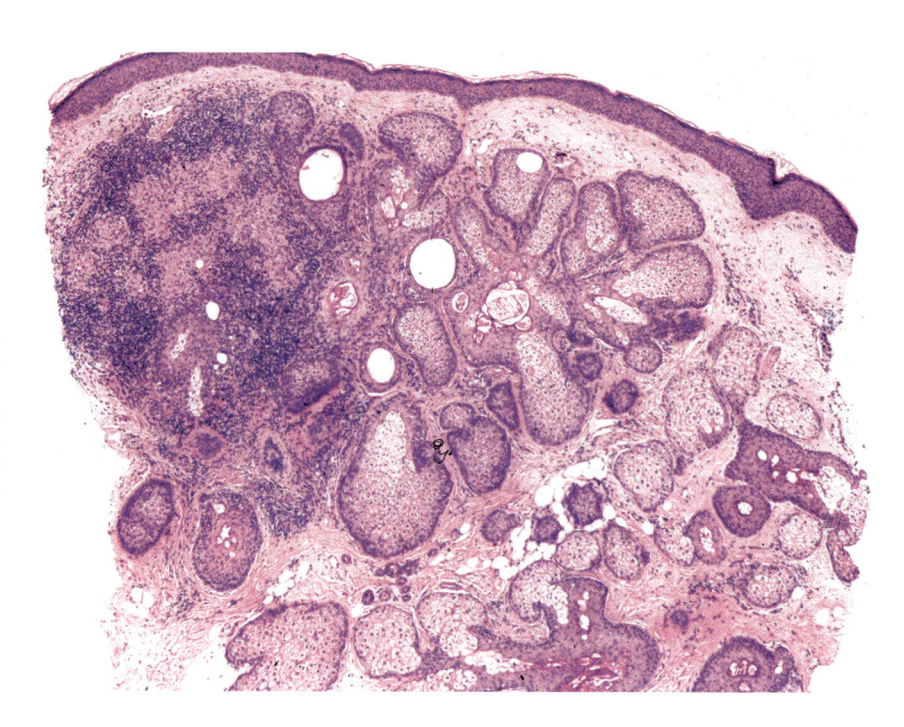

The pathognomonic lesion is a tiny papulopustule that is 2 or 3 mm in diameter. The small pustule surmounts the papule. There are no comedones in rosacea, which allows its differentiation from acne vulgaris. The late phases of rosacea are associated with erythema, edema, sometimes even lymphedema of the forehead, central face, and chin, and marked sebaceous hyperplasia (e.g., as in rhinophyma).

*Rosacea blepharitis* is a chronic conjunctival inflammation and episcleritis that may lead to *rosacea keratitis*. The latter is associated sometimes with corneal ulcers (30,31).

**Pathologic Findings.** There are three histologic components of rosacea, although their pathogenetic relationship remains unclear and they may not all be present in a given patient or biopsy specimen. The first two are noninflammatory: sebaceous hyperplasia and superficial vascular ectasia. The third is a perifollicular lymphohistiocytic infiltrate (figs. 14-18, 14-19) that occasionally is frankly granulomatous, mimicking the micropapular form of sarcoidosis. There is often associated follicular infundibular ectasia, and acutely inflamed lesions may show infundibular microabscess formation as well.

**Differential Diagnosis.** The differential diagnosis of rosacea includes acne vulgaris, infectious folliculitis, and infestation with *Demodex*. Seborrheic dermatitis and subacute lupus erythematosus both cause a malar rash that resembles rosacea. Micropapular sarcoidosis is usually differentiated from granulomatous forms of rosacea in serial sections or levels, since the former fails to show a peri-infundibular distribution, and there is no evidence in the epithelioid cells of lipidization often seen in rosacea.

**Treatment and Prognosis.** Metronidazole, sulfur lotions, and topical antibiotics are useful, but more marked disease best responds to tetracycline or minocycline therapy (32–35). In very severe cases, oral isotretinoin results in a favorable response (36).

## KERATOSIS PILARIS, INFLAMMATORY VARIANT

**Definition.** *Keratosis pilaris* occurs commonly in childhood, but as well in adult life, and presents as prominent hyperkeratotic papules in hair follicles (37,38). It is usually associated with ichthyosis vulgaris.

**Clinical Features.** The lateral aspects of the arms, thighs, and buttocks are most commonly affected by tiny, discrete, hyperkeratotic follicular papules. The lesions become more severe in winter months (probably due to occlusion).

**Pathologic Findings.** Keratosis pilaris is characterized by follicular infundibular hyperkeratosis. The keratotic plug often extends above

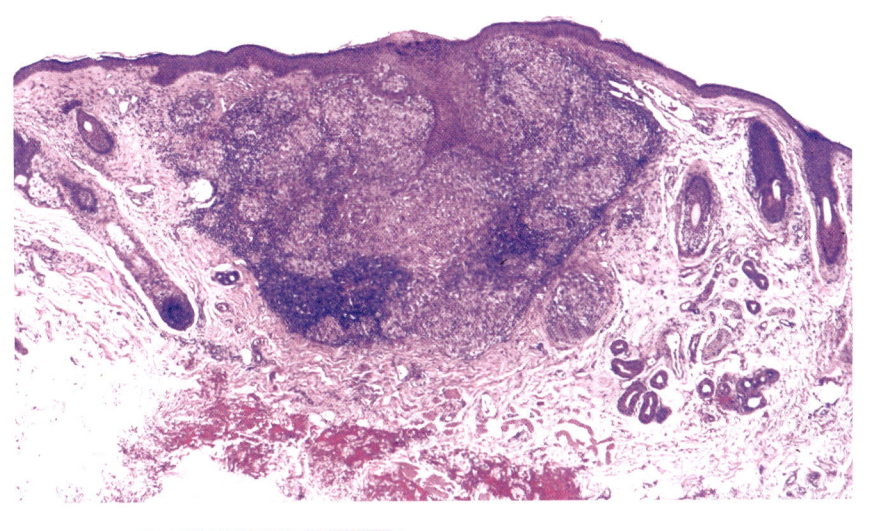

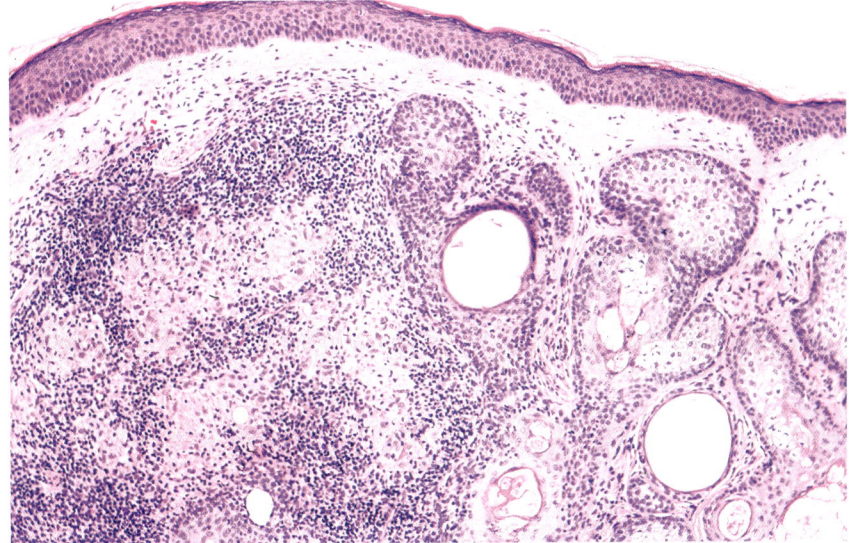

*Inflammatory Disorders with Primary Adnexal Alterations: Follicular Conditions*

**Figure 14-19**

**ACNE ROSACEA: GRANULOMATOUS VARIANT**

Top: The granulomas predominate, raising a differential diagnosis that includes superficial papular sarcoidosis.

Bottom: Higher magnification of lesion shown in figure 14-18; note the prominent non-necrotizing perifollicular epithelioid granulomas, a distribution distinct from superficial papular sarcoidosis that has no follicular association.

the infundibular orifice to form a spiculated "micro-horn" that is appreciated clinically as multiple sharp spines (fig. 14-20). The inflammatory component consists of an associated lymphocytic peri-infundibulitis.

**Differential Diagnosis.** The lesions are quite characteristic, and may be a manifestation of an ichthyosiform eruption.

**Treatment and Prognosis.** Usually, emollients are sufficient (39). In more advanced or refractory cases, some type of gel containing keratolytics, such as salicylic acid, as well as topical retinoids result in at least temporary amelioration of the disorder. The lesions are persistent and recurrent.

## EOSINOPHILIC PUSTULAR FOLLICULITIS

**Definition.** *Eosinophilic pustular folliculitis* is an idiopathic follicular eruption that is extremely pruritic. It characteristically affects the upper trunk, and at times, even the face and extremities (40–44). It is most commonly associated with human immunodeficiency virus (HIV) infection; however, it may occur in patients with no underlying disorder, in which case it is referred to as *Ofuji syndrome*.

**Clinical Features.** Eosinophilic pustular folliculitis occurs most commonly in patients with HIV infection and also in association with antiretroviral therapy. The lesions present as itching, 3- to 5-mm follicular papules that are

*Inflammatory Disorders of the Skin*

**Figure 14-20**

**KERATOSIS PILARIS**

The most superficial portion of the follicular infundibulum contains a dense keratotic plug that generally protrudes above the epidermal surface (not apparent here). An associated lymphoid infiltrate is seen, consistent with the inflammatory variant.

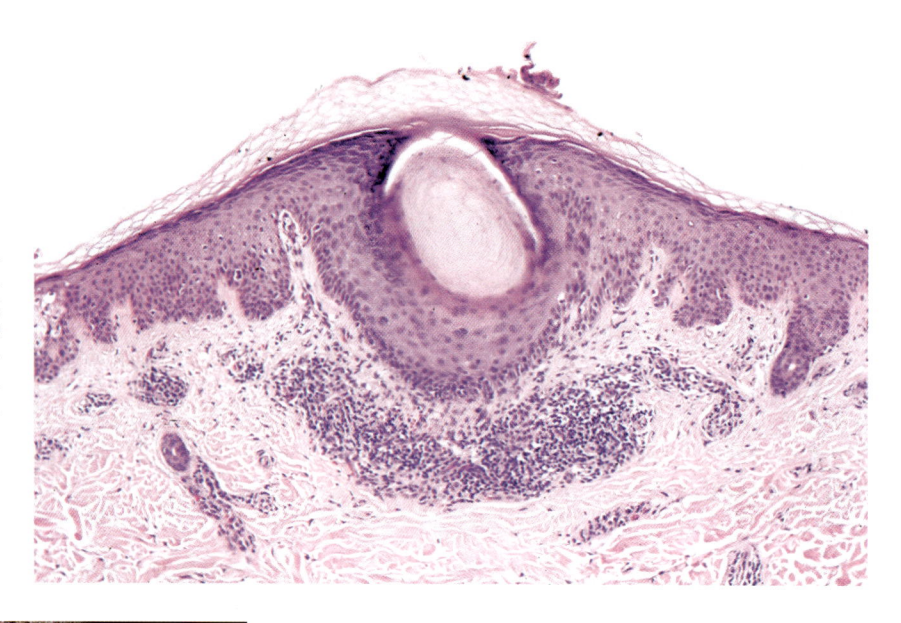

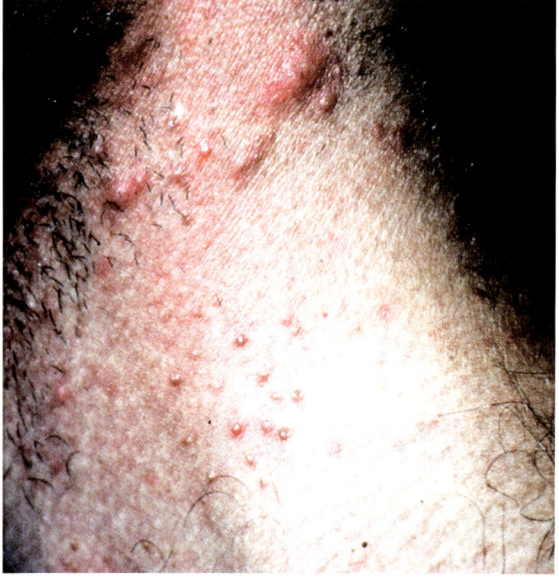

**Figure 14-21**

**EOSINOPHILIC PUSTULAR FOLLICULITIS**

There are numerous follicular papules involving the neck and beard area of this patient with human immunodeficiency virus (HIV).

erythematous and edematous, and sometimes reveal pustules (fig. 14-21). The patients may exhibit a few lesions, or hundreds, all of which are associated with prominent itching that is unresponsive to a variety of therapies.

The itching and scratching lead to secondary changes, including prurigo nodularis or lichen simplex chronicus. Postinflammation pigmentation is common. The lesions occur mainly on the trunk, but may affect the face and proximal extremities; in some patients, however, it is limited to the face. The course of this disorder is persistent and in patients who have the highly active antiretroviral therapy known as HAART, it is chronic; the symptoms persist unless treated.

**Pathologic Findings.** Histologically, there is acute perifolliculitis and folliculitis involving the infundibulum and sometimes the follicular isthmus (figs. 14-22–14-24). The inflammatory component is mixed, consisting of lymphocytes, histiocytes, neutrophils, and eosinophils, the latter of which may dominate the histologic picture in early lesions. Occasionally, a *Demodex* mite is documented in the region of the sebaceous duct, a finding of questionable pathogenetic significance.

**Differential Diagnosis.** Insect bites and other types of folliculitis, including bacterial, fungal, and *Demodex*-induced, and allergic contact dermatitis or atopic dermatitis are in the differential diagnosis.

**Treatment and Prognosis.** The treatment is directed toward the pruritic symptoms, and includes antihistamines and topical corticosteroids (45). Systemic agents include oral prednisone, oral isotretinoin, and even itraconazole in some cases. Some patients respond to ultraviolet B therapy (46).

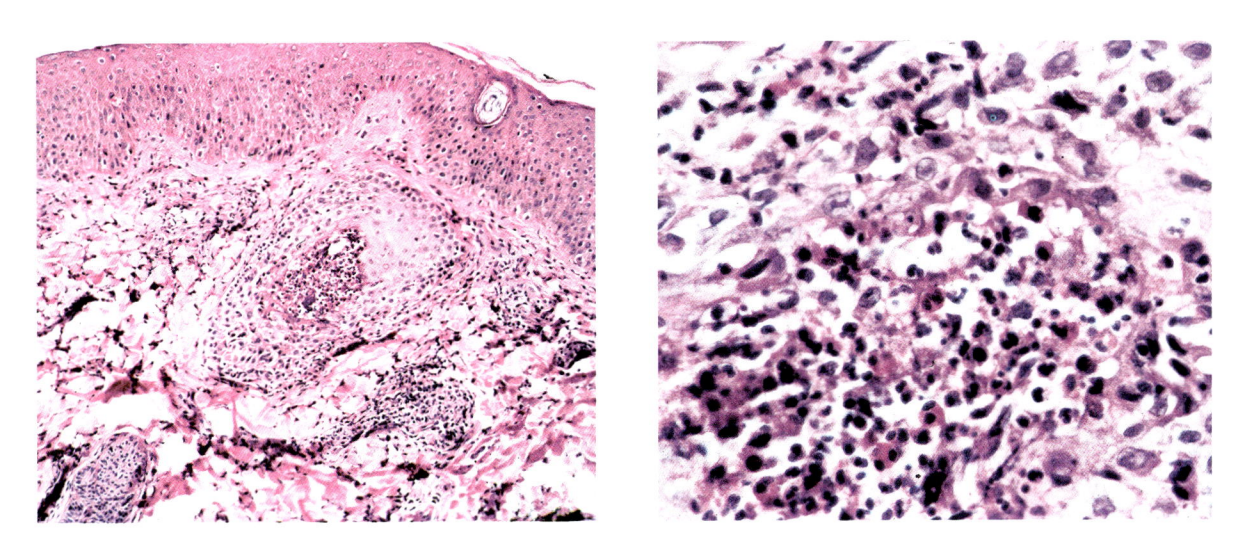

*Inflammatory Disorders with Primary Adnexal Alterations: Follicular Conditions*

Figure 14-22

**EOSINOPHILIC PUSTULAR FOLLICULITIS**

Left: There are discrete zones of inflammation centered on distorted hair follicles.
Right: At high magnification, a zone of follicular epithelium infiltrated and disrupted by aggregates of eosinophils and rare lymphocytes is seen.

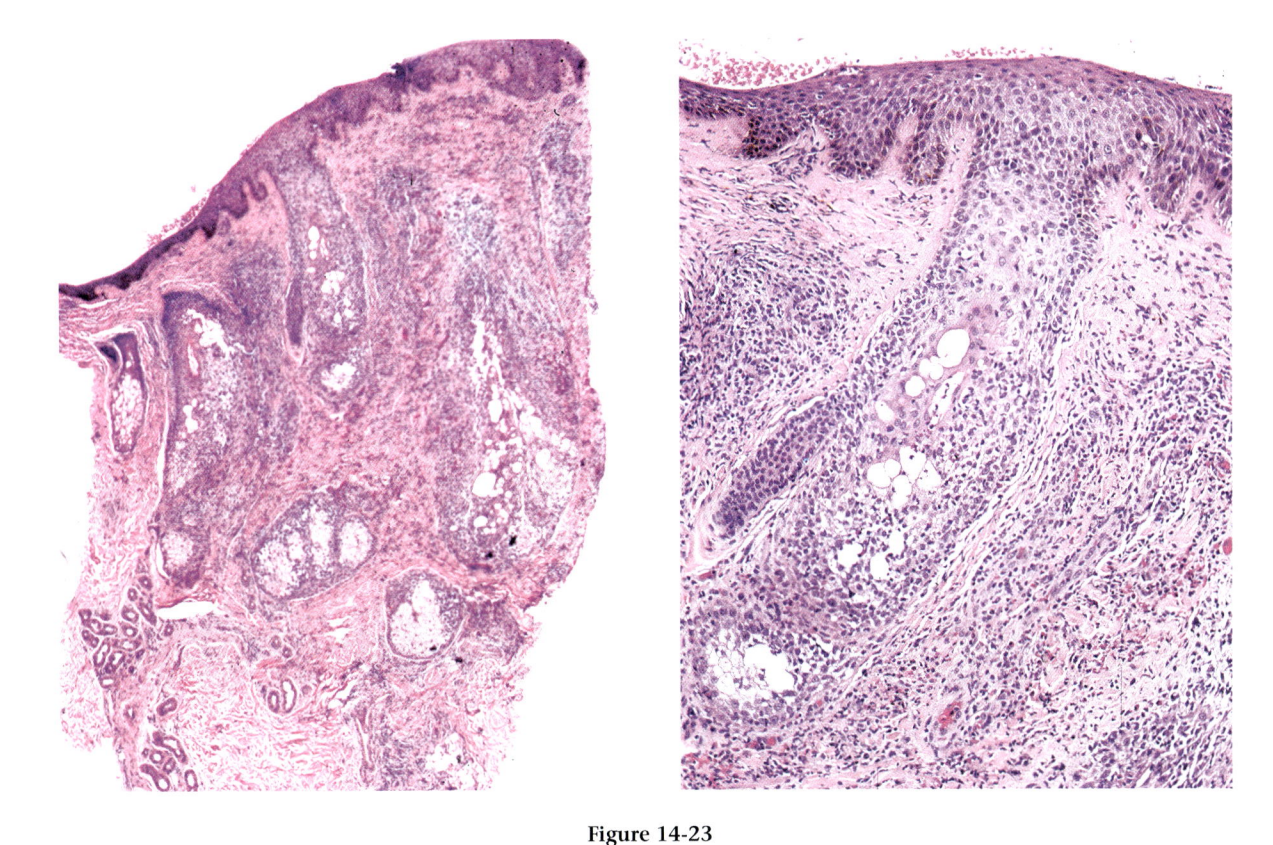

Figure 14-23

**EOSINOPHILIC PUSTULAR FOLLICULITIS: ADVANCED LESION**

Left: The follicular and perifollicular inflammatory infiltration involves most follicles.
Right: At higher magnification, the prominent mixed inflammatory infiltrate involves the upper and middle third of the hair follicle.

*Inflammatory Disorders of the Skin*

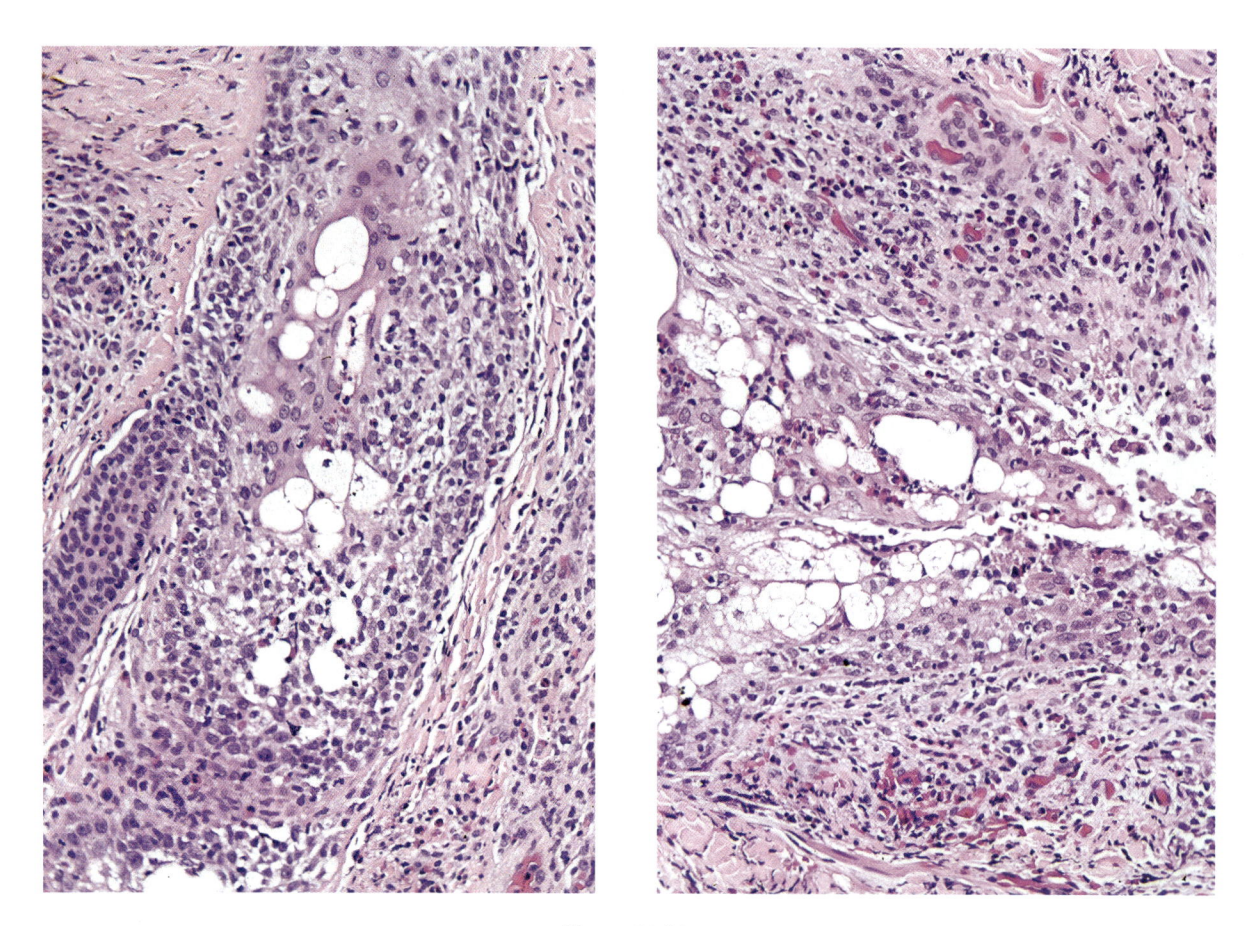

**Figure 14-24**

**EOSINOPHILIC PUSTULAR FOLLICULITIS: ADVANCED LESION**

Left: There is an admixture of inflammatory cells, with a predominance of lymphocytes.
Right: More eosinophils than would normally be anticipated in a lymphocyte-mediated folliculitis are seen focally within the hair follicles.

## PERFORATING FOLLICULITIS

**Definition.** *Perforating folliculitis*, considered one of the transepidermal elimination diseases, is associated with a chemical genesis or with some abnormality of the hair follicle. The exact etiology is unknown. True transepidermal elimination in this disorder does not occur.

**Clinical Features.** There is a striking papular eruption that is usually asymptomatic or at most pruritic. It occurs in both men and women equally in mid life, but lesions occur in adolescents as well. Principally, it affects the hairy portions of the extremities, and the buttocks and trunk. Individual lesions are prominent follicular papules, about 5 mm in average diameter, with a white keratin plug that emits a hair through the surface.

Lesions develop slowly or rapidly, and heal as a hypopigmented area or a depressed scar. Characteristically, lesions occur periodically over months or years and there are exacerbations and remissions.

**Pathologic Findings.** The primary finding is follicular infundibular hyperkeratosis, often associated with a distorted hair shaft. Perforation of the follicular canal results in extrusion of follicular contents into the surrounding dermis, eliciting an acute and chronic inflammatory reaction and focal degenerative alterations within the adjacent adventitia (fig. 14-25). Occasionally, elastic fibers and basophilic perifollicular debris find their way into the follicle through the site of perforation. Thus, the follicular contents may be extruded into the dermis, and basophilic dermal contents and cellular debris may enter the follicle.

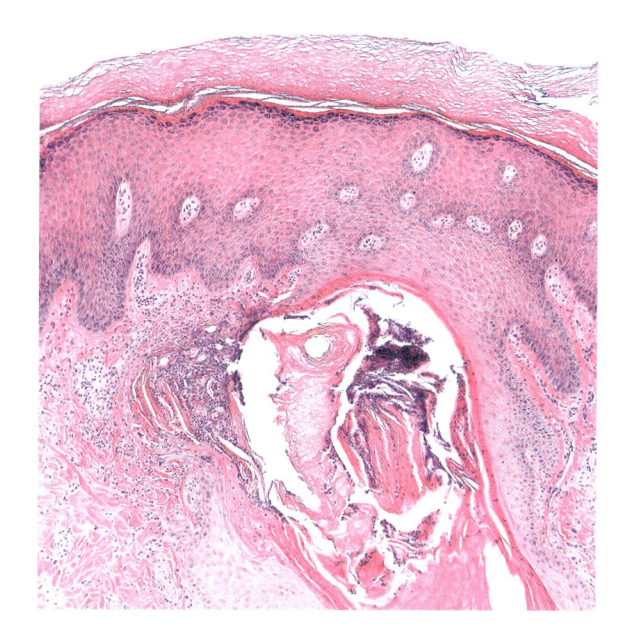

## Figure 14-25

**PERFORATING FOLLICULITIS**

The follicular infundibulum is plugged with keratotic material and basophilic debris. A zone of early perforation with inflammatory response is to the left of center.

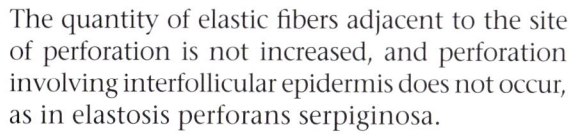

The quantity of elastic fibers adjacent to the site of perforation is not increased, and perforation involving interfollicular epidermis does not occur, as in elastosis perforans serpiginosa.

**Differential Diagnosis.** The differential diagnosis includes other types of folliculitis. Acne vulgaris should also be considered, but the distribution and the nature of the lesions, especially the absence of comedones, help separate this disorder from acne. The lesions of keratosis pilaris are usually not inflamed and do not perforate. Elastosis perforans serpiginosa and reactive perforating collagenosis have characteristic features, which allow for differentiation.

**Treatment and Prognosis.** Retinoid therapy and topical keratolytics are successful, as are retinoids with PUVA (psoralen with ultraviolet A).

## ALOPECIA AREATA

**Definition.** *Alopecia areata* is a type of nonscarring hair loss that occurs in a localized or generalized distribution (47–57). Children and young adults are more frequently affected, but it occurs at any time in life, and is equally distributed among the sexes.

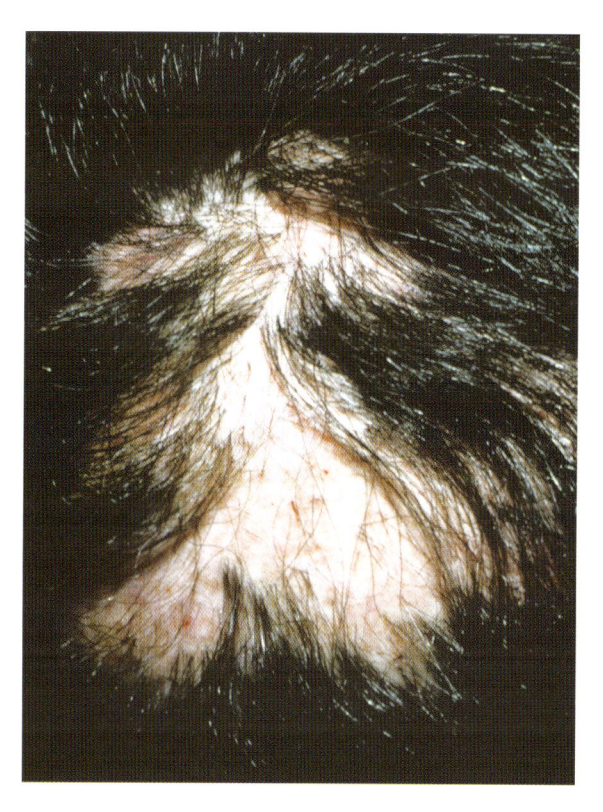

## Figure 14-26

**ALOPECIA AREATA**

There are geographic areas of hair loss, within which the hair shafts have characteristically tapered ends (sometimes referred to as "exclamation point" hairs).

**Clinical Features.** Alopecia areata affects approximately 1 to 2 percent of the population. The etiology of this disorder is unknown, but it appears to be immunologically mediated. The lesions begin over a few weeks to months and patches of alopecia appear. Lesions are usually asymptomatic, although there may be some redness around affected areas.

The area of alopecia, which can be discrete and coin-like or multifocal on the scalp, resolves with an irregular distribution of residual hair, leaving only normal skin at the site (fig. 14-26). The areas of alopecia appear sharply demarcated; however, with the use of a magnifying lens, broken off "stubby" areas, called "exclamation point hairs," are seen. Total alopecia of the scalp is called *alopecia totalis*. *Alopecia universalis* is a late stage of alopecia areata in which there is total loss of body hair. The disorder is associated with Hashimoto thyroiditis, myasthenia gravis, and vitiligo, implicating an autoimmune

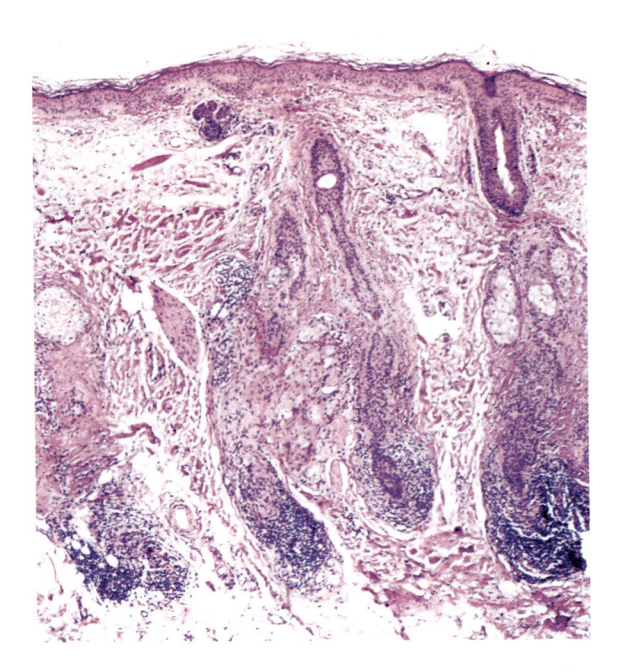

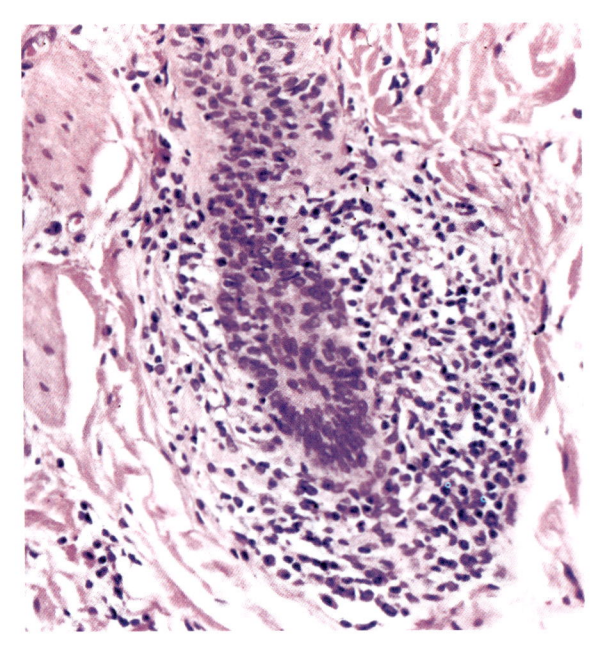

**Figure 14-27**

**ALOPECIA AREATA**

Left: There are intense lymphocytic infiltrates centered about the follicular bulbs in an early and active lesion.
Right: At high magnification, the lymphocytic infiltrate is characteristically centered about the remnants of an involuting follicular bulb (a pattern that has been likened to a "swarm of bees").

process. The dorsal nail plate may exhibit multiple, striking small depressions, resulting in the appearance of "hammered glass."

**Pathologic Findings.** Early lesions are the most informative, showing intense lymphocytic inflammatory infiltration about anagen hair bulbs, the characteristic "swarm of bees" pattern (figs. 14-27–14-29). As the lesions evolve, there is premature conversion of affected anagen follicles into catagen and telogen phases. Late lesions show miniaturization of terminal hairs and a paucity of anagen follicles.

**Differential Diagnosis.** The differential diagnosis includes other types of nonscarring alopecia, especially secondary syphilis, which can induce patchy areas on the scalp and other sites. Trichotillomania, traction alopecia, early lupus erythematosus, and androgenic alopecia, when localized, can mimic alopecia areata.

**Treatment and Prognosis.** Overall, more than 75 percent of treated patients regrow hair within a year. Therapy with intralesional steroids is most common; topical steroids are not as helpful. Anthralin is used as a second line agent, as is squaric acid. PUVA is employed but is associated with recurrence when discontinued. Systemic immunosuppression with prednisone or cyclosporine has been reported, but recurrence and systemic side effects limit the efficacy of this therapy (58–61). When the hair regrows, it is often white. Complete spontaneous resolution occurs in approximately a third of patients

## ANDROGENIC (PATTERN) ALOPECIA

**Definition.** *Androgenic (pattern) alopecia* is a common type of progressive hair loss that occurs as a genetically determined factor, as well as due to the action of androgens on genetically predisposed hair follicles of the scalp (62–69). This form of alopecia causes different patterns of alopecia in men and women, but it most commonly occurs as bitemporal recession in men (70,71).

**Clinical Features.** Androgenic (pattern) alopecia affects men much more commonly than women. Occurrence is any time after puberty, as early as the teenage years but most commonly in the fourth decade of life (72). In women, it usually occurs during or after menopause, in the sixth decade of life.

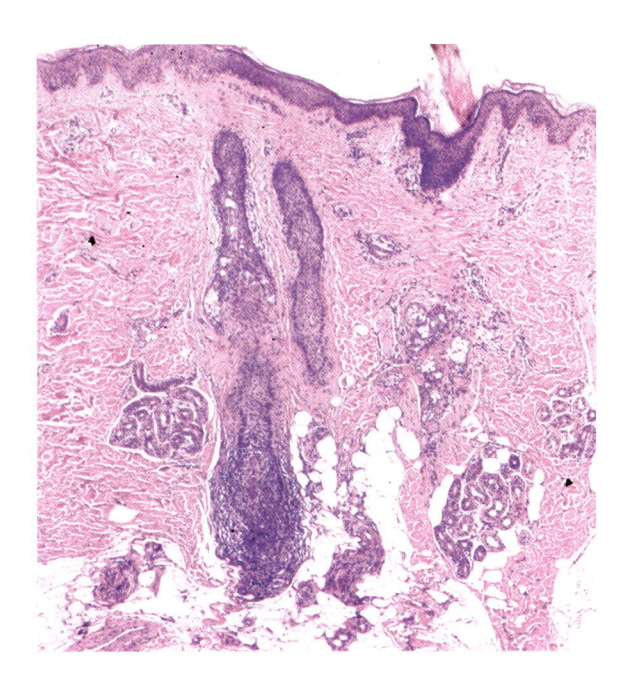

*Inflammatory Disorders with Primary Adnexal Alterations: Follicular Conditions*

**Figure 14-28**

**ALOPECIA AREATA**

Above: There is obvious diminution in anagen follicle density associated with a residual lymphocytic infiltrate involving the hair bulb, a clue to the underlying cause.

Right: The characteristic "swarm of bees" pattern is seen.

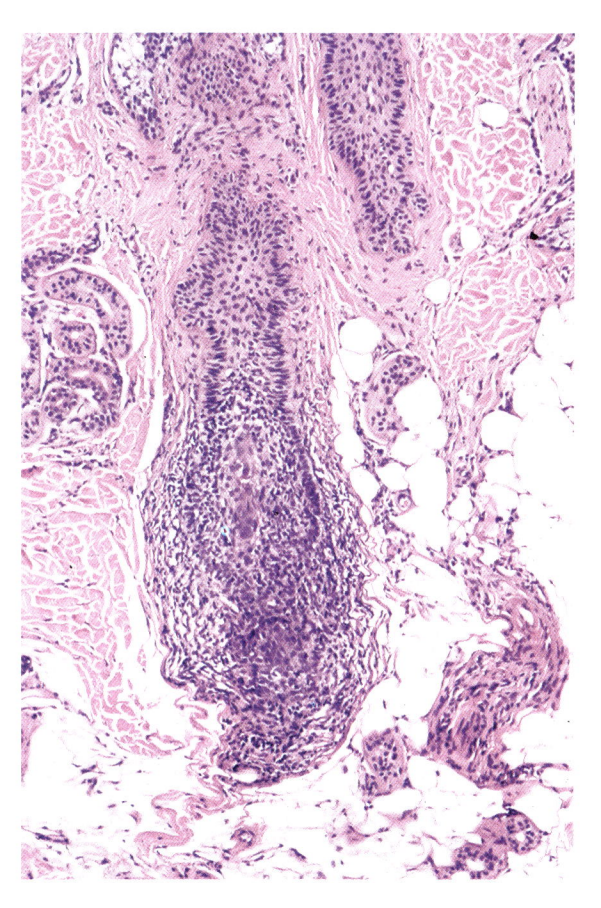

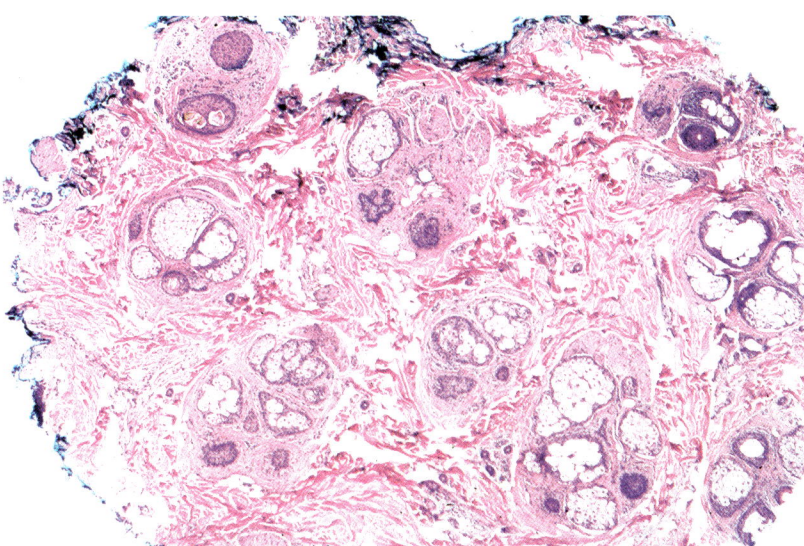

**Figure 14-29**

**ALOPECIA AREATA**

In a transverse section, increased numbers of telogen follicles with only scattered inflammatory cells, primarily lymphocytes, are associated with the involuted bulbs.

Androgenic (pattern) alopecia is inherited, probably as an autosomal dominant trait in men and as an autosomal recessive trait in women. The common bitemporal recession of the hairline in men is followed by loss of hair in the crown (fig. 14-30). In women, the pattern of loss is more central, without recession of the hairline or the crown bald spot. The hair loss is usually gradual, and only in severe cases are the patients aware of hair "falling out."

*Inflammatory Disorders of the Skin*

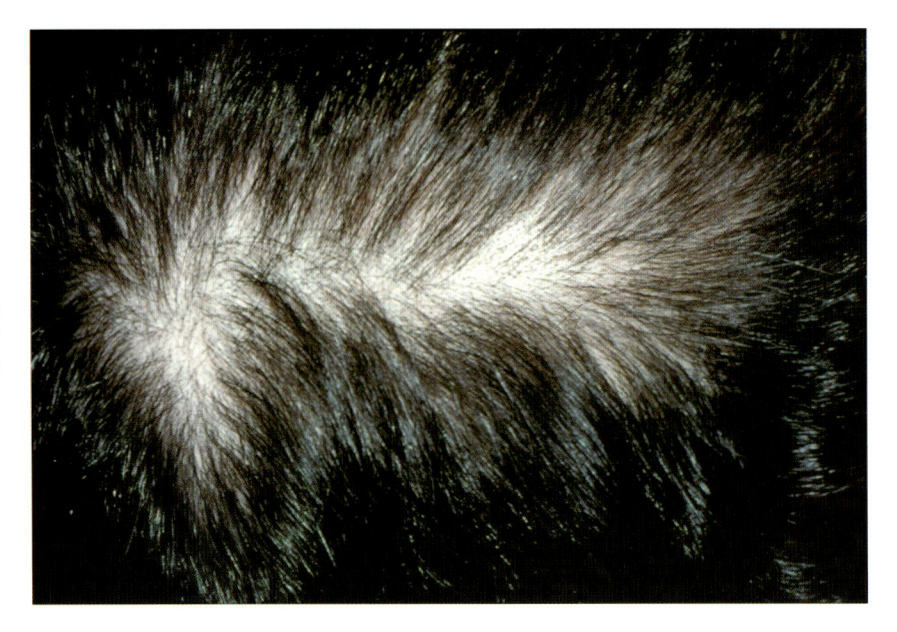

**Figure 14-30**

ANDROGENIC ALOPECIA

The thinning of the hair primarily involves the apex of the scalp in the absence of signs of active inflammation.

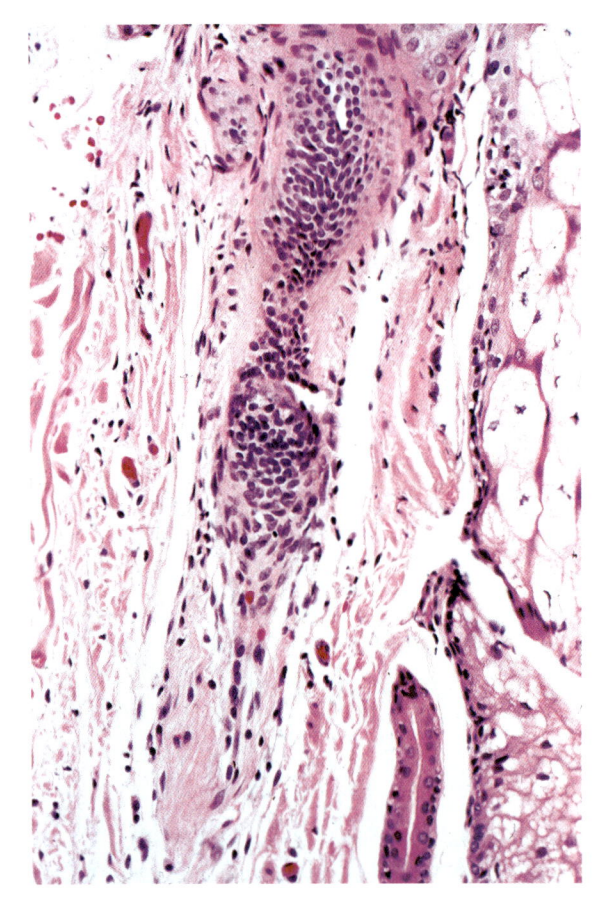

**Figure 14-31**

ANDROGENIC ALOPECIA

There is marked diminution in the caliber of this residual hair follicle.

There are no other typical lesions, although sometimes patients have seborrheic dermatitis. The hair characteristically becomes finer in texture, and there is a debate as to whether the hair gradually diminishes, or tapers, in size and diameter or whether it abruptly diminishes in diameter. Late stages show fine, delicate vellus (miniaturized) hairs, and eventually complete loss of the hair.

The lateral and posterior scalp in men is spared. In women, the hair loss in the male pattern of alopecia areas is less striking but more diffuse. Women who are affected in a predominantly male pattern must be examined to determine if there are any virilizing factors, but most women do not have endocrine abnormalities.

**Pathologic Findings.** The histologic alterations are subtle and highly variable as a consequence of stage and site of sampling. In early inflammatory lesions, there is a mononuclear infiltrate centered about the junction of the follicular infundibulum and the sebaceous duct. As the process progresses, occasional terminal hair follicles become replaced by vellus or rudimentary (miniaturized) anagen follicles (fig. 14-31). During this stage, fibrous tracts or "streamers" are conspicuous within the dermis, demarcating foci previously occupied by terminal follicles, and telogen follicles may appear more prominent. In areas of established alopecia, pronounced miniaturization of follicles and complete zones of terminal hair replacement by vellus follicles are seen. The sebaceous glands

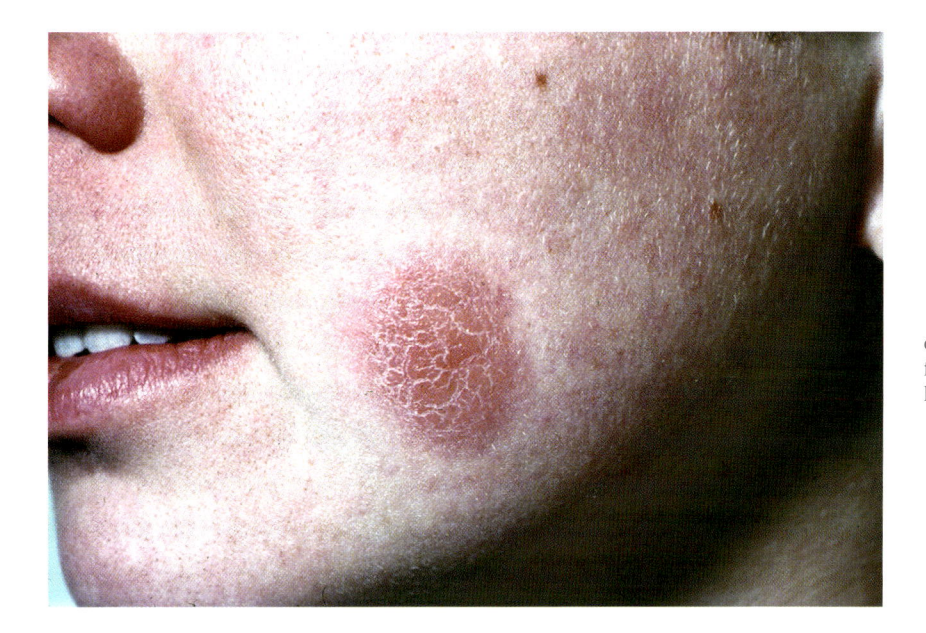

**Figure 14-32**

**ALOPECIA MUCINOSA**

There is a discrete plaque of erythema with prominent follicular ostia devoid of vellus hair shafts.

may appear more prominent, and inflammatory infiltrates are minimal. If inflammatory cells near the follicular bulge damage stem cells, normal regeneration may be impeded. Ultrastructural analysis has demonstrated that with disease progression there is thickening of perifollicular fibrous sheaths. This alteration of the normally delicate envelope surrounding the hair follicle may impede its normal descent into the deep dermis and subcutaneous fat, as the follicle cycles from telogen into a renewed anagen phase, thus providing a structural basis for androgenic alopecia.

**Differential Diagnosis.** The diffuse nonscarring alopecias, such as telogen effluvium, diffuse alopecia areata, or secondary syphilis, as well as endocrinopathies such as hypothyroidism, must be considered in the differential diagnosis, particularly in women, where characteristic pattern and history may be lacking. Associated dermatitis (e.g., seborrheic dermatititis) may be a complicating factor, and biopsies should also be carefully examined for such coexisting pathology.

**Treatment and Prognosis.** Currently, the most successful treatment is oral finasteride, which inhibits the conversion of testosterone to dihydrotestosterone (73–75). This drug does not have an affinity for androgen receptors, and therefore does not lead to changes in the usual actions of testosterone, such as normal libido and spermatogenesis. Currently, this drug is only approved for use in men (76). Minoxidil is also available and can be used concurrently with finasteride. There is no role for topical steroids unless an inflammatory, scarring alopecia coexists.

## ALOPECIA MUCINOSA

**Definition.** *Alopecia mucinosa* is associated with the deposition of acid mucopolysaccharides in the follicular epithelium (77,78). It is sometimes associated with distinctive disorders, one of the most significant of which is cutaneous T-cell lymphoma (79–81).

**Clinical Features.** Groups of red to flesh-colored follicular papules that may coalesce to form a raised plaque with a boggy feel to palpation characterize the lesions (fig. 14-32). When these occur in visibly hair-bearing areas, alopecia often signals onset. The lesions are single or multiple, and usually resolve after several months with regrowth of hair. If there is successful treatment of the underlying cause of the follicular mucinosis, such as cutaneous T-cell lymphoma, the hair regrows and the lesions subside. The plaques of follicular mucinosis are either chronic or self-healing.

Most cases of follicular mucinosis are not associated with systemic disease, but between 10 and 15 percent are associated with cutaneous T-cell lymphoma. Langerhans cell histiocytosis is also associated with follicular mucinosis, usually in children but rarely in adults. Chronic benign follicular mucinosis may go on to develop into mycosis fungoides. Angiolymphoid hyperplasia

*Inflammatory Disorders of the Skin*

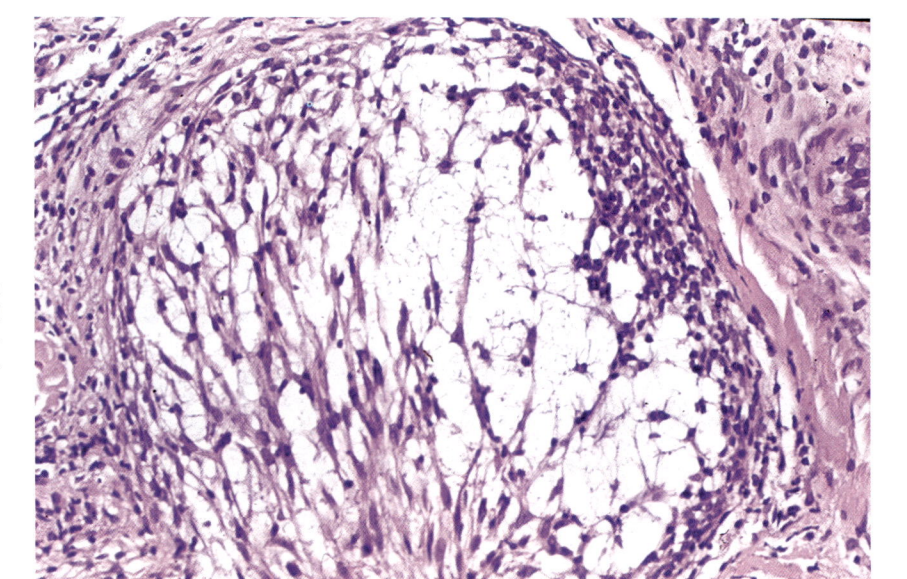

**Figure 14-33**

**FOLLICULAR MUCINOSIS**

There is striking deposition of mucin within the involved follicle associated with a perifollicular and intrafollicular lymphocytic infiltrate.

is also associated with this disorder. Therefore, all alopecia mucinosa lesions must be biopsied and if the lesions persist, rebiopsy and careful follow-up are necessary.

**Pathologic Findings.** Histologically, multiple hair follicles show mucin in the follicular epithelium, with variable infiltration by lymphocytes, histiocytes, and eosinophils. The mucin is pale blue-gray and tends to be intercellular, producing a spongiotic architecture (fig. 14-33). Follicular disruption and degeneration are also present. The presence of mucin is confirmed by staining with Alcian blue or colloidal iron.

**Differential Diagnosis.** Plaques that result in alopecia are in the clinical differential diagnosis, including cutaneous lupus erythematosus and early morphea. In nonhair-bearing skin, eczematous dermatitis, lymphocytic infiltrate of Jessner, and lymphoma cutis are considered. Extension of the inflammatory infiltrate into the overlying epidermis, cytologic atypia of the infiltrating lymphocytes, and lack of eosinophils are suggestive of cutaneous T-cell lymphoma as a cause of follicular mucinosis. In such cases, cell marker analysis and T-cell receptor gene rearrangement studies by polymerase chain reaction (PCR) are useful special diagnostic adjuncts. Follicular eczema is also in the differential diagnosis.

**Treatment and Prognosis.** The lesions that are benign and not associated with lymphoma spontaneously remit. They sometimes respond to topical potent corticosteroid application and even to injection of steroids. Rare reports show a benefit of dapsone and interferons (81a). When alopecia mucinosa is associated with lymphoma, antilymphoma therapy is effective. Lesions within T-cell dyscrasias respond to PUVA therapy, nitrogen mustard, and radiation.

## LUPUS ALOPECIA

**Definition.** Lupus erythematosus may produce discrete zones of hair loss, as well as diffuse thinning of scalp hair (*lupus alopecia*) (82–86). Rarely, the involvement is primarily or exclusively follicular, especially when lesions affect the head and scalp skin. These patients have a better prognosis than those with generalized forms of discoid lupus erythematosus, with lesser tendency for evolution into systemic disease.

**Clinical Features.** Discoid plaques of alopecia are associated with erythema and scaling (fig. 14-34). There are prominent comedonal plugs and associated retraction of follicular ostia. Scarring may be observed centrally as zones of hyperpigmentation with complete loss of follicular epithelium. There may also be areas of hypopigmentation and telangiectasia.

**Pathologic Findings.** The earliest alteration is a perivascular lymphocytic infiltrate with occasional admixed plasma cells at the dermal-follicular infundibular junction and often about eccrine coils (figs. 14-35, 14-36). There may be vacuolization and apoptosis of cells within the

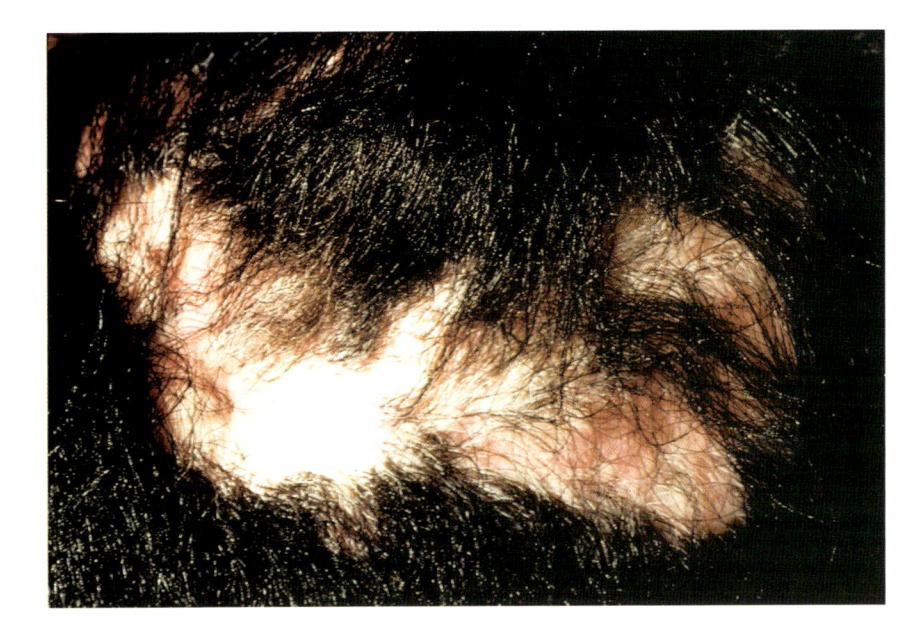

**Figure 14-34**

**LUPUS ALOPECIA**

Patchy hair loss is associated with zones of erythema, scarring, epidermal atrophy, and follicular keratotic plugging.

**Figure 14-35**

**LUPUS ALOPECIA**

There is a marked decrease in anagen hair density, evidence of follicular ectasia and keratotic plugging, atrophy of the epidermis and follicular epithelium, and a focally deep lymphoid inflammatory infiltrate involving follicles, neurovascular bundles, and eccrine coils.

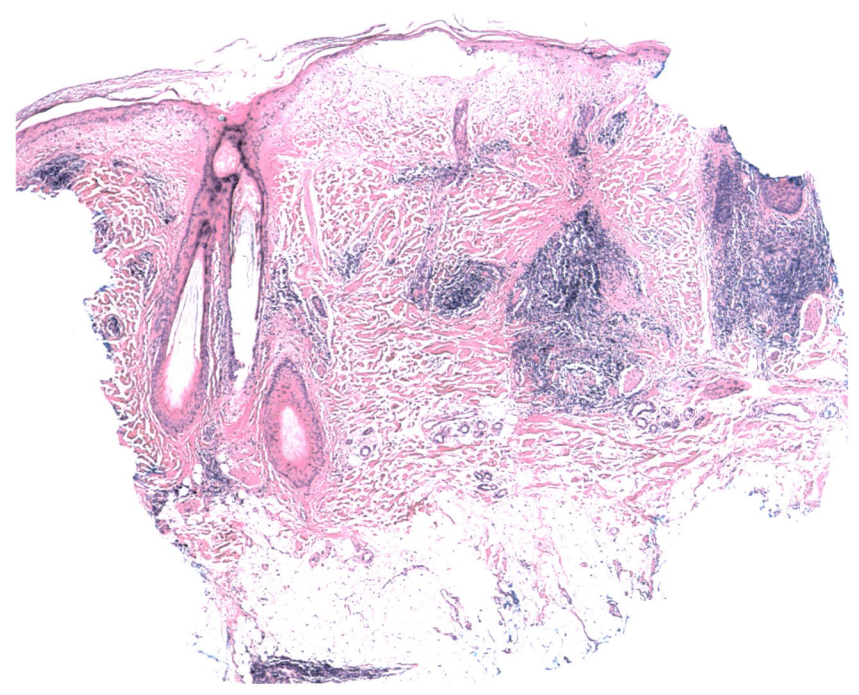

basal cell layer. The infundibular epithelium eventually becomes atrophic and hyperkeratotic, leading to ectasia and keratotic plugging of the follicular canal. The dermal-epidermal junction may also have interface changes, although the follicular pathology generally dominates the picture. Patchy perineurovascular, predominantly lymphocytic, infiltrates may be present within the superficial and deep dermis. Diffuse dermal mucin deposition is the rule. In advanced lesions, follicles destroyed by the extensive interface injury are replaced by dense bands of fibrosis with associated pigment incontinence and residual patchy lymphoid aggregates.

**Differential Diagnosis.** The primary differential diagnostic consideration is lichen planopilaris (see below for similarities and differences).

**Treatment and Prognosis.** Immunosuppressive agents (corticosteroids) are used most often, although the scarring alopecia is often

*Inflammatory Disorders of the Skin*

**Figure 14-36**

**LUPUS ALOPECIA**

A: A perifollicular interface lymphocytic infiltrate is associated with early keratotic plugging of the follicular infundibulum, epidermal atrophy, and focal interface changes along the dermal-epidermal junction.

B: There is prominent thickening of the basement membrane and mucin deposition within the underlying dermis. The epidermis is markedly thin.

C: The lymphoplasmacytic inflammatory infiltrate that surrounds the eccrine coil is a characteristic finding.

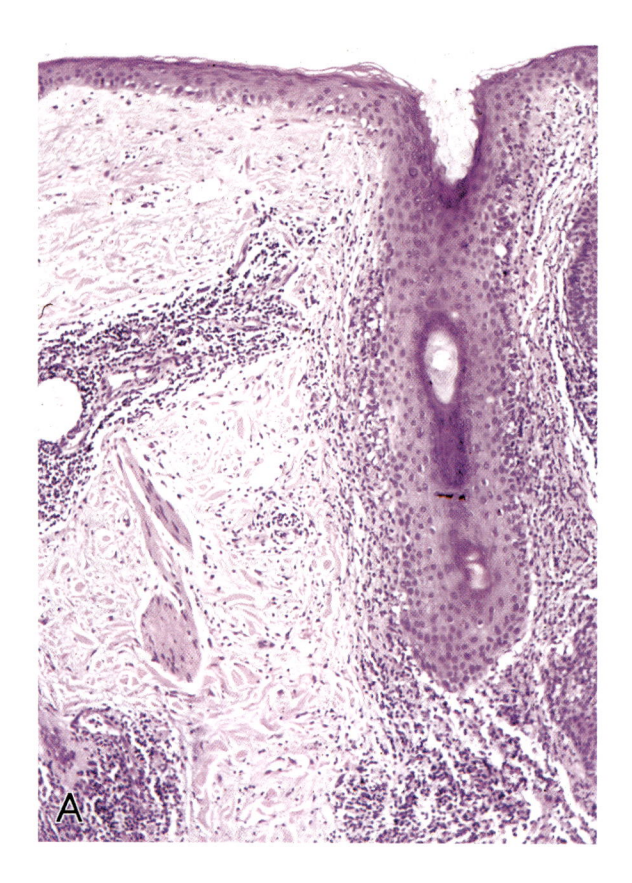

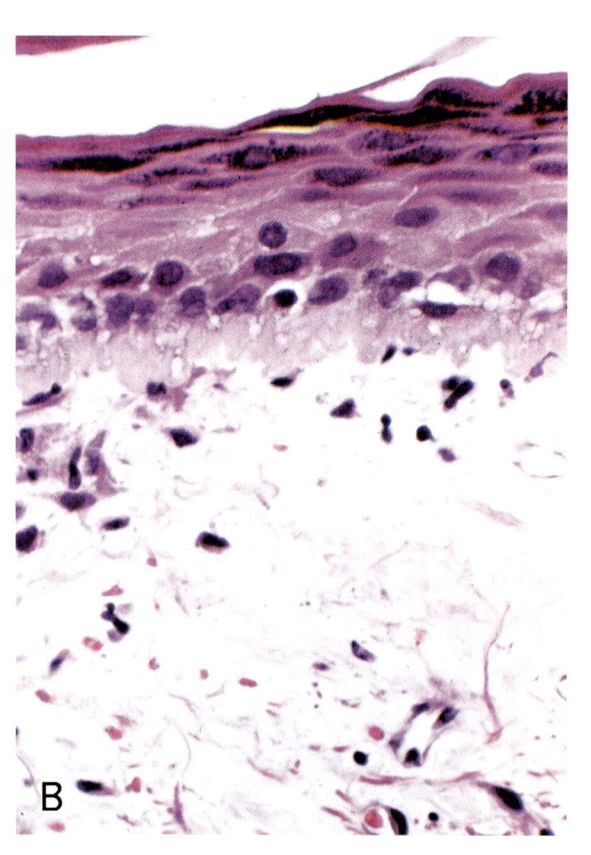

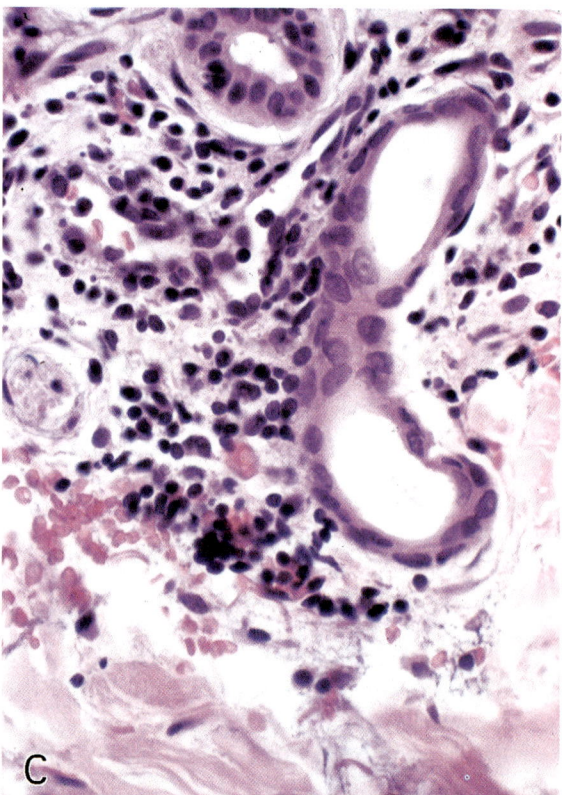

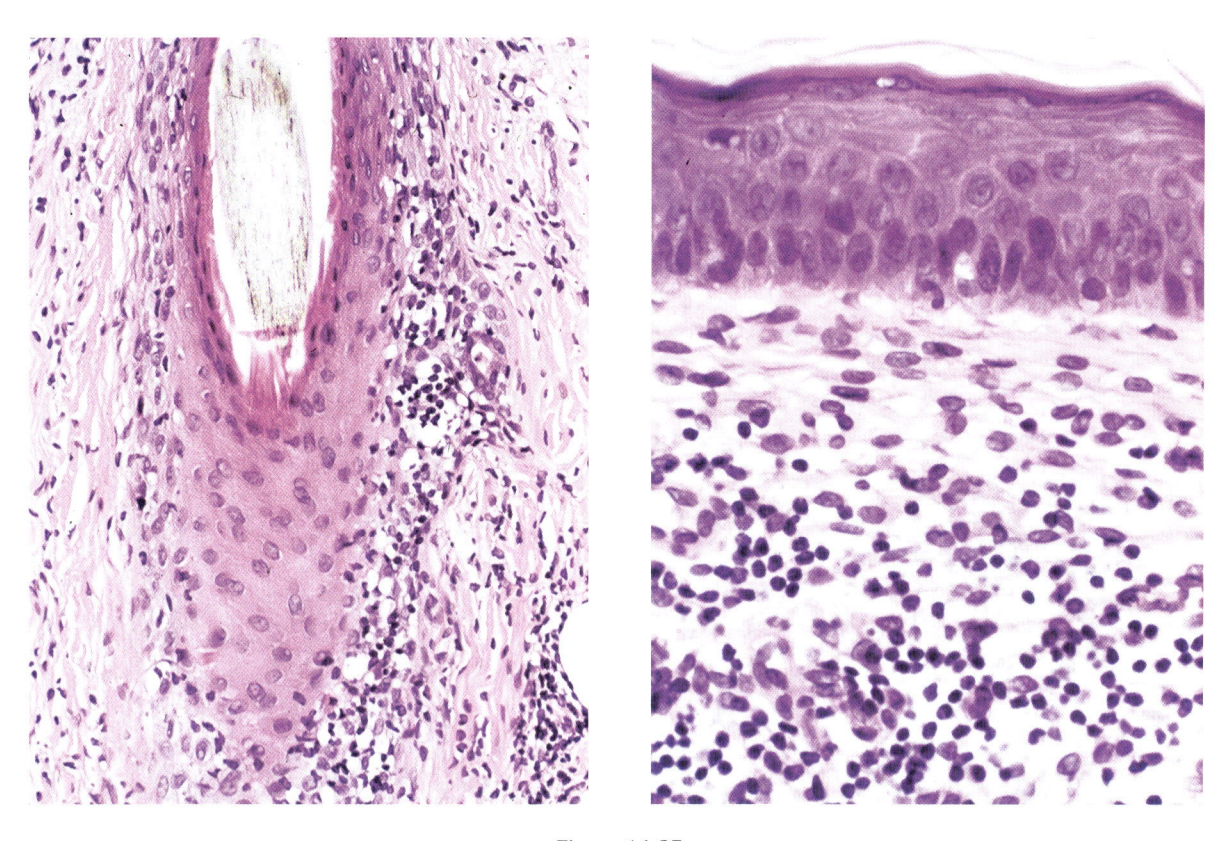

**Figure 14-37**

**LICHEN PLANOPILARIS**

Left: There is a band-like interface infiltrate of lymphocytes that surrounds the upper half of the hair follicle, resulting in chronic injury to the basal layer of the infundibulum. Unlike lupus alopecia, the infundibular epithelium is hyperplastic, not atrophic.

Right: Although the chronic interface injury to the intrafollicular epidermis has resulted here in atrophy, there is no evidence of thickening of the basement membrane, as would be anticipated in lupus alopecia.

progressive and may be extremely refractory to therapeutic management. Topical injection of steroids is sometimes helpful.

## LICHEN PLANOPILARIS

**Definition.** *Lichen planopilaris* is a form of follicular lichen planus that affects hair-bearing surfaces including the scalp, trunk, extremities, and intertriginous areas such as the axillae (87–92).

**Clinical Features.** On the scalp, lichen planopilaris appears as areas of hair loss within which intact hair follicles are surrounded by red to violaceous papules. These areas slowly enlarge, leaving in their wake zones of scarring and permanent hair loss. Lesions of lichen planopilaris and lichen planus affecting glabrous skin often coexist.

**Pathologic Findings.** There is a band-like inflammatory infiltrate composed of lymphocytes associated with the follicular infundibulum. Basal cells are often apoptotic or squamatized, with the former incorporated into the inflammatory infiltrate within the follicular adventitia as colloid bodies with pigment incontinence (figs. 14-37–14-40). The infundibular epithelium is generally acanthotic with hypergranulosis, and the infundibulum is filled with hyperkeratotic scale. Over time, perifollicular fibrosis develops, and the follicular epithelium is replaced by dense bands of collagen in a manner similar to end-stage lupus alopecia. A characteristic feature of lichen planopilaris is multifocal involvement of the follicle with the interface changes in contrast to lupus where the follicle is diffusely involved.

**Differential Diagnosis.** The primary entity in the differential diagnosis is lupus alopecia. Table 14-2 highlights some of the more helpful differential features. We have encountered examples

*Inflammatory Disorders of the Skin*

**Figure 14-38**

**LICHEN PLANOPILARIS**

The multiple foci of lymphocytic infiltration are preferentially centered about follicular infundibula.

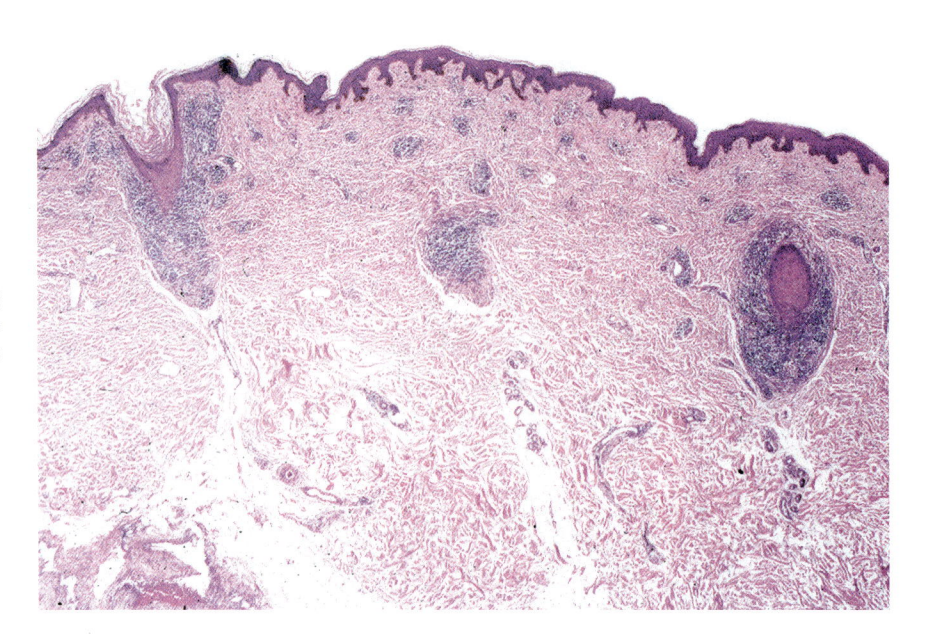

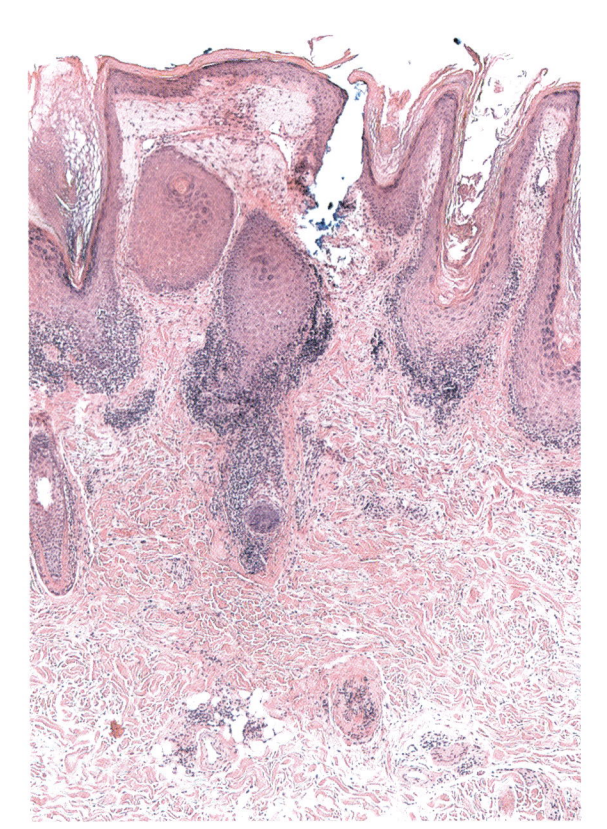

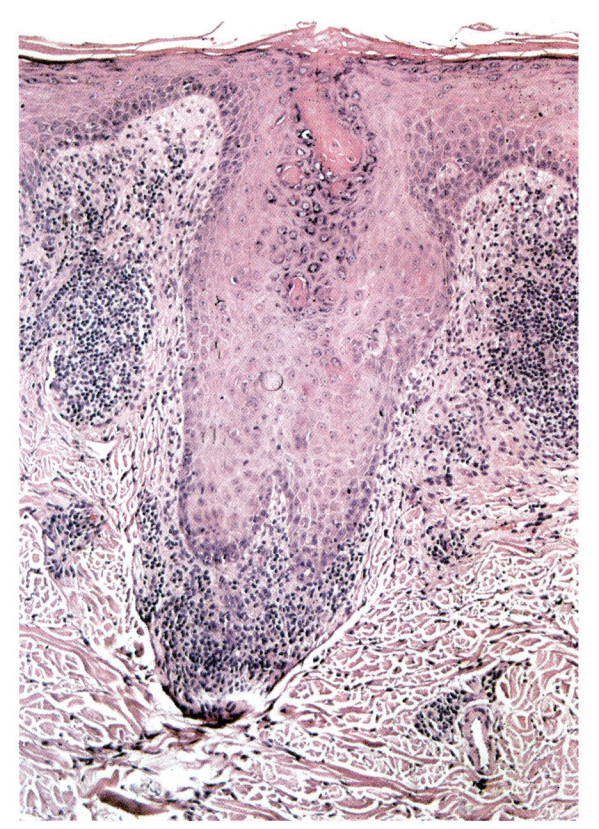

**Figure 14-39**

**LICHEN PLANOPILARIS**

Left There is a lymphocyte-mediated interface folliculitis with lichen planus-like thickening of the infundibular lining. Right: Although there is lymphocyte-mediated cytotoxic injury to the infundibular basal cell layer, unlike lupus, epithelial hyperplasia and hypergranulosis are present.

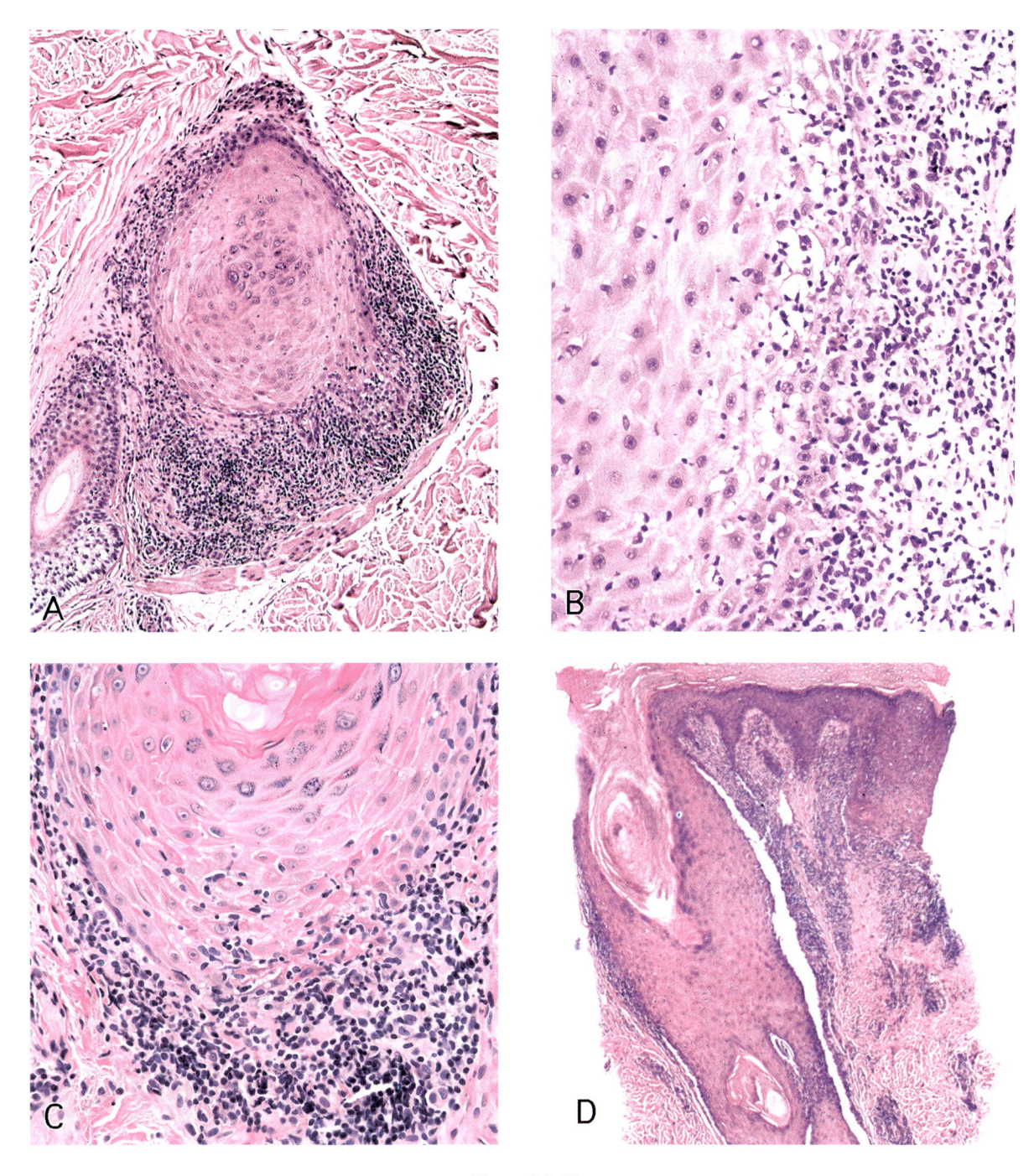

**Figure 14-40**
**LICHEN PLANOPILARIS**

A: In a horizontal section, the band-like lymphocytic infiltrate, follicular hyperplasia, and hypergranulosis required for the diagnosis are readily apparent.

B: At higher magnification, the infiltrative lymphoid response is associated with basal cell layer vacuolization, squamatization, and apoptosis.

C: The causative lymphocytic infiltrate is associated with the formation of colloid/apoptotic bodies at the follicular interface akin to the changes seen in lichen planus.

D: The marked follicular epithelial hyperplasia involving deeply situated anagen follicles must not be mistaken for well-differentiated invasive carcinoma.

of lichen planopilaris where endophytic follicular hyperplasia and distortion is so pronounced that a misdiagnosis of well-differentiated invasive squamous cell carcinoma is rendered. Biopsies of end-stage disease may be difficult to classify and, therefore, clinicians are always encouraged to sample regions in active evolution.

**Treatment and Prognosis.** Topical keratolytics and retinoids are often the first line of therapy. Systemic steroids, methotrexate, azathioprine, and cyclosporine are used as short-term management to ablate inflammation and prevent further hair loss. Once scarring ensues, hair does not grow back. Hair transplantation may be an option in these cases.

## TRAUMATIC AND SCARRING ALOPECIA GROUP

These conditions, differing in physical or inflammatory cause, all share common histopathologic features, and, therefore, are discussed together in this section.

### Trichotillomania

*Trichotillomania* is a nonscarring alopecia with a usually well-defined area of hair loss, often with an unusual shape (93–99). Twisting of scalp hair around the fingers especially, or pulling of scalp hair, results in the breakage of the hair. There are often some normal hairs scattered throughout the area affected.

This disorder responds at times to drugs that are useful in treating obsessive-compulsive patterns of behavior (100–104). At times, simply informing the patient of the cause of the problem helps eliminate the lesion (105).

### Traction Alopecia

The nonscarring *traction alopecia* is often related to using curlers or pulling of hair too tightly to produce a "ponytail" (106). The patterning of the alopecia provides a clue, as it follows along the lines of curler implantation or along a part line (fig. 14-41). The pulling of the hair posteriorly can result in unusual hairline alopecia that sometimes has a "moth-eaten" appearance.

Any type of trauma results in traction alopecia. For example, a headband that is tightly worn or a tight football helmet may cause ischemia. Occasionally, prolonged pressure on an area that results, for example, from a person in coma not being moved properly or a person during surgery having applied pressure for a period of time to a given area, can result in traction alopecia.

Traction alopecia may not be reversible but with early identification and discontinuation of the cause regrowth of hair may ensue. Proper handling of the patient in a coma, identification of the appropriate headgear, or use of a different type of styling appliance may result in reversal of the alopecia.

### Follicular Degeneration Syndrome

*Follicular degeneration syndrome,* previously been described as "hot comb alopecia," occurs most commonly in African Americans and was originally associated with the thermal effects of a hot comb (107). It results in patchy alopecia of the scalp that has distinctive clinical features (108).

Early discontinuance of the use of the hot comb results in regrowth of hair. Chronically induced lesions, however, show marked follicular destruction and are not reversible.

### End-Stage Scarring Alopecia

*Scarring alopecia* is caused by a variety of disorders that result in the destruction of the follicles by a fibrosing process. These include systemic diseases that affect the scalp including lupus erythematosus, morphea, lichen planus, pityriasis rubra pilaris, necrobiosis lipoidica, sarcoidosis, epidermolysis bullosa, and cicatricial pemphigoid. Radiation dermatitis and direct trauma from physical agents may also cause sufficient damage to produce

Table 14-2

DIFFERENTIAL DIAGNOSIS OF LUPUS ALOPECIA AND LICHEN PLANOPILARIS

| Feature | Lupus Alopecia | Lichen Planopilaris |
|---|---|---|
| Peri-infundibular infiltrate | Present | Present |
| Plasma cells | Present | Rare |
| Basal layer injury | Vacuolization | Colloid bodies, squamatization |
| Infundibular atrophy | Present | Absent |
| Infundibular acanthosis | Absent | Present |
| Dermal mucin | Present | Scant to absent |
| Perieccrine infiltrates | Present | Absent |
| Follicular destruction and scarring | Present | Present |

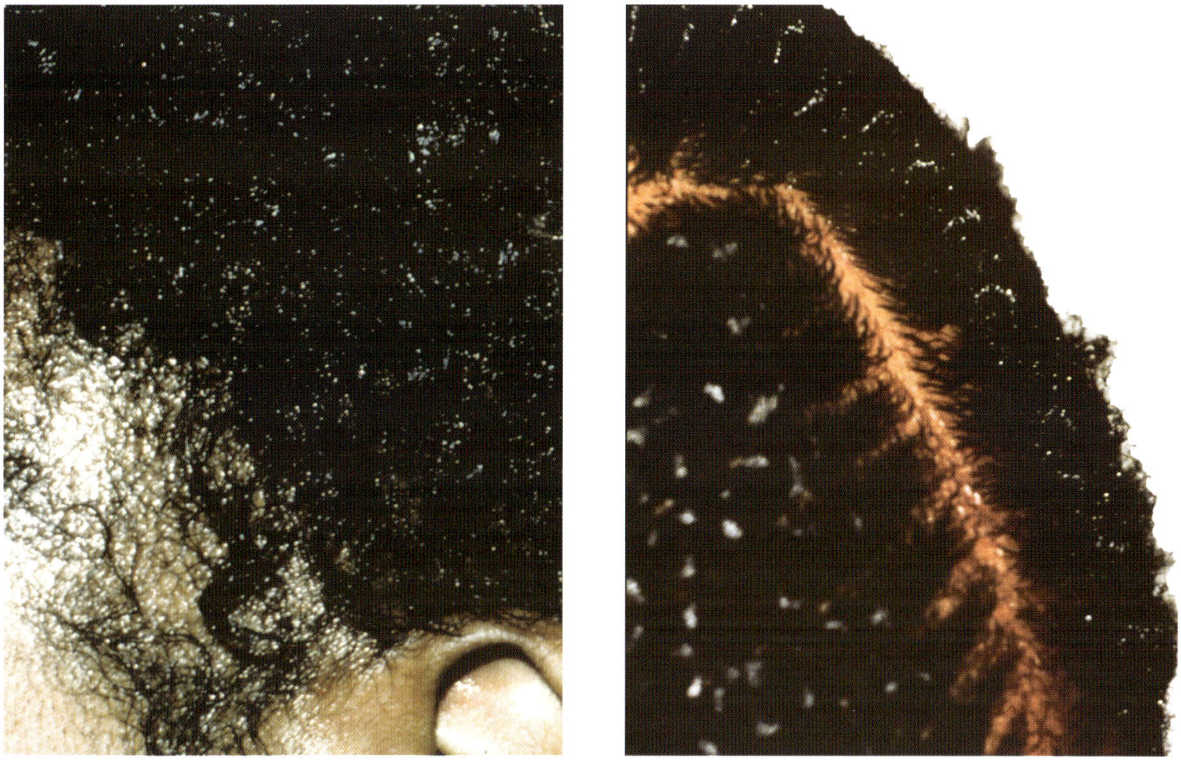

*Inflammatory Disorders with Primary Adnexal Alterations: Follicular Conditions*

Figure 14-41
**TRACTION ALOPECIA**
Widening of the parted hair is the result of chronic tension due to tight braiding.

scarring of the scalp. A variety of follicular syndromes, including folliculitis decalvans, follicular degeneration syndrome, pseudopelade, and dissecting perifolliculitis of the scalp are among other causes of this disorder.

Traumatic alopecia due to a variety of physical agents and insults produces similar histologic features, including fibrosis occupying sites of previous anagen follicles and foci indicative of the previous trauma that incited the destructive changes (figs. 14-42, 14-43). Inconspicuous zones of granulomatous inflammation, fragmented hair shafts within the granulomatous foci, twisted and contorted hair shafts within follicular canals, and melanin or hemosiderin within macrophages indicative of the destruction of pigmented follicular epithelium or remote hemorrhage are also present. In follicular degeneration syndrome, there may be premature thinning and attenuation of the follicular sheath epithelium and foci of extruded follicular contents into the adjacent dermis.

The differential diagnosis includes other forms of scarring alopecia, and this may be extremely problematic in end-stage lesions where fibrosis dominates the picture at the expense of residua of primary inflammatory (e.g., lupus or lichen planopilaris) or traumatic (e.g., trichotillomania or traction) causes.

Prevention of mechanical injury is the only treatment for traumatic alopecia. In cases where manipulation of the hair shaft has a psychological basis, counseling should be considered. Once follicular destruction and scarring have developed, there is no effective treatment short of hair transplantation. Treatment for other forms of scarring alopecia also depends upon the underlying cause: treatment of diabetes may resolve necrobiosis lipoidica and antiinflammatory agents may slow or prevent hair loss in cicatricial pemphigoid, sarcoidosis, and even in later stages of cytotoxic follicular injury progressing in the direction of end-stage scarring alopecia (so-called pseudopelade).

*Inflammatory Disorders of the Skin*

**Figure 14-42**

**TRAUMATIC ALOPECIA**

A: There is prominent perifollicular fibrosis, zones of scarring correlating with tracks occupied by preexisting follicles, and marked diminution in hair density. Occasional transverse sections representing anagen follicles within the subcutis appear to be uninvolved.

B: A twisted "corkscrew" hair remnant is present within the follicular infundibulum.

C: There is prominent fibrous thickening of the adventitial sheath of an involuting follicle.

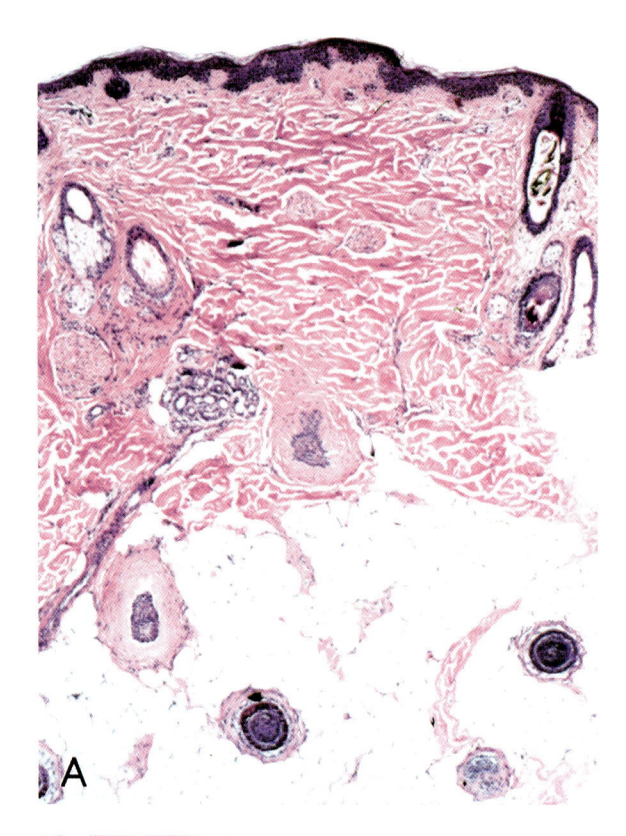

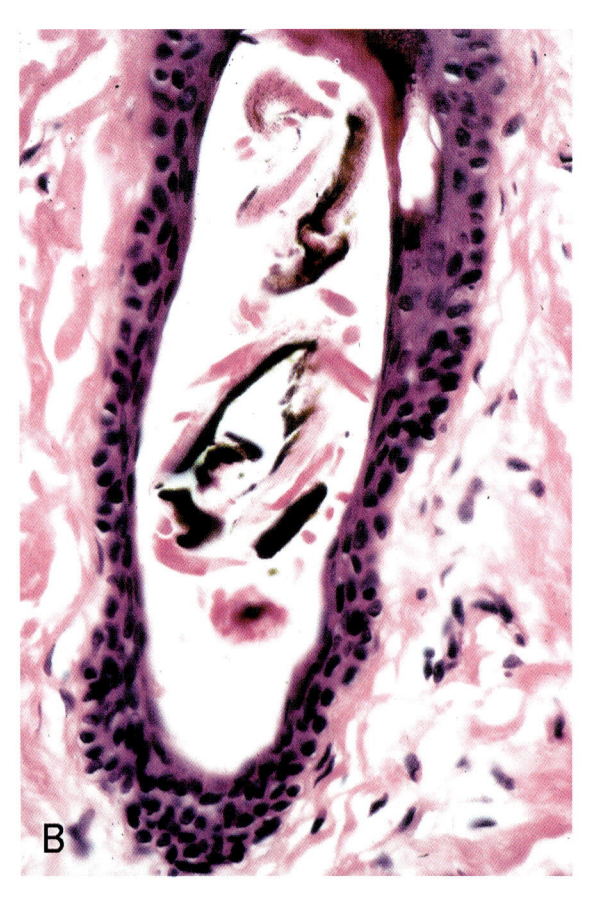

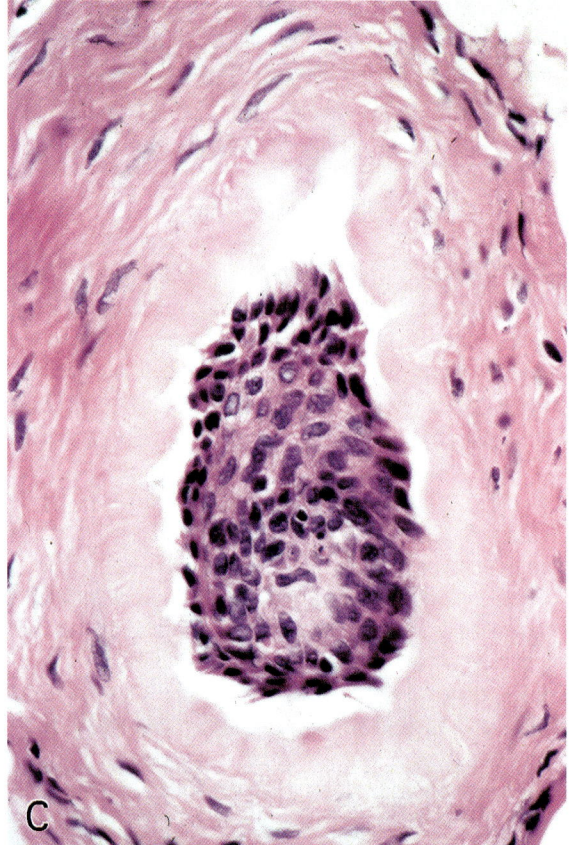

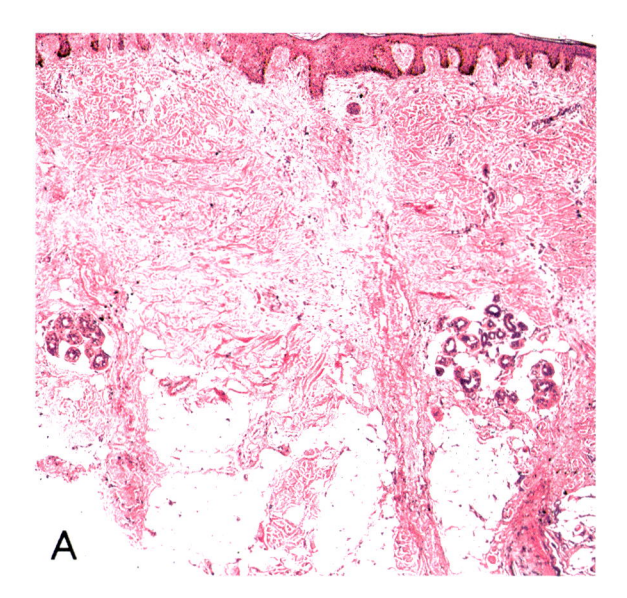

*Inflammatory Disorders with Primary Adnexal Alterations: Follicular Conditions*

**Figure 14-43**

**SCARRING ALOPECIA**

A: The dermis shows no evidence of previous follicles aside from finger-like zones of fibrosis that extend into subcutaneous fat.

B: At higher magnification, the zone fibrosis that extends into the subcutis contains a centrally hyalinized region, the remnant of the follicular glassy membrane.

C: In pseudopelade, rare appendages (a sebaceous gland and pilar muscle) surround fibrotic tracts in the absence of inflammation.

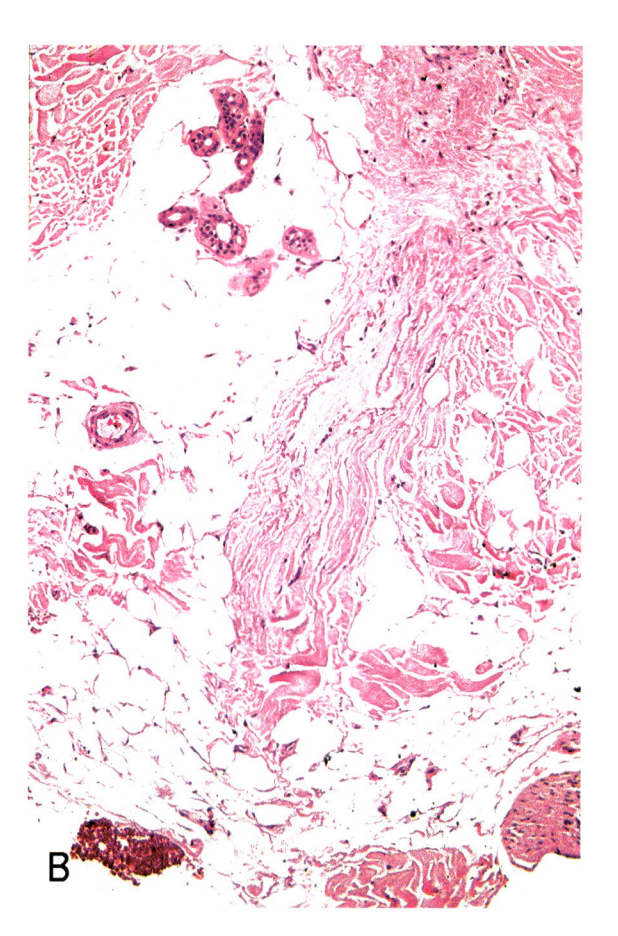

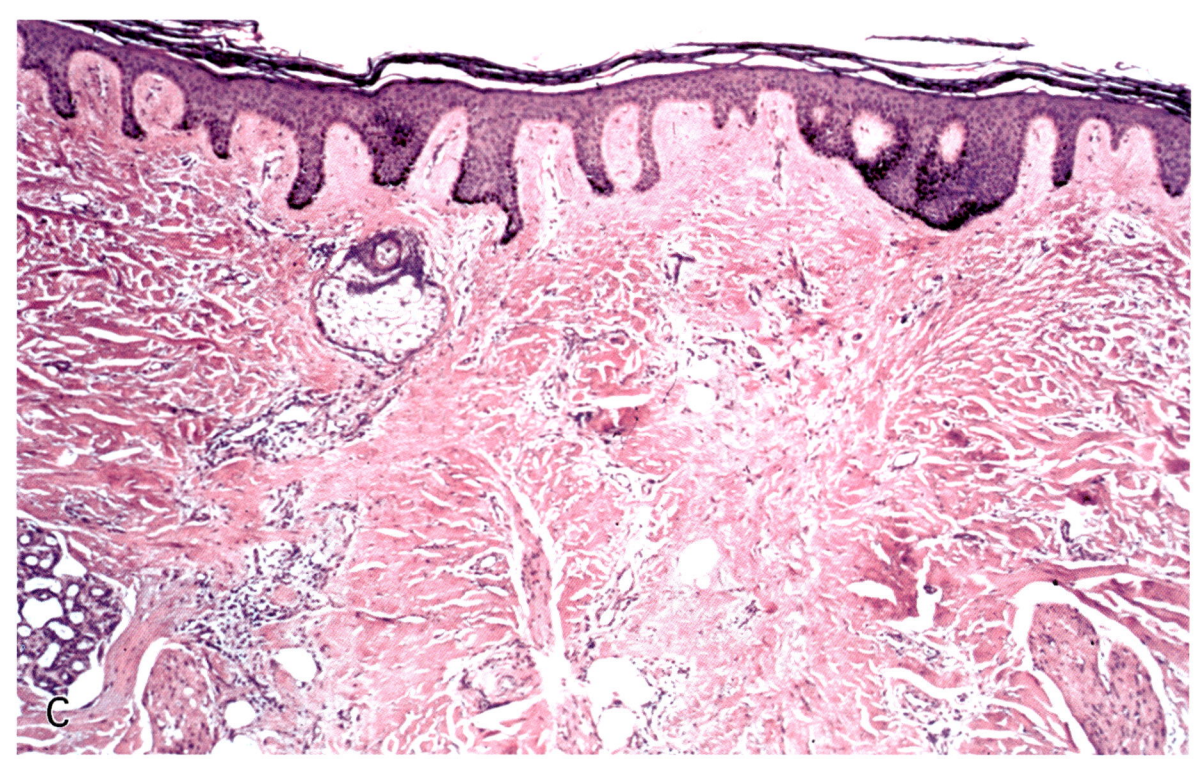

# REFERENCES

1. Bergfeld WF. The pathophysiology of acne vulgaris in children and adolescents, Part 1. Cutis 2004;74:92-7.
1a. Mirshahpanah P, Maibach HI. Models in acnegenesis. Cutan Ocul Toxicol 2007;26:195-202.
1b. Domashenko A, Gupta S, Cotsarelis G. Efficient delivery of transgenes to human hair follicle progenitor cells using topical lipoplex. Nat Biotechnol 2000;18:420-3.
1c. Cotsarelis G, Sun TT, Lavker RM. Label-retaining cells reside in the bulge area of pilosebaceous unit: implications for follicular stem cells, hair cycle, and skin carcinogenesis. Cell 1990;61:1329-37.
1d. Murphy GF, Lavker RM, Whitaker D, Korngold R. Cytotoxic folliculitis in GvHD. Evidence of follicular stem cell injury and recovery. J Cutan Pathol 1991;18:309-14.
2. Harper JC. An update on the pathogenesis and management of acne vulgaris. J Am Acad Dermatol 2004;51(Suppl):S36-8.
3. Pawin H, Beylot C, Chivot M, et al. Physiopathology of acne vulgaris: recent data, new understanding of the treatments. Eur J Dermatol 2004;14:4-12.
4. Oberemok SS, Shalita AR. Acne vulgaris, I: pathogenesis and diagnosis. Cutis 2002;70:101-5.
5. Webster GF. Acne vulgaris. BMJ 2002;325:475-9.
6. Webster G. Mechanism-based treatment of acne vulgaris: the value of combination therapy. J Drugs Dermatol 2005;4:281-8.
7. Jain S. Topical tretinoin or adapalene in acne vulgaris: an overview. J Dermatol Treat 2004;15:200-7.
8. Waugh J, Noble S, Scott LJ. Spotlight on adapalene in acne vulgaris. Am J Clin Dermatol 2004;5:369-71.
9. Dreno B. Topical antibacterial therapy for acne vulgaris. Drugs 2004;64:2389-97.
10. Haider A, Shaw JC. Treatment of acne vulgaris. JAMA 2004;292:726-35.
11. Leyden JJ. Antibiotic resistance in the topical treatment of acne vulgaris. Cutis 2004;73(Suppl):6-10.
12. Wolf JE Jr. Maintenance therapy for acne vulgaris: the fine balance between efficacy, cutaneous tolerability, and adherence. Skinmed 2004;3:23-6.
13. Leyden JJ. A review of the use of combination therapies for the treatment of acne vulgaris. J Am Acad Dermatol 2003;49(Suppl):S200-10.
14. Longshore SJ, Hollandsworth K. Acne vulgaris: one treatment does not fit all. Cleve Clin J Med 2003;70:670, 672-4, 677-8.
15. Webster G. Combination azelaic acid therapy for acne vulgaris. J Am Acad Dermatol 2000;43(Pt 3):S47-50.
16. Johnson BA, Nunley JR. Topical therapy for acne vulgaris. How do you choose the best drug for each patient? Postgrad Med 2000;107:69-70, 73-6, 79-80.
17. Luelmo-Aguilar J, Santandreu MS. Folliculitis: recognition and management. Am J Clin Dermatol 2004;5:301-10.
18. Al-Dhafiri SA, Molinari R. Herpetic folliculitis. J Cutan Med Surg 2002;6:19-22.
19. Ayers K, Sweeney SM, Wiss K. Pityrosporum folliculitis: diagnosis and management in 6 female adolescents with acne vulgaris. Arch Pediatr Adolesc Med 2005;159:64-7.
20. Foti C, Filotico R, Calvario A, Conserva A, Antelmi A, Angelini G. Relapsing herpes simplex-2 folliculitis in the beard area. Eur J Dermatol 2004;14:421-3.
21. Stulberg DL, Penrod MA, Blatny RA. Common bacterial skin infections. Am Fam Physician 2002;66:119-24.
22. Guay DR. Treatment of bacterial skin and skin structure infections. Expert Opin Pharmacother 2003;4:1259-75.
23. Gupta AK, Chaudhry MM. Rosacea and its management: an overview. J Eur Acad Dermatol Venereol 2005;19:273-85.
24. Powell FC. Clinical practice. Rosacea. N Engl J Med 2005;352:793-803.
25. Dahl MV. Rosacea subtypes: a treatment algorithm. Cutis 2004;74:21-7, 32-4.
26. Murphy G. Ultraviolet light and rosacea. Cutis 2004;74:13-6, 32-4.
27. Crawford GH, Pelle MT, James WD. Rosacea: I. Etiology, pathogenesis, and subtype classification. J Am Acad Dermatol 2004;51:327-41.
28. Millikan L. The proposed inflammatory pathophysiology of rosacea: implications for treatment. Skinmed 2003;2:43-7.
29. Rohrich RJ, Griffin JR, Adams WP Jr. Rhinophyma: review and update. Plast Reconstr Surg 2002;110:860-69.
30. Stone DU, Chodosh J. Ocular rosacea: an update on pathogenesis and therapy. Curr Opin Ophthalmol 2004;15:499-502.
31. Tanzi EL, Weinberg JM. The ocular manifestations of rosacea. Cutis 2001;68:112-4.
32. Wolf JE Jr. Present and future rosacea therapy. Cutis 2005;75(Suppl):4-7.
33. Pelle MT, Crawford GH, James WD. Rosacea: II. Therapy. J Am Acad Dermatol 2004;51:499-512.

34. Lowe NJ. Use of topical metronidazole in moderate to severe rosacea. Adv Ther 2003;20:177-90.
35. Rebora A. The management of rosacea. Am J Clin Dermatol 2002;3:489-96.
36. Zouboulis CC. Retinoids—which dermatological indications will benefit in the near future? Skin Pharmacol Appl Skin Physiol 2001;14:303-15.
37. Callaway SR, Lesher JL Jr. Keratosis pilaris atrophicans: case series and review. Pediatr Dermatol 2004;21:14-7.
38. Lateef A, Schwartz RA. Keratosis pilaris. Cutis 1999;63:205-7.
39. Gerbig AW. Treating keratosis pilaris. J Am Acad Dermatol 2002;47:457.
40. Ellis E, Scheinfeld N. Eosinophilic pustular folliculitis: a comprehensive review of treatment options. Am J Clin Dermatol 2004;5:189-97.
41. Lazarov A, Wolach B, Cordoba M, Abraham D, Vardy D. Eosinophilic pustular folliculitis (Ofuji disease) in a child. Cutis 1996;58:135-8.
42. Dupond AS, Aubin F, Bourezane Y, Faivre B, Van Landuyt H, Humbert PH. Eosinophilic pustular folliculitis in infancy: report of two affected brothers. Br J Dermatol 1995;132:296-9.
43. Camacho-Martinez F. Eosinophilic pustular folliculitis. J Am Acad Dermatol 1987;17:686-8.
44. Majamaa H, Vaalasti A, Vaajalahti P, Reunala T. Eosinophilic pustular folliculitis. J Eur Acad Dermatol Venereol 2002;16:522-5.
45. Ellis E, Scheinfeld N. Eosinophilic pustular folliculitis: a comprehensive review of treatment options. Am J Clin Dermatol 2004;5:189-97.
46. Misago N, Narisawa Y, Matsubara S, Hayashi S. HIV-associated eosinophilic pustular folliculitis: successful treatment of a Japanese patient with UVB phototherapy. J Dermatol 1998;25:178-84.
47. Alexis AF, Dudda-Subramanya R, Sinha AA. Alopecia areata: autoimmune basis of hair loss. Eur J Dermatol 2004;14:364-70.
48. Norris D. Alopecia areata: current state of knowledge. J Am Acad Dermatol 2004;51(Suppl):S16-7.
49. Hordinsky M, Ericson M. Autoimmunity: alopecia areata. J Investi Dermatol Symp Proc 2004;9:73-8.
50. McDonagh AJ, Tazi-Ahnini R. Epidemiology and genetics of alopecia areata. Clin Exp Dermatol 2002;27:405-9.
51. Randall VA. Is alopecia areata an autoimmune disease? Lancet 2001;358:1922-4.
52. Papadopoulos AJ, Schwartz RA, Janniger CK. Alopecia areata. Pathogenesis, diagnosis, and therapy. Am J Clin Dermatol 2000;1:101-5.
53. Duvic M, Nelson A, de Andrade M. The genetics of alopecia areata. Clin Dermatol 2001;19:135-9.
54. McElwee K, Freyschmidt-Paul P, Ziegler A, Happle R, Hoffmann R. Genetic susceptibility and severity of alopecia areata in human and animal models. Eur J Dermatol 2001;11:11-6.
55. Green J, Sinclair RD. Genetics of alopecia areata. Australas J Dermatol 2000;41:213-8.
56. Bertolino AP. Alopecia areata. A clinical overview. Postgrad Med 2000;107:81-5, 89-90.
57. Madani S, Shapiro J. Alopecia areata update. J Am Acad Dermatol 2000;42:549-66.
58. Price VH. Therapy of alopecia areata: on the cusp and in the future. J Invest Dermatol Symp Proc 2003;8:207-11.
59. Freyschmidt-Paul P, Happle R, McElwee KJ, Hoffmann R. Alopecia areata: treatment of today and tomorrow. J Invest Dermatol Symp Proc 2003;8:12-7.
60. Sehgal VN, Jain S. Alopecia areata: clinical perspective and an insight into pathogenesis. J Dermatol 2003;30:271-89.
61. Freyschmidt-Paul P, Hoffmann R, Levine E, Sundberg JP, Happle R, McElwee KJ. Current and potential agents for the treatment of alopecia areata. Curr Pharm Des 2001;7:213-30.
62. Hernandez BA. Is androgenic alopecia a result of endocrine effects on the vasculature? Med Hypotheses 2004;62:438-41.
63. Birch MP, Lalla SC, Messenger AG. Female pattern hair loss. Clin Exp Dermatol 2002;27:383-8.
64. Hoffmann R. Male androgenetic alopecia. Clin Exp Dermatol 2002;27:373-82.
65. Bolduc C, Shapiro J. Management of androgenetic alopecia. Am J Clin Dermatol 2000;1:151-8.
66. Sinclair RD, Dawber RP. Androgenetic alopecia in men and women. Clin Dermatol 2001;19:167-78.
67. Ellis JA, Harrap SB. The genetics of androgenetic alopecia. Clin Dermatol 2001;19:149-54.
68. Ramos-e-Silva M. Male pattern hair loss: prevention rather than regrowth. Int J Dermatol 2000;39:728-31.
69. Hogan DJ, Chamberlain M. Male pattern baldness. South Med J 2000;93:657-62.
70. Price VH. Androgenetic alopecia in women. J Invest Dermatol Symp Proc 2003;8:24-7.
71. Chartier MB, Hoss DM, Grant-Kels JM. Approach to the adult female patient with diffuse nonscarring alopecia. J Am Acad Dermatol 2002;47:809-18.
72. Price VH. Androgenetic alopecia in adolescents. Cutis 2003;71:115-21.
73. Burkhart CG, Burkhart CN. 5 alpha-reductase and finasteride in pattern alopecia and acne. J Drugs Dermatol 2004;3:363-4.
74. Libecco JF, Bergfeld WF. Finasteride in the treatment of alopecia. Expert Opin Pharmacother 2004;5:933-40.
75. Sinclair RD. Management of male pattern hair loss. Cutis 2001;68:35-40.
76. Redmond GP, Bergfeld WF. Treatment of androgenic disorders in women: acne, hirsutism, and alopecia. Cleve Clin J Med 1990;57:428-32.

77. LeBoit PE. Alopecia mucinosa, inflammatory disease or mycosis fungoides: must we choose? And are there other choices? Am J Dermatopathol 2004;26:167-70.
78. Anderson BE, Mackley CL, Helm KF. Alopecia mucinosa: report of a case and review. J Cutan Med Surg 2003;7:124-8.
79. Plotnick H, Abbrecht M. Alopecia mucinosa and lymphoma. Report of two cases and review of literature. Arch Dermatol 1965;92:137-41.
80. Boer A, Guo Y, Ackerman AB. Alopecia mucinosa is mycosis fungoides. Am J Dermatopathol 2004;26:33-52.
81. Boer A, Ackerman AB. Alopecia mucinosa or follicular mucinosis—the problem is terminology! J Cutan Pathol 2004;31:210-1.
81a. Meissner K, Weyer U, Kowalzick L, Altenhoff J. Successful treatment of primary progressive follicular mucinosis with interferons. J Am Acad Dermatol 1991;24(Pt 2):848-50.
82. Fabbri P, Amato L, Chiarini C, Moretti S, Massi D. Scarring alopecia in discoid lupus erythematosus: a clinical, histopathologic and immunopathologic study. Lupus 2004;13:455-62.
83. Miteva L. Alopecia: a rare manifestation of lupus vulgaris. Int J Dermatol 2001;40:659-61.
84. Inaloz HS, Chowdhury MM, Motley RJ. Lupus erythematosus/lichen planus overlap syndrome with scarring alopecia. J Eur Acad Dermatol Venereol 2001;15:171-4.
85. Annessi G, Lombardo G, Gobello T, Puddu P. A clinicopathologic study of scarring alopecia due to lichen planus: comparison with scarring alopecia in discoid lupus erythematosus and pseudopelade. Am J Dermatopathol 1999;21:324-31.
86. Crowley E, Frieden IJ. Neonatal lupus erythematosus: an unusual congenital presentation with cutaneous atrophy, erosions, alopecia, and pancytopenia. Pediatr Dermatol 1998;15:38-42.
87. Wiedemeyer K, Schill WB, Loser C. Diseases on hair follicles leading to hair loss part II: scarring alopecias. Skinmed 2004;3:266-9.
88. Gupta SN, Palceski D. Lichen planopilaris presenting as truncal alopecia: a case presentation and review of the literature. Cutis 2003;72:63-6.
89. Chieregato C, Zini A, Barba A, Magnanini M, Rosina P. Lichen planopilaris: report of 30 cases and review of the literature. Int J Dermatol 2003;42:342-5.
90. Mirmirani P, Willey A, Price VH. Short course of oral cyclosporine in lichen planopilaris. J Am Acad Dermatol 2003;49:667-71.
91. Mehregan DA, Van Hale HM, Muller SA. Lichen planopilaris: clinical and pathologic study of forty-five patients. J Am Acad Dermatol 1992;27:935-42.
92. Matta M, Kibbi AG, Khattar J, Salman SM, Zaynoun ST. Lichen planopilaris: a clinicopathologic study. J Am Acad Dermatol 1990;22:594-8.
93. Kuprevich CL, Nagra B, Rosenbaum R. Trichotillomania: a brief review. Del Med J 2005;77:253-7.
94. Tay YK, Levy ML, Metry DW. Trichotillomania in childhood: case series and review. Pediatrics 2004;113:494-8.
95. Nuss MA, Carlisle D, Hall M, Yerneni SC, Kovach R. Trichotillomania: a review and case report. Cutis 2003;72:191-6.
96. Papadopoulos AJ, Janniger CK, Chodynicki MP, Schwartz RA. Trichotillomania. Int J Dermatol 2003;42:330-4.
97. Hautmann G, Hercogova J, Lotti T. Trichotillomania. J Am Acad Dermatol 2002;46:807-21.
98. Bergfeld W, Mulinari-Brenner F, McCarron K, Embi C. The combined utilization of clinical and histological findings in the diagnosis of trichotillomania. J Cutan Pathol 2002;29:207-14.
99. Walsh KH, McDougle CJ. Trichotillomania. Presentation, etiology, diagnosis and therapy. Am J Clin Dermatol 2001;2:327-33.
100. Chamberlain SR, Blackwell AD, Fineberg NA, Robbins TW, Sahakian BJ. Strategy implementation in obsessive-compulsive disorder and trichotillomania. Psychol Med 2006;36:91-7
101. Walsh KH, McDougle CJ. Pharmacological strategies for trichotillomania. Expert Opin Pharmacother 2005;6:975-84.
102. van Minnen A, Hoogduin KA, Keijsers GP, Hellenbrand I, Hendriks GJ. Treatment of trichotillomania with behavioral therapy or fluoxetine: a randomized, waiting-list controlled study. Arch Gen Psychiatry 2003;60:517-22.
103. Stewart RS, Nejtek VA. An open-label, flexible-dose study of olanzapine in the treatment of trichotillomania. J Clin Psychiatry 2003;64:49-52.
104. Khouzam HR, Battista MA, Byers PE. An overview of trichotillomania and its response to treatment with quetiapine. Psychiatry 2002;65:261-70.
105. Bohne A, Keuthen NJ, Tuschen-Caffier B, Wilhelm S. Cognitive inhibition in trichotillomania and obsessive-compulsive disorder. Behav Res Ther 2005;43:923-42.
106. Hantash BM, Schwartz RA. Traction alopecia in children. Cutis 2003;71:18-20.
107. Sperling LC, Sau P. The follicular degeneration syndrome in black patients. 'Hot comb alopecia' revisited and revised. Arch Dermatol 1992;128:68-74.
108. Sperling LC, Skelton HG 3rd, Smith KJ, Sau P, Friedman K. Follicular degeneration syndrome in men. Arch Dermatol 1994;130:763-9.

# 15 APOCRINE AND ECCRINE CONDITIONS

## MILIARIA GROUP

**Definition.** Eccrine sweat duct occlusion is the basic cause of all types of *miliaria* (1,2). Whether or not the sweat leaks into the inflammatory tissue because of rupture of the ducts determines the type of inflammatory reaction. *Eccrine miliaria* is a disorder in which sweat is retained within the skin due to a variety of local factors.

**Clinical Features.** There are four types of miliaria. In *miliaria crystallina*, superficial noninflammatory vesicles rupture easily on trauma (3,4). *Miliaria rubra*, also known as *prickly heat,* is the presence of inflamed papules after repeated episodes of sweating in infants and adults, especially in an environment that is humid and hot (5,6). If the lesions become pustular, it is called *miliaria pustulosa* (7). The final type of miliaria, *miliaria profunda* (8), occurs after exposure to a very hot environment; for example, troops sent into the tropics develop miliaria profunda. The skin is covered with multiple papules that are reminiscent of goose flesh, or sometimes, no papules are evident. Ductal blockade results in rupture of the ducts and leakage of the sweat into the skin. Unless rapid adequate treatment is instituted, patients lose the cooling effect of sweating and may die of hyperthermia and hypersphyxia.

**Pathologic Findings.** Spongiotic vesicles arise in the intraepidermal and superficial dermal portions of the sweat duct (figs. 15-1, 15-2). In miliaria crystallina, the vesicle is subcorneal and confined to the intraepidermal duct. In

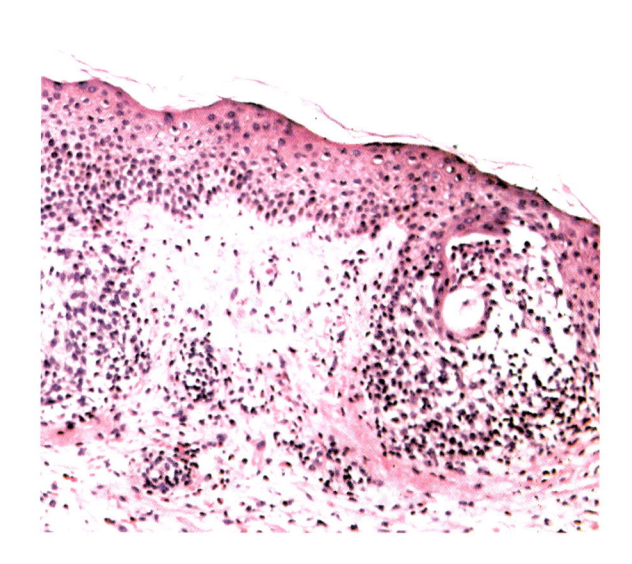

Figure 15-1

**MILIARIA**

Above: At scanning magnification, there is a brisk inflammatory infiltrate centered about the superficial portion of the eccrine ducts.

Right: At higher magnification, there is striking exocytosis of lymphocytes within the acrosyringium. A Langerhans cell microgranuloma is forming.

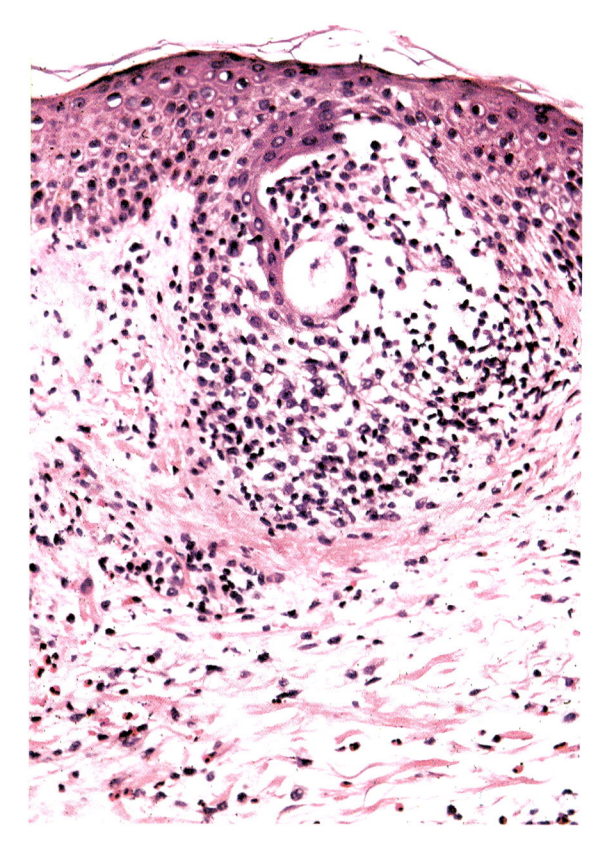

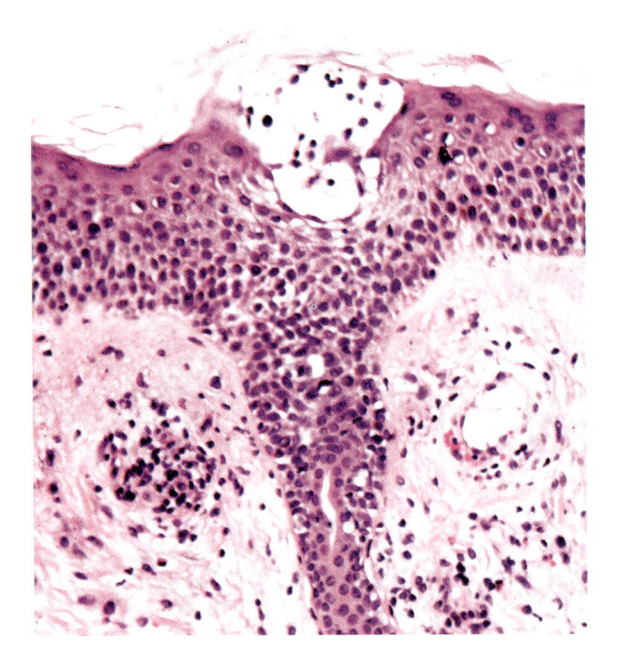

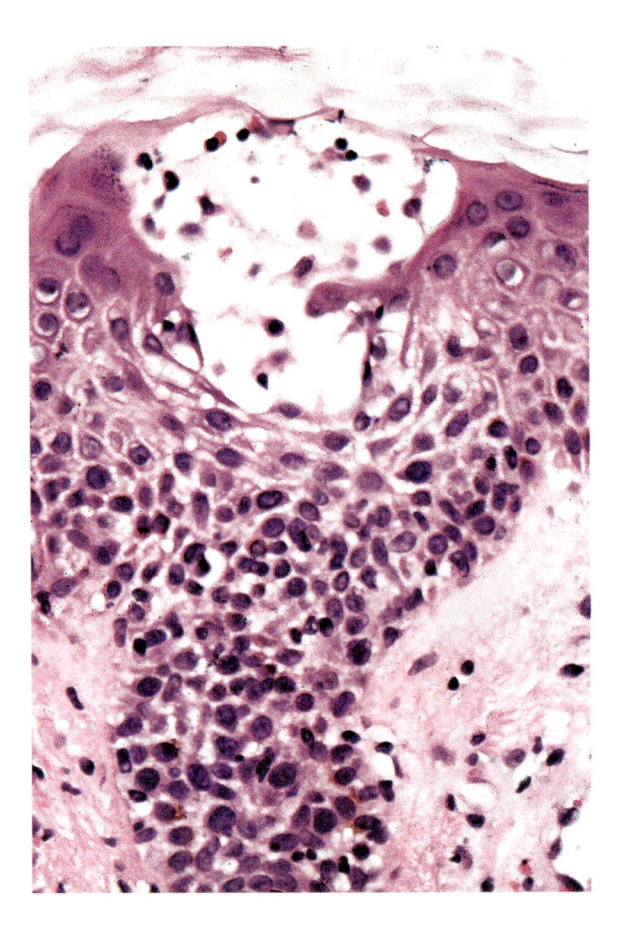

*Inflammatory Disorders of the Skin*

Figure 15-2
**MILIARIA: EARLY VESICLE FORMATION**
Above: The vesicle is forming in a subcorneal location directly above the eccrine duct.
Right: At higher power, the subcorneum contains mixed inflammatory cells in addition to fluid. Spongiosis is adjacent.

miliaria rubra, there is an associated periductular lymphocytic infiltrate, and the duct lumen may contain inspissated periodic acid–Schiff (PAS)-positive secretions. In miliaria profunda, there is a striking change in the eccrine gland: the cells form a syncytium in the acute phase. In extreme cases the sweat duct ruptures, with associated inflammation. Multiple biopsy levels may be required to detect these alterations.

**Differential Diagnosis.** Early contact dermatitis or cutaneous lymphangioma should be differentiated clinically from miliaria crystallina. Miliaria rubra, if involving the axillary areas, is similar to apocrine miliaria. If scattered on the skin, it also resembles erythema toxicum neonatorum in infants, especially when pustular. It can also resemble a drug reaction. The goose flesh appearance of miliaria profunda must be differentiated from other papular eruptions such as insect bite reactions, papular urticaria, or systemic hypersensitivity reactions, as to a drug.

**Treatment and Prognosis.** For miliaria crystallina, proper ventilation and cool compresses are usually sufficient. For miliaria rubra, a cool environment and a topical antiinflammatory lotion containing corticosteroids or menthol result in quick resolution of the lesions. In miliaria profunda, a cool environment and antiinflammatory agents are useful. If the patient becomes hyperthermic, immersion in cold water may be necessary. In order to counteract the vasoconstriction induced by rapid cooling, chlorpromazine is used. When the symptoms are severe, oral corticosteroids may be necessary.

## NEUTROPHILIC ECCRINE HIDRADENITIS

**Definition.** *Neutrophilic eccrine hidradenitis* primarily affects the eccrine secretory coil in association with drug therapy, particularly certain chemotherapeutic agents (9–16). It is a member of the family of neutrophilic dermatoses and dermatosis-like disorders.

**Clinical Features.** The lesions present as single to multiple, erythematous to purpuric papules, nodules, and plaques on the trunk and extremities. Acute myelogenous leukemia

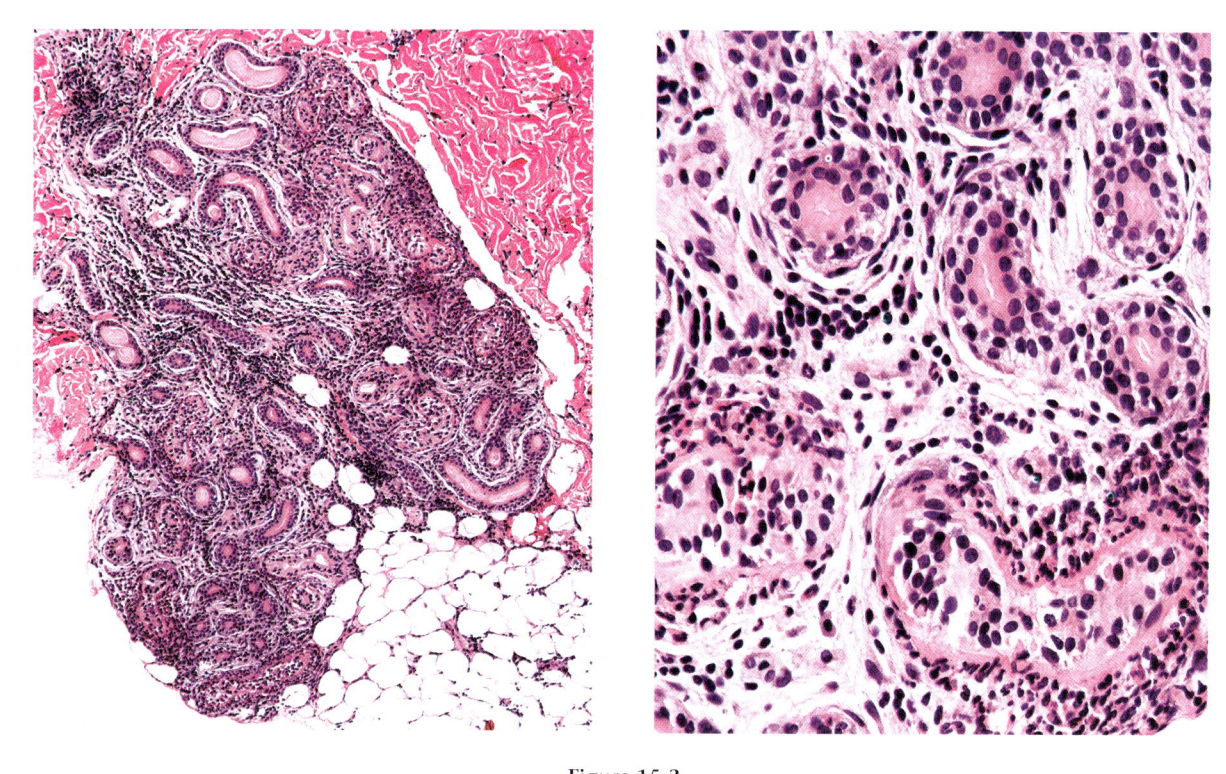

**Figure 15-3**

**NEUTROPHILIC ECCRINE HIDRADENITIS**

Left: At scanning magnification, a brisk inflammatory infiltrate is centered about the eccrine coil.
Right: At higher magnification, mixed inflammatory cells with a preponderance of neutrophils are evident.

associated with chemotherapy (cytosine arabinoside induction therapy) is often the setting. The lesions may occur during or months after chemotherapy. Neutrophilic eccrine hidradenitis is also associated with infection, specifically infection with gram-positive bacteria and dermatophytes. At present, there is no known association between neutrophilic eccrine hidradenitis and other forms of neutrophilic dermatosis associated with leukemia/lymphoma.

**Pathologic Findings.** The neutrophilic infiltration specifically involves the eccrine coil. Secondary secretory epithelial vacuolization and necrosis with neutrophils occur in the glands (figs. 15-3, 15-4).

**Differential Diagnosis.** The clinical differential diagnosis includes leukemia cutis, sepsis, vasculitis, and neutrophilic dermatosis. The histopathology is reasonably specific, however, and the primary diagnostic pitfall involves lack of recognition or awareness of this entity. Multiple levels may be required to identify the most characteristic alterations. Pure lymphocytic eccrine hidradenitis is generally associated with other diagnostic changes, as in pernio.

**Treatment and Prognosis.** Unlike the conditions in the clinical differential diagnosis, lesions may subside spontaneously. Nonsteroidal medication is useful for patients in discomfort. Similar to other neutrophilic dermatoses, topical or systemic steroids are needed in severe cases.

## HIDRADENITIS SUPPURATIVA

**Definition.** *Hidradenitis suppurativa* is characterized by draining sinuses and scarring in an apocrine distribution. Although a pathogenic role or relationship to apocrine glands has not been established, the disease has a striking predilection for the axilla, groin, and lower abdomen, sites of apocrine gland function (17).

**Clinical Features.** Patients present with painful nodules and follicular lesions in the above-mentioned regions. Acutely, the lesions are erythematous and edematous nodules and cysts (fig. 15-5). Scarring is seen with chronicity (fig. 15-6). Sinuses develop that may suppurate

*Inflammatory Disorders of the Skin*

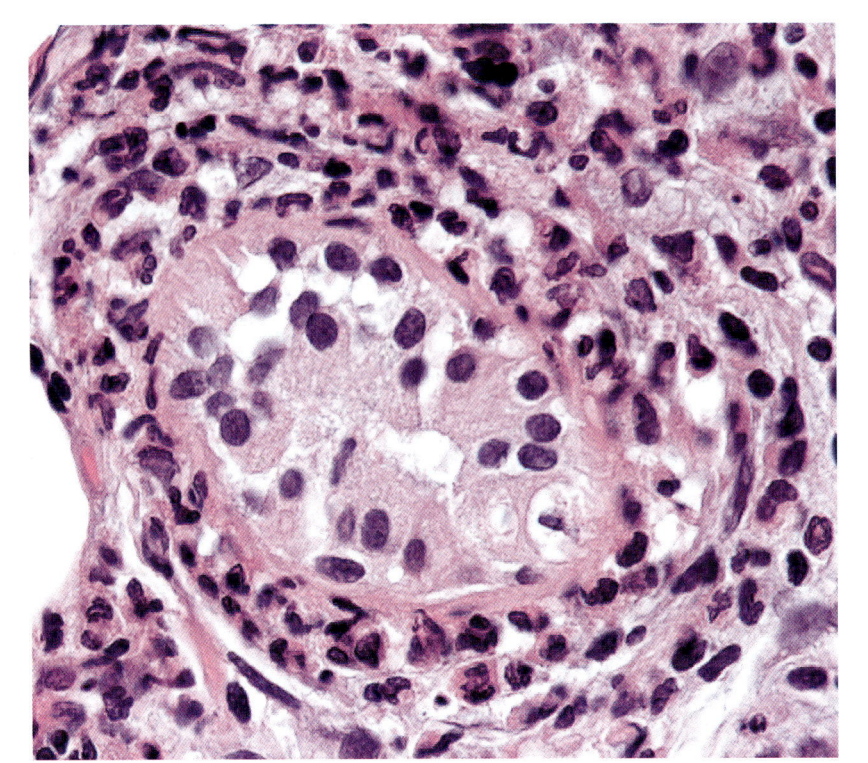

**Figure 15-4**
**NEUROPHILIC ECCRINE HIDRADENITIS**
The neutrophilic infiltrate is associated with vacuolar degeneration and necrosis of the secretory epithelial cells.

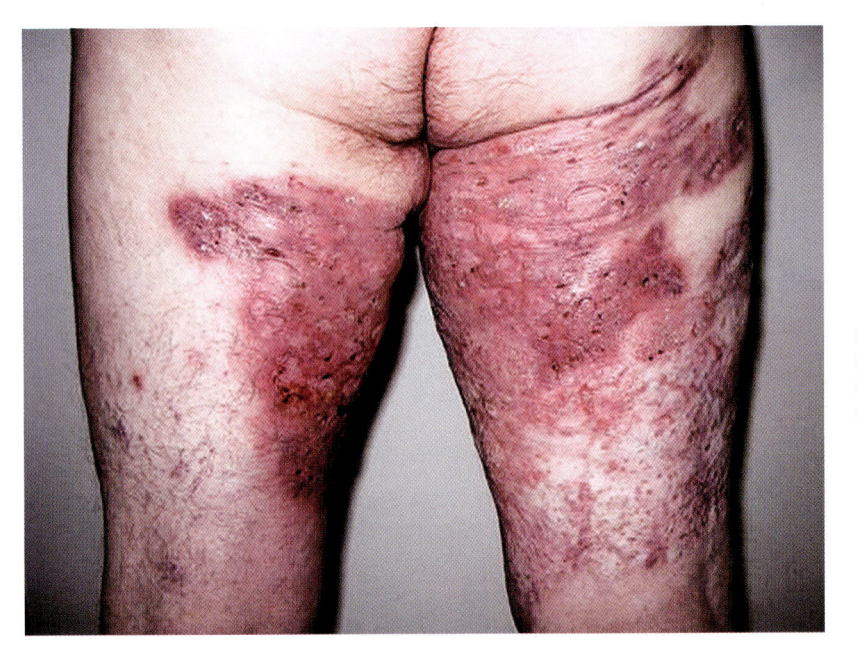

**Figure 15-5**
**HIDRADENITIS SUPPURATIVA**
This is a form of purulent and fibrosing folliculitis, rather than a disorder of sweat glands. Boggy erythematous plaques, often with draining sinuses, are produced.

and create a malodorous discharge. The disorder can occur as part of the so-called occlusion triad, which in addition includes acne conglobata and dissecting cellulitis of the scalp.

**Pathologic Findings.** The histopathology may not be diagnostic and clinicopathologic correlation is essential. In the acute phase, a dermal polymorphous infiltrate is noted, including neutrophils, lymphocytes, histiocytes, and rare eosinophils. Association of the infiltrate with apocrine glands is a secondary effect and is the exception rather than the rule. Eccrine glands may be involved. Deep abscesses may be noted and sinuses lined with squamous epithelium are

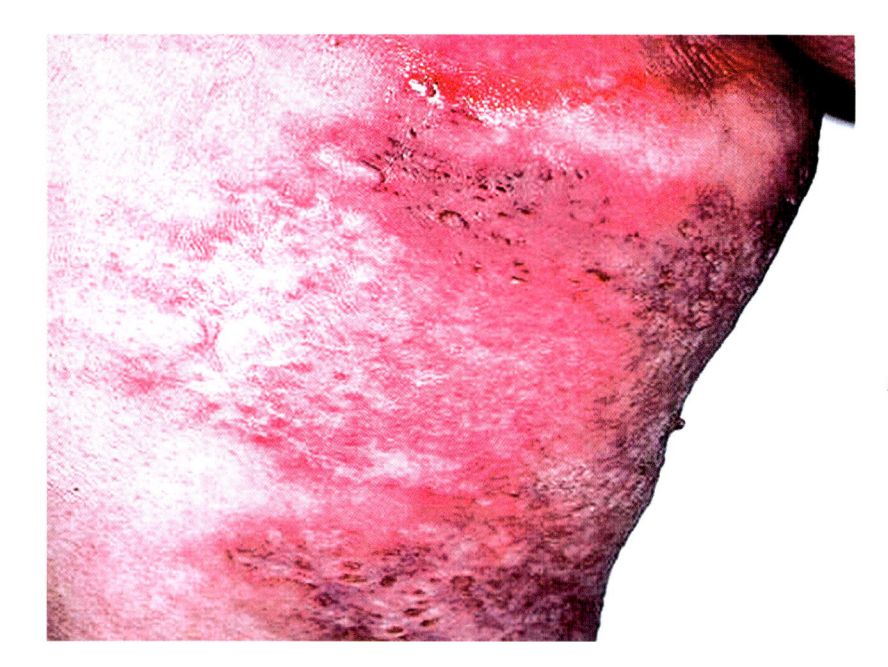

**Figure 15-6**

**HIDRADENITIS SUPPURATIVA**

The chronic manifestation of zones of scarring.

often present. Keratin production may incite a dense granulomatous reaction surrounding the sinuses and follicular structures. In the late stage, little to no inflammation is observed, and instead, fibrosis may be prominent around apocrine glands. Many consider hidradenitis suppurativa to represent an advanced and diffuse purulent form of folliculitis (see fig. 14-4) with prominent sinus tract formation and a predisposition for apocrine-rich areas.

**Differential Diagnosis.** Infection must be ruled out and appropriate stains for microorganisms should be obtained. Occasionally, the lesions become superinfected, and microbial colonization on histopathology does not exclude the diagnosis. Involvement of eccrine glands may suggest the diagnosis of eccrine miliaria but does not exclude hidradenitis.

**Treatment and Prognosis.** The disease may have a prolonged course (18). Initially, topical antibiotics, such as clindamycin, and topical retinoids are helpful. Oral antibiotics are used for both their antimicrobial and antiinflammatory functions when the disease flares. Oral retinoids have been used with variable success. Intralesional steroids are often more helpful than topical steroids for controlling the acute inflammation associated with hidradenitis. Systemic antitumor necrosis factor-alpha agents such as etanercept are effective in some cases (19). Cyclosporine, antiandrogens, and pentoxyphylline are also used. The prognosis is poor once patients have developed scarring. Most lesions have a chronic flaring and remitting course.

## APOCRINE MILIARIA

**Definition.** *Apocrine miliaria*, also known as *Fox-Fordyce disease*, is caused by inflammation and keratotic plugging of apocrine glands leading to pruritus and inflammation of involved areas of skin (20).

**Clinical Features.** Apocrine miliaria is a rare inflammatory disorder most commonly seen in adult females; rare cases have been reported in males. The main symptom is pruritus, which is often paroxysmal and related to emotional stress, weather changes, physical stimuli, or sexual activity. Apocrine-bearing areas of skin are involved, most commonly the axilla; however, anogenital, periareolar, and truncal areas are involved on rare occasion. Hair loss may be noted in areas affected by the disease.

**Pathologic Findings.** The acute inflammation of the apocrine glands and follicular infundibulum may extend to the dermis and deep subcutaneous layers. Apocrine glands may be dilated as secretions are entrapped by the inflammatory infiltrate. There may be follicular plugging, hyperkeratosis, and spongiosis of the follicular infundibulum as well as of the apocrine duct (21). Late lesions may show scarring surrounding apocrine glands. Necrosis is not a predominant feature. In very late-stage lesions, the apocrine glands may not be seen at all, having been replaced by scarring and fibrosis.

**Differential Diagnosis.** The diagnosis of apocrine miliaria is difficult to make in the absence of clinical information. Keratosis pilaris and pityriasis rubra pilaris may enter the differential diagnosis if apocrine glands are not present in the sections examined. Primary disorders of the hair follicle and follicular eczema may be entertained and microbiologic stains should be performed to exclude infection when indicated.

**Treatment and Prognosis.** The disease is treated with topical and intralesional steroids, as well as topical clindamycin and retinoids (22). Systemic steroids are useful for acute flares but their role in chronic therapy is limited. Oral retinoids have been used with variable success. Women respond to oral contraceptives. Spontaneous resolution has been documented after menopause (23).

## REFERENCES

1. Haas N, Henz BM, Weigel H. Congenital miliaria crystallina. J Am Acad Dermatol 2002;47(Suppl):S270-2.
2. Feng E, Janniger CK. Miliaria. Cutis 1995;55:213-6.
3. Haas N, Martens F, Henz BM. Miliaria crystallina in an intensive care setting. Clin Exp Dermatol 2004;29:32-4.
4. Anbu AT, Williams S. Miliaria crystallina complicating staphylococcal scalded skin syndrome. Arch Dis Child 2004;89:94.
5. Urbatsch A, Paller AS. Pustular miliaria rubra: a specific cutaneous finding of type I pseudohypoaldosteronism. Pediatr Dermatol 2002;19:317-9.
6. Donoghue AM, Sinclair MJ. Miliaria rubra of the lower limbs in underground miners. Occup Med (Lond) 2000;50:430-3.
7. Nanda S, Reddy BS, Ramji S, Pandhi D. Analytical study of pustular eruptions in neonates. Pediatr Dermatol 2002;19:210-5.
8. Kirk JF, Wilson BB, Chun W, Cooper PH. Miliaria profunda. J Am Acad Dermatol 1996;35(Pt 2):854-6.
9. Shih IH, Huang YH, Yang CH, Yang LC, Hong HS. Childhood neutrophilic eccrine hidradenitis: a clinicopathologic and immunohistochemical study of 10 patients. J Am Acad Dermatol 2005;52:963-6.
10. Headley CM, Ioffreda MD, Zaenglein AL. Neutrophilic eccrine hidradenitis: a case report of an unusual annular presentation. Cutis 2005;75:93-7.
11. Chng WJ, Thamboo TP. Unusual presentation of neutrophilic eccrine hidradenitis. Br J Dermatol 2004;151:507-8.
12. Mercader-Garcia P, Vilata-Corell JJ, Pardo-Sanchez J, Fortea-Baixauli JM. Neutrophilic eccrine hidradenitis in a patient with Behcet's disease. Acta Derm Venereol 2003;83:395-6.
13. Roustan G, Salas C, Cabrera R, Simon A. Neutrophilic eccrine hidradenitis unassociated with chemotherapy in a patient with acute myelogenous leukemia. Int J Dermatol 2001;40:144-7.
14. Keane FM, Munn SE, Buckley DA, Hopster D, Mufti GJ, du Vivier AW. Neutrophilic eccrine hidradenitis in two neutropaenic patients. Clin Exp Dermatol 2001;26:162-5.
15. Bachmeyer C, Aractingi S. Neutrophilic eccrine hidradenitis. Clin Dermatol 2000;18:319-30.
16. Combemale P, Faisant M, Azoulay-Petit C, Dupin M, Kanitakis J. Neutrophilic eccrine hidradenitis secondary to infection with Serratia marcescens. Br J Dermatol 2000;142:784-8.
17. Attanoos RL, Appleton MA, Douglas-Jones AG. The pathogenesis of hidradenitis suppurativa: a closer look at apocrine and eccrine glands. Br J Dermatol 1995;133:254-8
18. Shah N. Hidradenitis suppurativa: a treatment challenge. Am Fam Phys 2005:72:1547-52.
19. Cusack C, Buckley C. Etanercept: effective in the management of hidradenitis suppurativa. Br J Dermatol 2006:154:726-9.
20. Kamada A, Saga K, Jimbow K. Apoeccrine sweat duct obstruction as a cause for Fox-Fordyce disease. J Am Acad Dermatol 2003;48:453-5.
21. Macarenco RS, Garces SJC. Dilation of apocrine glands. A forgotten but helpful histopathological clue to the diagnosis of axillary Fox-Fordyce disease. Am J Dermatopathol 2009;31:393-7.
22. Miller ML, Harford RR, Yeager JK. Fox-Fordyce disease treated with topical clindamycin solution. Arch Dermatol 1995:131:1112-3.
23. Katsambas AD, Lotti TM. European handbook of dermatological treatments, 2nd ed. Berlin: Springer; 2003:52-3.

# Index*

## A

Acantholysis, epidermal, 10
Acantholytic dermatitis, 113, *see also under individual entities*
    Darier disease, 125
    diagnostic studies, 113
    Grover disease, 123
    Hailey-Hailey disease, 126
    herpes blisters, 129
    pathogenesis, 113
    pemphigus, 114
Acantholytic dyskeratosis, epidermal, 11
Acanthosis, epidermal, 8
Acanthotic dermatitis, 73, *see also under individual entities*
    chronic seborrheic dermatitis, 92
    halogen induced, 100
    hyperkeratosis lenticularis perstans, 98
    interface dermatitis, 103
    lichen simplex chronicus, 74
    mycotic infection induced, 100
    pityriasis rosea, 94
    pityriasis rubra pilaris, 89
    prurigo nodularis, 74
    psoriasiform nutritional disorders, 107
    psoriasiform stasis dermatitis, 97
    psoriasis, 78
        and AIDS, 89
        erythrodermic psoriasis, 88
        follicular psoriasis, 88
        pustular psoriasis, 87
        Reiter disease, 87
Acne fulminans, 433
Acne keloidalis nuchae, 434
Acne rosacea, 443
Acne vulgaris, 432
Acquired immunodeficiency syndrome (AIDS), **89**, 92, 204
    and chronic seborrheic dermatitis, 92
    and interface dermatitis, 204
        differentiation from acute graft-versus-host disease, 205
    and psoriasis, 89
Acquired perforating disorder of diabetes or renal failure, 259
Acquired vitamin B3 deficiency, 107
Acroangiodermatitis, 97
Acrodermatitis enteropathica, 107
Acropustulosis of infancy, 171
Acute cytotoxic dermatitis, 181, *see also* Interface dermatitis
Acute cytotoxic drug reaction, 200
    differentiation from other forms of interface dermatitis, 200
Acute febrile neutrophilic dermatitis, 339
Acute graft-versus-host disease, 188, **190**, 205
    differentiation from erythema multiforme, 188; from toxic epidermal necrolysis, 193; from AIDS-related interface dermatitis, 205
Acute lupus erythematosus, 226
Adipocytes, 27
Allergic contact dermatitis, **37**, 94
    clinical features, 37
    definition, 37
    differential diagnosis, 42; differentiation from chronic seborrheic dermatitis, 94
    pathologic findings, 39
    photoeczematous reaction, 38
    treatment and prognosis, 43
Alopecia androgenetica, 450
Alopecia areata, 449
Alopecia lupus, 454
Alopecia mucinosa, 453
Alopecia totalis, 449
Alopecia universalis, 449
Alpha-1-antitrypsin deficiency, and panniculitis, 422
Anatomy, normal, 1
Androgenetic alopecia, 450
Angiocentric dermatitis, **275**, **307**
    nonvasculitic, 275, *see also* Nonvasculitic angiocentric vasculitis
    vasculitic, 307, *see also* Vasculitic angiocentric vasculitis
Angioimmunoblastic lymphadenopathy involving skin, 332

---

*In a series of numbers, those in boldface indicate the main discussion of the entity.

Annular elastolytic giant cell granuloma, 363
Annular psoriasis, 79
Anthrax, 268
Aphthous stomatitis/mucositis, 261
　Behçet syndrome, 261
　herpetiform ulceration, 261
　major ulceration, 261
　minor ulceration, 261
Apocrine disorders, 467
Apocrine ducts, 20
Apocrine glands, 20
Apocrine miliaria, 471
Apoptosis, epidermal, 11
Arthropod bite reaction 48
Aspergillosis, 371
Atopic dermatitis, 39, **43**
Atrophic lichen planus, 214
Atrophie blanche, 319
Atrophy, epidermal, 10
Atypical pyoderma gangrenosum, 265
Auspitz sign, 78
Autosensitization spongiotic dermatitis, 47

## B

Bacterial pyoderma, 344
Bacterial vasculitis, 313
Balanitis circinata, 87
Basement membrane zone, 21
Behçet disease,
　and aphthous stomatitis, 261
　and erythema nodosum, 403
Benign familial pemphigus, 126
Blastomycosis, 373
Blastomycosis-like pyoderma, 344
Buerger disease, 322
Bullous disease of childhood, 156
Bullous fixed drug eruption, 158
Bullous impetigo, 171
Bullous lichen planus, **158**, 216
Bullous lichen sclerosis, 158
Bullous lupus erythematosus, 158, **226**
Bullous pemphigoid, 142
　Brunsting-Perry type, 144
　cicatricial pemphigoid, 142
　clinical features, 142
　differentiation from pemphigus vulgaris, 146
　　lichen planus pemphigoides, 142
　pathologic findings, 144
　treatment and prognosis, 147
Bullous vasculitis, 162

## C

*Candida albicans*, **172**, 373
　and pustular candidiasis, 172
Candidiasis, **172**, 373
Cat scratch disease, 270
Cervicofacial actinomycosis, 345
Chancroid, 271
Cheilitis granulomatosa, 356
Chloroma, 337
Chromomycosis, 371
Chronic eczematous dermatitis, differentiation from psoriasis, 86
Chronic graft-versus-host disease, 225
　epidermal type, 225
Chronic hand dermatitis, 45
Chronic necrolytic migratory erythema, 107
Chronic seborrheic dermatitis, 92
　AIDS related, 93
　differentiation from allergic contact dermatitis, 94; from psoriasis, 94
　sebopsoriasis, 92
Cicatricial pemphigoid, 142
Coccidioidomycosis, 371
Collagen, 24
Coma bullae, 163
Connective tissue panniculitis, 411
Contact dermatitis, 285
Crohn disease, 356
　metastatic granulomas, 357
Cryptococcal folliculitis, 436
Cryptococcosis, 371
Cutaneous necrotizing vasculitis, 307
　differentiation from urticarial vasculitis, 309
　Henoch-Schönlein purpura, 312
Cutaneous polyarteritis nodosa, 315
　macroscopic polyarteritis nodosa, 315
　microscopic polyarteritis nodosa, 315
Cytotoxic alteration, epidermal, 11
Cytotoxic dermatitis, **181**, 211, *see also* Interface dermatitis
　acute, 181
　subacute/chronic, 211, *see also* Lichenoid dermatitis
Cytotoxic drug reaction, 200

differentiation from other forms of interface dermatitis, 202

## D

Darier disease, 124, **125**
    differentiation from Grover disease, 124; from Hailey-Hailey disease, 126
Delayed hypersensitivity reaction, 286
Dermal contact dermatitis, 285
Dermal delayed hypersensitivity reaction, 286
Dermal microvascular unit, 22
Dermatitis herpetiformis, 153
    differentiation from subcorneal pustular dermatosis, 167
Dermatographism, 281
Dermatomyositis, **234**, 412
    differentiation from lupus erythematosus, **234**, 237
    panniculitis, 412
Dermatophytosis, 64
Desmosomes, 6
Discoid lupus erythematosus, 226
Drug-induced cytotoxic reaction, 200
    differentiation from other forms of interface dermatitis, 202
    fixed, 200
    generalized, 200
Drug-induced lichenoid reaction, 238
Drug-induced pemphigus, 119
Dyshidrotic eczema, 45
Dyskeratosis, epidermal, 10
Dysplastic lymphocytic vasculitis, 327

## E

Early psoriasis, 46
    differentiation from allergic contact dermatitis, 47; from seborrheic dermatitis, 47
    guttate psoriasis, 46
    papulosquamous eruption, 46
Eccrine disorders, 467
Eccrine glands, 20
Eccrine miliaria, 467
Ecthyma gangrenosum, 266
Eczema, *see* Spongiotic dermatitis
Eczematous stasis dermatitis, 58
Elephantiasis verrucosa nostra, 97
Elastosis perforans serpiginosa, 254
Electrical injury blisters, 166

Enzymatic panniculitis, 416
Eosinophilic cellulitis, 341
Eosinophilic fasciitis, **348**, 414
    and morphea, 348
    and panniculitis, 414
Eosinophilic panniculitis, 421
    differential diagnosis, 421
Eosinophilic pustular folliculitis, 445
Epidermal hyperplasia, 8
    retiform epidermal hyperplasia, 9
Epidermal acantholysis, 10
Epidermal acanthosis, 8
Epidermal atrophy, 10
Epidermal spongiosis, 10
Epidermis, 3, 8
    hyperplasia, 8
    normal anatomy, 3
Epidermolysis bullosa acquisita, inflammatory variant, 149
Erysipelas, 344
Erythema annulare centrifugum, 55, **295**
    deep variant, 295
Erythema chronicum migrans, 297
Erythema elevatum diutinum, 325
Erythema gyratum repens, 296
Erythema induratum, 404
Erythema multiforme, 158, **183**
    clinical features, 183
    definition, 183
    differentiation from graft-versus-host disease, 188; from other bullous diseases, 188
    erythema multiforme major, 185
    erythema multiforme minor, 184
    pathologic findings, 185
    Stevens-Johnson syndrome, 183
    toxic epidermal necrolysis, 183
    treatment and prognosis, 188
Erythema nodosum, 399
    clinical features, 399
    definition, 399
    differential diagnosis, 403
    pathogenesis, 400
    pathologic findings, 400
    treatment and prognosis, 404
    variants, 402
        in Behçet disease, 403
        subcutaneous nodular migratory panniculitis, 402

Erythema nodosum leprosum, 325
Erythema toxicum neonatorum, 169
Erythrodermic lichen planus, 215
Erythrodermic psoriasis, 88
Erythrodermic sarcoid, 353
Extracellular dermal matrix, 24

## F

Familial cold urticaria, 281
Fibrinoid necrosis, 275
Fixed drug eruption, 200
Flegel disease, 98
Fogo selvagem, 114
Foliaceus pemphigus, 114
Follicular degeneration syndrome, 460
Follicular disorders, 431, *see also under individual entities*
    acne rosacea, 440
    acne vulgaris, 432
    alopecia areata, 449
    alopecia mucinosa, 453
    androgenetic alopecia, 450
    animal models, 432
    diagnostic studies, 432
    follicular degeneration syndrome, 460
    infectious folliculitis, 436
    keratosis pilaris, 444
    lichen planopilaris, 455
    lupus alopecia, 454
    pathogenesis, 432
    perforating folliculitis, 448
    scarring alopecia, 460
    traction alopecia, 460
    trichotillomania, 460
Follicular eczema, 42
Follicular occlusion syndrome, 433
Follicular psoriasis, 88
Folliculitis, *see* Follicular disorders
Folliculitis decalvans, 434
Freeze blisters, 165
Friction blisters, 162
Fungal folliculitis, 439
Fungal infection and panniculitis, 422
Fungus and retiform epidermal hyperplasia, **100**, 102

## G

Gianotti-Crosti syndrome, 67
Giant cell arteritis, 322

Glucagonoma syndrome, 107
Glycocalyx, 6
Graft-versus-host disease, **190, 225**
    acute graft-versus-host disease, 190, *see also* Acute graft-versus-host disease
    chronic graft-versus-host disease, 225, *see also* Chronic graft-versus-host disease
Granulocytic dermatitis, 337
Granuloma annulare, 358
    nodular granuloma annulare, 358
    perforating granuloma annulare, 358
Granuloma faciale, 324
Granuloma inguinale, **271**, 373
Granuloma syphilis, 373
Granulomatous dermatitis, 337
Granulomatous response, **350, 371**
    to drugs and foreign substances, 350
    to infectious agents, 371
        differential diagnosis, 373
        organisms involved, 371
Granulomatous panniculitis, 423
Granulomatous vasculitis, 320
    Buerger disease, 320
    giant cell aortitis, 320
    temporal arteritis, 320
Grover disease, 123
    differentiation from Darier disease, 124
Guttate parapsoriasis of Juliusberg, 195
Guttate psoriasis, 45, 79

## H

Hailey-Hailey disease, 126
    differentiation from Darier disease, 126
Hair follicle, 17, 431
    inflammatory disorders, 431, *see also* Follicular disorders
Halogens, inducing psoriasiform reaction, 100
Hemidesmosome, 7
Henoch-Schönlein purpura, 277
Herald patch, 94
Hereditary angioedema, 281
Herpes folliculitis, 436
Herpes gestationis, **148**, 282
    differentiation from pruritic urticarial papules and plaques of pregnancy (PUPPP), **148**, 282
Herpesvirus, 129
Herpetic blisters, 129
Hepatobiliary disease, vesiculopustular eruption, 174

Hidradenitis suppurativa, 469
Histiocytic cytophagic panniculitis, 420
Histiocytic response to infectious agents, 370
Histochemical stains, 28
Histoplasmosis, 371
Hives, 278, *see also* Urticaria
Human immunodeficiency virus (HIV), and interface dermatitis, 204
Hydropic degeneration, epidermal, 12
Hyperkeratosis, 9
Hyperkeratosis lenticularis perstans, 98
Hyperorthokeratosis, 10
Hypertrophic lichen planus, 214
Hypogammaglobulinemia, 422

## I

Id reaction, 47
IgA pemphigus, 121, **167**
Immunofluorescence studies, 29
Immunohistochemical stains, 28
Impetigo, 167, **171**
    bullous impetigo, 171
    differentiation from subcorneal pustular dermatosis, 167; from staphylococcal scalded-skin syndrome, 172
    impetigo contagiosa, 171
    pathogenesis, 171
Impetigo contagiosa, 171
Indeterminate cells, 15
Infectious folliculitis, 436
    cryptococcal folliculitis, 436
    fungal folliculitis, 439
    herpes folliculitis, 436
    Pityrosporon folliculitis, 439
Infectious panniculitis, 423
Inflammatory linear verrucous epidermal nevus, differentiation from lichen striatus, 221
Inflammatory pityriasis rosea, 95
In situ hybridization studies, 29
Insect bite reaction, **48**, 197, 238
    differentiation from pityriasis lichenoides et varioliformis acuta, 197
    lichenoid, 238
Interface dermatitis, 103, 158, **181**, *see also under individual entities*
    acute graft-versus-host disease, 190
    and retiform epidermal hyperplasia, 103
    animal models, 183

    diagnostic studies, 183
    drug eruption, 200
        fixed, 200
        generalized, 200
    erythema multiforme group, 183
    human immunodeficiency virus associated, 204
    paraneoplastic pemphigus, 206
    pathogenesis, 181
    pathology, 181
    pityriasis lichenoides et varioliformis acuta, 195
    toxic epidermal necrolysis, 188
    with bullous lesions, 158
Interstitial dermatitis, 337, *see also* Nodular/interstitial dermatitis
Interstitial inflammatory reactions to infections, 371
Intestinal bypass syndrome, 171
Inverse pityriasis rosea, 95
Ischemia-induced vesiculobullous lesions, 162
    due to physical agents, 162
    due to primary vasculopathic injury, 162

## J

Jessner lymphocytic infiltrate, 299

## K

Keratinocytes, 1
    abnormal keratinization, 9
    histology, 1
    hyperplasia, 8
    ultrastructure, 6
Keratoderma blennorrhagicum, 87
Keratosis follicularis, *see* Darier disease
Keratosis pilaris, 444
Koebner phenomenon, 78
Kyrle disease, 253

## L

Lamellar ichthyosis, 109
Lamina densa, 21
Lamina lucida, 21
Langerhans cell, 14
Langerhans cell microgranuloma, **16**, 41
Large cell anaplastic lymphoma, differentiation from lymphomatoid papulosis, 332
Leishmaniasis, 373
Lepromatous leprosy, 374
Leprosy, 372

Leukocytoclastic vasculitis, *see Cutaneous necrotizing vasculitis*
Lichen aureus, 287
Lichen nitidus, 219
   differentiation from lichen planus, 222
Lichen planopilaris, 214, **457**
   differentiation from lupus alopecia, 460
Lichen planus, 142, 158, **211**
   associated with bullous pemphigoid, 142
   atrophic lichen planus, 214
   bullous lichen planus, **158**, 216
   differentiation from lichen nitidus, 222; from lichenoid immune reaction, 238
   drug related, 212
   erythrodermic lichen planus, 215
   hypertrophic lichen planus, 214
   lichen planopilaris, 214
Lichen planus pemphigoides, 142
Lichen sclerosus, 158, **243**
   bullous, 158
Lichen simplex chronicus, 74
   differentiation from psoriasis, **77**, 86
   pathogenesis, 76
   pemphigoid nodularis, 75
   pseudoepitheliomatous hyperplasia, 75
   syringometaplasia, 75
Lichen striatus, 220
   differentiation from inflammatory linear verrucous epidermal nevus, 221
Lichenoid dermatitis, 211, *see also under individual entities*
   chronic graft-versus-host disease, 225
   dermatomyositis, 234
   diagnostic studies, 211
   lichen planus, 211
   lichen sclerosis, 243
   lichen striatus, 220
   lichenoid immune response, 237
   lichenoid pigmentary purpura, 245
   lupus erythematosus, 226
   pathogenesis, 211
   pityriasis lichenoides chronica, 237
   secondary syphilis, 239
Lichenoid drug reaction, 238
Lichenoid immune response, 237
   differentiation from lichen planus, 238
Lichenoid insect bite reaction, 237
Lichenoid pigmentary purpura, 245

Lichenoid purpura of Gougerot-Blum, **245**, 287
Lichenoid secondary syphilis, 239
Linear IgA disease, 158
Lipodermatosclerosis, 419
Lipomembranous panniculitis, 420
Livedo reticularis, 319
Livedo vasculitis, 319
Luetic alopecia, 438
Lupus alopecia, 454
   differentiation from lichen planopilaris, 460
Lupus erythematosus, 158, **226**
   acute lupus erythematosus, 226
   alopecia, 454
   bullous lupus erythematosus, **158**, 226
   differentiation from dermatomyositis, 234; from polymorphous light eruption, 234
   discoid lupus erythematosus, 226
   lupus panniculitis, 226
   lupus profundus, 226
   necrotizing vasculitic lupus erythematosus, 226
   predominantly dermal type, 230
   subacute lupus erythematosus, 226
Lupus panniculitis, 226
Lupus pernio, 353
Lupus profundus, 226, 230, **409**
Lupus tumidus, 230
Lupus vulgaris, 372
Lymphocytic hidradenitis, 221
Lymphocytic vasculitis, 275, **327**
Lymphogranuloma venereum, 270
Lymphomatoid papulosis, 197, **329**
   differentiation from pityriasis lichenoides et varioliformis acuta, 197, 332
Lymphomatoid vasculitis, 327

# M

Melanocyte, 12
   histology, 12
   pigment incontinence, 14
   ultrastructure and immunohistochemistry, 13
Melanosome, 13
Melanosome complex, 7
Merkel cell, 16
Miescher cheilitis, 356
Migratory panniculitis, 422
Miliaria, 467
   apocrine miliaria, 471
   eccrine miliaria, 467

miliaria crystallina, 467
miliaria profunda, 467
miliaria pustulosa, 467
miliaria rubra, 467
Miliaria crystallina, 467
Miliaria profunda, 467
Miliaria pustulosa, 467
Miliaria rubra, 467
Mondor disease, 318
Morbilliform viral exanthem, 289
Morphea, **347**, 412
　eosinophilic fasciitis, 349
　morphea profunda, 349
　panniculitis, 412
Mucha-Habermann disease, *see* Pityriasis lichenoides et varioliformis acuta
Muckle-Wells syndrome, 281
Mucormycosis, 371
Munro microabscess, 82
Mycobacterial infection and panniculitis, 422

## N

Nail psoriasis, 80
Necrobiosis, 26
Necrobiosis lipoidica, 360
Necrobiotic xanthogranuloma, 365
Necrolytic migratory erythema, 109
Necrotizing vasculitis, **162**, 226
　and lupus erythematosus, 226
Neonatal pemphigus, 115
Nephrogenic systemic fibrosis, 367
Neutrophil-rich urticaria, 281
Neutrophilic eccrine hidradenitis, 468
Nodular/interstitial dermatitis, 337, *see also* under individual entities
　acute febrile neutrophilic dermatitis, 339
　annular elastolytic giant cell granuloma, 363
　bacterial pyoderma, 344
　cheilitis granulomatosa, 356
　cutaneous Crohn disease, 356
　diagnostic studies, 339
　eosinophilic cellulitis, 341
　granuloma annulare, 358
　granulomatous response, 350, 371
　morphea, 347
　necrobiosis lipoidica, 360
　necrobiotic xanthogranuloma, 366
　nephrogenic systemic fibrosis, 368
　pathogenesis, 338
　pyoderma gangrenosum, 342
　rheumatoid nodule, 362
　sarcoidosis, 350
Nodular granuloma annulare, 358
Nodular sarcoidosis, 353
Nodular vasculitis, *see* Erythema induratum
Nonvasculitic angiocentric dermatitis, 275, *see also under individual entities*
　animal models, 277
　dermal contact dermatitis, 285
　diagnostic studies, 276
　erythema annulare centrifugum, 296
　erythema chronicum migrans, 297
　erythema gyratum repens, 296
　Jessner lymphocytic infiltrate, 299
　morbilliform viral exanthem, 289
　pathogenesis, 276
　polymorphous light eruption, 294
　progressive pigmentary purpura, 287
　pruritic urticarial papules and plaques of pregnancy (PUPPP), 282
　reticular erythematous mucinosis, 288
　Still disease, 301
　urticaria, 278
Nutritional disorders and acanthosis, 107, see also Psoriasiform nutritional disorders

## O

Ofuji syndrome, 445

## P

Pancreatic panniculitis, 416
Panniculitis, 397
　alpha-1-antitrypsin deficiency, 422
　connective tissue panniculitis, 411
　diagnostic studies, 399
　eosinophilic fasciitis, 414
　eosinophilic panniculitis, 421
　erythema induratum, 404
　erythema nodosum, 399
　granulomatous panniculitis, 423
　histiocytic cytophagic panniculitis, 420
　hypogammaglobulinemia, 422
　infectious panniculitis, 422
　lipodermatosclerosis, 419
　lobular panniculitis, 398
　lupus profundus, 409

migratory panniculitis, 422
pancreatic panniculitis, 416
pathogenesis, 398
relapsing febrile nodular nonsuppurative panniculitis, 414
Rothman-Makai panniculitis, 422
septal panniculitis, 398
sclerema neonatorum, 416
subcutaneous fat necrosis of newborn, 417
Papular acrodermatitis of childhood, 67
Papular pityriasis rosea, 95
Papulosquamous eruption, psoriasis, 45
Parakeratosis, 9
Paraneoplastic pemphigus, 119, **206**
Parapsoriasis, 60
guttate parapsoriasis, 60
small plaque parapsoriasis, 60
superficial digitate dermatosis, 60
Pattern alopecia, 450
Pellagra, 107
Pemphigus, **114**, 167
clinical features, 114
clinicopathologic variants, 119
drug reaction pemphigus, 119
IgA pemphigus, 121
paraneoplastic pemphigus, 119
definition, 114
fogo selvagem, 114
foliaceus variant, 114
neonatal pemphigus, 115
pathologic findings, 116
pemphigus erythematosus, 116
pemphigus foliaceus, 167
pemphigus vegetans of Hallopeau, 115
pemphigus vegetans of Neumann, 115
pemphigus vulgaris, 114
treatment and prognosis, 122
Pemphigus erythematosus, 116
Pemphigus foliaceus, 167
Pemphigus vegetans of Hallopeau, 115
Pemphigus vegetans of Neumann, 115
Pemphigus vulgaris, 114, *see also* Pemphigus
differentiation from bullous pemphigoid, 146
Perforating dermatitis, 253, *see also under individual entities*
acquired perforating disorder of diabetes or renal failure, 259
elastosis perforans serpiginosa, 254
Kyrle disease, 253
reactive perforating collagenosis, 257
Perforating folliculitis, 448
Perforating granuloma annulare, 358
Perniosis, 328
Photoallergic dermatitis, 52
Photoeczematous reaction/eruption, 38, **52**
Photoeczematous spongiotic dermatitis, 38
differentiation from allergic contact dermatitis, 43
Phototoxic dermatitis, 52
Phytophotodermatitis, 38, 53
Pigmentary purpura, 287
Pityriasis lichenoides chronica, **196**, 197, 237
differentiation from pityriasis lichenoides et varioliformis acuta, 197
Pityriasis lichenoides et varioliformis acuta (PLEVA), 97, 159, **195**, 331
bullous, 159
chronic form, 196
differentiation from pityriasis rosea, 97; from insect bite reaction, 197; from lymphomatoid papulosis, 198, 332; from pityriasis lichenoides chronica, 197
Pityriasis rosea, 62, **94**
definition and clinical features, 94
differentiation from pityriasis lichenoides et varioliformis acuta, 97; from small plaque parapsoriasis, 97
herald patch, 94
inverse pityriasis rosea, 95
papular/inflammatory pityriasis rosea, 95
pathogenesis, 96
pathologic findings, 95
recurrent pityriasis rosea, 95
treatment and prognosis, 97
vesicular pityriasis rosea, 95
Pityriasis rubra pilaris, 87, **89**
differentiation from psoriasis, **87**, 91
Pityrosporon folliculitis, 439
Plaque-like mucinosis, 288
Polyarteritis nodosa, 277
Polymorphous light eruption, 52, **294**
Polymyositis, **234**, 412
panniculitis, 412
Polysaccharide ground substance, 25
Postherpetic granulomatous dermatitis, 422
Pressure bullae, 163
Prickly heat, 467

Primary irritant dermatitis, 37
    differentiation from allergic contact dermatitis, 42
Primary syphilis, 271
Progressive pigmentary purpura, 287
Progressive pigmentary purpuric dermatosis, 287
Prurigo nodularis, 74, *see also Lichen simplex chronicus*
Pruritic urticarial papules and plaques of pregnancy (PUPPP), 148, **282**
    differentiation from herpes gestationis, **148**, 282
Pseudoepitheliomatous hyperplasia, 75
Pseudofolliculitis barbae, 434
Psoriasiform cutaneous T-cell lymphoma, 109
Psoriasiform dermatitis, 73
Psoriasiform drug eruption, differentiation from psoriasis, 86
Psoriasiform lupus erythematosus, 109
Psoriasiform nutritional disorders, 107
    acrodermatitis enteropathica, 107
    chronic necrolytic migratory erythema, 107
    pellagra, 107
Psoriasiform reaction to halogens, 100
Psoriasis, **78**, 94, 167
    definition, 78
    clinical features, 78
    clinical variants, 79
        annular psoriasis, 79
        guttate psoriasis, 79
        nail psoriasis, 80
        psoriasis vulgaris, 79
        psoriatic erythroderma, 79
    differentiation from chronic eczematous dermatitis, 86; from lichen simplex chronicus, 86; from psoriasiform drug eruptions, 86; from pityriasis rubra pilaris, 87; from chronic seborrheic dermatitis, 94; from subcorneal pustular dermatosis, 167
    pathogenesis, 83
    pathologic findings, 81
    pathologic variants, 87
        and AIDS, 89
        erythrodermic psoriasis, 88
        follicular psoriasis, 88
        pustular psoriasis, 87
        Reiter disease, 87
    treatment and prognosis, 87
Psoriasis, early, *see Early psoriasis*
Psoriasis vulgaris, 79
Psoriatic erythroderma, **78**, 79

Pustular candidiasis, 172
Pustular folliculitis, 443
Pustular psoriasis, 87
Pustular vasculitis, 173, **313**
Pyoderma, bacterial, 344
Pyoderma gangrenosum, 263, **342**
    atypical pyoderma gangrenosum, 265

## R

Reactive perforating collagenosis, 257
Reiter disease, 87
Relapsing febrile nodular nonsuppurative panniculitis, 414
Reticular erythematous mucinosis, 288
Retiform epidermal hyperplasia, 9, **73**, 100, 103
    induced by mycotic infection, **100**, 102
    with interface dermatitis, 103
Rheumatoid nodule, 362
Rhinophyma, 443
Rhinosporidiosis, 371
Ritter disease, *see Staphylococcal scalded-skin syndrome*
Rocky Mountain spotted fever, 314
Rothman-Makai panniculitis, 422
Rupial secondary syphilis, 239

## S

Sarcoidosis, 350
Satellitosis, epidermal, 11
Scabies, 65
Scarring alopecia, 460
Schamberg disease, 287
Sclerema neonatorum 416
Scleroderma panniculitis, 412
Sebopsoriasis, 92
Seborrheic dermatitis, 47, **54**, 92
    chronic seborrheic dermatitis, 92, *see also Chronic seborrheic dermatitis*
    differentiation from allergic contact dermatitis, 47; from early psoriasis, 47
Secondary syphilis, 239
    rupial, 239
Senear-Usher syndrome, 116
Septic vasculitis, 313
Shulman syndrome, 414
Small plaque parapsoriasis, **60**, 97
    differentiation from pityriasis rosea, 97
Sneddon syndrome, 319
Sneddon-Wilkinson disease, *see Subcorneal pustular*

*dermatosis*
Solar urticaria, 52
Spongiform pustules of Kogoj, 82
Spongiosis, epidermal, 10
Spongiotic arthropod bite reaction, 48
Spongiotic dermatitis, 35, *see also under individual entities*
    allergic contact dermatitis, 37
    atopic dermatitis, 43
    clinical variants, 35
    dermatophytosis, 64
    diagnostic studies, 37
    dyshidrotic eczema, 45
    early psoriasis, 46
    eczematous stasis dermatitis, 58
    erythema annulare centrifugum, 55
    Id reaction, 47
    papular acrodermatitis of childhood, 67
    parapsoriasis, 60
    pathogenesis, 36
    photoeczematous eruption, 52
    pityriasis rosea, 62
    scabies, 65
    seborrheic dermatitis, 54
    spongiotic arthropod bite reaction, 48
    spongiotic drug eruption, 51
    toxic shock syndrome, 68
Spongiotic drug reaction 51
Sporotrichosis, 371
Staphylococcal scalded-skin syndrome, **159**, 172
    differentiation from impetigo, 172
*Staphylococcus aureus*, **159**, 171
    and impetigo, 171
    and scalded-skin syndrome, 159
Stasis dermatitis, 58, **97**
    acroangiodermatitis, 97
    elephantiasis verrucosa nostra, 97
Stevens-Johnson syndrome, 183
Still disease, 301
Stratum basalis, 4
Stratum corneum, 3
Stratum granulosum, 4
Stratum spinosum, 4
Streptococcal ecthyma, 267
*Streptococcus*, and impetigo, 171
Subacute lupus erythematosus, 226
Subacute nodular migratory panniculitis, 422
Subcorneal pustular dermatosis, 166
    differentiation from impetigo, 167; dermatitis herpetiformis, 167; pemphigus foliaceus, 167; from psoriasis, 167
Subcutaneous fat, 27
Subcutaneous fat necrosis of the newborn, 416, **417**
Subcutaneous migratory nodular panniculitis, 402
Superficial digitate dermatosis, 60
Superficial migratory thrombophlebitis, 318
Sweet syndrome, 339
Swimming pool granuloma, 372
Syphilis, **239**, **271**
    primary, 271
    secondary, 239
        rupial, 239
Syringometaplasia, 75

## T

Temporal arteritis, 322
Thermal/heat blisters, 163
Thromboangiitis obliterans, 322
Thrombogenic vasculopathy, 314
Tonofilaments, 7
Toxic epidermal necrolysis, 158, 183, **188**, 195
    differentiation from acute graft-versus-host disease, 189, 195
Toxic shock syndrome, 68
Traction alopecia, 460
Transient acantholytic dermatosis, *see Grover disease*
Transient neonatal pustular melanosis, 169
Trichotillomania, 460
Tuberculoid leprosy, 372
Tuberculosis, cutaneous, 372
Tularemia, 268

## U

Ulcerating infectious disorders, 266
Ulcerative dermatitis, 261, *see also under individual entities*
    anthrax, 268
    aphthous stomatitis, 261
    cat scratch disease, 270
    chancroid, 271
    ecthyma gangrenosum, 266
    granuloma inguinale, 271
    lymphogranuloma venereum, 270
    primary syphilis, 271
    pyoderma gangrenosum, 263
    staphylococcal ecthyma, 267

tularemia, 268
Ultrastructural studies, 29
Urticaria, 278
    acute, 278
    chronic, 278
    clinical features, 278
    definition, 278
    differential diagnosis, 281
    pathologic findings, 279
    treatment and prognosis, 282
    variants, 281
        dermatographism, 281
        familial cold urticaria, 281,
        hereditary angioedema, 281
        Muckle-Wells syndrome, 281
        neutrophil-rich urticaria, 281
        urticarial vasculitis, 281
Urticarial vasculitis, 277, 281, **313**
    differentiation from cutaneous necrotizing vasculitis, 309

## V

Varicella zoster virus, 132
Vascular plexus, 22
    deep, 22
    superficial, 22
Vasculitic angiocentric dermatitis, 307, *see also under individual entities*
    angioblastic lymphadenopathy, 332
    atrophie blanche, 319
    cutaneous necrotizing vasculitis, 307
    cutaneous polyarteritis nodosa, 315
    erythema elevatum diutinum, 325
    erythema nodosum leprosum, 325
    granuloma faciale, 324
    granulomatous vasculitis, 320
    livedo reticularis, 319
    livedo vasculitis, 320
    lymphocytic vasculitis, 327
    lymphoid papulosis, 329
    nodular vasculitis, 320
    pustular vasculitis, 313
    Rocky mountain spotted fever, 314
    septic vasculitis, 313
    superficial migratory thrombophlebitis, 318
    thrombogenic vasculopathy, 314
    urticarial vasculitis, 313
    Wegener granulomatosis, 322
Vasculitis, *see Vasculitic angiocentric dermatitis*
Vesicular pityriasis rosea, 95
Vesiculobullous/vesiculopustular dermatitis, non-acantholytic, 137, *see also under individual entities*
    acropustulosis of infancy, 171
    animal models, 142
    bullous disease of childhood, 156
    bullous pemphigoid, 142
    dermatitis herpetiformis, 153
    diagnostic studies, 140
    epidermolysis bullosa acquisita, 149
    erythema toxicum neonatorum, 169
    hepatobiliary disease eruption, 174
    herpes gestationis, 148
    IgA pemphigus, 167
    impetigo, 171
    intestinal bypass syndrome, 171
    ischemia related, 162
    linear IgA disease, 158
    pathogenesis, 139
    pustular candidiasis, 172
    pustular vasculitis, 173
    staphylococcal scalded-skin syndrome, 159
    subcorneal pustular dermatosis, 166
    transient neonatal pustular melanosis, 169
    with interface dermatitis, 158
Verrucous incontinentia pigmenti, 109

## W

Weber-Christian disease, 414
Wegener granulomatosis, 322
Wells syndrome, 341